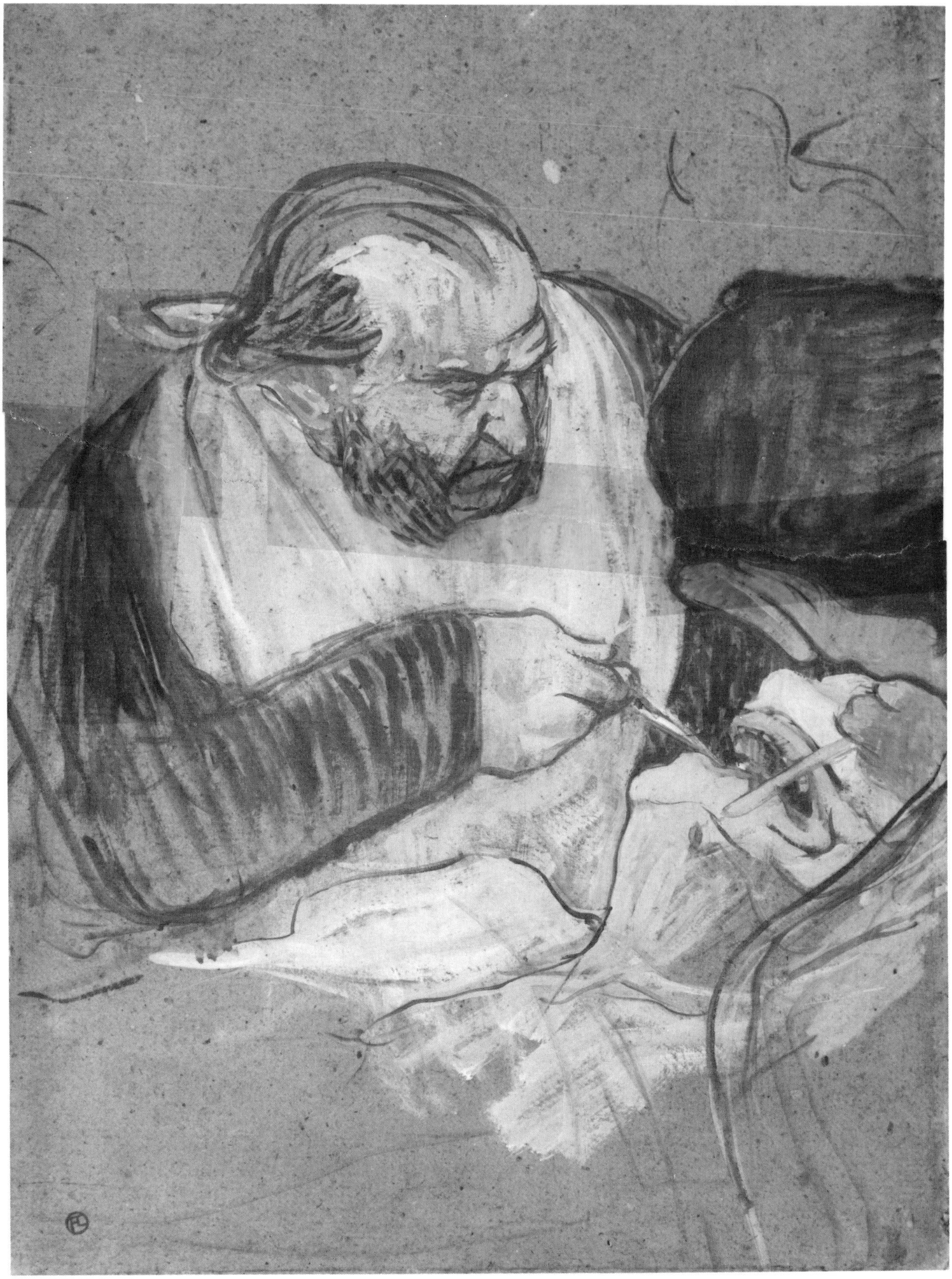

"Dr. Jules-Emile Pean" by Henri de Toulouse-Lautrec.
Reproduced by permission of the
Sterling and Francine Clark Art Institute,
Williamstown, Massachusetts.

HEAD AND NECK CANCER
Clinical Decisions and Management Principles

HEAD AND NECK CANCER
Clinical Decisions and Management Principles

DONALD G. McQUARRIE, M.D., Ph.D.

Professor of Surgery
University of Minnesota
Minneapolis V.A. Medical Center
Minneapolis, Minnesota

GEORGE L. ADAMS, M.D.

Associate Professor of Otolaryngology
University of Minnesota
Minneapolis V.A. Medical Center
Minneapolis, Minnesota

ALAN R. SHONS, M.D.

Professor of Surgery
Head, Division of Plastic Surgery
Case Western Reserve University
Cleveland, Ohio

GRAEME A. BROWNE, B.Sc., M.Sc. B.D.S., F.R.C.D.

Clinical Assistant Professor of Oral Surgery
University of Minnesota
Chief, Oral Surgery
Minneapolis V.A. Medical Center
Minneapolis, Minnesota

Illustrated by LORI McQUARRIE

YEAR BOOK MEDICAL PUBLISHERS, INC.
CHICAGO

0 9 8 7 6 5 4 3 2 1

Library of Congress Cataloging in Publication Data
Main entry under title:

Head and neck cancer.

Includes bibliographies and index.
1. Head—Cancer. 2. Neck—Cancer. I. McQuarrie, Donald G. [DNLM: 1. Head and Neck Neoplasms—diagnosis. 2. Head and Neck Neoplasms—therapy. WE 707 H43175]
RC280.H4H385 1985 616.99′491 85-8255
ISBN 0-8151-5848-3

Sponsoring Editor: Daniel J. Doody
Manager, Copyediting Services: Frances M. Perveiler
Production Project Manager: R. Allen Reedtz
Proofroom Supervisor: Shirley E. Taylor

This book is dedicated to our students, residents, and specialist fellows who continue to stimulate us, keep our outlook fresh, and make us look for better questions and more complete answers.

Preface

> The capacity of the human mind for formulating and solving complex problems is small compared with the size of problems . . . [encountered] in the real world.
>
> H. A. Simon (1957)[1]

WHY ANOTHER TEXTBOOK on head and neck malignancy? There are three reasons. First, this book was written to focus on decision-making in head and neck cancer. Our present-day knowledge is too incomplete to allow construction of rigid decision-making algorithms. But, structured logic is important where uncertainty exists. To provide some example decision maps, we attempted to gather some of the better available data, knowing that there would be a trade-off between completeness and pithy brevity. Second, we wanted to reemphasize the need for intercommunication among the medical disciplines that are involved in the care of patients with head and neck cancer. Future progress will come from less insular specialization. Third, by addressing our discussion to a phantom senior specialty fellow, we hoped to direct each chapter to significant, explicit questions that have been posed to us. It is hoped that this format will be more helpful than patronizing for the reader.

There are good atlases of head and neck anatomy and surgical techniques. Numerous texts describe malignant diseases of the head and neck in considerable detail. Many different therapies are presented and championed for comparable lesions. We felt the need to help fellows in training formulate some guiding principles for advancing through the areas of agonizing decision-making. The *Index Medicus* is increasing in actual weight at a logarithmic rate.[2] How can you sort out the many alternatives? Why do you use one therapy over another? What latitudes exist in selecting effective therapy, in the course of treatment, during surgery, and in office follow-up? In recent years, structured decision-making has gained popularity.[1, 3–7] We do advocate structured decision-making in head and neck cancer. However, it is essential that any such decision structures have enough latitude to accommodate patient individuality.

In a medical field with significant progress, today's decision structure may be altered at any future time by diagnostic or therapeutic advances. To paraphrase R. Varco, a stimulating University of Minnesota teacher,[8]

> The current half life of knowledge is short. One should not push for change just for the sake of change. But, *a fortiori*, without change, progress is impossible. There should be a climate or attitude which actively seeks new tightly reasoned ideas. These ideas might appropriately grow out of some basic controversies. Hopefully, the process of examination and improvement may evoke, and then animate the energy input which is critical to the pursuit of excellence.

In the brief history of head and neck cancer treatment detailed in chapter 1, it will be seen that progress in the field is agonizingly slow but steady. Medical leaders have provided the intellectual push for improvement. Surgical mortalities have fallen from 35% to about 1%.[9, 10] In 50 years the aggregate 5-year survivals for some tumors have increased from the miserable 10% range to 65%–75%. Reconstruction and rehabilitation have taken big strides with various specialized flaps and microsurgery. Radiation biology has become a precise science. Progress will stop if we cling to rigid doctrine. There must be an aggressive search for improvement.

On the other side of the coin, not everything that is new or different is necessarily better. Quantified data must be examined to separate true progress from enthusiastic advocacy. Our younger colleagues should be encouraged to keep that nice balance between retaining workable principles while they adjust to genuine progress or even assume a leading position in the development of the field. They should constantly weigh each decision and reject unquestioning acquiescence to therapeutic rituals and idiosyncrasies.

Each physician probably pursues a different intellectual route when he makes a clinical decision. Our patterns of thinking and medical care are synthesized from an eclectic selection of patterns of thinking adopted from senior role models, in person or in print. An experienced senior clinician may see a patient and rapidly make a correct decision. The appropriate logic may be obvious to him. The decision is made quickly. He does not consciously record the nuances or express the many subordinate questions that arise in a complex logic pattern. To an outsider, these decisions may appear to spring fully developed from some intuitive reservoir. We shouldn't be deceived. The decisions on the care of patients with head and neck malignancy have pursued long chains of questions. Our illustrations in subsequent chapters are an attempt to demonstrate the levels of complexity that are present and must be dealt with. The inherent questions must be precisely formulated, especially where risks, perceived utility, and end results may vary. We cannot lace our discussions with common logical fallacies or incorrect data. Each step in the patient's total care should fit into a coherent custom-made plan. If all parties are to be effective in the care of the patient, they must work from the same care plan. Precision of communication is also important.

Unfortunately, we must make decisions based on clinical data that have built-in errors and variance. It is at these points of uncertainty that a more structured analysis can be effective. Clear questions that can be placed in diagrams or posed in quantifiable probabilistic terms can set a logical agenda for the discussion. This is not to say that a period of emotionally stimulating, semirational, free associative discussion cannot be effective. Indeed, such occasions for interchange spark new ideas. They represent much of the fun of medicine. But when the time comes to unravel a tangled skein of clinical facts or to proceed with an expeditious care program, then uncluttered logic, good data, and structured decisions are required. Sometimes the right decision is that there are not enough data to support one course of action over another.

The book develops within a format that assumes that the reader wishes to make difficult decisions and cannot count on spontaneous inspiration. We have highlighted some of the common questions in head and neck cancer care. Each anatomical area discussed is presented in terms of selected data and options for care. We decided to plunge into controversial areas rather than tiptoe around them. At the outset, we know that clinicians in different settings who have had different experiences will have different ideas and slightly different approaches that are equally valid. We hope the differences stimulate an interest in the decision-making process rather than provoke obstinate dogmatism.

A definite effort was made to emphasize the need for humanistic warmth and personal concern for the patient. It must be incorporated into the decision-making process. Effective care cannot be conducted unless every decision considers the whole patient—his body, his family, his fears, his successes.

Finally, we admit we are all perpetual students. Our selection of questions and development of answers will hold our logic up to criticism in hopes that the reader will be piqued to refine our efforts.

The book was planned with three distinct divisions. The early chapters cover questions that are common to the care of many head and neck malignancies. These chapters focus on the general decision process for common head and neck cancer problems. The central chapters analyze the problems that arise in diagnosing and treating particular types of tumors within specific anatomical locations. Because of the detailed scope of the care of the lymphomas, and because they are the domain of the hematologist-oncologist, they are discussed only in the context of differential diagnosis. And because of the specialized nature of tumors confined to the globe of the eye, they were omitted. The final chapters examine important problems in postoperative complications, care of the uncured patient, and effective ward management and follow-up. The promise of immunology as a potential improvement for the future ends the book.

In preparing this book we have drawn on many sources that seemed to have applicable merit. We have tried to credit the sources accurately. Any effective text must be derivative of the previous work in the field. References, drawings, techniques, and judgments were gleaned from our view of what is applicable or important. Another set of authors would perhaps select other sources, have varying opinions, illustrate different techniques. We hope the reader will follow Paul's admonition to the Philippians (Philippians, Chap. 4, Verse 8):

> Finally, brethren, whatsoever things are true, whatsoever things are honest, whatsoever things are just, whatsoever things are pure, whatsoever things are lovely, whatsoever things are of good report; if there be any virtue, and if there by any praise, think on these things.

DONALD G. MCQUARRIE, M.D., PH.D.

GEORGE L. ADAMS, M.D.

ALAN R. SHONS, M.D.

GRAEME A. BROWNE, B.SC., M.SC., B.D.S., F.R.C.D.

1. Shoemaker P.J.H.: *Experiments on Decisions Under Risk: The Expected Utility Hypothesis.* Boston, Kluwer-Nijhoff Publishers, 1980.
2. Durack D.T.: The weight of medical knowledge. *N. Engl. J. Med.* 298:773–775, 1978.
3. Feinstein A.R.: *Clinical Judgment.* Baltimore, Williams & Wilkins Co., 1967.
4. Eiseman B., Wolkins R.S.: *Surgical Decision Making.* Philadelphia, W.B. Saunders Co., 1978.
5. Eiseman B.: *Prognosis of Surgical Disease.* Philadelphia, W.B. Saunders Co., 1980.
6. Beck J.R., Kassirer J.P., Pauker S.G.: A convenient approximation of life expectancy (the "DEALE"): I. Validation of the method. *Am. J. Med.* 74:883–888, 1982.
7. Beck J.R., Pauker S.G., Gottlieb J.E., et al.: A convenient approximation of life expectancy (the "DEALE"): II. Use in medical decision-making. *Am. J. Med.* 73:888–898, 1982.
8. Varco R.L.: Even in his own country a prophet is not without prophecies: On the occasion of the dedication of the Phillips-Wangensteen Research Laboratory. *Surgery* 87:253–257, 1980.
9. Absolon K.B., Rogers W., Aust J.B.: Some historical developments of surgical therapy of tongue cancer from the 17th to the 19th century. *Am. J. Surg.* 104:689, 1962.
10. Beahrs O.H.: Hayes Martin Lecture: Factors minimizing mortality and morbidity rates in head and neck surgery. *Am. J. Surg.* 126:443–451, 1973.

ACKNOWLEDGMENT

A number of the authors wish to express a formal "thank you" to MRS. MARY DREHER for her extra effort in processing and reprocessing large masses of the words. The same "thank you" goes to many other helpers in other offices.

Contributors

GEORGE L. ADAMS, M.D.
Associate Professor of Otolaryngology
University of Minnesota
Minneapolis V.A. Medical Center
Minneapolis, Minnesota

NORMAN T. BERLINGER, M.D., PH.D.
Assistant Professor of Otolaryngology
University of Minnesota
Minneapolis V.A. Medical Center
Minneapolis, Minnesota

GRAEME A. BROWNE, B.SC., M.SC., B.D.S., F.R.C.D.
Clinical Assistant Professor of Oral Surgery
University of Minnesota
Minneapolis V.A. Medical Center
Minneapolis, Minnesota

THEODOR B. GRAGE, M.D., PH.D.
Professor of Surgery
University of Minnesota
Minneapolis, Minnesota

JAMES T. LEE, JR., M.D., PH.D.
Assistant Professor of Surgery
University of Minnesota
Minneapolis V.A. Medical Center
Minneapolis, Minnesota

SEYMOUR H. LEVITT, M.D.
Professor and Head
Therapeutic Radiology
University of Minnesota
Minneapolis, Minnesota

CATHERINE C. LIMAS, M.D.
Associate Professor of Pathology
University of Minnesota
Chief, Anatomic Pathology
Minneapolis V.A. Medical Center
Minneapolis, Minnesota

ROBERT H. MAISEL, M.D.
Associate Professor of Otolaryngology
University of Minnesota
Chief, Otolaryngology
Hennepin County Medical Center
Minneapolis, Minnesota

DONALD G. MCQUARRIE, M.D., PH.D.
Professor of Surgery
University of Minnesota
Minneapolis V.A. Medical Center
Minneapolis, Minnesota

CHARLES E. MORROW, M.D.
Medical Fellow in Surgery
University of Minnesota
Minneapolis, Minnesota

MARK E. NESBIT, M.D.
Professor of Pediatrics
University of Minnesota
Minneapolis, Minnesota

MELODY J. O'CONNOR, M.D.
Assistant Professor of Surgery
University of Minnesota
Minneapolis V.A. Medical Center
Minneapolis, Minnesota

MARTIN M. OKEN, M.D.
Associate Professor of Medicine
University of Minnesota
Minneapolis V.A. Medical Center
Minneapolis, Minnesota

A.D.J. PEARSON, M.D., B.S., M.R.C.P., D.C.H.
Visiting International Fellow
Pediatric Oncology
University of Minnesota
Minneapolis, Minnesota

BARRY H. J. PRESS, M.D.
Medical Fellow in Surgery
University of Minnesota
Minneapolis V.A. Medical Center
Minneapolis, Minnesota

YASHODA RAO, M.D.
East Metro Radiation Therapy Center
St. Joseph's Hospital
St. Paul, Minnesota
Formerly
Assistant Professor
Therapeutic Radiology
University of Minnesota
Minneapolis V.A. Medical Center
Minneapolis, Minnesota

MICHAEL L. SCHWARTZ, M.D., PH.D.
Clinical Assistant Professor
University of Minnesota
Minneapolis V.A. Medical Center
Minneapolis, Minnesota

ALAN R. SHONS, M.D., PH.D.
Professor of Surgery
Head, Division of Plastic Surgery
Case Western Reserve University
Cleveland, Ohio

DALE C. SNOVER, M.D.
Assistant Professor of Pathology
University of Minnesota
Minneapolis, Minnesota

DAVID E. TUBMAN, M.D.
Chief, Neuroradiology
Abbott-Northwestern Hospital
Formerly Assistant Professor of Radiology
University of Minnesota
Minneapolis, Minnesota

Contents

1 / Objectives of Care in Head and Neck Malignancy

DONALD G. MCQUARRIE, M.D., PH.D.

PROGRESS IN the treatment of head and neck cancer has been associated with procedures that have never pleased the patient. The historical origins of surgical treatment are found in the brutalities of punishment, revenge, and torture of the early barbarian and theocratic societies. Hunerich the King of the Vandals demonstrated in 484 A.D. that a major part of the tongue could be removed from Christians by grabbing the mobile portion with a hook and slicing off as much as could be delivered to view. There were occasional survivors. The only technical advance was the addition of hot actual cautery. This allowed more tortured examples to survive. Early curative treatment for oral malignancy used the same techniques as the barbarians. The first published report of removing a tongue cancer came from Professor Machetti of Padua in 1664.[1] Reports of oral cancer before 1700 are rare because of diagnostic inaccuracy. Life span was short. Smoking was rare before 1700. Consequently, the incidence of squamous cancer was probably low.

The antemortem diagnosis of laryngeal and pharyngeal lesions was unusual. The Spanish singing master Manuel Garcia demonstrated in 1854 and 1855 that the larynx could be examined in bright sunlight with a small angled mirror on a long handle.[2] The professor of medicine at Strasburg, Adolph Kussmaul, who described "fearful dyspnea," developed the laryngoscope in 1869.[3] Sir Morell MacKenzie began doing direct laryngoscopy and esophagoscopy in London in 1869.[3] MacKenzie's interest in the larynx explains his involvement in Crown Prince Frederick's care some 20 years later.[4] Billroth's first laryngeal fissure operation was performed in 1870 on a patient with tuberculosis of the larynx. He then performed a series of laryngeal fissures for laryngeal malignancy, followed by a series of total laryngectomies, with no survivors.[2] Billroth had more success when he operated on 45 patients with cancer of the tongue, reporting 10 "cures."[1] By 1870 Bernhard Frankel of Berlin had successfully removed a laryngeal cancer from a Professor Julius Wiggers by serial transoral resections and a subsequent neck node removal. In 1885 Kocher and Butlin each reported removing lesions of the tongue through the floor of the mouth. Toulouse-Lautrec recorded Professor Pean (the inventor of a simple latching hemostat) performing oral procedures for cancer in 1891 (Fig 1–1). Toulouse-Lautrec misidentified the procedure.

The advances of anesthesia occurred with Crawford Long's cases in 1841, reported in 1849. W. T. G. Morton used ether anesthesia with success at Massachusetts General Hospital on Oct. 16, 1846. Examination, diagnosis, and minor procedures were made much simpler in 1859, when Albert Neimann isolated cocaine from the Peruvian cocoa leaf. Karl Koller of Vienna, later of New York, described the use of cocaine as a topical anesthetic in opthalmology in 1884. Halstead investigated cocaine injections for local anesthesia and reported 1,000 cases of its use in minor surgery in 1885.[2] Pathology was also evolving. As we will see below, Virchow was alive and active.

In the decade after 1885, three politically important figures had serious head and neck malignancies. Their diseases and the records of the treatments give us an insight into the medical thinking of the times.

CROWN PRINCE FREDERICK, SON OF WILLIAM I, EMPEROR OF GERMANY.—In a speech on the occasion of his father's 90th birthday, March 18, 1887, the 56-year-old Crown Prince was noted to be hoarse. A small lesion was found on the left vocal cord. It was cauterized three times. Pain and hoarseness persisted. Professor Ernst Bergman diagnosed malignancy on clinical grounds and planned an operation for May 21, 1887. There was a flurry of consultation involving Chancellor Bismark and the Crown Prince's Mother-in-Law, Queen Victoria. Surgery was postponed until Morell MacKenzie, then England's leading laryngologist, could be summoned. MacKenzie hadn't known the purpose of his mission and had to make a return trip to fetch his tools. Three biopsy samples were taken and submitted to Professor Rudolph Virchow. It is interesting that Virchow became the final arbiter, since he had been a fiery public adversary of Bismark and his militarism. Virchow could not demonstrate that Frederick's lesion was cancer. His reports were lengthy opinions of some 800 words each. After three equivocal biopsies, and with a knowledge of the results of available treatments, the Crown Prince refused any operation except tracheostomy. At that time 138 laryngectomies had been reported, with a 36% operative mortality. Only eight patients had survived more than 18 months. Prince Frederick's father, William I, died on March 19, 1888. Crown Prince Frederick became Kaiser Frederick III for a total of 90 days of progressive misery. He died at

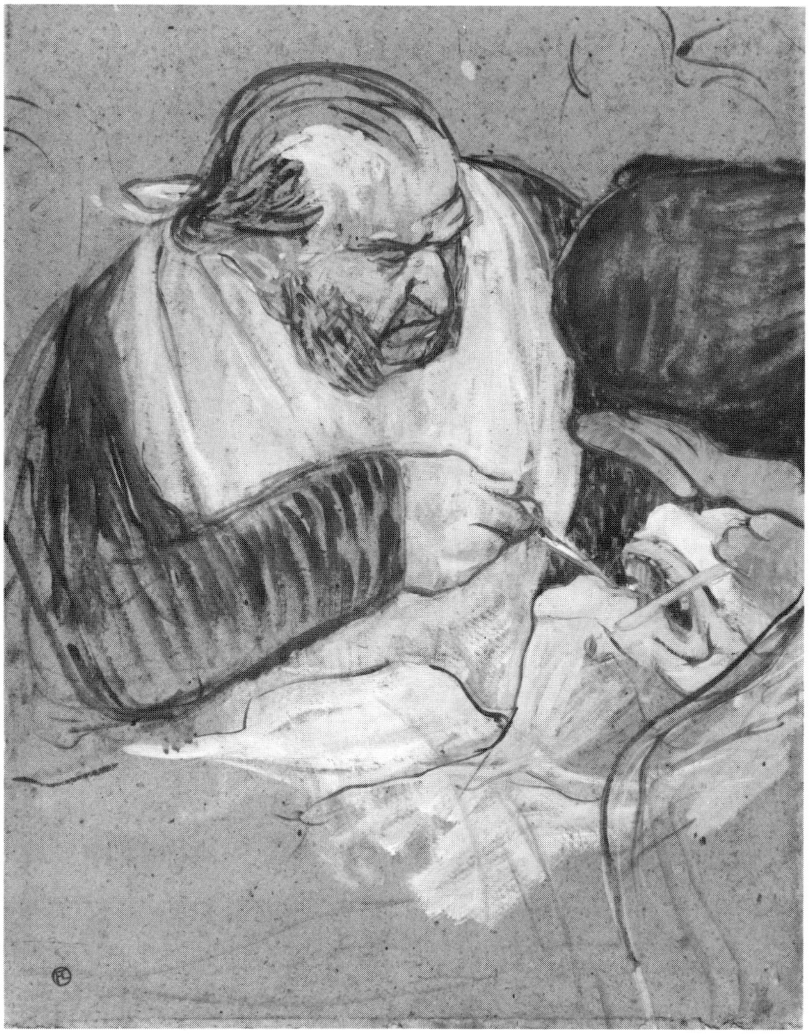

Fig 1–1.—The 1891 painting "Dr. Jules-Emile Pean," erroneously subtitled in some early reference works as "The Tracheotomy," by Henri de Toulouse-Lautrec (1864–1901). (Reproduced by permission of the Sterling and Francine Clark Art Institute, Williamstown, Massachusetts.)

San Remo on June 16, 1888. Frederick's son, William II, became Kaiser. In the years before his death, Frederick had made commitments to peace and friendship abroad and a progressive democracy at home. This attitude was not shared by his son, William II ("Kaiser Bill" of World War I). Because Frederick III's disease was potentially curable and was mismanaged by contemporary standards, there has been persistent speculation about whether successful treatment might have resulted if Professor Bergman had been allowed to operate as he recommended. If cure had been achieved, would it have altered the course of European history? No one is certain whether Frederick would have had different policies than Kaiser William II. The accounts are fascinating to read, and the events have been nicely summarized by McInnis et al.[4]

ULYSSES S. GRANT.—This American Civil War hero was the only President who *died* of cancer. Seven years after leaving office as President, he had a squamous carcinoma of the base of the tongue and/or anterior tonsillar pillar. The best description favors anterior tonsillar pillar. His first symptoms of sore throat and pain on swallowing were noted in June 1884. Dr. Schrady, one of his physicians, recognized the relationship between his heavy cigar smoking and the cancer. Limited surgical resection was technically possible.

Surgery was discussed and dismissed. All subsequent treatment was symptomatic. His terminal episodes with nocturnal near-suffocation, local pain, inability to eat, and progressive inanition were documented by his physician, Dr. John Hancock Douglas, and by the ex-President himself in written notes and memoirs. His death was typical of the drawnout tragic end of life of the uncured patient. He died on July 23, 1885. Unfortunately, his illness and death occurred in an atmosphere of personal financial ruin.[5]

THE SECRET OPERATION ON PRESIDENT GROVER CLEVELAND.—Treatment of President Cleveland's epidermoid cancer of the hard palate/maxillary antrum is exemplary of the glimmerings of surgical success in head and neck cancer. The President's cancer was found in mid-1893. The treatment took real medical courage. His care involved a team of three surgeons, two physicians, and a dentist. The group was headed by Dr. Joseph Decatur Bryant and included the noted neurosurgical pioneer, Dr. W. W. Keen. They operated on Cleveland on July 1, 1893, in an improvised secret setting aboard the yacht Oneida, anchored in Long Island Sound. The rotund, 250-pound, 57-year-old gouty President was given nitrous oxide and open-drop ether with local cocaine to supplement the anesthetics. The surgeons had battery-powered lighting and cautery. The operation lasted from 12:56 to 1:55 P.M. Without endotracheal respiratory control they did an extensive maxillectomy to the floor of the orbit. Because there was a suspicious margin, Cleveland was operated on for a second time on July 17 under the same conditions. A prosthesis was made to fill the palatal defect. Twenty-two days after the second operation Cleveland delivered a speech to Congress urging repeal of the Sherman Silver Act. He lived 15 years longer and died of what was probably a bowel obstruction with complications of "heart failure." His operation remained a partial secret until 1917, when Keen reported it.[6]

These cases near the beginnings of effective therapy of head and neck cancer illustrate how frequently errors in diagnosis and management were made. The first two cases chronicle the miseries of failed biopsies, partial treatment, therapeutic nihilism, and unsuccessfully treated disease. Cleveland's therapy demonstrated that effective no-nonsense treatment could return a patient to productive life. Unfortunately, partial futile treatment and hopeless resignation remained the norm for another 60 years.

By the 1900s, operations could be done on primary oropharyngeal lesions. Spread of disease to the neck nodes defeated most cures. In 1906, G. W. Crile described a systematic cervical lymphadenectomy.[7] His mortality for laryngectomy with cervical lymphadenectomy was 13%.

Progress in the surgical treatment of head and neck cancer seemed stymied by high mortalities from 1910 to 1930. This was due to aspiration, poor anesthesia, and the technical restrictions of blood loss and infection. Before antibiotics virtually eliminated a common scourge, hemolytic streptococcal cellulitis of the face (erysipelas) could produce devastation and death in 24–48 hours. Infectious spread produced septic cavernous sinus thrombophlebitis. Most such complications of the first half of the century are now rarities.

A second path of therapy had been evolving. On Nov. 8, 1895, Wilhelm Conrad Röntgen (1845–1923) made the discovery of x-rays. It was reported in the paper "Preliminary Communication to the President of the Physical-Medical Society of Wurzburg" on Dec. 28, 1895.[3] John Daniel used x-rays at Vanderbilt University in 1896 to produce skin reactions and loss of hair. The first reported response of skin cancers was later in 1896 by T. A. U. Sjögren and J. T. Seinbeck.[3] The Curies discovered radium in 1898. They also related its emanations to x-rays. W. A. Pusey in 1902, Nicholas Senn in 1903, and G. Dock in 1904 used x-rays to treat lymphomas. The surgeon Robert Abbe, of the Abbe-Estlander flap, was the first to implant radium directly into tumors in 1906. Both radium and external irradiation with x-rays became the mainstay in the treatment of the head and neck primary. Through the 1920s surgery was limited to excisions of lip lesions and an occasional oral lesion. Attempts to control metastatic neck node disease kept the neck dissection in common use.

In the history of head and neck cancer treatment, the experience of the charismatic Dr. Hayes Martin marks the leading edge of rapid progress in the 1930s and 1940s. Starting in the 1930s, Dr. Martin used H. Coutard's method of fractionated radiation doses to treat head and neck cancer.[8] He and his colleagues at New York Memorial Hospital pushed the radiation doses to the maximum allowable by the low-kilovoltage apparatus of the time.[9] The usual plan was to try to eliminate the cancer of the primary site with radiation. If the primary could be controlled, a lymphadenectomy was done. Control rates were poor. Skin damage and mucositis were frequent with the low-energy radiation sources. Disillusionment with x-ray treatment results began about the time that blood transfusion became routine. Endotracheal anesthesia (originally described in 1908 by Samuel Meltzer and John Auer, of the Rockefeller Institute) was finally being adopted for head and neck, thoracic, and general surgery. Sulfonamides and subsequent antibiotics helped control the scourge of *Streptococcus* and other pathogenic microbes. Hayes Martin[10] (Memorial Hospital, New York), Grant Ward[11] (Johns Hopkins Hospital, Baltimore), and James Barrett Brown (Washington Hospital, St. Louis) were leaders who developed composite operations that encompassed the primary oropharyngeal or laryngeal lesion with the contiguous tissues of a cervical lymphadenectomy. The pendulum swung from reliance on radiation therapy to extended resective surgery. The late 1940s saw lower operative mortalities and higher expectations for cure for many early head and neck cancers. A key to general progress was the dissemination of technical skills by the effective teaching of Hayes Martin and Grant Ward. Their pupils in turn became effective and inventive teachers with a keen interest in coordinated treatment and rehabilitation of head and neck cancer victims.

A. J. Kremen's 1956 report on a series of tongue cancers was typical of the post-World War II era. He reported a 68% 5-year tumor-free survival with 0% mortality.[12] This achievement in our local area made it apparent that temporizing treatment and fatalistic resignation were no longer acceptable.

The next decade brought an abrupt escalation in 5-year survival. Meanwhile, radiation therapy had not been standing still. The period of 1940–1960 ushered in a post-World War II interest in high-energy radiation sources. Megavoltage x-ray and cobalt sources offered predictable sparing of superficial tissues. The scientific refinements in radiation physics, radiobiology, and precise therapy planning were more important. These advances resulted in better local control of favorable lesions while reducing damage to skin, bone, and uninvolved tissues. Under the leadership of Grant Ward[13] and MacComb and Fletcher,[14] planned combinations of radiation therapy and surgery were explored. The variations of radiation dosage, surgical scope, timing, and sequence are still under investigation.

Chemotherapy had its origins in the late 1930s and during World War II. The effects of mustard gas analogues were being studied. Alfred Gilman, Louis S. Goodman, and Thomas F. Dougherty, then at Yale, had found that nitrogen mustard was cytotoxic for lymphoid tissues. After favorable results in transplanted mouse lymphosarcoma, the first human trial was made in 1942 on a young, nearly moribund male patient of Dr. Gustaf E. Lindskog. There was a dramatic early response of the lymphoma followed by a recurrence. Characteristic bone marrow suppression was also found.[15] This launched the search for thousands of potential drugs, bringing us to the era of modern chemotherapy for the treatment of malignancy. The addition of chemotherapy to surgery and irradiation places us in the framework of contemporary management of head and neck cancer.

HOW SIGNIFICANT A PROBLEM IS HEAD AND NECK CANCER IN THE UNITED STATES?

Table 1–1 lists the estimated number of new cases and number of deaths from head and neck cancer for 1984.[16] These data were developed by using 5-year distribution data from the National Cancer Institute SEER program from 1973–1979 and then correcting for 1984 population figures. The rates are increasing annually for squamous cell cancer. A more representative total is obtained by adding the 3,500 malignant melanomas of the head and neck (23% of all malignant melanomas) and the 1,200 soft tissue and bone tumors (estimated). Not included are eye, brain, lymphomas, and skin cancers. If we were to add all nonmelanoma skin cancers, the numbers would be grossly distorted, since about 400,000 new skin cancers were estimated to occur in 1984, of which 90% (360,000) would be expected to occur in the head and neck. In essence, the numbers can

TABLE 1–1.—NUMBERS OF HEAD AND NECK CANCERS AND FREQUENCY OF DEATH IN 1984*

SITE	ESTIMATED NEW CANCER CASES	ESTIMATED NO. OF CANCER DEATHS
Lip	4,900	175
Tongue	4,900	2,050
Salivary gland		700
Floor of mouth	9,800 (salivary gland, floor of mouth, other oral sites combined)	525
Other oral sites		1,600
Pharynx	7,900	4,300
Larynx	11,100	3,750
Thyroid	10,300	1,100
Head/neck melanoma	3,500†	1,200†
Head/neck bone and soft tissue	1,250†	500†
Total	53,550	15,950 (3.6% of cancer deaths)
Total cancers in U.S. population, 1984, all sites‡	870,000	450,000 (20.6% of all U.S. deaths)

*From Silverberg.[16] Reproduced by permission.
†Estimated allocation to head and neck area.
‡Does not include carcinoma in situ and nonmelanoma skin cancers.

be different depending on what is included as a head and neck cancer. For purposes of this text, the large or life-threatening cancers are the major concern.

Figure 1–2 gives a graphic perspective on head and neck cancers, their relative importance, and their appropriate distribution. Table 1–2 gives the absolute incidence and the relative incidence by site of all head and neck cancers.[17]

The right-hand column of Table 1–1 records an estimated 15,950 deaths from head and neck cancer in 1984. This implies that about one person in three who gets a significant head and neck cancer dies from it. We do know that thyroid cancer is compatible with very long survival. On the other hand, advanced pharyngeal cancer has a low 5-year survival.

In the aggregate, the treatment of squamous cell cancer of the head and neck is much more successful than the treatment of the other major tobacco-related disease, cancer of the lung. The Minneapolis Veterans Administration Hospital saw 2,352 lung cancer patients between 1947 and 1975. Only 632 were candidates for a curative resective attempt. At 5 years, 170 were alive, for a 27% operative cure rate but a miserable 7% overall survival.[18] Head and neck cancer does not reach the epidemic proportion of lung cancer (139,000 lung cancers per year, with 121,000 deaths in 1984, the annual rate is rising).

Squamous cell cancer constitutes at least 75% of head and neck cancers. Like other oroairway cancers, it tends to occur in the fifth and sixth decades of life. With thyroid cancer, connective tissue cancers, and parotid gland cancer, the peak incidence of the tumor is found in younger people.

WHAT ATTITUDES DO PATIENTS HAVE TOWARD TREATMENT OF HEAD AND NECK CANCER?

The peculiar problems of head and neck cancer must be considered in terms of physician attitudes, patient

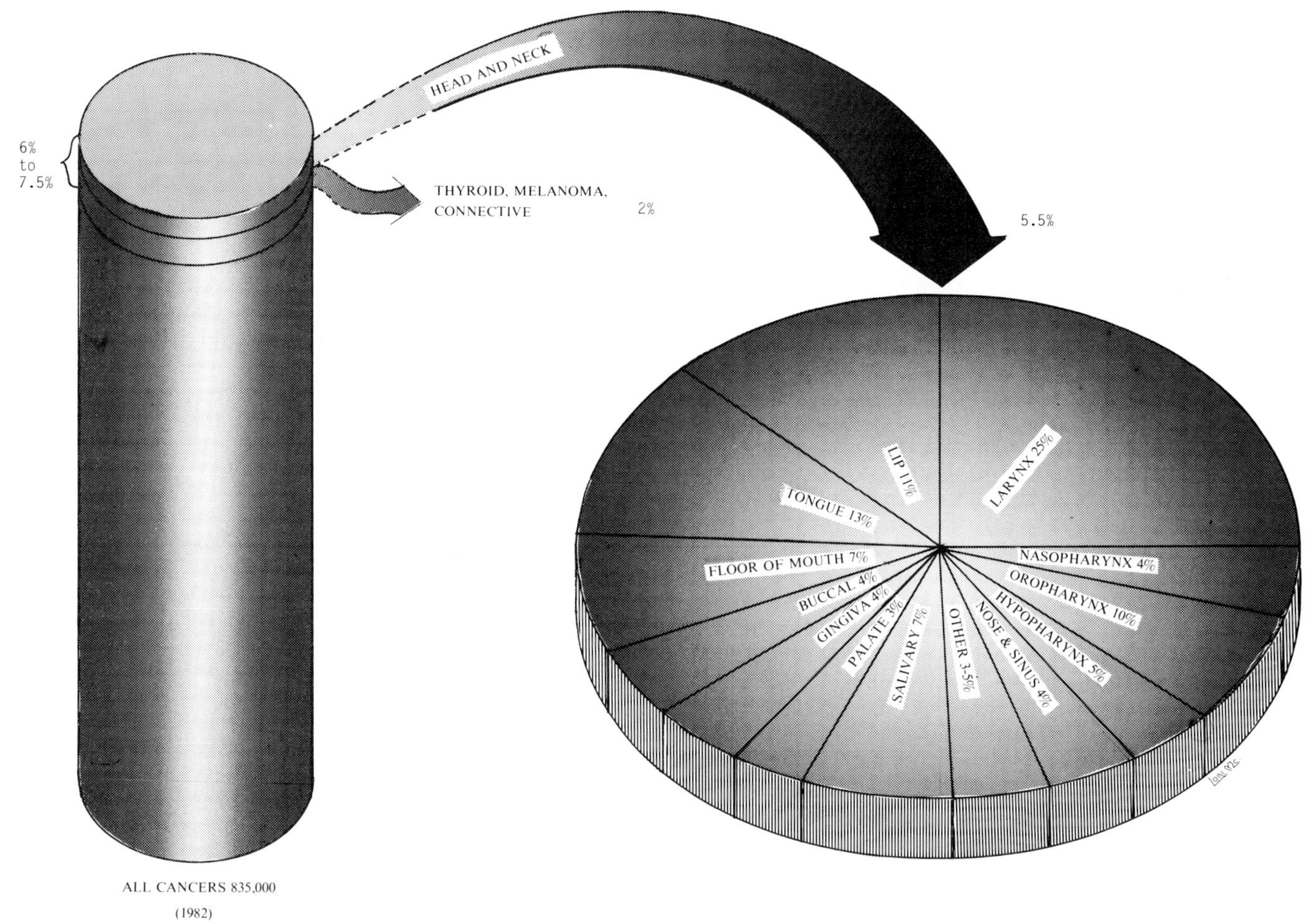

Fig 1–2.—The relative importance and distribution of head and neck cancer. Figure was constructed from 1982 SEER data. Exact percentages may differ slightly from percentages in the tables. The illustration does accurately reflect the relative importance of various sites.

TABLE 1–2.—DETAILS OF U.S. HEAD AND NECK CANCER INCIDENCE: DISTRIBUTED BY SITE*

SITE	RATE/100,000	% OF HEAD/NECK CANCERS	% OF ALL CANCERS
Lip	1.9	12	0.6
Tongue	2.1	13	0.7
Other oral:	2.8	17	0.9
Floor of mouth	(1.0)	(7)	(0.3)
Buccal	(0.7)	(5)	(0.2)
Gingival	(0.7)	(5)	(0.2)
Palate	(0.4)	(3)	(0.1)
Salivary gland	1.1	7	0.4
Total oral	**7.9**	**48**	**2.6**
Nasopharynx	0.6	4	0.2
Other pharynx	2.4	15	0.8
Larynx	4.2	25	1.4
Nose and Paranasal sinus	0.7	4	2
Cervical esophagus	0.35	15	0.8
Ear	0.15	1	0.1
Unknown primary	0.35	2	0.2
Total head/Neck	**16.12**	**100**	**5.5**
Expanded Head and Neck			
Thyroid	3.6		1.2
Soft tissue and bone (H/N)	0.5		.2
Melanoma (H/N)	1.3		.4
Total expanded	**22.6**		**7.3**

*From *Management Guidelines for Head and Neck Cancer.*[17] Some subcategories do not add precisely due to rounding errors.

attitudes, real and imagined disability or disfigurement, and loss of key functions of swallowing, speech, and vision. A better cure rate with aggressive treatment exacts its price in disability. There are good articles addressing the patient anxieties and attitudes.[19, 20] For treatment planning purposes there is no good way to measure a particular patient's assessment of risk versus disability. The rules and guidelines for compensation for disability probably indicate the features which a general population considers important. The following material is taken from *Social Security Regulations, Rules for Determining Disability and Blindness,* and the *Supplementary Manual on Development and Evaluation:*[21]

2202. Loss of Speech

Ordinarily, when an individual's impairment prevents effective speech, the loss of function is sufficiently severe so that an allowance under Listing 2.09 [total disability] is justified on the basis of medical considerations alone, unless such a finding is rebutted by work activity. To speak effectively, an individual must be able to produce speech that can be heard, understood, and sustained well enough to permit useful communication in social and vocational settings. These criteria are applicable to the production of speech whether by natural function of the voice mechanism or by the use of a prosthetic device.

Three attributes of speech pertinent to the evaluation of speech proficiency are: (1) audibility—the ability to speak at a level sufficient to be heard; (2) intelligibility—the ability to articulate and to link the phonetic units of speech with sufficient accuracy to be understood; and (3) functional efficiency—the ability to produce and sustain a serviceably fast rate of speech output over a useful period of time. When at least one of these attributes is missing, overall speech function is not considered effective.

2206. Facial Disfigurement

A. Facial disfigurement is difficult to evaluate when it cannot be measured objectively in terms of specific loss of function. In such instances, realistic consideration must be given to reduced job opportunities due to an abhorrent face, as well as residual physical capacity.
B. Although physical deformity without functional loss is seldom a basis for a finding of disability, severe facial disfigurement may prevent substantial gainful activity where the person's remaining capacity for employment limits him or her to occupations having major requirement for dealing with the public. . . .

The more detailed instructions for rating disability can be reviewed to give the physician a perspective on what the world at large considers crucial in head and neck disease and patient rehabilitation. It also clearly points out the information that is needed by insurance carriers and rating boards to establish that a patient is disabled.

These disabilities are further adjudicated on the basis of maximum sustained work capacity—heavy, sustained physical work, moderate work, or sedentary occupation. It is here that loss of spinal accessory nerve function is important. Any patient with a rapidly growing *uncured* cancer is disabled for the duration of survival, with few exceptions.

WHAT IS THE PRICE OF THERAPEUTIC FAILURE?

The major objectives of therapy are summarized in Figure 1–3. A trip through a terminal care ward shows what advanced treated and untreated squamous cell cancer looks like. The prime requirement of controlling the cancer should be kept in mind when one weighs options that may have cosmetic or functional consequence. Figure 1–4 is a brief diagram of the major options open to a patient with a T_2 squamous cell tongue cancer. Basically, such a patient ends up in one of two outcome categories, an agonizing death or a long period of survival with some disability. As one discusses therapeutic options it is necessary to keep in mind that untreated disease, or a compromised treatment that fails, may produce disabilities more horrible and miserable than any rational therapeutic option. Drooling, loss of speech, pain from nerve invasion,[22] muscular functional loss, inability to chew, and repellant appearance are all found in advanced and terminal cancer. In addition, there is relentless compression of the airway and esophagus. Open cancer is invariably infected and malodorous, bulky, and infiltrative, with a propensity to serum weeping and bleeding.

This point is belabored because one occasionally encounters well-meaning novices who counsel a patient with the potential for cure about his "right to die with dignity." It is the very same counselor who cannot tolerate a lack of cosmetic perfection and who is the first to back away and reject the patient with growing disfigurement and miseries.

A second basic error in judgment is perpetrated by medical professionals with little or no experience with head and neck cancer. With good intentions they may implant ideas of cure rates, therapeutic options, and lack of rehabilitation which they encountered in the decades past or which they extrapolate from a single advanced "case " There have been tremendous strides in functional and cosmetic preservation and restoration in the past 20 years. In looking at Figure 1–4, if the tumor growth can be arrested and the cancer eliminated, then a different set of options are possible. Frequently, the basic life-or-death options outlined in Figure 1–4 are lost or confused in "fog bombs" of erudite quotations and haggling over minutiae. If curative therapy is to be undertaken, a lazy or ill-advised compromise of thorough treatment for a minimal cosmetic benefit may cost the cure with *no net benefit*.

WHAT ARE THE COMMON ETIOLOGIES OF HEAD AND NECK CANCERS?

When we discuss etiology, we must first focus on squamous cell cancer. Squamous cell cancer of head and neck accounts for 66% of cancer occurrences and about 75% of cancer deaths. Oral cancer was not reported frequently in the West prior to 1700. The American colonists discovered that tobacco was a great cash crop. The use of tobacco increased further as cigarettes provided the merchants' dream product—"make it for a dime, sell it for a dollar, and hope it's habit-forming." Increased tobacco use was followed by an increase in oroairway cancers. The 1964 Surgeon General's report gave belated official notice of the obvious etiology.[23] Besides lung cancer, it reviewed the relationship of smoking to oral cancer up to that time. There were two prospective studies after the Surgeon General's report that defined the oral cancer mortality rates of smokers and nonsmokers.[24] The data are summarized in Table

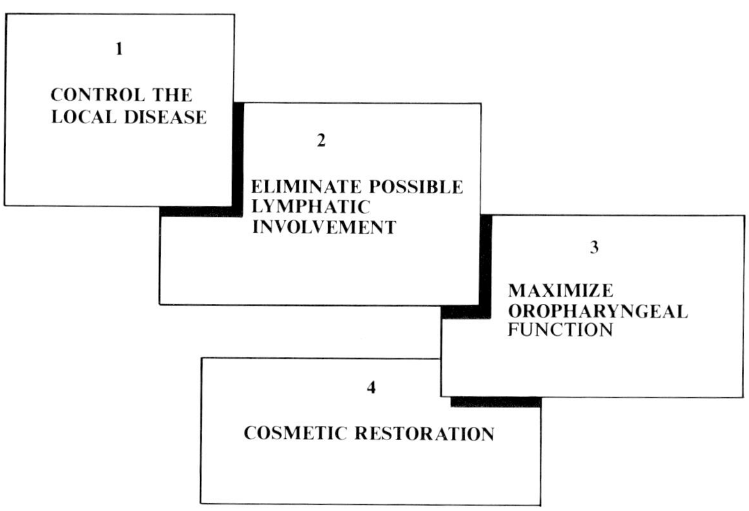

Fig 1–3.—Major objectives in the treatment of head and neck cancer, arranged by priority. Cosmetic reconstruction and rehabilitation require successful attention to the preceding priorities.

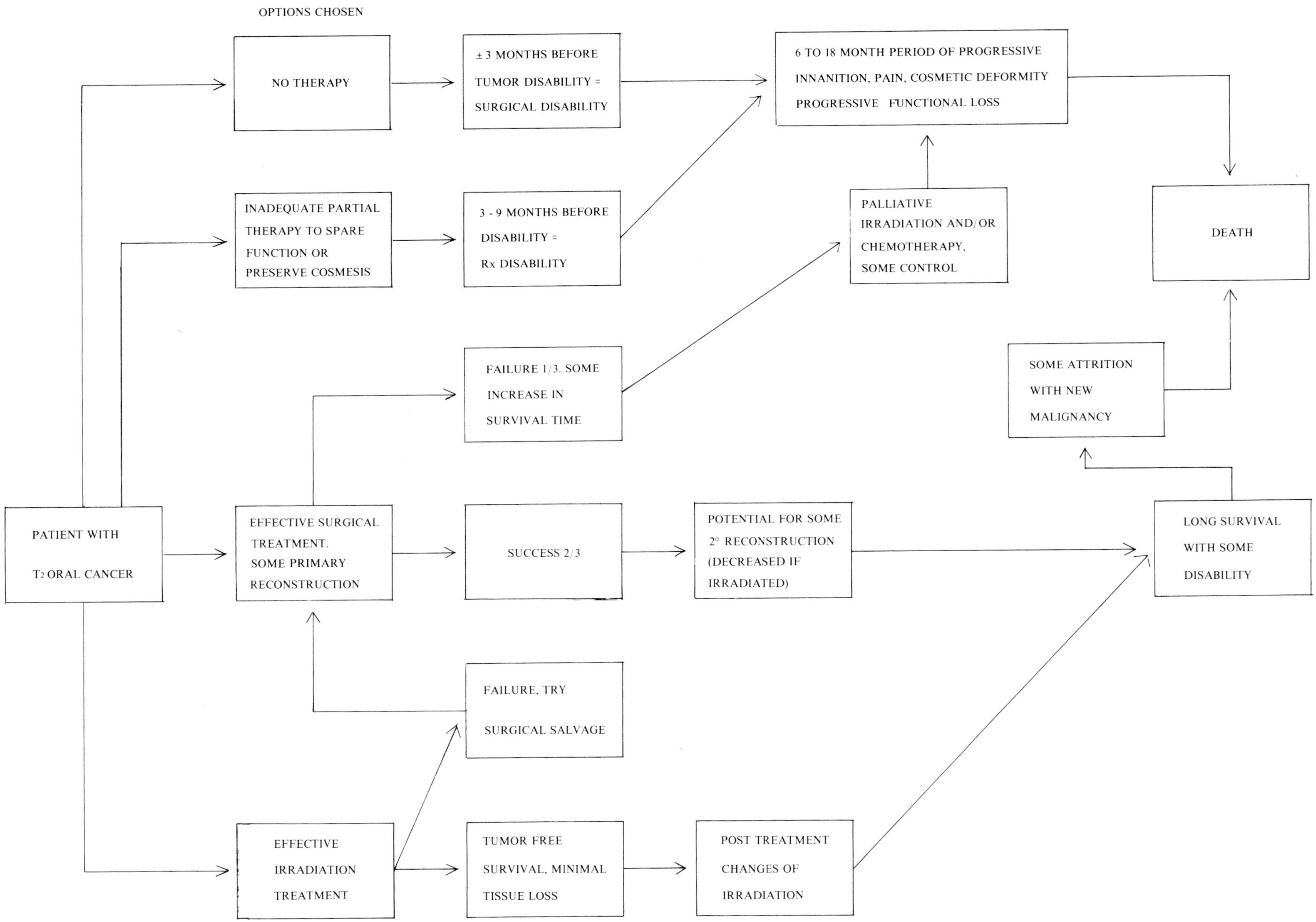

Fig 1–4.—General treatment options that may be followed in a patient with a potentially curable T_2 oral squamous cell cancer. Without therapy, or with inadequate therapy, the disability and functional loss from tumor growth soon exceed the disability from effective curative treatment.

1–3. Other studies confirmed the etiologic relationship.[25-28] In a population with many nonsmokers, Smart et al. reported a clear *reduction* of oropharyngeal cancer.[29] The rate was 43% below the national incidence where cigarette consumption per capita was 52% below national average. The duration and amount of smoking have been directly and positively correlated with oropharyngeal cancers.[30] Continued smoking increases the likelihood of second cancers.[31] Wynder and Wright also showed that the tars from tobacco smoke were more carcinogenic in mice than an extract from unburned tobacco.[32] Snuff chewers and tobacco chewers repetitively conduct a clear experiment when the quid of tobacco is placed in a specific oral locus. Tobacco produces a spatially corresponding epithelial response (frequently leukoplakia). In many patients who continue habitual use, a cancer develops in the exact spot.[33]

Outside of the United States and Western Europe, betel nut chewing in its classic form or with added tobacco is the most frequent cause of oral cancer. In India and Sri Lanka (Celon), oral cancer is estimated to cause as many as 50% of all major cancer deaths.[34] Betel nut chewing is common in India, Sri Lanka, Coastal East Africa, and Malasia. Two different plants are combined to make the chew, the seed of the areca palm (*Areca catechu*, fam. Palme) and the leaf of the betel pepper plant (*Piper betel*, fam. Piperaceae). The palm seed is husked, boiled, sliced, and dried. For use, it is wrapped in a betel pepper leaf with a small amount of slaked lime to liberate the active alkaloids and then chewed. The betel nut releases the chief alkaloid, arecoline. The arecoline produces profuse salivation. The leaf probably contains other alkaloid agents. A related plant, *Piper methysticum*, has known mild narcotic properties. If the habitués chew more, there is a higher incidence of oral cancer.[35] Adding tobacco potentiates the carcinogenicity.[36] A review correlates the habitual placement of the chew with the locus of the oral epithelial changes,[37] just as it correlates for snuff dippers in Scandinavia.[38] It's difficult to deny a relationship between oral cancer and tobacco use in the United States and betel nut chewing and/or tobacco use in Asia.

In the distant past, syphilis was thought to be a factor in oral cancer. The florid stomatitis and glossitis of the secondary phase of syphilis left a severely scarred mouth with focal areas of smoldering spirochetal inflammation. Separating this cause from the effects of tobacco is impossible. The rates of syphilis have fallen in the postantibiotic era. Martin reported in 1948 that 30% of his patients with head and neck cancer had syphilis, compared to 4% of the hospital population at large.[39] In our hospital, 12% of patients with oral cancer had a positive test for syphilis on admission during the 1935–1960 period. The current rate is negligible.

The isolated role of alcohol in squamous cell cancer is not clear. Virtually every alcoholic smokes. There is no question that alcoholism is common in head and neck cancer patients; one study of such patients found that 92% were drinkers and 62% were heavy drinkers.[40] Adjuvant carcinogenicity can be postulated to be due to poor oral hygiene, nutritional inadequacy, direct irritation, something related to cirrhosis, and postindulgence xerostomia.[40] Vogler et al. did not find a direct relationship between oral cancer and alcohol intake.[41] In summary, the etiologic effect of alcohol is not as defined as tobacco use. Clinical decisions must consider special operative risks in the alcoholic (see Chap. 5).

Finally, patients with achlorhydria and Plummer-Vinson (or Patterson-Kelly) syndrome have a higher incidence of pharyngeal cancer.[42] This could be related to nutritional deficiency or chronic iron deficiency. There are no clear data to support one relationship over another.

In summary, the great majority of oroairway squamous cell cancers are self-inflicted cancers.

The etiological risks of radiation exposure in thyroid cancer, the associated viral presence in nasopharyngeal

TABLE 1–3.—SMOKING AND OROPHARYNGEAL CANCER: EXCESS MORTALITY RATE WITH TOBACCO USE*

STUDY	TOBACCO TYPE	MORTALITY RATE RATIO† Age 45–64	Age 65–79	SITE
Hammond	Cigarettes	9.90	2.93	Oral
	Pipe/Cigar	4.94		
Dorn	Cigarettes	6.00		Buccal cavity
	Pipe/Cigar	4.00		
	Cigarettes	12		Pharynx
	Pipe/Cigar	3		

*From *The Health Consequences of Smoking*.[24]
†The number is the age-corrected ratio of: Observed mortality rate/100,000 with tobacco use divided by expected mortality rate/100,000

cancer, sinus cancers in furniture workers, and mutagenic effects of solar exposure in melanoma are discussed elsewhere in this volume.

HOW CAN HEAD AND NECK CANCER BE PREVENTED?

For the prevention of head and neck cancer, one message towers above all others—stop smoking! Most of us have been frustrated over many years by our inability to get heavy smokers to alter their habits. We are beginning to understand that smoking is not just a habituation but, more likely, an addiction wherein smoking causes the production and release of significant amounts of β-endorphins.[43] This now gives us hints about how to structure an effective "stop smoking" program. Such programs should encourage running, vigorous physical activity, and other steps that can be substituted to raise β-endorphin levels. As a priority, physicians must discourage tobacco use. The American College of Chest Physicians has produced a useful packet of informational materials (911 Busse Highway, Park Ridge, IL 60068). The packet is called "Doctor, you can really help patients stop smoking." It contains simple instructional aids and printed material with which one can give patients a sensible program. Similar informational aids can be obtained from the American Lung Association.

Some melanomas can be prevented. It is useful to remove moles from feet and friction areas. It is also necessary to reduce exposure to sunlight. It is tragic to see a fair-skinned, freckled, red-head sitting in the sun. The only tan produced is a confluence of the solar-activated freckles in a sea of sunburn. The data on melanoma in relation to fair skin and sun exposure are found in chapter 22.

IF PREVENTION CANNOT BE ACHIEVED, WHAT IS THE POTENTIAL CONTRIBUTION OF EARLY DETECTION?

Earlier detection of head and neck squamous cell cancers has the highest probability of increasing cure rates. A large part of the gain in survival in the past two decades can be traced to an increased proportion of earlier (T_1, T_2) lesions. Typically, 5-year tumor-free survival increases from 50% to 90% when laryngeal cancers are found at a T_1 stage rather than T_3. For the oral tongue, the difference is 35% versus 85% 5-year survival when T_3 is compared to T_1. The clinicians involved in treating head and neck cancers are *not* the clinicians seeing large groups of patients at risk. Those caring for head and neck cancer patients have a responsibility to teach, emphasize, exhort, and demonstrate to other health professionals the need for good oral and head and neck examinations. The usual perfunctory oral examination—"open up, say ah"—is worthless. A good examination as outlined in chapter 2 is easy and quick.

Who should receive special scrutiny?

1. Any smoker over 35 years of age.
2. Other tobacco (snuff, pipe, cigar) users. Increase suspicion with alcohol use.
3. Anyone with a husky voice.
4. Orientals with symptoms referable to nasal sinuses.
5. Anyone with a history of Plummer-Vinson syndrome.
6. A freckled fair-skinned person with heavy solar exposure.
7. Anyone with a history of head and neck irradiation.
8. Furniture workers.

Any epithelial lesion existing in the oropharyngeal or laryngeal areas for 2 weeks should be biopsied. Any lesion with equivocal histology that appears suspicious and persists should be rebiopsied or totally excised.

IF A HEAD AND NECK CANCER HAS BEEN FOUND, HOW DO YOU BEGIN TO PLAN TREATMENT?

If you approach a senior head and neck surgeon or radiation oncologist and ask, "How do you treat a squamous cell cancer of the floor of the mouth?", either one would look at you askance and not give a clear answer. They need to have a number of precise clinical dimensions to begin to match a particular patient to a spectrum of therapeutic options. We will look at the first decision requirement, adequately detailed patient data. Some of the elements are listed in Table 1–4.

A subquestion might be, "Why do you stage a head and neck cancer?" When cancer "cures" began to be regularly achieved, it became apparent that patients with early cancers did better than patients with advanced cancers. Each reporting group had its own system of classification. It was difficult to share experience in management and therapy without a common set of categories. The American Joint Committee for Cancer Staging and End Results Reporting was organized on Jan. 9, 1959 to develop a system of staging. Classifications have been made to agree as closely as possible to a parallel effort by the Union International Contre le Cancer (UICC).

The TNM staging system has undergone refinement and revision.[44] It may not be perfect, but it is very good. The system should be mastered by anyone par-

TABLE 1–4.—PATIENT INFORMATION NEEDED FOR EFFECTIVE CLINICAL DECISION-MAKING IN HEAD AND NECK CANCER

REQUIRED FOR CLINICAL STAGING:
- *Facts about the tumor:*
  - Exact location
  - Histologic type
  - Estimated degree of local invasion
  - Local behavior (e.g., exophytic or invasive)
  - Cytologic grade
  - Involvement of other structures
- *Local lymph node involvement:*
  - Location of all suspicious nodes
  - Size
  - Firmness
  - Degree of fixation to other structures
- *Distant Metastases*
  - Organ system involved
  - Degree of tumor replacement

PRESENCE OF COMPLICATING ILLNESS THAT MAY AFFECT:
- Anesthetic use or tolerance of surgery
- Radiation therapy (dose, location, or extent)
- Use of chemotherapeutic agents
- Design or use of rehabilitative surgical procedures
- Use of other medical supportive measure
- Sensitivities, bleeding, etc.
- Nutrition
- Immunity

SOME ESTIMATE OF PATIENT'S FUNCTIONAL PERFORMANCE STATUS (KARNOFSKY SCALE OR ECOG/INBROD SCALE)

PRESENCE OR ABSENCE OF SECOND CANCER

ticipating in the diagnosis, management, and postoperative care of head and neck cancer patients. An extracted booklet dealing only with head and neck sites is available from The American Joint Committee, 55 East Erie St., Chicago, IL 60611. The full staging manual is now published commercially.[45] There has been some controversy surrounding the staging. Platz et al. recently compared four staging schemes to see if they produced prognostically homogeneous categories.[46] Perfection was not obtained. There will be future revisions and refinements. Head and neck cancer care has been justifiably accused of being "stage struck." But staging is essential if any comparisons are to be made.

An essential element in staging is precise diagrammatic and written description of the data elements in Table 1–4. Preprinted forms containing the information lists and drawings for staging are available from Adria Laboratories, P.O. Box 16529, Columbus, OH 43216, attn. Mr. Larry Johnson. This is a set of unbound master copies which may be reproduced by photocopying for entry of patient data. They are easy to complete and insert into the patient record. The form set is free. An additional aid is to have preprinted forms or large rubber stamps with the anatomical drawings available in the office and ward. Where several disciplines may be consulting, accurate written and diagrammatic communication is needed.

When the facts are gathered, TNM staging is straightforward (Table 1–5). For each tumor site the T (tumor) and N (node) subdivisions are defined in the *Manual for Staging of Cancer*[45] and in the appropriate chapters of this book. The TNM system is directly adaptable to the old stage I, II, III, and IV grouping, as shown in Figure 1–5. Major problems arise in using the I, II, III, IV staging system since there are different prognostic categories in stage IV (shown by the shaded

TABLE 1–5.—DEFINITION OF STAGING TERMS

Three capital letters are used to describe the extent of cancer: *T* (tumor), *N* (nodes), and *M* (metastases)

Type of classification:
- c Clinical (diagnostic)
- s Surgical (evaluative)
- p Postsurgical treatment (pathologic)
- r Retreatment
- a Autopsy

This classification is extended by the following designations:

Tumor

T_X	Tumor cannot be assessed
T_0	No evidence of primary tumor
T_{IS}	Carcinoma in situ
T_1, T_2, T_3, T_4	Progressive increase in tumor size and local involvement

Nodes

N_x	Regional lymph nodes cannot be assessed clinically
N_0	Regional lymph nodes not demonstrably abnormal
N_1, N_2, N_3, N_4	Increasing degrees of demonstrable abnormality of regional lymph nodes

Metastases

M_x	Not assessed
M_0	No (known) distant metastasis
M_1	Distant metastases present Specify sites of metastasis

HISTOPATHOLOGY:

The histologic type of cancer

Grade (G)

G_1	Well differentiated
G_2	Moderately well differentiated
G_3, G_4	Poorly to very poorly differentiated; use whichever indicator is most appropriate (term or G+ number)

RESIDUAL TUMOR(R)

(This information does not enter into establishing stage of tumor but should be recorded on data form for use in considering additive therapy)

When the cancer is treated by definitive surgical procedures, residual cancer, if any, is recorded.

Residual tumor following surgical treatment:

R_0	No residual tumor
R_1	Microscopic residual tumor
R_2	Macroscopic residual tumor: Specify ________

Continued

TABLE 1–5.—*Continued*

HOST PERFORMANCE SCALE

The host performance status is determined at the time of clinical-diagnostic classification and recorded at subsequent times of classification as well as at each follow-up examination to measure the quality of life. The ECOG-Zubrod Scale or the Karnofsky Scale are used as outlined in (54).

HOST

H denotes the physical state (performance scale) of the patient considering all cofactors determined at the time of stage classification and subsequent follow-up examinations:

H_0	Normal activity
H_1	Symptomatic and ambulatory—cares for self.
H_2	Ambulatory more than 50% of time—occasionally needs assistance
H_3	Ambulatory 50% or less of time—nursing care needed
H_4	Bedridden—may need hospitalization

area in Fig 1–5). The gradations in stage III also need refinement. The TNM system with some subcategories is still the most helpful classification system for planning care and evaluating end-stage results.

AFTER PATIENT DATA ARE OBTAINED, HOW DOES A CLINICAL TEAM BEGIN TO DECIDE ON A TREATMENT PROGRAM?

This book will build an eclectic sample of decision-making algorithms. The purpose of any algorithm is to demonstrate how decisions *might* be made. They are not rigid protocols. The reader should seek refinements in both treatment options and logic patterns. Patient variation and the uncertainty of the effect of treatment will dictate wider variations. Our aim is to give the reader a crude road map to the appropriate factors that must be considered in order to arrive at minimally prejudiced clinical decisions. Kassirer and associates have found that physicians do not always pursue the orderly decision path they espouse.[47] Clinical problem-solving skills are reduced when specialists move beyond their area of expertise.[47, 48] Kassirer's studies show that clinicians learn thousands of combinations of diagnoses, diseases, treatments, and likely outcomes.[48] Their group's experience with a clinical simulation program (CONNIVER) established that experienced clinicians: (1) Rely heavily on guessing, (2) rapidly make initial hypotheses and plans based on skimpy data, (3) mentally test the plan or hypothesis for correctness, moving to a new hypothesis if necessary, (4) rarely begin with more than a few potential hypotheses or plans, (5) continuously pare the list by eliminating some possibilities and combining others into new options, and (6) usually associate one hypothesis or plan with others which are similar and with which it can be confused. Kassirer's group also found that the student or inexperienced physician has trouble making complex interrelated decisions and projecting risks accurately.[49] In the absence of vast experience or in the presence of unusual problems, one must still retreat to structured decisions to ensure that the patient will have the best chance at a favorable outcome.

There are times when a clinician's behavior suggests he is trying to avoid the responsibility of making a clear decision. He may stall with further inconclusive tests, needless consultation, or trials of inappropriate partial treatment. One must use adequate but not excessive or redundant data. The data that enter into the decision-making process must be sufficiently detailed to reflect the complexity of real-life circumstances.

To make a decision, there must be an intent to reach a decision. Then, diagrammatic or structured decision-making can be a helpful tool when one is out of an area of total familiarity.[50] Figure 1–6 begins to structure the gathering of facts. The process is basic to developing a plan as shown in Figure 1–7. The key to Figure 1–6 is to *make an explicit statement of the problems and questions that are posed.* After an initial flurry of fact gathering, the cycle can be repeated throughout the clinical management decision process.

In decision-making processes, there are three key features:

1. "The word risk is an 'absence of certainty.' Risk implies that there is a difference between a decision and its outcome. There is often a tendency to 'pay only for results [the desired outcome]' "[51]

2. In studies on equal risk in insurance, U.S. citizens consistently prefer to be exposed to low-probability, high-loss hazards than to high-probability, low-loss hazards, when the net loss to two large groups would be equal.[51] If this is extrapolated to head and neck cancer, the usual patient would prefer a 5%–10% chance of death in order to avoid deformity, rather than accept a sure deformity worth 5%–10% of his "quality of life" value at no risk of death.

3. Real-life decisions may be quite complex. An accurate statistical knowledge leads to decisions of higher quality. Figure 1–7 shows how rapidly treatment decisions become complex when treatment is contemplated for a head and neck cancer patient with complicating illness and strong personal preferences.

Each decision factor must be isolated and weighed on the basis of accurate patient data analyzed against the most reliable data of past experience. Chapter 5 examines decision tools for estimating risks and outcomes. Not all decision points are quantal yes-no decisions. Some have probability and preference grades that lead to weighting measures.

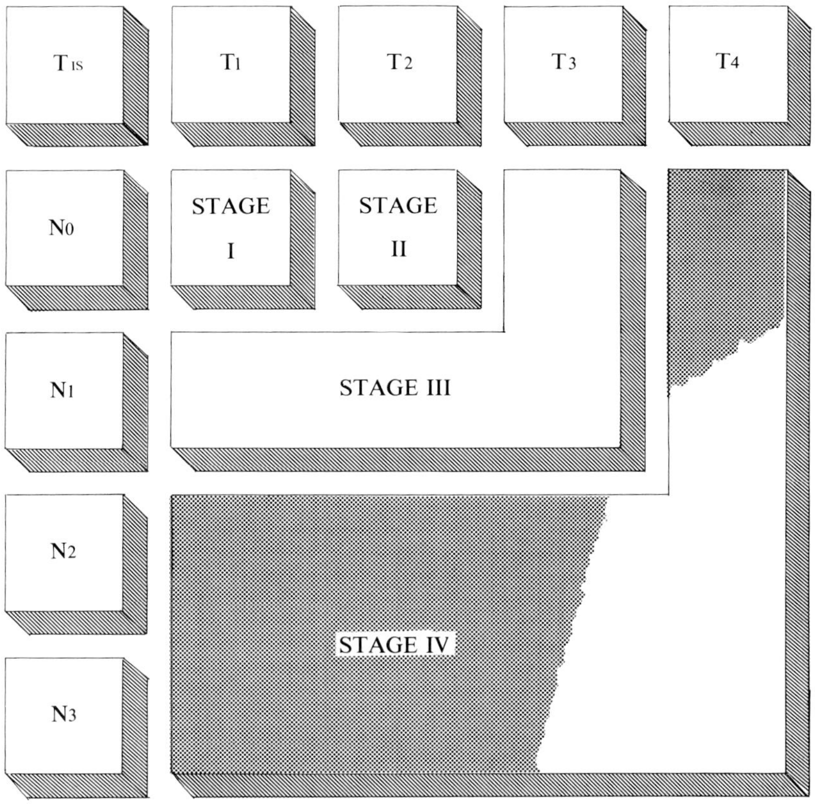

Fig 1–5.—The TNM staging scheme as it relates to the older stage I, II, III, and IV system. The latter is still used to group patients into presumed prognostic categories. There are many problems encountered in stage 4, as indicated by the length and breadth of the shaded area. Patients in these categories are clearly in better prognostic groups that those in the lower right-hand corner (T_4-N_3).

HOW CAN THE CLINICIAN EVALUATE PUBLISHED LITERATURE TO AID IN DECISION-MAKING?

To treat head and neck cancer, one must maintain a clear set of priorities and an ability to critically analyze published data. To quote George Higgins,[52]

> In the past times, and still too often today, medical therapies have emerged in a haphazard trial-and-error fashion, often to glittering and enthusiastic prominence, only to sink back into the ooze of obscurity when evaluated by the uncompromising eye of time. . . . The use of historic controls or comparisons based on dissimilar groups of patients, while somewhat better, still invites erroneous and haphazard conclusions, especially when buttressed by large but noncomparable numbers. When the therapeutic effect is great or the difference between therapies being compared is large, these methods have been satisfactory. . . . When the therapeutic difference is small, more precise methods are essential to reach valid conclusions.

Wide variations in reports of results in treating head and neck cancers may be due to any of the following:

1. Different patient populations being treated.
2. Changing mix of tumor stages or improved survival of control groups over different years.
3. Patients at different disease stages entered into groups. If there is no correction for pathologic findings, the clinical staging of neck nodes will have a 15% false positive rate and a 25% false negative rate. This would produce an inherent bias if a clinically staged group were compared with a pathologically staged group.
4. Comparison of heterogeneous groups with different anatomical components. For example, comparison incorporating the entire oropharynx would show a poorer 5-year survival than in a group with oral lesions only.
5. Different therapeutic techniques may be used over a period of time or in different institutions.
6. Errors in follow-up. A careful examination will find more recurrences than a letter questionnaire. If frequency of follow-up is increased, recurrence will be found earlier and the tumor-free interval will shorten.
7. Meaningless description of treatment effect. "Tumor is controlled" has no dimension as to time, location, and presence or absence of cervical nodal or dis-

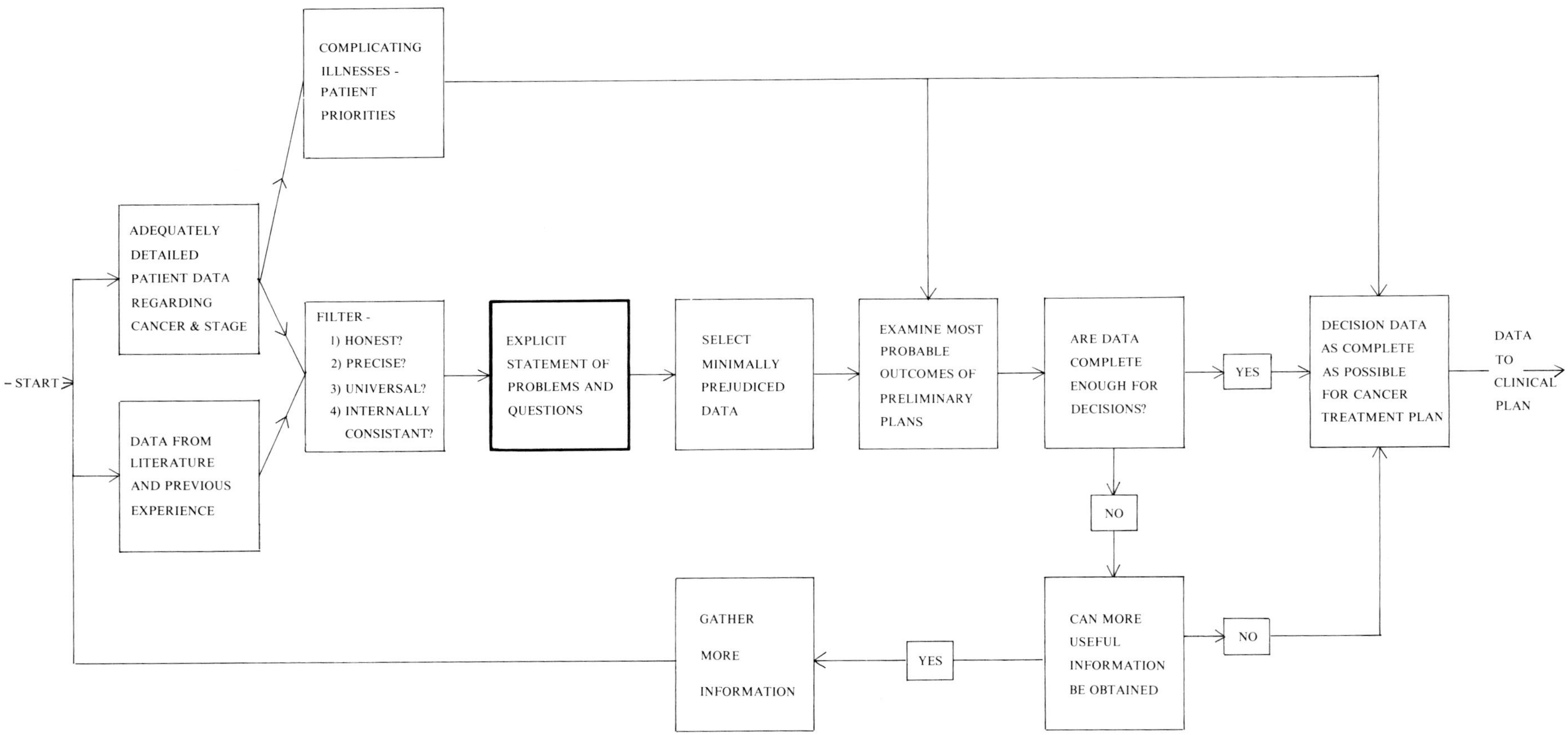

Fig 1–6.—The data-gathering cycle in clinical decision-making. The data must be intellectually filtered. One must explicitly examine the decision questions posed by the patient's disease. Several cycles are usually required. Continuous refinement can occur through the course of a patient's care.

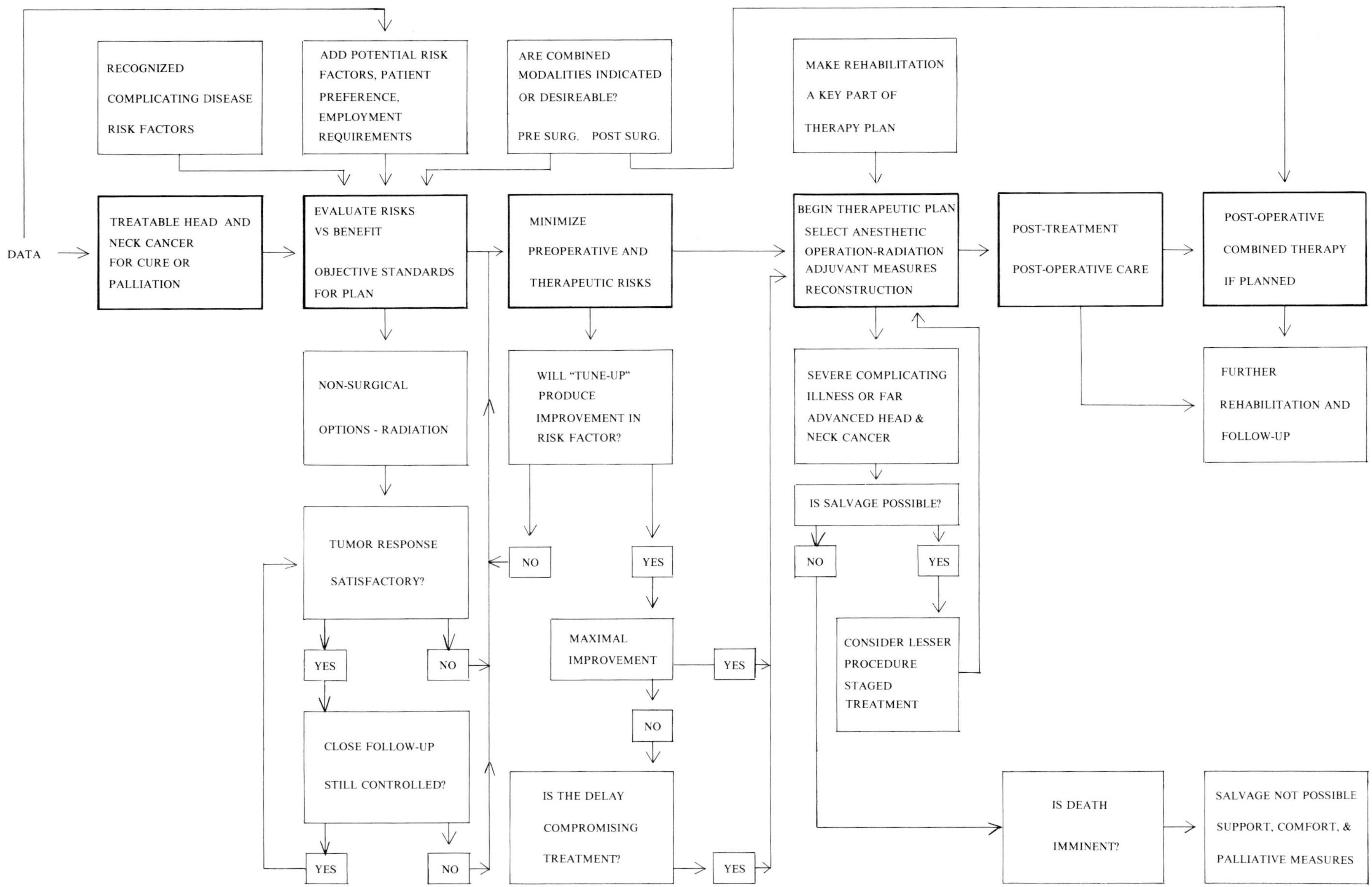

Fig 1–7.—The general clinical decision-making process in a structured form. The four elements in the top boxes must be incorporated into the treatment decisions. The main line of decisions (second row of boxes, heavily outlined) are further modified by decision factors that may require a longer period of evaluation and observation of clinical effect. The need to alter decisions as time passes adds an additional dimension to the scheme.

tant metastases. Furthermore, a transient response has rarely been translated to prolonged survival in most careful clinical trials.

8. Failure to correct for normal death rate. A selected group of younger patients with early cancers will have a longer composite survival, independent of treatment type.

9. It is likely that patients with oroairway squamous cell cancer continue to get subsequent cancers at a relatively fixed rate.[53]

Survival figures are more accurate when life-table methods as outlined in the cancer staging manual are used.[45] As early as 1731, the Reverend Stephen Hales (who first measured arterial pressure directly) observed, "since we are assured that the all-wise Creator has observed the most exact proportions of *number*, *weight*, and *measure*, in the make of all things; the most likely way, therefore, to get any insight into the nature of those parts of the creation, which come within our observation, must in all reason be number, weight, and measure."[54] We should add, "by the least biased methods." In giving weight to clinical evidence one would give more credence to a therapeutic test that eliminated confusing extra diseases as much as possible. The better study would randomly and prospectively allocate patients to treatment groups. Subsequent tests would confirm that there was a true randomization. Patients would be accurately staged, with the diagnosis and staging confirmed by pathologic review. Treatment would be consistently applied. Follow-up would be rigorous and frequent. Data would be gathered for a valid duration and would be sufficiently detailed; the analysis would be statistically tested.

Even a simple *retrospective* unrandomized study of our own evaluating T_1T_2 anterior tongue cancer (see Chap. 13) is seriously flawed despite best efforts at analysis. It would need random allocation of patients to one of two treatment programs. Where staging may be clinical versus pathologic between the two groups, where many patients fail follow-up, and where follow-up examinations are perfunctory, then a 15%–25% variant bias in survival data might be expected to occur. For the present, *the bulk of data for head and neck cancer treatment is seriously flawed.* We can look at aggregate trends from a number of sources and give greater weight to the minimally prejudiced probabilities rather than the most amazing unconfirmed data. When therapeutic differences are small, in the 5%–10% range, we must recognize that it takes many hundreds of patients in a controlled randomized trial to show a significant difference once the usual statistical variance in cancer survival is taken into account.

REFERENCES

1. Absolon K.B., Rogers W., Aust J.B.: Some historical developments of surgical therapy of tongue cancer from the 17th to the 19th century. *Am. J. Surg.* 104:689, 1962.
2. Wangensteen O.H., Wangensteen S.D.: *The Rise of Surgery from Empiric Craft of Scientific Discipline.* Minneapolis, University of Minnesota Press, 1978, pp. 181–184.
3. Castiglioni A.: *A History of Medicine,* ed. 2. New York, Alfred A. Knopf, 1947.
4. McInnis W.D., Egan W., Aust J.B.: The management of carcinoma of the larynx in a prominent patient, or did Morell MacKenzie really cause World War I? *Am. J. Surg.* 132:515–522, 1976.
5. Steckler R.M., Shedd P.: General Grant, his physicians and his cancer. *Am. J. Surg.* 132:508–514, 1976.
6. Morrells C.L. Jr.: New historic information on the Cleveland operations. *Surgery* 62:542–551, 1967.
7. Crile G.: Excision of cancer of the head and neck with special reference to the plan of dissection based on 132 operations. *JAMA* 47:1780–1786, 1906.
8. Coutard H.: Roentgen therapy of epitheliomas of the tonsillar region, hypopharynx and larynx from 1920 to 1926. *AJR* 28:313–331, 1932.
9. James A.G.: Hayes Martin Lecture: Control of head and neck cancer. *Am. J. Surg.*
10. Martin H.: Cancer of the head and neck. *JAMA* 137:1306–1315, 1366–1376, 1948.
11. Ward G.E., Edgerton M.T., Chambers R.B., et al.: Cancer of the oral cavity and pharynx and results of treatment by means of the composite operation (in continuity with radical neck dissection). *Ann. Surg.* 150:202–220, 1959.
12. Kremen A.J.: Results of surgical treatment of cancer of the tongue. *Surgery* 39:49–53, 1956.
13. Ward G.E.: Discussion of methods and results of treatment of cancer of the floor of the mouth, in *Symposium on Cancer of the Head and Neck.* New York, American Cancer Society, Inc., 1957.
14. MacComb W.S., Fletcher G.H.: Planned combination of surgery and radiation in treatment of advanced primary head and neck cancers. *AJR* 77:397, 1957.
15. Gilman A.: The initial clinical trial of nitrogen mustard. *Am. J. Surg.* 105:574–578, 1963.
16. Silverberg E.: Cancer statistics 1984. *CA* 34:9–23, 1984.
17. *Management Guidelines for Head and Neck Cancer.* Bethesda, Md., USDHEW NIH publication No. 80–2037, September 1979.
18. Mayer J.E., Ewing S.L., Ophoven J.J., et al.: Influence of histologic type on survival after curative resection for undifferentiated lung cancer. *J. Thorac. Cardiovasc. Surg.* 84:641–648, 1982.
19. Herzon F.S., Boshier M.: Head and neck cancer: Emotional management. *Head Neck Surg.* 2:112–118, 1979.
20. Cote L.: Psychosocial rehabilitation of the head and neck cancer patient. *Laryngoscope* 88(pt. 2, suppl. 8):93–94, 1978.
21. Social Security Regulations: *Rules for Determining Disa-*

bility and Blindness. Washington, D.C., Social Security Administration.
22. Carter R.L., Pittam M.R., Tanner N.S.B.: Pain and dysphagia in patients with squamous carcinomas of the head and neck. *J. R. Soc. Med.* 75:598–606, 1982.
23. U.S. Public Health Service: *Smoking and Health: Report of the Advisory Committee to the Surgeon General of the Public Health Service.* Washington, D.C., U.S. Department of Health, Education, and Welfare, Public Health Service publication No. 1103, 1964.
24. U.S. Public Health Service: *The Health Consequences of Smoking: A Public Health Service Review: 1967.* Washington, D.C., U.S. Department of Health, Education and Welfare, Public Health Service publication No. 1696, 1967.
25. Moore C.: Cigarette smoking and cancer of the mouth, pharynx, and larynx. *JAMA* 218:553, 1971.
26. Wynder E.L., Dodo H., Block D.A.: Epidemiologic investigation of multiple primary cancers of the upper alimentary and respiratory tracts. *Cancer* 24:730, 1969.
27. Wynder E.L.: Etiologic aspects of squamous cancers of the head and neck. *JAMA* 215:452, 1971.
28. Vincent R.G., Marchetta F.: The relationship of the use of tobacco and alcohol to cancer of the oral cavity pharynx and larynx. *Am. J. Surg.* 106:501, 1963.
29. Smart C.R., Lyon J.L., Skolnick M., et al.: Cancer of the head and neck in Utah. *Am. J. Surg.* 128:463, 1974.
30. Wynder E.L., Stellman S.D.: Comparative epidemiology of tobacco related cancers. *Cancer Res.* 37:4608, 1977.
31. Silverman S., Griffith M.: Smoking characteristics of patients with oral carcinoma and the risk of second oral primary carcinoma. *J. Am. Dent. Assoc.* 85:637, 1972.
32. Wynder E.L., Wright G.: Study of tobacco carcinogenesis: I. Primary fractions. *Cancer* 10:255–271, 1957.
33. Brown R.L.: Snuff dippers' intraoral cancer: Clinical characteristics and response to therapy. *Cancer* 18:2–13, 1964.
34. Shanta V., Krushnamuthi S.A.: Study of aetological factors in oral squamous cell carcinoma. *Br. J. Cancer* 13:(3)27, 1959.
35. Hirayama T.: An epidemiologic study of oral and pharyngeal cancer in Central and Southeast Asia. *Bull. WHO* 34:41–69, 1966.
36. Reddy D.G., Anguli V.C.: Experimental production of cancer with betel nut, tobacco and slaked lime mixture. *J. Indian Med. Assoc.* 49:315–318, 1967.
37. Singh A.D., Von Easen C.F.: Buccal mucosa cancers in South India: Etiologic and clinical aspects. *AJR* 96:6–14, 1966.
38. Pindborg J.J., Kenstrup G.: Studies in oral leukoplakias: II. Effect of snuff on oral epithelium. *Acta Derm. Venereol.* 43:271–276, 1963.
39. Martin H.: Cancer of the head and neck. *JAMA* 137:1306–1315, 1366–1376, 1948.
40. Keller A.Z.: Cirrhosis of the liver, alcoholism, and heavy smoking associated with cancer of the mouth and pharynx. *Cancer* 20:1015–1022, 1967.
41. Vogler W.R., Lloyd J.W., Milmore B.K.: A retrospective study of etiologic factors in cancer of the mouth, pharynx, and larynx, *Cancer* 15:246–258, 1962.
42. Wynder E.L., Hultberg S., Jacobsson F., et al.: Environmental factors in cancer of the upper alimentary tract: A Swedish study with special reference to Plummer-Vinson (Patterson-Kelly) syndrome. *Cancer* 10:470, 1957.
43. Chernick V.: The brain's own morphine and cigarette smoking: The junkie in disguise? *Chest* 83:2–3, 1983.
44. Chandler J.R., Guillamondegui D.M., Sisson G.A., et al.: Clinical staging of cancer of the head and neck: A new "new system." *Am. J. Surg.* 132:525–528, 1976.
45. Beahrs O.H., Meyers M.H. (eds.): *Manual for Staging of Cancer,* ed. 2. Philadelphia, J.B. Lippincott Co., 1983.
46. Platz H., Fries R., Hudec M., et al.: Carcinomas of the oral cavity: Analysis of various pretherapeutic classifications. *Head Neck Surg.* 5:93–107, 1982.
47. Kassirer J.P., Kuipers B.J., Gorry G.A.: Toward a theory of clinical expertise. *Am. J. Med.* 73:251–260, 1982.
48. Kassirer J.P., Garry G.A.: Clinical problem solving: A behavioral analysis. *Ann. Intern. Med.* 89:245, 1978.
49. Pauker S.G., Gorry G.A., Kassirer, J.P., et al.: Towards the simulation of clinical cognition: Taking a present illness by computer. *Am. J. Med.* 60:981, 1976.
50. Tribus M.: Making up the collective mind. *IEEE Spectrum,* October 1974, pp. 59–64.
51. Shoemaker P.J.H.: *Experiments on Decisions Under Risk: The Expected Utility Hypothesis.* Boston, Kluwer-Nijhoff Publishers, 1980.
52. Higgins G.A.: Clinical trials in surgery. *Surg. Rounds* 5:(9)28–35, 1982.
53. Humphrey E.W., Higgins G.A., Shields T.W.: The long-term survival of patients with visceral carcinoma. *Surg. Gynecol. Obstet.* 149:385–394, 1979.
54. Mann R.J.: The statistical way of inquiry of the Reverend Stephen Hales, 1677–1761. *Mayo Clin. Proc.* 53:191–194, 1978.

2 / Head and Neck Examination

Graeme A. Browne, B.Sc., M.Sc., B.D.S., F.R.C.D.

A comprehensive examination of the external surfaces of head and neck will cover 9% of the total body surface. We should also include the nasal, oral, pharyngeal, and hypopharyngeal regions. The dynamic nature of the tongue and other structures makes it difficult to measure the added surface. In young healthy adults at rest, the estimated additional surface would be equal to 4% of the total body surface area. Consequently, a good head and neck examination covers an area equivalent to 13% of the body surface.

To conduct a systematic and informative examination one must be familiar with head and neck regional anatomy and understand the functional anatomy and applied physiology of the upper aerodigestive tract. The ultimate objective of a successful examination is to detect a lesion in its earliest stage before the patient is aware of any symptoms of focal pathology. If we could achieve this goal, we could improve the survival of patients who develop malignancies. There would be less morbidity because ablative surgical fields would be smaller. In reality, many patients do not get early medical attention for a known lesion because of unfounded optimism, denial, fear, ignorance, or economics. When there is an opportunity, the examiner must actively seek to perform a full head and neck examination on vulnerable individuals. Therefore, the examiner must decide which asymptomatic patients are vulnerable on the basis of habits, age, clinical signs, and symptoms.

A patient who is seen for a regular dental checkup or who, for an unrelated medical reason, seeks an opinion, also should be given a head and neck screening evaluation to establish the state of health of this region. An adult with abnormal physical findings or symptoms referable to the head and neck must be filtered through the "diagnostic sieve" in which *neoplasia is a probable diagnosis until excluded* by complete resolution or a tissue diagnosis.

Preventive medicine and dentistry *can* be practiced within the scope of family practice. Patients should be told of the risks they are taking with tobacco use. The clinician can decrease patients' ignorance about the genesis of most oroairway cancers. Some patients will seek help with behavior modification to reduce or to eliminate the consumption of tobacco along with alcohol. Should this fail, careful clinical supervision in the hope of early detection must suffice.

The clinician should undertake examination of the oral cavity with the same diagnostic enthusiasm and diligence as he might perform a rectal examination. A diagnostic parallel exists between these orifices: both are primary sites of pathology and both require digital examination and some effort and instrumentation to inspect. Yet many avoid examination of the mouth, with the idea that it is the domain of dentists to examine. It is the clinical responsibility of dentists and primary care physicians to conduct meaningful head and neck examinations and to thoughtfully interpret their findings.

If an appropriate examination by the family dentist or physician detects an early lesion, then timely referral of a patient to an interested and trained head and neck specialist will likely result in an adequately treated neoplasm. The head and neck specialist will be held to a higher standard of thoroughness. Too frequently there is delay in establishing a tissue diagnosis or in rendering the appropriate therapy.

The fact that the patient is a woman is no guarantee that an oral lesion is benign. Social acceptance of the use of tobacco and alcohol by women has produced a precipitous increase in the incidence of oral cancer. The rate is rapidly approaching the observed incidence for men. Gender is no longer important in assessing the risk of developing an oroairway malignancy; rather, the key issue is that of personal habits that contribute to the development of neoplasms in the mouth, pharynx, lungs, and bladder.

Prevention is making slow progress. Early detection of head and neck cancers could be improved at the primary care level. Self-examination for the easily observed oral areas is superior to chance observation, or to waiting until a large detectable mass causes altered sensation or impediments to function. For breast and testicular cancer, some mortality reduction has shown the value of self-examination. The mouth is more difficult to self-examine than these other organs. Nevertheless, clinicians should continue to emphasize that tobacco causes cancer and point out the need for oral self-examination and teach some simple early warning signs to vulnerable patients. The areas of vulnerability in the mouth are illustrated in chapter 13.

HOW DO YOU CONDUCT A THOROUGH PHYSICAL EXAMINATION OF THE HEAD AND NECK?

Inspection and palpation are the principal modes of clinical examination of the head and neck. The examiner should be familiar with the gross appearance of various lesions. *A Color Atlas of Oral Cancer*, by Burkhardt and Maerker, is recommended as a companion piece to this text.[1] The color illustrations could not be improved. The atlas correlates gross appearance with histology.

It is difficult to overemphasize the need for careful palpation during an examination. The subtley of many muscosal changes and the difficulty of examining each area of the mouth and pharynx limit the adequacy of a cursory bedside examination. With poor light, poor exposure, and poor position, only the most overt oral pathology will be identified. The apparent low yield of mucosal lesions found on bedside examination should not discourage the clinician from thoroughly scrutinizing the oropharynx or from asking a consultant well versed in the head and neck region to review any aberrant findings.

The following sections contain a plethora of suggestions and maneuvers. The number of steps should not discourage you. A thorough examination can be conducted in much less time than it takes to read about it. With careful observation, almost all of the cranial nerve functions can be evaluated during the course of the routine examination. Visual and functional information are coordinated. A simple setup makes the examination easy. A searching attitude, good light, good position, and simple maneuvers are the keys to early detection. Examination of the larynx and hypopharynx is discussed in chapter 16. Additional hints and guides are found in other specific chapters.

Technique for a Good Examination

In a comprehensive examination, the patient should be seated with the head and shoulders in the position of anatomical rest. This gives a relaxed and balanced posture for the patient. A comfortable patient allows the clinician to rapidly inspect the surface contours, the skin color, and the range of motion of the head, neck, and thorax. Muscle tension will make the task more difficult. The bulk of a tight muscle will mask contiguous or subjacent masses. Vascular pulsations will often be obscured by overlying contracting muscle. Visibility is often limited in the oral cavity by tensing of the muscles of mastication in the floor of the mouth, tongue, and the buccal area. The patient should be kept cooperative. On the positive side, voluntary muscle contraction can help define the difference between a superficial location of a mass with respect to the underlying working muscle.

Inspection is improved if the examiner is at a slightly higher level than the patient. The examiner should be able to continually inspect different areas without pausing to change the patient's position. The perfunctory and almost ritualistic use of the disposable wooden tongue and cheek blade that prefaces inspection of the uvula and tonsillar regions is not adequate for finding oro-airway neoplasms. Included in the armamentarium

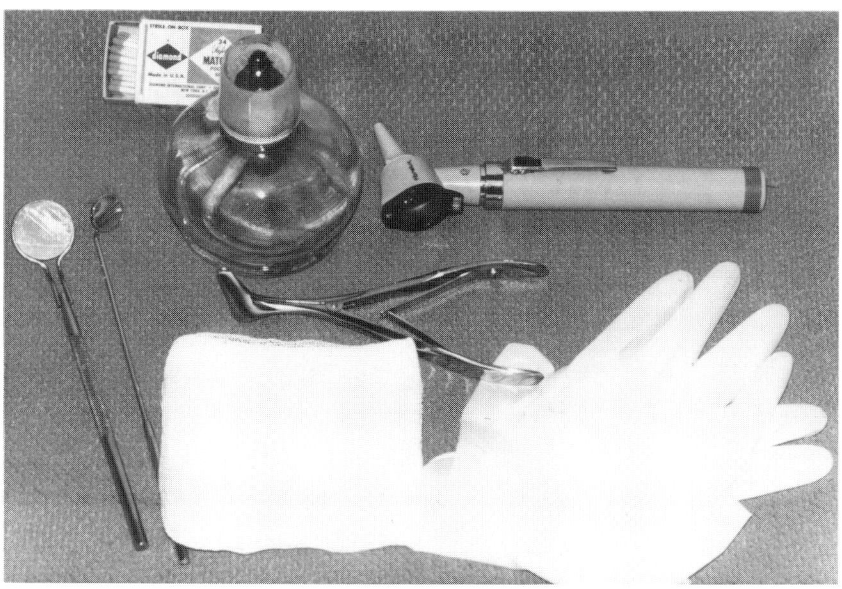

Fig 2–1.—Basic armamentarium for a general head and neck examination includes a laryngoscopy mirror, a dental mirror, 4 × 4 inch gauze, examination gloves, a nasal speculum, an otoscope, and an alcohol burner.

for a routine head and neck examination are (1) a dental mirror, (2) a laryngoscopy mirror, (3) an alcohol burner or warm running water, (4) several 4 × 4-inch gauzes, (5) a nasal speculum, (6) an otoscope, and (7) examining gloves (Fig 2–1).

Color-corrected illumination is best provided by a dental light. Red and blue areas of the spectrum should be reduced to improve the visual identification of mucosal color changes.

Physical Inspection by Site

EXTERNAL REGIONS OF THE HEAD AND NECK

The patient should remove spectacles, neck tie, and toupé to allow examination of the areas covered by these items. Hearing aids are left in position and operating until the ears are examined. This helps the patient maintain comprehension of the procedure. Dental prostheses should be kept in the mouth until that facet of the examination is done. The clinician should be sensitive to any patient embarrassment when prosthetics and articles of apparel must be divested. Privacy may be required.

Simple anterior inspection of facial and cervical regions will allow gross appreciation of regional symmetry. This may be supplemented with comparative lateral tangential views that may highlight the presence of neck or facial masses. Canthal form and position, dissimilar size of ophthalmic fissures, presence of epiphora, nares conformation, and range of motion of the mandible should be assessed. A simple examination of the intertriginous areas of the nasolabial fold, medial and lateral canthus, and behind the ears will frequently disclose an unsuspected cutaneous malignancy in the older sun-exposed person. A differential temperature gradient may be detected as unilateral facial flushing. This finding in conjunction with meiosis and ptosis is indicative of Horner's syndrome. The condition may be precipitated by Pancoast's tumor or cervical lymphadenopathy secondary to inflammatory or malignant infiltration. A posterior look at the pinna, retromandibular region, and mastoid process will occasionally disclose a parotitis posterior, cervical adenopathy, or a superficial adenoma of the parotid gland. Lateral inspection of the anterior and posterior cervical triangles will occasionally disclose vascular pulsations, or neck masses that are derived from embryologic branchial clefts, pharyngeal pouch, laryngocele, carotid body tumor, the thyroid gland, or an aggregation of lymph nodes due to metastases. Granulomatous lymph node disease is rare today and is almost always due to atypical tuberculosis. Malignant lymphadenopathy may be primary, from diseases such as Hodgkin's disease, or secondary, from metastatic disease of the head and neck or of the thorax and abdomen. A delphian node (encased in the deep cervical fascia in the midline anterior to the thyroid isthmus) from carcinoma of the thyroid or from subacute thyroiditis is readily distinguishable by location on palpation from Virchow's (or Troisier's) node (an enlarged supraclavicular node).

Inspection of the temporomandibular joint during its range of motion may disclose a limitation of translation. Trismus is a sign of deep tumor invasion or deep-seated perimandibular infection. Because of this, trismus will require further investigation to establish a diagnosis. Masses located deep to the sternocleidomastoid often cause restriction of cervical rotation away from the involved side with the pathology. Limited cervical extension may be due to bony spine disorders, local inflammatory irritation of the fascia or muscle, or invasive neoplastic space-occupying lesions.

The thoracic inlet, or thoracic retroclavicular ledge, must be included in the evaluation by noting restriction or change in the usual ventilatory excursions that may reflect tissue fixation by inflammatory or malignant processes. Because of the anatomical characteristics of lymphatic flow via the thoracic or subclavian ducts, abdominal or thoracic malignant disease may be initially detected by the enlargement of Virchow's node. More often, this node is on the left side deep to the sternocleidomastoid muscle. A Pancoast tumor may manifest as a readily visible mass in the root of the neck that is associated with arm pain from invasion of the lower brachial plexus roots.

PALPATION OF THE EXTRAORAL REGIONS OF THE HEAD AND NECK

Skillful palpation provides the clinician with a substantial amount of corroborative information. A lesion may be described in terms of its size, shape, consistency, texture, mobility, extent of fixation, relation to contiguous structures, and pulsations (is the mass expansile or is the pulsation transmitted?). One should consciously observe if a mass is crepitant or fluctuant, the extent of local temperature gradients, or if manipulation evokes exquisite pain, tenderness, or sharp neuropathic pain.

Palpation of the head and neck is best conducted from the rear of the patient who is seated in a relaxed, upright posture at a level of convenience for the examiner. This position provides simultaneous comparison of paired contralateral structures (Fig 2–2). A regionally systematic stepping with the palpating hands will provide maximal information yield, if muscle spasm or pain is not incurred during the examination. If tenderness or pain is expected, the specific area should be examined last to sustain patient cooperation.

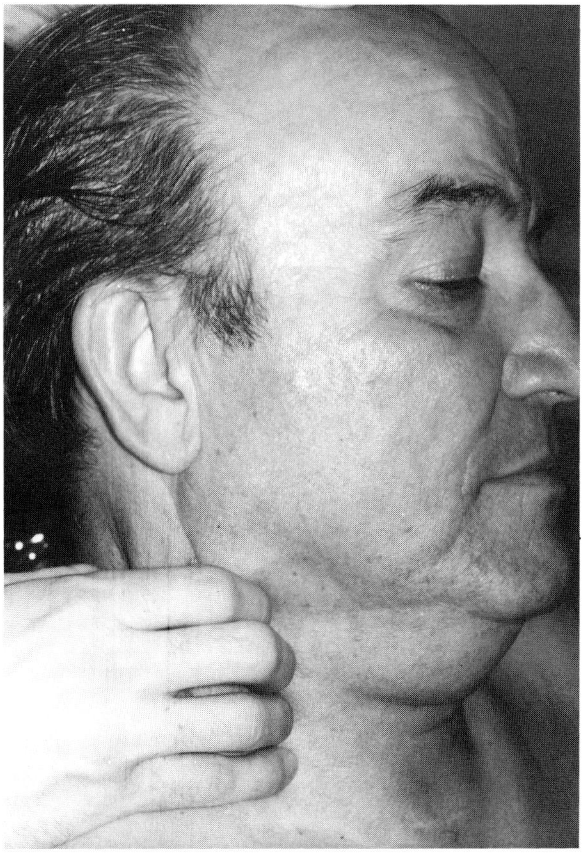

Fig 2–2.—Examination of the sternocleidomastoid region. The patient's head is laterally rotated and if necessary the cervical spine is slightly flexed to relax the muscle. The palpating fingers gently retract the muscle, facilitating examination of contents of this region. The examiner carefully notes the presence of lymphadenopathy associated with the deep descending cervical chain, or at a lower level, a Virchow's node. Pharyngeal masses may lie concealed by scar unless this area is actively examined. *Caution*—Carotid vascular plaques may be dislodged by aggressive manipulation.

The palpation portion of the physical examination begins at the thoracic inlet, passes through the base of the posterior cervical triangles and then moves upward within the anatomical confines of this triangle to the apex at the superior nuchal line. The inverted anterior cervical triangles are palpated from the apex below at the sternoclavicular junction and suprasternal notch, to their bases located at the inferior border of the mandible.

It is important to interrupt the simultaneous bilateral manual palpation to displace the sternocleidomastoid muscle posteriorly and laterally (see Fig 2–2). This displacement is readily accomplished by having the nonexploring hand flex and laterally rotate the cervical spine to a degree that permits the palpating hand to adequately feel the area under the sternocleidomastoid. Note that the accessory cervical group of lymph nodes is deep to the middle third of this muscle.

Cervical lymphadenopathy may be secondary to an inflammatory or malignant process, or both. Mucosal ulceration may occur during the progress of an oropharyngeal carcinoma. It then becomes secondarily infected. There may be superimposition of inflammation on the usually painless, malignant or metastatic lymph nodes. In a clinical examination, no reliable interpretation can be given to tender nodes, since they may be harboring malignant cells.

When a mass compatible with an enlarged node is found in the neck, a detailed knowledge of regional lymphatic afferent and efferent flow is essential to find a possible oropharyngeal carcinoma (Fig 2–3). It should be remembered that a sarcoma usually spreads via hematogenous routes rather than the lymphatic routes as seen with carcinoma. When the site of the primary neoplasm is known, the more frequent regional lymph drainage areas are examined with care. Clinical staging of malignancy requires evaluation of primary tumor size, the existence of regional node involvement, and evidence of distant spread of the neoplasm. This information is crucial for the clinical decision-making process and management of neoplasia. Understanding lymphatic afferent pathways will also assist in finding the probable origin of isolated malignant neck masses (see Chap. 25). Figures 2–4 through 2–11 show some of the common areas of nodal metastases from various primary sites.

Palpation of the trachea and larynx is performed from the rear of the patient. Lack of infrahyoid muscle adhesions and persistence of lateral freedom to displacement suggest the absence of grossly infiltrating cancer. Thyroid gland palpation is performed by light simultaneous bilateral digital examination. Form, consistency, and evidence of tenderness should be noted on palpation. This organ may be better examined by having the patient swallow several times while the clinician is palpating the organ. The pretracheal fascia which splits to envelop the thyroid gland and trachea allows a smooth gliding upward displacement of the thyroid structures with the hyoid bone during the first phase of deglutition. Retrosternal thyroid lobes or nodules may rise and be easy to feel in the lower neck when the patient is actively swallowing.

Occasionally a prominent carotid bulb is misidentified as a lymph node, particularly if the bulb wall has undergone dystrophic calcification that reduces elasticity. The usual pulsatile transmitted wave form is damped out. The lack of vertical mobility will help differentiate the carotid bulb from regional lymph node or another mass.

A chemodectoma of the carotid body can be moved

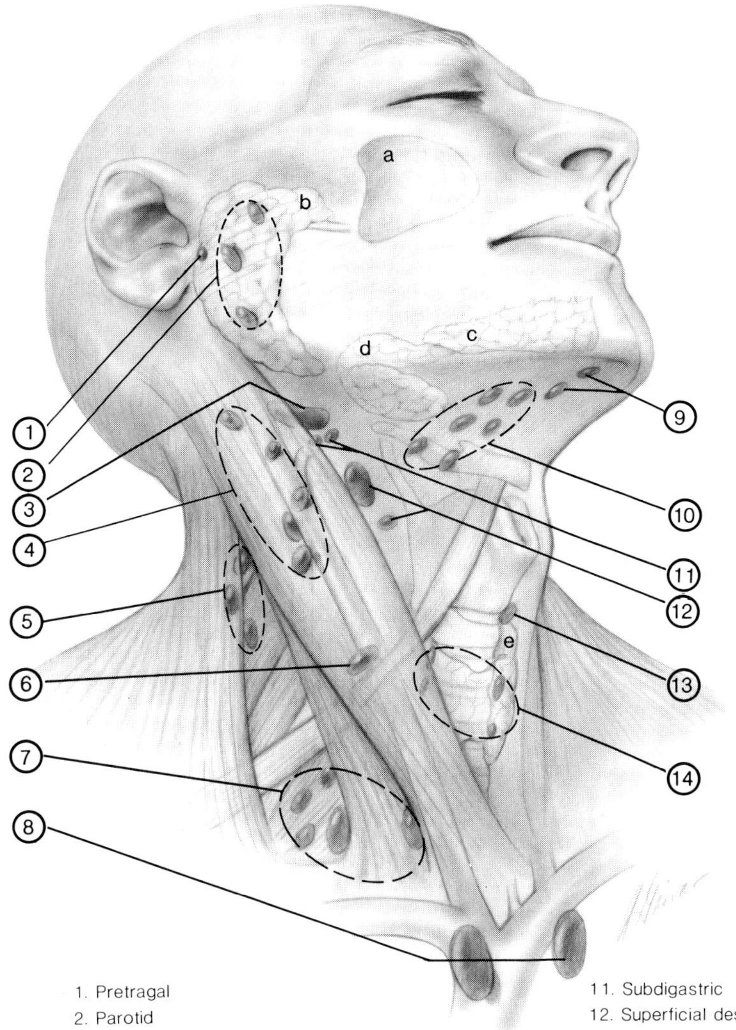

1. Pretragal
2. Parotid
3. Jugulodigastric
4. Upper deep cervical
5. Nodes of accessory nerve
6. Jugulo-omohyoid
7. Inferior deep cervical
8. Upper anterior mediastinal
9. Submental
10. Submandibular
11. Subdigastric
12. Superficial descending cervical
13. Delphian
14. Tracheoesophageal
15. Retropharyngeal (not pictured)

a. Maxillary sinus
b. Parotid gland
c. Sublingual gland
d. Submandibular gland
e. Thyroid

Fig 2–3.—Regional lymphatic nodal stations: surface markings and locations.

forward and backward on lateral play in the carotid artery, but it will not move cephalad-caudad.

It may be clinically difficult to differentiate regional structures from nodes in the submandibular triangle. Occasionally the submandibular glands show variations in contour and texture secondary to sialadenoses. These firm areas may be incorrectly identified as fixed nodes. Deep palpation may permit the clinician to outline the body and superficial process of the gland, which may extend down to the digastric sling (Fig 2–12). Bimanual intraoral/extraoral palpation is essential to defining masses in the area (Fig 2–13). Bimanual intraoral/extraoral palpation also assesses floor of the mouth thickness and defines intervening structures with more precision. External auditory canal patency, condylar shape, and condylar function and tenderness on palpation during mandibular function must be assessed. The tops of the ears should be felt for cutaneous irregularities or thin cutaneous malignancies. The medial canthal region, infraorbital, maxillary, and nasal regions are palpated for asymmetry, for evidence of obstruction, and for altered sensation over these regions. The presence of active pathology is assumed if one or more of these conditions exist.

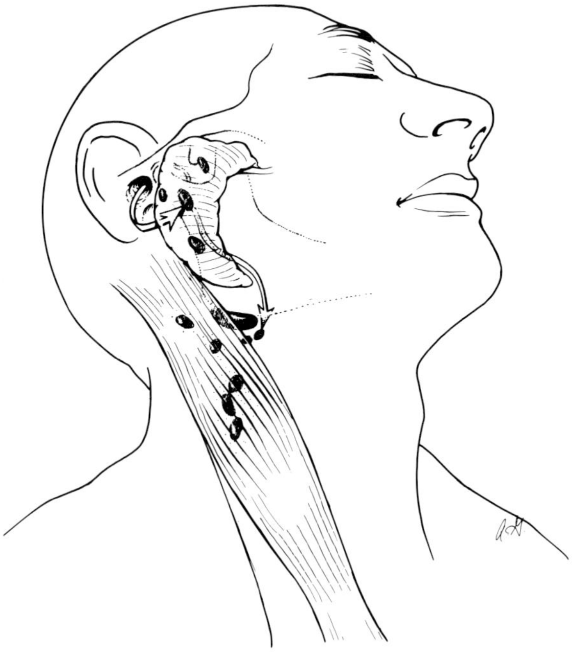

Unilateral

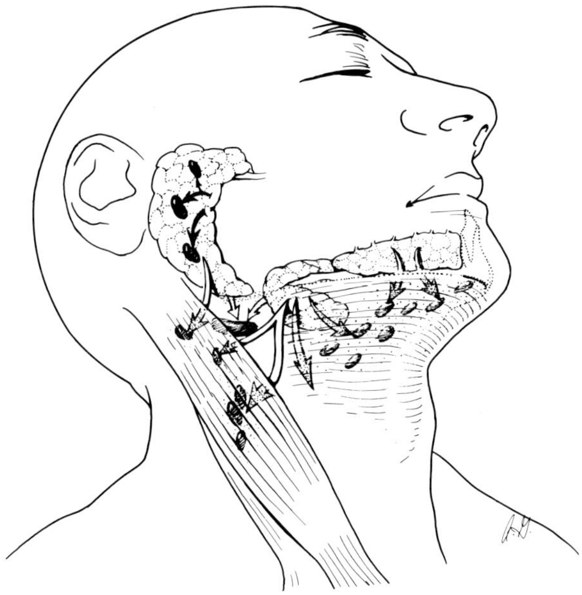

Unilateral

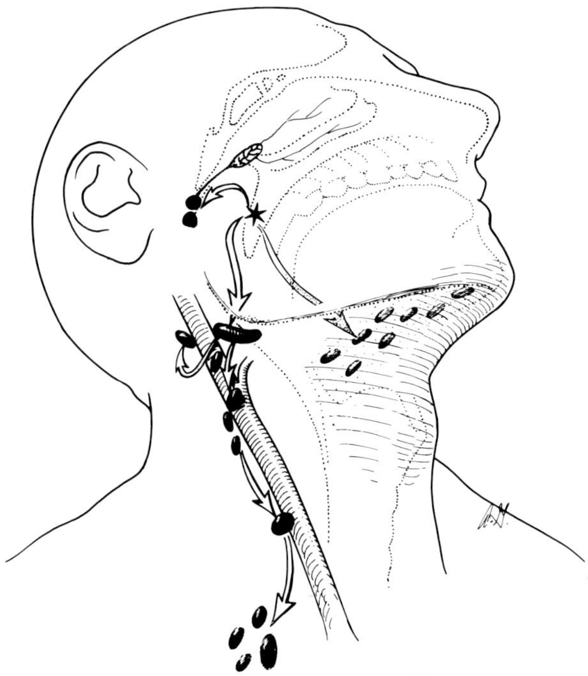

Unilat./Bilateral

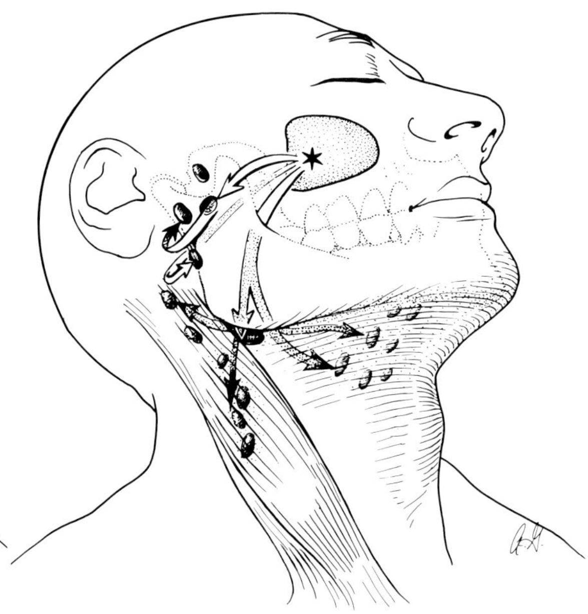

Unilateral

Fig 2–4 (top left).—External auditory canal: primary lymphatic nodal stations in the preauricular and parotid-subdigastric areas.

Fig 2–5 (top right).—Primary lymphatic nodal stations: drainage from major salivary glands.

Fig 2–6 (bottom left).—Nasopharynx primary and secondary lymphatic nodal stations. Note potential for bilateral dissemination. Disease frequently spreads to the posterior cervical node(s).

Fig 2–7 (bottom right).—Maxillary sinus: primary and secondary lymphatic nodal stations. Note that posterior medial lesions may disseminate bilaterally.

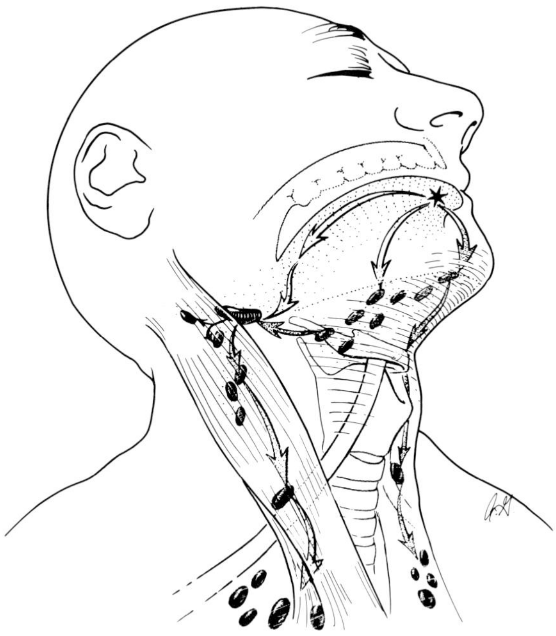

Bilateral

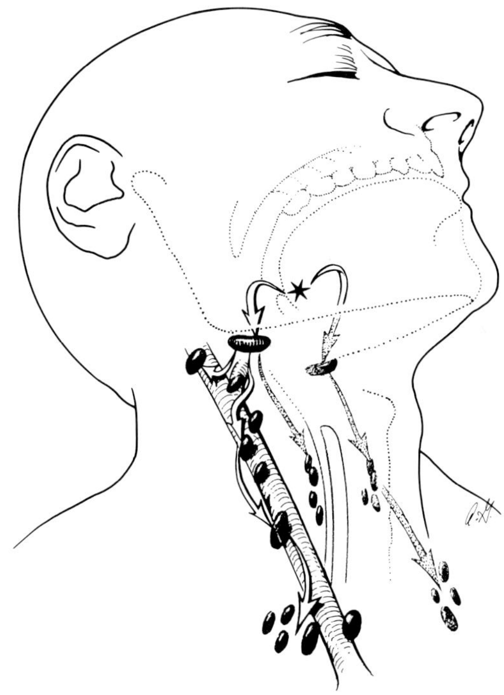

Bilateral

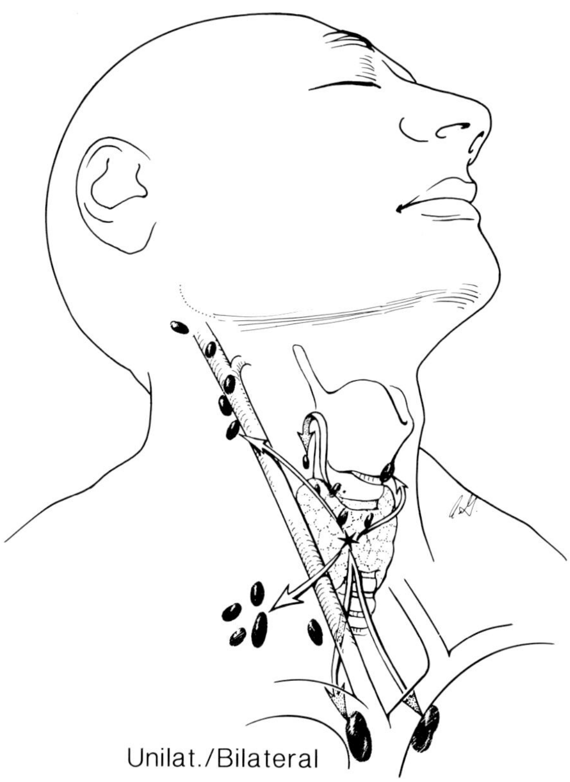

Unilat./Bilateral

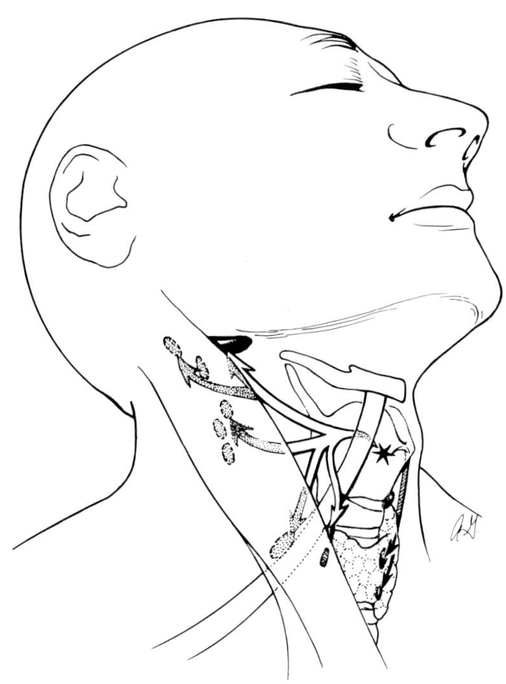

Bilateral

Fig 2–8 (top left).—Anterior tongue and floor of the mouth primary and secondary lymphatic nodal stations.

Fig 2–9 (top right).—Posterior third of tongue and hypopharynx primary and secondary lymphatic nodal stations. Bilateral nodal spread is frequent.

Fig 2–10 (bottom left).—Thyroid gland. Primary and secondary lymphatic nodal stations in lower neck and paratracheal areas. Note potential for bilateral dissemination.

Fig 2–11 (bottom right).—Larynx. Primary and secondary lymphatic nodal stations.

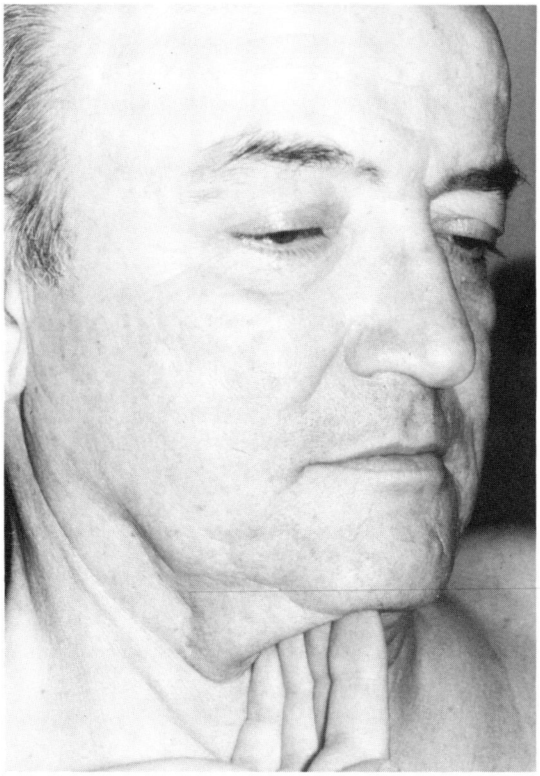

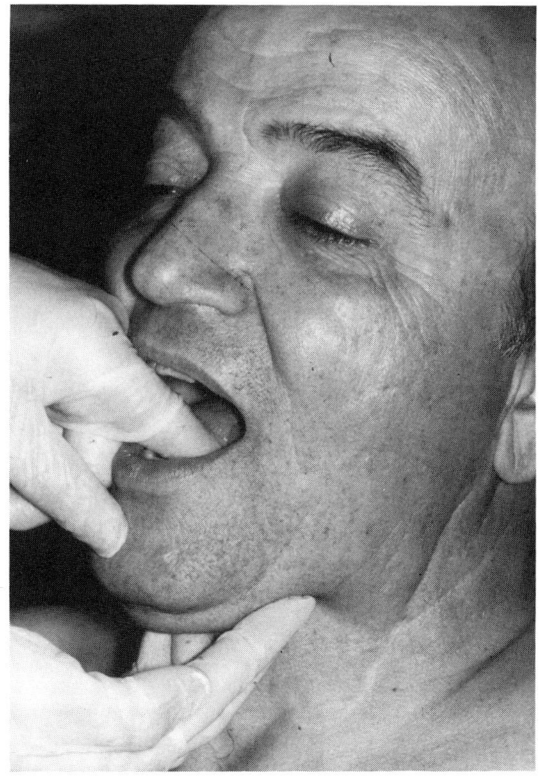

Fig 2–12 (left).—Submental triangle. Digital examination allows palpation of submandibular gland. Firm midline placement of the fingers, between the anterior digastrics, followed by a lateral rolling action toward and against the inferior border of the mandible, enables palpation of regional lymph nodes.

Fig 2–13 (right).—Bimanual digital examination of the floor of the mouth. Firm reciprocating palpation between the intraoral and extraoral examining fingers provides essential comparative clinical information between anterior and posterior aspects and between opposite sides of the floor of the mouth and the contents of the submandibular and submental triangles. The tongue *must* also be palpated in this manner, although this picture does not show this being done.

EXAMINATION OF THE NOSE

The external examination of the nose looks for septal asymmetry. The skin of the nose and the nasolabial folds are examined and palpated for superficial cutaneous lesions.

EXAMINATION OF THE ORAL CAVITY

Tandem inspection and bimanual palpation (see Fig 2–13) provides a rapid but thorough examination of the oral cavity. A systematic pattern of integrated regional examinations followed routinely for all patients will avoid the occasional oversight of pathology. For convenience, it is suggested that the examination of the oral cavity commence with inspection and palpation of the lips, noting the symmetry, size, quality, and integrity of the vermillion borders. Actinic mucosal changes are noted almost exclusively on the lower lip. While examining lesions of this type, it should be borne in mind that communicable diseases may be contracted by the unwitting clinician who fails to wear protective gloves or finger cots on his exploring hands. Any concern for loss of tactile sensations while wearing gloves is overcome by drying the mucosa that is under inspection. Removal of sialomucins overlying a region of altered texture will improve the perception of tactile differences that may exist between normal and abnormal mucosa. In addition, inspection of this area of pathology will disclose an altered light reflex consistent with a nonuniform surface, implying structural mucosal change.

TECHNIQUE OF EXAMINING THE TONGUE, FLOOR OF MOUTH, AND POSTERIOR ORAL CAVITY

The posterior regions of the oral cavity cannot be examined in patients that exhibit prominent gag reflexes. The gag reflex can sometimes be inhibited with topical anesthetic mouth rinses or topical anesthetic sprays. Premature application of the anesthesia will impair a good neurologic evaluation. The agents may be rapidly absorbed systemically when there is hyperemic or ulcerated mucosa.

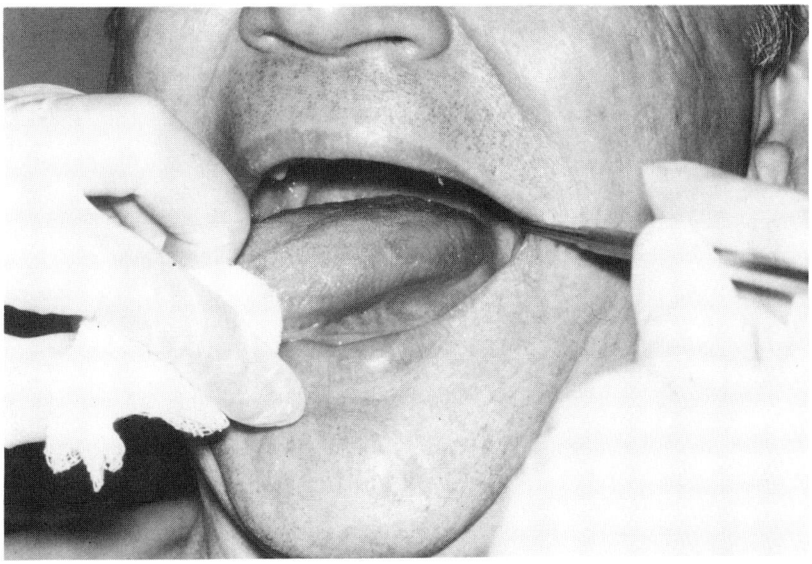

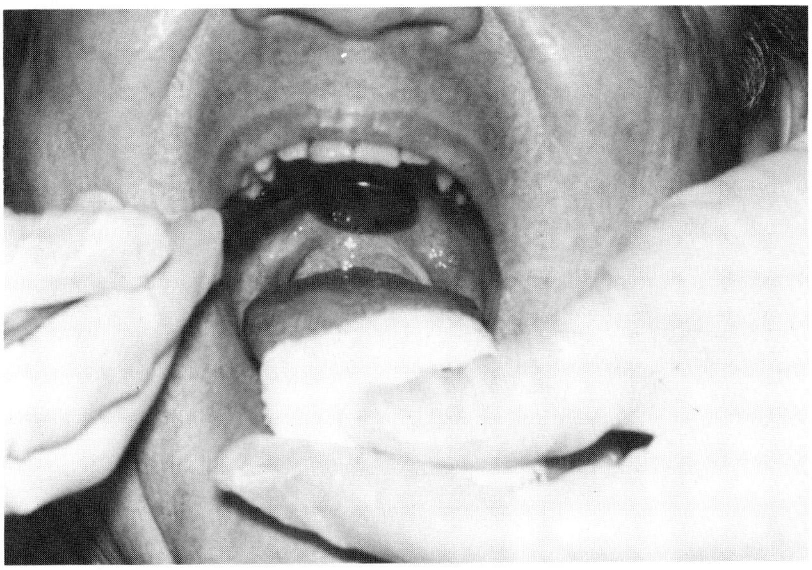

Fig 2–14 (top).—Examination of the tongue. Anterior traction and displacement to the contralateral side greatly facilitate direct observation of the posterior lateral border of the tongue and its contiguous surfaces, including the root of the anterior pillar of fauces and the posterior alveolingual sulcus. Gentle retraction of the oral commissure further aids observation.

Fig 2–15 (bottom).—Indirect examination of oral cavity—hypopharynx. Anterior tongue traction facilitates observation of the posterior third of the tongue, the palatine tonsillar fossae, the posterior pharyngeal wall, the valleculae, and the laryngeal aditus. For examination of more posterior structures, the angled mirror is placed beneath the uvula and the soft palate is displaced upward. Cord function is checked by having the patient say "EEE." Pharyngeal functional symmetry is checked with a swallow.

Examination of the tongue is best accomplished on the protruding tongue. Additional traction is applied to the tongue tip, which is wrapped with gauze. This maneuver offers free visual and tactile access to the posterior third of the tongue and its lateral borders (Fig 2–14). The alveolingual sulcus may also be freely examined.

To avoid an extensive gag reaction, the clinician should palpate each side of the tongue separately and explain to the patient what he is doing.

It is important to place the second hand on the lateral neck just beneath the mandible so that any mass will be palpated between two hands. This technique is especially helpful when palpating the anterior floor of the mouth and the alveolar ridge area to see if a tumor is fixed to the mandible, or to determine if the submandibular gland or the nodes in this region are enlarged. Bimanual palpation not only allows the surface configuration of the lesion to be determined but also provides some assessment of the depth or extent of any tumor infiltration.

Mirror examination should be used for the base of tongue, hypopharynx, nasopharynx, and larynx (Fig 2–15). For physicians who are not accustomed to using mirrors, various endoscopic devices are available that permit indirect visualization of these structures. Even if there is an obvious tumor on the floor of the mouth, it is still essential to examine the hypopharynx and larynx carefully because of the high incidence of second primary malignancies.

Squamous cell carcinoma generally presents as a painful, ulcerating lesion. It may bleed easily on palpation and initially extends along the surface mucosa before becoming deeply infiltrative.

Adenocarcinoma, on the other hand, begins in the submucosal tissue and therefore does not ulcerate unless biopsied late in the course of the disease. Adenocarcinoma presents as a smooth, rounded mass that is seldom tender. Adenocarcinoma also has a propensity for developing at the junction of the hard and soft palate adjacent to the midline or in the tongue and buccal mucosa.

Squamous cell carcinoma occurs most commonly along the anterolateral border of the mobile portion of the tongue. In addition to the ulcerating tumor, there may be a surrounding zone of what appears to be a white flake-like mucosa, described as leukoplakia. The center of the ulcer frequently contains yellow-white squamous epithelial debris.

The second most frequent site for the development of squamous cell carcinoma is the floor of the mouth adjacent to the frenulum of the tongue. Since this tumor lies near the midline, it will frequently involve the opening of the submandibular (Wharton's) duct.

Squamous cell carcinoma next most commonly arises in the tonsillar area, or the area between the last molar and the tonsillar fossa (the retromolar trigone). While squamous cell cancer may originate in the true tonsil, it develops more commonly along the tonsillar pillars and extends into the soft palate region or the base of the tongue. Commonly the tumor presents at the junction of the anterior tonsillar pillar and the lateral tongue.

Cancers developing in the posterior third of the tongue—that is, posterior to the circumvallate papillae—may reach considerable size before being recognized. These cancers infiltrate deeply into the tongue before causing any overlying ulceration. Pain may be referred to the ear (referred otalgia) and may be present only during swallowing. Because direct examination with a tongue blade or indirect examination with a mirror may not reveal the tumor, the diagnosis depends on palpation. The index finger should be carefully pressed along the posterolateral border of the tongue. An area of ulceration or extreme pain that is palpated in a patient with referred otalgia is strongly suggestive of a tumor.

Indirect laryngoscopy is conducted with the examiner holding the tongue forward with a gauze sponge. A bare light bulb is placed behind the patient and a focused head mirror conducts the light source to an angle laryngeal mirror in the back of the throat. The mirror is heated to prevent fogging. The mirror examination should include the back of the tongue, the vallecula, the parts of the hypopharynx that are visible, and the larynx. The studies can be assisted by additional examination with a fiberoptic nasolaryngoscope.

Observation of soft palatal symmetry and function should be followed by sweeping palpation to detect low nasopharyngeal masses.

THE NASAL AIRWAY

Examination of the nasal airway is performed with the aid of a nasal speculum and an adequate light source. The atrium and alar-labial junction are inspected for evidence of epithelial discontinuity or a mass lesion. Beyond the rima naris, the inferior turbinate covers the orifice to the nasolacrimal duct and plica lacrimalis. The medial wall of the nasal cavity formed by the nasal septum may exhibit deviations, spurs, or fenestrations.

Generally, this is the end of a routine examination of the nose unless there are other symptoms or findings referable to the nose, nasopharynx, or paranasal sinuses. Further examination requires more elaborate techniques. Careful inspection of the conchae is difficult to perform. Topical application of cocaine 4% (with proper premedication and precautions) will provide local anesthesia, vasoconstriction, mucosal shrinkage, and euphoria, all of which facilitate examination. Fiberoptics are an essential aid for complete inspection and biopsy in clinically difficult regions of the nasopharynx. Changes in nasal airway patency with accompanying stained mucous secretions must be regarded as ominous and justify careful examination of the nose and prompt additional studies of the paranasal sinus (see Chap. 17).

THE EXTERNAL EAR

The ear examination includes inspection and palpation of the lateral and medial surfaces of the pinna. It is essential to remove spectacles, hearing aids, and similar devices to perform a complete examination. An otoscope is used to examine the external auditory canal and tympanic membrane. Cerumen must be removed with care to avoid tympanic membrane perforation or bleeding from a lesion. The posterior auditory canal wall near the anulus is a common site for malignancy. Lymphatics from the ear drain to the preauricular, mastoid, subparotid, and subdigastric nodes. Lesions of the anterior canal metastasize to the pretragal or parotid nodes. Hyperesthesia over the posterior wall of the external auditory canal (Hitselberger's sign) in association with an ipsilateral peripheral facial nerve weakness, diminished facial sensation, and impaired oculomotor function suggest the presence of an acoustic neuroma. Squamous cell or basal cell carcinoma of the ear are the most frequently encountered lesions (see illustrations in Chap. 21).

LYMPH NODES

A detailed knowledge of the lymphatic system and the regions that provide afferent relays from specific regions of the head and neck is required to stage a neoplasm. Clinical staging based on the TNM system is the best system available to describe the extent of node involvement by the malignancy. However, there are definite errors when the clinical stage is compared with the pathologic stage. The specificity and sensitivity of the physical examination for detecting cervical node metastases are discussed and diagramed in chapter 9.

WHAT ARE THE KEY ELEMENTS IN THE NEUROLOGIC EXAMINATION OF THE HEAD AND NECK?

Many of the required observations for cranial nerve and otoneurologic testing are made during the course of the routine examination with simple conscientious observation. The clinician must train himself to observe pharyngeal, tongue, and vocal cord function. A brief outline of specific function would include the following:

OLFACTORY NERVE.—The olfactory nerve is checked by presenting simple familiar odors such as coffee or vanilla to one nostril while the other is held closed.

OPTIC NERVE.—The optic nerve is checked by reading a visual acuity chart and doing the simple checks of peripheral visual fields. If a defect is suspected, a formal study of visual fields is made with ophthalmologic testing equipment. Careful inspection of the fundus should be part of every examination.

OCULOMOTOR, TROCHLEAR, AND ABDUCENS NERVES.—The oculomotor, trochlear, and abducens nerves are tested by pupillary reflexes and a check for full range of eye motion. The examiner should ask specifically about diplopia.

TRIGEMINAL NERVE.—The trigeminal nerve carries sensation from the face. The examiner should look for an absent corneal reflex. Blinking will occur when the cornea is touched with a wisp of cotton. This does not occur when the sclera is touched.

FACIAL NERVE.—The facial nerve controls the muscles of facial expression. The examiner should ask the patient to grin, grimace, show teeth, pucker the lips, close the eyes tightly, open the eyes fully.

AUDITORY NERVE.—The auditory nerve is evaluated by a gross assessment of hearing and differential perception of bone conductance of a tuning fork. The cochleovestibular components also mediate balance. Vertigo is a definitive symptom. Nystagmus, past pointing, gait, and tandem standing abnormalities may signal vestibular disorders. CNS disorders that cause changes in proprioception and coordination may mimic vestibular disease.

GLOSSOPHARYNGEAL NERVE.—The glossopharyngeal nerve supplies sensation to the pharynx and is responsible for the gag reflex. The gag reflex should be checked when inspecting the pharynx. An absent gag reflex is a common end result of basilar artery vascular disease.

VAGUS NERVE.—The vagus nerve innervates the muscles of the soft palate (except tensor palatini), pharynx and larynx. One should examine carefully for symmetric effective motion of these muscular components.

SPINAL ACCESSORY NERVE.—The spinal accessory nerve can be tested by having the patient shrug his shoulders against resistance.

HYPOGLOSSAL NERVE.—The hypoglossal nerve provides motor innervation to the tongue. The examiner should look for unilateral atrophy or fasciculation and check for inability to protrude the tongue. The tongue turns toward the side of weakness or deficit on forced protrusion.

A reasonably effective neurologic examination of the cranial nerves can be done during the course of other observations. The examiner should discipline his final thinking to go through the 12 item checklist to be sure the observations were made and noted.

WHAT HISTORY, HABITS, SYMPTOMS, AND SIGNS SHOULD ALERT THE EXAMINER TO THE POSSIBILITY OF AN EXISTING HEAD AND NECK MALIGNANCY?

The most common error in diagnosis is to ascribe a nonneoplastic cause to a mass in the neck or to a persisting "sore" on the side of the tongue or floor of the mouth. Time after time, an enlarged cervical mass has been treated for a long period with antibiotics without the doctor or dentist having once performed a careful oropharyngeal examination. After acute incision or trauma the tongue will heal in 5–7 days. Aphthous or herpetic lesions have a self-limiting 10-day time course in an immunocompetent person. Any lesion persisting more than 2 weeks should immediately be suspected as malignant.

A history of a nonhealing ulcer or mass that has undergone progressive changes in size is suggestive of a neoplastic process, particularly when there is no history of regional trauma. Altered sensation, altered sense of smell, decreased function, hemorrhage, sialorrhea, fetor oris, dysphagia, dysphonia, sudden loss of denture retention, and the need for frequent denture periphery recontouring are all suggestive of local manifestations of a neoplasm.

Occupational health hazards are seen with furniture workers, arc welding and glass blowing, in which the risk of developing aerodigestive tract malignancy is greater than in other occupations. Social habits of chewing or smoking tobacco, chronic consumption of alcohol, chewing slaked lime or betel nuts, or the consumption of very spicy foods are known to produce oral carcinoma. Ethnic differences exist in the frequency of certain head and neck cancers. For example, Scandinavian women with Plummer-Vinson syndrome tend to develop pharyngeal malignancy more readily than those who do not have the syndrome. Chinese from the southern provinces, Hong Kong, or Singapore have a high propensity for developing nasopharyngeal tumors. HLA differences have been thought to be responsible for the incidence of this neoplasm. On the other hand, Chinese now living in the United States whose early immediate origins were from these high-incidence regions do not reflect the expected frequency of nasopharyngeal neoplasms when compared to their Southeast Asia–dwelling counterparts. Epstein-Barr virus is implicated in the genesis of nasopharyngeal tumors. In final analysis, tobacco use is far and away the most common cause of oropharyngeal cancer. Heavy or long duration of use should automatically trigger a suspicion of malignancy.[2]

Poor oral hygiene and local dental or denture trauma appear to have some relationship to the development of squamous cell carcinoma of the buccal mucosa, lip, tongue, floor of mouth, alveolar process, and palate. A common precursor is a white patch in the immediate vicinity of the trauma. It is suggested that the white patch (leukoplakia) will histologically change from hyperkeratosis, acanthosis, and dyskeratosis to carcinoma in situ, which will then become invasive. De novo genesis from within a white patch is a possibility. The frequent progression of chronic trauma–white patch–cancer has been noted in some studies.

What Is the Diagnostic Significance of Leukoplakia and White Patches?

The term leukoplakia has frequently implied premalignancy wherever it has been used. There has been a conceptual parallel established between cancer and leukoplakia of the vulva, uterine cervix, urinary bladder, and renal pelvic mucosa. Unfortunately, this historically malevolent connotation has been applied to any oral mucosal changes that appear white. Thus, "leukoplakia" has been loosely applied to white patches of the oral cavity along with the implication of oral mucosal premalignancy. The general pathologic criteria for leukoplakia, dyskeratosis, dysplasia, and early cancer are discussed in detail in chapter 4.

All that the examiner sees is a whitish patch of varying subtlety. It is important to know that not all white patches of oral mucosa possess many of the histologic stigmata of dyskeratosis. Therefore, "leukoplakia" should be reserved for referring to a white plaque that has no other known etiology (e.g., lichen planus, white sponge nevus, lues, chemical burns, and other stomatitides). Leukoplakia should simply denote the existence of a white mucosal patch of unknown etiology, and judgment about the neoplastic potential should be reserved.

The clinical problem is to intercept the 5% of white patches that will be contiguous with squamous cell cancer or subsequently undergo malignant transformation. One may think of leukoplakia as a garden in which cancer may grow or be growing undetected. It is the precancerous nature of some of these lesions that makes it necessary to monitor and investigate the lesion.

Leukoplakia takes on a wide range of clinical appearances ranging from nonpalpable and faintly translucent to elevated, roughened, opaque, white palpable plaques.[3–5] The reader is again referred to the illustrations in *A Color Atlas of Oral Cancers.*[1] Two classes of leukoplakia can be identified: (1) chronic leukoplakia, which persists unchanged for 10–20 years as a thinner diffuse plaque, and (2) acute leukoplakia, which develops rapidly over weeks to months. The latter form often becomes thick and papillomatous or ulcerates; it is more *apt* to contain changes of malignancy. Plaques that change in appearance or show fissuring deserve prompt biopsy. A reddish irritated-appearing area with a partially or completely circumferential patch of leukoplakia is particularly ominous. These changes often portend malignant change.

Another question arises in tracking suspected evolving leukoplakia: what is the impact of multiple incisional biopsies on leukoplakia? Can the trauma of repeated biopsy tip the balance and precipitate neoplastic change in previously benign mucosal leukoplakia? We are not able to answer these questions at this time. Intuitive reasoning would suggest that (1) incisional biopsies may fail to sample in a malignant area, and therefore a type I sampling error would have been committed; (2) the mechanism that caused leukoplakia to develop in previously normal epithelium is unknown. We speculate that the germinal layer of epithelium is responding to some focal noxious stimulus. Whether this is intrinsic or extrinsic to the tissue is sometimes unknown. An intrinsic stimulus could be an aberrant local cell line in which loss of cell communication has occurred, causing limited loss of contact inhibition. Local tissue and humoral factors, including chalones, may limit the activity of this clone until the intrinsic equilibrium is shifted, e.g., by immunosuppression, low T_3 syndrome or malnutrition. A number of immunopathologic studies have been conducted. The results of such studies are tantalizing because they suggest that immunologic adjustments are associated with carcinomatous transformation. The studies to date do not clearly establish that these carcinomatous changes are due to prior immunologic factors. Extrinsic stimuli are much easier to identify. There is no doubt about the etiology of leukoplakia in snuff chewing, where the quid (a known carcinogen) is kept in direct contact with the abnormal mucosa. The problems of localized leukoplakia with continued exposure to carcinogens of known potency make a white patch an ominous problem.

Because of the problems in assuring accurate early diagnosis, I have adopted the liberal use of mucosal stripping to manage smaller suspicious areas of oral leukoplakia in an institutional clinical practice. Mucosal stripping is a means of:

1. Obtaining an excisional biopsy.
2. Debriding the region of abnormal-appearing mucosa down to the corium and resurfacing with normal regional mucosa, or allowing secondary intention healing to take place in the absence of any obvious inciting factors (jagged teeth, traumatic dental flanges).
3. Reducing the incidence of leaving undiagnosed precancerous leukoplakia in place. Many patients do not comply with follow-up and do not stop using tobacco products. Figure 2–16 shows a schema of management of oral leukoplakia.

What Is the Significance of Red Patches and Erythroplasia?

The incidence of malignant change occurring in mucosa is significantly greater with red plaques than with white plaques.[3, 6] About one fourth to one half of malignant erythroplakic patches have some adjacent leukoplakia. These red patches are referred to as erythroplasia. They are best seen if the mucosa is dried and viewed under a color-corrected lamp. *All red patches should be biopsied without hesitation.* One exception exists, and that is when "erythroplasia" is noted on the midline dorsum of the tongue. It is essential to avoid removing a superficially placed functioning lingual thyroid gland that may occur in the area anterior to the sulcus terminalis. A radionuclide scan will confirm the presence or absence of a normal cervical thyroid gland.

Clinically, erythroplasia has a well-defined perimeter, without induration or elevation. It is often painless but may have a burning sensation on touching it. These lesions do mimic focal inflammatory lesions.

The significance of the red patch is discussed further in chapter 13.

In summary, it is *essential* to biopsy all red patches, with one notable exception (see above). It is *desirable* to remove all acute leukoplakias by stripping and, by so doing, obtaining an excisional biopsy specimen. Periodic supervision with incisional biopsy appears to be adequate for follow-up of soft, unfissured, stable chronic leukoplakias in *nonsmokers* since these generally have a low annual rate of conversion to malignancy.

What Do You Do if a Biopsy Specimen Shows Dysplasia?

Dysplasia is a term that is used both clinically and formally in histopathology (see chap. 4). In histopathology, dysplasia reflects a loss of individual cell uniformity and tissue architecture. Dysplasia is usually reversible if the surgeon can completely remove identifiable inciting factors. With continued exposure to carcinogens, dysplasia may proceed irreversibly to anaplasia. The mechanism responsible for the change from reversible to irreversible (dysplastic to anaplastic) is not known.

In a limited study we tried to answer some of the preceding questions about early superficial epithelial changes in human tissues from representative areas of acanthosis, dyskeratosis, carcinoma in situ, and squamous cell carcinoma of the oral cavity. Vital dyes were used to identify round cells. Specific red cell adherence was used to ascertain the presence of tissue isoantigen. Specific fluorescein isothiocyanate conjugated antiglobulins were used to evaluate the nature of any immunologically detectable antigenic alterations that may be present in the dysplastic, anaplastic, and superficially malignant tissues.

Observations made from this study included the following:

1. There was a positive correlation between lymphocytosis and histologic changes associated with malignancy.

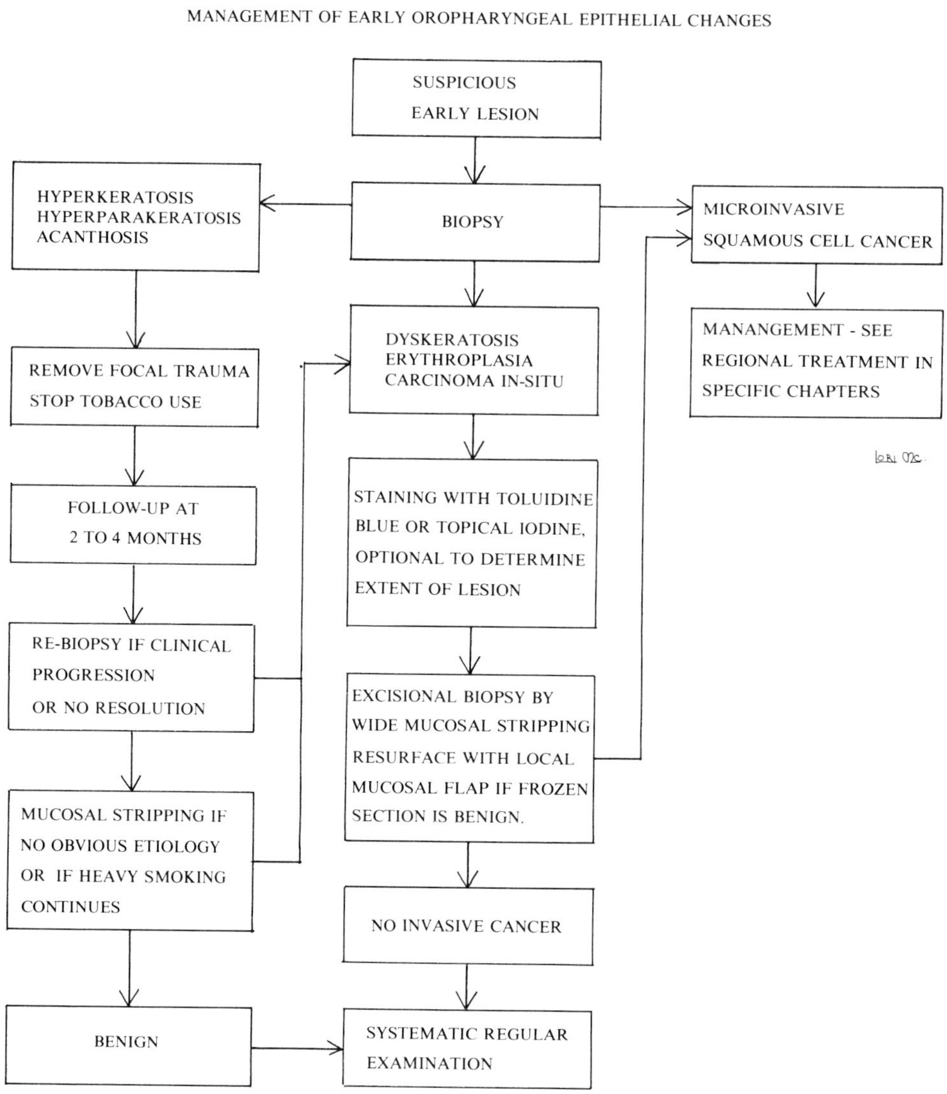

Fig 2–16.—Approach to managing early oral epithelial changes.

2. Tissue isoantigens are lost with malignancy.

3. Nonmalignant tissue specimens contained IgG and IgM. Malignant oral tissue specimens contained IgA and C3 complement fraction(s).

4. Dyskeratotic oral tissue contained IgA, IgG, and C3.

5. Any lymphocytic infiltrate depolarizes from the germinal epithelial layer between the rete pegs in carcinoma in situ and early invasive squamous cell carcinoma, suggesting loss of "information" with which the cells align themselves along the histologically altered interface; or blocking factors may be generated to increase the spatial relationship described above.

Such findings by ourselves and others are tantalizing and suggest that the future may hold a better explanation for the progressive change to malignancy. There may be some hope of separating the "stable" lesion from the "unstable" lesion with predictable reliability. For the present, biopsy is the strong tool.

WHAT SHOULD WE DO TO MANAGE AND FOLLOW-UP OROAIRWAY EPITHELIAL CHANGES?

Several attempts have been made to promote screening tests that would aid the clinician. Staining techniques can be used in conjunction with a thorough clinical examination to help identify leukoplakia, erythroplasia, or malignancy. Three techniques are (1) toluidine blue (tolonium), (2) topical iodine (Schiller test), and (3) secretory IgA titer of saliva.

Toluidine blue is a basic metachromatic nuclear stain

which may be applied to a specific area or used as a mouth rinse. The rinse technique has been reported to be useful in highlighting second synchronous oropharyngeal neoplasms. It will detect areas of erythroplasia that may otherwise be clinically overlooked and therefore left undiagnosed. This screening modality has a 2.0% false negative rate (type I error) with direct application of the stain to a cancer, while the rinse technique has a 5.9% false negative rate. False positive rates of 9.3% with the direct stain technique and of 7.4% with the rinse technique have been reported.

In an effort to reduce the false positive rate due to inflammation, the lesion should be restained 10–14 days following detection. Etiologic factors thought to be responsible for the inflammatory response should be removed during this period. *A clearly indicated biopsy should not be delayed* in order to differentiate the suspected character of the tissue on the basis of its mordancy, whether the lesion is inflammatory or neoplastic. Since a type I sampling error is reported to range from 2% to 5.9%, the clinician must vigorously ascertain the histopathology of the mucosa. *Obtain a prompt and adequate tissue diagnosis.*

In the Schiller test, a solution of iodine and potassium iodine is applied to atypical mucosal cells; neoplastic cells that are devoid of glycogen fail to stain, but nonneoplastic normal mucosa stains deeply. Atypical cells are depleted of glycogen, which is the site of iodine fixation. Hyperplasia and dysplasia are associated with a positive Schiller test (no stain uptake). Therefore, this test is not diagnostic but suggests the presence of malignancy.

It has been reported that secretory IgA (S-IgA) levels in salivary samples are elevated in squamous cell carcinoma of the oral cavity and oropharynx.[7] S-IgA, therefore, has been proposed as a potentially useful tumor marker. Theoretically, S-IgA measurement would provide a general screening method to aid in the detection of aerodigestive tract mucosal neoplasia. The required 2–3 ml of saliva is readily obtained. An inverse relationship exists between salivary flow rate and the concentration of salivary IgA. No correlation exists between serum IgA and salivary IgA concentrations. Cancer patients with recurrence have greater salivary IgA levels than do patients with their first malignancy. Patients who have been free of clinically detectable malignant disease show a persistently elevated serum IgA level but a return to normal levels of salivary IgA. Evidence of recurrent disease or of a second primary neoplasm may be related to the appearance of a spike in the salivary S-IgA titer. The present clinical usefulness and reliability of immunologic tests for oropharyngeal cancer are still under evaluation.

HOW DO YOU DOCUMENT EPITHELIAL CHANGES FOUND ON EXAMINATION?

The management of a patient with visible oroairway epithelial changes requires information obtained from biopsy. A brief algorithm is shown in Figure 2–16.

It is crucial to have complete, accurate clinical notes and drawings. They should pinpoint the exact location, dimensions, appearance, and texture of the lesion. The documentation should note any altered sensation or pain or tenderness associated with the region. Good quality anatomical drawings must be used to plot location. A standardized series of diagrams provides the clinician with a rapid topographical record that surpasses his own artistic skills. Several examples are given in this text and are used in the staging manual.

Radiographic studies should be supplemented with clinical photographs, taken with the aid of a macrolens that is color corrected for reds/blues. Lip and tongue retractors will substantially improve photographic quality. The photographs are also obtained in order to make later comparisons of the mucosal appearance.

WHEN A WORRISOME BUT NONMALIGNANT LESION IS PRESENT, HOW CAN IT BE MANAGED?

When the dentist or oral surgeon is part of a coherent multidisciplinary team, there may be maneuvers and treatments he can use to see if the observed pathology can be reversed. When the initial examination reveals mucosal changes opposite a focal source of trauma, it is important to remove the local irritant (broken tooth, rough filling, denture flange with calculus, overextended denture flanges, pipe stem, etc.). Commonly, inflammatory mucosal changes resolve in 7–10 days. Reevaluation following this period should be helpful in (1) clinically differentiating traumatic lesions from neoplastic lesions and (2) reducing the area of inflammation and the degree of inflammation that may accompany a mucosal neoplasm. Resolution of an inflammatory component will give the clinician an optimum site selection for biopsy. Concomitantly, subtle changes in the tissue may be easier for the pathologist to interpret without a florid substrate of acute inflammation.

Long-term supervision of noncancerous but suspicious mucosal changes depends on successfully establishing a mucosal environment that is free of factors thought to be associated with neoplasia. The key element is behavior modification to avoid tobacco use and alcohol consumption. Additional steps may include removing focal mechanical irritations such as broken dentition or a denture flange, or by making dental restorations; cleaning accumulated accretions from natural teeth or prosthodontic appliances; and improving oral hygiene. Failure to refrain from the use of tobacco products and to maintain oral hygiene predisposes to continued mucosal neoplasia. If lesions persist, biopsy (incision vs. excision) is required.

WHAT IS THE BEST WAY TO BIOPSY THE SUSPICIOUS MUCOSAL LESION?

Earlier discussion presented the need for adequate timely biopsy. The decision value of repeated small incisional biopsies is unquestionably better than not taking any biopsy of mucosal abnormalities. In clinical practice the biopsy must yield enough information that a clear decision can be made.

The first problems concern the area to be sampled: Where are the most representative sites? A small focal lesion can be easily excised in toto. An extensive area of mucosal change will require a thorough experience with the range of normal mucosal appearances. The clinician develops that knowledge by doing numerous careful examinations. Regional difficulties in identifying abnormalities occur at the lateral border of the posterior one third of the tongue, the junction of the anterior pillar of the tonsillar fauces and the tongue, the sublingual carunculi, the mucogingival junction, the uvula, and the posterior pharyngeal wall. Wiping the mucosa dry will aid in making reliable identification of existing mucosal changes. Staining techniques may help.[8]

Prior or repeated biopsies will cause a progressive change in the mucosal characteristics due to inflammation and cicatrix formation. The postbiopsy healed surface contour is likely to be confluent but irregular. The early color changes from surgery will temporarily mask intrinsic changes associated with the primary pathology. Later the maturing scar will have an opalescent hue that may cause clinical concern over an apparently progressive "leukoplakia."

There is a haunting theoretical concern that repeated surgical trauma to an area of mucosa may accelerate some sort of focal change. What is the effect of repeated surgical insult on dysplastic epithelium? No data are available.

When multiple biopsy specimens are taken at one session, each specimen must be accurately oriented, labeled, and precisely mapped in the record. With this information the clinician can plan the limits of the treatment field.

In most instances, the problems cited above may be eliminated for oral lesions by performing an excisional biopsy in the form of mucosal stripping. The specific problems of the tonsil, larynx, and hypopharynx are discussed in chapters 14 and 16. A margin of about ½ cm should be included to provide sufficient leeway to accommodate the clinically indistinct margin. Margins will be difficult to obtain in areas of the buccal aspect of the posterior mandibular alveolar ridge, the palatal raphe, and circumferentially to existing natural teeth unless mucoperiosteal stripping is performed. The single specimen can be pinned on cardboard, labeled, oriented, and tagged with ease, permitting accurate identification of specific areas of histopathology. The specimen should be placed in an adequate-sized container for fixation so that crumpling is avoided. Handling of the biopsy specimen is discussed in chapter 4. The removal of all clinically abnormal-appearing mucosa provides the region with a "fresh start;" resurfacing of the denuded submucosa or connective tissue can be done with a free mucosal graft or a mucosal flap from healthy-appearing tissue. Resurfacing will decrease postoperative discomfort, reduce recovery time, and preserve the appearance or function of the region. In contrast, a split-thickness skin graft will confuse clinical follow-up because of the altered appearance and texture at the mucosa-skin interface. Healing by secondary intention is satisfactory only for small areas in which mucosal stripping was performed (e.g., palate). Significant cicitricial contracture will occur if the lip and cheek have had wide full-thickness stripping without resurfacing. When multiple or large areas are to be stripped, it may be practical to stage the procedure in order to minimize morbidity. The area of greatest clinical concern should be stripped first.

Electrocautery and a laser excision probably cause enough "sauté artifact" at the margins to produce problems with histopathologic interpretation, particularly where margins are under question.

The capricious use of silver nitrate sticks and other caustic substances applied to ulcerative mucosal lesions or mucosal changes is mentioned to be condemned. The clinician will occasionally fall victim to a presumptive clinical diagnosis of aphthous ulcer and start the topical application of silver nitrate only to be distressed with the belated realization of the true nature of the original lesion. Cauterization denies the patient the opportunity for early tissue diagnosis since usually no biopsy is obtained. Often the patient will continue to treat himself. There is a role for the judicious use of sclerosing agents to reduce pain in the management of *proved* recurrent aphthous stomatitis.

All too often one sees patients in whom long-term wide-spectrum antibiotics have been used empirically to treat mucosal changes that mimic ulcerative gingivostomatitis. In general, a rapid response should be expected within days if appropriate therapeutic agents, including topical dilute H_2O_2, are used to treat periodontal gingivostomatitis. A Gram stain can provide further coroborative information. If the condition persists in a florid state for more than 5 days, it would be clinically wise to perform a biopsy.

Patients who complain of "sore throats" and swollen cervical lymph nodes and in whom empirical antibiotics have been unsuccessful should *not* be provided with different antibiotics or an extended supply, just in case "the strain of bacteria is resistant." It is essential that these patients have appropriate cultures and be given a thorough head and neck examination. If indicated, endoscopy is included to search for the etiology of the patient's complaint(s). A high index of suspicion must be developed in order to minimize clinical oversight and to avoid misdiagnosing a benign cause for a malignant process.

WHAT ARE SOME USEFUL TECHNIQUES FOR BIOPSYING THE ORAL CAVITY?

Excisional biopsy is usually performed if the lesion is thin, focal, well circumscribed (usually not exceeding 1.5 cm in diameter), and accessible. The patient should be cooperative and aware of the nature of the procedure. Analgesics will be required for modest postoperative discomfort.

Incisional biopsies are done for large ill-defined mucosal lesions or those that involve hard tissues. Incisional biopsies should include a section of the junction of solid abnormal tissue and contiguous normal-appearing tissue. The sample should not be taken from large central areas of necrosis. The necrotic cells do not provide the clinically important information that is obtained from the margin of an ulcerative lesion. The depth of a mucosal biopsy need only include the corium in continuity with the mucosa to establish the cardinal criterion for malignancy, invasion deep to the lamina propria. Injudicious use of sutures for coaptation of mucosa or lesion edges after an incisional biopsy is often an exercise in futility when the adjacent tumor tissue is friable. Sutures may transport malignant cells deeply from an otherwise superficial mucosal abnormality. A general principle is to avoid suturing incisional biopsy wounds. To minimize mucosal spreading after biopsy, the clinician should select a long axis for an elliptical incisional or excisional biopsy that will not be at right angles to the usual mucosal stress lines.

Regional sensory nerve blockade or ring block provides satisfactory surgical anesthesia. Regional nerve blockade should be employed where clinically possible to avoid theoretical iatrogenic deep seeding of tumor cells with infiltration or ring block. Care must be exercised in avoiding distortion of the biopsy site, which may be caused by rapid infiltration, excessive volume, or infiltration into the biopsy site, leading to separation of the mucosa from connective tissue.

Other biopsy techniques include:

- Fine needle aspiration
- Large needle aspiration
- Curettage
- Punch biopsy
- Exfoliative cytology

Needle aspiration biopsy is suitable for low-viscosity fluids within a mass. It is performed to obtain information on the color, consistency, cytology, volume, and coagulation potential (see Chap. 19). Needle biopsy is sometimes advocated, but, except for the thyroid, it merely provides corroborative information and rarely gives enough information to alter the decision process (see the discussion of needle biopsy of "unknown" neck masses in Chap. 25).

Needle core biopsy is uncommonly used for the oral cavity. It can be useful when it is performed well in the proper circumstances. Poor sampling might occur if portions of lymph nodes, adjacent normal tissue, or minimally affected tissue are obtained. This technique is used for percutaneous biopsy of a mass to confirm recurrent disease or metastases in a patient with known malignancy.

Biopsy by curettage is the usual method for intraosseous lesions of the mandible and maxilla.

Punch biopsy is usually undertaken when formal incisional techniques cannot be performed, such as for lesions on the surface of the tonsil or the nasopharynx, due to limited regional access. Crushing and distortion of the specimen are common when a small biopsy cup is used. An adequate-sized cup should be used. Obtaining multiple samples from the area under investigation will make it more likely that one will be of satisfactory diagnostic quality.

Exfoliative cytology has not provided the same level of reliability in the diagnosis of oropharyngeal malignancy as it has for uterine, cervical, and vaginal malignancies. The constant mechanical debridement of tissue by the saliva, tongue, and cheeks does not allow the accumulation of exfoliated malignant cells, such as occurs in the female reproductive tract or other body recesses. Exfoliative cytology is not a substitute for biopsy.

REFERENCES

1. Burkhardt A., Maerker R.: *A Color Atlas of Oral Cancers.* Chicago, Year Book Medical Publishers, Inc., 1981.
2. Graham S., Dayal H., Rohrer T., et al.: Dentition, diet, tobacco, and alcohol in the epidemiology of oral cancer. *JNCI* 59:1611–1623, 1977.
3. Banoczy J., Sugar L.: Longitudinal studies in oral leukoplakias. *J. Oral Pathol.* 1:265–272, 1972.

4. Waldron C.A., Shafer W.E.: Leukoplakia revisited: A clinico-pathologic study of 3256 oral leukoplakias. *Cancer* 36:1386–1392, 1975.
5. WHO Collaborating Center for Oral Precancerous Lesions: Definition of leukoplakia and related lesions: An aid to studies on oral precancer. *Oral Surg.* 46:518–539, 1978.
6. Mashberg A.: Erythroplasia: Earliest sign of asymptomatic oral cancer. *J. Am. Dent. Assoc.* 96:615–620, 1978.
7. Watanabe T., Inglehart J.D., Bolognesi D.P., et al.: Secretory immune response to oropharyngeal cancer. *Surg. Forum* 32:548–551, 1981.
8. Helsper J.T.: Staining techniques: Screening tests for oral cancer, in Baker H.W., et al. (eds.): *Oral Cancer,* an American Cancer Society Professional Education Publication. American Cancer Society, Inc., 1973.

3 / Newer Techniques for the Radiographic Diagnosis of Head and Neck Malignancy

DAVID E. TUBMAN, M.D.

RADIOLOGIC IMAGING is now able to provide an accurate representation of normal and pathologic anatomy of the head and neck. Accurate mapping of lesions of these regions can be performed when clinical and radiologic findings are correlated, thereby allowing a precise treatment plan.[1] Decisions as to resectability, radiation field margins, possible prognosis, and preservation of function may be made with a greater degree of accuracy than in the past. A summary of suggested studies is given in Table 3–1.

While greater precision is now possible in diagnosis, this is not without the penalty of relatively high radiation dose and financial cost. Therefore, the efficacy of examinations is an important concept which should be remembered in the investigation of these patients. This chapter attempts to provide a basis for allowing an informed choice of examination.

PARANASAL SINUSES

The initial examination of all patients with suspected paranasal sinus disease should be plain radiography. Soft tissue mass and bone destruction may be assessed in the sinuses as well as in the nasal cavity, nasopharynx, and skull base. Further investigation of this region should be performed with computerized tomography (CT) rather than conventional tomography.

High resolution CT scanning at present provides superior bony resolution when compared to conventional tomography. The added advantage of CT is the superb soft tissue depiction. Bony plates running parallel to the axis of the beam may be seen as soft tissue densities due to partial volume averaging with adjacent air or soft tissue.[2, 3] Coronal or sagittal scans may be necessary. Low resolution scanners often demonstrate cartilaginous or very thin bony walls as areas of dehiscence, particularly if the region is not in the plane of section. Thinly collimated high resolution scans may be necessary to demonstrate intact bony structures.

Axial scanning, with or without coronal and sagittal reconstruction, is usually performed as the initial examination. Intravenous (IV) contrast medium is given to delineate intracranial extension and to determine the cause of opacification of other paranasal sinuses. A large nasal cavity mass may occlude multiple ostia. Even though the majority of paranasal sinus carcinomas do not enhance with contrast media, despite their relative hypovascularity, there is a tendency for an increase in density to equal that of the surrounding musculature—a whole body of opacification effect. Sinuses containing secretions do not increase in density. The hypodensity of the occluded sinus does not absolutely rule out the presence of tumor. Biopsy is usually necessary for definitive proof.[4]

Scans are obtained through the entire sinus architecture into the sella turcica, middle fossa, and orbits. If subtle extension into the orbital floor or middle cranial fossa is suggested, either computer reconstruction of the axial data or direct coronal scanning is performed.

The extrasinus spread of maxillary sinus carcinoma influences the surgical approach. The important areas to assess are the orbits, intracranial cavity, infratem-

TABLE 3–1.—ALGORITHM FOR INVESTIGATION OF HEAD AND NECK MALIGNANCY

SITE	FIRST STUDY	CONFIRMING STUDY
Paranasal sinuses	Plain films	CT
Nasopharynx	CT	
Temporal bone	Conventional tomography or high resolution CT	
	Acoustic neuroma	Contrast-enhanced CT; if negative, CO_2 cisternography
Salivary glands	Parotid mass	Contrast-enhanced CT scan; if dense parotid gland, CT-sialography
Larynx	Contrast-enhanced CT	
Cervical region	Contrast-enhanced CT	

poral and pterygopalatine fossae, nasal cavity, and nasopharynx (see illustrations in chap. 17 showing areas of spread).[3]

Tumors in the maxillary antrum may extend in virtually any direction. The spread is usually related to the site of origin of the tumor and the anatomical areas of weakness in the sinus walls. In the case of adenoidcystic carcinoma, perineural extension is a common feature.[2]

Bony destruction of the antral walls is easily demonstrated, with soft tissue density seen outside the confines of the sinus. An increase in the width of the skin of the cheek suggests dermal lymphatic invasion. Destruction of the posterior wall of the sinus is usually associated with extension into the lucent fat pad situated between the sinus wall and the lateral pterygoid and temporalis muscles. Assessment of the pterygopalatine fossa is based on demonstrating obliteration of the normal flat planes found in this region, which is associ-

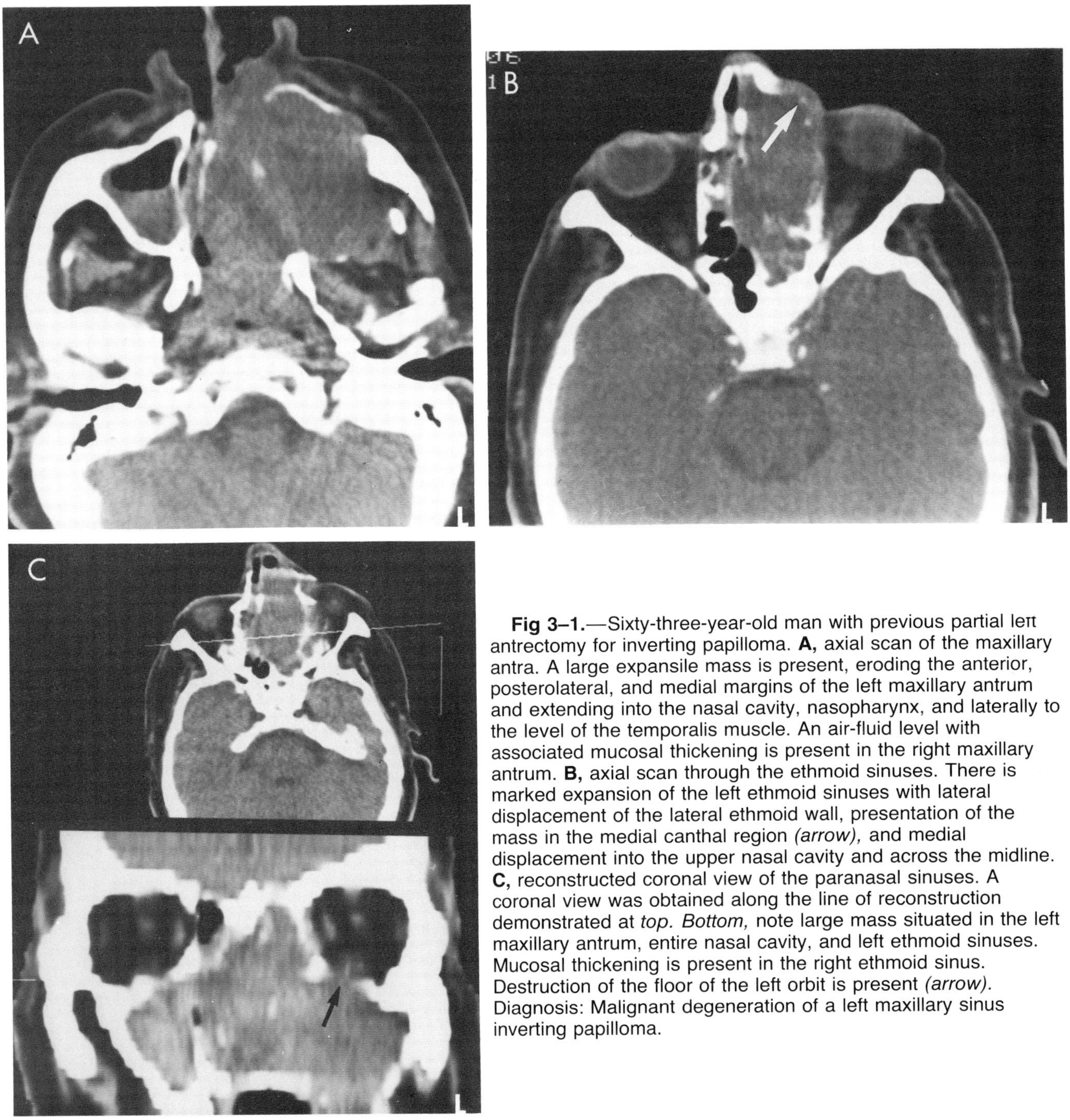

Fig 3–1.—Sixty-three-year-old man with previous partial left antrectomy for inverting papilloma. **A,** axial scan of the maxillary antra. A large expansile mass is present, eroding the anterior, posterolateral, and medial margins of the left maxillary antrum and extending into the nasal cavity, nasopharynx, and laterally to the level of the temporalis muscle. An air-fluid level with associated mucosal thickening is present in the right maxillary antrum. **B,** axial scan through the ethmoid sinuses. There is marked expansion of the left ethmoid sinuses with lateral displacement of the lateral ethmoid wall, presentation of the mass in the medial canthal region *(arrow),* and medial displacement into the upper nasal cavity and across the midline. **C,** reconstructed coronal view of the paranasal sinuses. A coronal view was obtained along the line of reconstruction demonstrated at *top. Bottom,* note large mass situated in the left maxillary antrum, entire nasal cavity, and left ethmoid sinuses. Mucosal thickening is present in the right ethmoid sinus. Destruction of the floor of the left orbit is present *(arrow).* Diagnosis: Malignant degeneration of a left maxillary sinus inverting papilloma.

ated with destruction of the adjacent posterior antral wall or pterygoid plates. This posterior extension indicates spread beyond the limits of current surgical resection (Fig 3–1).

Accurate assessment of orbital and middle fossa extension is best made with direct coronal scanning with IV contrast. Extension may occur through the inferior orbital fissure to the orbital apex, cavernous sinus, and middle cranial fossa. Antral tumor may spread to the ethmoid sinus and then through the medial orbital wall, or to the cribriform plate region into the anterior cranial fossa (Fig 3–2).

Carcinoma of the ethmoid, sphenoid, and frontal sinuses may grow intracranially or into the orbit. Axial scanning with IV contrast enhancement usually depicts these masses well. They are considerably less common than tumors in the maxillary antrum.

Assessment of the postoperative changes within a sinus may be difficult. To address this problem, Som et al. suggested a protocol consisting of a baseline scan at 6–8 weeks postoperatively and follow-up examinations at 4- to 6-month intervals thereafter for 3 years.[5] In their group of 18 patients, recurrent tumors in three of four patients were clinically occult and detected only by CT.

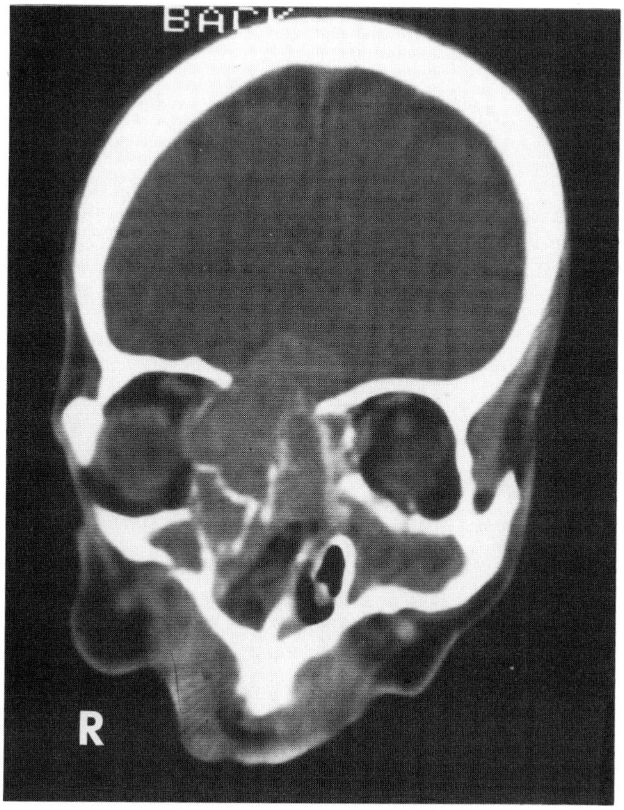

Fig 3–2.—Seventy-year-old man with a nasal mass. A direct coronal scan following infusion of contrast medium demonstrates a large mass in the ethmoid and nasal regions with lateral extension into the right orbit and superior extension through the cribriform plate-orbital roof region to displace the gyri recti of the frontal lobes. The mass extends inferiorly into the right aspect of the nasal cavity. Bilateral opacity of the maxillary antra on axial views was less dense than the intranasal mass, indicating maxillary ostial blockage. Diagnosis: Esthesioneuroblastoma.

After partial or radical maxillectomy, the lining of the cavity should be smooth. Postradiation mucosal changes and chronic sinusitis cause uniform mucosal thickening. Any nodularity or focal swelling is considered abnormal and consistent with recurrence (Fig 3–3).[5]

NASOPHARYNX AND OROPHARYNX

There are two clinical indications for radiologic examination of the nasopharynx. (1) In patients with a diagnosed nasopharyngeal mass, the airway component, deep extension, orbital, base of the skull, and paranasal sinus invasion may be demonstrated. (2) In patients with an unknown head and neck tumor, radiologic imaging of the nasopharynx along with the pyriform sinuses and base of the tongue is of considerable importance in the search for a primary.[6] Presently, the only examination that will provide evidence of soft tissue and bone disease in the nasopharyngeal and paranasopharyngeal regions is CT.

CT scans are performed in axial and, if needed, coronal projections. IV contrast medium should be given to assess intracranial extension. Scans from the middle cranial fossa to the epiglottis are usually sufficient.

The airway portion of the nasopharyngeal mass is easily demonstrated. On occasion, a large mass in the adult airway may be confused with malignancy. Usually, if the parapharyngeal spaces are normal bilaterally, the mucosal masses represent hypertrophy of the lymphoid tissue. Differentiation between lymphoid tissue and neoplastic mass may be obtained by scanning the patient with the mouth open or during a modified Valsalva maneuver. The fossae of Rosenmüller will distend and the eustachian tubes become more filled with air in the case of plastic lymphoid tissue.[2] With neoplasm, there is no change in airway margins with these maneuvers.

Asymmetry of the nasopharyngeal airway is common, but the adjacent paranasopharyngeal spaces are usually very symmetric.[6] For a nasopharyngeal mass to enter the paranasopharyngeal space, it must cross the dense pharyngobasilar fascia, which forms the boundaries of the nasopharynx. Thus, any asymmetry of the paranasopharyngeal spaces, particularly when associated with a nasopharyngeal mass, indicates either malignancy or aggressive infection. Hemorrhage and edema may obliterate this space; therefore, scanning must be conducted prior to biopsy or surgery. Postirradiation

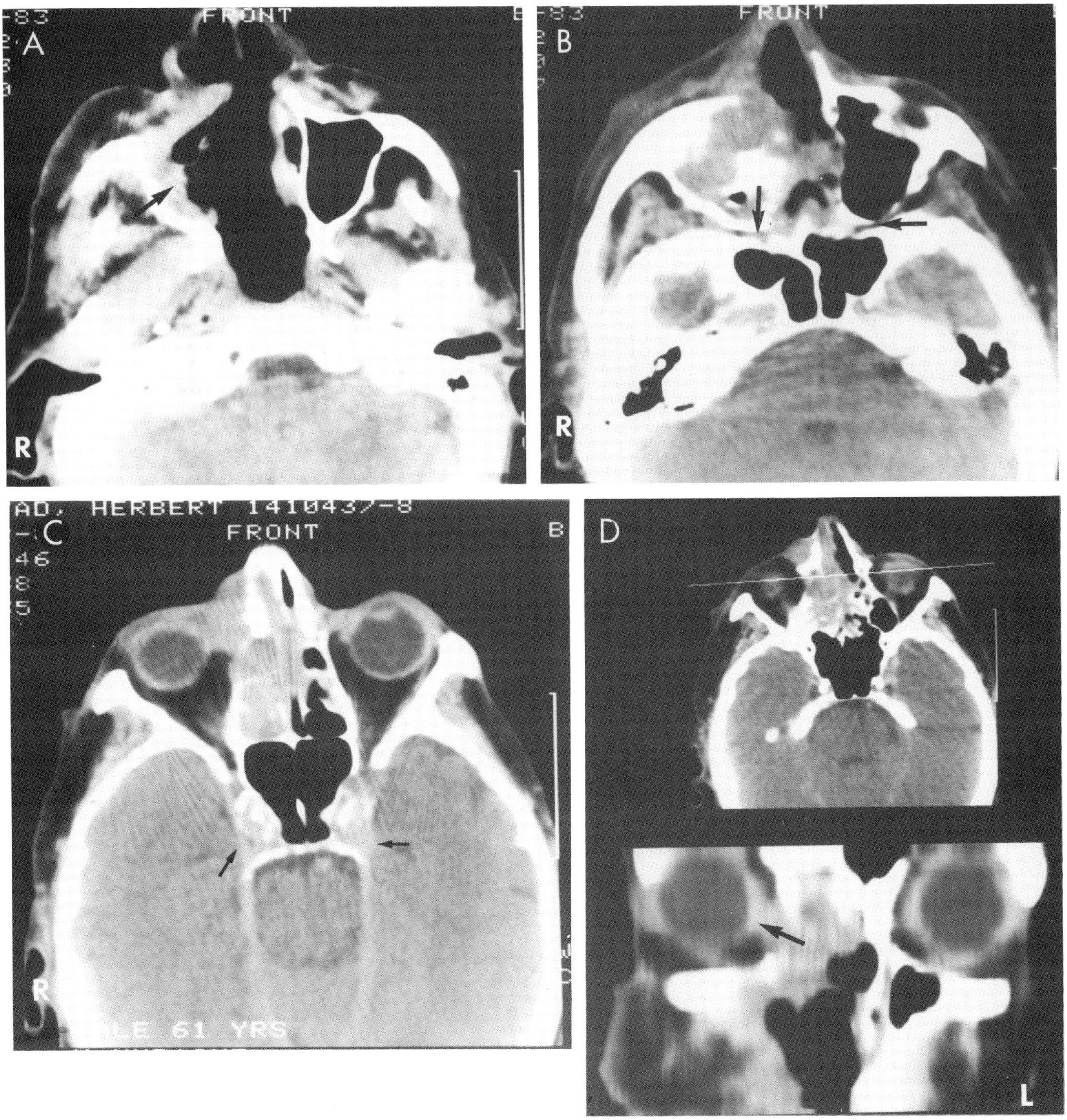

Fig 3–3.—A 65-year-old man with previous partial right antrectomy for squamous cell carcinoma. Presenting symptoms were a left nerve VI palsy and right cranial nerve VI paresis. **A, B,** and **C** are axial scans. **A,** considerable irregularity of the soft tissue margins of the right partial antrectomy cavity is present *(arrow)*. **B,** soft tissue extends into the right nasal cavity, across the midline to the medial wall of the left antrum, posteriorly into the superior reaches of the nasal pharynx, and into the right pterygopalatine fossa *(vertical arrow)*. The normal fat-containing left pterygopalatine fossa is indicated *(horizontal arrow)*. **C,** there is superior soft tissue extension into the right ethmoid sinuses and nasal cavity, with destruction of the medial orbital wall and extension into the medial and inferior aspects of the right orbit, subtly compressing and encasing the right globe. The normal smooth lateral contour of the right cavernous sinus is indicated *(oblique arrow)*. The irregular margin of the left cavernous sinus *(horizontal arrow)* indicates tumor extension to this region, likely through the superior reaches of the ptergyopalatine fossa and inferior orbital fissure. **D,** reconstructed coronal view. Lobulated tumor is present in the right antrectomy cavity, extending superiorly into the right ethmoidal sinus and nasal cavity. The mass extends superolaterally into the medial orbit with attachment to the medial aspect of the globe *(arrow)*. Diagnosis: Recurrent squamous cell carcinoma of the maxillary antrum.

edema and fibrosis may produce the same changes (Fig 3–4).

Nasopharyngeal carcinoma may be shown to extend inferiorly to the oropharyngeal space, superiorly to the petrous apex, laterally into the infratemporal fossa, and even contralaterally.[2] Bone destruction may involve the pterygoid plates and the skull base, with intracranial extension. Tumor may also extend intracranially along the carotid artery and occasionally along nerve sheaths.[2] Lymph node metastases are common and may be unilateral or bilateral. Nodes larger than 1.5 cm in diameter and of homogeneous density or with a low-density necrotic center probably are metastatic.

Juvenile nasopharyngeal angiofibromas are investigated with contrast-enhanced axial and coronal CT followed by angiography if surgery is contemplated. These lesions appear to originate in or near the sphenopalatine foramen and grow into the bony channels in the region of this foramen.[7] Lateral extension occurs through the pterygomaxillary fissure into the infratemporal fossa. Superior extension occurs through the foramina at the base of the skull into the cavernous sinus and medial cranial fossa. Medial extension is usually into the nasopharynx. Extension into the maxillary sinus may occur either from the pterygopalatine fossa or from the medial nasal component of the tumor.

Usually these tumors enhance markedly and homogeneously, although occasional cases may have central lucency. Lesions that may enhance markedly and therefore may be confused with angiofibromas are lymphoepitheliomas, fibrous dysplasia,[8] and inflammatory polyposis.

The angioarchitecture of angiofibromas is characteristic, with dilated reticulated arteries and a dense tumor blush seen in the venous phase. The lesions are often supplied by the internal maxillary and ascending pharyngeal branches of the external carotid artery as well as by intracavernous branches of the internal carotid artery (Fig 3–5).[7]

CT has been able to demonstrate lesions in patients who present with symptoms and signs consistent with head and neck cancers but with normal mucosa. The site of origin and the deep extension of these lesions may be well shown.[10] Both enlarged lymph nodes and deep lesions of the head and neck may be easily biopsied via fine needle aspiration,[11, 12] if such a technique is indicated, with or without CT guidance.

TEMPORAL BONE

High resolution CT is gradually replacing conventional tomography for investigation of the temporal

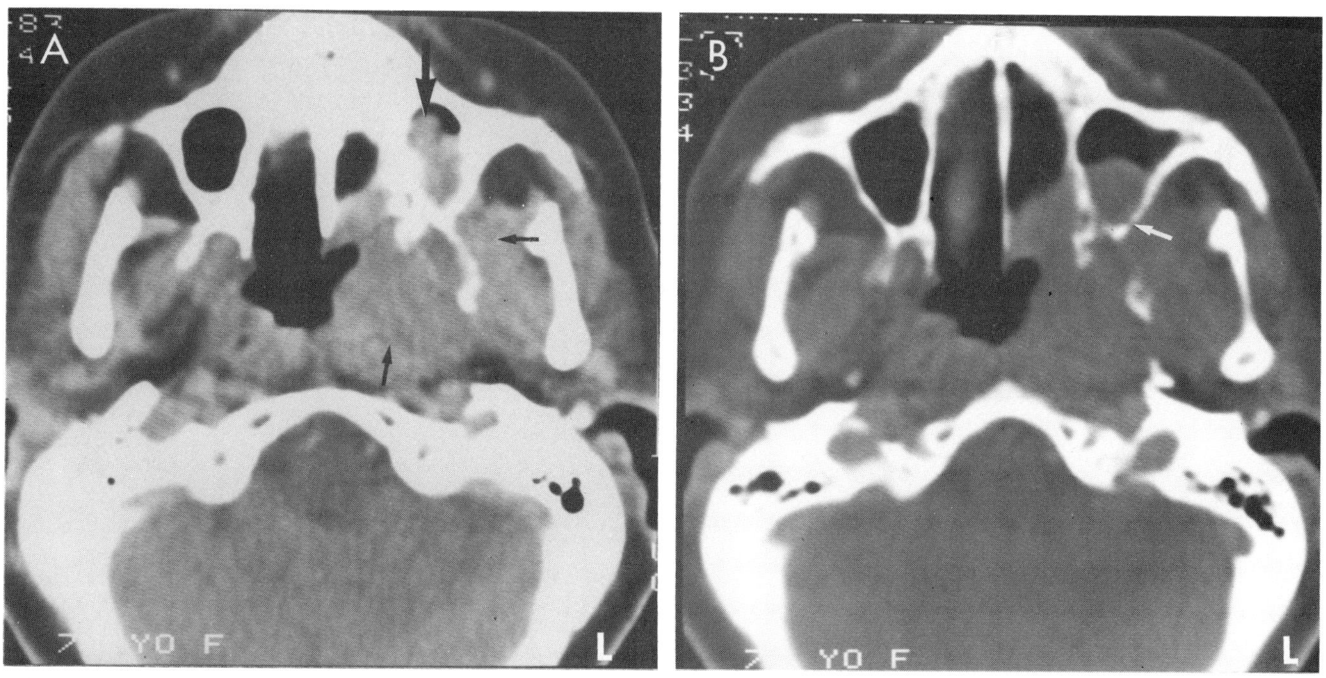

Fig 3–4.—Seventy-year-old woman with left facial pain. **A,** axial scan. A left nasopharyngeal mass *(arrows)* is present with lateral extension into the paranasopharyngeal space to the level of the lateral pterygoid muscle, and anterior extension into the posterior left nasal cavity and the left maxillary antrum. **B,** axial scan inferior to Figure 4,**A.** Bone windows. There is permiative destruction of the medial and posterolateral walls of the left maxillary antrum as well as of the pterygoid process. Tumor is present in the infratemporal fossa, surrounding both the temporalis and lateral pterygoid muscles. Diagnosis: Nasopharyngeal carcinoma with extension into the paranasopharyngeal space, left maxillary antrum, posterior nasal cavity, and infratemporal fossa.

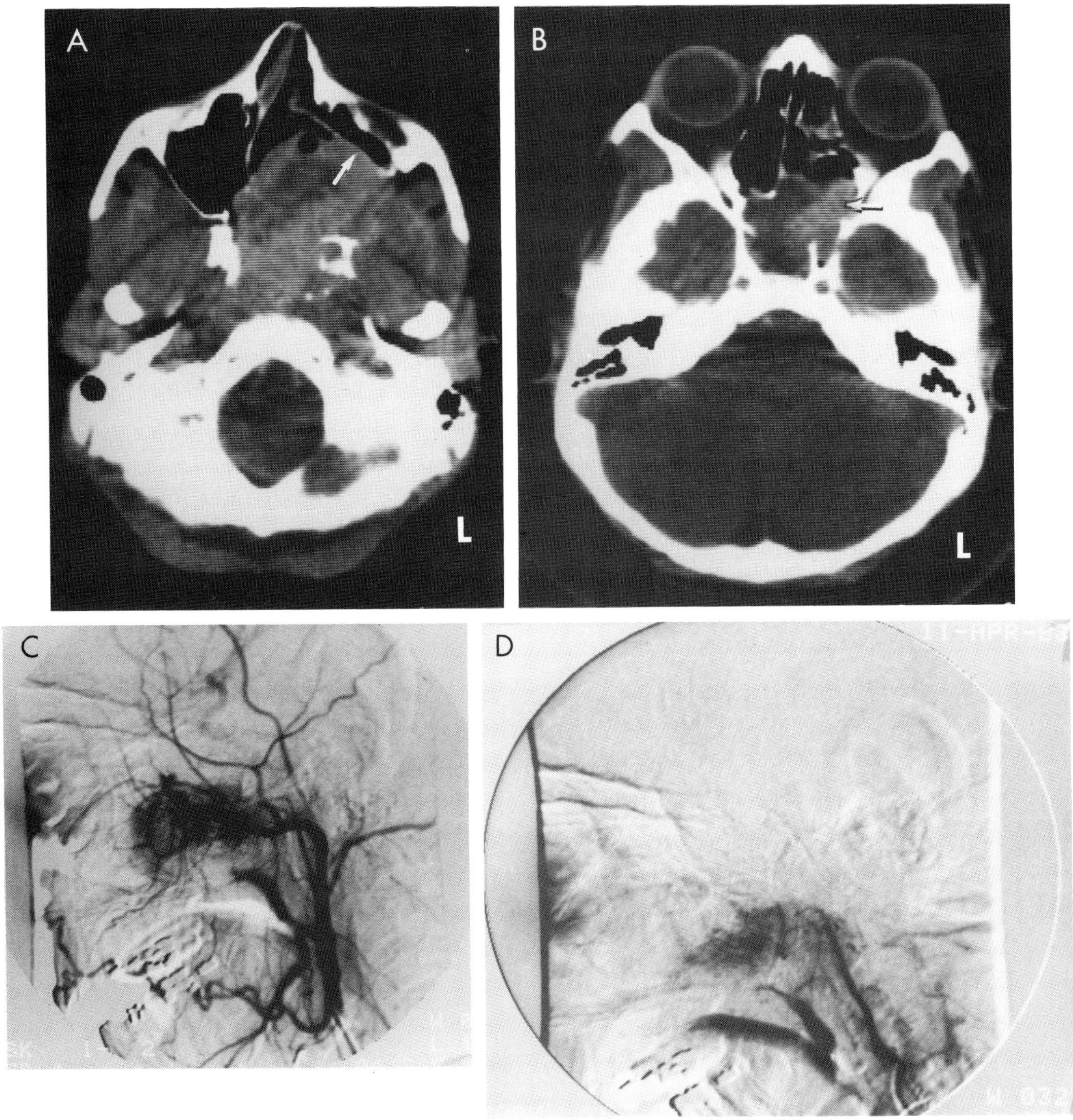

Fig 3–5.—Fifteen-year-old boy with multiple episodes of epistaxis. **A,** axial contrast-enhanced CT scan of the nasopharynx. A large irregularly enhancing nasopharyngeal mass is present with a marked widening of the left pterygopalatine fossa and extension into the infratemporal fossa. There is marked anterior displacement of the posterior wall of the left maxillary antrum *(arrow).* Lucency is present in the mid-aspect of the mass. **B,** axial CT scan of the sphenoid sinus. An enhancing mass *(arrow)* is present in the left aspect of the sphenoid sinus, extending from the superior aspect of the left pterygopalatine fossa. The remainder of the sphenoid sinus is opaque due to ostial blockage. **C,** left external carotid lateral digital angiogram. A hypervascular mass is present in the nasopharynx and infratemporal fossa and is supplied by the internal maxillary artery. **D,** left ascending pharyngeal lateral digital angiogram. The ascending pharyngeal arteries supply the inferior and posterior aspects of the hypervascular mass. *(Continued)*

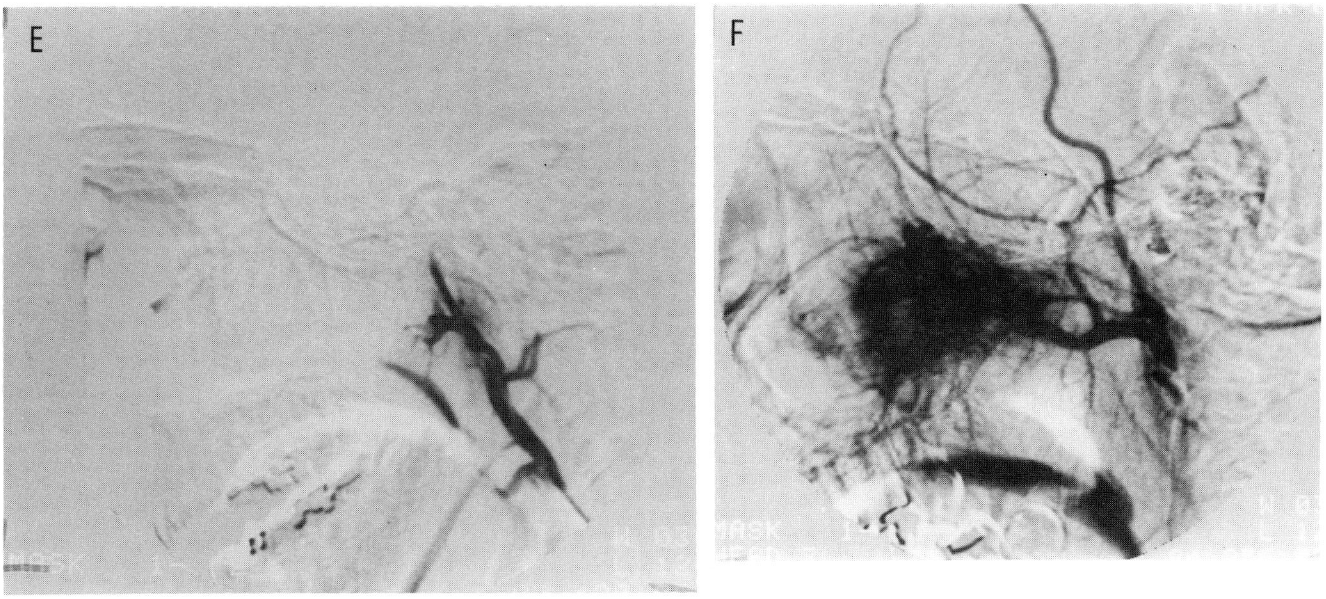

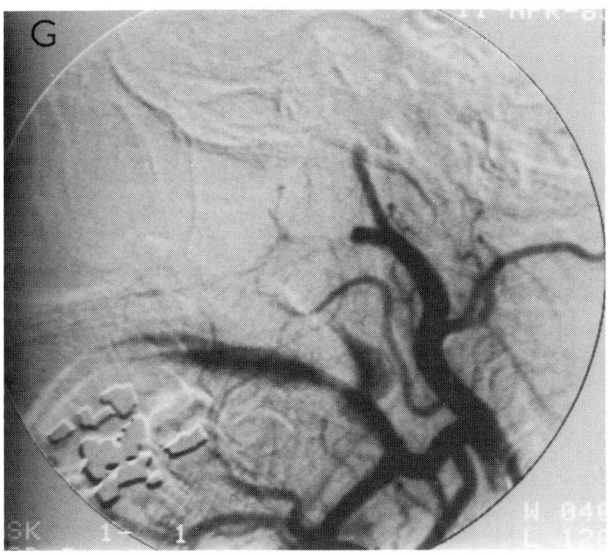

Fig 3–5 cont.—**E,** left external carotid angiogram following Ivalon embolization. There is occlusion of multiple branches of the external carotid artery without opacification of the nasopharyngeal mass. **F,** lateral view, right external carotid digital angiogram. The hypervascular mass is supplied by the right internal maxillary artery. **G,** lateral view, right external carotid digital angiogram obtained following embolization. The superior temporal and internal maxillary arteries are occluded. Diagnosis: Juvenile nasopharyngeal angiofibroma.

bone.[13] The ability to satisfactorily image bone and soft tissue components simultaneously compensates for the slight loss of resolution of some CT scanners. For example, those scanners with the best available resolution can routinely visualize the stapes and often the stapedius muscle, demonstrating far better resolution than conventional tomography.

Tumors presenting in the cerebellopontine angle cistern are the most common neoplasms of the temporal bone. Acoustic neuromas (75%–91%), meningiomas (3.1%), and epidermoid tumors (2.4%) are the most common tumors.[14] Lesions arising in the adjacent clivus (chordomas, chondromas) and brain (pontine gliomas, ependymomas, medulloblastomas) as well as vascular malformations and arachnoid cysts may all present in this region. In a patient thought to harbor a neoplasm, the most efficacious radiologic examination is a high resolution, infused CT examination of the posterior fossa. Any suspected malignant lesion in this area must be distinguished from the more common, cytologically benign lesions. If audiologic testing suggests the presence of an eighth nerve lesion, the CT scan is immediately followed by a carbon dioxide gas cisternogram of the appropriate internal auditory canal.[2, 15]

Differentiating meningiomas from acoustic neuromas in the cerebellopontine angle may not always be possible. In general, meningiomas show increased density on noninfused studies and produce hyperostosis of the adjacent petrous bone and edema in the adjacent brain. Meningiomas often have a sessile attachment to the petrous bone and are usually not centered at the internal auditory canal.

Epidermoid tumors and arachnoid cysts are nonenhancing, cerebellopontine angle lesions that are easily differentiated from acoustic neuromas and meningiomas. Neuromas of the trigeminal nerve appear as bilobed enhancing lesions in the region of Meckel's cave and the adjacent brain stem.[16]

Glomus jugulare tumors are seen on CT scans as enhancing lesions situated in the jugular fossa, usually with well-demarcated destruction. They may extend distally along the jugular vein for a considerable distance and proximally into the posterior fossa. Angiography may be utilized to demonstrate the vascular supply to these lesions, particularly if preoperative embolization is considered. The venous drainage of the cerebral hemisphere should be assessed at the time of angiography so that a decision may be made whether to sacrifice the transverse sinus at surgery.[1, 17] Glomus tympanicum tumors of the middle ear have been demonstrated by high resolution CT. Angiography may also show the extent of this lesion if high resolution CT is not available (Fig 3–6).

Rhabdomyosarcoma of the middle ear cavity is a rare tumor.[18] This lesion demonstrates the importance of utilizing IV contrast in examining lesions of the head and neck regions. Intracranial extension, which is common, will not be appreciated if the contrast study is not performed. The tumor will be the same density as the cerebellum on the noncontrast study. Enhancement of the tumor on the contrast study allows demonstration of the lesion against the background of the nonenhancing cerebellum.[19] These tumors may extend to the posterior middle fossa or infratemporal region, with considerable bone destruction.

SALIVARY GLANDS

The demonstration of normal and pathologic anatomy of the salivary glands can be performed utilizing sialography, CT, or combined CT-sialography.

Demonstration of calculus or ductal disease is best performed with plain film or xeroradiographic sialography. Evaluation for suspected neoplastic disease should consist of an initial CT scan with IV contrast and, if needed, CT-sialography.

CT scans are obtained from the level of the external auditory canal inferiorly to the hyoid bone, so as to include the jugulodiagastric nodes. IV contrast is useful in differentiating lymph nodes from vessels in the neck.

Parotid masses are usually seen on CT scans as areas of increased density compared to the surrounding hypodense parotid parenchyma.[20] Tumor location, infiltrative patterns, extraglandular extension, and associated lymphadenopathy are well shown (Fig 3–7).

The morphological patterns seen in parotid tumors on CT are the following:

1. Round, well-defined pattern. These are usually benign tumors, such as Warthin's tumor and oncocytoma.
2. Lobulated, well-defined pattern. These are more aggressive lesions that are occasionally recurrent, such as pleomorphic adenoma.
3. Infiltrating, poorly defined pattern. These poorly marginated lesions often show extension beyond the gland. Carcinomas make up the majority of this group.[21]

It is important to note that in high-density parotid glands, tumors may be isodense and therefore not seen with infused CT.[22] If the gland is noted to be of high density, CT-sialography is indicated following the initial CT scan (Fig 3–8).

Masses in the parapharyngeal or paranasopharyngeal space may be characterized as to origin due to the presence of an intact fat plane between the mass and the deep lobe of the parotid gland. This fat plane is produced by the fat and fascia forming the reflection of the deep cervical fascia about the medial aspect of the deep lobe of the parotid gland.[23]

CT is useful in demonstrating the approximate position of the facial nerve.[24, 25] The nerve itself cannot be imaged, but its relationship to the base of the skull and venous anatomy may be demonstrated.

The position of the submandibular gland tends to make clinical examination highly accurate. Extension of masses in the submandibular gland into the lateral low-density fat plane adjacent to the tongue is well shown by CT.[26] Because of the relative frequency of malignancy in this gland (50%) versus the parotid gland (20%), most submandibular gland masses are removed, usually without radiologic investigation.[2]

LARYNX

The radiologic techniques for investigation of laryngeal disease include plain films, tomography, positive contrast laryngography, and CT. Plain films and tomography are cheap and noninvasive but provide little useful information. Positive contrast laryngography allows the best radiologic assessment of the mucosal surfaces and will demonstrate the physiology of the larynx. Deep infiltration must be inferred. Much of the information gained simply duplicates that obtained from direct laryngoscopy. CT provides a good view of cartilage destruction and deep extension of tumors with associated lymphadenopathy. The examination is easily performed, and with present-generation fast scanners, some physiologic information can be obtained.[27]

CT scanning of the larynx is done with the patient supine and the neck slightly hyperextended. The gantry is angled to provide true axial views of the larynx. Multiple scans are performed from the base of the tongue

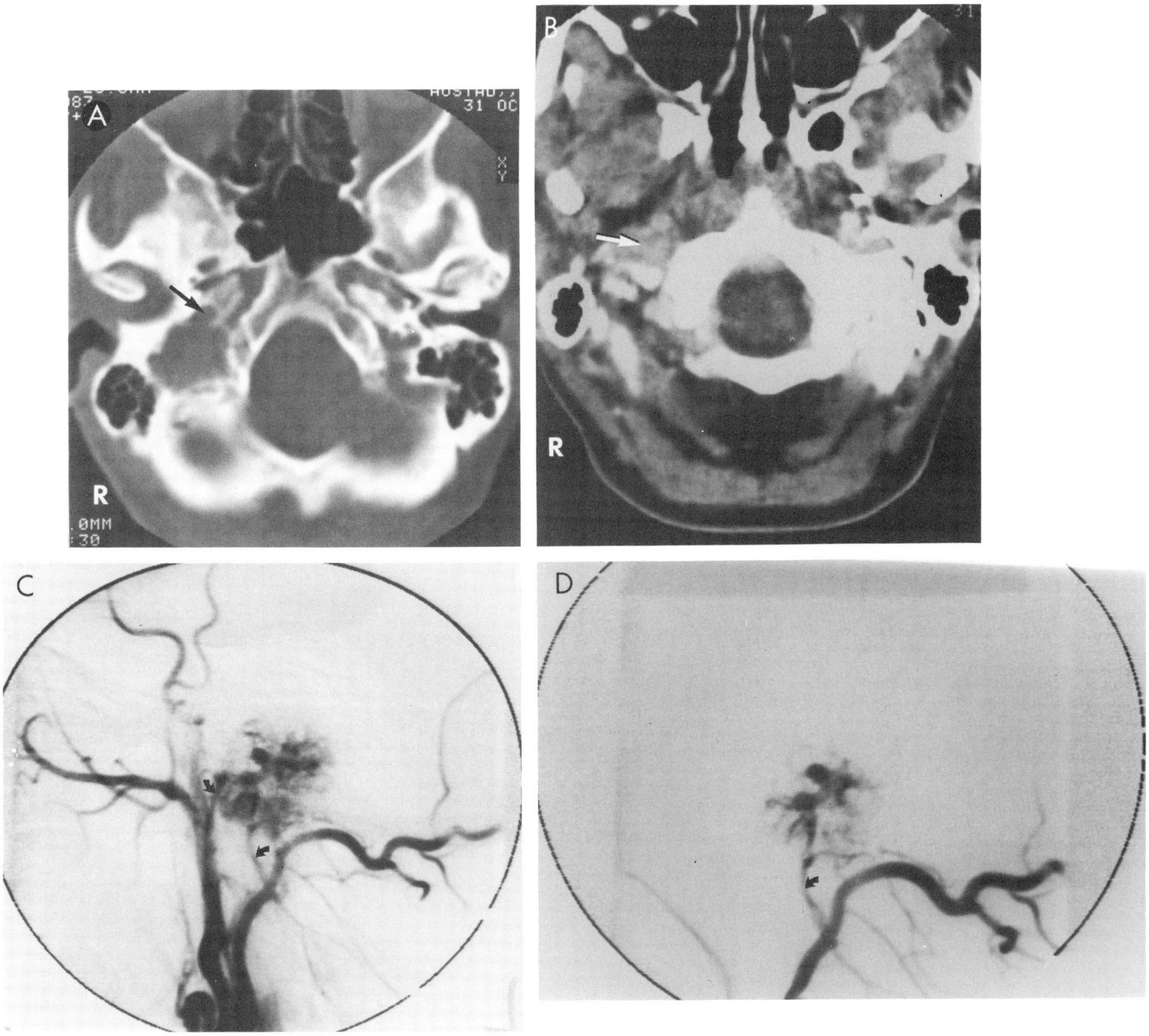

Fig 3–6.—Thirty-three-year-old woman with right cranial nerve XII palsy. **A,** axial view of skull base. A destructive lesion with irregular margins is present immediately posterior to the right carotid canal *(arrow)* at the site of the jugular foramen. **B,** contrast-enhanced axial scan at the level of the hypoglossal canals. An enhancing mass is present posterior to the right internal carotid artery *(arrow).* On this rotated scan, the exocranial aspect of the hypoglossal canal is immediately craniad to this level. **C,** lateral view, right external carotid digital angiogram. An enlarged inferior tympanic branch *(vertical arrow)* of the right ascending pharyngeal artery is seen supplying the anterior aspect of a hypervascular mass in the hypotympanum. An enlarged stylomastoid branch *(horizontal arrow)* of the right occipital artery is seen supplying the component of the vascular mass situated in the jugular fossa. **D,** lateral view, selective right occipital artery digital angiogram. The hypertrophied stylomastoid branch of the right occipital artery is noted supplying the posterior and inferior aspect of a jugular fossa mass. Characteristic irregular hypervascularity is present. Diagnosis: Glomus jugulare tumor with inferior extension and compression of the right nerve XII; interestingly, a jugular foramen syndrome was not present.

to slightly below the cricoid cartilage. Scans are performed with a 3-mm collimator in 3-mm increments to provide high-quality thin section axial pictures with satisfactory sagittal and coronal reconstructed views. If necessary, selected scans are then performed with phonation to assess vocal cord movement. IV contrast is infused to allow differentiation of lymphadenopathy from vascular structures. Intimate knowledge of the anatomy and anatomical variants of this region is exceedingly important. An excellent review of CT anat-

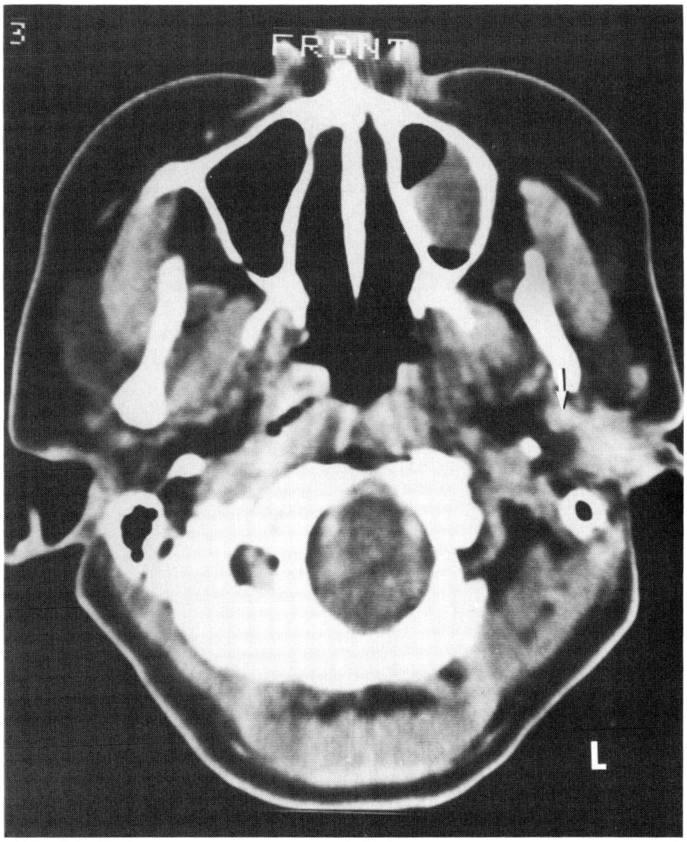

Fig 3–7.—Axial scan of the parotid glands. An irregular hyperdense mass is present in the posterior aspect of the left parotid gland with encasement of the retromandibular vein *(arrow)* and posterior extension to involve the subcutaneous fat and skin of the inferior aspect of the left ear. There is no extension into the paranasopharyngeal space. The dome of a mucous retention cyst is present in the left maxillary antrum. Diagnosis: Mucoepidermoid carcinoma of the left parotid gland involving the superficial and deep lobes.

omy of the larynx has been published by Mancuso and Hanafee.[2]

Tumors in the larynx have been divided according to their sites of origin into supraglottic, glottic, and subglottic.[28] All tumors may become transglottic by spread along the mucosa or through deep tissue planes. Tumors arising in the anterior third of the vocal cords tend to spread across the anterior commissure to the contralateral true cord.[2] Only 1–2 mm of tissue should be identified at the anterior commissure level of the true cords in the normal larynx.[29] Therefore, more tissue seen in this region is indicative of tumor extension. Spread may occur to the thyroid cartilage or paralaryngeal space and from this region become transglottic. Tumors arising in the middle to posterior third of the true cords spread laterally to the paralaryngeal space, posterolaterally between the thyroid and cricoid cartilages, and posteriorly to involve the cricoarytenoid joint.[9] Displacement and erosion of the arytenoid and cricoid cartilages may be demonstrated. The tumor may also extend into the posterior commissure area and superiorly into the aryepiglottic folds. Inferior extension to the subglottis often occurs along the mucosa and less often in the paralaryngeal space lateral to the conus elasticus. The mucosa of the cricoid region is well applied to the inner margin of the cricoid, and any soft tissue seen in this region is indicative of tumor extension.[2]

Tumors of the false cords and aryepiglottic folds are often deeply infiltrative into the parapharyngeal space with superior extension to the epiglottis.[9] At the false cord level, the petiolus of the epiglottis and thyroepiglottic ligament will produce some soft tissue density in the pre-epiglottic space (Fig 3–9).

Soft tissue abnormalities may be produced by fibrosis, edema, and tumor.[9] At present, it is difficult to differentiate between these processes. Therefore, CT scanning should be performed prior to the biopsy.

Epiglottic tumors may be suprahyoid or infrahyoid in location.[2] Infrahyoid tumors of the epiglottis enter the pre-epiglottic space, whence they may spread inferiorly to the vocal cords or laterally to the paralaryngeal space. The epiglottic or paralaryngeal space involvement is depicted as replacement of the normal low-density fat-containing area by soft tissue density. Pyriform sinus involvement may be well demonstrated as obliteration of the normal architecture, particularly if the modified Valsalva maneuver is used.

Suprahyoid tumors usually spread along the lateral pharyngoepiglottic fold to the lateral pharyngeal wall and along the glossoepiglottic fold to the base of the tongue. Thickening of these folds may be well demonstrated by CT.

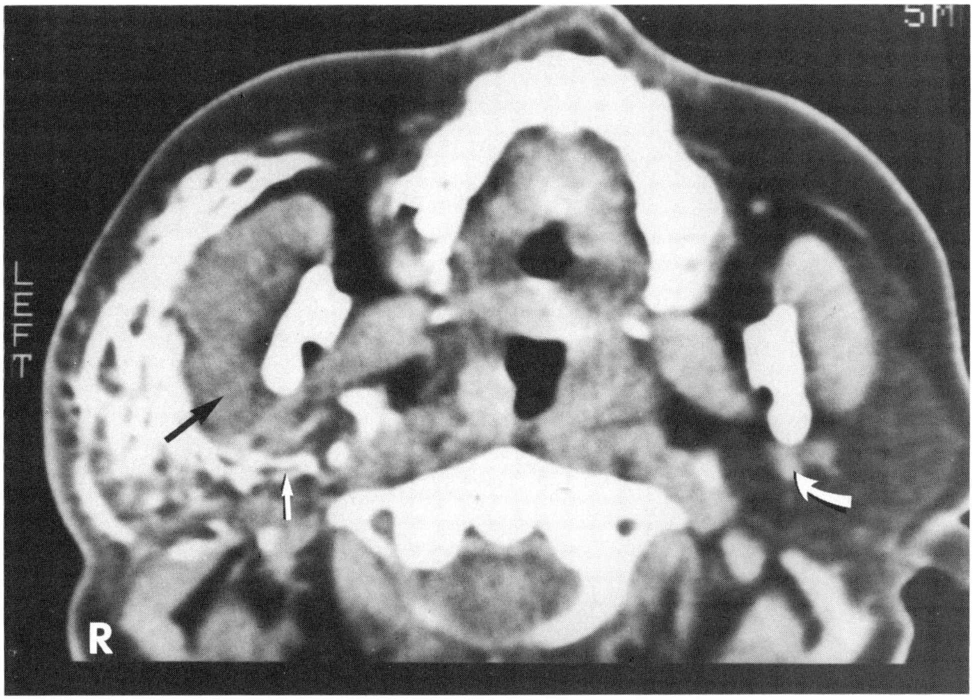

Fig 3–8.—Forty-two-year-old woman with right facial fullness. A CT-sialogram following injection of dilute water-soluble contrast in the right parotid duct demonstrates a soft tissue mass *(large arrow)* situated immediately posterior to the right masseter muscle and extending posteriorly to engulf the retromandibular veins. The deep lobe of the right parotid gland is displaced posteriorly and compressed *(small arrow)*. The normal hypodense left parotid gland with normal retromandibular veins *(curved arrow)* may be compared to the sialogram. Diagnosis: Papillary carcinoma of the deep portion of the superficial lobe of the right parotid gland with extension into the deep lobe.

The thyroid cartilage may be buckled, spread, fractured, tethered, or destroyed by either a remote or adjacent tumor.[2] Paramedial thinning and irregular calcification as well as asymmetric positioning may all give the artifactual appearance of cartilage destruction. When the tumor is predominantly positioned below the apex of the arytenoid cartilage and is more than 16 mm in diameter, a high probability of laryngeal cartilage invasion exists. The customary sites for invasion of the thyroid cartilage are at the anterior commissure level and at the junction of the anterior one fourth and posterior three fourths of the thyroid lamina due to penetrating collagen bundles in the perichrondrium, producing areas of focal weakness. The initial site of invasion of the cricoid and arytenoid cartilage is at the cricoarytenoid joint. Invasion may also occur at the attachments of the cricothyroid and cricotracheal membranes.[30]

NECK MASSES

Cervical Lymph Nodes

Evaluating the extent of malignant disease of the head and neck requires assessment of the primary neoplasm as well as metastatic lymph node involvement. CT scanning allows depiction of normal and abnormal lymph nodes, often demonstrating clinically occult nodal involvement. The use of IV contrast enhancement causes vascular opacification, which aids in the differentiation of soft tissue densities. Findings that suggest abnormal lymph nodes include the following:

1. A nonenhancing mass larger than 1.5 cm in a lymph node–bearing area may be found to be reactive and neoplastic nodes.
2. A peripherally dense, centrally lucent mass in a node-bearing area, particularly one larger than 1.5 cm in diameter. Peripheral enhancement is usually uniform in thickness in neoplastic disease and thick and irregular in inflammatory disease (Fig 3–10).
3. Obliteration of fascial planes in the node-bearing areas in the nonoperated and nonirradiated neck may be found in both neoplastic and inflammatory disorders. In neoplastic disease, the fascial plane obliteration may be due to direct extension of the primary disease into the adjacent tissues or extension beyond the capsule of involved lymph nodes (Fig 3–11).
4. Three or more contiguous nodes measuring 8–15 mm in diameter which are ill defined. Nonneoplastic disease may produce a similar picture. While

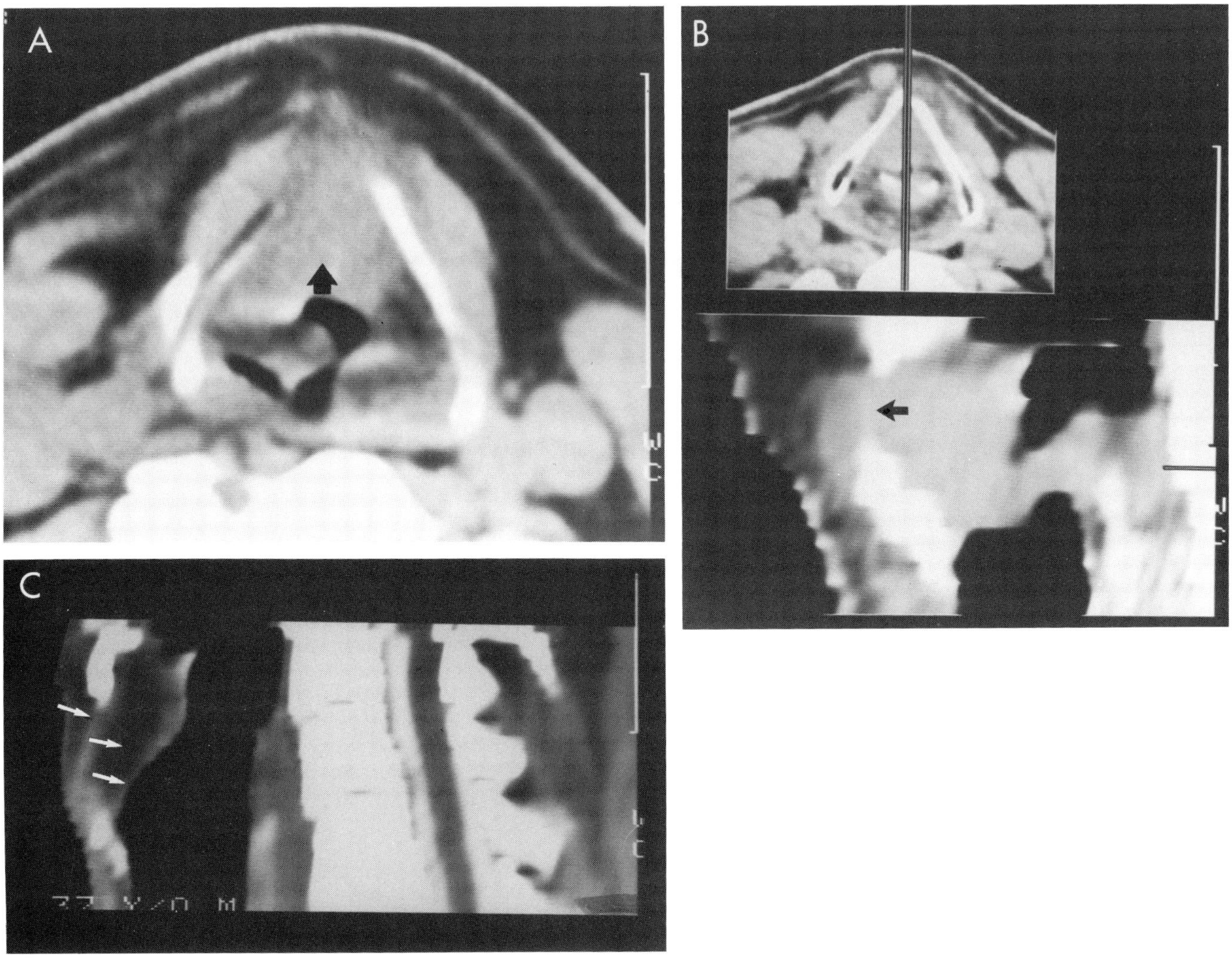

Fig 3–9.—Seventy-six-year-old alcoholic smoker with hoarseness. **A,** axial CT scan through the pre-epiglottic space. A large soft tissue mass is noted replacing the fat of the pre-epiglottic space and extending anteriorly through the thyrohyoid membrane into the soft tissues of the neck. Both aryepiglottic folds are thickened. **B,** sagittal reconstruction through the larynx. The large pre-epiglottic space mass extends anteriorly through the thyrohyoid membrane. Posteriorly, thickening of the aryepiglottic folds is seen. **C,** lateral sagittal reconstruction of the normal pre-epiglottic space. Thyrohyoid membrane, pre-epiglottic space, and epiglottis (anterior to posterior *arrows*) are demonstrated.

false positives will occur with these criteria, the history and physical findings provide some indication of the proper diagnosis.[30, 31]

Localized Cervical Masses

Localized pulsatile masses in the neck are best assessed with digital IV angiography followed by CT.

Oblique and anteroposterior (AP) digital fluoroscopic views of the neck following right atrial injection will demonstrate cervical carotid aneurysms, displacement by masses, the characteristic appearance of carotid body paragangliomas, and a normal, laterally situated internal carotid artery. CT performed after digital angiography is useful in delineating the margins of the masses and related adjacent structures.

Neuromas and carotid body tumors may be easily differentiated by digital angiography. The relatively avascular neuroma, usually arising in the cervical sympathetic ganglion or neuroma situated in the carotid sheath, characteristically displaces the carotid artery anteriorly and medially, and the jugular vein posteriorly and occasionally anteriorly (Fig 3–12).

CT of neuromas demonstrates a peripherally enhancing mass which, over time, may become homogeneously enhancing. These lesions are usually centered more craniad than the carotid bifurcation. Erosion of the intravertebral canal may occur if the lesion arises from one of the cervical peripheral nerves.

Paragangliomas of the neck are usually of carotid body origin and therefore occur at the carotid bifurca-

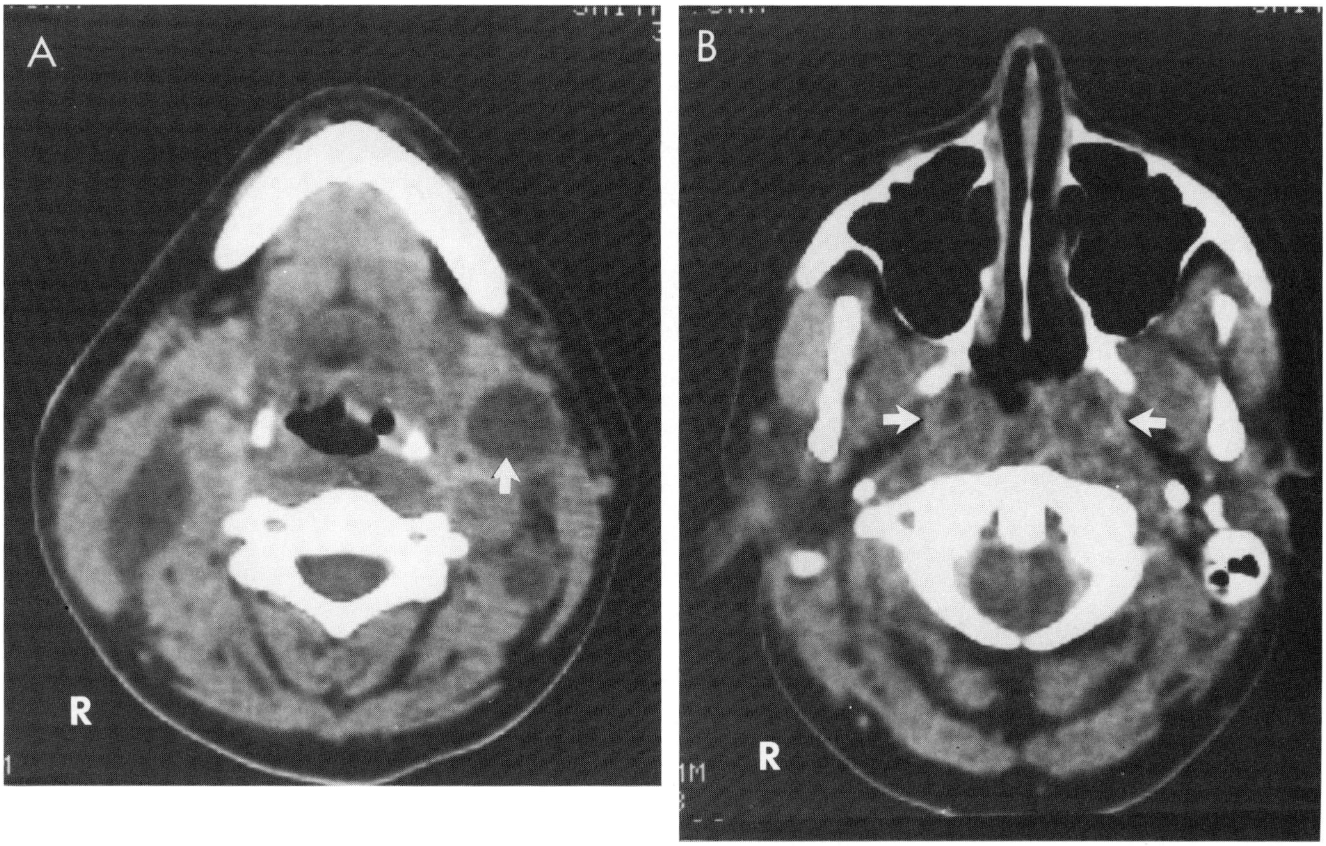

Fig 3–10.—Thirty-three-year-old woman with right neck mass. **A,** noncontrast axial CT scan through C3. Low-density masses are evident deep to the sternocleidomastoid muscles bilaterally. A relatively thick-walled left jugulodigastric node is present *(arrow).* **B,** noncontrast axial CT scan through C1. An irregular bilateral nasopharyngeal mass *(arrows)* extends laterally into the paranasopharyngeal spaces and into the nasopharyngeal airway. Diagnosis: Nasopharyngeal carcinoma with metastatic cervical lymphadenopathy.

tion. Bowing of the external and internal carotid arteries about a very vascular mass is characteristically seen on angiography. An intense centrally enhancing mass is seen on CT, usually at the hyoid level. These lesions may be multifocal and may arise in the tympanic bone, ganglion nodosum of the vagus nerve, larynx, orbit, nodes, or aortic arch (Fig 3–13).

Other lesions, usually nonpulsatile, that must be considered in the differential diagnosis of the lateral neck mass include lymphadenopathy of inflammatory etiology, malignant lymphoma from metastatic tumor, brachial cleft cyst, and salivary gland tumors. All of these masses are characteristically hypovascular and are usually seen only as mass lesions on the CT scan. They do not show abnormal enhancement.[34]

ANGIOGRAPHY

Angiography of head and neck lesions is used primarily to assess the arterial supply to lesions which have a propensity to be highly vascular, and as a mapping procedure prior to embolization. Juvenile nasopharyngeal angiofibromas, paragangliomas, glomus jugulare, tympanicum and vagale tumors, meningiomas of the skull base, and angiodysplasias to the head and neck may all be imaged by CT, but angiography is essential to provide information on the angioarchitecture of these lesions.

There has been considerable success in the ablation of abnormal vasculature using multiple embolic materials. High-quality angiographic studies are a prerequisite for identification of the vascular pedicles to abnormal areas. As well, identification of anatomical variants, such as origin of the ophthalmic artery from the middle meningeal artery, is essential in planning a safe embolization procedure.

Currently, the aim of embolization procedures is to occlude the abnormal vessels at the capillary level, thereby preventing the formation of collateral vasculature from nonoccluded vessels. This may be done by injecting multiple very small particulate emboli or liquid embolic agents such as silicone or isobutyl-2-cyanoacrylate. The particulate and liquid embolic agents are flow-guided into the appropriate areas following selective catheterization of the most distal feeding arteries. With particulate emboli, an end point is reached

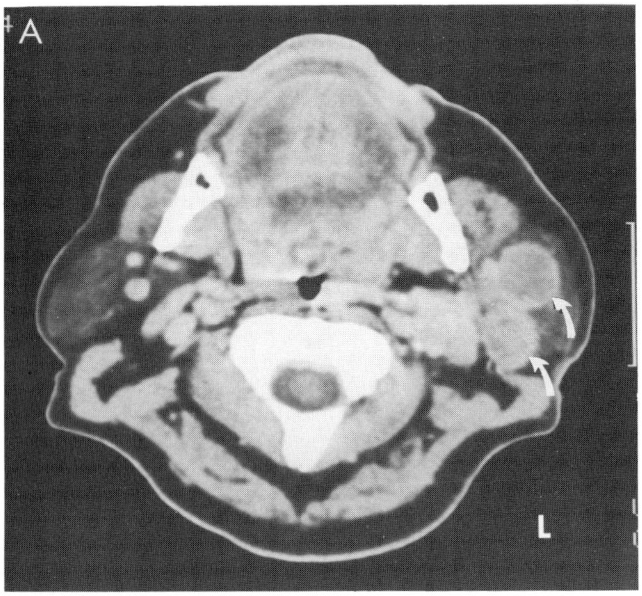

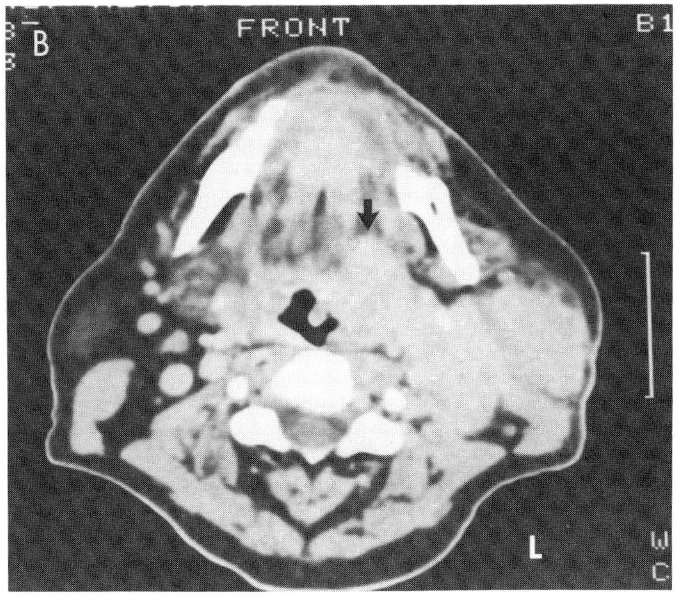

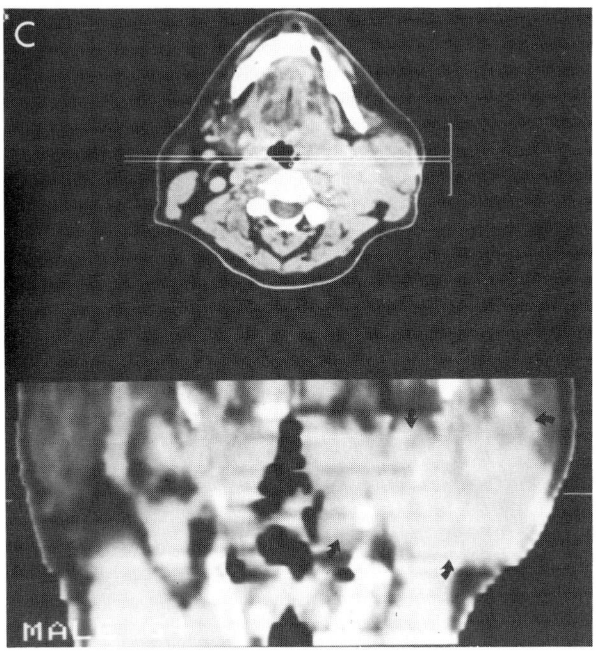

Fig 3–11.—Sixty-six-year-old man with left parotid and pharyngeal masses. **A,** axial CT scan through the parotid glands. Two peripherally dense, centrally lucent masses are noted displacing to the inferior aspect of the left parotid gland and displacing the lateral carotid artery. **B,** axial CT scan through the tongue base. A large left oropharyngeal mass is noted with anterior extension into the lateral fat space of the tongue *(arrow)* and lateral extension into the neck. **C,** reconstructed coronal view through the neck. The confines of the pharyngeal-parotid mass can be demonstrated *(arrows).* The mass extends inferiorly into the paralaryngeal space *(medial arrow),* and superiorly into the inferior aspect of the parotid gland. Diagnosis: Massive lymphadenopathy from squamous cell carcinoma, thought to originate in the base of the tongue.

when antegrade flow is extremely slow but not stopped. This slight antegrade flow allows deposition of emboli into the external carotid artery without reflex and disastrous complications in the internal carotid distribution.

Recently the development of digitalized radiology has provided a rapid, high resolution angiographic technique.[32] Digital IV subtraction angiography may be utilized as a screening procedure for vascular disease of the head and neck. A right atrial injection of contrast media followed by imaging of the appropriate areas allows a good view of major vascular anatomy. With good quality arterial and venous phases, it is possible to rule out sizable glomus jugulare tumors, particularly with venous occlusion, presentation of the carotid artery in the middle ear cavity, high position of the jugular bulb, and dural arteriovenous malformation of the transverse sinus/jugular fossa region.

Digital arterial subtraction angiography, utilizing a low-dose selective arterial contrast injection, provides a very high resolution, exquisite subtraction study of large as well as small vessels.[33] This technique is particularly important for lesions of the temporal bone where misregistration of conventional film angiograms often obliterates small vasculatures. Because of the instantaneous image presentation, digital arterial subtraction has become an important adjunct in embolization pro-

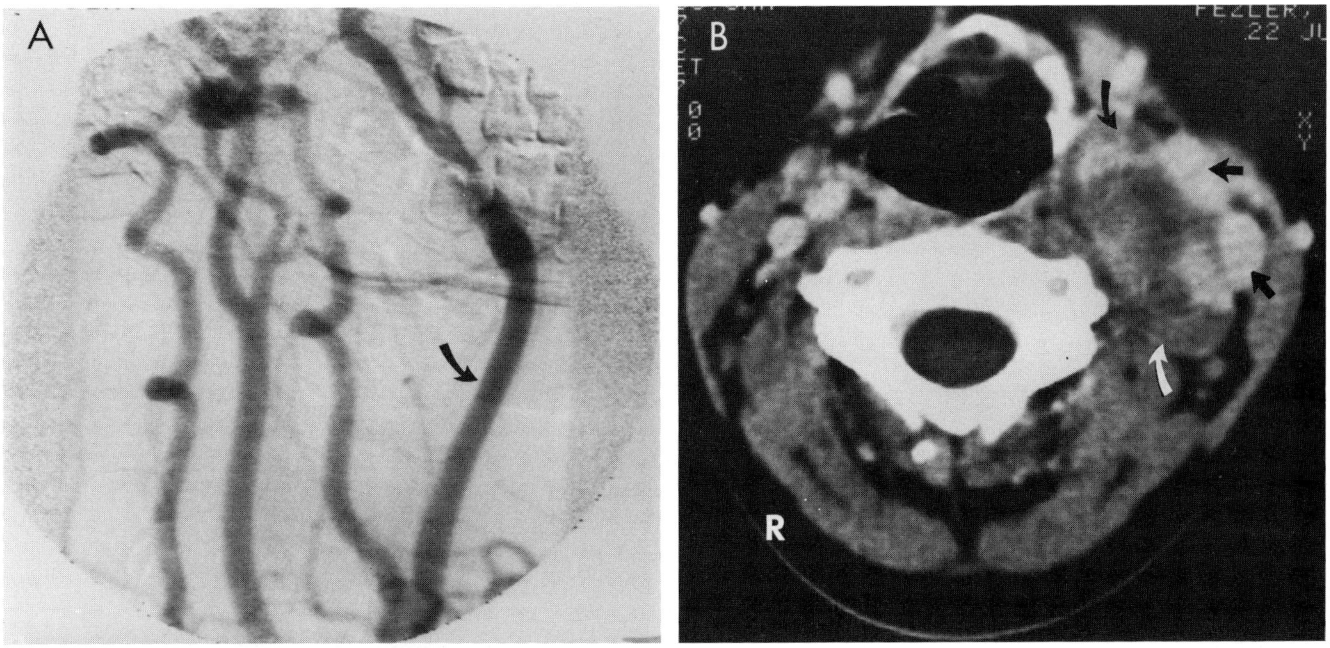

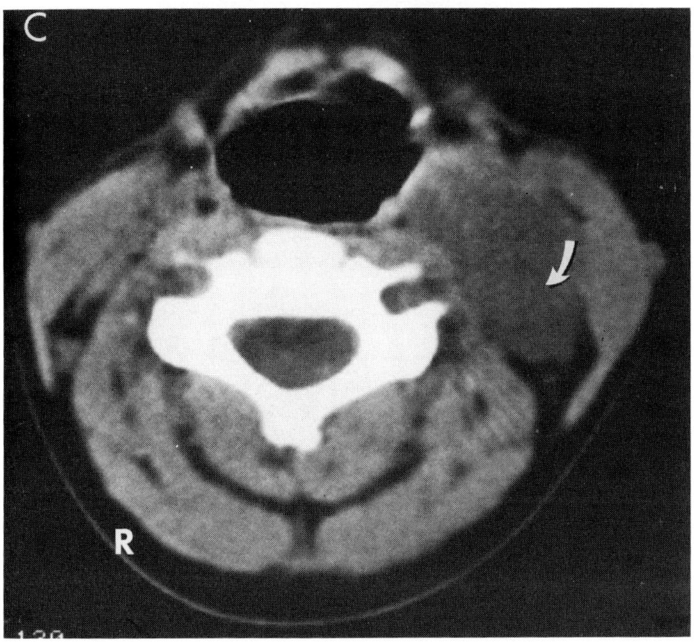

Fig 3–12.—Six-year-old boy with left neck mass, noted following trauma. **A,** oblique digital venous angiogram of the neck. The left common carotid artery *(arrow)* is markedly displaced anteriorly. **B,** axial CT scan at the level of the hyoid bone obtained immediately following the digital angiogram. A large left neck mass *(curved arrows)* is present displacing the left internal jugular vein *(oblique arrow)* and the common carotid bifurcation *(horizontal arrow)* regions anteriorly and laterally. Irregular marginal enhancement of this mass is present. **C,** non-contrast-enhanced axial CT scan. An oblong hypodense mass is noted situated deep to the sternocleidomastoid muscle in the left paraspinal region. Lateral and anterior displacement of the carotid artery and jugular vein is consistent with a medial carotid sheath mass, likely a neuroma. Diagnosis: Ganglioneuroma.

cedures, where the efficacy of embolization and assessment of occlusion of normal branches can be rapidly and safely assessed.

TECHNICAL CONSIDERATIONS

There is considerable variation in scanning parameters and therefore in density and spatial contrast resolution among the various available scanners.

As a rule, older generation scanners cannot provide the thinly collimated, high resolution, movement-free scans that newer scanners are able to produce. The ability to produce multiple slices in a short period of time is important in terms of patient comfort. Due to the complex anatomy of the head and neck, thin collimation or "slices" is important in order to satisfactorily separate contiguous small anatomical structures. The ability to demonstrate minute anatomy, such as the ossicular chain, is an example of what is meant by high spatial resolution. The ability to differentiate subtle differences in density, i.e., between the white and gray matter in the brain, is an example of what is meant by high density resolution. To satisfactorily image the vocal chords and adjacent paralaryngeal space, thin slices,

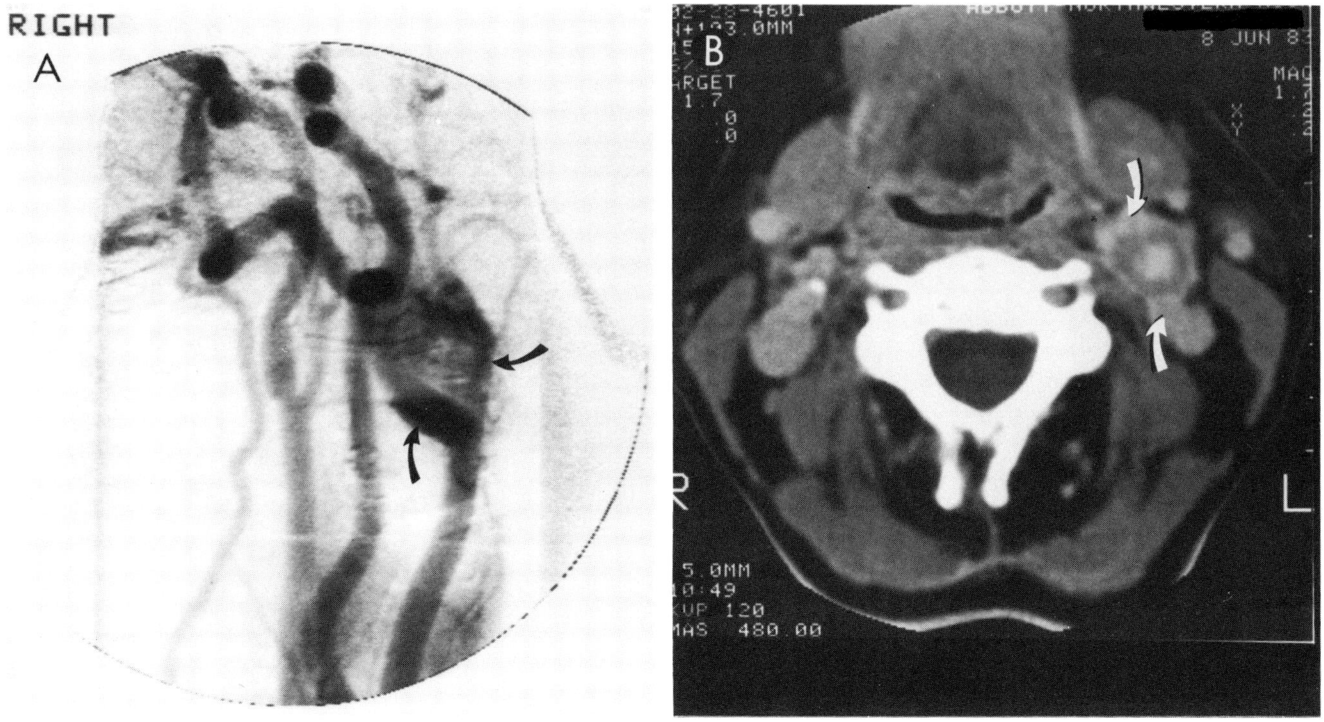

Fig 3–13.—Thirty-two-year-old woman with left neck mass. **A,** oblique intravenous digital angiogram. A hypervascular mass is present at the bifurcation of the left common carotid artery displacing the internal carotid *(vertical arrow)* posteriorly and the external carotid *(horizontal arrow)* anteriorly. **B,** axial CT scan through the carotid bifurcation. A centrally dense, peripherally lucent mass is present displacing the left internal carotid artery posteriorly *(bottom arrow)* and the external carotid artery anteriorly *(top arrow).* The hypervascularity of the mass on the digital angiogram and its position are characteristic of a paraganglioma. Diagnosis: Carotid body paraganglioma.

high density and spatial resolution are all necessary to demonstrate the chord anatomy and the fatty paralaryngeal space.

The ability of a CT scanner to provide adequate images should be assessed by all physicians prior to patient referral. Useless or misleading information may be obtained from scanners unable to provide acceptable resolution.

IV contrast administration is utilized in CT scanning for two purposes. First—and most useful in head and neck scanning—is to delineate the normal vascular structures. A low-dose, continuous infusion of contrast material permits prolonged visualization of the vessels throughout the course of the study.

The second use of contrast enhancement is to demonstrate the vascularity of lesions against a background of normally less enhancing normal anatomy. Bolus technique is utilized to produce initial high levels of contrast medium, followed by a continuous drip for vascular delineation. Extension of head and neck lesions intracranially may be visualized due to the difference between the amount of enhancement seen in the abnormal lesion versus the lesser amount of enhancement seen in the normal brain. Intracerebral metastatic lesions are seen after IV contrast administration due because of leakage of contrast medium across an abnormal blood-brain barrier.

A comparison of the radiation dosage of various examinations of the head and neck demonstrates the relatively high dose required by conventional tomography, compared to CT (Table 3–2). Due to the narrowly collimated beam of CT, the patient's gonadal dose is exceedingly small. The more widely collimated beam of conventional tomography produces a gonadal dose

TABLE 3–2.—RADIATION DOSAGE AND HOSPITAL CHARGE FOR HEAD AND NECK RADIOLOGIC EXAMINATIONS

EXAMINATION	DOSAGE (Rad)	COST ($)
Conventional angiogram: AP and lateral films × 3 angiographic runs (48 films)	10	1,000
Digital venous angiogram: 4 filming sequences (40 images)	6	295
Digital arterial angiogram: 4 filming sequences (40 images)	6	343
CT with contrast: 20 scans	3	220
Conventional tomograms: 10 films each, AP and lateral views (total, 20 films)	6	125
Plain films of paranasal sinuses	.5–1	49

which is at least one-half the target radiation dose.

Digital angiography radiation doses are approximately two-thirds those of conventional film examinations. Digital arterial techniques also allow rapid recognition of incorrect catheter placement or slippage, in some instances saving the patient from unnecessary radiation exposure.

The technical costs cited in Table 3–2 are for an individual hospital and will vary with different institutions.

REFERENCES

1. Wiet R.J., Kazan R., Sacy G.: Skull base mapping. *Laryngoscope* 92:515–523, 1982.
2. Mancuso A., Hanafee W.B.: *Computed Tomography of the Head and Neck.* Baltimore, Williams & Wilkins Co., 1982.
3. Parsons C., Hodson N.: Computed tomography of paranasal sinus tumors. *Radiology* 132:641–645, 1979.
4. Bilaniuk L.T., Zimmerman R.A.: Computed tomography in evaluation of the paranasal sinuses. *Radiol. Clin. North Am.* vol. 20, No. 1, March 1982.
5. Som P.M., Shugar J.M.A., Biller H.F.: The early detection of antral malignancy in the postmaxillectomy patient. *Radiology* 143:509–512, 1982.
6. Mancuso A.A., Bohman L., Hanafee W.B., et al.: Computed tomography of the nasopharynx: Normal and variants of normal. *Radiology* 137:113–121, 1980.
7. Bryan R.N., Sessions R.B., Horowitz B.L.: Radiographic management of juvenile angiofibromas. *Am. J. Neuroradiol.* vol. 2, No. 2, March/April 1981.
8. Shaffer K., Houghton V., Farley G., et al.: Pitfalls in the radiographic diagnosis of angiofibroma. *Radiology* 127:425–428, 1978.
9. Hanafee W.B.: Radiology of the pharnyx and larnyx, in *Radiology of the Ear, Nose and Throat.* Philadelphia, W.B. Saunders Co., 1981.
10. Mancuso A.A., Hanafee W.N.: Elusive head and neck carcinomas beneath intact mucosa. *Laryngoscope* 93, February 1983.
11. Miller D., Ervin T., Weichselbaum R., et al.: The differential diagnosis of the mass in the neck: A fresh look. *Laryngoscope* 91:140, 1981.
12. Templer J., Perry M.C., Davis W.E.: Metastatic cervical adenocarcinoma from unknown primary tumor. *Arch. Otolaryngol.* 107:45–47, 1981.
13. Taylor S.: The petrous temporal bone (including the cerebellopontine angle). *Radiol. Clin. North Am.* vol. 20, No. 1, March 1982.
14. Brackmann D.E., Bartels L.J.: Rare tumors of the cerebellopontine angle. *Otolaryngol. Head Neck Surg.* 88:555–559, 1980.
15. Kricheff I.I., Pinto R.S., Bergeron R.T., et al.: Air-CT cisternography and canalography for small acoustic neuromas. *Am. J. Neuroradiol.* 1:57, 1980.
16. Robertson W.D., Nugent R.S., Lapointe J.S., et al.: Computed tomographic scanning of the cerebellopontine angle and the internal auditory canal. *J. Otolaryngol.* vol. 2, No. 5, 1982.
17. Hesselink J.R., Davis K.R., Taveras J.M.: Selective arteriography of glomus tympanicum and jugular tumors: Techniques, normal and pathologic arterial anatomy. *A.J.N.R.* 2:289–297, 1981.
18. Valvassori G.E., Buckingham R.A.: Radiology of the temporal bone, in Hanafee W.B. (ed.): *Radiology of the Ear, Nose and Throat.* Philadelphia, W.B. Saunders Co., 1981.
19. Tubman D.E.: Use of contrast infusion in cranial extracerebral computed tomography. *J. Can. Assoc. Radiol.* September 1980.
20. Carter B.L., Karmody C.S., Blickman Jr., et al.: Computed tomography and sialography: 2. Pathology. *J. Comput. Assist. Tomogr. Suppl.* 1:46–53, 1981.
21. Kassell E.E.: CT Sialography: Part II. Parotid masses. *J. Otolaryngol.* vol. 2, suppl. 12, December 1982.
22. Sone S., Higashihara T., Morimoto S.: CT of parotid tumors. *Am. J. Neuroradiol.* 2:143–147, 1982.
23. Kassell E.E.: Parapharyngeal and deep lobe parotid tumors. *J. Otolaryngol.* vol. 2, suppl. 12, December 1982.
24. Kassell E.E.: CT Sialography: Part I. Introduction, technique, anatomy and variants. *J. Otolaryngol.* vol. II, suppl. 12, December 1982.
25. Som P.M., Biller H.F.: The combined CT-sialogram. *Radiology* 135:387–390, 1980.
26. Larsson S.G., Mancuso A.A., Hanafee N.: Computed tomography of the tongue and floor of the mouth. *Radiology* 143:493–500, 1982.
27. Gamsu G., Well W.R., Shallit J.B., et al.: CT in carcinoma of the larynx and pyriform sinus: Value of phonation scans? *AJR* 136:577–584, 1981.
28. Cocke E.W., Wang C.C.: Cancer of the Larnyx: Part I. Selecting optimum treatment. *Cancer* 26:194–200, 1976.
29. Silverman P.M., Korobkin M.: Pictorial essay: High resolution computed tomography of the normal larynx. *AJR* 140:875–879, 1983.
30. Archer C.R., Yeager V.L., Herbold D.R.: Computed tomography versus histology of laryngeal cancer: Their value in predicting laryngeal cartilage invasion. *Laryngoscope* 93, February 1983.
31. Reede D.L., Bergeron R.T.: CT of cervical lymph nodes. *J. Otolaryngol.* 11:411–418, 1982.
32. Kinney S.E., Modic M.T., Starnes D., et al.: Digital subtraction angiography in lesions of the head and neck. *Laryngoscope* 92:557–561, 1982.
33. Brant-Zawadski M., Gould R., Norman D., et al.: Digital subtraction cerebral angiography in intra-arterial injection: Comparison with conventional angiography. *Am. J. Neuroradiol.* 3:593–600, 1982.
34. Silver A.J., Ganti S.R., Hilal S.K.: The carotid region: Normal and pathologic anatomy on CT. *Radiol. Clin. North Am.* 22:219–238, 1984.

4 / Decisions in the Pathologic Diagnosis of Head and Neck Cancers

Catherine C. Limas, M.D.

The major objectives of this chapter are (1) to enhance the simple skills necessary to obtain and handle correctly biopsy materials, (2) to create an understanding of how the pathologist can best assist the therapist, (3) to improve the quality of communication between the therapist and the pathologist by understanding the significance of commonly used terms, and (4) to describe the major categories of neoplasms of the head and neck area. Some of the material overlaps with that presented in other chapters, but an accurate pathologic diagnosis is fundamental to all head and neck cancer treatment. Hence, an early categoric discussion is important to the other chapters.

HISTOLOGIC CONFIRMATION

Obtaining and Submitting Material for Histologic Confirmation

WHEN SHOULD A TISSUE DIAGNOSIS BE OBTAINED?

Always before administering decisive therapy, whether it is extensive surgical resection, radiation, or chemotherapy.

Whenever the extent of a malignant lesion must be assessed prior to therapy or the adequacy of resection margins is in doubt.

Whenever recurrence or metastasis of a malignant lesion is suspected.

Whenever any "lesion" is removed from the human body for therapeutic or cosmetic reasons.

Whenever a "lesion" is encountered incidentally during surgery and is not amenable to biopsy after the surgical incision is closed.

WHAT MATERIAL IS OBTAINED FOR BIOPSY?

Material for morphological diagnosis may be obtained by removing a sample of tissue or cells from the suspicious lesion. Whole tissue samples are used for histologic diagnosis ("histos" = tissue), while detached cells are utilized for cytologic diagnosis.

The biopsy tissue specimen can be removed by a variety of methods, depending on a number of indications which are briefly discussed in this section. Following is a list of commonly used types of biopsies:

Excisional	Needle (cutting) core
Incisional	Shave
Punch	Curettage

A variety of methods also exist for obtaining samples of cells from a lesion. Thus, one may collect exfoliated cells, detach the cells from the surface of a lesion with a brush or by touching the lesion with a slide, or aspirate the cells through a fine needle into a syringe. Following is a list of most frequently used cytologic sampling methods:

Exfoliated cells	Touch preparations
Brushings	Needle (thin) aspiration
Washings	

The choice of the procedure depends on:

1. The location of the lesion.
2. The size of the lesion.
3. The suspected nature of the lesion.
4. The special studies required for differential diagnosis.
5. The time limitations and patient's discomfort.
6. The expertise of the persons obtaining and evaluating the material and facilities available.

In general, biopsies permit the study of both the cells and their relationship to the surrounding tissues and thus provide information about the malignant or benign nature of the lesion as well as the presence of invasion. Procedures providing cytologic preparations cause less discomfort, require less equipment, and may be faster than biopsies. The cytologic preparations, however, permit the study of cells only and therefore are unsuitable for evaluating the presence of invasion and for discriminating between certain benign and well-differentiated malignant tumors.

Specific examples of the use of each of these procedures will be given in the specific chapters. At this point, the following general remarks are made: For easily accessible lesions, e.g., in the skin or on mucosal surfaces, excisional or incisional biopsy is recommended.[1] Excisional biopsy is more suitable for small lesions with grossly well-defined borders. Incisional biopsy is indicated for large lesions, lesions with ill-defined borders, or lesions so located that only a very minute amount of tissue can be excised without significant damage or deformity. For masses located deep within the tissues, needle core biopsy may be superior to incisional biopsy. Before one proceeds with a cutting needle biopsy, the anatomical location, e.g., proximity to large vessels, must be thoroughly evaluated in order to avoid serious complications. In this setting, needle aspiration may be equally adequate provided that persons experienced in the preservation and evaluation of such material are available.

A list of the major indications of each method is provided in Table 4–1. As an example of factors influencing the choice of one method over another we consider here a neck mass. If the patient has a well defined palpable node with no previous history of malignancy, and if the workup for a cryptic primary source is negative (see chapt. 25), then it is better to excise the node and submit it fresh to the pathologist, who will decide how to process it further, depending on the gross, frozen section, or touch preparation findings. If the mass is large, ill defined, and/or adherent to other structures, a needle biopsy is more appropriate. A similar mass in a patient with a previous well-established diagnosis of cancer in the head and neck area may be adequately evaluated by needle aspiration. In summary, there are no strict rules, but the surgeon and the pathologist must be in close consultation to arrive at the most accurate diagnosis with the least risk and discomfort to the patient.

TABLE 4–1.—MAJOR INDICATIONS FOR BIOPSY AND CYTOLOGIC SAMPLING

METHOD OF SAMPLING	INDICATION
Biopsy	
Excisional	Easily accessible, small lesion with grossly well-defined borders
Incisional	Easily accessible, large lesion and/ or ill-defined borders
Punch	Easily accessible, superficial lesion usually in the skin
Shave	Easily accessible, superficial lesion occupying large surface area, e.g., vermillion border of lip
Curettage	Lesions of skin or mucosal surfaces which are either superficial and multifocal, e.g., basal cell carcinoma of skin, or which cannot be clearly visualized and localized, e.g., in paranasal sinuses
Needle	Deeply seated, large lesions
Cytology	
Exfoliative	Lesions inaccessible without instrumentation from which spontaneously shed cells accumulate in easily collectable secretions, e.g., sputum
Washings and brushings	Mucosal lesions in deep viscera that are poorly visualized and/or ill defined grossly
Touch preparation	Easily accessible surface lesions, e.g., erosions, blisters; under certain circumstances may substitute or complement the frozen section procedure
Needle aspiration	Deeply seated solid or cystic masses

WHERE DO YOU BIOPSY A LESION?

Of course, the answer to this question is, where the best diagnostic material will be obtained. The best diagnostic material is the tissue sample which provides the most information about the nature and extent of a lesion. Therefore, when biopsying a lesion one must use observation, knowledge, and judgment. First, one must make a thorough gross examination of the lesion by inspection and palpation; second, one must make a reasonable differential diagnosis on clinical grounds and recall a little of the pathology of the entities to be differentiated; third, one must use common sense. For example, a 0.5-cm mucosal ulceration surrounded by an indurated zone 1 cm wide is found in the oral cavity of a 60-year-old man. The differential diagnosis includes malignancy, and the biopsy specimen should enable the pathologist to confirm or exclude this possibility, define the type of malignancy, and interpret invasion. A superficial biopsy from the periphery of this lesion may yield normal mucosa or mucosa with dysplasia or carcinoma in situ, while a biopsy from the ulcer crater may yield necrotic debris and inflammatory exudate (Figs 4–1 and 4–2). It stands to reason that the sample most accurately representing the lesion must be at the interface of the ulcer and the induration and must include tissue deep to the mucosa. Multiple site biopsies may be necessary when the lesion is large or when a tumor with great variability in its components is suspected (e.g., salivary gland tumors). More specific examples will be given in the appropriate chapters. In general, the following are useful guidelines. Sample the area(s) with gross characteristics most representative of the lesion, and include superficial and deep tissue to facilitate evaluation of the relationship of the lesion to the surface epithelium and of the depth of invasion.

HOW DO YOU HANDLE AND SUBMIT THE BIOPSY?

Every effort should be made to preserve the tissue sample in excellent condition. A perfect sample may become useless because of ignorance or carelessness in handling; unfortunately, this is a common cause of unsatisfactory, uninterpretable specimens. Everybody in the medical field is aware that tissues are sensitive to mechanical, thermal, osmotic, and chemical trauma, but they often do not seem to apply this basic knowledge to tissue specimens. Tissues or cells to be used for histologic diagnosis should not be crushed, cauterized, frozen and thawed, placed in water or other hypotonic solutions, dehydrated or stored without fixatives which

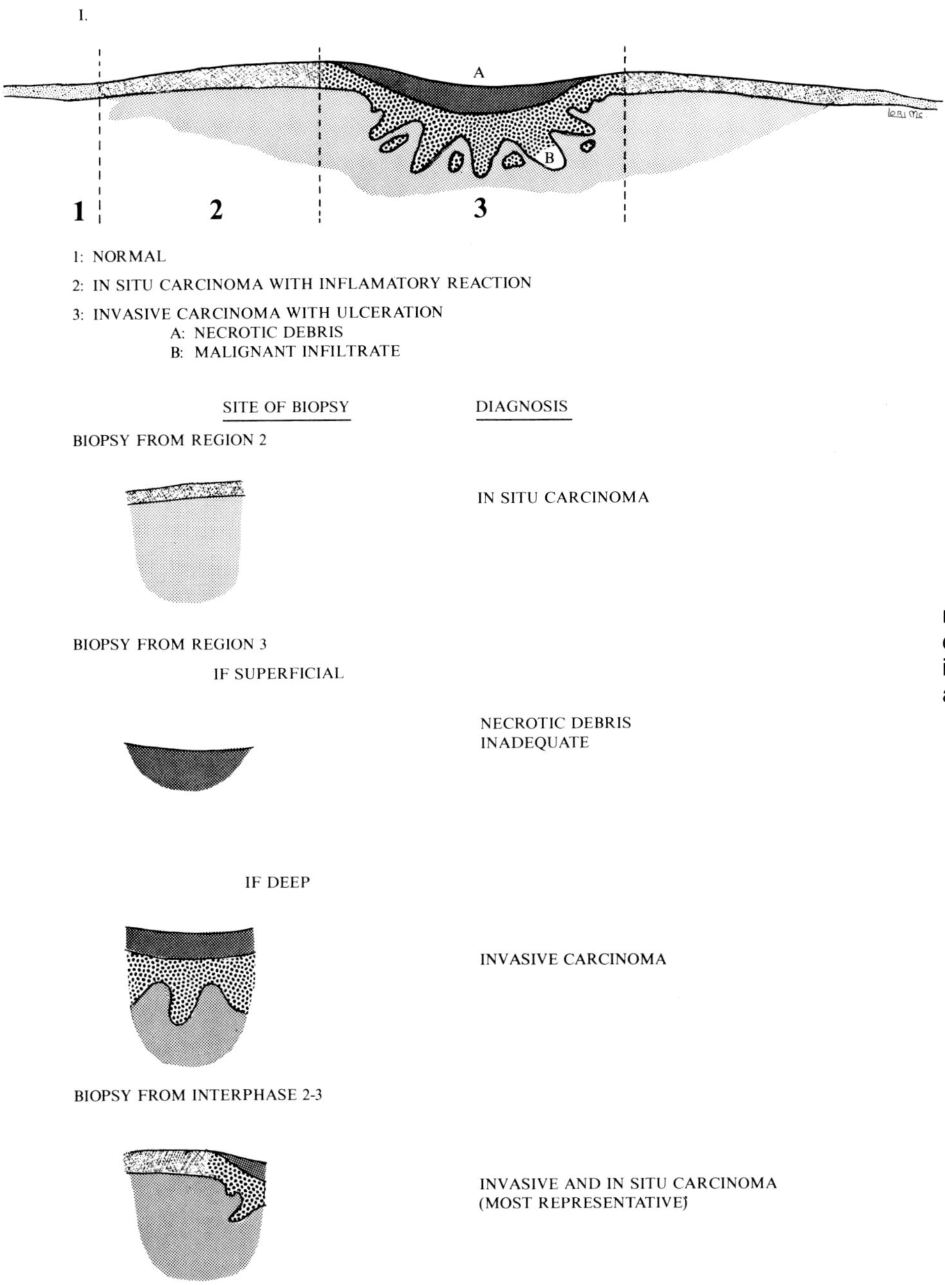

Fig 4–1.—The typical zones that may occur in a squamous cell cancer. This stresses the importance of appropriate and adequate biopsy.

prevent autolysis. Once severed from the body, specimens left exposed to the air will dehydrate quickly and numerous artifacts will appear. Small tissue fragments and cytologic material are extremely sensitive to dehydration artifacts.

The specimen may be submitted in the fresh state or in fixative.

Fresh tissue must be submitted when an immediate diagnosis using the frozen section procedure is required. Some special studies require fresh tissue for diagnosis. The tissue must be placed immediately in a physiologic solution or on a *smooth* cloth *presoaked* with a physiologic solution. It is common sense that fresh tissue will stick to dry gauze, which makes small fragments hard to retrieve without crushing. Unfortunately, because of bad habit, this is the way most specimens are submitted to the pathology laboratory.

It is preferable to submit large resection specimens in the fresh state, unless several hours' delay is anticipated prior to the pathologic examination. In the latter case, the specimen must be placed in a large container with plenty of fixative so that the specimen can be fully expanded and completely covered. If the specimen tends to float, the surface should be covered with a cloth or other absorbent material (cotton, paper, etc.)

2. ACTUAL MICROPHOTOGRAPH

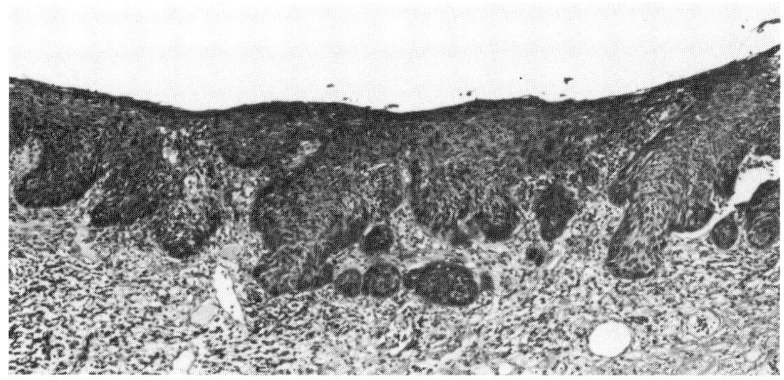

THE GOOD LARGE BIOPSY SHOWS MICROINVASIVE SQUAMOUS CELL CARCINOMA WITH SURROUNDING IN-SITU CARCINOMA

Fig 4–2.—Actual photomicrographs of a biopsy specimen similar to the example shown in Figure 4–1 except there is only microinvasive squamous cell carcinoma with a bordering area of carcinoma in situ.

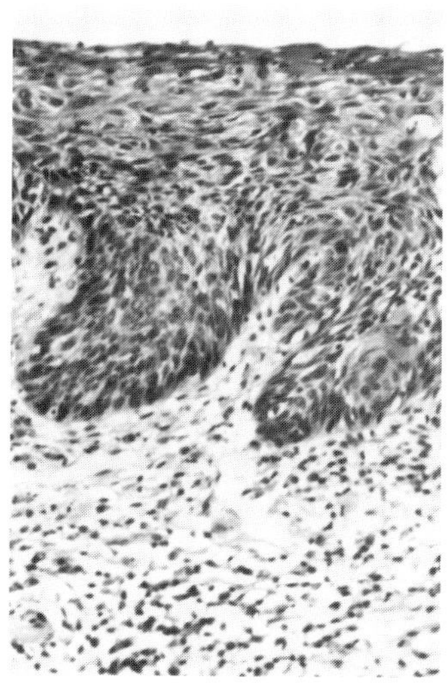

A BIOPSY FROM THE PERIPHERY WOULD ONLY SHOW THE IN-SITU CARCINOMA AND MISS THE INVASIVE COMPONENT

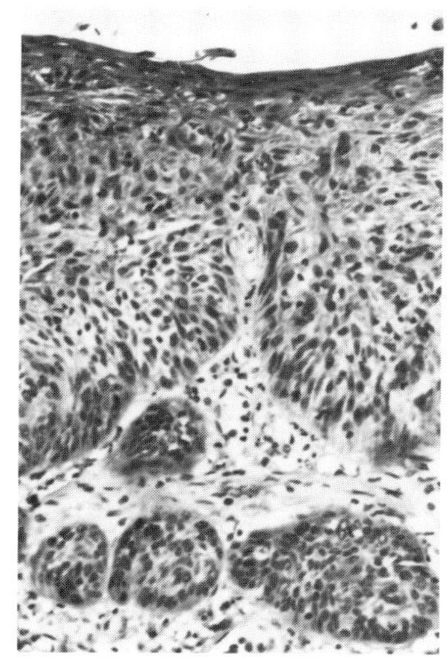

A SAMPLE FROM THE CENTER WOULD SHOW ONLY THE INVASIVE CARCINOMA AND MISS THE SURROUNDING AREA OF IN-SITU CARCINOMA.

soaked in fixative. Again, because of bad clinical practices, large specimens are often received tightly stuffed in disproportionally small containers without space left for fixative.

When only routine pathologic examination is required, the specimen is submitted in a fixative solution supplied by the pathology laboratory. The most common fixative is 10% buffered Formalin. This fixative has been most satisfactory for all usual histologic preparations but does not actually preserve all substances found in tissues. Also, it is not ideal for ultrastructural studies or for evaluating cytologic details in lymphomas. Therefore, if one of the above considerations is significant for the diagnosis, the pathologist must be consulted in advance so that the proper fixative is used. The container with the fixative must always be at hand when the biopsy is performed so that the tissue is placed in it immediately.

A most important task in the conduct of a biopsy is to *label the specimen.* A clinician and patient who have gone through all the steps to obtain an appropriate biopsy will be absolutely frustrated if the specimen is rejected by the laboratory because of inappropriate labeling. Inadequate identification is a good reason for withholding any pathologic report because errors in such a simple issue may harm one or more patients, depending on the situation. A most unfortunate reality is that often it cannot be determined whose task it was to write the identifying information on the requisition form and on the specimen container. To avoid such catastrophes, somebody must be made responsible, and if it is someone other than the surgeon, his (her) name must be on the form.

WHAT CLINICAL INFORMATION DO YOU GIVE THE PATHOLOGIST?

To answer this question the surgeon must resolve two issues:

1. What do I expect the pathologist to tell me?
2. How does the pathologist go about in responding to my expectations?

The surgeon expects the pathologist's report to state whether the process is neoplastic or not, benign or malignant, metastatic or primary, and to be specific about the histologic classification and depth of invasion. Although on several occasions the pathologist may be able to provide these specifics with minimal clinical information, quite often the degree of accuracy of a pathologist's report reflects the detail and accuracy of the clinical data made available. The microscopic appearance of many lesions is not always pathognomonic, especially if one considers the sampling limitations, the secondary phenomena obliterating the primary cellular changes, and the overlapping histopathologic characteristics in diverse diseases. The information needed to clarify all these issues must accompany every specimen. Often the only clinical information on the requisition is: "lesion in mouth, rule out cancer"—a short but pointless statement. An equally short statement, like "firm mass 2 × 2 cm on right side of tongue," would have made a few helpful points.

In order to make the best of a good pathologist, the head and neck surgeon should communicate information which he certainly possesses when he obtains a biopsy and which usually includes the following:

1. Site of biopsy specified (e.g., "right side of tongue," instead of the ill-defined "oral cavity"). This is helpful in evaluating the biopsy because of peculiarities in the histology, patterns of tissue reactivity, and neoplasms in certain anatomical locations.

2. Size of lesion. This may prove significant in judging the adequacy of sampling and avoiding false negative results (e.g., the differential diagnosis between papilloma and verrucous carcinoma is facilitated by knowing the approximate size of the lesion).

3. Number of lesions. This helps to guide the differential diagnosis since some processes are characteristically multifocal.

4. Gross appearance (e.g., mass, ulcer, white or red patch). Numerous examples can be given emphasizing the importance of gross appearance. Often the gross description helps to determine whether a biopsy is adequate or not. For example, if a mass deep in the floor of mouth is described and the biopsy contains only dysplastic mucosa, the sampling is inadequate for defining the nature of the mass, which may be anything from an inflamed salivary gland to cancer. Similarly, if a rough, red mucosal area with central ulceration is described and the biopsy shows carcinoma in situ only, one should suspect that only the peripheral area was sampled, and a more advanced invasive component may be present in the ulcerated center that might have been missed.

The pathologist should note any such discrepancies and make the appropriate comments in writing so that the patient may be reevaluated prior to decisive therapy.

5. Radiologic or other laboratory data. These are useful for the interpretation of lesions involving bones and endocrine organs and for the differential diagnosis of hematologic-lymphoreticular malignancies.

6. History of neoplasia in other organs. This is important for excluding metastatic lesions or lesions associated with systemic diseases. For example, an undifferentiated malignant tumor in the neck area will be worked up differently if the patient has a history of melanoma.

7. Previous radiation therapy involving the site of biopsy. Most of the time an experienced pathologist will suspect that the tissue has been irradiated. Occasionally, however, irradiation changes may be misinterpreted if there is no warning to that effect in the clinical information.

8. Age and sex of the patient. These may facilitate the differential diagnosis, particularly when one is evaluating metastatic lesions from unknown primaries.

9. Other clinical data such as duration, pain, and so forth are less significant, given their subjectivity.

In practice, most of the pertinent information may be given within a couple of lines: e.g., "65-year-old male, ulcer with indurated base, 2 × 2 cm, midline floor of mouth, around 6 months." Or, "50-year-old female, right thyroid, well-defined cold nodule 3 × 2 cm, symptomless; radical mastectomy 1976."

WHEN IS A FROZEN SECTION DIAGNOSIS NEEDED?

Immediate pathologic diagnosis by the frozen section procedure must be requested when a decision on treatment or adequacy of resection margins is to be made while the patient is in the operating room. Frozen section diagnosis may also be required in order to ascertain the adequacy of biopsies from lesions in anatomical locations which are not easily accessible (e.g., biopsy samples obtained from intracranial lesions or at exploratory laparotomies). When resection margins are to be microscopically assessed, the tissue must be submitted fresh, as described above. When properly utilized, frozen section diagnosis is a significant contribution to the improvement of surgical patient care. In the great majority of cases (over 95%)[2] the pathologist can make within minutes the following differential diagnoses using hematoxylin-eosin-stained frozen sections: Is the lesion neoplastic or not; benign or malignant; epithelial, mesenchymal, or lymphoreticular. More specific subclassification is usually (75%–80%) possible when the neoplasm is well or moderately well differentiated. The classification of poorly differentiated malignancies must await the study of multiple sections of well-fixed tissues. Special workup sometimes includes histochemistry and electron microscopy.

The frozen section procedure is not suitable for the study of excessively fatty or calcified tissues. Many artifacts are created by freezing and thawing the tissues. The portions used for frozen sections have poor morphological preservation when subsequently fixed in Formalin for routine preparations. Previously frozen specimens are absolutely useless for ultrastructural studies. Therefore, before requesting the frozen section, one must make sure that the pathologist will be able to use this technique to answer the most pertinent questions raised. If this is not possible, additional tissue must be submitted for routine preparations, electron microscopy, and whatever else is needed.

Evaluation of Tissue Specimens

WHAT ARE THE ISSUES TO BE RESOLVED BY HISTOLOGIC EXAMINATION?

Prior to obtaining a tissue sample the surgeon must have a clear idea of what he (she) wants to know and what the probability is of getting the answers in the pathology report. This is fundamental for a proper response to each of the questions raised in the previous section. With an ideal specimen examined under light microscopy the pathologist can accomplish:

1. Differentiation between neoplastic and nonneoplastic processes with only a rare exception (99.9%).
2. Differentiation between benign and malignant neoplasms with very few exceptions (98%).
3. Definition of the broad histologic category (e.g., carcinoma, sarcoma, lymphoma) in the great majority of cases (95%).
4. Definition of the presence or absence of invasion in the great majority of mucosal and skin cancers (95%).
5. Classification of a neoplasm into a specific histologic type, e.g., squamous cell cancer, adenocarcinoma, liposarcoma, rhabdomyosarcoma, etc., in the majority of cases (85%).
6. Differentiation between primary and metastatic malignancies in the majority of cases (90%).
7. Grade of cytologic malignancy, whenever pertinent.
8. Definition of the primary site of a metastatic malignancy from the histology and clinical data in most cases (80%), and from the histology alone in some cases (50%).
9. Definition of the pathologic stage.
10. Evaluation of the involvement of resection margins.

Techniques such as electron microscopy, histochemistry, and immunochemistry will increase the accuracy of pathologic diagnosis for items 3, 5, and 8. Extended techniques are not useful in improving the pathologic interpretation for any of the other items.

When dealing with malignancies which show no differentiation by light microscopy, the basis of histologic classification is not well defined. To study all undifferentiated tumors by electron microscopy, immunochemistry, and so forth is impractical and of questionable scientific and clinical merit. Such studies are pertinent in *selected* cases when very specific answers are sought, such as the differential diagnosis of metastatic melanoma or thyroid medullary carcinoma from a poorly differentiated primary tumor.

WHAT IS THE SIGNIFICANCE OF PATHOLOGIC STAGE AND GRADE?

Some confusion exists concerning the significance and prognostic value of grading as compared to staging of malignancies. Grade and stage are two distinct concepts which are useful in predicting the clinical course and are therefore expected to show good correlation with each other. However, there are fundamental differences between these two concepts which must be clearly borne in mind for their most effective clinical utilization. The grade assigns a degree of *malignant potential* depending on the *cytologic characteristics* of the neoplasm. The stage describes the apparent *extent of tumor* growth and spread at *a given time* in its evolution. A high *stage* means that there is a heavy load of tumor cells and/or that the tumor has metastasized. A high *grade* implies that the neoplasm is of the rapidly growing variety with invasive properties and has the potential for rapid advance to a high stage in the near future.

There is some overlap in some cancers in the prognostic significance of stage and grade from a statistical point of view. The message conveyed by each one of

carcinomas, and fibromatoses). Exclusion of margin involvement by in situ carcinoma or dysplasia requires microscopic examination.

The extent of sampling for frozen sections depends on the type of specimen, the nature of the process, and the procedure to be immediately performed. For example, if the surgeon wants to proceed immediately with a definitive reconstructive procedure, every effort should be made to avoid a false negative report. Under such circumstances the frozen section diagnosis is the definitive pathologic evaluation and errors due to incomplete examination are unacceptable.

There are two major approaches in requesting pathologic examination of resection margins:

1. The surgeon selects and submits separately tissue samples from the margins.

2. The resected specimen is submitted to the pathologist, who samples the margins as needed.

For extensive resections both methods are often used in combination. The surgeon does the initial sampling of the margin in order to define how extensive a procedure is needed or what modifications are required. Once these decisions are made on the basis of the frozen section report, the resection is carried out and the entire margin is examined by the pathologist. Additional frozen sections may or may not be requested. It is important that the surgeon mark the areas from which the initial samples were taken so that duplications, potentially leading to false positive results, may be avoided.

Proper orientation of the specimen is essential for communicating the results of margin examination. Some specimens contain anatomical structures which permit orientation without additional markings. Many specimens, however, need some kind of marking, which is very easily accomplished with a suture, small clip, or ink. The marking should not distort the margin and should be as remote as possible from crucial areas so that the pathologic examination is not compromised. It is sufficient to mark one margin as long as adequate information for identifying the anatomical location is given. For example, place a suture at one margin of a skin ellipse and write on the requisition form: "Left side of nose; suture at superior margin."

The technique for sectioning the resection margin varies from institution to institution, specimen to specimen, and even from margin to margin of the same specimen. For this reason, the way a specific margin was sectioned must be clearly described in the pathologist's report. To avoid confusion, especially when more than one person is involved in the processing of the specimen (e.g., the pathology fellow describes the gross appearance and the staff pathologist makes the final diagnosis), it is recommended that Polaroid photographs of the specimen be taken. The photographs are then marked to show where the sections were taken (Fig 4–3).

A common practice is to paint the margin with India ink and then cut the sections perpendicularly through the margin toward the lesion or through the entire width of the specimen into the opposite margin. This technique, however, is not always applicable, and for some specimens it is far from ideal. Generally, large specimens with extensive or irregular margins are handled differently from small specimens. It is not always possible to examine microscopically the entire margin. Such an endeavor is probably superfluous for most large specimens. Figure 4–3 illustrates these general principles. Specifics concerning the resection margins of certain specimens will be mentioned in the appropriate chapters.

INTERPRETATION OF THE HISTOLOGIC DIAGNOSIS

Understanding Terms Commonly Used in the Pathologist's Report

Effective decision-making involves intercommunication. For head and neck cancer, it is essential that the use of terms be as precise as possible. The following sections try to clarify commonly used (and misused) terms.

WHAT ARE REACTIVE CHANGES?

The expression "reactive changes" is often used to describe morphological deviations from the normal which result from tissue reaction to injury. Such changes are a response to injury, often protective for the tissues, and should regress when the injurious stimuli are eliminated. In this category belong three very frequent processes: regeneration, hyperplasia, and metaplasia.

Regenerating tissues consist of young, not fully differentiated cells with increased mitotic activity. These characteristics occasionally cause problems in the differential diagnosis from neoplasia.

Hyperplasia denotes an increase in the number of cells which differentiate and perform their intended function. Mitotic activity is very variable but always limited to the cell layers from which the tissue normally proliferates. For example, hyperplastic squamous epithelium has more cell layers than normal, has mitoses only in the deep basal layer, and the frequency of mitoses may be normal or increased, depending on the phase of evolution of hyperplasia. Hyperplastic surface epithelia may expand downward, pushing onto the subjacent tissues, or upward, forming plaques or papillary projections. Thus, marked hyperplasia may be difficult

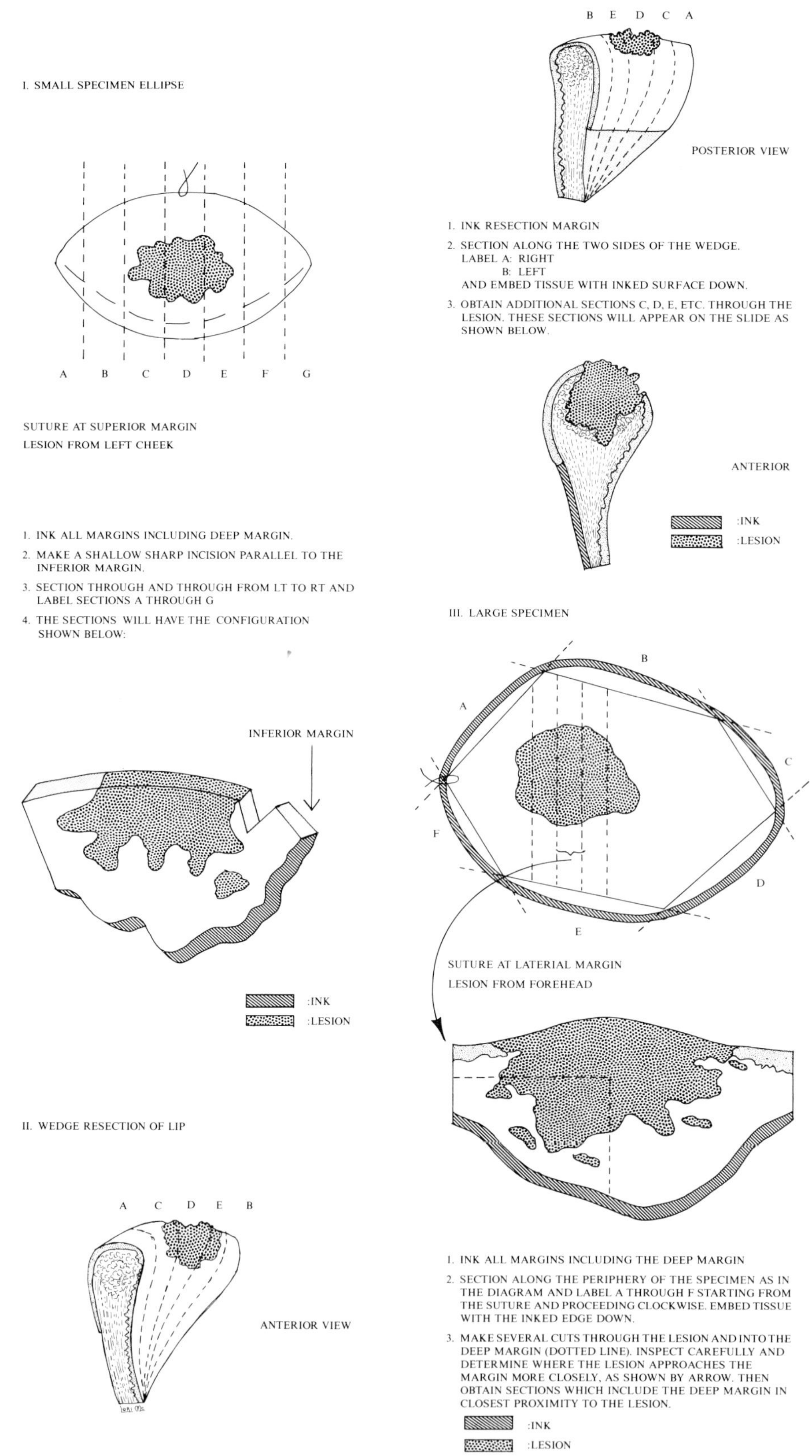

Fig 4–3.—Some methods of studying a pathologic specimen, identifying the borders for completeness of excision, and studying the major portions of the identifiable lesion.

to distinguish from neoplasia. Indeed, the cutoff point between hyperplasia and neoplasia is not well defined morphologically and problems of semantics are common. For example, the distinction between squamous papilloma and papillary hyperplasia is often arbitrary.

Metaplasia is an acquired process in which a mature, differentiated tissue is replaced by another tissue which is also mature. The replacement tissue shows a different type of specialization. This phenomenon usually affects surface epithelial (e.g., change from ciliated to squamous epithelium), but it also occurs in other tissues (e.g., osseous metaplasia in the connective tissue of scars). Metaplasia is usually a reactive process which enables the cells to survive in an altered environment. Therefore, whenever metaplasia is found, a significant change in the cell milieu may be assumed. In this respect, metaplasia may be a herald of more abnormalities to come and is often found in tissues harboring dysplasia and neoplasia.

HOW ARE THE TERMS "ATYPIA" AND "DYSPLASIA" USED?

Atypia means deviation from the typical structure and *dysplasia* means "not well-formed" structure. The structure affected may be the nucleus, the cytoplasm, the cell arrangement, or combinations of these elements. In essence, these terms are synonymous and do not necessarily imply an autonomous or progressive process such as neoplasia.

Atypia usually applies to a more general concept irrespective of tissue type and is frequently employed in the description of neoplastic cells. For example, it is often stated that benign neoplasms show little cellular atypia while malignant ones consist of highly atypical cells.

Dysplasia is almost exclusively applied to epithelia. Dysplasia was originally used to describe a spectrum of abnormalities in the exfoliative cytology of surface epithelia. Therefore, when referring to *surface epithelia*, the term "dysplasia" is appropriate.

The deviation from typical structure varies in extent and severity and must be graded as to whether it is mild, moderate, or severe. Mild dysplasia is associated with reactive changes and regresses when the noxious stimuli are eliminated. Moderate dysplasia may also be a reversible morphological expression of tissue reaction to injury. For example, viral infections, irradiation, and drugs affect the mitotic processes and produce cellular atypia in several tissues. Severe dysplasia is seemingly beyond the scope of a reactive phenomenon and denotes altered cell differentiation, disordered cellular interaction, and an inappropriately high cell turnover rate.

Severe dysplasia does not have a clear connotation of a progressive, autonomous process but implies a higher risk for coexisting or subsequent malignancy.[4, 5] Expressions such as "premalignant," "preneoplastic," or "borderline" lesion should not be used in either the pathology report or the surgeon's communication to the patient. When severe dysplasia is found, the entire anatomical area should be scrutinized to exclude the presence of malignancy, but by no means should the case be viewed as if there is or will be an irrevocable progression. Very little hard data exist about the natural history of epithelial dysplasia in the upper aerodigestive tract.

There are no strict criteria in grading dysplasia. In general, several morphological features are simultaneously assessed and an overall grade is assigned. The most important features to be assessed are preservation of architectural arrangement, maturation or differentiation of individual cells, nucleocytoplasmic ratios, nuclear details, and the frequency and distribution of mitoses.

HOW SHOULD THE TERMS "NEOPLASIA," "TUMOR," AND "MALIGNANCY" BE USED, AND WHAT ARE THE CRITERIA OF MALIGNANCY?

There are inconsistencies in the use and interpretation of these terms. The ambiguity is partly attributable to an inherent vagueness in the definitions of the processes to which these terms refer. In addition, the prognostic implications originally attached to these terms are no longer indiscriminantly applicable to individual patients. Nowadays it has become imperative to further clarify these terms in order to place prognosis and therapy in a realistic perspective.

The term "neoplasia" signifies an autonomous, persistent, and seemingly purposeless cell proliferation. Accumulation of neoplastic cells often results in obvious deformation and "tumor." Thus, the descriptive term "tumor" may be used for some neoplasms but should not substitute for the term "neoplasia" in general. Neoplasms that remain localized are referred to as "benign," while those capable of metastatic spread are designated as "malignant." Whenever the metastatic potential has already been expressed, there can be no doubt about the use of the term "malignant neoplasm" or "malignancy" and its prognostic implications. If metastases are not demonstrable at the time of clinical presentation, the sine qua non criterion for malignancy must be replaced with a number of criteria that are exclusively morphological and usually associated with malignancy. There is no single morphological criterion that consistently predicts biologic behavior. The pathologist notes a constellation of structural abnormalities and makes a judgment based on a large body of experience built up over many years of careful observations.

The criteria of malignancy pertain to three major

structural aspects of neoplasia: (1) The relationship of neoplastic cells to preexisting tissues (e.g., invasion (see below), (2) cytologic details (e.g., chromatin abnormalities), and (3) the rate of growth (e.g., mitotic activity). The weight that each of these three aspects contributes to a particular diagnosis will vary with the anatomical location, the histologic type of the neoplasm, and even with the age of the patient. A thorough understanding of a catalogue of facts is necessary to appreciate the limitations of certain techniques of specimen procurement.

In lay language, malignant neoplasms are referred to as "cancers." Cancer is not a term used in the pathologist's report but rather is a word used to signify a poorly understood abnormal state of body cells believed to be incurable and fatal if not controlled. In reality, our knowledge today suggests that neither the etiology nor the clinical course of malignant neoplasms should be viewed from this narrow angle. There is such great diversity in the treatment response and outcome among various malignant neoplasms that classifying a neoplasm as malignant without further elaboration is of little value for the management of a given patient. For example, the statement "cancer of the thyroid" is not an acceptable diagnosis because it encompasses a wide spectrum of possibilities, from a low-grade papillary carcinoma with over 70% 20-year survival to an advanced undifferentiated carcinoma with less than 20% 2-year survival.[6] The highly specialized terminology of the histopathologic report should be communicated to the patient using carefully chosen words that do not create undue pessimism or unwarranted expectations.

WHAT DO THE TERMS "INVASION" AND "MICROINVASION" SIGNIFY?

The relationship of the neoplastic cells to the surrounding tissues is an important morphological criterion of biologic potential. Benign neoplasms usually show a high degree of cellular cohesiveness and form well-circumscribed masses separated from the adjacent tissues by a discrete capsule. Malignant neoplasms always display signs of reduced cellular cohesiveness and some evidence of dispersion within adjacent tissues which results in poor demarcation. The dispersion of malignant cells among preexisting structures is called invasion (or infiltration). Invasion may vary from extremely diffuse to very focal. Neoplasms with a diffusely infiltrative growth pattern are more difficult to eradicate by narrow local excision. Such neoplasms are often highly malignant because they also invade lymphatics and vascular channels to give early metastases. However, there are many examples of neoplasms which do not metastasize or do so rarely, but recur locally due to their infiltrative growth pattern (e.g., dermatofibrosarcoma protuberans, fibromatosis). The terminology used to define this type of neoplasia is unsatisfactory. Some pathologists classify these infiltrative, locally recurring growths as benign[7] and some as low-grade malignancies.[8]

Well-encapsulated neoplasms have grossly apparent margins. Local excision suffices for their eradication. Exceptions to this rule do exist. For example, the apparently encapsulated pleomorphic adenomas (mixed tumor) of salivary glands often have microscopic extensions beyond the capsule which form the nidus for multifocal recurrence when the tumor is treated by either enucleation or a very conservative local excision. Still, pleomorphic adenomas are classified as benign and the extensions through the capsule are not referred to as "invasion." On the other hand, focal microscopic breaks through the capsule of a follicular thyroid neoplasm that otherwise lacks cytologic criteria of malignancy signify metastatic potential and suffice to categorize the neoplasm as low-grade malignancy.[9]

In some organs (or tissues) the presence of invasive growth can be easily assessed while in others this assessment is difficult and somewhat subjective. For example, it is easy to assess invasion in neoplasms arising from surface epithelial linings which are delineated by a continuous basement membrane. In this case, invasion is defined as a break through the basement membrane and extension of neoplastic cells into the subjacent tissues. The invasion may be extensive and obvious at first glance or it may be limited to a microscopic focus where few neoplastic cells have just penetrated the basement membrane. A focal, minor invasion is called *microinvasion* and must be distinguished from overt invasion because it has a more favorable prognosis and is often treatable with more conservative means.[10] Occasionally, the pathologist may suspect microinvasion that is not objectively interpretable due to complicating factors. For example, whenever intense inflammatory infiltrate obscures the delineation of basement membrane or whenever an irregularly thickened surface epithelium has been sectioned tangentially, the assessment of minor invasion becomes quite tenuous. In such instances, some pathologists elect to use less specific terminology, such as "superficial" squamous cell carcinoma, which denotes a hesitancy to commit oneself to either "in situ" or "microinvasive." The surgeon confronted with such a diagnosis should understand that the lesion is not overtly invasive but that a minor degree of invasion may be present.

HOW DOES "CARCINOMA IN SITU" DIFFER FROM EITHER OVERT MALIGNANCY OR DYSPLASIA?

The term "carcinoma in situ" was introduced to define a very special situation in which the lining epithelium of an organ is replaced by cells with overt cytologic criteria of malignancy without evidence of invasion. In other words, invasion—the most consistent morphological criterion of malignancy—is absent. This fact has caused some controversy about the use of the term "carcinoma," which denotes a malignant epithelial neoplasm.[11, 12] The term "intraepithelial neoplasia" has been proposed as more appropriate. I prefer to use the expression "carcinoma in situ," which is familiar to physicians and adequately describes the histopathologic picture. Carcinoma in situ is a morphological entity distinct from either overt malignancy or dysplasia. There are uncertainties about the clinical evolution of carcinoma in situ in most anatomical locations with the exception of the uterine cervix, which has been the subject of several well-organized longitudinal studies. Data for the oral cavity, larynx, and pharynx show a high frequency of carcinoma in situ juxtaposed with invasive lesions.[13, 14] This close association is subject to various pathophysiologic interpretations with quite diverse practical consequences. The notion that carcinoma in situ is the preinvasive phase (stage 0) of malignant neoplasia has received wide acceptance, but whether it is also an irreversible or progressive process is still debatable.[15, 16] There is an impasse in the argument about the nature of the in situ carcinoma: metastases do not occur prior to the invasive stages, and therefore the hallmark of malignant biologic behavior is never present and will never appear if the lesions are treated while in the in situ stage. Nevertheless, whenever carcinoma in situ is diagnosed, the entire anatomical area should be thoroughly reexamined and additional biopsy specimens obtained. In this manner coexisting invasive malignancies can be detected in relatively early stages when they are still amenable to treatment. Also, additional foci of in situ carcinomas may be discovered and promptly treated. Preventive measures must also be taken in the hope of delaying or, possibly, eliminating the evolution of remaining transformed cells into invasive stages. For example, further exposure to noxious agents (most commonly tobacco products) must be avoided. In this context *carcinoma in situ* has a connotation similar to *severe dysplasia*. It is not clear whether distinction between carcinoma in situ and severe dysplasia is significant for clinical management and prognosis. This issue will never be resolved if pathologists do not discriminate between the two morphological entities. Unfortunately, the criteria of malignancy that are required to make the distinction are not strict enough. The terms severe dysplasia and carcinoma in situ are being inconsistently applied. The surgeon and the pathologist must develop an understanding of each other's definitions of the terms as applied to specific examples.

UNDERSTANDING SPECIFIC TERMINOLOGY

What are the major categories of neoplasms of epithelial derivation in the head and neck, and what are their characteristics most relevant to clinical practice?

The great majority of head and neck neoplasms are of epithelial derivation. In particular, the squamous epithelium of the skin and upper aerodigestive tract is the source of over 80% of carcinomas in this region.[17] In general, malignant neoplasms of epithelial origin are designated as carcinomas. Their benign counterparts are called papillomas, when exophytic, and adenomas, when they form deep-seated solid masses. Carcinomas are classified primarily on the basis of morphological evidence of differentiation into various types of normal epithelium. Thus, one may use the following scheme, which is simple and easy to memorize:

1. *Undifferentiated*, when the neoplastic cells are recognized as epithelial but no further differentiation is apparent by usual morphological techniques.
2. *Differentiated*, when some degree of differentiation toward known cell types is apparent, e.g.:
   - Basal cell carcinoma
   - Squamous cell carcinoma
   - Adenocarcinoma
   - Mixed cell type (mucoepidermoid, adenosquamous)
   - Other specialized differentiation (e.g., thyroid, parathyroid, neuroendocrine)

UNDIFFERENTIATED CARCINOMAS.—Undifferentiated carcinomas are often subclassified depending on cell size and/or shape: e.g., small cell (oat, lymphocyte-like), intermediate (polygonal, fusiform), large cell type. The histogenesis of undifferentiated carcinomas is largely speculative. Some, but not all, small cell types contain electron-dense neuroendocrine-type granules, and may derive from neural crest elements. Large cell types may show poorly developed squamous or glandular-secretory characteristics when examined with the electron microscope. The distinction between small and large cell types is clinically relevant because of significant differences in the response to systemic chemotherapy. Primary small cell undifferentiated carcinomas are very rare in the head and neck. Whenever such a diagnosis is based on biopsy specimens from neck masses the possibility of metastasis from a lung primary must be considered and excluded by thorough workup prior to any radical surgery.

DIFFERENTIATED CARCINOMAS

BASAL CELL CARCINOMAS.—Basal cell carcinomas occur in the skin of the face more often than in any other region.[18] They consist of cells which closely resemble the basal layer of stratified squamous epithelium. Their existence in organs other than skin is questionable. Basaloid forms of neoplasms have been described in the parotid and larynx, but the natural course in these locations is not comparable to that of cutaneous basal cell neoplasms. Several histologic subtypes are recognizable on the basis of cell arrangement and interaction with the stroma (solid, cystic, adenoid, morphea-like). Some subtypes have a rather characteristic clinical picture and are worth noting in the pathology report. Occasionally, basal cell carcinomas contain large amounts of melanin (pigmented basal cell carcinoma) and may grossly resemble melanomas, from which they can be easily differentiated by histologic examination. Gross evaluation of the resection margins for basal cell carcinoma is often unreliable due to the invasive growth pattern, which results in considerable lateral spread beneath normal epidermis. Microscopic examination of frozen sections is required and is particularly valuable when basal cell carcinomas are located in areas such as the face, where the surgeon can not afford to be too generous in the extent of resection.

SQUAMOUS CELL CARCINOMA.—Squamous cell carcinomas are by far the most common malignant neoplasms of the head and neck. The term "epidermoid" is sometimes used in lieu of "squamous." Epidermoid, meaning epidermis-like, is a descriptive term and not as accurate as "squamous" in denoting the histogenesis of these carcinomas. The growth pattern is extremely variable, ranging from exophytic (verrucous type) to invasive with diffuse tissue induration and/or ulceration. The growth pattern is prognostically significant: the invasive pattern is associated with greater recurrence rate, most probably because of inability to obtain completely uninvolved resection margins.[19] Recurrences sometimes occur even when the margins have been reported as negative.[20] One must realize that the margins of large resection specimens from the oral cavity and pharynx cannot be completely examined microscopically and small focal extensions may be missed. Metachronous neoplasia may be another plausible explanation for some recurrences.

The hallmark of squamous differentiation is the presence of well-formed desmosomal attachments and intracytoplasmic bundles of keratin tonofilaments. Depending on the degree of expression of these characteristics, squamous cell carcinomas are classified as well, moderately, and poorly differentiated.[21] The term "nonkeratinizing" is sometimes used to denote the absence of obvious keratinization on light microscopy. However, if the neoplasm is indeed squamous, there will be intracytoplasmic keratin demonstrable by electron microscopy and immunochemistry (immunoperoxidase reaction for keratin). Therefore, the term "nonkeratinizing" is confusing and is better avoided. Such carcinomas are best designated as poorly differentiated. Squamous cell carcinomas may be graded, usually into four grades (1 through 4).[22] Those of low grade (1–2) are also well differentiated and less prone to metastasize early. They are regarded as more curable by local excision if treated prior to achieving a large size. Histologically, these low-grade squamous cell carcinomas closely resemble the marked hyperplasia such as may develop around chronic ulcers (pseudoepitheliomatous hyperplasia).

The term "keratoacanthoma" has been used to describe a type of squamous neoplasia of the skin which presents a rather characteristic gross pattern and has been reported to undergo spontaneous regression.[23] Histologically, these growths are low-grade squamous cell carcinomas.[24] They are usually small (< 2 cm), well defined, and easily resectable in their entirety. The most reasonable approach in the management of such lesions is to perform an excisional biopsy with a clear margin, which will be curative for a low-grade cutaneous carcinoma in the majority of cases. Simply taking a biopsy of the lesion and then waiting for it to regress is not wise. A good number of cases recur[25] and may follow the usual course of more invasive squamous carcinoma and eventually require extensive surgery. The diagnosis of keratoacanthoma, implying a benign process, should never be based on gross inspection or on a small nonexcisional biopsy specimen of the lip. Extension of growth or lymphatic involvement is too high a risk to take while waiting for spontaneous resolution in order to avoid a minimal excision of a lesion.

High-grade (3 and 4) squamous carcinomas show little evidence of differentiation and have a higher implied metastatic potential. The probability of cure by local surgical excision alone is reduced, even if the primary lesion is resectable, because of the early occurrence of lymphatic dissemination.

In general, the local recurrence rate for all squamous cell carcinomas is predictable when the resection margins are involved.[26] Therefore, it is advisable to carefully assess the extent of the growth prior to definitive surgery and to obtain intraoperative histologic evaluation of the margin. It is also advisable to histologically assess the extent of the lesion prior to preoperative irradiation. The frequency of margin involvement increases in resections performed following irradiation because the radiation-induced changes modify the structure of the tissues and makes it harder to grossly define the boundaries of the neoplastic infiltrate.

Types of squamous cell neoplasms peculiar to certain anatomical locations.—In addition to the above general classification, there are a number of histologic variants that tend to be topographically specialized.

Lymphoepithelioma (Schmincke tumor) is a morphological variant of poorly differentiated squamous cell carcinoma which occurs in the nasopharynx. On light microscopy it may be difficult to differentiate from large cell lymphoma. The correct interpretation may necessitate ultrastructural examination, which clearly reveals its squamous derivation.[27]

Spindle cell squamous carcinoma is a rare variant characterized by fusiform malignant cells and an associated intense proliferation of stromal fibroblasts. It resembles mesenchymal spindle cell malignancy (sarcoma) and for this reason is sometimes referred to as "pseudosarcomatous," "carcinosarcoma," or "pleomorphic carcinoma." This variant is found in the hypopharynx and larynx and may pose a diagnostic problem for those unaware of its existence. Electron microscopic examination demonstrates squamous characteristics in many of the fusiform cells. A polypoid and an infiltrative variant have been described. The polypoid form has a better prognosis.[29]

Verrucous carcinoma is a morphological variant of low-grade squamous cell carcinoma which occurs in the oral cavity, larynx, and nasal fossa. It is characterized by a bulky exophytic growth pattern (verruca-wart-like) and a very high level of differentiation. The neoplastic cells resemble closely the fully mature squamous epithelium. Cytologic atypia is minimal. The diagnosis of carcinoma can be made only by demonstrating invasion of deep tissues. Superficial biopsies of such lesions are often inadequate because they do not permit evaluation of stromal invasion. A good gross description of the lesion by the surgeon or endoscopist is very important in guiding the pathologist. For example, if a large cauliflower-like tumor was seen and the small superficial biopsy shows a squamous papilloma, the pathologist should suspect the possibility of a verrucous carcinoma and should request a deeper, larger biopsy specimen which is likely to demonstrate the invasion, if present. As a low-grade malignancy, verrucous carcinoma grows locally and may reach large dimensions prior to lymphatic dissemination.[30, 31] Therefore, if diagnosed while still resectable, this type of neoplasia can be cured by an adequate surgical excision. Some published data suggest that radiation adversely affects the course of such carcinomas;[32] however, this observation remains debatable[33] (see chapter 13).

Florid papillomatosis is a term used to define a disease condition of the upper aerodigestive tract characterized by multifocal exophytic proliferations of the mucosal squamous epithelium. Neither invasion of deep tissues nor cytologic malignancy is detectable. The natural course, however, is not compatible with either hyperplasia, a self-limiting process, or benign neoplasia, which can be controlled by local excision. The morphologically benign epithelial growths recur[34] and may eventually acquire or be associated with the morphological and biologic characteristics of malignant neoplasia,[35] although such transformation remains doubtful.

Inverted papilloma is a morphological type of neoplasia involving the epithelium of the nasal cavity and paranasal sinuses. It is characterized by a downward (inverted) proliferation of very cohesive, sharply delineated squamous epithelium without cytologic evidence of malignant potential. The characteristic growth pattern results in downward, undersurface extension which is considered distinct from "real" stromal invasion. The clinical course is not typical of benign neoplasia because recurrences are very frequent and an association with frankly malignant process has been reported by several authors, who, however, disagree as to the nature of such association.[36]

ADENOCARCINOMAS.—Adenocarcinomas are infrequent in the head and neck; most arise from glands and few from surface epithelium. For example, the major and minor salivary glands, the lacrimal, ceruminous, and skin adnexal glands, and occasionally the columnar epithelium of the upper airways may be the primary site of an adenocarcinoma in this area. Carcinomas arising in the thyroid and parathyroid glands are usually considered separately from the common group of adenocarcinomas. Numerous histologic patterns of adenocarcinomas have been recognized in various anatomical locations. The general characteristic is the arrangement of cells in glandular structures and/or the production of secretion. Either of these characteristics may be obvious on routine light microscopic examination in the usual case with well to moderately differentiated adenocarcinomas. The diagnosis of poorly differentiated adenocarcinomas may require either histochemical studies for the demonstration of mucinous secretions or electron microscopic study for the visualization of intercellular junctional complexes, secretory vacuoles, or granules. The mucinous secretion may be predominantly extracellular (e.g., colloid or mucinous carcinoma), intracellular (e.g., signet ring carcinoma), or both intracellular and extracellular. The neoplasias of the skin, adnexae, and salivary glands present a large spectrum of histologic patterns which are beyond the scope of this chapter. The major salivary gland tumors are discussed in chapter 20. Minor salivary and mucous gland neoplasms may arise at any level of the upper aerodigestive tract but are most common in the oral cavity, particularly in the palate. Their histologic classification follows that applied to major salivary glands and the frequency of malignancy varies in different series, the larger series showing that over 50% of minor salivary gland neoplasms are malignant,[37] with the predominant histologic type being adenoid cystic carcinoma.[38]

Adenocarcinomas of the surface epithelium of the upper respiratory tract originate most often in the paranasal sinuses. They are usually classified into three morphological patterns: sessile, papillary, and mucoid alveolar. There is significant difference in the prognosis to make this distinction clinically meaningful.[39] Adenocarcinomas of the oropharynx and larynx are rare and arise exclusively from mucous or minor salivary glands. Most are adenocarcinomas (not otherwise specified); the remaining are adenoid cystic and mucoepidermoid and, very rarely, oncocytic.

MIXED TYPES OF CELLULAR DIFFERENTIATION.—When both squamous and glandular (or secretory) differentiation is found within the same neoplasm, the terms adenosquamous and mucoepidermoid are usually employed to describe the phenomenon of variable differentiation. Such neoplasms are uncommon, with the exception of salivary glands. The extent to which each component participates will vary; usually the neoplasm is graded on the basis of the predominant component. Low-grade mucoepidermoid carcinomas are often cystic and can be mistaken for benign lesions. Grading of mucoepidermoid carcinomas is clinically significant.[40–42]

WHICH ARE THE MAJOR CATEGORIES OF NONEPITHELIAL NEOPLASMS IN THE HEAD AND NECK AREA?

There are many types of tissues other than epithelium in the head and neck, and each may give origin to neoplasms. These can be roughly classified, according to their derivation, into mesenchymal, neural, complex, and indeterminate. Further subclassification yields a very large number of categories, each of which encompasses several morphological variants of benign and malignant neoplasms. The resultant nomenclature of nonepithelial neoplasia is very complex and difficult to memorize if not utilized frequently. Furthermore, inconsistencies in terminology have created confusion, and over the years several terms have been used for the same entity by different authorities. In general, an attempt was made to classify these diverse neoplasms according to the tissue of origin as specifically as possible. Sometimes this so-called histogenetic approach is stretched too far. Claims to specific embryogenetic derivation may be based on traces of a substance found in otherwise unidentifiable cells. Presently, the practical therapeutic importance of such an endeavor is not readily apparent.

Regardless of histogenesis, most of these neoplasms could be graded on the basis of morphological criteria very similar to those applied to epithelial neoplasms. Malignant mesenchymal neoplasms are designated as sarcomas (fibrosarcoma, osteosarcoma, liposarcoma, etc.). Occasionally the biologic potential can not be determined morphologically. For example, most pathologists agree that absence of malignant criteria in hemangiopericytomas does not guarantee a nonmetastatic behavior.[43] In contrast, severe cellular atypia in superficial cutaneous fibroxanthomas is of no clinical consequence.[44]

It was mentioned previously that some neoplasms, although lacking significant metastatic potential, have a highly invasive growth pattern and require extensive resections to achieve clear margins and prevent uncontrollable local disease. The terminology applied to such locally destructive neoplasms is particularly inconsistent. They are sometimes classified as low-grade malignancies (e.g., fibromatosis may be referred to as low-grade or differentiated fibrosarcoma).[45] However, other similarly persistent and locally invasive neoplasms are classified as benign (e.g., myxoma of the jaw, intramuscular lipoma).[46]

Despite such inconsistencies, nonepithelial neoplasms are subject to the general principles of morphological interpretation. Thus, invasive growth patterns, cytologic atypia, frequency of mitoses, size of tumor, and extent of necrosis are quite reliable criteria in most instances.

Since most nonepithelial neoplasms are large, deeply seated, and lack discrete borders, exfoliative cytology, punch biopsy, shave and excisional biopsies are not appropriate. Needle aspiration or core or incisional biopsies are most often utilized. Material removed by needle from the center of a large tumor may not be interpretable because of the central necrosis which often occurs in large neoplastic masses. More than one area should be sampled by moving the needle in various directions. The adequacy of the material may be assessed by examining frozen sections or touch preparations or smears requiring only few minutes. If necessary the diagnostic procedure could be repeated in the same session.

The very rich blood supply in some of these neoplasms adds significant risk to the biopsy procedure, especially when the location does not permit good control of hemorrhage. In some instances, angiographic studies may be needed prior to any tissue disruption, such as when a large carotid body paraganglioma is suspected.[47]

Superficial biopsies are often nondiagnostic and may even be misleading. For example, a superficial biopsy from a nodule in the tongue may show severe epithelial hyperplasia suspicious for well-differentiated squamous cell carcinoma while the underlying process is indeed a benign granular cell tumor.

The age of the patient is particularly significant in the differential diagnosis of mesenchymal tumors. For example, embryonal rhabdomyosarcoma is a relatively common neoplasm of the head and neck in children but is not usually included in the differential diagnosis in adults.

The following may duplicate some of the discussion in chapter 24, but nonepithelial neoplasms are briefly listed here to clarify the diagnostic spectrum:

Fibrous tissue derivation

Fibromatosis: Consists of well-differentiated fibroblasts and abundant collagen. Malignant cytologic criteria are absent, but the growth pattern is infiltrative and recurrence is frequent. Metastases do not occur. A number of variants have been described according to location, age, and morphology. Postirradiation fibromatosis may have atypical nuclear features. History of irradiation to the involved area is necessary for differential diagnosis.

Fibrosarcoma: Consists of atypical fibroblasts and variable amounts of collagen. The degree of atypia, cellularity, and mitotic activity determines the malignancy grade, but the age of the patient is also an important factor. The growth pattern is infiltrative and recurrences are common. The metastatic potential depends on the grade. Children less than 5 years old have a better prognosis than older subjects with similar tumor morphology.[49] In addition to their usual location in soft tissues, fibrosarcomas may occur in the jaw bones.[50]

Fibrohistiocytic derivation

Benign histiocytoma, fibrous histiocytoma (xanthogranuloma, dermatofibroma, subepidermal nodular fibrosis) are curable by local excision.

Malignant fibrous histiocytoma:

Low-grade (dermatofibrosarcoma protuberans): The growth pattern is infiltrative; local recurrences are frequent, but metastases are extremely uncommon.[51]

High-grade: It is usually located in deep tissues, has overt cytologic malignant criteria and infiltrative growth pattern, and gives distant metastases.

Exception: Atypical fibroxanthoma is a clinicopathologic variant of fibrous histiocytoma of the skin which shows severe cytologic atypia but has no malignant potential and is cured by local excision.[44] It is small, usually less than 2 cm, and superficially located in the dermis of sun-exposed or irradiated skin.

Adipose tissue derivation

Benign lipoma: Usually located in the subcutis and consists of well-differentiated, mature adipocytes. Rarely, it may arise in the oral cavity.[52] Spindle cell lipoma is a variant occurring in the region of neck which is occasionally misinterpreted as malignant.[53]

Liposarcoma: Several morphological variants exist that also differ in their biologic behavior. The well-differentiated variant tends to recur locally but has minimal metastatic potential. Although it may appear well defined, it requires wide excision. The myxoid variant is the most common. It occurs deep within soft tissues and gives a false impression of encapsulation but it is locally invasive and recurs. It has little metastatic potential. The round cell and pleomorphic types of liposarcoma have high metastatic rates.[54] Typically liposarcomas arise from deeply seated tissues. In the head and neck region they may arise in the subcutaneous fat[55] and oral cavity.[56]

Muscle derivation

Benign leiomyoma: A rare tumor in the region of head and neck which may originate from the arrectores pilorum in the skin and occasionally in the tongue.

Leiomyosarcoma: Also very rare in the head and neck. Cases have been reported in the paranasal sinuses and in the oral cavity.[57]

Benign rhabdomyoma: A very rare neoplasm occurring in the oral cavity and pharynx.[58]

Rhabdomyosarcoma: Of the various morphological types, the embryonal is more common in the head and neck of children less than 6 years old. The orbit, nasopharynx, and larynx are the most frequent sites of origin. It is highly malignant but responds to combined therapy.[59] The alveolar type is very rare in the head and neck and is also highly malignant (see chapter 24).

Osseous and cartilaginous derivation

Osteosarcoma: May occasionally arise in the bones of the jaws, especially the mandible.[60] Case reports of osteosarcomas primary in the soft tissues of the larynx exist.[61]

Ossifying fibroma: This benign tumor has been described in the bones of the face and may pose problems in its differential diagnosis from fibrous dysplasia and osteosarcoma.[62]

Benign chondroma: May originate from bones or may develop within the soft tissues of the nasopharynx and larynx. It consists of well-differentiated, predominantly hyalinized cartilage without nuclear atypia.[63]

Chondrosarcoma: Few cases have been reported in

the nasal cavity, the sinuses, nasopharynx, or larynx.[60] Chondrosarcomas may be graded on the basis of morphological malignant criteria. Grade 1 chondrosarcomas may be confused with benign chrondromas. The prognosis depends on location, size, and grade. Complete resection with clear margins is required. Otherwise they recur, and most patients die of uncontrollable local disease.[64] Metastases rarely occur (about 8%).

Exception: Cartilaginous tumors of the larynx usually have a more favorable course than would be expected from their morphology. They usually arise in the subglottic region from the cricoid.[65]

Hematopoietic-lymphoreticular derivation

Lymphomas: Lymph nodes in the nead and neck region are often involved by all types of malignant lymphomas. The classification of lymphomas is revised frequently and is beyond the scope of this text. The bones, soft tissues, and mucosae may also be primary sites of lymphomas. Burkitt's lymphoma has a high predilection for these regions. The tonsils and oropharyngeal and pharyngeal lymphoid tissue are common sites for primary extranodal lymphomas. Concomitant cervical lymphadenopathy may be present.[66]

The term lymphoepithelioma has been used for poorly differentiated carcinomas of the nasopharynx which contain many reactive lymphocytes. The malignant cells are epithelial, with ultrastructural features of squamous differentiation.[27]

Plasmocytoma: Neoplasms of plasma cells occur not only in the bones but also in the soft tissues of head and neck, e.g., in the oral and nasal cavities, nasopharynx, and larynx. They may be part of disseminated multiple myeloma or present as solitary lesions. Most extraosseous solitary plasmocytomas evolve into disseminated disease, although this may take many years.[67]

Vascular derivation

Benign hemangioma: This may be primary in the skin, mucosa, or soft tissues. Subglottic hemangioma occurs typically in infants, while in adults the typical location is on or above the glottis.[68]

Depending on the size of vascular channels, benign hemangiomas are distinguished as capillary, cavernous, or venous. Several distinct histologic types have been recognized in addition to the main categories. The most common of these are:

Angiofibroma. This is characteristically located in the posterior lateral wall of the roof of the nose and has distinct clinical presentation and morphology. It consists of vessels and fibrous stroma and has an invasive growth pattern. The course is variable; it may regress spontaneously or may recur and become locally destructive.[69] Malignant transformation has been described following irradiation.[70]

Glomus tumor (glomangioma). This may be found occasionally in the nasal cavity and is a benign neoplasm.

Hemangiopericytoma. This is a rare neoplasm which may occur in the nasal cavity and paranasal sinuses. It consists of branching, small vascular channels surrounded by spindle cells which lie outside the endothelial basement membranes. The biologic behavior is hard to predict. Local recurrence is common and metastases may develop.[43]

Benign lymphangioma. Most benign proliferations of lymphatic vessels are congenital. They may be cystic (cystic hygroma of the neck) or may diffusely infiltrate the soft tissues, resulting in massive enlargement of organs (macroglossia, macrochelia).

Angiosarcoma. The head and neck of elderly individuals are often the primary site of this rare neoplasm. The neoplastic cells show endothelial differentiation, form irregular anastomosing channels, and pile up, projecting into the lumina. This is a malignant neoplasia which recurs and eventually spreads to lymph nodes and lungs. Except for the skin, the nasal cavity and paranasal sinuses may be the site of origin.[71] Angiosarcoma of the thyroid is a controversial entity.

Kaposi's sarcoma. This is also a malignant neoplasm of vascular origin which has a predilection for immunodeficient subjects.[72] The lesions are multiple and may occasionally involve the head and neck.

Neural Derivation

Neurofibroma: A benign tumor affecting skin, mucosae, or deep tissues. Multiple plexiform neurofibromas are characteristic of Recklinghausen's disease.

Neurilemmoma: A benign encapsulated neoplasm which compresses but does not infiltrate the nerve of origin. It may be enucleated without resecting the nerve. The histology is usually very distinct, with nuclear palisading and organoid structures. It may undergo extensive cystic degeneration.

Malignant schwannoma (neurofibrosarcoma): Essentially a malignant neurofibroma. The diagnosis must be supported by identifying the nerve of origin or residual neurofibroma or by evidence of von Recklinghausen's disease. The course is characterized by recurrences and distant metastases.[73]

Olfactory neuroblastoma (esthesioneuroblastoma): A unique neoplasm that arises from neuroepithelium in the roof of the nasal fossa and, very rarely, in paranasal sinuses. It consists of small uniform oval cells and fibrillary matrix. Neurofilaments and dense-core cytoplasmic granules (neurosecretory) are seen on electron microscopy. It is highly infiltrative, often extending into the sinuses, nasopharynx, orbit, and brain. It may metastasize to lymph nodes and lung. The differential diagnosis includes rhabdomyosarcoma and lymphoma.[74]

Ectopic glioma

Paraganglioma (nonchromaffin, chemodectomma):

- Carotid body tumor. A benign neoplasm with only rare exceptions of malignant course.
- Glomus Jugularae. A locally destructive, nonmetastasizing tumor.
- Glomus of larynx. A rare benign tumor of the subglottic region.

Neoplasms of the Odontogenic Apparatus

Ameloblastoma: Usually involves the mandible and is characterized by the presence of ameloblasts and stellate reticulum. It recurs but does not give distant metastases.[75]

Ameloblastic fibroma: A benign neoplasm that differs from ameloblastoma because of the abundant mesenchymal component. It responds favorably to simple curettage.[76]

Adenomatoid and calcifying epithelial odontogenic tumors are benign but the latter may recur.

Ameloblastic carcinoma and ameloblastic fibrosarcoma are the malignant counterparts of ameloblastoma and ameloblastic fibroma, respectively.

Odontoma: A benign neoplasm that may occasionally be locally aggressive. Morphology is helpful in determining the aggressive potential.[77]

Myxoma of the jaw: Believed to be odontogenic, involves the maxilla or mandible. It is locally destructive and may recur.[78]

Melanocytic Derivation

Benign nevocellular nevi: These very common lesions of the skin are classified into junctional, compound, and intradermal, depending on the location relative to the dermal-epidermal junction.

Malignant melanoma: see chapter 22.

Blue nevus: Consists of spindle dermal melanocytes and may arise in the skin or mucosa.[79]

Cellular blue nevus: Consists of very cellular nodules of dermal melanocytes and may become locally destructive.[80]

Malignant melanoma: see chapter 22.

Miscellaneous

Granular cell tumor: A proliferation of benign cells which have abundant, finely granular, eosinophilic cytoplasm. The granules stain PAS positive and correspond to lysosomes. The histogenetic derivation of these cells is uncertain. It has been suggested that they derive from myocytes, schwann cells, or from various types of cells through a peculiar degenerative process. The tongue is the most common site of origin, followed by the skin. The larynx is among other organs less frequently involved. The overlying epithelium often becomes markedly hyperplastic and may contribute to misdiagnosis of epithelial neoplasia. Granular cell tumors are benign, with very few exceptions.[81]

Synovial sarcoma: A malignant neoplasm of mesenchymal derivation which shows differentiation toward synovial membrane. It does not usually arise from preformed synovium and, as a rule, is not found within joints. The neck region is one of the sites where this rare neoplasm has been reported with some frequency.[82] Morphologically it is characterizied by a biphasic pattern (epithelium-like and fibroblast-like cells). The prognosis of head and neck synovial sarcomas is similar as in other anatomical locations.

Chordoma: A neoplasm originating from notochordal rests and characterized histologically by large "physalipherous" cells embedded in abundant mucoid stroma. About 30% arise in the area of the spheno-occipital synchondrosis. They may extend into the nasopharynx, nasal cavity, and antrum. Rarely, growth may extend into the cervical vertebrae. Prognosis is poor due to the difficulty of achieving complete excisions. A high frequency of recurrence is typical.[83]

REFERENCES

1. Giunta J., Meyer I., Shklar G.: The accuracy of the oral biopsy in the diagnosis of cancer. *Oral Surg.* 28:552, 1969.
2. Dehner L.P., Rosai J.: Frozen section examination in surgical pathology: A retrospective study of one year experience comprising 778 cases. *Minn. Med.* 60:83, 1977.
3. American Joint Committee on Cancer: *Staging of Cancer of Head and Neck Sites and of Melanoma.* Chicago, American Joint Committee on Cancer, 1980.
4. Cawson R.A.: Premalignant lesions of the mouth. *Br. Med. Bull.* 31:164, 1975.
5. Pindborg J.J., Defrary D.K., Mehta F.S.A.: A follow-up study of 61 oral dysplastic precancerous lesions in Indian villagers. *Oral Surg.* 43:383, 1977.
6. Woolner L.B., Beahrs O.H., Black B.M., et al.: Thyroid carcinoma: General considerations and follow-up data on 1181 cases, in Yung S., Inman D.R. (eds.): *Thyroid Neoplasia: Proceedings of the Second Imperial Cancer Research Fund Symposium.* New York, Academic Press, 1968, p. 51.
7. Rosai J.: In *Surgical Pathology.* St. Louis, C.V. Mosby Co., 1981.
8. Stout A.P.: Juvenile fibromatosis. *Cancer* 7:953–978, 1954.
9. Rosai J.: In *Surgical Pathology.* St. Louis, C.V. Mosby Co., 1981, p. 357.
10. Batsakis J.G.: *Tumors of the Head and Neck: Clinical and Pathological Considerations.* Baltimore, Williams & Wilkins Co., 1979.
11. Smith C.: Carcinoma in situ. *Am. J. Dermatopathol.* 1:145, 1979.
12. Ackerman A.B.: Carcinoma in situ. *Am. J. Dermatopathol.* 1:147, 1979.
13. Slaughter D.P., Southwick H.W., Smejkal W.: "Field cancerization" in oral stratified squamous epithelium: Clinical implications of multicentric origin. *Cancer* 6:963, 1953.
14. Bauer W.C.: Concomitant carcinoma in situ and invasive carcinoma of the larynx. *Can. J. Otolaryngol.* 3:533, 1974.
15. Shafer W.G.: Oral carcinoma in situ. *Oral Surg.* 39:227, 1975.
16. Hampel H.: Preinvasive carcinoma: Recent results. *Cancer Res.* 44:53, 1974.
17. Jesse R.H.: In Suen J.Y., Myers E.N. (eds.): *Cancer of the Head and Neck: General Considerations.* New York, Churchill Livingstone, 1981, p. 1.
18. Jansen G.T., Westbrook K.C.: In Suen J.Y., Myers E.M. (eds.): In *Cancer of the Head and Neck: General Considerations.* New York, Churchill Livingstone, 1981, p. 212.
19. Batsakis J.C.: In *Tumors of the Head and Neck: Clinical and Pathological Considerations.* Baltimore, Williams & Wilkins Co., 1979, p. 153.
20. Looser K.G., Shah J.P., Strong E.W.: The significance of "positive" margins in surgically resected epidermoid carcinomas. *Head Neck Surg.* 1:107, 1978.
21. Bauer W.C.: Varieties of squamous carcinoma: Biologic behavior. *Front. Radiat. Ther. Oncol.* 9:164, 1974.
22. Broders A.C.: Carcinoma grading and practical application. *Arch. Pathol. Lab. Med.* 2:376, 1926.
23. Finley A.G.: Kerato-acanthoma. *Aust. J. Dermatol.* 2:144, 1954.
24. Lever W.F., Schaumberg-Lever G.: In *Histopathology of the Skin,* ed. 6. Philadelphia, J.B. Lippincott Co.
25. Rook A., Kexdel-Vegas R., Young J.A.: Recurrences in kerato-acanthoma. *Med. Cutan. Iber. Lat. Am.* 11:17, 1967.
26. Lee J.G.: Detection of residual carcinoma of the oral cavity, oropharynx, hypopharynx and larynx: A study of surgical margins. *Trans. Am. Acad. Ophthalmol. Otolaryngol.* 78:948–949, 1974.
27. Svoboda D.J., Kirchner F.R., Shanmugaratnam K.: The fine structure of nasopharyngeal carcinomas, in Muir C.S., Shanmugaratnam K. (eds.): *Cancer of the Nasopharynx.* Copenhagen, Munksgaard, 1967, p. 163.
28. Lichtiger B., Mackay B., Tessmer C.F.: Spindle-cell variant of squamous carcinoma: A light and electron microscope study of 13 cases. *Cancer* 26:1311, 1970.
29. Friedel W., Chambers R.G., Atkins J.P.: Pseudosarcoma of the pharynx and larynx. *Arch. Otolaryngol.* 102:286, 1976.
30. Fonts E.A., Greenlaw R.H., Rush B.F., et al.: Verrucous squamous cell carcinoma of the oral cavity. *Cancer* 23:152, 1969.
31. Biller H.F., Ogura J.H., Bauer W.C.: Verrucous cancer of the larynx. *Laryngoscope* 81:1323, 1971.
32. Kraus F., Perez-Mesa C.: Verrucous carcinoma: Clinical and pathological study of 105 cases involving oral cavity, larynx and genitalia. *Cancer* 19:26, 1966.
33. Rider W.D.: Toronto experience of verrucous carcinoma of the larynx, in Alberti P.W., Bryce D.P. (eds.): *Workshops From the Centennial Conference on Laryngeal Cancer.* New York, Appleton-Century-Crofts, 1976, p. 460.
34. Rock J.A., Fisher E.R.: Florid papillomatosis of the oral cavity and larynx. *Arch. Otolaryngol.* 72:593, 1960.
35. Samitz M.H., Ackerman A.B., Lantis L.R.: Squamous cell carcinoma arising at the site of the oral florid papillomatosis. *Arch. Dermatol.* 96:286, 1967.
36. Batsakis J.G.: In *Tumors of the Head and Neck: Clinical and Pathological Considerations.* Baltimore, Williams & Wilkins Co., 1979, pp. 135–136.
37. Chandhry A.P., Vickers R.A., Gorlin R.J.: Intraoral minor salivary gland tumors: An analysis of 1414 cases. *Oral Surg.* 14:1194, 1961.
38. Spiro R.H., Koss L.G., Hajdu S.L., et al.: Tumors of minor salivary origins: A clinicopathologic study of 492 cases. *Cancer* 31:117, 1973.
39. Batsakis J.G., Holtz F., Sneper R.H.: Adenocarcinoma of the nasal and paranasal cavities. *Arch. Otolaryngol.* 77:625, 1963.
40. Foote F.W. Jr., Frazell E.L.: Tumors of the major salivary glands. *Cancer.* 6:1065, 1953.

41. Healey W.V., Perzin K.H., Smith L.: Mucoepidermoid carcinoma of salivary gland origin: Classification, clinical-pathologic correlation and results of treatment. *Cancer* 26:368, 1970.
42. Spiro R.H., Huvos A.G., Berk R., et al., Mucoepidermoid carcinoma of salivary gland origin: A clinicopathologic study of 367 cases. *Am. J. Surg.* 136:461, 1978.
43. Hajdu S.I.: *Pathology of Soft Tissue Tumors.* Philadelphia, Lea & Febiger 1979, p. 385.
44. Dahl I.: Atypical fibroxanthoma of the skin. *Acta Pathol. Microbiol. Scand.* [A] 84:183, 1976.
45. Butler J.J.: Fibrous tissue tumors: Nodular fascitis, dermatofibrosarcoma protuberans, and fibrosarcoma, grade I, desmoid type, in *Tumors of Bone and Soft Tissue.* Chicago, Year Book Medical Publishers, Inc., 1965, p. 397.
46. Dionne C.P., Seemayer T.A.: Infiltrating lipomas and angiolipomas revisited. *Cancer* 34:720, 1974.
47. Batsakis J.G.: In *Tumors of the Head and Neck: Clinical and Pathological Considerations.* Baltimore, Williams & Wilkins, 1979, p. 373.
48. Rosai J.: In *Surgical Pathology.* St. Louis, C.V. Mosby Co., 1981, pp. 1417–1418.
49. Soule E.H., Pritchard D.J.: Fibrosarcoma in infants and children: A review of 110 cases. *Cancer* 40:1711, 1977.
50. Van Blarcom C.W., Masson J.K., Dahlin D.C.: Fibrosarcoma of the mandible. *Oral Surg.* 32:428, 1971.
51. Taylor H.B., Helwig E.B.: Dermatofibrosarcoma protuberans: A study of 115 cases. *Cancer* 15:717, 1962.
52. Hatziotis J.C.: Lipoma of the oral cavity. *Oral Surg.* 31:511, 1971.
53. Enzinger F.M., Harvey D.A.: Spindle cell lipoma. *Cancer* 36:1852, 1975.
54. Kindblom L.G., Angervall L., Svendsen P.: Liposarcoma: A clinicopathologic, radiographic and prognostic study. *Acta Pathol. Microbiol. Scand. Suppl.* 253, 1975.
55. Sauk J.J. Jr.: Liposarcoma of the head and neck. *J. Oral Surg.* 29:38, 1971.
56. Badeu E., Newmay R.: Liposarcoma of the oropharyngeal region: Review of the literature and report of two cases. *Oral Surg.* 44:889, 1977.
57. Farman A.G., Kay S.: Oral leiomyosarcoma: Report of a case and review of the literature pertaining to smooth muscle tumors of the oral cavity. *Oral Surg.* 43:402, 1977.
58. Di Sant'Agnese P.A., Knowles D.M.: Extracardiac rhabdomyoma. *Cancer* 46:780, 1980.
59. Maurer H.M.: Rhabdomyosarcoma in childhood and adolescence. *Curr. Probl. Cancer* 2:3, 1978.
60. Garrington G.E., Scofield H.H., Cornyn J., et al.: Osteosarcoma of the jaws. *Cancer* 20:377, 1967.
61. Dalun L.J., Schaefer S.D., Carder H.M., et al.: Osteosarcoma of the soft tissue of the larynx. *Cancer* 42:2343, 1978.
62. Langdon J.D., Rapidis A.D., Patel M.F.: Ossifying fibroma—one disease or six? An analysis of 39 fibro-osseous lesions of the jaws. *Br. J. Oral Surg.* 14:1, 1976.
63. Chaudhry A.P., Robinovitch M.R., Mitchell D.F., et al.: Chondrogenic tumors of the jaws. *Am. J. Surg.* 102:403, 1961.
64. Fu Y.-S., Perzin K.H.: Non-epithelial tumors of the nasal cavity, paranasal sinuses and nasopharynx: A clinicopathologic study. *Cancer* 34:453, 1974.
65. Goethals P.L., Dahlin D.C., Devine K.D.: Cartilaginous tumors of the larynx. *Surg. Gynecol. Obstet.* 117:77–82, 1963.
66. Freeman C., Berg J.W., Cutler S.J.: Occurrence and prognosis of extranodal lymphomas. *Cancer* 29:252, 1972.
67. Fu Y.-S., Perzin K.H.: Nonepithelial tumors of the nasal cavity, paranasal sinuses and nasopharynx: A clinicopathologic study. X malignant lymphomas. *Cancer* 43:611, 1979.
68. Ferguson G.B.: Hemangioma of the adult and of the infant larynx. *Arch. Otolaryngol.* 40:189, 1944.
69. Neel H.B., Whicker J.H., Devine K.D., et al.: Juvenile angiofibroma: Review of 120 cases. *Am. J. Surg.* 126:547, 1973.
70. Batsakis J.G., Klopp C.T., Newman W.: Fibrosarcoma arising in a "juvenile" nasopharyngeal angiofibroma following extensive radiation therapy. *Am. Surg.* 21:786, 1955.
71. McClatchey K.D., Batsakis J.G., Rice D.H.: Angiosarcoma of the maxillary sinus: Report of a case. *J. Oral Surg.* 34:1019, 1976.
72. Klepp O., Dahl O., Stenwig J.T.: Association of Kaposi's sarcoma and prior immunosuppressive therapy: A 5 year material of Kaposi's sarcoma in Norway. *Cancer* 42:2626, 1978.
73. D'Agostino A.N., Soule E.H., Miller R.H.: Primary malignant neoplasm of nerves (malignant neurilemmoma) in patients without manifestations of multiple neurofibromatosis. *Cancer* 16:1003, 1963.
74. Kahn L.B.: Esthesioneuroblastoma: A light and electron microscopic study. *Hum. Pathol.* 5:364, 1974.
75. Mehlisch D.R., Dahlin D.C., Masson J.K.: Ameloblastoma: A clinicopathologic report. *J. Oral Surg.* 30:9, 1972.
76. Gorlin R.J., Meskin L.H., Brodey R.: Odontogenic tumors of man and animals: Pathological classification and clinical behavior. A review. *Ann. NY Acad. Sci.* 108:722, 1963.
77. Baden E.: Odontogenic tumors. *Pathol. Ann.* 6:475, 1971.
78. White D.K., Chen S.Y., Molinac A.M., et al.: Odontogenic myxoma: A clinical and ultrastructional study. *Oral Surg.* 39:901, 1975.
79. Harper J.C., Waldroy C.A.: Blue nevus of palate. *Oral Surg.* 20:145, 1965.
80. Rodriguez H., Ackerman L.V.: Cellular blue nevus. *Cancer* 21:393, 1968.
81. Al-Sarraf M., Loud A.V., Vaitkevicius V.K.: Malignant granular cell tumor: Histochemical and electron microscopic study. *Arch. Pathol.* 91:550–558, 1971.
82. Roth J.A., Enzinger F.M., Tanneubaum M.: Synovial sarcoma of the neck: A follow-up study of 24 cases. *Cancer* 35:1243, 1975.
83. Dahlin D.C., MacCarty C.S.: Chordoma: A study of 59 cases. *Cancer* 5:1170, 1952.

5 / Assessing Pretreatment Systemic Risk Factors: The Effect on Treatment Decisions

DONALD G. MCQUARRIE, M.D., PH.D.

Who shall decide, when doctors disagree, and soundest casuists doubt like you and me

Alexander Pope (1688–1744) Epistle iii to Lord Bathurst

PREOPERATIVE DECISION-MAKING is more than selecting one therapy over another therapy. Chapter 1 began the approach to clinical decision-making in head and neck cancer. This chapter discusses in detail the process of making difficult choices using a decision tree. Each treatment for head and neck cancer patient has its own requirements for time, anesthesia, and costs. Mortality, morbidity, and deformity are altered by each choice. The discussion in this chapter assumes a general knowledge of surgical and anesthetic risk factors. There are unique aspects of treatment risks in head and neck cancer patients that set these patients apart from the usual cancer patient. There is a good news-bad news dichotomy. The good news is that treatment of head and neck cancer does not carry the risk that treatment of thoracic and abdominal visceral cancer does. The risk criteria for major general surgery cannot be transferred directly to head and neck surgery. The bad news is that patients with head and neck cancer are usually older and beset with more cardiovascular, pulmonary, hepatic, and nutritional disease. Several key risk factors will be examined and analyzed. A structured method of examining risk is presented as just one of several possible models for decision-making. A preoperative decision must reflect wide variations of real risks and allow for "quality of life" estimates.

WHAT RISK FACTORS POSE PARTICULAR PROBLEMS IN TREATING HEAD AND NECK CANCER PATIENTS?

A categorical list would include the following:

1. Advanced age with a decline in the functional reserves of the heart, lung, kidney, and general neurologic functions[1, 2].
2. High rate of atherosclerosis:
   a. Coronary artery disease
   b. Cerebral vascular disease
   c. Peripheral vascular disease
3. Respiratory disease:
   a. Acute airway obstruction
   b. Chronic obstructive pulmonary disease
   c. Second primary oroairway cancer
4. Effects of alcoholism:
   a. Acute toxic or withdrawal symptoms
   b. Cirrhosis of the liver
   c. Alcoholic CNS degeneration and/or peripheral neuropathy
   d. Malnutrition
   e. Acute alcoholic gastritis and/or peptic ulcer
   f. Decreased synthesis of vitamin K–dependent blood clotting factors secondary to (b)
5. Nutritional deficiencies:
   a. Calories—weight loss
   b. Protein—muscle wasting
   c. Vitamins B, C, K (relative)
   d. Trace elements, Mg^{++}
6. Poor oral hygiene:
   a. Periodontal sepsis
   b. Caries
7. Impaired immune mechanisms due to malnutrition, chemical toxicity, and/or tumor
8. Fluid and electrolyte abnormalities:
   a. Chronic low sodium syndrome
   b. Low potassium
9. Unrepaired anemia
10. Need for emotional support
11. Other diseases

The risks of complicating diseases have to be factored into the well-known risks of treatment by anesthesia and surgery. One cannot assume that radiation therapy is totally risk free. It adds its own particular set of acute and late risks. Ballantyne reported a 6% late mortality in nasopharyngeal cancer patients (Table 5–1).[3] Larson et al. found a 40%–70% incidence of severe late radiation sequelae in oral and oropharyngeal sites in their review of the M. D. Anderson Hospital experience.[4] Multidrug chemotherapy carries the risk of direct lethal toxicity and later septic sequelae in the immunocompromised phase (see Chap. 8).

IS THE SURGICAL MORTALITY RISK OF A MAJOR HEAD AND NECK CANCER RESECTION COMPARABLE TO THE RISK OF OTHER SURGICAL PROCEDURES?

Beahrs set an enviable standard of 908 consecutive head and neck surgical cases with one death (0.1%).[5] Many other groups have reported a 30-day operative mortality of 1%–2%.[6–8] In our own patients, mortality

TABLE 5–1.—FATAL COMPLICATIONS IN 218 PATIENTS COMPLETING RADIATION THERAPY FOR NASOPHARYNGEAL CARCINOMAS*

FATAL COMPLICATIONS†	NO.
Stricture of pharynx	1
Spinal cord myelopathy	5
Necrosis with fatal hemorrhage	3
Nerve paralysis	2
Brain abscess	1
Radiation-induced cancer	1
Total	13/218 = 6% mortality

*Data abstracted from Ballantyne.[3]
†Complications occurred from 1½ months following irradiation to years later. The majority occurred in the first 2 years. It should be emphasized that complications are increased by the difficult location and the need to treat the nasopharyngeal cancer aggressively.

TABLE 5–2.—POSTOPERATIVE DEATH (30-DAY) IN HEAD AND NECK CANCER PATIENTS*

STUDY, YEAR	DEATHS/TOTAL NO. OF CASES	INSTITUTION	CAUSE OF DEATH: CARDIOVASC.	AIRWAY OR PULMONARY	HEMORRHAGE	HEPATIC	RENAL	OTHER AND UNSPECIFIED
O'Brien and Catlin,[9] 1965	4/122 (3%)	Memorial Hosp., New York	1		1		2	
Ruffine and MacComb,[10] 1966	6/180 (2%)	M. D. Anderson Hosp.		2	2			2
Kremen,[11] 1967	0/49 (0%)	Private						
Beahrs,[5] 1973	1/908 (0.1%)	Mayo		1				
Robbins et al.,[12] 1975	7/100 (7%)	Vancouver Gen.		6‡	1			
Joyce and McQuarrie,[13] 1976	2/178 (1%)	Univ. of Minn.	1			1		
Shedd and Calamel,[14] 1976	4/228 (2%)	Roswell Park		1	1			2§
Mendelson et al.,[15] 1976	3/307 (1%)	Mayo	2		1			
Total	2072 (1.3%)		4	10	6	1	2	4
Ward et al.,[16]† 1959	18/577 (3%)	Johns Hopkins	*Causes of death not specified*					
Spiro and Strong,[17] 1973	3/333 (1%)	Memorial Hosp., New York						
Shaw and Tollefson,[18] 1974	15/352 (4%)	Memorial Hosp., New York						
Chu and Strawitz,[19] 1978	10/271 (4%)	Fox Chase						

*Data were selected to represent different cancer sites and medical centers.
†Include to give an older series
‡Airway obstruction, 3 acute aspiration, 2 pneumonia
§Pulmonary embolism

has been 1% for the past decade. There is an anecdotal experience to suggest that head and neck surgery does not have the metabolic, respiratory, or cardiovascular impact of intra-abdominal or thoracic surgery. Acute surgical mortality risk is low (Table 5–2). At 24–48 hours, the patient is usually near general preoperative vigor. Pulmonary and cardiovascular events dominate the postoperative complications. Lethal hemorrhage in the postoperative period is almost always a consequence of tissue necrosis in areas of previous irradiation.

In selecting treatment, the induction of anesthesia poses the first risk. Anesthesiologists have been pioneers in defining risk categories. The widely used Dripps-American Society of Anesthesiologists (ASA) grouping is based on the general physical status of the patient, as follows:

Class I—A normal healthy patient undergoing elective operation.

Class II—A patient with mild systemic disease.

Class III—A patient with severe systemic disease that limits activity but is not incapacitating.

Class IV—A patient with incapacitating systemic disease that is a constant threat to life.

Class V—A moribund patient who is not expected to survive 24 hours with or without an operation.

The suffix "E" is used if the operation is an emergency.

The Dripps-ASA classification has been clinically used and analyzed. In a review of 68,388 different operations, Vacanti et al. found a direct correlation between higher classification and a higher 48-hour mortality (Table 5–3).[20] In most studies of postoperative deaths, there is a heavy representation of cardiac-related causes. Lewin et al. studied a group of "high-risk" elderly patients in 1970.[21] They found that all

TABLE 5–3.—MORTALITY RATES (WITHIN 48 HOURS) FOR EACH ASA PHYSICAL STATUS CLASS*†

PHYSICAL STATUS	ANESTHETIC PROCEDURES (N)	DEATHS (N)	MORTALITY (%)
I	50,703	43	0.08
II	12,601	34	0.27
III	3,626	66	1.8
IV	850	66	7.8
V	608	57	9.4
Total	68,388	266	0.39

*Data taken from Vacanti et al.[20]
†Mortality from elective and emergency operations performed in 11 U.S. Naval Hospitals, July 1964 to June 1966.

deaths occurred in patients in Dripps-ASA classes III, IV, and V. After refining the risk estimates in terms of measured preoperative physiologic parameters, Lewin et al. found that a measure of cardiac performance (left ventricular stroke work) and a measure of respiratory effectiveness (A − a gradient) were better predictors of complications and death. Their high-risk groups were:

A—Good ventricular function, low A − a Do_2 gradient: 10% mortality.
B—Good ventricular function, high A − a Do_2 gradient: 22% mortality.
C—Poor ventricular function, low A − a Do_2 gradient: 45% mortality.
D—Poor ventricular function, high A − a Do_2 gradient: 71% mortality.

The duration of a procedure has been related to operative mortality. In 587 patients with known heart disease who underwent different types of noncardiac surgery, Steen et al. found a direct linear correlation of reinfarction with the duration of anesthesia.[22] The rate calculates to a 2.57% increase in likelihood of reinfarction per hour of surgery. Therefore, a 6-hour procedure would have a 15.4% reinfarction rate. Obviously, head and neck patients will have longer procedures, but does that 6-hour period contain the same physiologic events as the 6 hours required for a thoracotomy, an aneurysmectomy, or a lesion that has produced septic peritonitis? The analysis needs further refinement. Stein et al.[22] did analyze their cases further, as shown in Table 5–4. Extracavitary surgery, such as head and neck surgery, is clearly safer than an operation within one of the major body cavities. Nachlas had shown that mastectomy, another extracavitary procedure, did not pose the high risk that accompanies laparotomy or thoracotomy.[23] Skinner and Pierce had no deaths in high-risk cardiac patients undergoing head and neck surgery, while those undergoing cholecystectomy had a 12% mortality, and the mortality from gastric resection was much higher.[24] Intraperitoneal procedures had a 29% overall mortality in these very ill patients with heart disease. Other factors minimizing systemic impact of head and neck surgery are the following:

1. Lower levels of anesthesia and muscle relaxants are required.
2. Precise hemostasis is easy to maintain.
3. There is no pressure or traction on lung, liver, or heart.
4. There is little impairment of respiratory bellows.
5. Ileus is infrequent and of short duration.
6. There is no need for bed rest.
7. External nutrition can resume in 24–48 hours.

TABLE 5–4.—RELATION OF MYOCARDIAL REINFARCTION TO DURATION OF ANESTHESIA IN 587 PATIENTS (WITH PREVIOUS MYOCARDIAL INFARCTION) UNDERGOING NONCARDIAC SURGERY*

GROUP	SITE: Intrathoracic and Upper Abdominal	SITE: Other
	Anesthesia < 3 Hours	
No. of pts.	68	329
Reinfarcts	4 (5.9%)	12 (3.6%)
	Anesthesia > 3 Hours	
No. of pts.	107	78
Reinfarcts	17 (15.9%)	3 (3.8%)

*Data derived from Steen et al.[22]

Head and neck cancer surgery should carry a significantly lower risk than intracavitary procedures in comparable patients. The data of Table 5–2 confirm the low mortality. Some retrospective series reach farther into the past than others; consequently the mortality may be higher. Authors reporting low mortalities have exercised considerable attention to detail and judgment. Dr. Beahrs' Hayes Martin Lecture on minimizing morbidity and mortality is well worth a trip to the library.[5] To achieve low mortalities, the surgeon must promptly recognize and treat complications.

WHAT GENERAL PREOPERATIVE STRATEGIES CAN BE EFFECTIVE IN MINIMIZING OPERATIVE RISKS?

One way clinicians evaluate risk is to mentally run through a large number of logically assembled scenarios of anticipated events. They see if they can produce the panoply of answers for all of the "worst case" problems. The more experienced the surgeon, the larger the number of cliff-hangers he may anticipate. One must look carefully for risk factors that can be reduced or eliminated with preoperative care. About one third of our head and neck cancer patients need detoxification, nutritional supplementation, and oral hygiene. Another third have a complicating disease that can usually be improved. Frequent complicating preoperative illness was found in 79 consecutive patients with cancer of the tongue.[25] These problem diseases are listed in Table 5–5. The list includes diseases that complicate both surgery and anesthesia.

Priority of attention must be given to complications that cause postoperative death (see Table 5–2). Hemorrhage is a leading cause of death. Where details are available, the pattern was typically heavy irradiation (usually more than 6 months previously), infection and/or wound breakdown, an exposed irradiated carotid artery, focal vascular necrosis, hemorrhage. This sequence is best avoided by planning an operation that protects the vessel with viable tissue. If the complication occurs, management is prompt (see Chap. 27).

The next most common problem is respiratory death due to aspiration, airway occlusion, or pneumonia in the heavy smoker with advanced chronic obstructive lung disease and/or wasted respiratory musculature.

Cardiovascular problems are as frequent as respiratory complications. Sudden cardiac death and lethal arrhythmias are a constant threat. Renal and hepatic problems contribute an occasional death.

ACQUIRED HEART DISEASE IS A COMMON PROBLEM IN ASSESSING RISKS AND PLANNING A TREATMENT PROGRAM. HOW MUCH DOES HEART DISEASE INFLUENCE ALTERNATIVES?

Known or unrecognized heart disease is common in any elderly population. We obtained a computer-interpreted electrocardiogram (ECG) in 200 consecutive patients over 50 years old admitted to the hospital for noncardiac reasons. Forty percent of the patients had an abnormal ECG. (Two patients with injury current were sent directly to ICU.) Twenty percent of the 200 were known to have abnormal ECGs. *Therefore, an equal number of abnormal ECGs were totally unsuspected.* The subsequent admitting history failed to elicit evidence of significant heart disease.

TABLE 5–5.—COMPLICATING PREOPERATIVE ILLNESSES IN 79 CONSECUTIVE PATIENTS WITH CANCER OF THE TONGUE*

COMPLICATION	N
Peptic ulcer (bleeding, perforation, or gastrectomy in the past)	12
Laennec's cirrhosis (chemically or biopsy proved)	11
Heart disease (previous infarct, significant valvular disease, failure)	6
Alcoholic neuropathy	5
Concurrent carcinoma	3
Active tuberculosis†	3
Pernicious anemia	3
Severe hypertension	3
Other diseases requiring hospitalization (diabetes, etc.)	5

*Disease was entered if patient had been hospitalized for it in recent past. No patient had more than two diseases entered.
†In patient's treated earlier in series.

Acquired heart disease is always a potential risk. When we know it is present, a modern workup can define past damage down to the left ventricular ejection fraction. It is much harder to predict tomorrow's cardiac event. Recognizing that a patient has significant heart disease concomitant with a certainly lethal malignancy is only the first step on the way to a decision. A flood of questions are triggered. Myocardial infarct? When? Angina pectoris present? How often? What provokes it? Congestive heart failure now or in the past? Patient on medications? What medications? Will an anesthetic be tolerated? How long? What are other treatment options? Radiation? Cryotherapy? Can we get the patient in better shape? Key question—Can we tidy up our decision-making process? Yes!

Rogers reviewed the anesthetic management of patients with heart disease.[26] Newer data have made it easier to select anesthetics and provide supportive measures such as pacemakers.

The data in Tables 5–3 and 5–4 combined with the ASA classification give us a beginning guide. More refinement is needed. A first step is to recognize that there is a greater likelihood of postoperative death if the patient has had a myocardial infarct in the past 6 months.[22, 27, 28] In Steen's series, patients operated on within 3 months of a myocardial infarct had a 27% reinfarction rate. Those operated on 3–6 months later had a reinfarction rate of 11%, and after 6 months the rate stabilized at 4%–5%.[22] Although the data of Table 5–4 suggest less risk for head and neck surgery, the reinfarction rate undoubtedly increases with proximity to the first infarction. There are additional discriminating features which are important. Goldman et al. studied 1,001 consecutive major operations, of which 231 involved the head and neck.[28] In that series of patients, 103 had dyspnea of cardiac origin, 69 had classic angina pectoris, 69 had atypical chest pain, 280 were hypertensive, 58 had documented hyperlipidemia, and 23 had aortic stenosis. Many other features were present and recorded. Of the 1,001 patients, 19 died in the postoperative period from cardiac disease. Forty others died of noncardiac causes. Thirty-six had pulmonary edema; 12 had ventricular tachycardia but did not die. Weighted multifactorial calculations produced a "point" scoring system that would have predicted fatality in their patients. This system is shown in Table 5–6. An important lesson Goldman et al. stress is that 28 of the possible 53 "points" are potentially controllable with optimum preoperative care. Thus, there is an opportunity to lower operative risk, if time allows. The general death rates for coronary heart disease are shown in

TABLE 5–6.—ESTIMATION OF CARDIAC RISK FOR MAJOR NONCARDIAC SURGERY PATIENTS*

CRITERIA	"POINTS"
History	
Age > 70 yr	5
MI in previous 6 mo.	10
Physical examination	
S_3 gallops or jugular vein distention	11
Important valvular aortic stenosis	3
Electrocardiogram	
Rhythm other than sinus or premature atrial contractions or last preop. ECG	7
>5 PVCs/minute documented any time preoperatively	7
General status	
$Po_2 < 60$ mm Hg, $PCo_2 > 50$ mm Hg, $K^+ < 3$ or $HCO_3^- < 20$ mEq/L, BUN > 50 or Cr. > 3.0 mg/dl, abnormal SGOT, signs of chronic liver disease, or patient bedridden from noncardiac cause	3
Operation	
Intraperitoneal, intrathoracic, or aortic operation	3
Emergency operation	4

RECOMMENDATIONS:
>26 points: life-saving procedures only.
13–25 points: sufficient cardiac risk to warrant preoperative cardiac consultation and in-hospital improvement of cardiac function.
<13 points: less risk.

*Modified from Goldman et al.[28] See original publication for more detail.

Table 5–7.[29] We now appreciate the tremendous additive effect of heavy smoking on coronary artery disease. The data on cardiac risk from smoking reported in two large studies are combined in Table 5–8.[30, 31]

HOW CAN WE WEIGH POTENTIAL THERAPEUTIC RISKS AGAINST THE THREAT OF KNOWN MALIGNANT DISEASE?

The final objective is to achieve the longest survival of life with enough quality to be acceptable to the patient. The data we have developed so far can be used to select therapy by several judgmental systems. One of the more objective methods has been advanced by Beck et al.[32, 33] It is well worth considering in detail as an example of structured clinical decision-making. It

TABLE 5–8.—RELATIVE RISK OF CORONARY ARTERY DISEASE AND CIGARETTE SMOKING IN MEN IN THE UNITED STATES: RISK RATIO, SMOKERS/NONSMOKERS*

STUDY, AGES (YR)	NO. OF CIGARETTES SMOKED/DAY			
	0	<20	20	>20
Framingham Heart Study				
45–54	1.00	1.29	1.67	2.15
55–64	1.00	1.15	1.32	1.51
65–74	1.00	1.12	1.24	1.39
Western Collaborative Group Study				
39–49	1.00	1.29	1.56	1.95
50–59	1.00	1.33	1.77	2.35

*Data from Kannel et al.[30] and Rosenman et al.[31]

also emphasizes the need for clear, reliable, detailed data.

Beck and co-workers estimate a patient's specific life expectancy as an outcome of various therapeutic choices. They have presented analyses that corroborate the assumption that survival with most diseases follows a simple declining exponential function.[32] This was found by Humphrey et al. to be true for other malignancies, including lung cancer.[34] An exponential curve is probably valid over a 5- to 10-year interval. Beck et al. used the exponential curve assumption in a method called the *declining exponential approximation of life expectancy* (DEALE).[33] This allows us to use clinically available data (life expectancy, 5-year survival, survival curves, or median survival) to arrive at an estimate of average life expectancy for a particular patient when we evaluate different therapeutic options. The method employs some symbols and simple mathematics. A pocket calculator with an *ln* function gives an answer in seconds. It seems worthwhile to abstract the method from Beck's more detailed discussions.

First the method, then an example. Even healthy persons have a finite average life expectancy (LE) based on their age, sex, and race. For our use, expected years of life and expected deaths per 1,000 population are shown in Table 5–9.[35] From these figures we extract the life expectancy for age, sex, and race (LE_{ASR}).

TABLE 5–7.—RISK ESTIMATES IN ISCHEMIC HEART DISEASE: DEATH RATE PER 100,000 IN THE U.S., 1977*

AGE (YR)	WHITE M	WHITE F	NON-WHITE M	NON-WHITE F
35–44	59.8	11.1	91.3	36.6
45–54	266.9	56.5	315.9	144.7
55–64	715.1	216.9	786.3	423.0
65–74	1642.8	704.8	1435.5	945.8
Age-adjusted rate	264.7	119.0	245.3	152.3

*Selected data from Braunwald.[29] Reproduced by permission.

TABLE 5–9.—EXPECTATION OF LIFE AND EXPECTED DEATHS, BY RACE, SEX, AND AGE: 1980*

AGE IN 1980 (YEARS)	EXPECTATION OF LIFE IN YEARS					EXPECTED DEATHS PER 1,000 ALIVE AT SPECIFIED AGE				
		WHITE		BLACK			WHITE		BLACK	
	TOTAL	MALE	FEMALE	MALE	FEMALE	TOTAL	MALE	FEMALE	MALE	FEMALE
At birth	73.7	70.7	78.1	63.7	72.3	12.66	12.33	9.69	23.35	19.49
10	64.9	61.9	69.1	55.6	64.1	.20	.20	.17	.34	.24
20	55.3	52.4	59.4	46.0	54.3	1.25	1.83	.58	2.38	.74
21	54.4	51.5	58.4	45.2	53.3	1.32	1.91	.58	2.76	.84
22	53.5	50.5	57.4	44.3	52.4	1.36	1.96	.57	3.06	.93
23	52.5	49.6	56.5	43.4	51.4	1.37	1.95	.57	3.25	1.01
24	51.6	48.7	55.5	42.5	50.5	1.36	1.90	.57	3.35	1.09
25	50.7	47.8	54.5	41.7	49.5	1.34	1.84	.57	3.43	1.17
26	49.7	46.9	53.6	40.8	48.6	1.32	1.78	.57	3.54	1.26
27	48.8	46.0	52.6	40.0	47.7	1.31	1.73	.58	3.65	1.34
28	47.9	45.1	51.6	39.1	46.7	1.31	1.69	.59	3.80	1.40
29	46.9	44.2	50.6	38.3	45.8	1.31	1.67	.62	3.98	1.46
30	46.0	43.2	49.7	37.4	44.8	1.33	1.65	.64	4.16	1.52
31	45.1	42.3	48.7	36.6	43.9	1.35	1.64	.68	4.35	1.60
32	44.1	41.4	47.7	35.7	43.0	1.38	1.65	.72	4.54	1.69
33	43.2	40.4	46.8	34.9	42.1	1.43	1.69	.77	4.75	1.81
34	42.2	39.5	45.8	34.1	41.1	1.50	1.75	.83	4.98	1.94
35	41.3	38.6	44.9	33.2	40.2	1.59	1.83	.90	5.23	2.09
36	40.4	37.6	43.9	32.4	39.3	1.69	1.93	.98	5.51	2.27
37	39.4	36.7	42.9	31.6	38.4	1.81	2.06	1.07	5.82	2.47
38	38.5	35.8	42.0	30.8	37.5	1.96	2.21	1.17	6.16	2.73
39	37.6	34.9	41.0	29.9	36.6	2.12	2.38	1.28	6.55	3.02
40	36.7	34.0	40.1	29.1	35.7	2.31	2.59	1.41	6.97	3.34
41	35.7	33.0	39.1	28.3	34.8	2.53	2.83	1.55	7.44	3.68
42	34.8	32.1	38.2	27.5	33.9	2.77	3.11	1.71	7.98	4.05
43	33.9	31.2	37.3	26.8	33.1	3.04	3.43	1.89	8.63	4.43
44	33.0	30.3	36.3	26.0	32.2	3.35	3.79	2.09	9.36	4.85
45	32.1	29.4	35.4	25.2	31.4	3.68	4.19	2.31	10.14	5.29
46	31.3	28.6	34.5	24.5	30.5	4.04	4.64	2.55	10.97	5.76
47	30.4	27.7	33.6	23.8	29.7	4.44	5.15	2.82	11.88	6.24
48	29.5	26.8	32.7	23.0	28.9	4.89	5.72	3.10	12.88	6.74
49	28.7	26.0	31.8	22.3	28.1	5.38	6.36	3.42	13.95	7.26
50	27.8	25.2	30.9	21.6	27.3	5.91	7.05	3.76	15.10	7.81
51	27.0	24.3	30.0	21.0	26.5	6.48	7.80	4.13	16.29	8.40
52	26.1	23.5	29.1	20.3	25.7	7.09	8.60	4.52	17.52	9.04
53	25.3	22.7	28.2	19.7	24.9	7.72	9.46	4.92	18.76	9.72
54	24.5	21.9	27.4	19.0	24.2	8.39	10.38	5.34	20.03	10.45
55	23.7	21.2	26.5	18.4	23.4	9.10	11.37	5.80	21.35	11.22
56	22.9	20.4	25.7	17.8	22.7	9.88	12.44	6.31	22.74	12.04
57	22.2	19.6	24.8	17.2	22.0	10.74	13.61	6.87	24.23	12.93
58	21.4	18.9	24.0	16.6	21.3	11.69	14.89	7.51	25.85	13.91
59	20.6	18.2	23.2	16.0	20.5	12.73	16.27	8.22	27.59	14.96
60	19.9	17.5	22.4	15.5	19.8	13.84	17.75	9.00	29.44	16.12
61	19.2	16.8	21.6	14.9	19.2	15.04	19.34	9.83	31.36	17.33
62	18.5	16.1	20.8	14.4	18.5	16.32	21.10	10.72	33.32	18.52
63	17.8	15.4	20.0	13.9	17.8	17.69	23.06	11.64	35.27	19.66
64	17.1	14.8	19.2	13.4	17.2	19.17	25.21	12.63	37.26	20.79
65	16.4	14.2	18.5	12.9	16.5	20.75	27.51	13.69	39.30	21.92
70	13.2	11.3	14.8	10.5	13.4	30.94	41.84	21.19	52.53	31.90
75	10.4	8.8	11.5	8.3	10.7	45.74	61.92	33.74	69.56	44.80
80	7.9	6.7	8.6	6.3	8.2	69.01	91.49	55.55	94.62	64.63
85 and over	5.9	5.0	6.3	4.5	6.1	1,000.00	1,000.00	1,000.00	1,000.00	1,000.00

*From *Statistical Abstract of the United States 1984.* Ed. 104. U.S. Dept. of Commerce—Bureau of the Census

LE_{ASR} is reciprocally related to an average mortality rate, $\bar{\mu}_{ASR}$, $\bar{\mu}_{ASR} = \frac{1}{LE_{ASR}}$. Mortality increases with age and tends to double every 8 years. For a mixed U.S. population, an approximate LE can be calculated without a table:

LE = 69.5 − (0.80 × Age) for ages 20–70 years.

LE = 51.9 − (0.55 × Age) for age > 70 years.

There is a direct reciprocal relationship of life expectancy to average mortality:

$$\bar{\mu}_{ASR} = \frac{1}{LE} \text{ and } LE = \frac{1}{\bar{\mu}_{ASR}} \quad \text{(Equation 1)}$$

It is easy to see that a subpopulation with a severe specific disease will have an average mortality that exceeds that of the general population. This increased mortality risk can be expressed as:

$\bar{\mu}_D$ = Average excess mortality due to disease D.

A person with disease D would have a compound average mortality ($\bar{\mu}_C$) risk of:

$$\bar{\mu}_C = \bar{\mu}_{ASR} + \bar{\mu}_D \quad \text{(Equation 2)}$$

For someone with disease D, the life expectancy then becomes:

$$LE = \frac{1}{(\bar{\mu}_{ASR} + \bar{\mu}_D)} \quad \text{(Equation 3)}$$

The problems can be extended for more than one disease:

$$LE = \frac{1}{(\bar{\mu}_{ASR} + \bar{\mu}_{D1} + \bar{\mu}_{D2} \ldots)} \quad \text{(Equation 4)}$$

If the two values of LE are compared for a treated and untreated patient with similar risks, how can we use the therapeutic efficiency (E) of an operation or treatment? Therapeutic efficiency can vary from 0 to 1, where 1 indicates that the treatment or operation completely eliminates deaths caused by the disease and 0 indicates that the treatment or operation is totally ineffective.

The disease-specific mortality would be calculated as follows,

$$\text{Disease-specific mortality (treated)} = \bar{\mu}_D(1 - E)$$

Here, the more effective the treatment (E is larger), the smaller the mortality rate ($\bar{\mu}_D$). Several therapies (E_1, E_2 . . .) can be evaluated separately.

Operative or therapeutic mortality data can also be included. Mortality (M) may vary from 1 to 0, where 1 indicates 100% operative or treatment mortality and 0 indicates no operative or treatment mortality.

The mortality will be directly reflected in life expectancy, so the effect of mortality (with operation or treatment) equals:

$$LE\ (1 - M)$$

Average life expectancies can be compared for different therapies which have different mortalities (M_1, M_2 . . .).

Finally, LE can be reduced by the direct loss of useful living time as a consequence of hospitalization or therapeutic morbidity. If an operation has a short-term morbidity (STM) of 4 weeks, this is subtracted directly from LE as .08 year.

Sometimes there is a long-term disability (LTD), for example, loss of speech. If this is estimated at 20% of a patient's quality of life value, then the value of LE is reduced by using (1 − LTD) as a multiplier:

$$LE(1 - LTD) = LE\ (1 - .20) = LE \times .80$$

for our example.

In combining various terms to define LE for a patient with D_1 and D_2 in which D_1 could be treated with a therapeutic efficiency of E, a mortality of M, a long-term morbidity of LTD, and a short-term morbidity of STM, then an expanded expression is:

$$LE = \left[\frac{1}{\bar{\mu}_{ASR} + \bar{\mu}_{D1}(1 - E) + \bar{\mu}_{D2}} \times (1 - M)(1 - LTD)\right] - STM \quad \text{(Equation 5)}$$

By now, the perceptive reader has seen that the method is simple if a good estimate(s) of $\bar{\mu}_{D1}$, $\bar{\mu}_{D2}$ . . . are available. Unfortunately, very few papers accurately calculate excess mortality from a particular disease. Beck et al. show in detail how we may use available mortality and survival statistics to arrive at $\bar{\mu}_D$ estimates that are free of competing independent diseases.[33] There are several sources for obtaining excess mortality for some common diseases.[35, 36] Since it is difficult to keep such data at hand, there are five principal ways to estimate $\bar{\mu}_D$ (excess mortality due to the disease D):

1. A rare author may actually calculate the *excess mortality rate*. It will be stated in this form: "With disease D, the additional risk (corrected for age, sex and race) of death is X/1,000/year." This is converted to a decimal fractional value between 0 and 1; thus, 24/1,000/year becomes $\bar{\mu}_D = 0.024$.

2. Most survival data are *compound mortality rates* ($\bar{\mu}_C$). They are reported in this form: "With disease D, the mortality risk is X/1,000/year." Here we must subtract the normal age-, sex-, and race-specific mortality:

$$\bar{\mu}_D = \bar{\mu}_C - \bar{\mu}_{ASR} \quad \text{(Equation 6)}$$

Thus, for 65-year-old white male with disease D, $\overline{\mu}_C$ = 95/1,000/years, and an LE_{ASR} of 14.0 years,

$$\overline{\mu}_{ASR} = \frac{1}{LE_{ASR}} = 0.071$$

$$\overline{\mu}_D = 0.095 - 0.071 = 0.024$$

3. *Five-year survivals*[5] are commonly reported. Two-, three-, or ten-year survivals can also be used for *t* in equation 7 below. Unless the reported survival numbers are rare examples of ASR-corrected statistics, they represent a compound mortality. The form usually used is "The probability of surviving 5 years ($t = 5$) with disease D is 5/100." Then ($s = 5$):

$$\overline{\mu}_C = -\frac{1}{t}\,\ell n\left(\frac{s}{100}\right) \quad \text{(Equation 7)}$$

Marvelously, almost all pocket calculators will give an instant value for ℓn of N as well as direct reciprocals. If we use a 65-year-old white man with disease D for which the 5-year survival is 65%, then from equation 7,

$$\overline{\mu}_C = -\frac{1}{5}\,\ell n\ .65 = 0.0862$$

and from equation 6,

$$\overline{\mu}_D = \overline{\mu}_C - \overline{\mu}_{ASR} = 0.0862 - 0.071 = 0.0152$$

4. *Median Survival* is reported as the years of survival for 50% of the cohort with disease D. Again, this is usually a compound survival figure. Another way of stating survival is, "The probability of surviving *t* years with disease D is 0.50." This is calculated using equations 1, 6, and 7. Assuming a disease with a 3.5-year median survival in a 60-year-old man, then:

$$\overline{\mu}_{ASR} = \frac{1}{17.2} = .0581$$

$$\overline{\mu}_C = \frac{1}{3.5}\,\ell n\ (.50) = \frac{1}{3.5}(-\ 0.693) = .198$$

$$\overline{\mu}_D = \overline{\mu}_C - \overline{\mu}_{ASR} = 0.198 - 0.0581 = 0.140$$

5. Finally, accurate survival graphs can be used to get a survival *(s)* at 5 years or some other time *(t)*. Again, one must distinguish whether it is a compound mortality rate ($\overline{\mu}_C$) or an age-corrected value. $\overline{\mu}_D$ is obtained as in (3) or (4) above.

Table 5–10 summarizes the simple data needed to calculate LE.

AN EXAMPLE OF THE USE OF THE DEALE METHOD OF ESTIMATING AVERAGE LIFE EXPECTANCY WITH DIFFERENT THERAPIES AND DIFFERENT RISKS

A 60-year-old white man is found to have a thin T_2N_1 cancer of the middle third of the tongue. He had a myocardial infarct 6 months ago. He now has stable angina pectoris responding well to medications, i.e., he conducts activities of daily living without pain. He is known to have diffuse two-vessel coronary disease (distal left anterior descending and right coronary lesions).

TABLE 5–10.—DATA NEEDED TO CALCULATE PATIENT SPECIFIC LIFE EXPECTANCY ON A SPECIFIC TREATMENT PROGRAM

1. Age, sex, and race of patient. This is used to find:
2. Age-, sex-, and race-specific life expectancy (LE_{ASR}):

$$\overline{\mu}_{ASR} = \frac{1}{LE_{ASR}}$$

3. Principal disease (D_1):

   $\overline{\mu}_{D_1}$ with one treatment program T_1 (data obtained from one of five sources listed in text) ________.
   $\overline{\mu}_{D_1}$ with any other treatment program T_2, T_3 . . . being considered ________.

4. Risk of other diseases (complicating illnesses):

   $\overline{\mu}_{D_2}$ ________, $\overline{\mu}_{D_3}$ ________, . . .

   These may be modified by the efficiencies of planned treatment.
5. Expected mortality rate for treatments considered:

   M_{T_1} = ________ [convert to survival multiplier (1 − M).]
   M_{T_2} = ________.

6. Estimate direct survival time lost due to therapy and period of convalescence.

   Short-term morbidity (STM) in terms of days/365 or weeks/52 = ________.

7. Calculate a long-term disability quality of life weighting factor (LTD). A reduction in quality of life = a multiplier of (1 − LTD) × percent reduction in quality of life (estimate).

For the example, we will use 5-year NED survival values of 55% for composite resection and 40% for irradiation treatment.

The data needed are the following:

- Age, sex, race (50-year-old white man).
- $\bar{\mu}_{ASR} = 0.0581$ (calculated as 1/LE, from Table 5–9).
- Cancer is D_1. If 5-year NED survival is 55% for surgery and 40% for irradiation, then:
- $\bar{\mu}_{D1}$ (Surg.) $= \left(-\frac{1}{5}\, ln\ 0.55\right) - \bar{\mu}_{ASR} = \bar{\mu}_C - \bar{\mu}_{ASR} = 0.0615$
- $\bar{\mu}_{D1}$ (Rad.) $= \left(-\frac{1}{5}\, ln\ 0.40\right) - \bar{\mu}_{ASR} = \bar{\mu}_C - \bar{\mu}_{ASR} = .1252$
- Heart disease is D_2 (natural survival, from Table 5–11, = 88% 5-year survivors with this coronary disease pattern). This is an example where the more carefully defined data in Table 5–11 improve the quality of the decision.

$$\bar{\mu}_{D_2}\ (\text{Surg.}) - \left(-\frac{1}{5}\, ln\ 0.88\right) - .0581 = .0256$$

- M for composite resection = 4% (pessimistic estimate from Table 5–2).
- STM (short-term morbidity) from both treatments is about 0.12 years.
- LTD (long-term disability) of a hemiglossectomy for impairment of speech could be estimated as 10% of quality of life.
- LTD (long-term disability) of irradiation is estimated as minimal.

TABLE 5–11.—EXPECTED CARDIAC MORTALITY: MEDICAL TREATMENT ONLY WITH RADIOLOGICALLY DEFINED CORONARY ARTERY DISEASE*

DISEASE EXTENT†	MORTALITY Annual (%)	5-year (%)
Normal arteriogram	0	0
Single-vessel obstruction		
Left main obstruction:	15–25	70
LAD	2–4	10–20
RCA	1–2	2–8
CIRC	0–1	0–2
Two-vessel obstruction		
LAD + RCA or		
CIRC	7–10	35–50
Before FSP		40
After FSP		12
RCA + CIRC	3–6	15–30
Three-vessel obstruction	10–12	50–60

*Adapted from Humphries J.O.: Expected course of patients with coronary artery disease, in Rahimtoola S.H. (ed.): *Coronary Bypass Surgery*. Philadelphia, F.A. Davis Co., 1977.

†LAD, left anterior descending artery; RCA, right coronary artery; CIRC, left circumflex artery; FSP, first septal perforating artery.

Then (from equation 5):

$$\text{Disease and treatment-specific LE} = \left[\frac{1}{\bar{\mu}_{ASR} + \bar{\mu}_{D1} + D_2} \times (1 - M) \times (1 - LTD)\right] - STM$$

$$\text{For surgery, LE} = \left[\frac{1}{.0581 + .0615 + .0256} \times .96 \times .90\right] - .12 = 5.84 \text{ years.}$$

$$\text{For irradiation LE} = \left[\frac{1}{.0581 + .1252 + .0256} \times 1 \times 1\right] - .12 = 4.67 \text{ years.}$$

$$M = 0 \quad LTD = \text{nil for irradiation}$$

However, some of the irradiated patients may require subsequent surgical salvage to achieve the 40% 5-year survival rate. They will have an operative survival of .96 for M, and $\bar{\mu}_{D1}$ will be somewhere between 0.1252 and .0615. LE_{Surg} will still be greater than LE_{Rad} unless $\bar{D}_1$ (irrad.) can be improved.

The system emphasizes the need for accurate, tumor stage–specific survival data. The analysis places dimensions on the complicating disease. Complicating disease does not enter as an "I'm worried about it" nebulous feature.

In an extension of the example, we may add an additional disease, D_3, such as Laennec's cirrhosis, Child's class B, with moderate ascites. From tables given later in this chapter we see, that the 3-year survival is about 26%.

$$\bar{\mu}_{D3} = \bar{\mu}_{CD_3} - \mu_{ASR} = \left(-\frac{1}{3}\, ln\ 0.26\right) - .0581 = .3909$$

If this is added as D_3 to the example above and the operative mortality estimate is increased modestly from 4% to 7%, then:

$$LE_{Surg} = 1.44 \text{ years}$$
$$LE_{Rad} - 1.55 \text{ years}$$

Essentially there is no anticipated difference in average survival, even though strong arguments might be easy to generate. At this point it is necessary to go to the dark clinical arts and try to determine whether the liver disease is easily controllable with a period of abstinence, diet, and judicious diuresis. Is the patient willing to stop drinking in order to move up from a Child's B risk to an A risk? Will he stop alcohol intake in the postoperative period? Much of the decision-making can be reassessed to improve the average life expectancy if there are clinical improvements.

This system, and the example provided, do show that decision-making in complex cases cannot be made without good data and an objective analysis. The patient in the last example would be hard to evaluate without a few minutes with paper, pencil, and some simple data tables. When the analysis has been made, it guides management and the exercise of individualized judgment.

WHAT IS THE RISK OF INTRACRANIAL OR CAROTID OCCLUSIVE DISEASE?

One sometimes encounters patients with an oropharyngeal carcinoma who have also recently had a stroke, a transient ischemic attack, or an asymptomatic carotid bruit. It is a particular dilemma when the occlusion is on the side of involved nodes; however, noninvasive ultrasound, hemodynamic monitoring, and digital subtraction angiography have helped to detect correctable lesions. If the carotid endarterectomy is done first, the area might be seeded. If the stenosis is not treated, a fixed stroke or death may result.

What are the risks? Wishnant and co-workers studied TIAs in Rochester, Minnesota.[37] Their data are adapted in Table 5–12. This is in rough agreement with the data obtained in 178 patients in a trial of aspirin therapy who were followed up by Fields et al. (Table 5–13).[38] The general risks of asymptomatic bruits and TIAs have been reviewed elsewhere.[39] The operative risks appear to be small for noncardiac surgery. Unfortunately, good data dealing specifically with extracavitary noncardiac

TABLE 5–12.—PROGNOSIS OF PATIENTS WITH AND WITHOUT ANTICOAGULANT TREATMENT AFTER THEIR FIRST TRANSIENT ISCHEMIC ATTACK*

TREATMENT GROUP	% PROBABILITY OF SURVIVING, BY YEAR		
	Yr 1†	Yr 3	Yr 5
Anticoagulation (N = 80)	90	80	66
No anticoagulation (N = 118)	85	74	60
Survival of general population corresponding in age and sex	95	87	75

*Adapted from Wishnant et al.[37]
†There is a slightly lower risk of stroke in the first month; otherwise there is no significant difference between treatment groups.

TABLE 5–13.—COMPLICATIONS IN CEREBRAL ISCHEMIA: CUMULATIVE PROBABILITIES OF DEATH, NONFATAL STROKE OR RETINAL INFARCTION, BY TIME SINCE ENTRY INTO THE STUDY*

TIME (MO.)	CUMULATIVE PROBABILITY OF EVENT	
	Aspirin	Placebo
6	0.085	0.173
12	0.126	0.220
18	0.168	0.271
24	0.194	0.271

*Adapted from Fields et al.[38] χ^2 over all intervals: $P = 0.18$.

surgery in the setting of carotid stenosis could not be found. For most head and neck surgery, blood loss and hemodynamics can be maintained stable through the operation; consequently, we have treated the malignancy first. Where carotid endarterectomy has been required, it has been easily accomplished after the neck flaps have healed. Admittedly, it is tempting to do an indicated endarterectomy while the carotid is laid out in a lymphadenectomy, but the combined risk of infection, spread of tumor, and possible orocutaneous fistula with a new vascular suture line does not balance against the small risk of cerebrovascular accident.

HOW DO RESPIRATORY PROBLEMS AFFECT OPERATIVE RISKS?

Thoracic surgeons have taken the lead in defining the operative risks of pulmonary disease. Chest surgery alters the musculature, compliance, and amount of functioning pulmonary parenchyma. Head and neck surgery does not. Head and neck surgery *does* deal with the most critical element, the upper airway. As seen in Table 5–2, about a third to half of the surgical mortality is traceable to airway complications. The tumors may directly obstruct the airway. Therapy may alter swallowing and laryngeal protective reflexes and function. Heavy smoking leaves a residue of emphysema. Age reduces lung function. Table 5–14 shows that smoking is the real villain, not age.[40] A smoker with a two-pack-a-day habit for 20 years can be expected to have a 50% chance of moderate pulmonary emphysema and a 15% chance of severe pulmonary impairment. Late-stage chronic obstructive pulmonary disease (COPD) with cor pulmonale is associated with the higher operative mortality (Table 5–15). The data derived from Skinner and Pierce[24] show that the overall mortality of operations in patients with cor pulmonale is high (50%). If the figures are recalculated for extracavity surgery, the rate is only one-fifth that of intrathoracic or intra-abdominal surgery (bottom half Table 5–15).

TABLE 14.—AVERAGE DEGREE OF EMPHYSEMA IN NONSMOKERS AND CURRENT SMOKERS (1,443 MEN)*†

AGE (YR)	SUBJECTS WHO NEVER SMOKED	PIPE OR CIGAR	CIGARETTE SMOKERS <½ Pack	½–1 Pack	1–2 Packs	>2 Packs
<60	0.05	0.75	1.23	1.48	1.86	2.01
60–69	0.10	0.86	1.52	2.24	2.30	2.28
>70	0.11	1.06	1.55	2.12	2.37	2.50

*Condensed from Auerbach et al.[40]
†Morphologically defined changes found at autopsy. 0 = normal lung; 4 = severe advanced emphysema.

Dyspnea can be due to any of the following:

1. Tumor obstruction causing air flow resistance:
   Mass in airway
   Acute edema in oropharyngeal area
   Inspisated secretions, blood, serum, or necrotic tumor debris
2. COPD:
   With anoxia
   With hypercarbia
   With associated heart failure
3. Aspiration:
   Due to disordered swallowing or laryngeal function
   Tube feeding
   Gastrostomy feeding
4. Weakness of respiratory musculature from malnutrition
5. Previous pulmonary or other intrathoracic surgery
6. Acute pulmonary infections
7. Combinations of the above

Baseline impairment of pulmonary function makes the patient much more vulnerable to minimal complications arising from pneumonia, pulmonary embolism, aspiration, tracheostomy, or anesthesia. When there is minimal pulmonary functional reserve, a trivial complication becomes deadly. Again, the good therapist seeks quantification and assiduously protects the pulmonary function. The high-risk patient can be identified in a number of ways (Table 5–16). Thoracic surgeons have tried unsuccessfully to use computer techniques for multifactorial analysis in order to accurately predict operative mortality.[41] For head and neck surgery we must still look to FEV_1 (a volume of 600–800 cc is required for an effective cough), Po_2 exchange, evidence of CO_2 retention, and a composite pulmonary cardiovascular evaluation with an exercise test, locally called the

TABLE 5–15.—NONCARDIAC SURGICAL MORTALITY IN FUNCTIONALLY SYMPTOMATIC PATIENTS WITH CHRONIC PULMONARY DISEASE (CPD) WITH AND WITHOUT COR PULMONALE; PATIENTS ALSO HAD ACQUIRED HEART DISEASE*

DISEASE	TOTAL NO. OF CASES	OVERALL MORTALITY	BY OPERATION Cases	Mortality
Intrathoracic and Intra-Abdominal Operations				
CPD without cor pulmonale	75	20%	27	37%
CPD with cor pulmonale	24	29%	12	50%
Extrathoracic and Extra-Abdominal Operations				
CPD without cor pulmonale	48		(5)	10.4%
CPD with cor pulmonale	12		(1)	8%

*Adapted from Nachlas.[23]

TABLE 5–16.—INDICATIONS OF PULMONARY PROBLEMS

1. Inspiratory stridor, tachypnea.
2. Any elevation of Pa_{CO_2} above 46 mm Hg is abnormal and indicates severe abnormalities in the distribution of ventilation and perfusion.
3. Pa_{O_2} on room air:

Mild	>85 mm Hg:	Probably OK.
	75–80 mm Hg:	Mild but not unusual risk in the absence of other systemic findings. Usually this can be improved by stopping smoking, etc.
Moderate	<70 mm Hg:	Determine the cause and attempt to improve before surgery.
Severe	<50 mm Hg:	Big problems.

4. Data from spirometry can be compared with data from individuals of same age weight and height known to be free of disease. This nomogram is available in reference 43.
5. FEV_{1sec}

Mild	3 L:	OK.
	2 L:	Impaired.
Moderate	1–2 L:	Severe impairment.
Severe	<800 cc:	Will have trouble clearing secretions.

   This value is important, since it takes about 600–800 cc of air moving through an adult male trachea in 1 second to produce an effective cough that clears airway secretions.
6. Cor pulmonale with mean pulmonary artery pressure > 30 mm Hg on right heart catheter or Swan-Ganz catheter measurement.
7. Exercise tolerance (treppen-sprechen test): A measure of cardiopulmonary and skeletal muscular function.

0	Extremely poor risk: 10% + mortality; unable to walk on level without dyspnea.
1	Poor risk: Able to climb one flight of stairs with severe dyspnea.
2	Below average risk: Able to climb two flights of stairs with dyspnea.
3	Moderate risk: Able to climb two flights of stairs with some dyspnea. Unable to count to 20 on one breath.
4	Good risk: Able to climb two flights of stairs with minimal dyspnea. Counts to 20 on one breath.

"treppen-sprechen" or "stepping-talking" test, outlined in Table 5–16. One must look for the ominous predictor of CO_2 retention, since many patients build the CO_2 level slowly and become tolerant to the soporific effects.[42] A chronic disease patient may be ambulatory with a Pco_2 of 90 mm Hg. The prudent surgeon would regard a patient in any of the "severe" categories in Table 5–16 as having only a 50% likelihood of 1-year survival and an operative mortality approaching 5%–10% for a longer head and neck procedure. The major problem is intolerance of minor respiratory complications in the postoperative period. This judgment becomes critical in deciding for or against partial laryngeal or hypopharyngeal resections that may lead to chronic aspiration.

DOES LIVER DISEASE AFFECT OPERATIVE RISK AND SURVIVAL?

Head and neck cancer patients have a high frequency of alcoholism, as discussed in chapter 1. There is no question that alcoholism is deleterious to general health. Advanced Laennec's cirrhosis is a deadly disease even if no operative procedure is done. In the controlled studies of therapy for ascites, hepatic encephalopathy, and bleeding varices, there are nonoperative groups which confirm the rapid lethal attrition. The patients with Laennec's cirrhosis and ascites shown in Table 5–17 demonstrate a typical exponential decay curve, with one of five patients surviving 5 years after the diagnosis has been made.[44]

Ratnoff and Patek[45] described the same general curve.[46] The mortality holds for most categories of portal cirrhosis.[47] The widely used Child's classification is given in Table 5–18. When the cirrhosis is expressed as portal hypertension, there is a less than even chance that the patient will survive 3 years (see Table 5–18).[48] When surgery is considered, this poor survival has to be considered in the decision-making process. The problem with such a classification is the lack of definition of the morphologic type of the liver disease. Acute

TABLE 5–17.—PROGNOSIS IN ASCITES*

	SURVIVAL (%)	
YEARS OF OBSERVATION	Surgically Treated	Medically Treated
0	100	100
1	55	46
2	40	32
3	31	29
4	23	25
5	23	17

*Derived from Welch et al.[44]

TABLE 5–18.—PROGNOSIS IN LAENNEC'S CIRRHOSIS WITH VARICES: SURVIVAL IN SURGICALLY TREATED AND MEDICALLY TREATED GROUPS, STRATIFIED BY CHILD CLASS*

	LAB AND CLINICAL DATA				3-YEAR SURVIVAL (%)	
CHILD CLASS	Bilirubin (mg/dl)	Albumin (gm/dl)	Nutrition	Ascites	Surgery	Medical
A	<2	>3.5	+ +	−	61	52
B	2–3	3–3.5	+	+	21	26
C	>3	<3	−	+ +	27	40

*From Zieve.[48] Reproduced by permission.

alcoholic hepatitis may be rapidly progressive and lethal. A fatty liver may show remarkable recovery with 30 days of abstinence and good nutrition. A scarred, shrunken liver may have no recovery potential. Zieve has discussed the interrelationships.[48] There is much overlap, as is evident in Figure 5–1. Preoperative preparation in the hospital has proved to be the best index in deciding therapy. In advanced liver disease, the vitamin K–dependent hepatic factors of the clotting cascade may be reduced. A rapid recovery with nutrition and minimal vitamin K supplement presages the ability of liver function to improve. Recovery and survival after cancer treatment also depend on the physician's or surgeon's effort at employing his qualities as a shaman to induce the patient to enter an effective alcoholism treatment program.

In rare instances, one may encounter a head and neck cancer patient with acute viral or drug-induced hepatitis. It is generally agreed that greatest risks occur during the early icteric phase. If one waits until the patient is anicteric, then risks are reduced. There are no available data for extracavitary surgery. An early study by Harville and Summerskill showed that the four deaths in 58 patients (42 viral, 16 drug hepatitis) occurred in deeply icteric patients who had had abdominal exploration to rule out correctable obstruction.[49]

WHAT IS THE RISK OF HEAD AND NECK SURGERY FROM AGE ALONE?

It is difficult to get pure data separated from complicating diseases. In general, the very elderly (> 80 years) arrive at that age by being durable. A number of studies have shown that operative death in the elderly following head and neck surgery (within 30 days) is higher than in younger patients, but not prohibitively so.[50–52] Jun et al. reported the Memorial Sloan-Kettering experience with 159 patients over 80 years of age.[52] In 152 surgical procedures on 133 patients there were 7 hospital deaths (5.3% mortality). There was an average 41-month survival for all surgically treated patients. Treatment eliminated the cancer in 68% of patients. In general, age as a single factor is not a contraindication to treatment of a head and neck malignancy.

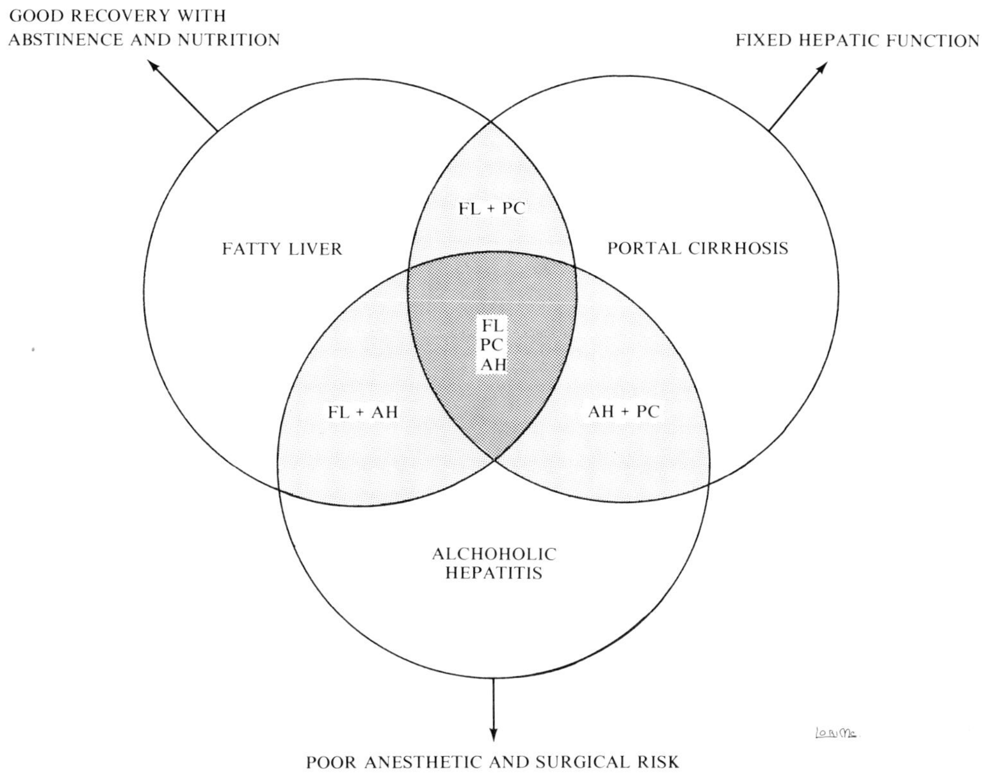

Fig 5–1.—Interrelationship of different morphological types of alcoholic cirrhosis. There is a variable degree of overlap. (From Zieve.[48] Reproduced by permission.)

WHAT PREOPERATIVE FLUID AND ELECTROLYTE CHANGES SIGNAL AN INCREASED OPERATIVE RISK?

Many head and neck cancer patients have complicating diseases (see Table 5–6). All of these diseases may alter water and electrolyte homeostasis. Problems with deglutition and nutrition alter body composition and fluid intake. Some of these are discussed below.

CHRONIC LOW SODIUM SYNDROME.—Chronic low sodium syndrome is commonly seen. With nutritional inadequacy, there is a loss of lean body mass. This is a combination of cell loss and protein depletion of remaining cells, particularly from muscle cells. With loss of the osmotically active protein molecules in cells there is a lower intracellular osmolality, in the range of 260–270 mOsm/L instead of the usual 290–295 range. The body behaves as though the "osmostat" were set at a lower level.[53]

Since Na^+ is the major determinant of extracellular fluid volume, free water will be retained and cross membranes to maintain osmotic balance. Patients may be tolerating serum Na^+ levels of 125–130 mEq/L without the significant neuromuscular symptoms that usually occur if the serum Na^+ is abruptly lowered to the same level. If one attempts to raise the serum sodium level by giving exogenous Na^+, the Na^+ transiently raises the osmolality of the extracellular fluid. Water leaves the cell to restore osmotic equilibrium, and the extracellular space expands. If the salt load is high, edema is produced. The treatment of chronic low Na^+ syndrome should avoid water and Na^+ loading. Restore positive nitrogen balance by enteral or parenteral nutrition, or control any septic and catabolic mechanisms, as discussed in chapter 11. Studies of total parenteral nutrition (TPN) in cancer patients have demonstrated that protein repletion is difficult to achieve in actual practice.[54]

HYPERNATREMIA.—Hypernatremia can occur when enteral feedings are administered without sufficient free water (see Chap. 27).

HYPOKALEMIA.—Starvation reduces the intracellular K^+ proportionately to protein loss. This depletion can amount to as much as one fourth to one third of the total exchangeable K^+ pool. Some other causes of low K^+ are listed in Table 5–19. On a long-term basis, low K^+ can produce a renal tubular nephropathy which of itself increases potassium loss. When a patient is volume depleted or dehydrated, aldosterone secretion increases. Renal sodium conservation results, but renal K^+ loss is increased.

TABLE 5–19.—COMMON MECHANISMS OF HYPOKALEMIA

Inadequate intake
GI loss
Vomiting
Diarrhea
Laxative use
Excessive urinary loss
Diuretics
Tubulointerstitial renal disease
Renal tubular acidosis
Magnesium deficiency
Bartter's syndrome
Transcellular shifts (acute)
Chronic nutritional depletion

TABLE 5–20.—OPERATIVE AND POSTOPERATIVE PROBLEMS ARISING FROM POTASSIUM DEPLETION

Neuromuscular
Adynamic ileus
Muscular weakness (including respiratory muscles)
Rhabdomyelolysis
Encephalopathy
Cardiac
ECG changes
Arrhythmias
Myocardial necrosis—fibrosis
Renal
Concentrating defect; hypokalemic tubular nephropathy
Chronic renal failure
Metabolic
CHO intolerance
Alkalosis

Hypokalemia can produce major problems (Table 5–20). Preoperative correction is needed. Persistent hypokalemia will be associated with intraoperative arrhythmias, skeletal muscle weakness and myocardial function limitation, prolonged depolarization after muscle relaxants, easy toxicity to digitalis alkaloids, etc.

WHAT SHOULD BE CONCLUDED FROM THIS CHAPTER?

Some data are available that allow modest quantification of the surgical risk for head and neck cancer patients. There are good methods for comparing various treatments in patients with these complications. Often, coexisting disease can be improved with simple and judicious pretreatment and perioperative management. The wise clinician does not have a "routine" management but uses careful analysis to individualize the decision-making process.

REFERENCES

1. Cape R.: *Aging: Its Complex Management.* Hagerstown, Md., Harper & Row, 1978.
2. Siegel J.H., Chodoff P.: *The Aged and High Risk Surgical Patient: Medical, Surgical, and Anesthetic Management.* New York, Grune & Stratton, 1976.
3. Ballantyne A.J.: Late sequellae of radiation therapy in cancer of the head and neck with particular reference to the nasopharynx. *Am. J. Surg.* 130:433–436, 1975.
4. Larson D.L., Lindberg R.D., Lane E., et al.: Major complications of radiotherapy in cancer of the oral cavity and oropharynx: A 10-year retrospective study. *Am. J. Surg.* 146:531–536, 1983.
5. Beahrs O.H.: Factors minimizing mortality and morbidity rates in head and neck surgery. *Am. J. Surg.* 126:443–451, 1973.
6. Spiro R.H., Huvos A.G., Strong E.W.: Cancer of the parotid gland: A clinicopathologic study of 288 cases. *Am. J. Surg.* 130:452–459, 1975.
7. Razack M.S., Silapasvang S., Sako K., et al.: Significance of site and nodal metastases in squamous cell carcinoma of the epiglottis. *Am. J. Surg.* 136:151–155, 1978.
8. Razack M.S., Sako K., Marchetta F.C., et al.: Carcinoma of the hypopharynx: Success and failure. *Am. J. Surg.* 134:489–491, 1977.
9. O'Brien P.H., Catlin D.: Cancer of the cheek. *Cancer* 18:1392–1398, 1965.
10. Ruffine C.D., MacComb W.S.: Bilateral neck dissections: Analysis of 180 cases. *Cancer* 19:1503–1508, 1966.
11. Kremen A.J.: Surgical management of cancer of the tongue. *Surg. Clin. North Am.* 47:1125–1129, 1967.
12. Robbins R.E., Budden M.K., MacDougal J.A.: Analysis of mortality and morbidity in 100 composite resections for oral carcinoma. *Am. J. Surg.* 130:178–179, 1975.
13. Joyce L.D., McQuarrie D.G.: Application of contemporary reconstructive techniques in head and neck surgery for oral-facial cancers. *Surgery* 80:373–378, 1976.
14. Shedd D.P., Calamel P.M.: Head and neck cancer surgery in the aged and high risk patient: General considerations, in Seigel J.H., Chodoff P.D. (eds.): *The Aged and High Risk Surgical Patient.* New York, Grune & Stratton, 1976.
15. Mendelson B.C., Woods J.E., Beahrs O.H.: Neck dissection in the treatment of carcinoma of the anterior two-thirds of the tongue. *Surg. Gynecol. Obstet.* 143:75–80, 1976.
16. Ward G.E., Edgerton M.T., Chambers R.G., et al.: Cancer of the oral cavity and pharynx and results of treatment by means of the composite operation. *Ann. Surg.* 150:202–220, 1959.
17. Spiro R.H., Strong E.W.: Discontinuous partial glossectomy and radical neck dissection in selected patients with epidermoid carcinoma of the mobile tongue. *Am. J. Surg.* 126:544–546, 1973.
18. Shaw J.P., Tollefson H.R.: Epidermoid carcinoma of the supraglottic larynx. *Am. J. Surg.* 128:494–499, 1974.
19. Chu W., Strawitz J.G.: Results in suprahyoid, modified radical and standard radical neck dissections for metastatic squamous cell carcinoma: Recurrence and survival. *Am. J. Surg.* 136:512–515, 1978.
20. Vacanti C.J., VanHouten R.J., Hill R.C.: A statistical analysis of the relationship of physical status to post-operative mortality in 68,388 cases. *Anesth. Analg.* 49:564–566, 1970.
21. Lewin I., Lerner A.G., Green S.H., et al.: Physical class

and physiologic status in the prediction of operative mortality in the aged sick. *Ann. Surg.* 174:217–231, 1971.
22. Steen P.A., Tinker J.H., Tarhan S.: Myocardial reinfarction after anesthesia and surgery. *JAMA* 239:2566–2570, 1978.
23. Nachlas M.M.: Influence of arteriosclerotic heart disease on surgical risk. *Am. J. Surg.* 101:447, 1965.
24. Skinner J.F., Pierce M.L.: Surgical risk in the cardiac patient. *J. Chron. Dis.* 17:57, 1964.
25. McQuarrie D.G.: Fluids and electrolytes, in Paparella M.M., Shumrick D.A. (eds.): *Otolaryngology*, ed. 2. Philadelphia, W.B. Saunders Co., 1980, chap. 27.
26. Rogers M.C.: Anesthetic management of patients with heart disease. *Mod. Concepts Cardiovasc. Dis.* 52:29–33, 1983.
27. Tarhan S., Moffitt E.A., Taylor W.F.: Myocardial infarction after general anesthesia. *JAMA* 220:1451–1454, 1972.
28. Goldman L., et al.: Multifactorial index of cardiac risk in non-cardiac surgical procedures. *N. Engl. J. Med.* 297:845–850, 1977.
29. Braunwald E.: *Heart Disease*. Philadelphia, W.B. Saunders Co., 1980.
30. Kannel W.B., McGee D., Gordon T.: A general cardiovascular risk profile: The Framingham Study. *Am. J. Cardiol.* 38:46, 1976.
31. Rosenman R.H., Brand R.J., Sholtz R.I., et al.: Multivariate prediction of coronary heart disease during 8.5 year follow-up in the Western Collaborative Group Study. *Am. J. Cardiol.* 37:903, 1976.
32. Beck J.R., Kassirer J.P., Pauker S.G.: A convenient approximation of life expectancy ("The DEALE"); I. Validation of the method. *Am. J. Med.* 73:883–888, 1982.
33. Beck J.R., Pauker S.G., Gottleib J.E., et al.: A convenient approximation of life expectancy ("the DEALE"): II. Use in medical decision making. *Am. J. Med.* 73:889–897, 1982.
34. Humphrey E.W., Keehn R.J., Higgins G.A. Jr., et al.: The long term survival of patients with visceral carcinoma. *Surg. Gynecol. Obstet.* 149:385–390, 1979.
35. *Vital Statistics of the United States* (annual). Washington, D.C., U.S. National Center for Health Statistics.
36. Singer R.B., Levinson L.: *Medical Risks*. Lexington, Mass., D.C. Heath Publishers, 1976, p. 9–21.
37. Wishnant J.P., Matsumoto N., Elvebach L.R.: The effect of anticoagulant therapy on the prognosis of patients with transient ischemic attacks in a community. *Mayo Clin. Proc.* 48:844–848, 1973.
38. Fields W.S., Lemak N.A., Frankowski R.F., et al.: Controlled trial of aspirin in cerebral ischemia. *Stroke* 8:301–315, 1977.
39. Machleder H.I.: Strokes, transient ischemic attacks and asymptomatic bruits. *West. J. Med.* 130:205–217, 1979.
40. Auerbach O., Garfinkel L., Hammond E.C.: Relation of smoking and age to findings in lung parenchyma: A microscopic study (1824 cases). *Chest* 65:29–35, 1974.
41. VonNostrand D., Kjelsberg M.O., Humphrey E.W.: Pre-resectional evaluation of risk from pneumonectomy. *Surg. Gynecol. Obstet.* 127:306–312, 1968.
42. McQuarrie D.G.: A kinetic concept of carbon dioxide narcosis. *Ann. Thorac. Surg.* 4:205–217, 1967.
43. Boren H.C., Kory R.C., Syner J.C.: The Veteran's Administration-Army Cooperative Study of Pulmonary Function: II. The lung volume and its subdivisions in normal men. *Am. J. Med.* 41:96 1966.
44. Welch H.F., Welch C.S., Carter J.H.: Prognosis after surgical treatment of ascites: Results of side-to-side shunt. *Surgery* 56:75–82, 1964.
45. Ratnoff O.D., Patek A.J.: The natural history of Laennec's cirrhosis of the liver. *Medicine* 21:207, 1950.
46. Douglas B.E., Snell A.M.: Portal cirrhosis: An analysis of 444 cases. *Gastroenterology* 15:407, 1950.
47. Resnick R.H., Iber F.L., Ishihara A.M., et al.: A controlled study of the therapeutic portocaval shunt. *Gastroenterology* 67:843–857, 1974.
48. Zieve L.: Alcoholic hepatitis in the context of alcoholic liver disease, in Najarian J.S., Delaney J.P. (eds.): *Surgery of the Liver, Pancreas and Biliary Tract*. New York, Stratton Intercontinental Medical Books, 1975, pp. 405–417.
49. Harville D.D., Summerskill W.H.J.: Surgery in acute hepatitis: Causes and effects. *JAMA* 184:257–261, 1963.
50. Beahrs O.H.: Geriatric patients with head and neck problems. *Am. J. Surg.* 100:813–817, 1969.
51. Jovan L.D., John H.W.: Predictions of outcome of surgery and anesthesia in patients over 80. *JAMA* 242:2301–2306, 1979.
52. Jun M.Y., Strong E., Saltzman E.I., et al.: Head and neck cancer in the elderly. *Head Neck Surg.* 5:376–382, 1983.
53. Andreoli T.E., Grantham, J.J., Rector F.: *Disturbances in Body Fluid Osmolality*. Bethesda, Md., American Physiological Association, 1977.
54. McCanley R.L., Brennan M.F.: Serum albumin levels in cancer patients receiving total parenteral nutrition. *Ann. Surg.* 197:305–309, 1983.

6 / General Principles of Primary and Late Reconstructive Surgery

Alan R. Shons, M.D., Ph.D.

HOW DO YOU ANTICIPATE THE NEED FOR RECONSTRUCTIVE PROCEDURES?

A reconstructive procedure is required when a defect following tumor excision cannot be closed by primary approximation of the tissue margins without functional or aesthetic compromise. When a large defect is created on the surface of the skin, the intraoral lining, or the bony facial framework, some type of reconstructive procedure will be required. An initial evaluation of the patient must include a careful estimate of adequate tumor margins to achieve curative removal of the specimen. If an intraoral cancer is invading the skin of the cheek, it is obvious that the resultant defect will require both intraoral lining and skin coverage for closure. If the tumor is fixed to the mandible a segmental mandibulectomy will be required. This poses the additional problem of mandibular reconstruction. It is necessary to custom design each repair from a spectrum of options.

HOW DOES THE NEED FOR RECONSTRUCTION BECOME INCORPORATED IN THE TREATMENT PLAN?

The initial therapy plan for the patient must provide for reconstruction after the cancer-bearing area has been ablated. The surgeon must be aware of the *best* reconstructive options for the potential defect that will be created. In all procedures it is important that the surgeon also have in mind a second or "fallback" reconstructive option should the procedure of choice prove to be impossible at operation or should the primary reconstruction fail in the operative or postoperative period. The extirpative operation should be planned with the reconstructive procedure in mind. However, under no circumstances should the reconstructive procedure take precedence over the need for curative operation. Frequently the planned tumor excision requires a more extensive resection to encompass the cancer. This forces a change in reconstructive plans. The surgeon must alter his primary plan or decide to employ one or two additional reconstructive options besides the primary reconstructive procedure of choice. The surgeon must keep as many options as possible available. Incisions for the tumor resection should be designed to accommodate the anatomy of all anticipated reconstructive procedures. Direct local or distant flap transfers may require a delay procedure prior to the definitive operation. The need for preparation of flaps must be anticipated so that the delay procedures are accomplished properly before the major resection.

HOW DOES PREOPERATIVE AND/OR POSTOPERATIVE RADIATION THERAPY AFFECT YOUR PLANNED RECONSTRUCTION?

The adverse effect of irradiation on tissue vascularity is the primary factor to be considered when radiation therapy is used before or after reconstructive procedures. After the initial inflammatory response, which lasts 4–6 weeks following irradiation, the degree of vascular sclerosis and interstitial fibrosis is directly related to time from irradiation and to the delivered dose.

There are several guideposts for surgical planning when a patient is given preoperative radiation therapy. Early after irradiation in the 5,000–6000-rad range, wound healing is reasonably good up to about 6 months. After that, reliability of wound healing deteriorates. The collateral blood flow, essential to flap survival, drops precipitously. Tissue planes may be obscured by the irradiation. Dissection around critical structures may be difficult. Incisions in the irradiated area should be planned to minimize damage to the vascular input. As an example, bipedicled parallel incisions (see Chap. 9) should be used for the neck dissection rather than alternative incisions which may create a unipedicle cervical flap. Tissue from any irradiated area should not be used for local transfer reconstructive procedures. Select an alternative donor site outside of the irradiated tissue.

Reconstructive procedures should be chosen to provide full-thickness, vascularized soft tissue coverage of critical areas in patients who will receive postoperative radiation therapy. Full-thickness flap coverage is more durable after irradiation than split-thickness graft coverage. Well-vascularized axial pattern flaps transferred directly or by free microvascular anastomoses withstand irradiation better than random pattern flaps.

The certainty or probability of postoperative radiation therapy is a relative contraindication to attempting complex bone reconstruction procedures in which the osseous vascularity may be tenuous. If bone reconstruction is required, vascularized bone grafts rather than free nonvascularized bone grafts are preferred. Generous soft tissue coverage must be provided over a bone area that will receive radiation therapy.

WHAT ARE THE PRIORITIES IN RECONSTRUCTION?

Reconstruction should be planned to involve the least number of procedures in the shortest possible time. Immediate one-stage reconstruction at the time of resection is most desirable. It can be achieved in many cases. Because a substantial number of head and neck patients will inevitably develop local-regional recurrence, the operative and reconstructive intervals should be as short as possible in order to provide the maximum quality of remaining life for the patient.

There are certain principles that must be adhered to when a reconstructive procedure is integrated with the extirpative procedure: any area of exposed brain must be covered with dura or a dural substitute and a full-thickness skin flap; the carotid artery must be protected by adequate skin coverage (i.e., at least full-thickness flap coverage); the eye must be protected by appropriate eyelid reconstruction; the mediastinum must be sealed off and the innominate artery protected; and complete skin and mucosal coverage must be provided for the oropharynx with provision for adequate oral continence.

From the above conditions it should be clear that the primary reconstructive procedure should be extensive and virtually all-encompassing. Certain other procedures can and should be relegated to a second-stage or delayed operation. Aesthetic reconstruction of the nose, ear, eyelid, and eyebrow is best done as a second-stage operation. In some areas such as the nose, reconstruction may involve a complex multistage flap procedure. One must be certain that tumor removal is complete prior to undertaking the definitive reconstructive procedure. Accordingly, it is frequently advisable to remove the tumor and await permanent section pathologic confirmation of tumor-free margins prior to proceeding with reconstruction.

WHAT ARE THE OPTIONS FOR COVERAGE TISSUE?

The multiple options for tissue coverage are discussed below. They are presented in a roughly ascending order of complexity. In general, the least complex method should be considered first.

Split-Thickness Skin Graft

Coverage with split-thickness skin grafts requires vascularized underlying subcutaneous tissue or muscle. Split-thickness skin grafts are frequently used for intraoral lining. Experience will rapidly show that accurate apposition and immobilization of intraoral split-thickness grafts with stents and packs may be challenging. Approximation of an unbroken skin graft with underlying suction catheters can sometimes be done.

Split-thickness grafts should not be used for coverage applied directly to bone, major vessels, or nerves. Skin grafts do not provide adequate coverage of areas where there will be underlying secondary bony reconstruction. Split-thickness skin grafts provide the least durable coverage for areas of planned postoperative radiation therapy. The surface produced by split-thickness skin graft coverage can be acceptable if the soft tissue recipient site is carefully contoured. Minor surface irregularities are common in areas of healed split-thickness skin graft coverage. An attempt should be made to resurface aesthetic units in a uniform manner when grafting the face (Fig 6–1).

Moderate thickness (12/1,000–15/1,000) split grafts are used for the face. Excellent quality large grafts can be harvested with the hand-driven Reese dermatome or the electric Padgett dermatome. The upper chest and back are the preferred donor sites for color match for the face. Grafts that are taken from the thigh are likely to develop hyperpigmentation. The grafts are used as an unbroken sheet graft. The graft is immobilized with a stent dressing.

Full-Thickness Skin Graft

Full-thickness skin grafts incorporate the entire dermal layer of skin. Full-thickness skin grafts are more slowly vascularized than are split-thickness skin grafts. Full-thickness skin grafts provide a coverage that more closely resembles normal skin texture than does a split-thickness skin graft. A full-thickness skin graft has the following advantages over a split-thickness skin graft: there is less tendency to hyperpigmentation postoperatively; there is less tendency for the graft to contract; the cover is more pliant and durable in friction and flexion areas; and there is less tendency to develop a smooth shiny surface. Full-thickness skin grafts can provide excellent resurfacing for the lower eyelids, nose, and lower lips. The preferred donor site is the retroauricular area. The donor site should be centered in the retroauricular sulcus. A graft as large as 4 × 5 cm can be obtained by using the skin of the posterior aspect of the ear and the adjacent mastoid area. The donor site is closed primarily. The harvesting of grafts 2.5 × 5 cm will produce a minimal change of the postauricular sulcus. The postauricular sulcus will be reduced in depth if a maximum-sized graft is obtained. The supraclavicular area is an alternate full-thickness skin graft donor area for facial coverage. Larger grafts can be taken from the supraclavicular area to cover aes-

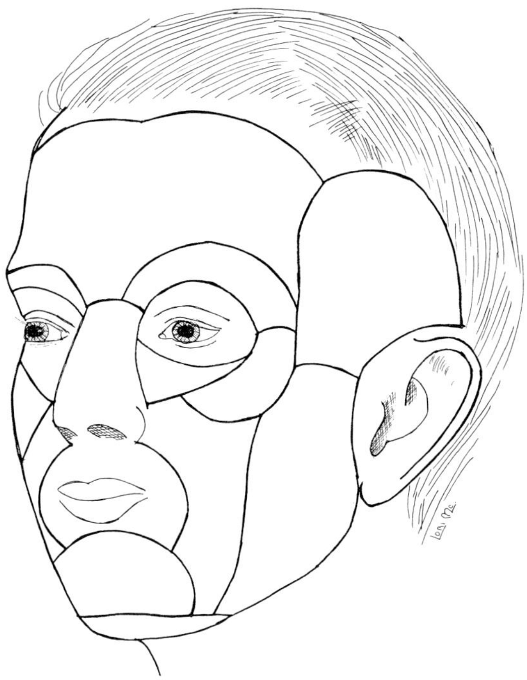

Fig 6–1.—Aesthetic units of the face. The margins of skin grafts or flaps should correspond to margins of aesthetic units.

thetic units such as the forehead or cheeks. The donor site is closed primarily. A wide scar will develop from primary closure of the supraclavicular donor site in virtually all patients; therefore the area should be avoided in women.

Mucosal Grafts

Buccal mucosal grafts can be used for free graft transfer within the oral cavity. Buccal mucosa can also be used for conjunctival coverage. Local flaps of the mucosa can be transferred within the oral cavity or rotated or advanced for lip coverage.

Free grafts of split-thickness skin, full-thickness skin, or mucosa must be securely immobilized in the postoperative period. We have found stent dressing immobilization very satisfactory. Adaptic gauze is placed over the graft and a bulky layer of absorbent cotton is then tied over the graft using interrupted stent sutures of 4–0 nylon. Sheets of absorbent cotton are cut to the size of the graft, soaked in saline, and placed onto the graft without being rung out. The stent sutures are then sequentially tied while the saline-soaked cotton is molded over the graft. When this technique is used, the stent gently conforms to the defect to secure the graft. The stent dressing is left in place for 5–7 days for split-thickness skin grafts and for 7–10 days for full-thickness skin grafts or mucosal grafts. It is important to remember that full-thickness skin or mucosal grafts heal slowly. They should be protected from minor trauma for a few days after stent removal.

Tongue Flaps

The tongue has been used to reconstruct a wide variety of intraoral and lip defects.[1] Operations which sacrifice a large segment of the tongue for surface coverage are largely unwarranted today. The functional loss is not justified in view of the large repertoire of other coverage options. One common exception may be the case in which a defect in the anterior floor of the mouth remains after tumor excision with adequate tongue bulk and external submental soft tissue. The tongue may be used for closure after tumor resection as a temporary measure to avoid a more complex coverage procedure. A minor secondary tongue release can be accomplished later (3–4 months) by freeing the tongue and covering the resultant defect with a split-thickness skin graft. This creates a new sulcus. In one other application, the tongue flap may be the procedure of choice for reconstruction of localized vermillion defects.[2] There is no significant functional loss since the amount of tissue is small. An excellent cosmetic appearance of the lip can be achieved.

Full-Thickness Flaps

Full-thickness flaps that include skin and subcutaneous tissue must be used for the repair of full-thickness defects of the cheek and lip. Full-thickness flap coverage is necessary over the carotid and for coverage of skeletal reconstruction. Full-thickness flap coverage is desirable in areas that will be subjected to radiation therapy.

Full-thickness flaps can be classified according to vascular anatomy. A random pattern or cutaneous flap receives a blood supply from arteries which lie deep to the muscle and send perpendicular perforating arteries to the interconnecting subdermal plexus of the skin. An axial pattern flap receives its blood supply from a direct cutaneous artery which courses above the muscle on the deep surface of the subcutaneous tissue.

Full-thickness skin flaps may also be classified as to their point of origin. There are direct local flaps, direct distant flaps, and distant flaps transferred by microvascular anastomoses. Direct local flaps lie adjacent to the defect and provide the best tissue match. They are the flap of choice for small defects. Direct local flaps are more easily executed in the older patient in whom the skin is slack. Direct local flaps are of two types; flaps that rotate about a pivot point (rotation and transposition flaps) and advancement flaps. A rotation flap is a semicircular skin flap that rotates about a pivot point. The donor area is closed by direct suture or skin graft. The line of greatest tension in a rotation flap extends from the pivot point to the leading edge of the flap (Fig 6–2,A). A transposition flap is a rectangular segment of skin that is turned on its pivot point to cover a defect.

A back-cut can be employed to gain additional mobility of the flap. A back-cut must be used judiciously because in order to be effective it must necessarily impinge on the vascular base of the flap (Fig 6–2,B). Advancement flaps are moved directly into the defect without lateral movement or rotation (Fig 6–2,C). Advancement flaps are rarely used in the head and neck area since foreward advancement is limited in most instances and the resulting linear scars are often unsightly. Figure 6–3 illustrates the use of superiorly and inferiorly based transposition flaps for cheek coverage. Figure 6–4 illustrates the use of a transposition flap for the coverage of a forehead defect. The use of transposition flaps in lip reconstruction is illustrated in chapter 12.

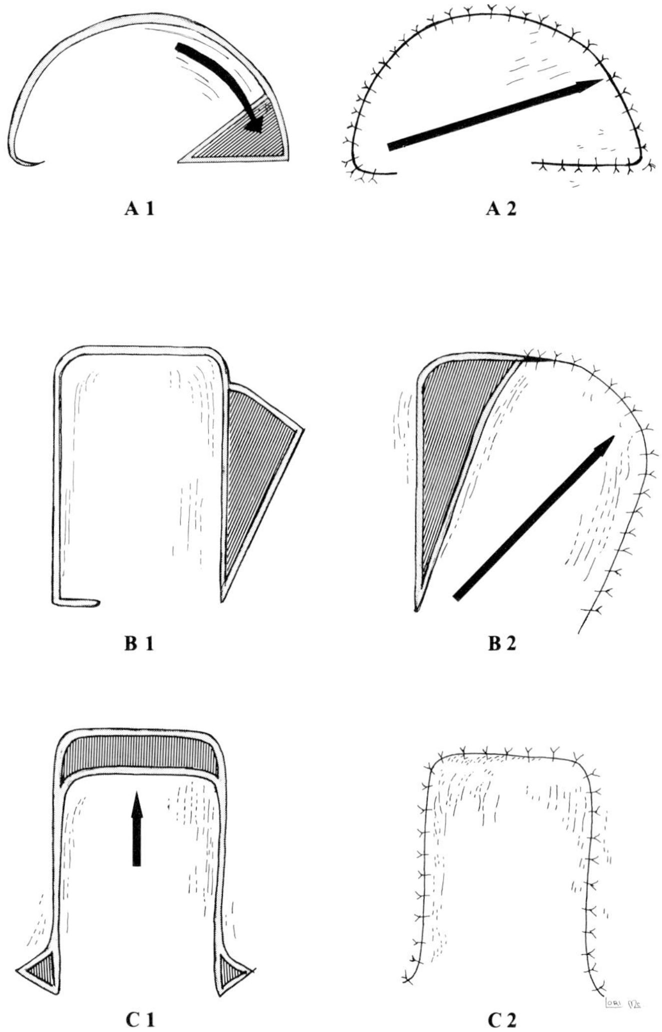

Fig 6–2.—Direct local flaps. **A,** rotation flap. *Arrow* in *2* indicates line of greatest tension. **B,** transposition flap. *Arrow* in *2* indicates line of greatest tension. **C,** Advancement flap. Closure at base *(1)* is facilitated by bilateral excision of Burow's triangles.

Specific Local Flaps

LATERAL CERVICAL FLAP

Lateral cervical tissues can provide cheek and lateral intraoral pharyngeal wall coverage. A superiorly based lateral cervical skin flap 6 cm wide and 12 cm long (Fig 6–5) will provide cheek coverage. The flap can be rotated 180° to bring the epidermal side inward, providing intraoral coverage by the creation of an intentional pharyngocutaneous fistula which is closed 3–4 weeks later (see Chaps. 13 and 14). The flap is raised with the underlying platysma muscle. This is a random pattern flap based on the rich dermal vascular plexis of the cervical area. This skin flap is less reliable than axial pattern skin flaps such as the forehead and deltopectoral flap, which will be discussed later. A delay procedure is advisable if the flap is to be extended beyond the 2:1 length to width ratio. Reliability can be enhanced by widening the base. The cervical flap is quite utilitarian for immediate reconstruction. We found it simple, reliable, and cosmetically acceptable in a reported series of 22 patients and in numerous subsequent patients.[3]

Owens suggested a modification of the lateral cervical flap to include the underlying sternocleidomastoid muscle.[4] The sternocleidomastoid muscle has a double origin from the manubrium and clavicle and inserts into the mastoid process and occipital bone. The muscle has a segmental pattern blood supply, but a dominant branch of the occipital artery enters near the insertion of the muscle and will usually support the entire muscle.[5, 6] The inclusion of the muscle as a carrier has improved the reliability of the flap when the underlying sternocleidomastoid muscle is not removed during the tumor resection.

MEDIAN FOREHEAD FLAP

The median forehead flap is useful for coverage of nasal defects that are extensive but only subtotal (Fig 6–6).[7] It is also useful for medial orbital defects. The median forehead flap receives its blood supply from the paired supratrochlear arteries. The flap is raised by two parallel vertical incisions over the forehead, extending from the hairline to the root of the nose. The vertical incisions are joined at the hairline. The incisions are deepened down to but not through the pericranium, to a point just above the nasofrontal angle. The incision is then continued only superficially through skin so that the integrity of the supratrochlear vessels is preserved. The flap is turned down and inset into the nasal defect. A flap 2 cm in width can be obtained and still allow primary closure of the donor area. Wider flaps will require the development of bilateral forehead transposition flaps to close the defect. At 18–21 days following inset, the flap pedicle is divided. The unused portion of the pedicle is returned to its original position and inset

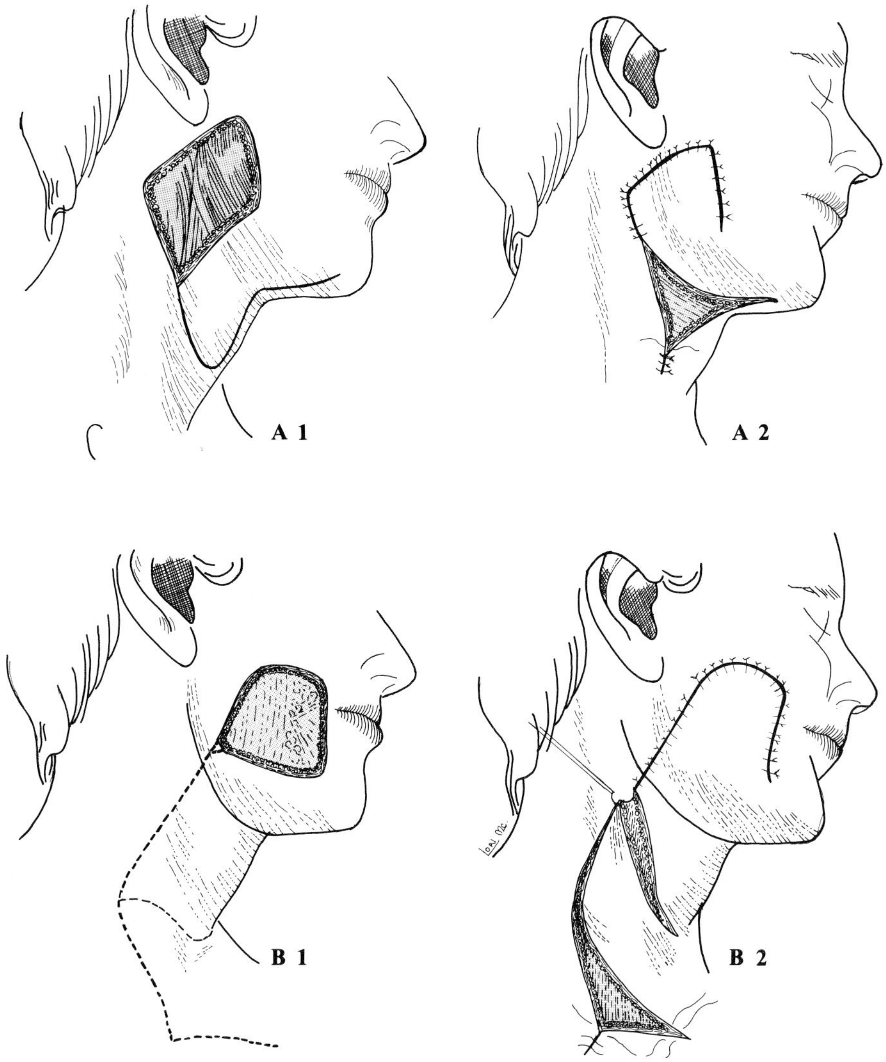

Fig 6–3.—Transposition flaps for cheek coverage. **A,** superiorly based cervical transposition flap. **B,** inferiorly based cervical transposition flap.

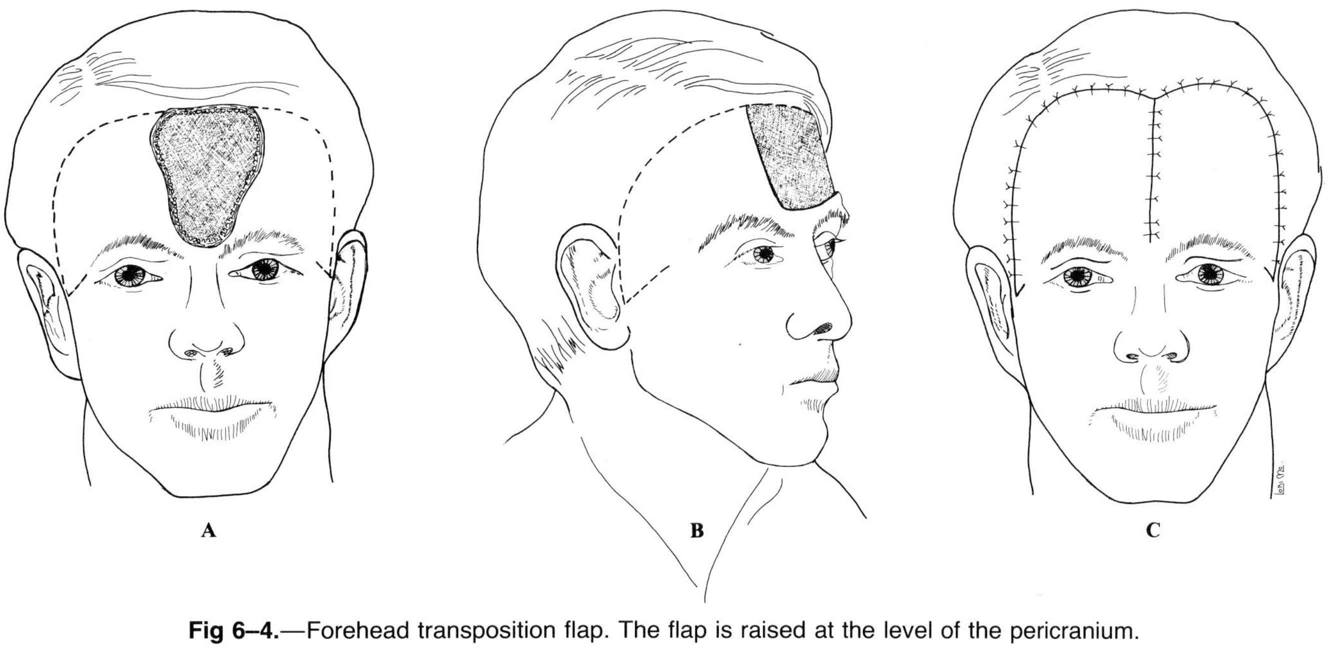

Fig 6–4.—Forehead transposition flap. The flap is raised at the level of the pericranium.

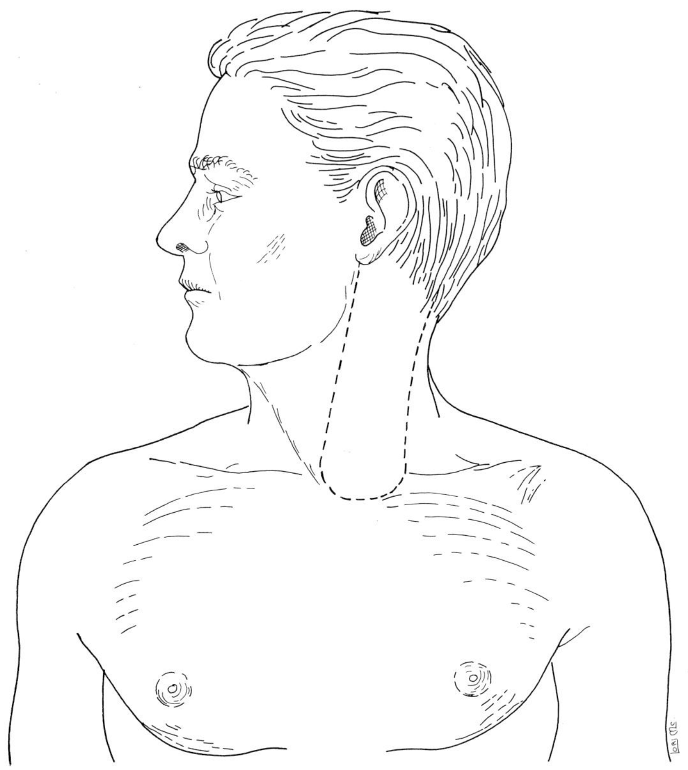

Fig 6–5.—Lateral cervical flap. The flap may contain platysma muscle or include the underlying sternomastoid muscle.

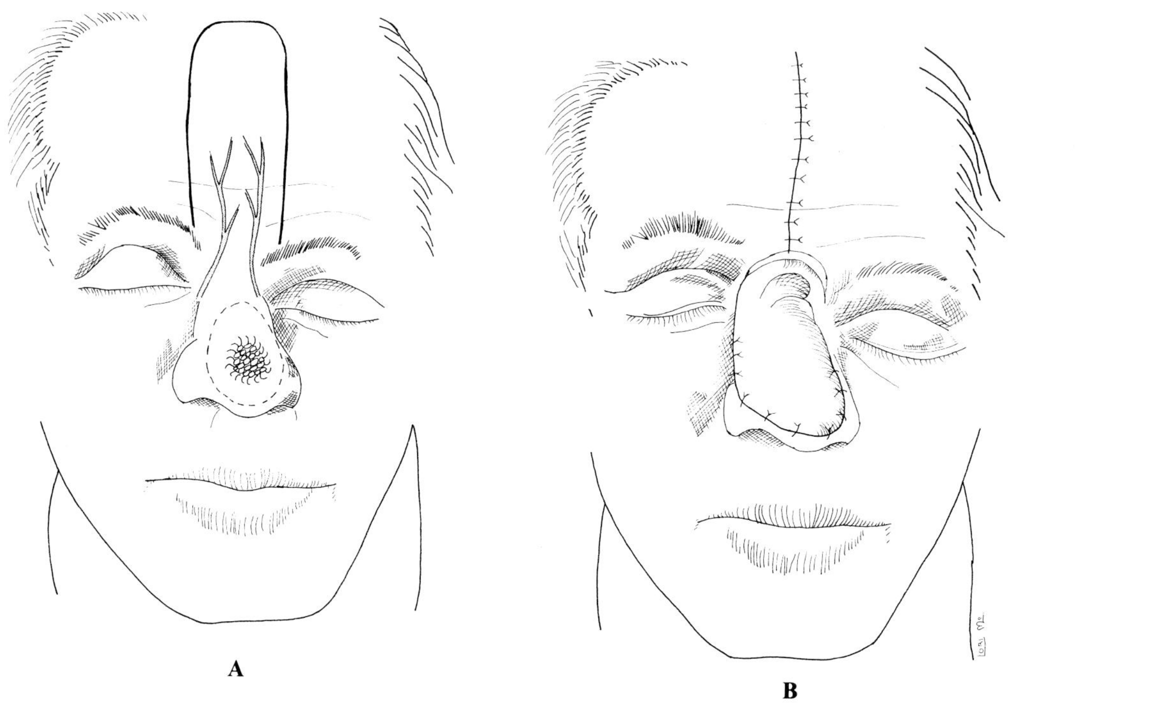

Fig 6–6.—Median forehead flap. **A,** flap is based on the paired supratrochlear arteries. **B,** flap is rotated 180° into the nasal defect. The donor site is closed primarily.

into the nasofrontal area. Narrowing of the intraeyebrow distance is alleviated by the secondary insetting of the base of the pedicle flap.

TOTAL FOREHEAD FLAP

The forehead flap can provide coverage for lateral cheek and lateral pharyngeal wall defects (Fig 6–7). It is difficult to make this flap reach the midline floor of the mouth. The total forehead flap has a long and useful history; however, at present there are relatively few occasions when this technique is a method of first choice. McGregor stimulated interest in the versatility of this flap.[8] Its several areas of application have been described by others.[9–11] A reconstructive technique should not create a greater deformity than the one which is being reconstructed. The forehead flap donor site is very apparent and does represent a significant cosmetic deformity. When you are desperate for full-thickness coverage, deformity may be a lesser consideration.

The forehead flap is based on the superficial temporal artery with a minor input from the posterior auricular artery. Both are branches of the external carotid artery. This flap should not be considered if the ipsilateral external carotid artery has been sacrificed in the tumor resection or has been given a heavy dose of irradiation. Pulsatile forward flow in the temporal artery can be confirmed by Doppler technique should there be any question. The flap should encompass the entire forehead, with the margins of the flap following the eyebrow and forehead hairlines. The flap is raised at the level of the pericranium. The vascularity of the distal portion of the flap may be tenuous, and therefore a delayed procedure is advisable. The flap is introduced into the mouth by a 180° medial rotation and the creation of a subcutaneous tunnel lying between the flap pedicle and the lateral surface of the zygomatic arch. The most direct path into the intraoral space is to pass the flap deep to the zygomatic arch. This space is narrow, so compression of the flap beneath the arch will frequently compromise the blood supply. Don't try it. A forehead flap can be lined with a split-thickness skin graft placed on the surface of the frontalis muscle in the initial portion of the delayed procedure. Thus, the flap can be used for both external and intraoral surface lining. The flap pedicle is divided 3 weeks postoperatively and the base is returned to be inset into the temporal area. A split-thickness sheet graft is used to cover the forehead donor area.

SCALPING FLAP

The scalping flap is reliable for coverage of full-thickness defects of the orbit and nasal area. The technique allows transposition of the lateral forehead skin to the midface area. Much of the incision of the scalping flap is within the hair-bearing area and thus is hidden. The donor area on the lateral forehead is a relatively inconspicuous location. The scalping flap is one of very few techniques suitable for total nasal reconstruction (Fig 6–8).[12]

Careful measurements of the defect to be covered are transferred to the lateral portion of the forehead. The incisions for the carrier portion of the scalping flap extend from the lateral border of the outlined donor area

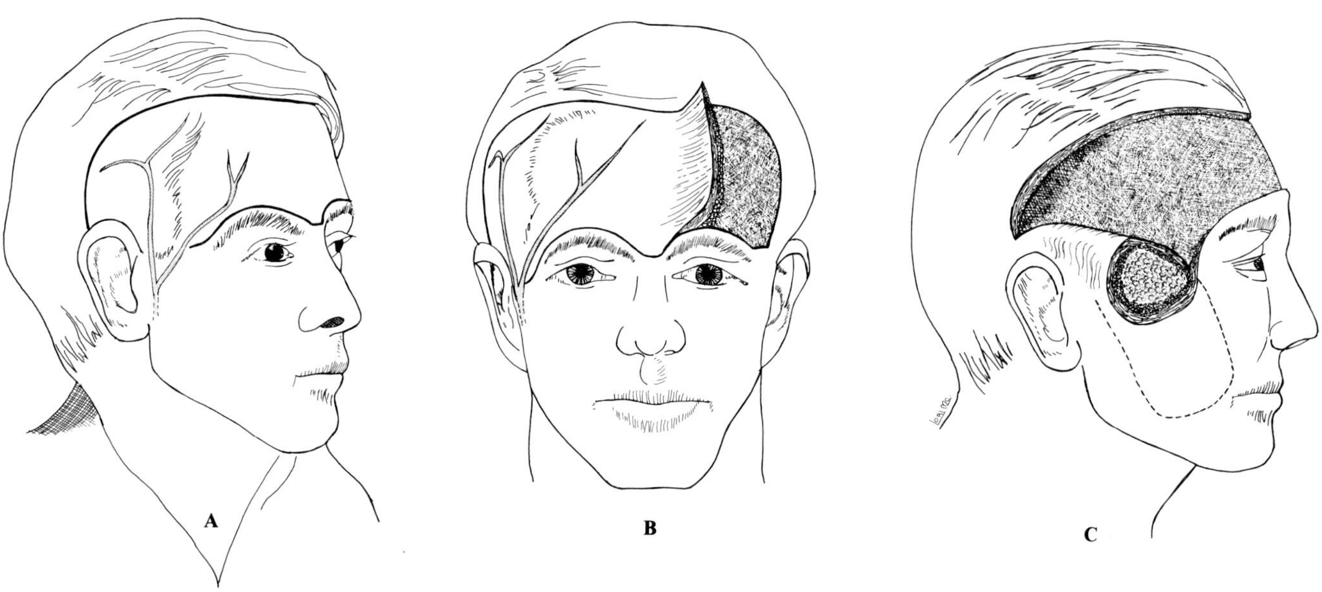

Fig 6–7.—Total forehead flap. **A,** the flap is based on the superficial temporal artery. **B,** the flap is raised in a plane superficial to the pericranium. **C,** the flap is turned intraorally through a subcutaneous tunnel that is superficial to the zygomatic arch.

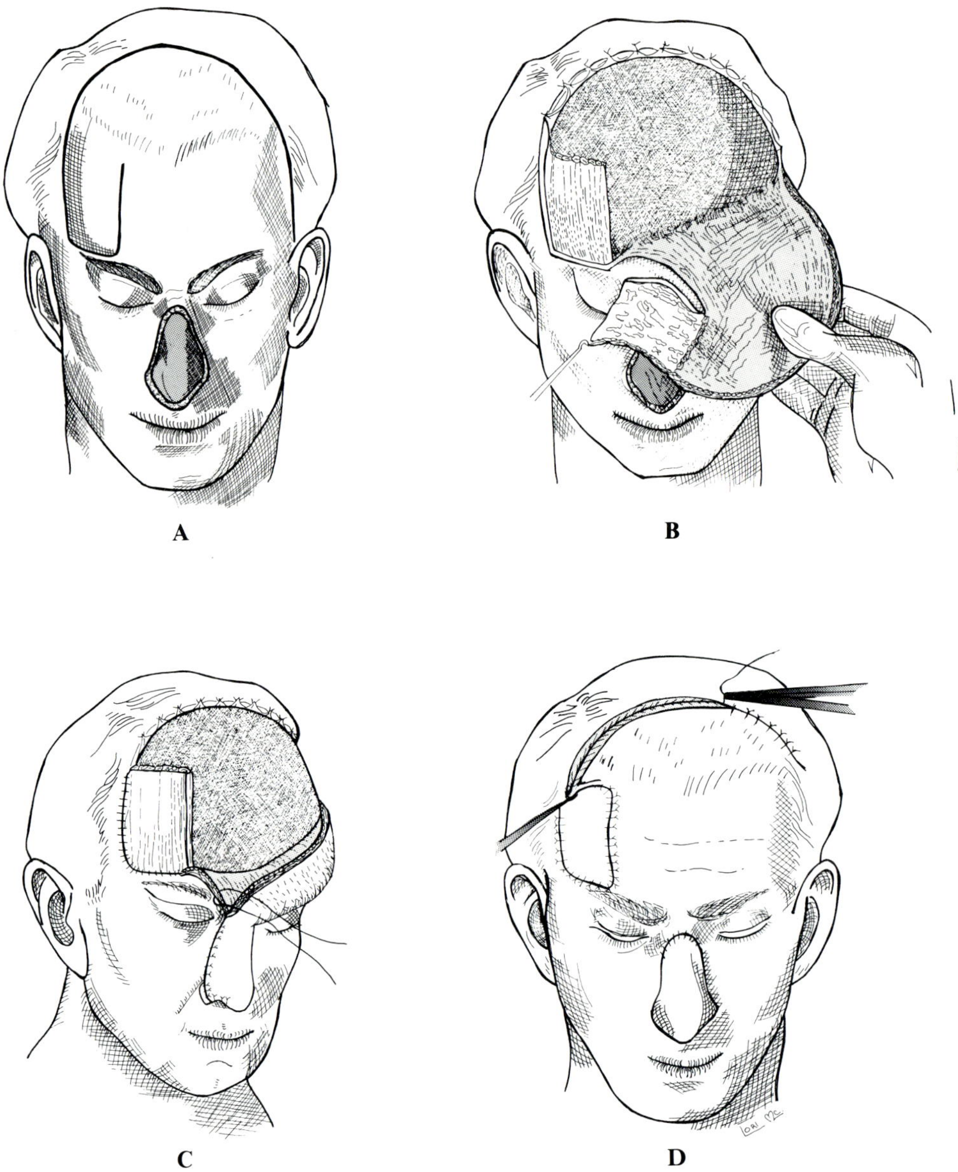

Fig 6–8.—Scalping flap. **A,** the door site is outlined in the lateral forehead. **B,** frontalis muscle is preserved in the donor area. The remaining flap is elevated in a plane superficial to the pericranium. **C,** the flap is tubed. **D,** 3 weeks later the pedicle is divided and the flap sutured into its original position. A retroauricular full-thickness skin graft covers the lateral forehead donor area.

superiorly and transversely across the midportion of the scalp to the superior auricular area on the contralateral scalp (see Fig 6–8,A). The area of skin to be transposed into the defect is elevated at a plane deep to the subcutaneous tissue and superficial to the underlying frontalis muscle. The remaining flap is raised at a plane superficial to the pericranium and deep to the frontalis muscle (see Fig 6–8,B). The flap is sutured into the recipient site and the flap base is tubed, producing an overhanging roll of skin in the area of the contralateral eyebrow (see Fig 6–8,C). The donor area is dressed with bacitracin ointment and telfa gauze. Three weeks following inset, the pedicle flap is divided and the scalp unrolled and sutured into its original position. At this time the donor defect in the lateral forehead area is covered with a full-thickness retroauricular graft which will provide an excellent pigment and texture match for the normal forehead skin (see Fig 6–8,D). Delay of the forehead flap is not necessary. A delayed procedure can be performed if lining tissue or stabilizing cartilage grafts are desired. For a delayed procedure the lateral forehead area is elevated 10 days prior to the reconstructive procedure and split-thickness skin or cartilage is attached to the subcutaneous tissue surface of the flap. The margins of the flap are resutured to allow healing of the implanted tissues.

TRAPEZIUS MYOCUTANEOUS FLAP

The trapezius myocutaneous flap can be used for coverage of the lower cheek and lateral lower neck area. This flap is based on the portion of the underlying trapezius muscle that originates from the thoracic vertebrae and seventh cervical vertebra. The primary blood supply of the muscle is the transverse cervical artery (Fig 6–9).

The flap is outlined by parallel vertical incisions placed lateral to the vertebral column and medial to the scapula. The flap extends to the lower border of the origin of the trapezius muscle. Flap elevation is begun by division of the origin of the trapezius muscle medially and division of the muscle distally. This is followed by careful separation of the trapezius muscle from the rhomboid muscle in the area of the scapula. The donor defect is closed primarily.[13]

Regional Flaps

DELTOPECTORAL FLAP

The deltopectoral flap is based medially and extends transversely over the upper anterior chest. This flap has an axial pattern blood supply (Fig 6–10).[14-16] The flap can be moved to cover all of the anterior head and neck area below the supraorbital ridge. It can be folded to provide both intraoral and cheek lining. In a delayed procedure, the deep surface can be covered with a split-thickness skin graft to provide both intraoral and external coverage. It is a thin, hairless, pliable flap which provides tissue with a satisfactory texture. The major disadvantage is that the pigmentation of the flap tends to be much lighter than the normal skin of the face. The flap is supplied by perforating branches of the internal mammary artery through the first, second, third and fourth interspaces. The vessels course laterally superficial to the pectoralis fascia. A secondary axial blood supply of the flap is provided by a branch of the thoracoacromial trunk and a branch of the first portion of the axillary artery entering the skin on the deep surface of the infraclavicular triangle. The vascular pattern of the flap is random lateral to the cephalic vein groove.

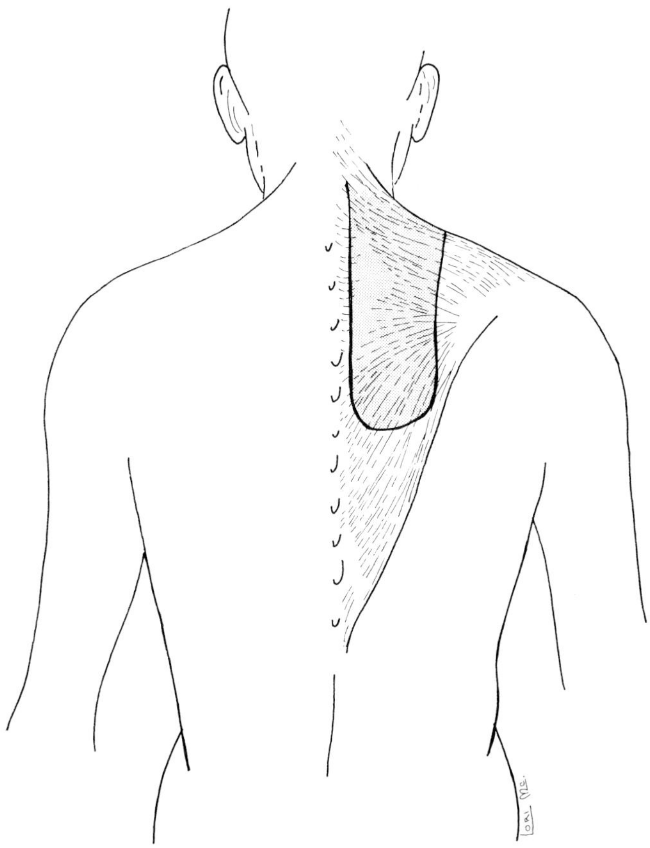

Fig 6–9.—Trapezius myocutaneous flap. The flap contains a medial component of the trapezius muscle.

A deltopectoral flap is designed with the superior margin just inferior to the clavicle. The incision parallels the course of the clavicle. The inferior margin of the flap is outlined parallel to the superior margin and crosses the axilla at the apex of the anterior axillary fold. It is the unusual pliancy of the periaxillary tissue which facilitates rotation of the deltopectoral flap. A flap which extends to the midlateral portion of the shoulder can be elevated without a preliminary delay procedure. In the shoulder area the flap is raised deep to the subcutaneous tissue and superficial to the underlying deltoid fascia. Medial to the cephalic vein groove the flap is raised with the underlying pectoral fascia to prevent injury to the axial vessels.

A lateral extension of the flap can be incorporated distally by using tissue along the anterior aspect of the arm. An arm extension would require preliminary delay of the flap in the shoulder area. The delay consists of outlining and elevating the portion of the flap that extends over the shoulder. In addition, the delay incision in the superior margin of the flap should be made to the level of the thoracoacromial trunk, which is divided.

When the flap is mobilized for use, the chest wall donor area is covered with a meshed split-thickness skin graft. The proximal portion of the flap is tubed to provide a closed wound. After 3 or more weeks, the pedicle is divided. This division is done only after adequate vascularization at the recipient site is assured by gentle constriction of the pedicle with a Penrose drain. The proximal portion of the flap can be unrolled and returned to the chest wall defect after removal of some of the split-thickness skin graft. The final result is an area of split-thickness skin graft coverage in the shoul-

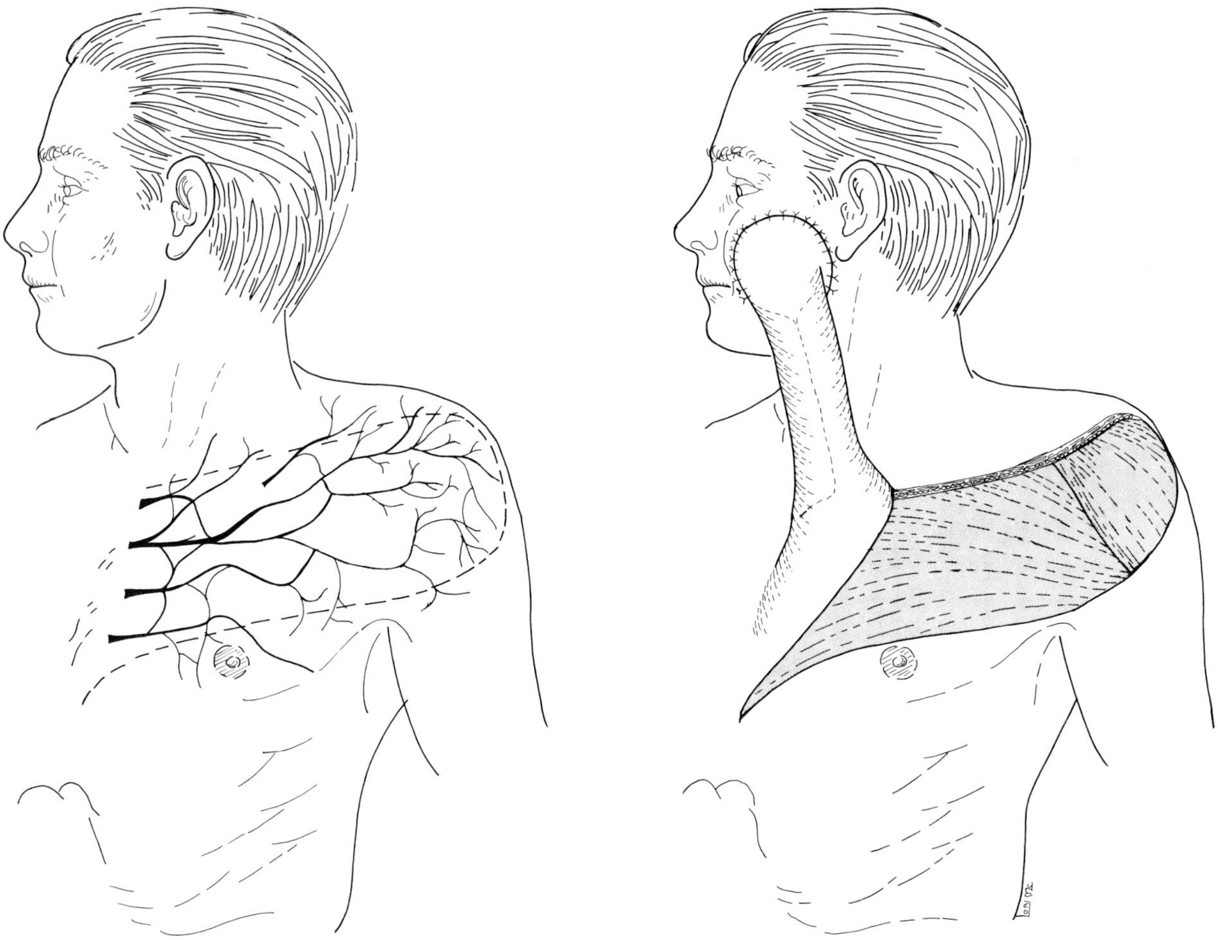

A B

Fig 6–10.—Deltopectoral flap. **A,** principal blood supply is axial pattern vessels which are perforating branches of the internal mammary artery through first, second, third, and fourth interspaces. **B,** the flap can be raised without delay to the midlateral shoulder area. The proximal portion of the flap is tubed. Additional variations of use are illustrated in chapter 14.

der area equivalent to the head and neck area covered in the reconstructive procedure.

The flap is extremely reliable and will tolerate manipulation without vascular compromise. We have had problems with the flap only in instances where external compression had been applied to the base area of the pedicle. In addition, we have noted problems in the use of the flap for the closure of long-standing orocutaneous fistulas. In two cases massive oral contamination led to infection and partial necrosis of the flap.

PECTORALIS MAJOR MYOCUTANEOUS FLAP

The pectoralis major myocutaneous flap is an alternative to the deltopectoral flap for coverage of lower face, intraoral, and anterior cervical defects (Fig 6–11).[17, 18] A skin island carried on the pectoralis major muscle is transposed to the defect. The pectoralis major muscle originates from the clavicle, sternum, and first seven ribs. It inserts into the bicipital groove of the humerus. The major blood supply is the thoracoacromial artery, a branch of the axillary artery. The skin territory which can be carried to the head and neck area for reconstruction overlies the muscle between the nipple and the sternum from the fifth to the eighth ribs (see Fig 6–11). The skin island can be extended inferiorly 3–4 cm based on a random pattern dermal plexis (shaded area in Fig 6–11,A). The distal extension has tenuous vascularity.

The flap is elevated by first outlining and incising the skin island. As an option, the upper skin and soft tissue may be raised as a deltopectoral flap. The inferior attachments of the muscle are divided and the retropectoral space is entered. The sternal and humeral attachments of the muscle are divided. In most cases the

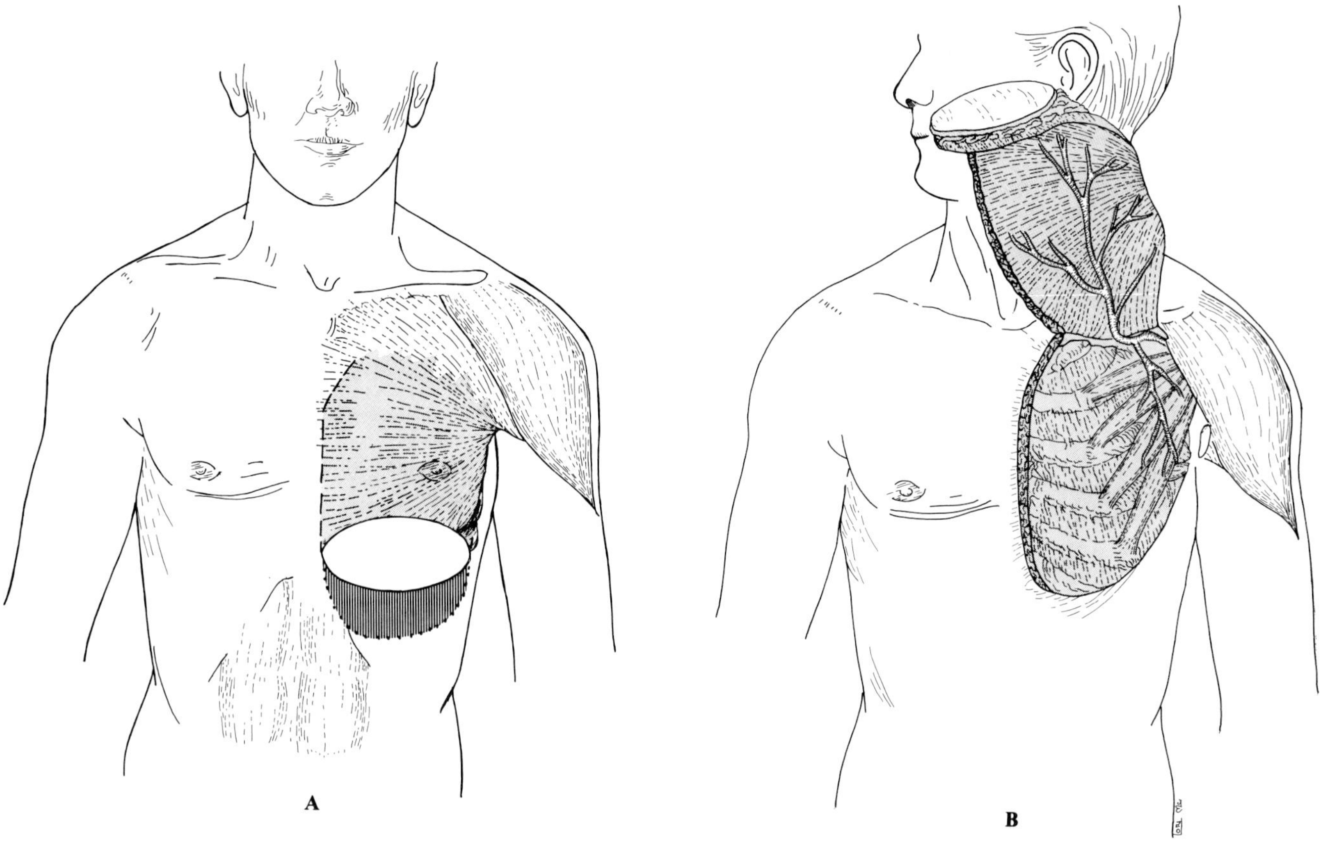

Fig 6–11.—Pectoralis major myocutaneous flap. **A,** a skin island overlying ribs 5–8 is carried on the underlying pectoralis muscle. *Shaded area* below the skin island is the possible lower extension. The overlying skin and soft-tissue between the skin island and the clavicle may be raised in the form of a deltopectoral flap as in Fig 6–10,A in order to preserve the option of an available secondary flap. **B,** the major vascular pedicle is the thoracoacrominal artery. Its use in oral closure is illustrated in chapters 14 and 15.

clavicular attachments of the muscle also will be divided with the muscle, which leaves the flap pedicled only on the thoracoacromial vessels. Great care must be taken to visualize the vascular supply and protect it from tension and injury during the course of the dissection. If a radical neck dissection has been performed the muscle is placed subcutaneously. In this position, it will provide contour restoration to the neck. If a radical neck dissection has not been performed, the muscle bulk may present a problem when placed in the subcutaneous position. An alternative is to place the muscle superficial to the skin and plan for a division of the muscle pedicle 3–4 weeks later. If the muscle pedicle is left outside the cervical skin in anticipation of the planned division at a second stage, a difficult wound care problem is created.

Experimental studies show better oxygenation of transferred tissues with a myocutaneous flap compared to a random flap.[19] This is accomplished by a trade for more potential technical complications. We believe that for routine frequent use, the pectoralis myocutaneous flap is no more reliable than the deltopectoral flap. The thoracoacromial vessels are easily injured. The skin supplied with the pectoralis major muscle unit has the same pigment and texture as the deltopectoral flap. The muscle bulk of the pedicle can add the advantage of contour restoration of the neck. Used in this way, the technique is a one-stage reconstruction (see Chaps. 13 and 14). In many applications the bulk of the muscular pedicle is a disadvantage that may lead to an unsightly fullness of the neck if it is left in the subcutaneous position. The myocutaneous flap may have its best use when transposed to a bacteriologically contaminated site.

LATISSIMUS DORSI MYOCUTANEOUS FLAP

The latissimus dorsi myocutaneous flap is currently the procedure of choice for myocutaneous flap breast reconstruction. The use of the flap has been extended to reconstruction problems of the head and neck area

(Fig 6–12).[20, 21] Though it is the least convenient of regional flaps for head and neck reconstruction, the advantages of the posteriorly placed chest wall donor incision make the flap an alternative choice in selected patients.

The latissimus dorsi muscle originates from the lower six thoracic vertebrae and inserts into the intertubercular groove of the humerus. The principal blood supply of the muscle is the thoracodorsal artery, with secondary input from perforators in the posterior midline. A skin island is designed in the area of the lower one third of the muscle, usually overlying the 10th to the 12th ribs. Through an incision in the midlateral position of the chest wall, the posterior midline and inferior origins of the muscle are divided and the muscle is mobilized (see Fig 6–12,A). It is usually necessary to detach the humeral insertion to allow the muscle mass to be transposed superiorly into the head and neck area. A long vascular pedicle allows much freedom of movement in the axillary area.

The latissimus dorsi myocutaneous unit has the same advantages and disadvantages related to the muscle bulk as does the pectoralis major myocutaneous unit. The posterior chest wall skin island is a rather poor color and texture match for the skin of the face.

MICROVASCULAR FREE FLAPS

Skin flaps or myocutaneous flaps transferred to the head and neck area by *microvascular anastomoses* can provide external surface coverage similar to the regional flaps described above. Useful donor sites for microvascular flaps have included the groin,[22] scapula,[23] upper arm,[24] latissimus dorsi, and tensor fascia lata.[25] We believe that microvascular free flaps in the head and neck area should be used to provide large areas of coverage which would not be possible by local or regional flap techniques. The complexity of the procedure and the poor color match of the transplanted tissues are significant disadvantages. Microvascular intestinal free flaps, however, are the procedure of choice for the restoration of esophageal continuity after esophagopharyngectomy and have wide application for intraoral coverage (see Chap. 16). This technique will be discussed below.

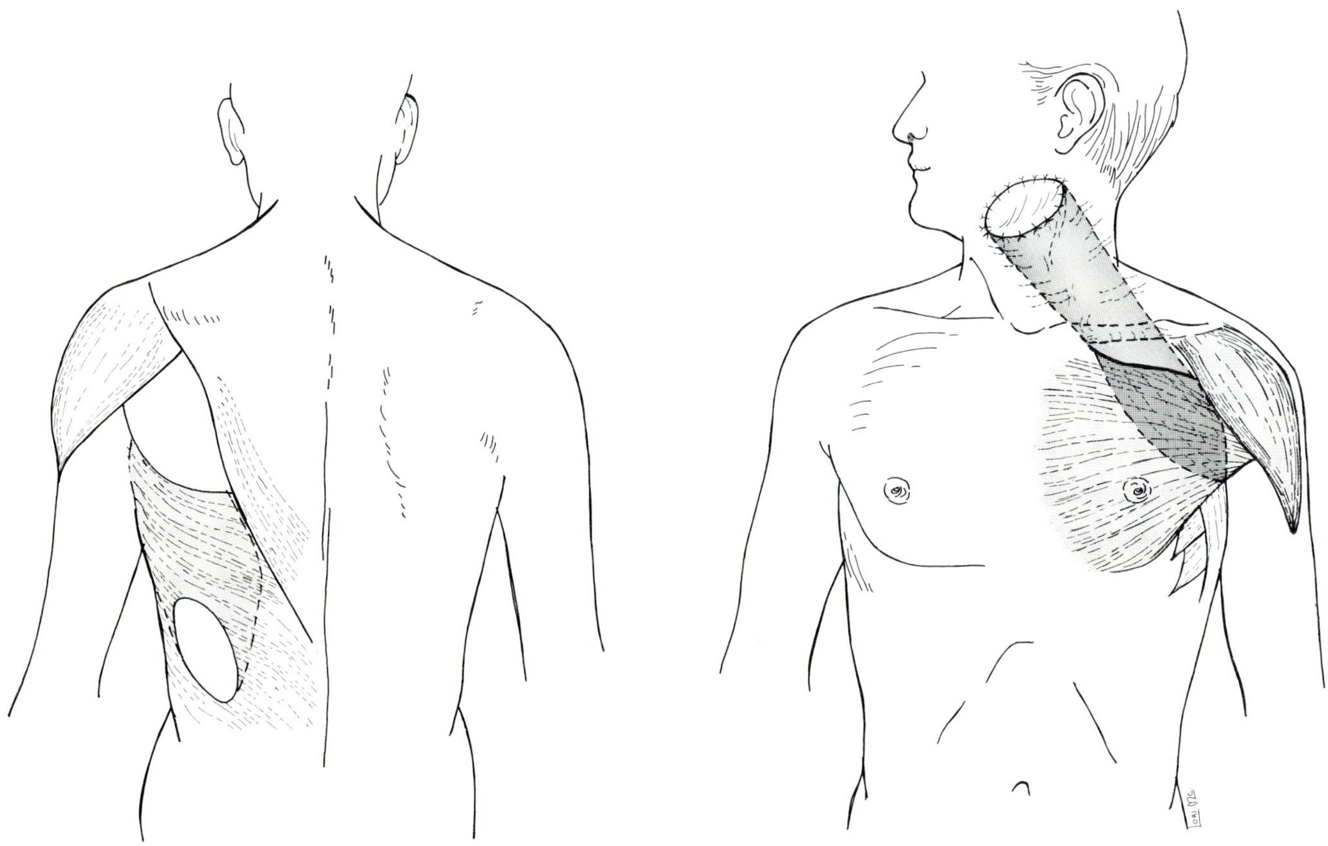

A B

Fig 6–12.—Latissimus dorsi myocutaneous flap. **A,** a skin island is outlined over the lower portion of the muscle. The donor site is closed primarily. **B,** the muscle is passed superficial or deep to the pectoralis and subcutaneously in the neck.

WHAT ARE THE OPTIONS FOR REPLACEMENT OF BONE LOSS?

Any technique of bone reconstruction has a primary requirement of adequate soft tissue coverage. Bone grafts of any type must be placed in a sterile, adequately vascularized, soft tissue bed if they are to survive in the long term and restore contour.

Nonvascularized Bone

Grafts of iliac crest or rib can be used for cranial and facial reconstruction. Nonvascularized bone grafts only survive by the ingrowth of vascularity from the surrounding tissues. Free nonvascularized bone grafts will *not* survive if they are placed in a heavily irradiated tissue bed. Unfortunately, the revascularization and long-term volume maintenance of nonvascularized bone grafts are unpredictable. Some bony resorption is inevitable so that contours must be overcorrected at the time of grafting. Since bone resorption is unpredictable, optimum contour restoration will usually require more than one operative procedure.

The ilium is an excellent source of both cancellous and cortical bone. The thickest area of the iliac crest is the anterior third between the anterior superior iliac spine and tubercle of the crest. With the skin retracted medially, an incision is made overlying the crest. This will allow the final position of the incision to fall lateral to the crest. The incision is carried to the periosteum and the periosteum is reflected. If a single table of cortical bone is desired, the inner table is exposed and a segment of the inner table can be removed by vertically sectioning the crest with osteotomies. Underlying cancellous bone can be removed as needed. The outer surface of the ala is also exposed if full thickness of cortical bone is required. Periosteal elevation is easier over the inner surface of the ilium. The iliac crest contour should be maintained by preserving a partial thickness of the crest. A suction drain is placed in the wound after the removal of large grafts. Fascial attachments overlying the iliac crest must be securely reconstructed in wound closure. The patients typically have significant discomfort and pain on walking for several days postoperatively.

Split-rib grafts are most useful for cranial and orbital reconstruction. Two different approaches may be used to obtain rib grafts. An incision is made anteriorly overlying the seventh rib when only a small segment of rib is required. Large defects that require several ribs require a larger posterolateral thoracoplasty approach. An incision is made parallel to the seventh rib from the scapula to the anterior axillary line. The latissimus dorsi muscle is divided and the lower edge of the trapezius muscle is raised. The fibers of the serratus anterior muscle are split anteriorly. A fascial plane is developed which allows access to the second through tenth ribs. Segments of alternate ribs can be removed. The periosteum is closed carefully with a running suture. The chest wall musculature is repaired in layers. The most common complication of rib graft harvest is a pneumothorax requiring short-term chest tube placement.

WHAT ARE THE OPTIONS FOR MANDIBLE RECONSTRUCTION?

Reconstruction of the mandible is the most common bony structural problem encountered in head and neck surgery. The need for mandible reconstruction depends on the size of the defect, the extent of distortion of the residual tissues, functional loss, and disfigurement. The restoration of bone continuity is not necessary if the defect is a short segment posterior to the mental foramen. Adequate soft tissue coverage will restore proper anatomical spatial relationship to the mandibular fragments and prevent contraction of adjacent tissues. Splints of Kirschner wires through Silastic blocks can be used as a temporary measure to maintain space during soft tissue healing.[26] When the tumor resection includes the anterior mandibular arch, significant disability will result from lack of lingual and pharyngeal support. Salivary incontinence, speech defects, and facial deformity will be aggravated (see Chap. 13). Patients with anterior segment mandible resection are candidates for some type of mandible reconstruction.

Nonvascularized Bone

Bone grafts of either iliac bone or rib may be used. Whole carved segments can be fashioned from iliac blocks.[27] Alternatively, individual segments of iliac bone can be wired together or threaded on Kirschner wires to conform to the defect with the intervening spaces packed with bone chips.[28] Bendable bone plate and screws are also used for stability. This is rarely successful when defects exceed 4 cm.

Vascularized Bone

The use of vascularized bone segments transferred by microvascular techniques presents an attractive option in mandibular reconstruction. Microvascular transplantation of an anterior rib segment supplied by periosteal vessels has been described.[29] Incorporation of the first metatarsal within a dorsalis pedis free flap has been successfully used.[30] The iliac crest based on the deep circumflex iliac artery is currently the most useful vascularized bone graft for mandibular reconstruction. An overlying skin island may be taken with the underlying bone graft to provide skin coverage as well.[31] The donor site dissection for the free iliac graft is difficult. The patients complain bitterly about postoperative pain.

The use of vascularized or nonvascularized bone grafts for mandible reconstruction requires secure immobilization during the period of healing. This can be accomplished with intermaxillary fixation if teeth are present and the maxillary arch is preserved. Acrylic splints secured to the stable arch structure are used if teeth are absent. The use of the external-internal Morris biphase appliance allows secure immobilization of the mandibular segment without oral occlusion.[32] If soft tissue coverage is adequate, then bendable plates can be used to achieve stability with screws.

Distant Myo-Osseous Bone Transfer

The pectoralis major muscle flap can be used as a carrier for the transfer of a vascularized rib segment. A medial segment of the fifth rib can be included with the myocutaneous flap for mandible reconstruction.[33] This procedure has been illustrated by Maisel and Adams.[34] Vascularity of the rib is maintained by a rather tenuous attachment of the pectoralis major, primarily to the medial cartilaginous extension of the rib. A lateral pectoral composite flap based on the lateral component of the pectoralis major muscle and lower border of the pectoralis minor muscle has been used with success in primary mandible reconstruction in difficult irradiated sites. The advantage of this flap is that the attachment of the carrier muscle to underlying full-thickness rib is more secure.[35]

Local Myo-Osseous Bone Transfer

One of the more common defects is the loss of the midpoint of the arch because of direct cancer invasion. Typically a 4- to 6-cm defect is produced when a segmental mandibulectomy must be done (see Chap. 13). In our group, Dr. Brown has pioneered a very useful local myo-osseous tissue advancement that can be accomplished without extensive distant transfer of bone. The technique is illustrated in Figures 6–13, 6–14 and 6–15. The upper portions of the masseter and pterygoid muscles are freed from the mandible, leaving complete attachment to the lower 1–1½ cm of remaining horizontal ramus. The horizontal ramus is sectioned horizontally in its long direction. The lower strip of horizontal ramus is advanced anteriorly as far as possible and angled inward. The fragments are then firmly secured with wire. In seven patients there has been only two failures of union.[36]

Bone Chips

Cancellous bone stabilized in a perforated metal device can be used for mandible reconstruction. Early techniques involved the use of metal trays for stabilization. Trays of Vitallium or titanium packed with cancellous autogenous bone have been moderately successful.[37] The most frequent problems have been intraoral erosion with exposure of the prosthesis. If infection occurs, then the prosthesis must be removed before ade-

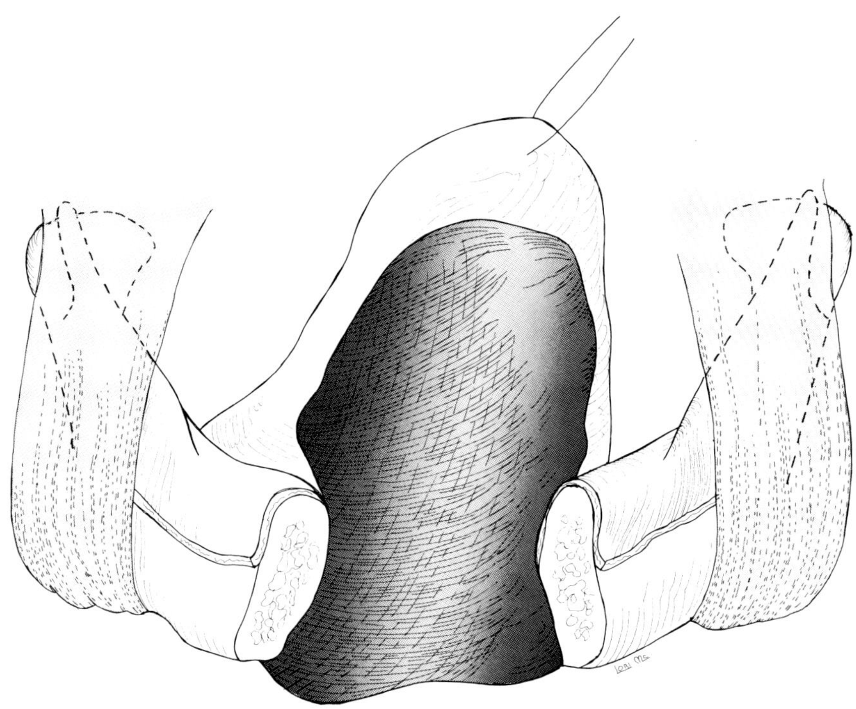

Fig 6–13.—The large anterior mandibular defect remaining after removal of a floor of the mouth cancer that invaded the mandible.

LARGE ANTERIOR MANDIBULAR DEFECT

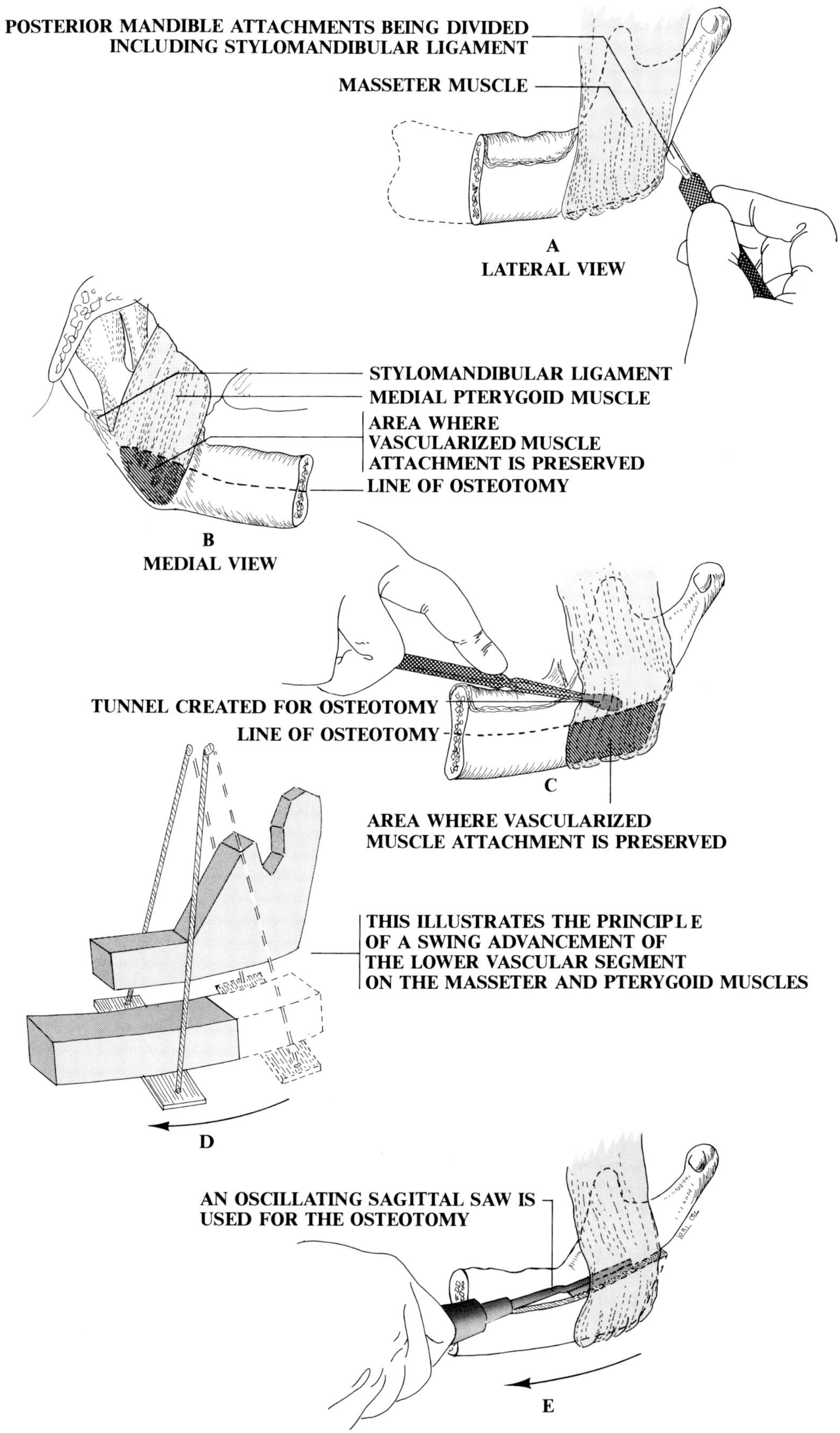

Fig 6–14.—Creation of a lower segment of mandible that is pedicled on the muscular attachments of the masseter and pterygoid muscles. The lower portion of the drawing shows the principle of forward swing of the free lower segment.

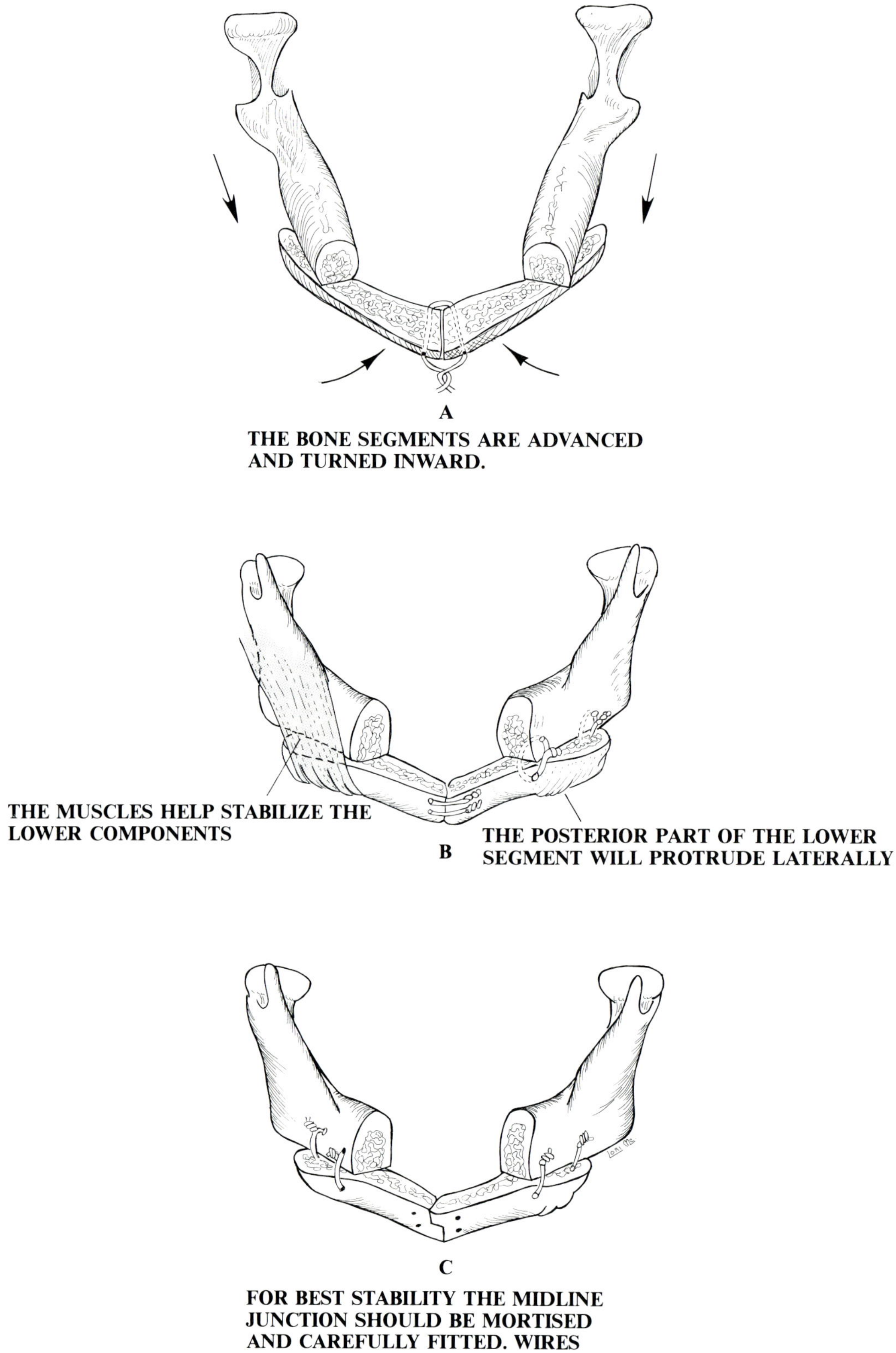

Fig 6–15.—Rotation and methods of securing the bilatually advanced lower segments of the mandible.

quate stabilization is achieved. This necessitates regrafting. A similar technique using a dacron-urethane prosthesis has been reported with a much higher success rate due to better acceptance of the dacron-urethane material by surrounding soft tissue.[38] A reduced failure rate of only 3% in 32 cases and a complication rate of 9% compares very favorably when compared to an earlier series of Vitallium prostheses in which a 16% failure rate and a 37% complication rate were noted.[39]

HOW CAN ESOPHAGEAL CONTINUITY BE RESTORED?

A variety of techniques have been employed for the reconstruction of the cervical esophagus. Various local and regional flaps have been used with indifferent success. Free jejunal transplantation is currently the technique of choice. Jejunal interposition may be combined with local or regional flap techniques for skin coverage.

The ablative surgery is carried out with preservation of recipient vessels, usually a branch of the external carotid and external jugular vein. A segment of jejunum is then easily harvested through a small laparotomy. The jejunal mesentery is thin. The vascular pedicle is short. End-to-end arterial and venous anastomoses can be constructed. The technique is useful in heavily irradiated areas because the transplanted jejunum brings its own normal distributive vasculature with it. A full-flow vascular supply is established. The transplanted jejunum maintains excellent motility and pliability. We have found the technique of value in our institution.[40] The disadvantage of the technique is the sensitivity of the intestine to warm ischemia. Swift, meticulous microsurgical technique is essential. The transplanted intestinal mucosa usually has a temporary hypersecretory phase.[41, 42] The surgeon must prepare to deal with the abundant secretions for several days after surgery. The technique is shown in Figure 16–15.

The technique of small bowel transplantation has been applied to the coverage of oropharyngeal defects with excellent success. Reuther et al.[43] reported one graft loss in 30 cases. The jejunal mucosa provided coverage with characteristics similar to oropharyngeal mucosa. The free transplant avoids the problems of cicatrix, induration, desquamation of epidermal layers, and hair growth that are seen with skin flaps. The technique can provide well-vascularized tissue over oral areas of mandibular reconstruction.

WHAT SECONDARY IMPROVEMENTS CAN BE MADE?

Scar Revision

Local and regional flap transposition may result in a scar that crosses areas of movement and maximum tension. Simple Z-plasty techniques can be used 6–12 months postoperatively to revise areas of scar tension when healing is complete. The base of a transposed flap may present an irregular contour due to partial folding of the flap base. Although it is tempting, revision of these areas at the time of flap transposition should not be done. The immediate revision will always produce some compromise of the vascular input to the base of the flap. Excision of the areas of irregularity can be done with safety at a later date once healing of the flap is complete.

Flap Revision

Full-thickness pedicle flaps or free microvascular flaps are often too prominent after healing is completed, due to excess subcutaneous tissue that is transferred with the flap. Vigorous defatting of such flaps at the time of transfer is risky. Secondary defatting can be done easily once the peripheral healing of the flap is secure. It is wise to perform defatting procedures in a conservative fashion and plan on more than one stage. It is easy to remove a little extra tissue in a second procedure. It is impossible to replace the tissue if too much is removed initially.

REFERENCES

1. Guerrero-Santos J.: Tongue flaps, in Grabb W.C., Myers M.B. (eds.): *Skin Flaps.* Boston, Little, Brown & Co., 1975, p. 201.
2. Rees T.D., Tabbal N., Aston S.J.: Tongue-flap reconstruction of the lip vermillion in hemifacial atrophy. *Plast. Reconstr. Surg.* 72:643, 1983.
3. Shons A.R., McQuarrie D.G.: Cervical-pectoral flaps in the treatment of advanced oral cancer. *J. Surg. Oncol.* 7:213, 1975.
4. Owens H.: Compound neck pedicle designed for the repair of massive facial defects: Formation, development and application. *Plast. Reconstr. Surg.* 15:369, 1955.
5. Littlewood M.: Compound skin and sternomastoid flaps for repair in extensive carcinoma of the head and neck. *Br. J. Plast. Surg.* 20:403, 1967.
6. Ariyan S.: One stage reconstruction for defects of the mouth using a sternomastoid myocutaneous flap. *Plast. Reconstr. Surg.* 63:618, 1979.
7. Kazanjian V.H.: The repair of nasal defects with the median forehead flap: Primary closure of the forehead wound. *Surg. Gynecol. Obstet.* 83:37, 1946.
8. McGregor I.A.: The temporal flap in intraoral cancer: Its use in repairing the post-excisional defect. *Br. J. Plast. Surg.* 16:318, 1963.
9. Hoopes J.E., Edgerton M.T.: Immediate forehead flap repair in resection for oral pharyngeal cancer. *Am. J. Surg.* 112:527, 1966.
10. Millard D.R. Jr.: Forehead flap in immediate repair of head, face, and jaw. *Am. J. Surg.* 108:508, 1964.
11. Smalley J.J., Cunningham M.P.: Forehead flap rotation

to protect carotid artery. *Plast. Reconstr. Surg.* 49:96, 1972.
12. Converse J.M.: Clinical applications of the scalping flap in reconstruction of the nose. *Plast. Reconstr. Surg.* 43:247, 1969.
13. Bertoli J.A.: Trapezius-musculotaneous island flap in the repair of major head and neck cancer. *Plast. Reconstr. Surg.* 65:16, 1980.
14. Bakamjian V.Y.: A two-stage method for pharyngoesophageal reconstruction with a primary pectoral skin flap. *Plast. Surg.* 36:173, 1965.
15. Bakamjian V.Y., Long M., Rigg B.: Experience with the medially based deltopectoral flap in reconstructive surgery of the head and neck. *Br. J. Plast. Surg.* 24:174, 1971.
16. McGregor I.A., Jackson I.T.: The extended role of the deltopectoral flap. *Br. J. Plast. Surg.* 23:173, 1970.
17. Ariyan S.: The pectoralis major myocutaneous flap: A versatile flap in reconstruction in head and neck. *Plast. Reconstr. Surg.* 63:73, 1979.
18. Ariyan S., Cuouno C.B.: Use of the pectoralis major myocutaneous flap for reconstruction of large cervical, facial or cranial defects. *Am. J. Surg.* 140:530, 1980.
19. Gottrup F., Firmin R., Hunt T.K., et al.: The dynamic properties of tissue oxygen in healing flaps. *Surgery* 95:527–536, 1984.
20. Quillen C.G.: Latissimus dorsi myocutaneous flaps in head and neck reconstruction. *Plast. Reconstr. Surg.* 63:664, 1979.
21. Barton F.E., Spicer T.E., Byrd H.S.: Head and neck reconstruction with the latissimus dorsi myocutaneous flap: Anatomic observations and report of 60 cases. *Plast. Reconstr. Surg.* 71:199, 1983.
22. Haarii D., Ohmori K., Torii S., et al.: Microvascular free skin flap transfer. *Clin. Plast. Surg.* 5:239, 1978.
23. Barwick W.J., Goodkind D.J., Serafin D.: The free scapular flap. *Plast. Reconstr. Surg.* 69:779, 1982.
24. Dolmans S., Guimberteau J.C., Baudet J.: The upper arm flap. *J. Microsurg.* 1:162, 1979.
25. Caffee H.H., Asokan R.: Tensor fascia lata myocutaneous free flaps. *Plast. Reconstr. Surg.* 68:195, 1981.
26. McQuarrie D.G.: Immediate functional restoration of the mandible after surgical treatment of advanced oral cancer: A simple prosthesis. *Arch. Surg.* 102:447, 1971.
27. Manchester W.M.: Immediate reconstruction of the mandible and temporomandibular joint. *Plast. Reconstr. Surg.* 18:291, 1965.
28. Millard D.R.: Immediate reconstruction of the lower jaw. *Plast. Reconstr. Surg.* 35:60, 1965.
29. Serafin D., Villarreal-Rios A., Georgiade N.G.: A rib containing free-flap to reconstruct mandibular defects. *Br. J. Plast. Surg.* 30:263, 1977.
30. Rosen I.B., Bell M.S.G., Barron P.T., et al.: Use of microvascular flaps including free osteocutaneous flaps in reconstruction after composite resection for radiation-recurrent oral cancer. *Am. J. Surg.* 138:544, 1979.
31. Taylor G.I., Townsend P., Corlett R.: Superiority of the deep circumflex iliac vessels as the supply for free groin flaps: Clinical work. *Plast. Reconstr. Surg.* 64:745, 1979.
32. Baumgarten R.S., DesPrez J.D.: The Morris biphase external splint for mandibular fixation. *Plast. Reconstr. Surg.* 50:66, 1972.
33. Ariyan S.L.: The viability of rib grafts transplanted with periosteal blood supply. *Plast. Reconstr. Surg.* 65:140, 1980.
34. Maisel R.H., Adams G.L.: Osteomyocutaneous reconstruction of the oral cavity. *Arch. Otolaryngol.* 109: 731–734, 1983.
35. Little J.W., McCulloch D.T., Lyons J.R.: The lateral pectoral composite flap in one-stage reconstruction of the irradiated mandible. *Plast. Reconstr. Surg.* 71:326, 1983.
36. Brown G.A.: Personal communication, 1984.
37. Boyne P.J., Zarem H.: Osseous reconstruction of the resected mandible. *Am. J. Surg.* 132:49, 1976.
38. Schwartz H.C.: Mandibular reconstruction using the Dacron-Urethane prosthesis and autogenous cancellous bone: A review of 32 cases. *Plast. Reconstr. Surg.* 73:387, 1984.
39. Cannole P.W., Terry B.C., Kelly J.F.: Late care (reconstruction-rehabilitation), in Kelly J.F. (ed.): *Management of War Injuries to the Jaw and Related Structures.* Washington, D.C., Naval Medical Research Institute, U.S. Government Printing Office, 1977, pp. 105–153.
40. Grage T.B., Click C.A.: Use of revascularized ileocolic autografts for primary repair after pharyngolaryngoesophagectomy. *Am. J. Surg.* 136:477, 1978.
41. Hester T.R., McConnel F., Nahai F., et al.: Reconstruction of cervical esophagus, hypopharynx and oral cavity using free jejunal transfer. *Am. J. Surg.* 140:487, 1980.
42. McConnel F., Hester T.R., Nahai F., et al.: Free jejunal grafts in reconstruction of pharynx and cervical esophagus. *Arch. Otolaryngol.* 107:476, 1981.
43. Reuther J.F., Steinau H., Wagner R.: Reconstruction of large defects in the oropharynx with revascularized intestinal grafts: An experimental clinical report. *Plast. Reconstr. Surg.* 73:345, 1984.

7 / General Principles of Radiation Therapy for Head and Neck Malignancy

YASHODA RAO, M.D. / SEYMOUR LEVITT, M.D.

THE DISCOVERY of x-rays by Roentgen and of radium by the Curies at the end of the 19th century became the stepping stone for the development of clinical radiation therapy. In the early part of this century, superficial roentgen therapy (250 to 400-kV machines) and radium needles were used to treat both benign and malignant diseases. Modern radiation equipment became available only in the last 40–50 years. Telecurie therapy using radium and, later, cobalt sources preceded the development of linear accelerators, which produce photon and electron beams with energies ranging from 4 to 25 MeV. Particle radiation (neutrons, protons, pi mesons), hyperthermia, and radiation modifiers are some of the latest developments (in the last two decades) in clinical radiation therapy and offer further hope for improving the management of cancer patients.

Intracavitary treatment of oropharyngeal lesions was attempted in the early part of this century. Sievert[1] in 1933 published the design of an apparatus which permitted the treatment of head and neck cancer with a degree of accuracy hitherto unattainable.[2] The availability of megavoltage in the last four decades is responsible for the important role radiation therapy is taking in the multidisciplinary management of head and neck cancers.

To arrive at a better understanding of the effect of radiation on neoplastic tissue, it is essential to know the physical properties of the different radiation beams that are available as well as the interaction of ionizing radiation with normal and malignant cells. The following section reviews the principles of radiation biology and physics necessary for a basic understanding of radiation therapy. The goal is enhanced communication for effective decision-making and the management of head and neck cancers.

WHAT IS THE BASIC MECHANISM BY WHICH RADIATION CAUSES CELL DEATH?

A major difference between tumor cells and normal cells is the capacity of tumor cells to proliferate indefinitely. The desired end result of radiation therapy is to halt this uncontrolled cancer cell replication by damaging critical targets. The exact mechanism of cell killing by radiation is not well understood. Two different theories exist. Radiation can act directly and cause irreversible damage to the chemical structure of targets such as DNA. Radiation can also interact indirectly with atoms or molecules in the cell (i.e., water) to produce free radicals like the hydroxyl radical. Such radicals are highly reactive and damage the critical targets.

WHAT IS A CELL SURVIVAL CURVE, AND WHAT ARE THE DIFFERENT FACTORS THAT MODIFY IT?

When mammalian cells are exposed to radiation, the surviving cell number decreases as the dose is increased. Cell survival curves are obtained by plotting the dose on a linear scale and the surviving fraction of cells on a logarithmic scale. Because deposition of radiation energy and infliction of radiation damage are random events, the survival curve is an exponential function of dose on the semilog graph.

Figure 7–1 shows typical survival curves for mammalian cells exposed to radiation. As the dose of radiation increases, the probability of cell killing also increases, up to a certain limit. The increasing probability of cell death is indicated by the presence of the initial shoulder on the survival curve for x- and γ-rays. The shoulder is followed by a straight or almost straight line, and the slope of this line is dependent on the radiosensitivity. The dose of radiation required to reduce the number of cells to 37% of their former value (1/e) is called the 37% dose slope, or D_0. For densely ionizing radiation like α particles and neutrons, there is no shoulder, and the survival curve is almost a straight line.

HOW DOES OXYGEN MODIFY RADIATION EFFECT?

The survival curves obtained when mammalian cells are exposed to x-rays in the presence and absence of oxygen show that the dose of radiation required to kill the same number of cells under hypoxic conditions is far greater than the dose required under aerated conditions. The ratio of the hypoxic to the oxygenated dose of radiation needed to achieve the same biologic effect is called oxygen enhancement ratio (OER). The value

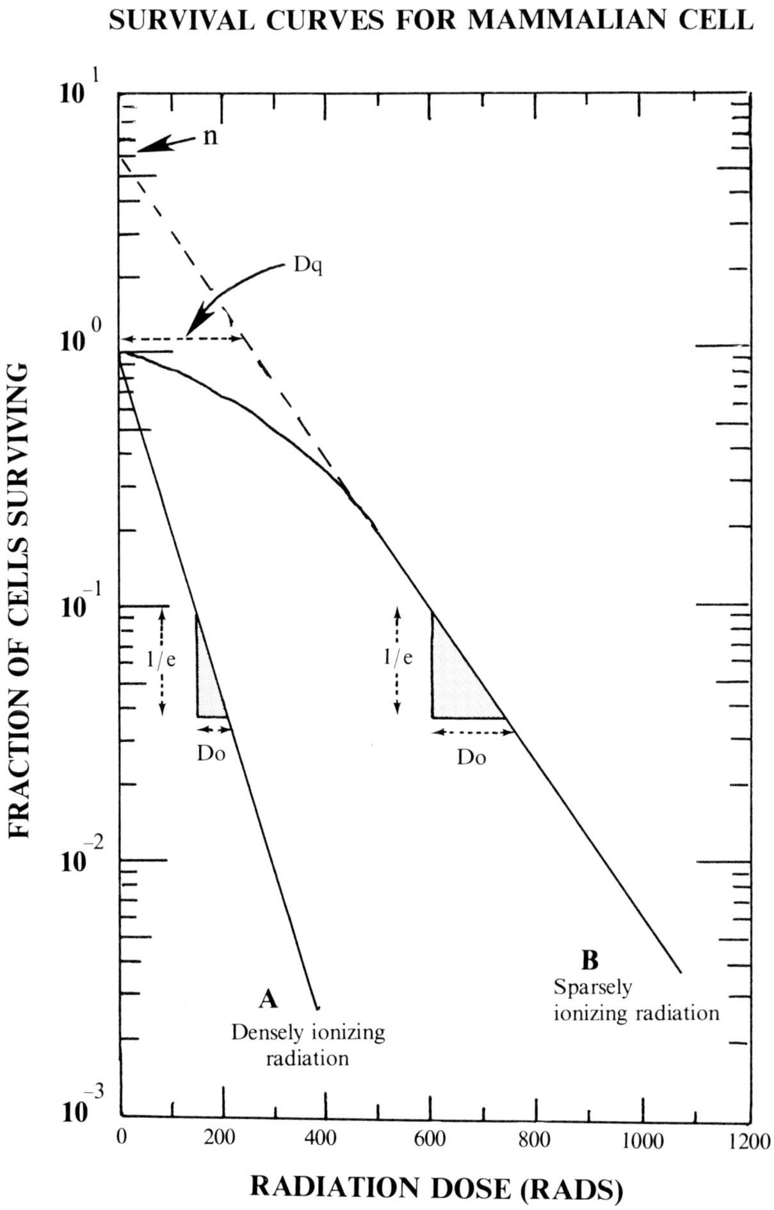

Fig 7–1.—Typical survival curves for mammalian cells exposed to either densely ionizing radiation (α particles and neutrons) or sparsely ionizing radiation (x-rays or γ-rays). For densely ionizing radiation, the response is a straight line. For sparsely ionizing radiations, there is a "shoulder" which may be specified in terms of a quasithreshold dose, Dq. The shoulder can also be characterized by extrapolating the straight part of the curve to *n*. The slopes of the straight portion of the curve can be described by the dose (D_0) required to reduce the cell population by 1/ln (to about 37% of the previous value). (Figure redrawn from Hall E.J.: *Radiology for the Radiobiologist.* Hagerstown, Md., Harper & Row, 1973.)

of OER varies with the type of radiation, but it is about 2.5–3.0 for 250-kV x-rays. The maximum OER is found with x-rays and γ-rays, which are sparsely ionizing radiation, whereas a densely ionizing radiation like α particles has very little oxygen effect and the OER is 1. The precise mechanism of the oxygen effect is not understood. Experiments have shown that the partial pressure of oxygen affects the level of free radicals that are responsible for biologic damage in the cells; that is, more toxic radicals are produced by radiation in the presence of oxygen. Oxygen must be present *during* irradiation to have a potentiating effect on cell death.

CAN HYPERBARIC OXYGEN OVERCOME THE PROBLEM OF HYPOXIC CELLS IN RADIATION THERAPY?

Attempts have been made to eliminate or minimize the problem associated with the presence of radioresistant hypoxic cells in tumors by allowing patients to breathe pure oxygen at a pressure of 2 or 3 atm during irradiation. None of the clinical trials have shown any advantage of hyperbaric oxygen over conventionally fractionated radiation in air.[3, 4]

WHAT IS THE BENEFIT OF FRACTIONATED RADIATION AS COMPARED TO SINGLE-DOSE TREATMENT?

There are several reasons why it is preferable to fractionate the irradiation dose. (1) There is a differential repair capacity between malignant cells and normal tissue. Radiation can cause immediate irreversible lethal changes in some cells. In other cell populations, damage may be sublethal, so that repair of cells occurs within a few hours after the irradiation. In the intervals between delivery of fractionated irradiation, both cancer cells and normal tissue cells may repair their sublethal damage. However, the repair potential of tumor cells might be less than that of normal tissue because of basic metabolic differences, or because there are suboptimal conditions in the intratumor environment, i.e., hypoxia. (2) Fractions of tumor cell population are hypoxic and thus radioresistant. In the intervals between treatment the hypoxic cells may undergo reoxygenation and become sensitive to subsequent radiation. (3) The normal tissue starts to repopulate faster than tumor cells during the intervals between treatment. For these reasons, greater damage occurs in tumor cells than in normal cells during the course of fractionated irradiation.

WHAT ARE RADIATION MODIFIERS?

Extensive research has been done to identify chemical agents that either (1) selectively potentiate radiation effects on cancer cells without affecting normal tissue, or (2) protect normal tissue without similarly protecting the tumor cells. These agents are called "radiation sensitizers" or "protectors," respectively.

RADIATION PROTECTORS.—Sulfhydryl compounds are the most common group of radiation protectors used. The chemical WR-2721 was reported to selectively protect normal tissues against the effects of irradiation. It has been intensively investigated for its ability to protect normal tissues like skin, salivary glands, and oral mucosa in the treatment of head and neck tumors. Unfortunately, the clinical benefit achieved with the use of this compound appears to be limited.[5]

RADIATION SENSITIZERS.—These are chemical agents that selectively sensitize tumor cells to radiation, as compared to normal cells, in a dose that is below the toxicity level. Halogenated pyrimidines like 5-bromodeoxyuridine (BUDR) and 5-iododeoxyuridine (IUDR) have been tried both experimentally and clinically as radiosensitizers without any marked beneficial results.[6–8]

HYPOXIC CELL SENSITIZERS.—These are chemical agents that can selectively sensitize hypoxic cells to radiation. If the radioresistant hypoxic cells in a solid tumor are selectively radiosensitized, then local control of tumor by radiation therapy can be significantly improved. Since the early 1960s a number of compounds have been tried, both in vitro and in vivo. Metronidazole (Flagyl) and, more recently, misonidazole (RO–07–0582) have been shown to produce significant sensitization of tumor cells to radiation in a variety of animal tumor models. Misonidazole has been used as a radiation sensitizer in multiple clinical trials. The limiting factor to clinical use is the neurotoxicity that occurs when the drug is given in multiple doses. To date no significant benefits are noted in any of these studies, but it is probably too early to conclude any definite results.[9]

WHAT IS THE ROLE OF HYPERTHERMIA IN THE TREATMENT OF HEAD AND NECK CANCER?

Experimental studies with cells have shown that concomitant heating potentiates the action of radiation in cell killing.[10–14] Hyperthermia is also selectively lethal to radiation-resistant cells such as S phase cells.[15] Cells that are in a low pH environment, as in necrotic tissue, are sensitive to heat. They are also nutritionally deprived and are especially heat sensitive.[16, 17] It is believed that greater hyperthermia damage occurs in cancer cells than in normal tissue because the tumors reach a higher temperature because there is sluggish heat dissipation by tumor blood flow, and also because the heat makes the microenvironment in tumors more acidic and nutritionally deprived. A number of methods have been used to produce localized heating. These include (1) a hot water bath, (2) extremity perfusion, (3) microwave heating, (4) radiofrequency, and (5) ultrasound heating. The problem with any of these methods is to adequately heat the tumor volume and accurately measure and control the temperature attained within the cancer. Maximum potentiation of radiation by hyperthermia occurs when it is given within a short period, either before or after irradiation. However, in order to increase therapeutic gain, heat is usually given 1–5 hours after irradiation.[18–20] At present, a number of centers have been treating patients with combined hyperthermia and radiation. When used for superficial malignancies, the combined treatment has been shown to enhance the therapeutic efficiency of radiation for local control.[21–24] Cancer in the head and neck area is usually accessible for local hyperthermia and radiation. When 15 patients with N2N3 multiple cervical nodes from head and neck cancer were treated with multiple episodes daily of fractionation radiation therapy, 85% achieved a complete response when radiation was combined with hyperthermia, compared to 46% of patients treated with multiple daily fractions of radiation and 30% of patients treated with conventional fractionation.[25]

WHAT ARE THE PHYSICAL PROPERTIES OF X-RAYS?

X-rays are electromagnetic radiation. X-rays are produced by high-energy electrons interacting with atoms. In any x-ray tube, a high voltage is used to accelerate electrons across the gap between the filament (or cathode) and the target (or anode). The electrons thus acquire kinetic energy. On reaching the target the electrons interact with the atoms in the target. The positive charge on the nucleus may deflect the electron from its path or stop it completely, causing it to lose kinetic energy in the form of photons. The electromagnetic radiation produced is termed bremsstrahlung.

The energy of the photon is measured in kiloelectron volts (keV) or megaelectron volts (MeV). Gamma rays are also photons, but they originate from within the nucleus of the atom as a result of radioactive decay process. When X- and γ-radiation beams interact with the tissues the resulting energy is absorbed by the tissues. The quantity of energy absorbed by the tissue is called the absorbed dose. The unit of absorbed dose is the rad (radiation absorbed dose) and equals 100 ergs of energy absorbed per gram of the material.

When a beam of low-energy x-rays reaches a patient, the maximum absorbed dose is at the skin surface, but for cobalt 60 and multimillion-volt x-rays, the maximum dose builds up deeper in the subcutaneous tissue (e.g., 0.5 cm for ^{60}Co, 1 cm for 4-MV x-rays, 2.5 cm for 10-MeV x-rays), thereby sparing the skin surface and subcutaneous tissue from an excessive dose (Fig 7–2).

The plot of absorbed dose along the central axis of the radiation field into the tissue is called the central axis depth dose curve, and the values are expressed as percentages of the dose at the depth of peak dose. The points of the equal percentage dose in a radiation field may be joined together to form a series of isodose curves that are used extensively in the treatment planning.

WHAT ARE THE DIFFERENT TYPES OF RADIATION?

Radiation used in the treatment of cancer patients can be of different types. The most common form of radiation used is photon beams. These are x-rays produced by different machines capable of generating beams of energy ranging from 50 kV to 20–30 MV (see Fig 7–2). The second most common form of radiation used is electron beams. Gamma rays from different sources of radioactive material are also used in techniques such as in brachytherapy. Particle radiation with neutrons, protons, and pions is still in the early stage of clinical investigation.

WHAT ARE THE DIFFERENT SOURCES OF RADIATION USED IN THE TREATMENT OF HEAD AND NECK CANCERS?

KILOVOLTAGE MACHINES.—Low-energy radiation from 50 kV to about 400 kV is generated by these x-ray machines. These were the earliest x-ray machines used in the treatment of cancer. Since the advent of cobalt and linear accelerators, orthovoltage machines have had limited use. The x-rays have poor penetrating qualities. Therefore, low-energy x-rays are used primarily in the treatment of superficial tumors like skin and lip cancers, and occasionally for boost radiation for oral cavity lesions, using intraoral cones.

COBALT 60.—The most commonly available high-energy radiation source is ^{60}Co. Unlike x-ray machines, which produce radiation with electrical energy, this machine has a source of radioactive cobalt which produces γ-rays of an average energy of 1.2 MV. Cobalt radiation has skin- and bone-sparing properties but delivers adequate radiation to the neck nodes and primary tumor. Cobalt is one of the most commonly used radiation sources for the treatment of head and neck cancer.

LINEAR ACCELERATORS.—These are megavoltage x-ray machines that produce radiation in the range of 4–20 MV x-ray. Electrons are accelerated to higher velocities, thereby acquiring higher energy levels. These electrons can be directed to strike a target to produce a high-energy photon beam, or the beam can be allowed to exit directly from the machine to give an electron beam. To adequately treat neck nodes, 4- to 6-MV x-rays are most commonly used. The higher energy x-rays tend to spare more of skin and superficial tissue. For the same reason they also spare superficially situated tumors or neck nodes. Very high energy x-rays in the range of 10–25 MV are used for very deep-seated tumors such as those located deep in the thorax and pelvis.

ELECTRON BEAM RADIATION.—The great advantage of electron beam irradiation is the rapid dose buildup and sharp dose falloff beyond a certain depth. Examples of percentage depth dose curves for different energy electron beams are shown in Figure 7–3. The surface dose is at or near the maximum dose, so there is little skin-sparing effect. For sites where a sharp cutoff in

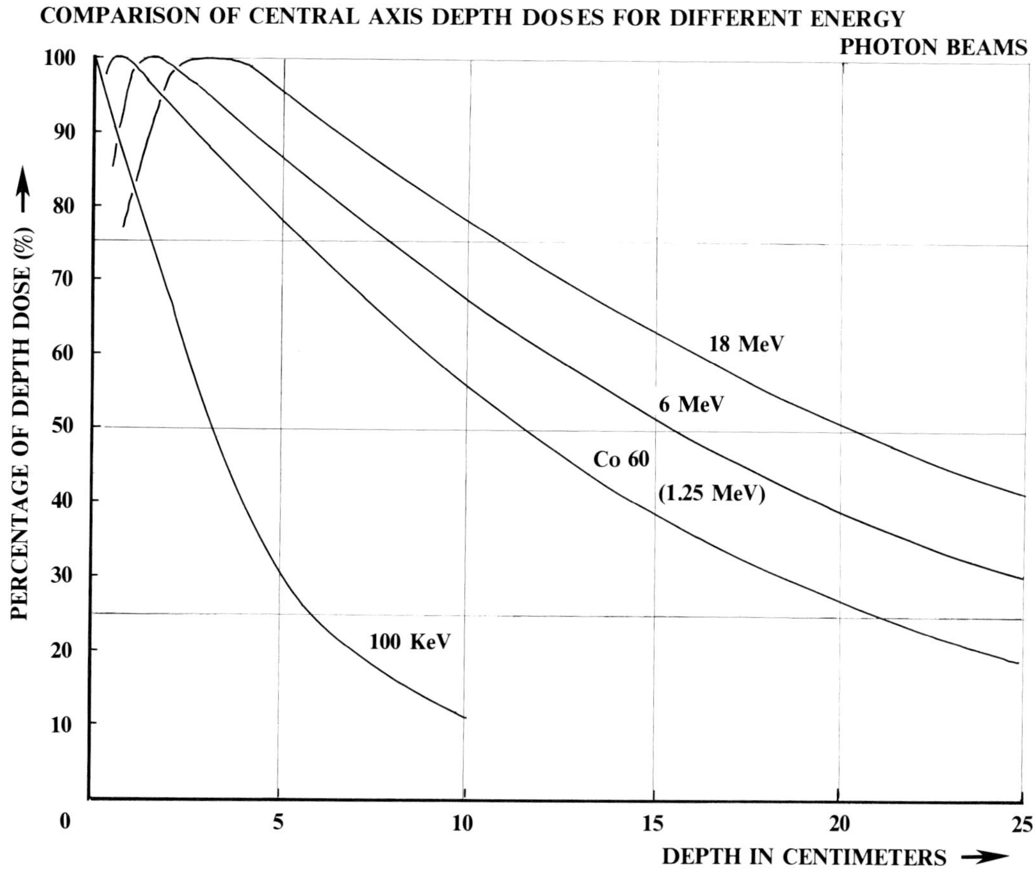

Fig 7–2.—Depth of tissue penetration for four photon beams of different energy is plotted against percentage of depth dose reaching various tissue depths. The dose delivered at the tissue surface is greatest with lower energy sources. Higher energies are required for tissue penetration.

dose is required beyond the tumor, electron beam irradiation offers distinct advantages over photon beam irradiation. Electron beams in the range of 4–15 MV are used in the treatment of head and neck tumors. The clinical uses of electron irradiation are as follows:

1. Elective radiation to one side of the neck to 5,000 rad.
2. Radiation to the neck following a recurrence that is limited to neck nodes.
3. Radiation of posterior cervical lymph nodes.
4. Boost radiation to residual disease in the posterior cervical chain following photon radiation that has reached spinal cord tolerance (4,500–5,000 rad).
5. Boost radiation to residual disease in the neck following a full course of irradiation.
6. Superficial cancers such as skin and lip cancers.
7. Boost radiation to an accessible primary cancer through an intraoral cone.[26]

PARTICLE RADIATION.—The particle radiation sources that are of interest for clinical use are fast neutrons, negative pions, α particles (helium nuclei), and heavy ions like carbon, neon, argon and protons. Each of these particle species has different physical and radiobiologic characteristics when compared to photon or electron beams. The dose distribution patterns of negative pions, heavy ions, and protons are more favorable than those obtained with photons or neutrons. The average loss of energy per unit length of path of radiation is termed linear energy transfer (LET). The main advantage of many of these particle radiations is their high LET values. The biologic effectiveness of high LET radiation in cell killing is less dependent on the cellular oxygen level at the time of radiation. The cells are less capable of repair of radiation damage. Sensitivity of cells is not as dependent on the position of the cell in the cell replication cycle for high LET radiation. Certain particles have the additional property of maximum ionization at the end of the path, called the Bragg peak, and the dose rapidly decreases beyond the peak. If the Bragg peak of the radiation is centered in the tumor volume, then the maximum dose of radiation can be delivered to the center of the cancer, with decreased radiation to the normal surrounding structures.

Catterall from Hammersmith Hospital, London, in a prospective randomized trial of patients with advanced

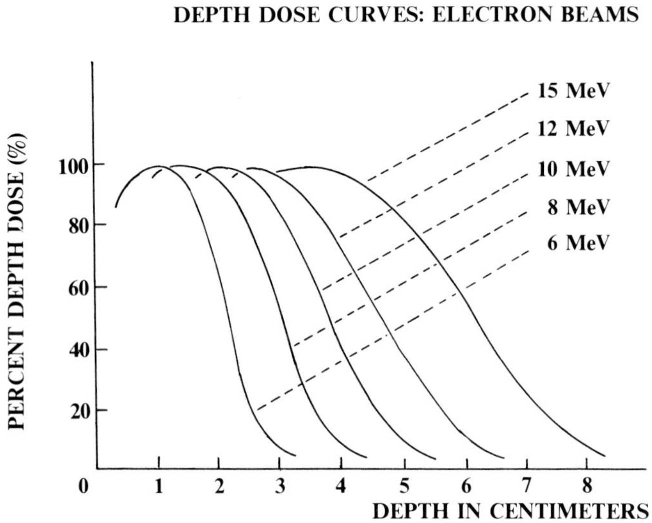

Fig 7–3.—Percentage depth dose curves for electron beams of increasing energy.

head and neck cancer treated with fast neutron therapy, has shown a clear and statistically significant superiority of local, regional control of the cancer when compared to photon beam radiation treatment.[27] Similarly, the M. D. Anderson Hospital conducted a randomized clinical trial comparing (1) mixed schedule irradiation using two neutron and three photon fractions per week with (2) standard photon irradiation for inoperable squamous cell carcinoma of head and neck. Actuarial analysis showed superior local control and survival rates with mixed schedule irradiation over photon irradiation only in the first 2 years.[28] Suit et al.[29] have reported promising results in the treatment of choroidal melanoma, sarcomas abutting CNS structures, and head and neck cancers using proton beam radiation. The use of these highly sophisticated and expensive methods of radiation is still in its infancy. At present, a large number of clinical trials are under way both in Europe and in the United States to assess the possible benefits and problems of particle radiation.

INTERSTITIAL RADIATION.—The main advantage of an interstitial radioactive implant compared to external beam radiation is the ability of the implant to deliver high doses of radiation in and near the tumor with a rapid decrease of dose toward the outside volume. Radium 226 has traditionally been an important γ-ray source for interstitial implantation to treat head and neck cancer. It is used in the form of rigid needles. Radium has the singular disadvantage that installation of the needles requires an excessive exposure dose to physicians, nurses, and other personnel. Recently the exposure has been reduced by the use of radium substitutes and afterloading techniques. The most commonly used afterloading removable implants are the special nylon ribbons that contain radioactive iridium seeds (Ir 192). Under anesthesia, 17-gauge hollow stainless steel guides are implanted in the tumor volume. Plastic implant tubes are inserted into these guides and the guides are then removed. This leaves the plastic tubes in the implant area. The nylon ribbons with iridium seeds are loaded into the plastic tubes and left in place for sufficient time to deliver the planned dose to the tumor volume. Interstitial radiation is used mainly as a boosting technique in most head and neck cancers except when the lesion is very small, easily accessible for implants, and has a predictably low incidence of node metastases. Intracavitary radiation treatment of nasopharyngeal cancer uses cesium 137 in an adapted endotracheal tube carrier.

HOW IS RADIATION TREATMENT PLANNED AND DELIVERED DAILY?

Radiation treatments are usually given 5 days a week (Monday through Friday) with a daily fraction of 175–200 rad. The total dose of curative radiation for head and neck cancer ranges from 6,500 to 7,500 rad. Only in cases of metastatic disease or when treatment volume is very small will a higher daily dose be used. Fewer larger fractions require an appropriate reduction in total tumor dose. The normal tissue tolerance to radiation is better with small daily fractionation and a protracted course of treatment.

The tumor control and radiation injury to the normal tissue are closely related to total tumor dose, total treatment time, number of daily fractions and dose per fraction. This is expressed mathematically as the "time dose fractionation" (TDF). This value is often helpful in comparing different radiation schedules in terms of their biologic effects on tumor and normal tissues.[30, 31]

Curative radiation for head and neck cancer requires meticulous treatment planning. Immobilization of patients for treatments, duplication of treatment fields each day, and an appropriate reduction in field size are important considerations for delivering a high dose of radiation to the tumor volume yet limiting the irradiation to adjacent normal tissues to tolerable doses. Precise planning is accomplished by use of a simulator and a computer. A simulator is an x-ray machine that is built to match the physical specifications of the treatment machine. The initial treatment fields are set up under the simulator, and radiographs of these fields are obtained (Figs 7–4 and 7–5). These films are used to localize tumor volume and to identify the relative position of critical normal structures (e.g., spinal cord) for future technique modification or reduction of field size. On all

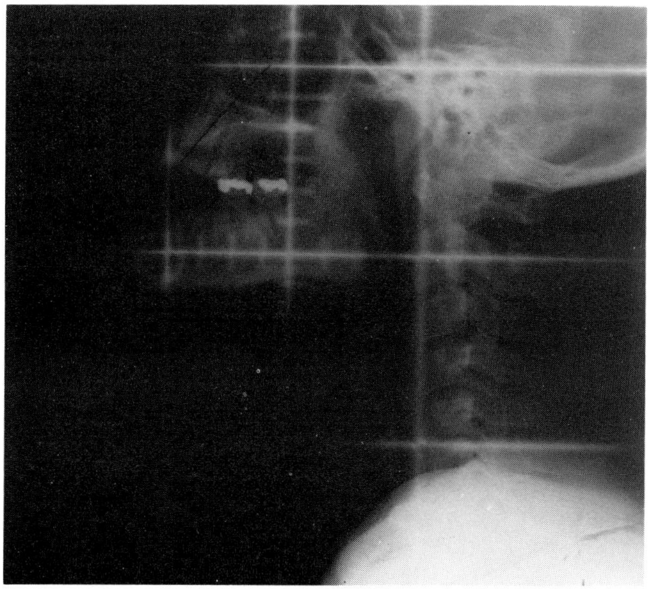

Fig 7–4.—Film from the radiation simulator showing the area for a lateral neck field.

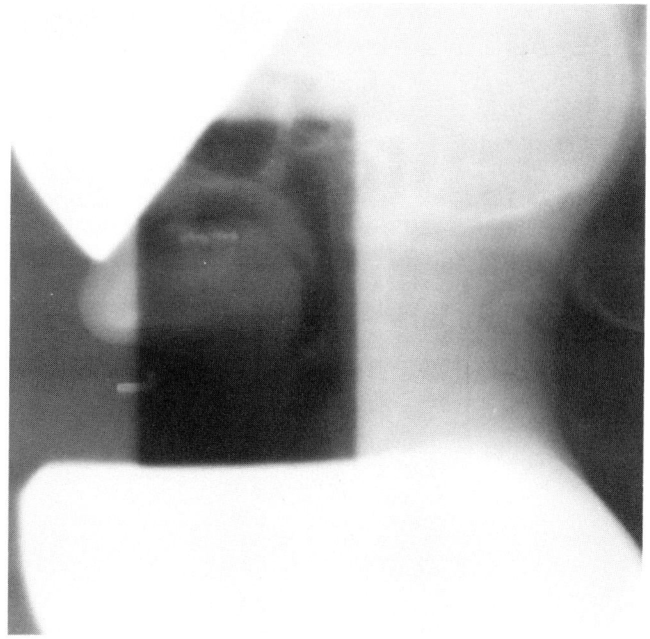

Fig 7–6.—"Port film" taken at the time of treatment to verify the position and accuracy of the treatment field.

patients in whom cure is the goal, a contour of the treatment area is taken to get the cross-sectional view of the patient in a plane passing through the tumor. In many centers, these data can be directly digitized from an appropriate CT scan cross section. This information is fed into the computer and isodose curves within and surrounding the tumor volume structures are obtained for evaluation of radiation dose distribution. The port films (radiographs taken with the treatment beam) are taken during the actual treatment to document the actual area of radiation treatment (Fig 7–6).

Most commonly used treatment portals are parallel opposed lateral neck fields (Fig 7–7). These fields are used to treat primary lesions of the nasopharynx and midline lesions of the oropharynx, larynx, and hypopharynx that are associated with bilateral neck node metastases. The lower neck is treated with a single anterior supraclavicular field. When opposing neck fields are used there is usually a significant variation of tissue thickness between the level of oropharynx and the level of the larynx. This will cause a nonhomogeneous dose distribution in the treatment volume. This problem is overcome by using metal wedges or custom-made compensators, which compensate for the missing tissue (Fig 7–8). The parallel opposed beams deliver a fairly uniform dose of radiation to the treatment volume and the dose is calculated at the midline depth. Treatment fields are modified at 4,500 rad (spinal cord tolerance) to boost the primary and neck nodes to a higher dose, using either reduced fields, electron beam, intraoral cone, interstitial radiation, or wedge pair setups.

Wedge pair technique (for a full course of radiation)

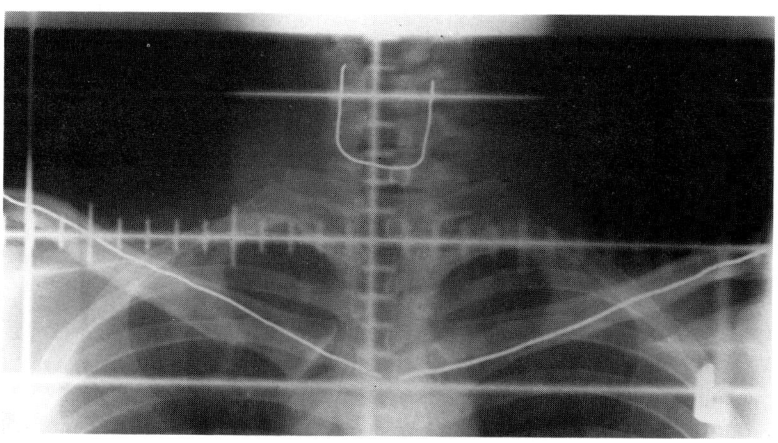

Fig 7–5.—Film from the radiation simulator showing an anterior supraclavicular radiation field setup. The area below the clavicular marker will be shielded as will the laryngeal area.

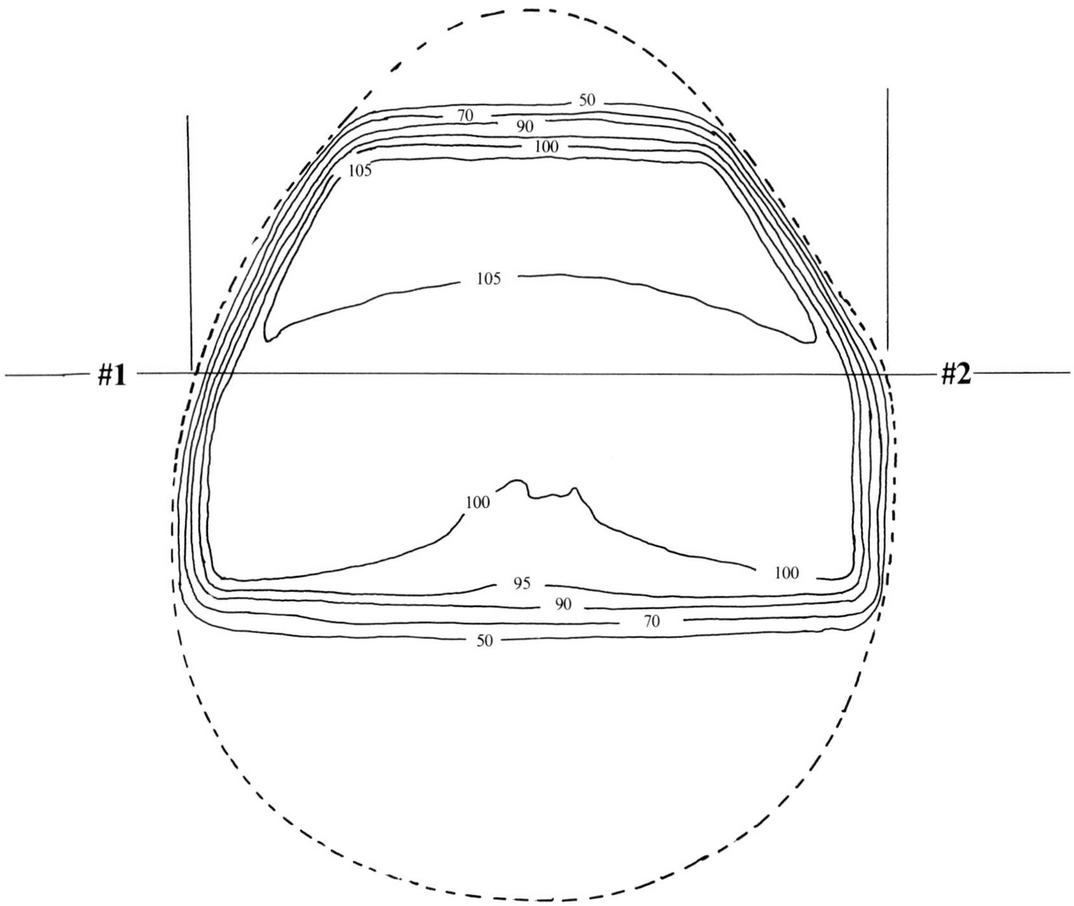

Fig 7–7.—Parallel opposed lateral neck fields (isodose distribution).

is mainly used for eccentrically situated lesions like those in the salivary gland, maxillary sinus, tonsillar fossa, and buccal mucosa and for which the incidence of metastasis to the contralateral neck node is very low. To spare the normal structures in the opposite neck, radiation beams are directed at the same surface or at adjacent surfaces at 60°–90° angles. If these fields are irradiated without wedges (wedge-shaped metal pieces), the perpendicular arrangement produces a highly nonuniform dose distribution. When appropriate wedges are interposed in the beams to attenuate them at the thick ends, the area of beam intersection receives a uniform dose (Fig 7–9).

WHAT IS THE ROLE OF RADIATION THERAPY IN THE MANAGEMENT OF LYMPH NODE METASTASES IN HEAD AND NECK CANCER?

Metastatic disease in the neck may be microscopic (subclinical or occult, without palpable lymph nodes) or gross, involving enlarged nodes. The treatment varies with each situation and must be individualized. Chapter 9 discusses irradiation management of cervical node metastases in more detail.

HOW EFFECTIVE IS IRRADIATION IN THE MANAGEMENT OF OCCULT NECK METASTASES, AND WHAT ARE ITS ADVANTAGES OVER ELECTIVE NECK DISSECTION?

The incidence of subclinical metastatic disease in the neck nodes ranges from 10% to 40%, depending on the site and stage of the primary lesion. The selection of method of treatment of neck node metastases is controversial and often depends on the medical specialty that is responsible for the care of the patient. Other major determinants are the planned treatment of the primary lesion and the anticipated reliability of patient follow-up. Subclinical disease can be treated by elective neck dissection or elective neck irradiation. At present, there are no randomized studies supporting the superiority of either for N_0 or N_1 necks (Fig 7–10).

The first report strongly advocating elective neck irradiation (ENI) was published in 1963.[32] Million et al. analyzed 281 cases of squamous cell carcinoma of the nasopharynx, tonsillar fossa, and base of the tongue for causes of failure by site, after *elective* neck irradiation. In only one case did a new node appear in a neck field.

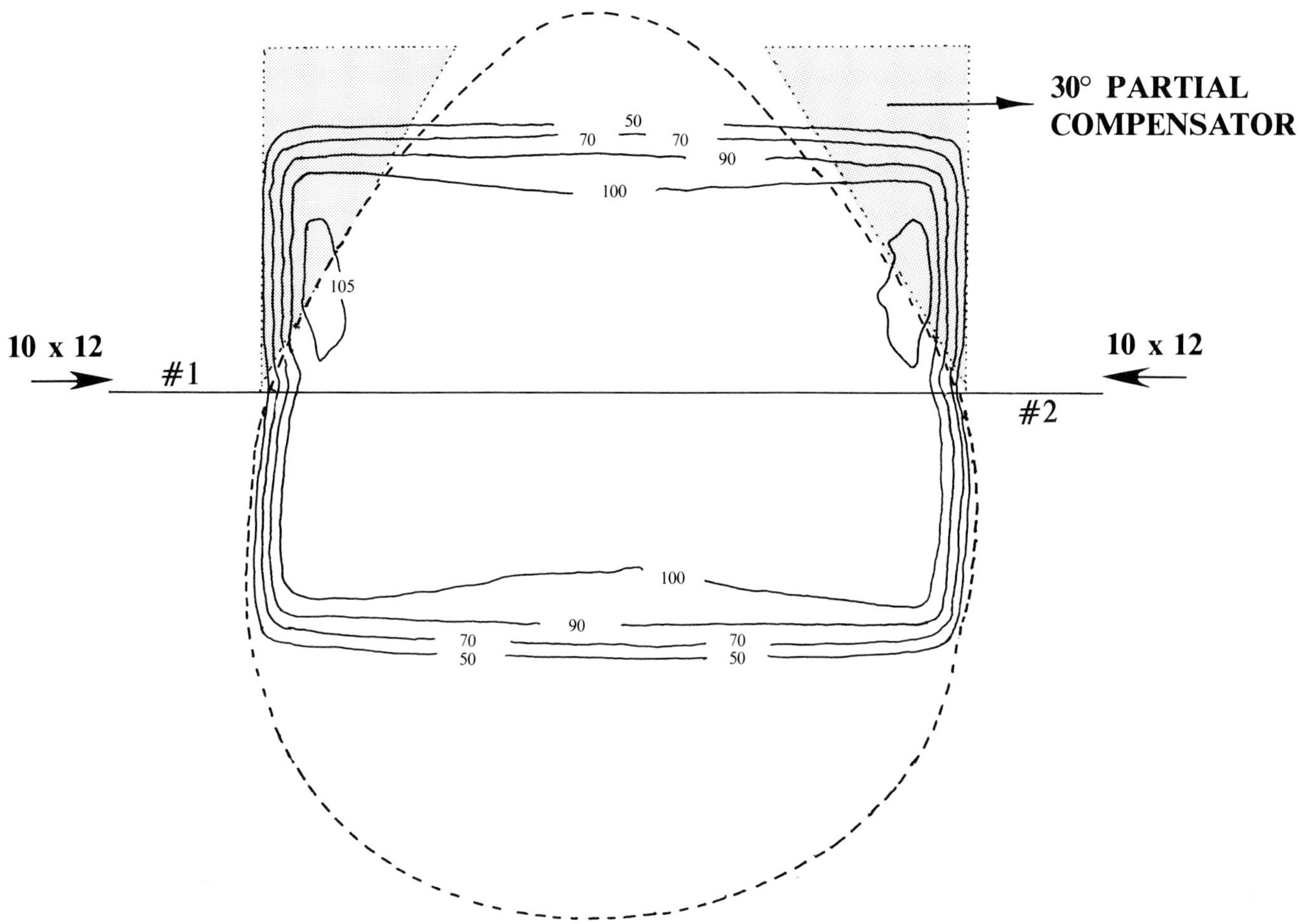

Fig 7–8.—Parallel opposed lateral neck fields (isodose distribution with 30° partial compensators).

Fletcher has shown elective neck irradiation to 4,500–5,000 rad (delivered over 4½–5 weeks) to be at least 95% efficient in eradicating subclinical squamous carcinoma metastatic to the lymph nodes.[33] Similar results have been reported by several other workers, which justifies the use of radiation for control of subclinical metastatic disease.[34–37]

There are two clinical applications of the above data.[38]

1. Elective irradiation of clinical uninvolved areas when the primary site is treated by irradiation alone.
2. Elective irradiation of clinically uninvolved areas in preoperative and postoperative irradiation.

The mortality from elective neck dissection ranges from 1% to 3%, depending on patient selection varying somewhat in different clinical series. The morbidity from elective neck dissection includes scars, cosmetic changes in neck shape, and occasional accessory nerve paralysis when a conservation dissection is not done. If the lesion is midline and there is therefore a greater chance of bilateral neck metastasis, then the complication rate increases with staged or simultaneous bilateral neck dissection.

Prophylactic neck irradiation is associated with no mortality and minimal morbidity. Irradiating both sides of the neck (along with the primary lesion) to 4,500–5,000 rad in 4½–5 weeks produces temporary dermal irritation, transient mucositis, moderate xerostomia, and clinically undetectable subcutaneous fibrosis.

WHAT ARE THE KEY POINTS ONE SHOULD CONSIDER BEFORE SELECTING ELECTIVE NECK IRRADIATION OR DISSECTION, WHEN BOTH MAY BE EQUALLY EFFECTIVE MODES OF TREATMENT FOR OCCULT METASTASES IN THE NECK?

1. Head and neck cancers with N_0 neck have 10%–40% chance of occult metastases in the neck.

2. The incidence of occult metastases increases with increasing stage of the primary tumor and also with tumors of certain anatomical location.

3. Midline lesions such as those in the base of

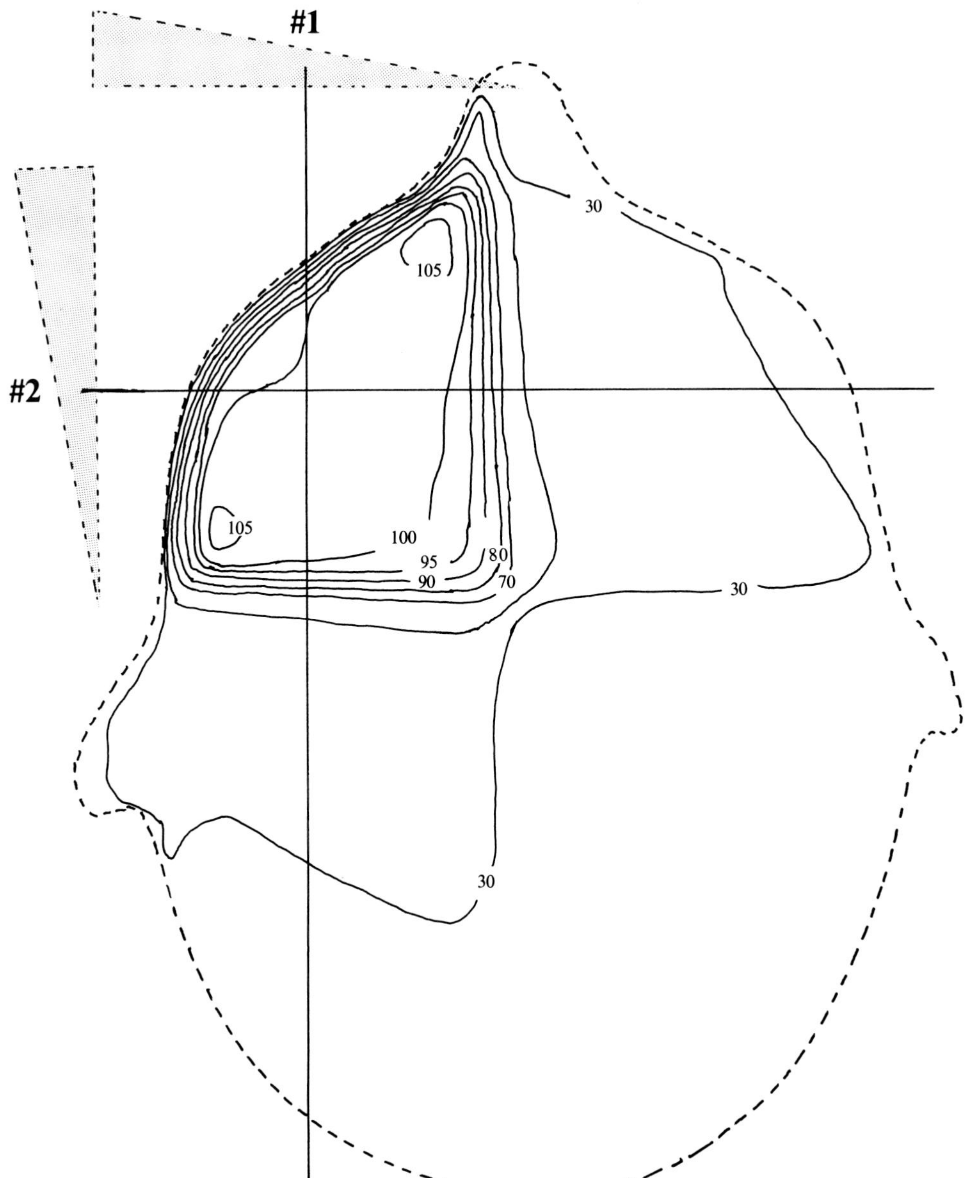

Fig 7–9.—Wedge pair setup (45°) for maxillary sinus radiation treatment.

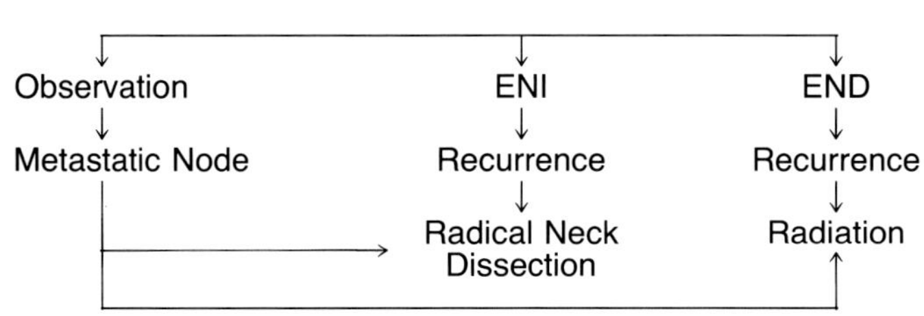

Fig 7–10.—Selecting treatment of the clinically negative neck, either by elective neck irradiation *(ENI)* or by elective neck dissection *(END)*.

tongue, the posterior pharyngeal wall, and the nasopharynx have a higher incidence of bilateral neck metastasis, mandating treatment to both sides of the neck.

4. The early treatment of subclinical disease influences the subsequent incidence of distant metastasis.

5. Small primary lesions of the head and neck (e.g., T_1 lesion of the glottis, tonsillar fossa, or mobile tongue) can be controlled effectively with either irradiation or surgery. In such cases one should consider the benefit of preservation of normal anatomy.

6. If radiation seems to be equally effective in controlling the primary site and the occult neck metastases, there would be no reason to divide the treatment of the entire disease into a radiotherapeutic approach to the primary tumor and surgery for the occult neck metastases, or vice versa.

7. When a single treatment modality is used for both the primary tumor and the neck metastases, the alternate treatment method can be reserved for salvage of recurrent disease.

8. Since all primary lesions in the nasopharynx are treated with radiation and since lymph node metastases are equally radiosensitive, radiation to both sites is the choice of treatment for nasopharyngeal carcinomas.

WHAT IS THE ROLE OF RADIATION IN TREATMENT OF CLINICALLY POSITIVE METASTATIC NECK DISEASE?

Until 1960, radical neck dissection was the time-honored method of treatment for clinically detectable metastatic neck nodes. A classic lymphadenectomy was performed without regard to the site of the primary cancer or the location and stage of the metastatic neck node. In the last two decades therapeutic attitudes have changed. Head and neck oncologists are more in favor of combining surgery and radiation. There are two main factors responsible for this change: (1) In most series, there are some local recurrences in the neck following radical neck dissection only. It would be desirable to reduce this rate further. (2) There is a perceived effectiveness of combined radiation and surgery in controlling advanced stage neck metastases.

WHAT IS THE RATIONALE FOR COMBINED TREATMENT FOR METASTATIC NECK DISEASE?

The natural history of cancer cells is to grow and infiltrate the surrounding tissues, the lymphatic channels, blood vessels, muscles, and perineural tissue. Also, as tumor size increases, the supporting normal connective tissue and blood vessels are incapable of supplying the tumor with oxygen and nutrients. Hence, the central part of the tumor mass becomes hypoxic and eventually necrotic, while the peripheral infiltrating viable tumor remains well oxygenated. The role of surgery in combined treatment is to remove the bulk of the hypoxic, necrotic tumor mass. The surgical failures occur when not all of the microscopic disease is removed despite a radical procedure. The objective of preoperative or postoperative radiation is to eliminate the oxygenated radiosensitive peripheral tumor cells. The two treatment modalities are intended to be complementary in their attack on the cancer.

HOW EFFECTIVE ARE COMBINED TREATMENTS IN CONTROLLING CLINICALLY POSITIVE NECK METASTASES?

In a 1969 study, Strong reported cancer recurrence within the dissected neck to be 36.5%. When the nodes were positive at multiple levels, the recurrence rate increased to 71%.[39] He concluded that low-dose (2,000 rad in five treatments) radiation to the neck followed promptly by radical neck dissection for epidermoid carcinoma of the head and neck area produced a significant reduction in the subsequent cervical recurrence rate without increasing morbidity and mortality.

Later, Jesse and Fletcher retrospectively studied 311 patients with squamous cell carcinoma of the oral cavity, supraglottic larynx, and hypopharynx who survived 24 months with the primary lesion controlled. The recurrence rate in the neck for surgically treated group was 14% for N_1, 26% for N_2, and 34% for N_3 stages, as compared to 2%, 11%, and 25%, respectively for those who received combined treatments with surgery and radiation.[40]

There are several prognostic factors related to the frequncy of recurrent disease in the neck. *Control of the primary* is an essential factor for control of neck nodes. A recurrence in the previously treated neck with no recurrence of the primary tumor is rarely encountered.[41] When the primary lesion in the head and neck is controlled, control of N_1 and N_2 neck metastases is frequently achieved if irradiation is combined with radical neck dissection.[42] *Extranodal spread of the cancer* into the connective tissue is another factor responsible for recurrent disease in the neck.[43] Patients with extranodal spread and no preoperative fixation of the lymph nodes experience a significantly lower rate of recurrence in the neck when radical neck dissection is combined with postoperative radiotherapy.[41] *The size and number of positive nodes* in the neck also influence the rate of control of neck disease. Radiation alone is usually sufficient to control an N_1 neck node, but surgical dissection should be combined with irradiation for N_2 and N_3 disease.[44–46] *Involvement of multiple neck nodes*, especially the lower cervical and supraclavicular lymph nodes, carries a poor prognosis. Adjunctive chemotherapy with surgery and radiation are used in such cases as a palliative measure. Patients with advanced neck disease on the ipsilateral side have an increased chance of occult metastases in the contralateral neck. Preoperative or postoperative radiation is one option for treating a contralateral clinically negative neck in order to prevent recurrent disease on the opposite side.

WHAT ARE THE DIFFERENT WAYS THE COMBINED TREATMENTS CAN BE USED FOR THE CONTROL OF CLINICALLY POSITIVE NECK METASTASES?

The planned combination of radiation and surgery may involve either preoperative or postoperative radiation along with radical neck dissection. Preoperative radiation entails delivering 5,000 rad over 5–6 weeks to the primary and the neck nodes, including all the potential areas of microscopic extension of the disease. The optimum interval between preoperative radiation and surgery varies according to the cell type and the anatomical location of the tumor. For most head and neck cancers a 3- to 4-week delay following completion of radiation is minimal, and 6 weeks is probably optimal. Any further delay before surgery may increase the chance of tumor regrowth. Preoperative radiation may also be given in high daily doses over a short period (400 rad/day for 5 days), followed immediately by a planned surgical procedure. This form of treatment has shown no advantage over the conventional method and in fact is less preferred radiobiologically. Postoperative radiation should be no less than 5,000 rad to the entire surgical area, with a boost to 6,000 rad to the tumor bed area. This should include the entire surgical field plus elective inclusion of the clinically uninvolved lymphatics. Postoperative radiation should be started 4–6 weeks after surgery. Delayed postoperative radiation can lead to repopulation of malignant cells and gross tumor recurrence.[47]

IS PREOPERATIVE OR POSTOPERATIVE RADIATION PREFERRED IN THE TREATMENT OF NECK METASTASES?

The choice between preoperative and postoperative radiation depends on the location of the primary cancer and the location and stage of any neck metastases. The aim of combined treatment is to achieve maximal local control with minimal morbidity and acceptable functional and cosmetic results. The decision should be made jointly by surgeons and radiation therapists before initiation of any form of definitive treatments. Clinical data from the M. D. Anderson Hospital have shown that local-regional control rates are identical with 5,000–6,000 rad given either preoperatively or postoperatively.[48] The definitive study trying to answer this question has been the randomized study of the Radiation Therapy Oncology Group. Patients with squamous cell carcinoma of the oral cavity, oropharynx, supraglottic larynx, hypopharynx, and maxillary sinus were allocated randomly to preoperative radiation or postoperative radiation. The results showed no difference in local-regional control or ultimate duration of survival of patients with oral cavity and oropharynx lesions using preoperative or postoperative radiation. For patients with supraglottic laryngeal and hypopharyngeal lesions, surgery and postoperative radiation produced fewer complications and appeared to be better tolerated than did preoperative radiation followed by surgery.[49]

WHAT ARE THE ARGUMENTS IN FAVOR OF PREOPERATIVE RADIATION?

1. In experimental animals, implantation of tumor cells that had been exposed to subtumoricidal doses of radiation was associated with a decreased frequency of tumor growth.[50]
2. Manipulation during surgery may promote distant metastasis by dislodging cancer cells into the bloodstream. Preoperative radiation can theoretically decrease the viability of these cells for implantation at distant sites. In a *retrospective* study from the M. D. Anderson Hospital, the incidence of distant metastasis in patients with T_3 or T_4 and N_2 or N_3 cancer of the head and neck was 33.3% in patients who received postoperative radiation, as compared to 16.7% when radiation was given preoperatively.[51] This was not supported by the results in the randomized controlled study of the Radiation Therapy Oncology group.[49]
3. The effectiveness of radiation depends on oxygenation of the involved tissue. Patients in whom the arterial supply has been surgically disrupted might have less oxygenated residual tumor with a reduced ability to respond to radiation if it is given postoperatively.
4. If preoperative radiation reduces the tumor volume, then a questionably resectable tumor may be converted to one that is definitely resectable.

WHAT ARE THE ARGUMENTS IN FAVOR OF POSTOPERATIVE RADIATION?

1. Since the bulk of residual tumor is significantly less in the postoperative patient, radiation to the smaller tumor volume would be more effective.
2. The true extent of the tumor can be defined during surgical exploration. Pathology studies refine the exact stage of the disease. Radiation can then be given only to those patients who would be likely to benefit from it.

3. Postoperative radiation can be precisely targeted to known areas of positive margins to help retard or prevent local recurrence if there is known residual disease left behind.

4. Surgical resection is technically easier and postoperative healing is more assured in unirradiated tissue.

5. Patients with extensive disease in the head and neck that requires laryngectomy, partial pharyngectomy, esophagectomy, and extensive flap reconstruction do have a wider range of reconstructive options with a higher degree of success in unirradiated tissues. There are fewer difficulties or septic complications after extensive surgery when the tissues are normal.

WHAT ARE THE IMPORTANT FACTORS TO BE CONSIDERED FOR COMBINED TREATMENTS?

1. In general, combined therapy is proposed for advanced disease with T_3T_4 primary and/or N_2 or N_3 neck nodes.

2. Preoperative or postoperative radiation is equally effective in most cases. The decision to select a particular course would depend on the patient's general condition, the extent of the primary and the neck metastases, and the type of surgery planned.

3. Often it is necessary to modify either radiation or the surgical procedure in order to keep the morbidity at an acceptable level.

4. Gross shrinkage of cancer should not tempt the surgeon to perform a less radical resection than was planned before starting definitive treatments.

WHAT IS THE BEST WAY OF MANAGING PRIMARY LESIONS IN HEAD AND NECK CARCINOMAS?

The following general descriptions present the radiotherapist's approach to different sites. Close consultation and multidisciplinary involvement in treatment planning will result in a tailored plan for each patient. There are several factors one must consider before attempting any curative treatment for head and neck carcinomas. (1) The site of origin of the primary lesion and its relationship to the adjacent important structures. (2) The necessity of preserving the anatomy of the primary site for useful function (i.e., larynx for voice production; tongue for speech and deglutition; the glottic and epiglottic tissues for prevention of aspiration of food, etc.). (3) Stage of the primary disease. (4) Stage of any accompanying neck disease. (5) General performance of the patient or a medical history that contraindicates extensive surgical procedures. (6) The reliability of the patient for follow-up. (7) The patient's strong wishes. (8) Occupational needs. (9) Most important, the likelihood that disease-free survival will be achieved by the chosen modality of treatment when weighed against the expected morbidity and mortality from that modality. (See the evaluation schemes discussed in Chap. 5).

Radiation and surgery both play an important complementary role in the management of head and neck cancers. As a general rule, patients with early stage disease (T_1N_0, T_1N_1, and T_2N_{0-1}) have equally good ultimate survival whether treated by radiation or surgery, with each modality adding salvage potential to the other. Some patients with deep-seated infiltrating T_3T_4 lesions have associated bone and muscle involvement and advanced cervical lymph node metastases. Such lesions are not suitable for radical surgical procedures, nor do they respond well to radiation treatments alone. Patients with stage II and stage III disease are most benefited by preoperative or postoperative radiation combined with surgery. For patients with advanced disease (T_4N_3), with or without distant metastases, any form of treatment is mainly for palliation. Such patients are often physically debilitated and will not tolerate radical procedures. Radiation is given only to control local symptoms like pain, bleeding, ulceration, and necrosis of the tumor through the skin. Even in such cases, a minimum of 6,000–7,000 rad is needed for local reduction of the disease. The patient and the family should be aware of the limited benefits, the prolonged course, and the side effects of such palliative treatment.

Because definitive treatments for cancer in each anatomical location are discussed in separate chapters, the following discussion addresses only general points pertinent to radiation treatment of different primary sites.

Oral Cavity

This includes carcinoma of the floor of the mouth, anterior two thirds of the tongue, buccal mucosa, hard and soft palate, and gingiva. Early (T_1T_2) lesions of this area can be adequately treated both by radiation and by surgery. If the lesion is superficial, away from bone, less than 2 cm in diameter, and without any neck nodes, interstitial radiation can be used for definitive treatment. If the lesion is T_2N_0, external radiation is given to include the primary site in the oral cavity along with the immediately adjacent submandibular and upper anterior cervical lymph nodes. After 5,000 rad has been given to this field, the primary site is boosted to 7,000–7,500 rad using an iridium implant or an intraoral cone. This reduces the morbidity from irradiating the entire oral cavity and the adjacent salivary glands to the full 7,000–7,500-rad dose of radiation.[52, 53] Moderately advanced superficial lesions (T_2T_3–N_0) of the uvula, soft palate, and anterior tonsillar pillar respond well to a full course of external radiation treatment.[54, 55] In contrast, T_2T_3 lesions of the floor of the mouth and anterior tongue often invade deep into the muscles and adjacent mandible and present with neck metastases. These tumors are best treated with combined radiation and surgery.[56, 57]

If superficial lesions of the floor of mouth, soft palate, buccal mucosa, and tonsil are treated by preoperative radiation, then, by the end of 4,500–5,000 rad, it is often difficult to detect any visible tumor for surgical resection. Therefore, the margins of such tumors should be tatooed before starting radiation so that one can subsequently resect the entire tumor bed area during surgery.

Oropharynx

This includes carcinoma of the tonsil, base of the tongue, valeccula, and lateral pharyngeal walls. Early carcinoma of the tonsil (T_1T_2-N_0) has a high local control rate with external beam radiation.[58–60] Advanced T_3T_4 tonsillar lesions often involve the adjacent mandible and soft tissue and metastasize to the regional lymph nodes. The reported superiority of results achieved with combined treatment support the value of combined treatment in advanced oropharyngeal lesions.[56, 61–63] Early carcinoma of the base of the tongue is asymptomatic. By the time the diagnosis is made, the tumor is most often well advanced, with infiltration of deep muscles of the tongue and bilateral cervical lymph nodes. Although small superficial lesions are well controlled just by a full course of radiation alone, most of the advanced oropharyngeal lesions will require combined treatments.[64, 65]

The oropharynx is rich in lymphatics. The incidence of either occult or clinical meatastases in the neck is high. Radiation ports should include the primary and bilateral neck nodes, including posterior cervical nodes. Interstitial implants are very difficult to use in these sites.

Larynx

The most common tumor of the larynx is squamous cell carcinoma of the true vocal cords. Since a small tumor will cause hoarseness, cancers are detected at an early stage. The true cords have limited lymphatic channels; therefore the incidence of cervical lymph node metastasis is low with an early glottic lesion. The radiation treatment for a limited glottic cancer employs a small field (5 × 5 cm or 6 × 6 cm) to cover the primary site only. When the tumor extends beyond the glottis (T_2 lesions), the chance of lymph node metastasis increases. Treatment fields should include the immediate draining nodes (subdigastric) along with the primary. Wedges and partial compensators are used to produce uniform dose distribution across the treatment volume. The treatments are well tolerated, and a local control rate of 95% in T_1 and 75%–80% in T_2 lesions makes radiation the treatment of choice. Although conservative surgery can produce similar survival results, the voice is preserved better by radiation treatment. Salvage surgery is highly effective for radiation failures.[66–68] When there is impaired cord mobility (T_3 and T_4 lesions) the chance of node metastasis and deep infiltration of tumor increases and the cure rate by radiation alone decreases. Surgery becomes the major therapy, with irradiation as an adjunctive combined treatment.[69–71]

Because of the abundant supply of lymphatics, supraglottic lesions have a predictably high incidence of lymph node metastases, often bilaterally. Because of this lymphatic spread, radiation fields should include both the primary lesion and the cervical lymph nodes bilaterally. Except for early lesions (best treated by high-dose radiation[72, 73]), preoperative or postoperative radiation combined with surgery has produced the best reported survival results.[74–76]

It is important to include the tracheostomy stoma in the radiation field, especially when a pretreatment tracheostomy is required because of respiratory obstruction or when there is transglottic tumor, since a pretreatment tracheostomy carries a high incidence of tracheal recurrence.

Hypopharynx

The most common carcinoma in the region is from the piriform sinus, followed by posterior pharyngeal wall lesions. Carcinomas arising in the postcricoid areas are rare. Often hypopharyngeal cancers are poorly differentiated carcinomas. They remain asymptomatic until they infiltrate the surrounding structures and present with neck node metastases.

Posterior pharyngeal wall lesions are usually large tumors and infiltrate deeply, along the retropharyngeal space. Because of the area of invasion and spread to retropharyngeal nodes, posterior pharyngeal cancers are nearly always unresectable. A full course of radiation is given, in the knowledge that it is largely palliative. Radical neck dissection is reserved for patients in whom the primary is controlled but who have residual disease in the neck following a full course of radiation. Large fields of radiation from the base of the skull to the upper cervical esophagus, including the cervical nodes bilaterally, is necessary for local control of posterior pharyngeal cancer.[77–80]

Most carcinomas of the piriform sinus are advanced lesions. If they are operable, combined treatment with radiation and surgery is most commonly used.[81, 82] Because an extensive surgical procedure is required (laryngopharyngectomy), preoperative radiation is avoided because it has a higher complication rate than does postoperative radiation treatment.[83–85] Only small superficial lesions that do not infiltrate the larynx or the thyroid cartilage (with early neck disease, T_1N_{0-1}) are controlled by radiation alone.[86–88] Radiation fields should be large enough to include the primary lesion and the cervical and retropharyngeal lymph nodes. The inferior margin of the field should be extended to include the upper cervical esophagus and trachea.

Nasopharynx

The nasopharynx is considered a blind spot and the patients often have extensive neck metastases when they are seen for the first time. Because of the anatomical location of nasopharynx, surgical resection cannot ablate this disease. Radiation treatment is the mainstay of therapy for this disease (chapter 15 discusses treatment in detail).

Paranasal Sinus

Cancers in this location are frequently advanced by the time they are discovered, with extension to local soft tissue structures and bone. These tumors are best treated by a combination of radiation and surgery.[89–91] The results are similar whether radiation is given preoperatively or postoperatively.[92, 93] Because of the rarity of cervical lymph node metastases, routine elective treatment (either with radiation or surgery) of the clinically negative neck is not indicated.[94] Radiation treatment fields should include the ipsilateral paranasal sinuses and orbit, depending on the extent of the local disease. Complicated multiple field setups, including the use of wedges, are necessary to deliver a uniform dose across the tumor volume while sparing important structures (cervical spine, lens, optic nerve) from high doses of radiation.

Salivary Glands

The majority of malignant tumors arise in the parotid and submandibular salivary glands. Surgery is the primary method of treatment. Postoperative radiation to the tumor bed area is used as an adjunct either because of the presence of known residual disease or because of an anticipated high rate of local recurrence following surgery.[95–98] Irradiation is used in the following situations:

1. Residual known cancer remaining following surgical resection (tumor left behind or positive resection margin).
2. Invasion of the gland capsule, involvement of lymphatics, or proximal perineural lymphatics.
3. Metastatic disease in the lymph nodes (N_2, N_3).
4. Involvement of deep lobe of the parotid with high-grade lesions.
5. High-grade lesions (i.e. high grade mucoepidermoid, squamous cell, undifferentiated, adenoid cystic, and adenocarcinomas.)
6. Postoperative radiation treatments are designed to cover the tumor bed area, including the known route of local extension of the tumor and the regional lymph nodes. The areas are treated to 6,000 rad.

HOW CRITICAL IS GOOD DENTAL CARE IN PATIENTS RECEIVING RADIATION TREATMENT FOR HEAD AND NECK CANCER?

The deleterious effects of radiation therapy in patients with head and neck cancer include (1) oral mucositis, (2) progressive periodontal disease, (3) reduced salivary secretion causing xerostomia, (4) increased incidence of dental caries, and (5) the most serious problem, osteoradionecrosis of the mandible. Most of the major dental problems are discussed in detail by Dr. Browne in chapter 11. Comprehensive dental care programs in several major centers have reported definite benefit from application of fluoride gel in the prevention of postirradiation dental caries.[99, 100]

All patients are seen in the dental department for careful evaluation prior to irradiation treatment. There is thorough examination of the teeth, gums, mandible, and maxilla. If necessary, there is correct fitting of the prosthesis in edentulous patients. If salivary function and quality are adequate, if the teeth are excellent or can be easily restored with one or two fillings, if there is no gingivitis or periodontitis, if the alveolar bone is not atrophic, and if the patient will be absolutely compliant to a life-long care ritual, then a preventive fluoride program can be undertaken. Unfortunately, most patients with oral cancer cannot meet the criteria. If few, or most, of the teeth are beyond repair, partial or complete extraction of them prior to radiation is done. Meticulous alveolectomy following extraction of the teeth is necessary for primary mucosal closure over the bone. Depending on the extent of the dental extraction, an appropriate waiting time is needed for complete healing of the extraction site before radiation treatment can be started. Inadequate healing before treatment can lead to osteoradionecrosis at the extraction site.

Periodic dental examination is necessary following radiation for the early detection of dental caries, periodontal disease, or a maladjusted prosthesis. Conservative treatments are often effective in these cases. Edentulous patients should not have dental prostheses fitted for about 1 year following radiation treatments. Then, the decision to use prostheses is based on the condition of the tissues and the qualities of the saliva.

A thorough dental program for head and neck cancer patients undergoing radiation therapy has helped in retention of teeth in selected patients and has reduced the incidence of postradiation osteoradionecrosis to 1%–2%.[101]

WHAT IS THE ROLE OF ADEQUATE NUTRITIONAL SUPPORT IN TOLERANCE OF HEAD AND NECK RADIATION?

Just as discussed for surgery patients in chapter 11, the irradiation patient has problems with nutritional adequacy. The association of high incidence of head and neck cancer with tobacco and alcohol abuse is well known. Consequently, most of the head and neck cancer patients have nutritional deficits prior to any treatments. Radiation treatments further compromise the nutritional status by affecting the normal tissue in and around the oral cavity and oropharynx. Irritation of the mucous membrane in these areas causes sore mouth, sore throat, and odynophagea. Impairment of taste and salivary secretion is another major side effect of radiation and are responsible for poor nutritional intake in these patients. Most patients receiving full courses of radiation to the head and neck area lose about 10 pounds during the treatment period.[102, 103]

At the beginning of the radiation, a dietician will be able to advise the appropriate diet that is tolerated by the patients. Use of food supplements and nasogastric tube feedings become essential if the weight loss is severe (≥ 5 lb). Optimal nutritional support in head and neck cancer patients allows more patients to tolerate radiation treatments and almost all of them to complete the full planned course.

WHAT ARE THE SIDE EFFECTS AND COMPLICATIONS OF RADIATION TREATMENTS?

When radiation is given to an area, it affects both tumor tissue and the normal tissues surrounding the tumor. The side effects of radiation are the expected reactions of normal tissue to radiation. With conservative management, the acute effects usually subside within a few weeks following completion of treatments. Late radiation complications, on the other hand, are due to excessive doses of radiation to some of the normal tissues. The late tissue changes may affect functions or may produce permanent damage that requires more than conservative treatment. Radiation complications can lead to considerable morbidity and occasionally death.

The usual side effects and complications of radiation are as follows:

Skin

The early or acute skin changes consist of erythema, hyperpigmentation, dry desquamation, and occasionally islands of moist desquamation in skin folds. Depending on the radiation dose, loss of hair in the treatment area can be temporary or permanent. Treatment for skin irritation consists of keeping the skin dry, avoiding local trauma (shaving or using irritating skin preparations), and maintaining skin oils with lanolin-based creams, with or without hydrocortisone creams. With megavoltage beams (x-ray beams with skin-sparing effects), skin reaction subsides by 4–6 weeks following completion of treatments.

Chronic, delayed reactions consist of skin atrophy, subcutaneous fibrosis, and delayed healing.

Mucous Membrane

Irritation (erythema, membranous mucositis) of the mucous membrane of the oral cavity and oropharynx is unavoidable during radiation treatments to these areas. This will cause pain, odynophagia, and dysphagia. This problem is aggravated by loss of taste and xerostomia. Management is discussed in chapter 11.

Salivary Glands

Radiation xerostomia depends on the extent of inclusion of salivary glands and the total radiation dose. Radiation-induced xerostomia can be quite disabling. In patients receiving full dose by curative radiation (to 7,000 rad) to the oral cavity and/or oropharynx, dry mouth can be permanent. Artificial salivary substitutes are helpful in keeping the mouth moist temporarily.

Taste

Radiation of oropharynx causes loss of taste, but most often this does not remain permanent following completion of treatments.

Larynx

The glottis is included in the radiation field when laryngeal and hypopharyngeal carcinomas are treated with radiation. The acute radiation reaction is more marked if the larynx is directly involved with tumor than if it is included in the pharyngeal lesions. By the third or fourth week of treatment there is increasing hoarseness. Treatments are conservative, with avoidance of smoking, rest of vocal cords, and the use of topical anesthetics. If there is no persistent edema, symptoms subside within a few weeks following the end of the treatments.

Laryngeal edema persisting over months after completion of treatments is a major radiation complication. Edema is often associated with recurrent disease. Persisting edema is ominous and effort should be made to exclude recurrent cancer. If the biopsy is negative (which often happens because recurrent disease is often found in deeper tissues), patients should be treated with steroids and antibiotics. If the patient continues to have hoarseness and significant pain, laryngectomy may be recommended in spite of the absence of histologic confirmation of recurrent cancer. The incidence of laryngeal edema increases directly with dose as the minimum tumor dose exceeds 7,000 rad delivered over 8 weeks. Laryngeal edema also increases proportionately with the field size and with an increased daily tumor dose.[104] Every effort should be made to avoid laryngeal edema and chondritis by meticulous treatment planning.

Ears

Early side effects of radiation treatments are dryness of the skin over the pinna and within the ear canal. Serous otitis media is commonly seen. Patients complain of earache or fullness in the ears. The otitis usually subsides with conservative management. Late effects on the middle and inner ear are infrequent. Complications are seen only when a full dose is delivered to the tumors in deeper structures in this region.

Eyes

The eye is usually shielded from the direct field of radiation except in tumors of the nasal cavity, nasopharynx, and paranasal sinuses. When there is evidence of involvement of the bony orbit, it is necessary to include either a part or all of the orbit in the full dose of radiation ports. A variety of complications is seen. Radiation effects on conjunctiva and cornea are minimized when radiation is delivered with the patient's eyes wide open, using a direct anterior field. The skin-sparing effects of megavoltage radiation also spares the conjunctiva and cornea from high-dose effects. Transient xerophthalmia, erythema, and edema of the conjunctiva and cornea are seen. If there is added infection and abrasive trauma, then punctate keratosis, corneal ulceration, and edema may lead to a permanent visual complication. A radiation-induced cataract may be seen if the lens is in a high-dose field of radiation. Such a cataract may require extraction. Severe radiation-induced complications producing blindness will occur only if the posterior part of the eye receives a high dose of radiation (> 6,000 rad). Three factors have been described for the etiology of radiation retinopathy: (1) macular and retinal degeneration, (2) optic nerve atrophy, and (3) central retinal artery thrombosis.[105] Radiation retinopathy is a late complication and occurs 2–5 years following the treatments. The incidence of radiation retinopathy is dependent on both high total dose and larger daily fraction size.[106] Despite occasional visual complications, one should not compromise the dose to the orbit when cure is attempted for definite orbital involvement. Orbital invasion with cancer will grow relentlessly and produce predictable blindness in most patients unless death supervenes.

Endocrine

The radiation fields used for treatment of laryngeal and hypopharyngeal carcinomas include the thyroid gland in the full dose of radiation. Similarly, for nasopharyngeal and paranasal sinus tumors, one must cover the hypothalamic-pituitary axis in the treatment ports. A large number of patients that are so irradiated will develop endocrine deficiencies that might include hypothalamic deficits, primary pituitary deficiencies, and primary hypothyroidism.[107, 108] It is important to have long-term general medical follow-ups of these patients because the endocrine complication may appear quite late (2–6 years) following treatments.

Bone

One of the major complications of head and neck radiation is osteoradionecrosis. The management and specific incidence is discussed in the chapter on complications (see Chap. 27). Osteoradionecrosis of the mandible is seen when high-dose radiation includes the mandible in the field used for treatment of oral cavity and oropharyngeal lesions. Local pain and swelling are the initial symptoms. This is followed by an area of exposed bone in the oral cavity. Several factors have been shown to correlate with the incidence of osteoradionecrosis,[109–112] as described below.

Total Radiation Dose.—Necrosis is rarely seen below a dose of 6,000 rad. The incidence increases sharply with doses above this level.

Mandibular Invasion.—Tumors that are adherent to or invading the mandible have a higher incidence of necrosis as compared to the tumors that are more remotely located. The larger tumors necrose, leaving the bone vulnerable to infection by oral organisms.

Dental Conditions.—Patients who are dentulous have 2.6 times the risk of developing osteoradionecrosis than those who are edentulous. Comprehensive judicious dental care has greatly reduced the incidence of bone necrosis.

Radiation Technique.—The risk of bone necrosis is greatest when an interstitial implant is used as the sole radiation source, less with the combination technique, and least with external beam irradiation alone.

Mandibular necrosis can be treated conservatively with antibiotics, good oral hygiene, and maintenance of adequate nutrition. Healing is very slow. If persistent pain disables the patient, surgical removal of the bone may become necessary (see Chap. 27).

Cervical Spinal Cord

The cervical spine may be included in the radiation field while treating nasopharyngeal cancer paranasal sinus cancer (ethmoids) or posterior neck nodes. If the dose to the spine is limited to 5,000 rad delivered over 5 weeks, no acute reaction is seen and the incidence of late cervical myelitis is extremely low. If higher doses cross the spinal cord, transverse myelitis may result. This is one of the areas where the radiation therapist's skill in computer-supported treatment planning, precise dosimetry, and simulator assistance are required.

REFERENCES

1. Sievert R.M.: The new apparatus for teleradium treatment used at radiumhemmet. *Acta Radiol.* 14:197–206, 1933.
2. Lederman M.: The early history of radiotherapy: 1895–1939. *Int. J. Radiat. Oncol. Biol. Phys.* 7:639–648, 1981.
3. Glassburn J.R., Brady L.W., Plenk H.P.: Hyperbaric oxygen in radiation therapy. *Cancer* 39:751–765, 1977.
4. Henk J.M.: Does hyperbaric oxygen have a future in radiation therapy? *Int. J. Radiat. Oncol. Biol. Phys.* 7:1125–1128, 1981.
5. Yuhas J.M.: Efficacy testing of WR-2721 in Great Britain or everything is black and white at Gray Lab. *Int. J. Radiat. Oncol. Biol. Phys.* 9:595–598, 1983.
6. Bagshaw M.A., Doggett R.L.S.: A clinical study of chemical radiosensitization. *Front. Radiat. Ther. Oncol.* 4:164–173, 1969.
7. Sano K., Nagai M., Arai T., et al.: Follow-up results of BUDR therapy of malignant brain tumors, in *Proceedings of the Fourth European Congress of Neurosurgery.* Amsterdam, Excerpta Medica, International Congress Series No. 272, 1972.
8. Goffinet D.R., Kaplan H.S., Donaldson S.S., et al.: Combined radiosensitizer infusion and irradiation of osteogenic sarcoma. *Radiology* 117:211–214, 1975.
9. Phillips T.L., Wasserman T.H., Stetz J., et al.: Clinical trials of hypoxic cell sensitizers. *Int. J. Radiat. Oncol. Biol. Phys.* 8:327–334, 1982.
10. Ben Hur E., Elkind M.M., Bronk B.V.: Thermally enhanced radio-response of cultured Chinese hamster cells: Inhibition of repair of sublethal damage and enhancement of lethal damage. *Radiat. Res.* 58:38–51, 1974.
11. Leith J.T., Miller R.C., Gerner E.W., et al.: Hyperthermic potentiation: Biological aspects and application to radiation therapy. *Cancer* 39:766–778, 1977.
12. Li G.C., Evans R., Hahn G.M.: Modification and inhibition of repair of potentially lethal x-ray damage by hyperthermia. *Radiat. Res.* 67:491–501, 1976.
13. Dewey W.C., Hopwood L.E., Sapareto S.A., et al.: Cellular responses to combination of hyperthermia and radiation. *Radiology* 123:463–474, 1977.
14. Robinson J.E., Wizenberg M.J.: Thermal sensitivity and effect of elevated temperature on the radiation sensitivity of Chinese hamster cells. *Acta Radiol.* 13:241–248, 1974.
15. Westra A., Dewey W.C.: Variation in sensitivity to heat shock during the cell cycle of Chinese hamster cells in vitro. *Int. J. Radiat. Oncol. Biol. Phys.* 19:467–477, 1971.
16. Gerweek L.E.: Modification of cell lethality at elevated temperatures: pH effect. *Radiat. Res.* 70:224–235, 1977.
17. Hahn G.M.: Metabolic aspects of the role of hyperthermia in mammalian cells in activation and their relevance to cancer treatment. *Cancer Res.* 34:3117–3123, 1974.
18. Alcieri A.A., Hahn E.W., Kim J.H.: The relationship between the time of fractionated and single dose of radiation and hyperthermia on the sensitization of an in vivo mouse tumor. *Cancer* 36:893–903, 1975.
19. Gerner E.W., Connor W.G., Boone M.L.M., et al.: The potential of localized heating as an adjunct to radiation therapy. *Radiology* 116:433–439, 1975.
20. Hahn E.W., Alcieri A.A., Kim J.H.: Increased cures using fractionated exposure of x-irradiation and hyperthermia in the local treatment of Riddgeway osteogenic sarcoma in mice. *Radiology* 113:119–202, 1974.
21. Scott R.S., Johnson R., Kowal H., et al.: Hyperthermia in combination with radiotherapy: A review of five years' experience in the treatment of superficial tumors. *Int. J. Radiat. Oncol. Biol. Phys.* 9:1327–1333, 1983.
22. Manning M.R., Cetas T., Miller R.C., et al.: Clinical hyperthermia. *Cancer* 49:205–216, 1982.
23. Perez C.A., Kopecky W., Rao V.D., et al.: Local microwave hyperthermia and irradiation in cancer therapy: Preliminary observations and directions for future clinical trials. *Int. J. Radiat. Oncol. Biol. Phys.* 7:765–772, 1981.
24. Maror J.B., Hahn G.M.: Combined radiation and hyperthermia in superficial human tumor. *Cancer* 46:1986–1991, 1980.
25. Arcangeli G., Barni E., Cividalli A., et al.: Effectiveness of microwave hyperthermia combined with ionizing radiation: Clinical results on neck node metastases. *Int. J. Radiat. Oncol. Biol. Phys.* 6:143–148, 1980.
26. Wang C.C., Doppke K.P., Biggs P.J.: Intra-oral cone radiation therapy for selected carcinomas of the oral cavity. *Int. J. Radiat. Oncol. Biol. Phys.* 9:1185–1189, 1983.
27. Catterall M.: Results of neutron therapy: Differences, correlations and improvements. *Int. J. Radiat. Oncol. Biol. Phys.* 8:2141–2144, 1982.
28. Maor M.H., Hussey D.H., Barkley T.H., et al.: Neutron therapy for head and neck cancer: II. Further follow up on the M. D. Anderson TAMVEC randomized clinical trial. *Int. J. Radiat. Oncol. Biol. Phys.* 9:1261–1265, 1983.
29. Suit H., Goitein M., Munzenrider J., et al.: Evaluation of the clinical applicability of proton beams in definitive fractionated radiation therapy. *Int. J. Radiat. Oncol. Biol. Phys.* 8:2199–2205, 1982.
30. Orton C.G., Ellis F.: A simplification in the use of N.S.D. concept in practical radiotherapy. *Br. J. Radiol.* 46:529–537, 1973.
31. Goitein M.: The computation of time dose and fractionation factors for irregular treatment schedule. *Br. J. Radiol.* 47:665–669, 1974.
32. Million R.R., Fletcher G.H., Jesse R.H.: Evaluation of elective irradiation of the neck for squamous cell carcinoma of the nasopharynx, tonsillar fossa and base of tongue. *Radiology* 80:973–988, 1963.
33. Fletcher G.H.: Clinical dose response curve of human malignant epithelial tumors. *Br. J. Radiol.* 46:1–12, 1973.

34. Million R.R.: Elective neck irradiation for T_xN_O squamous carcinoma of the oral tongue and floor of mouth. *Cancer* 34:149–155, 1974.
35. Bagshaw M.A., Thompson R.W.: Elective irradiation of the neck in patients with primary carcinoma of the head and neck. *JAMA* 217:456–458, 1971.
36. Rabuzzi D.D., Chang C.T., Sagerman R.H.: Prophylactic neck irradiation. *Arch. Otolaryngol.* 106:454–455, 1980.
37. Horiuchi J., Adachi T.: Some consideration on radiation therapy of tongue cancer. *Cancer* 28:335–339, 1971.
38. Fletcher G.H.: Elective irradiation of subclinical disease in cancer of the head and neck. *Cancer* 29:1450–1454, 1972.
39. Strong E.W.: Preoperative radiation and radical neck dissection. *Surg. Clin. North Am.* 49:271–276, 1969.
40. Jesse R.H., Fletcher G.H.: Treatment of the neck in the patients with squamous cell carcinoma of the head and neck. *Cancer* 39:868–872, 1977.
41. Bartelink H., Breur K., Hart G.: Radiotherapy of lymph node metastasis in patients with squamous cell carcinoma of the head and neck region. *Int. J. Radiat. Oncol. Biol. Phys.* 8:983–989, 1982.
42. Northrup M., Fletcher G.H., Jesse R.H., et al.: Evaluation of neck disease in patients with primary squamous cell carcinoma of the oral tongue, floor of mouth and palatine arch and clinically positive neck nodes neither fixed nor bilateral. *Cancer* 29:23–30, 1972.
43. Snow G.B., Annyas A.A., Van Slooten E.A., et al.: Prognostic factors of neck node metastasis. *Clin. Otolaryngol.* 7:185–192, 1982.
44. Jesse R.H., Lindberg R.D.: The efficacy of combining radiation therapy with a surgical procedure in patients with cervical metastasis from squamous cancer of the oropharynx and hypopharynx. *Cancer* 35:1163–1166, 1975.
45. Decroix Y., Ghossein N.A.: Experience of the Curie Institute in treatment of cancer of the mobile tongue: II. Management of the neck nodes. *Cancer* 47:503–508, 1981.
46. Schneider J.J., Fletcher G.H., Barkley H.T. Jr.: Control by irradiation alone of nonfixed clinically positive lymph nodes from squamous cell carcinoma of the oral cavity, oropharynx, supraglottic larynx and hypopharynx. *AJR* 123:42–48, 1975.
47. Vikram B.: Importance of the time interval between surgery and postoperative radiation therapy in the combined management of head and neck cancer. *Int. J. Radiat. Oncol. Biol. Phys.* 5:1837–1840, 1979.
48. Fletcher G.H.: Basic principles of the combination of irradiation and surgery. *Int. J. Radiat. Oncol. Biol. Phys.* 5:2091–2096, 1979.
49. Snow J.B., Gelber R.D., Kramer S., et al.: Randomized preoperative and postoperative radiation therapy for patients with carcinoma of the head and neck: Preliminary report. *Laryngoscope* 90:930–945, 1980.
50. Powers W., Plamer L.A.: Biological basis of preoperative radiation treatment. *AJR* 102:176–192, 1968.
51. Merino O.R., Lindberg R.D., Fletcher G.H.: An analysis of distant metastases from squamous cell carcinoma of the upper respiratory and digestive tracts. *Cancer* 40:145–151, 1977.
52. Puthawala A.A., Syed N.A.M., Neblett D., et al.: The role of afterloading iridium (Ir^{192}) implant in the management of carcinoma of the tongue. *Int. J. Radiat. Oncol. Biol. Phys.* 7:407–412, 1981.
53. Wang C.C., Boyer A.L., Mendiondo O.: Afterloading interstitial radiation therapy. *Int. J. Radiat. Oncol. Biol. Phys.* 1:365–368, 1976.
54. Chung C.K., Constable W.C.: Squamous cell carcinoma of the soft palate and uvula. *Int. J. Radiat. Oncol. Biol. Phys.* 5:845–850, 1976.
55. Gelinas M., Fletcher G.H.: Incidence and cause of local failure of irradiation in squamous cell carcinoma of the facial arch, tonsillar fossa and base of the tongue. *Radiology* 108:383–387, 1973.
56. Hamberger A.D., Fletcher G.H., Guillamondegui O.M., et al.: Results of advanced squamous cell carcinoma of the oral cavity and oropharynx treated with combined megavoltage radiation therapy and surgery. *Radiology* 119:433–438, 1976.
57. Marks J.E., Lee F., Freeman R.B., et al.: Carcinoma of the oral tongue: A study of patient selection and treatment results. *Laryngoscope* 91:1548–1559, 1981.
58. Perez C.A., Purdy J.A., Breaux S.R., et al.: Carcinoma of the tonsillar fossa. *Cancer* 50:2314–2322, 1982.
59. Tong D., Laramore G.E., Griffin T.W., et al.: Carcinoma of the tonsillar region. *Cancer* 49:2009–2014, 1982.
60. Fayor J.V., Lampe I.: Radiation therapy of carcinoma of the tonsillar region. *AJR* 111:84–94, 1971.
61. Shrewsbury D., Adams G.L., Duvall A.J., et al.: Carcinoma of the tonsillar region: A comparison of radiation therapy with combined preoperative radiation and surgery. *Otolaryngol. Head Neck Surg.* 89:979–985, 1981.
62. Maltz R., Shumrick D.A., Aron B.S., et al.: Carcinoma of the tonsil: Results of combined therapy. *Laryngoscope* 84:2172–2180, 1974.
63. Rolander T.L., Everts E.C., Shumrick D.A.: Carcinoma of the tonsil: A planned combined therapy approach. *Laryngoscope* 81:1199–1207, 1971.
64. Roll J., Rozenbom C.V., Thawley S., et al.: Squamous carcinoma of the base of the tongue. *Cancer* 47:333–342, 1981.
65. Blumberg A.L., Fu K., Phillip T.L.: Results of treatment of carcinoma of the base of the tongue: The UCSF experience 1957–1976. *Int. J. Radiat. Oncol. Biol. Phys.* 5:1971–1976, 1979.
66. Harwood A.R., Hawkins N.V., Rider W.D., et al.: Radiotherapy of early glottic cancer. *Int. J. Radiat. Oncol. Biol. Phys.* 5:473–476, 1979.
67. Mittal B., Rao D.V., Marks J.E., et al.: Role of radiation in the management of early vocal cord carcinoma. *Int. J. Radiat. Oncol. Biol. Phys.* 9:997–1002, 1983.
68. Sung D.I., Chang C.H., Harisiadis L., et al.: Primary radiotherapy for carcinoma in situ and early invasive carcinoma of the glottic larynx. *Int. J. Radiat. Oncol. Biol. Phys.* 5:467–472, 1979.

69. Mittal B., Marks J.E., Ogura J.H: Transglottic carcinoma. *Cancer* 53:151–161, 1984.
70. Mendenhall W.M., Million R.R., Sharkey D.E., et al.: Stage T_3 squamous cell carcinoma of the glottic larynx treated with surgery and/or radiation therapy. *Int. J. Radiat. Oncol. Biol. Phys.* 10:357–363, 1984.
71. Kaplan M.J., Johns M.E., Clark D.A., et al.: Glottic cancer. *Cancer* 53:2641–2648, 1984.
72. Wang C.C.: Megavoltage radiation therapy for supraglottic carcinoma: Results of treatment. *Radiology* 109:183–186, 1973.
73. Bataini J.B., Ennuyer A., Poncet P., et al.: Treatment of supraglottic carcinoma by radical high dose radiotherapy. *Cancer* 33:1253–1261, 1974.
74. Fu K.K., Eisenberg L., Dedo H.M., et al.: Results of integrated management of supraglottic carcinoma. *Cancer* 40:2874–2881, 1977.
75. Flynn M.B., Jesse R.H., Lindberg R.T.: Surgery and radiation in the treatment of squamous cell carcinoma of the supraglottic larynx. *Am. J. Surg.* 124:477–481, 1972.
76. Goepfert H., Jesse R.H., Fletcher G.H., et al.: Optimal treatment for the technically resectable squamous cell carcinoma of the supraglottic larynx. *Laryngoscope* 85:14–32, 1975.
77. Wang C.C.: Radiotherapy management of carcinoma of the posterior pharyngeal wall. *Cancer* 27:894–896, 1971.
78. Moez-Mendez R.T., Fletcher G.H., Guillamondegui O.M., et al.: Analysis of the results of irradiation in treatment of squamous cell carcinoma of the pharyngeal wall. *Int. J. Radiat. Oncol. Biol. Phys.* 4:579–585, 1978.
79. Marks J.E., Freeman R.B., Lee F., et al.: Pharyngeal wall cancer: An analysis of treatment results, complications and pattern of failure. *Int. J. Radiat. Oncol. Biol. Phys.* 4:587–593, 1978.
80. Talton B.M., Elkon D., Kim J.A., et al.: Cancer of the posterior pharyngeal wall. *Int. J. Radiat. Oncol. Biol. Phys.* 7:597–599, 1981.
81. Marks J.E., Kurnik B., Powers W.E., et al.: Carcinoma of the pyriform sinus: An analysis of treatment results and pattern of failure. *Cancer* 41:1008–1015, 1978.
82. El Badawi S.A., Goepfert H., Fletcher G.H., et al.: Squamous cell carcinoma of the pyriform sinus. *Laryngoscope* 92:357–364, 1982.
83. Vandenbrauch C., Sancho H., Lefur R., et al.: Results of a randomized clinical trial of preoperative irradiation versus postoperative irradiation in the treatment of tumors of the hypopharynx. *Cancer* 39:1445–1449, 1977.
84. Donald P.J.: Complications of combined therapy in head and neck carcinomas. *Arch. Otolaryngol.* 104:329–332, 1978.
85. Arriagada R., Eschwege F., Cachin Y., et al.: The value of combined radiation with surgery in the treatment of hypopharyngeal and laryngeal cancers. *Cancer* 51:1819–1825, 1983.
86. Bataini P., Brugere J., Bernier J., et al.: Results of radical radiotherapeutic treatment of carcinoma of the pyriform sinus. *Int. J. Radiat. Oncol. Biol. Phys.* 8:1277–1286, 1982.
87. Million R.R., Cassisi N.J.: Radical irradiation for carcinoma of the pyriform sinus. *Laryngoscope* 91:439–450, 1981.
88. Ahmad K., Fayos J.V.: High dose radiation therapy in carcinoma of the pyriform sinus. *Cancer* 53:2091–2094, 1984.
89. Cheng V.S.T., Wang C.C.: Carcinomas of the paranasal sinuses. *Cancer* 40:3038–3041, 1977.
90. Lee F., Ogura J.H.: Maxillary sinus carcinoma. *Laryngoscope* 91:133–139, 1981.
91. Bush S.E., Bagshaw M.A.: Carcinoma of the paranasal sinuses. *Cancer* 50:154–158, 1982.
92. Jesse R.H.: Preoperative versus postoperative radiation in the treatment of squamous carcinoma of the paranasal sinuses. *Am. J. Surg.* 110:552–556, 1965.
93. Yu-Hua H., Gui-Yi T., Yu-Qin Q., et al.: Comparison of pre and postoperative radiation in the combined treatment of carcinoma of maxillary sinus. *Int. J. Radiat. Oncol. Biol. Phys.* 8:1045–1049, 1982.
94. Pezner R.D., Moss W.T., Tong D., et al.: Cervical lymph node metastases in patients with squamous cell carcinoma of the maxillary antrum: The role of elective irradiation of the clinically negative neck. *Int. J. Radiat. Oncol. Biol. Phys.* 5:1977–1980, 1979.
95. Guillamondegui O.M., Byers R.M., Luna M.A., et al.: Aggressive surgery in treatment for parotid cancer: The role of adjunctive postoperative radiotherapy. *Am. J. Roentgenol. Radium Ther. Nucl. Med.* 123:49–54, 1975.
96. Fu K.K., Leibel S.A., Levine M.L., et al.: Carcinoma of the major and minor salivary glands. *Cancer* 40:2882–2890, 1977.
97. Shidnia H., Hornback N.B., Hamaker R., et al.: Carcinoma of major salivary glands. *Cancer* 45:693–697, 1980.
98. McNaney D., McNeese M.D., Guillamondegui O.M., et al.: Postoperative irradiation in malignant epithelial tumors of the parotid. *Int. J. Radiat. Oncol. Biol. Phys.* 9:1289–1295, 1983.
99. Daley T.E., Diane J.B.: *Management of dental problems in irradiated patients.* Houston, Texas, The University of Texas M. D. Anderson Hospital and Tumor Institute, 1972, pp. 1–43.
100. Hariot J.C., Schraub S., Bone M.C., et al.: Dental preservation in patients irradiated for head and neck tumors: A 10 year experience with topical fluoride and a randomized trial between two fluoridation methods. *Radiother. Oncol.* 1:77–82, 1983.
101. Hariot J.C., Bone M.C., Ibrahim E., et al.: Systematic dental management in head and neck irradiation. *Int. J. Radiat. Oncol. Biol. Phys.* 7:1025–1029, 1981.
102. Chencharick J.D., Mossman K.L.: Nutritional consequences of the radiotherapy of head and neck cancer. *Cancer* 51:811–815, 1983.
103. Donaldson S.S.: Nutritional consequences of radiotherapy. *Cancer Res.* 37:2407–2413, 1977.
104. Fu K.K., Woodhouse R.J., Quincy J.M., et al.: The significance of laryngeal edema following radiotherapy of carcinoma of the vocal cord. *Cancer* 49:655–658, 1982.
105. Shakovsky L.J., Fletcher G.H.: Retinal and optic nerve complication in a high dose irradiation technique of eth-

moid sinus and nasal cavity. *Radiology* 104:629–634, 1972.

106. Nukissa N., Rubin P., Strohl R., et al.: Ocular and orbital complication following radiation therapy of paranasal malignancies and review of literature. *Cancer* 51:980–986, 1983.
107. Samaan N.A., Vieto R., Schultz P.N., et al.: Hypothalamic pituitary and thyroid dysfunction after radiotherapy to the head and neck. *Int. J. Radiat. Oncol. Biol. Phys.* 8:1857–1867, 1982.
108. Shafer R.B., Nutall F.O., Pollack K.: Thyroid function after radiation and surgery for head and neck cancer. *Arch. Intern. Med.* 135:843–846, 1975.
109. Bedwinek J.M., Shukovsky L.J., Fletcher G.H., et al.: Osteonecrosis in patients treated with definitive radiotherapy for squamous cell carcinomas of the oral cavity and naso and oropharynx. *Radiology* 119:665–667, 1976.
110. Cheng V.S.T., Wang C.C.: Osteoradionecrosis of the mandible resulting from external megavoltage radiation therapy. *Radiology* 112:685–689, 1974.
111. Murray C.G., Herson J., Daley T.E., et al.: Radiation necrosis of the mandible: A 10 year study. Part I. Factors influencing the onset of necrosis. *Int. J. Radiat. Oncol. Biol. Phys.* 6:543–548, 1980.
112. Morrish R.B., Chan E., Silverman S., et al.: Osteonecrosis in patients irradiated for head and neck carcinoma. *Cancer* 47:1980–1983, 1981.

8 / Chemotherapy in the Treatment of Head and Neck Cancer

MARTIN M. OKEN, M.D.

WHAT ARE THE GENERAL PRINCIPLES OF CHEMOTHERAPY?

CHEMOTHERAPY for head and neck cancer differs in two fundamental respects from regional treatment by surgery and radiotherapy. First, chemotherapy reaches tumor cells throughout the body. Second, it can be administered in widely varying treatment schedules ranging from a brief single treatment course to extended treatment programs that may exceed a year in duration. While cumulative toxicity is dose-limiting for some drugs such as bleomycin and Adriamycin, in general, chemotherapy may be administered repeatedly for as long as it is effective and needed.

The goal of chemotherapy is to eliminate as many cancer cells as possible by selectively killing them with drugs while sparing normal tissues. Although the specificity of chemotherapeutic agents for cancer cells does not yet approach that of antibiotics for most bacterial pathogens, several drugs currently available for head and neck cancer are capable of killing tumor cells at pharmacologic dose levels that are reasonably well tolerated by the patient. A central concept underlying most chemotherapy is the cell kill hypothesis.[1] This includes the following principles: (1) a single cancer cell can multiply and eventually kill the host; (2) survival and ability to respond to chemotherapy are inversely related to the numbers of viable tumor cells; (3) generally a direct relationship exists between the dose of a drug and its ability to kill tumor cells; and (4) a given dose of drug will kill a constant fraction of tumor cells regardless of the number present prior to therapy. These principles imply that cytotoxic chemotherapy is likely to be most effective in eradicating tumor cells when given at the maximum tolerated dose and when administered while the tumor is still relatively small. Tumor cells with persistent resistance to chemotherapy appear to develop through somatic mutation in direct proportion to tumor cell number.[2] Furthermore, tumor growth follows Gompertzian kinetics so that the initial exponential growth is gradually replaced by an exponential retardation of growth as the overall tumor burden increases. These principles are consistent with the concept that sensitivity to chemotherapy varies inversely with tumor burden.

WHAT PROGNOSTIC FACTORS SHOULD BE CONSIDERED IN PLANNING CHEMOTHERAPY?

Several prognostic factors are recognized to have an effect on the response to chemotherapy for squamous cell head and neck cancer. The performance status and nutritional state of the patient are particularly important. Bedridden or malnourished patients, particularly those exhibiting marked weight loss, are frequently unable to tolerate chemotherapy. Furthermore, they are less likely to have tumor regression. Attention should be given to maintaining adequate nutrition before and throughout chemotherapy in order to minimize toxicity and to permit the administration of an adequate course of treatment (see Chap. 11). It is not clear, however, whether intensive nutritional programs involving hyperalimentation can produce further improvement in response rates. The importance of tumor burden has already been mentioned. Patients with bulky primary tumors or tumors with extensive lymph node spread and patients with advanced stage IV disease, particularly those with widespread visceral metastases, are less likely to derive sustained benefit from chemotherapy than are patients with smaller primary lesions and less extensive lymph node involvement.

Several studies have shown that tumor site might affect results with a given regimen. For example, in a recent controlled study of adjuvant chemotherapy in stage III and IV regional head and neck cancer, patients with hypopharyngeal cancer experienced significantly longer survival than those with oral cavity lesions.[3] In contrast, another study reviewed the results of methotrexate therapy for advanced head and neck cancer and found that patients with oral and oropharyngeal tumors had the highest response rates.[4] Although a consistent pattern is not yet apparent, it is important to stratify patient entry to ensure a balanced distribution of patients by tumor site in each of the treatment arms when clinical trials are designed to compare two or more regimens.

The degree of tumor differentiation may also be an important factor but requires further definition. Here the effect is likely to be greater on survival time than on response rate.

One of the most important prognostic variables is

prior treatment status. Prior radiation therapy appears to lower the response rates to chemotherapy by 20%–30%. This may relate in part to an impaired blood supply in the previously irradiated tumor. Patients who have had prior chemotherapy also have markedly reduced tumor response rates to subsequent chemotherapy, largely due to primary and acquired resistance to the drugs.

Other treatment considerations are important. The effects of chemotherapeutic agents are profoundly influenced by the functional status of the kidneys, liver, bone marrow, heart, and lungs. The ability of these systems to metabolize, excrete, and withstand the toxic effects of chemotherapeutic drugs must be carefully considered in arriving at a therapeutic strategy for each individual. Another important factor is the motivation and compliance of the patient. Many chemotherapeutic regimens are complex, and most require considerable cooperation and active participation by the patient. Inability to cooperate can be a critical contraindication to chemotherapy.

HOW IS RESPONSE TO CHEMOTHERAPY EVALUATED?

In patients with measurable tumor at the start of chemotherapy, response is measured by the degree of regression of the tumor. Clinically and pathologically documented disappearance of all detectable cancer represents a *complete response*. If a complete response is observed but is not confirmed by rebiopsy it is sometimes useful to qualify it as a *clinical complete response*. A decrease by at least 50% in the sum of the products of the long diameter and its perpendicular for each lesion represents a *partial response* if there is some residual tumor but no area of a local increase or the appearance of a new tumor mass. A 50% increase in the tumor or the development of new areas of disease represents objective *disease progression*. It is useful to specify response for the primary tumor, lymph nodes, and distant metastases as well as the overall response. It must be appreciated that objective response can be very difficult to evaluate when there is edema or induration in tissues in regions that have been previously irradiated or operated upon. In some patients a CT scan will be more objective than physical examination in gauging the degree of response. A careful evaluation of the response status is critical for making a decision to continue a regimen, to alter the treatment, or to discontinue it.

WHAT ARE THE CURRENT STRATEGIES INCORPORATING CHEMOTHERAPY?

The only *established* use of chemotherapy in squamous cell head and neck cancer is for the palliative treatment of metastatic or recurrent disease (Table 8–1). Objective responses can be obtained in up to 60% of patients with palliative treatment. Both complete and partial responses are likely to relieve symptoms and improve the patient's quality of life until relapse occurs. With the most effective currently available regimens, complete responses can be obtained in 15%–20% of patients. These appear to be the only responses associated with a demonstrable improvement in survival.

A more novel approach for the use of chemotherapy is to include it as part of a multimodality program directed at cure of local or regional disease (see Table 8–1). Such programs must still be considered experimental. Combined multimodal treatment of squamous carcinoma may hold considerable promise for the next likely advances in the treatment of head and neck cancer as it has in childhood rhabdomyosarcoma (see Chap. 24). The three main multimodal strategies utilizing chemotherapy for head and neck squamous cell cancer are listed in Table 8–1. Each is based on a different biologic concept. Advanced local-regional head and neck cancer has a high rate of local or distant recurrence. Chemotherapy administered prior to surgery can reduce the gross tumor mass and technically facilitate the surgery. Reduction of the tumor size may also make it more susceptible to irradiation. Theoretically, chemotherapy could diminish the amount of viable but hypoxic tumor and alter the growth kinetics.

When certain agents are administered simultaneously with radiation therapy, they act as radiosensitizers by increasing radiation-induced ionizations in hypoxic tumor tissue that is otherwise radioresistant. Some chemotherapeutic agents may inhibit DNA repair in sublethally irradiated cancer cells. The intent of most current radiosensitization regimens is to improve the

TABLE 8–1.—STRATEGIES FOR THE USE OF CHEMOTHERAPY IN HEAD AND NECK CANCER

Palliative
For recurrent regional disease
For metastatic disease
Primary multimodal treatment for cure or long-term disease control
Chemotherapy prior to surgery or radiation therapy to reduce tumor burden
Chemotherapy simultaneous with radiotherapy as a radiosensitizer
Postoperative adjuvant chemotherapy

regional control obtained by radiation of unresectable lesions.

The multimodality approach utilizing adjuvant postoperative or postirradiation chemotherapy is directed mainly at the cure of clinically undetected micrometastases that might be present at the time of local therapy. It is postulated that the micrometastases may be considerably more sensitive to chemotherapy immediately after regional therapy, when they are small and cryptic, rather than later, when they have grown to clinically detectable size.[5]

WHAT MAJOR CHEMOTHERAPEUTIC AGENTS ARE USED FOR THE TREATMENT OF HEAD AND NECK CANCER?

The major drugs used to treat squamous cell head and neck cancer are methotrexate, cisplatin, bleomycin, and 5-fluorouracil (5-FU). For certain nonsquamous cancers Adriamycin is used. The role of other drugs, including cyclophosphamide, hydroxyurea, vincristine, vinblastine, and mitomycin C, remains more uncertain.

Methotrexate

Methotrexate has been more extensively studied than any other chemotherapeutic agent in head and neck cancer. It inhibits dihydrofolate reductase, thereby interfering with thymidine production. Ultimately DNA synthesis is altered. Methotrexate is usually administered IV or IM at 40–60 mgm/m^2/week. When used as part of combination chemotherapy regimens, it is given at less frequent intervals. Although methotrexate can be given orally, this route has not been extensively utilized in head and neck cancer. Response rates of 30% are regularly observed with methotrexate in series of patients with metastatic disease or tumor recurrence following surgery and/or radiotherapy. The effectiveness of methotrexate in head and neck cancer has *not* been appreciably improved by using high-dose protocols with leucovorin rescue[6, 7] or by using intra-arterial infusion. The major dose-limiting toxicities of standard-dose methotrexate are stomatitis and myelosuppression with neutropenia, thrombocytopenia, and megaloblastic anemia. Methotrexate is principally excreted in its active form in the urine during the first 12 hours after administration. Therefore, when patients have impaired renal function, methotrexate should be avoided or used at reduced dosage.

Cisplatin

Cisplatin is a heavy metal coordination compound. It is the only inorganic compound currently used for the chemotherapy of head and neck cancer. It binds to DNA, forming intrastrand and interstrand crosslinks which may be related to its clinical activity. The level of cytotoxic activity in head and neck cancers is comparable to that obtained with methotrexate. Single-dose cisplatin is administered IV at 50–120 mg/m^2 every 3–4 weeks. Five-day divided dose regimens have also been utilized. The drug is often given by bolus injection but may be administered by infusions ranging in duration from 15 minutes to 1 more more days. Cisplatin causes no mucositis but it does produce mild myelosuppression. Problems with nausea and vomiting, nephrotoxicity, hypomagnesemia, and ototoxicity can be severe. Regimens utilizing metoclopramide, dexamethasone, haloperidol, or droperidol have been developed to help control cisplatin-induced vomiting. Cisplatin should be avoided in patients with a creatinine clearance rate less than 50 ml/min. At cisplatin doses above 40 mg/m^2, the risk of nephrotoxicity can be effectively countered with vigorous hydration supplemented with diuresis using mannitol, furosemide, or both. Several effective schedules have been published for the prevention of cisplatin nephrotoxicity.[8–10] In one regimen particularly designed for outpatient therapy cisplatin is administered as an IV bolus 30 minutes after starting a 2-hour infusion of 2 L of 5% dextrose in 0.45% sodium chloride containing 10 mEq KCl/L. Furosemide, 40 mg, is given IV at the start of the infusion, followed by 12.5 gm of mannitol as an IV bolus immediately prior to the cisplatin.[8] Adequate hydration must be maintained through the 24-hour period preceding cisplatin administration. Nephrotoxic drugs such as aminoglycoside antibiotics should be avoided.

Bleomycin

Bleomycin is actually a mixture of bleomycin peptides derived from *Streptomyces verticillus*. It is an antitumor antibiotic that results in DNA strand sission. The effectiveness of bleomycin in head and neck cancer appears to be less than that of methotrexate or cisplatin. Bleomycin yields a 15%–20% incidence of brief objective response in most clinical trials. This drug exhibits very little myelotoxicity and is therefore quite suitable for incorporation into combination chemotherapy programs. The usual doses of bleomycin range from 5 to 15 units/m^2 administered IM or IV every 1–3 weeks. It may also be administered as a constant IV infusion over 5–7 days at doses of 10–15 units/m^2/24 hours. Bleomycin causes fever in some patients. Cumulative dose-related mucocutaneous toxicity does occur. *The major dose-limiting toxicity of bleomycin is pulmonary fibrosis.* To minimize the incidence of this potentially lethal toxicity, cumulative doses of 200 units/m^2 should not be exceeded. Furthermore, the drug should be avoided in patients who have severe preexisting compromise of pulmonary function.

5-Fluorouracil

This pyrimidine antimetabolite causes thymidylate synthetase inhibition. Through this mechanism it blocks DNA synthesis. Although 5-FU is frequently given in courses of 500 mg/m^2 bolus for other nonsquamous cell solid tumors, the most promising mode of administration of 5-FU in squamous cell head and neck cancer is as a 120-hour continuous IV infusion of 1,000 mg/m^2/day (see Table 8–4). It is usually combined with cisplatin in chemotherapy cycles that are repeated every 3 weeks. The main toxicities of 5-FU are mucocutaneous (especially stomatitis and diarrhea) and myelotoxicity. The bone marrow suppression appears to be less severe when 5-FU is administered by continuous infusion than when it is given by IV bolus.[11]

Adriamycin

The main role for Adriamycin in head and neck cancer appears to be in the treatment of nonsquamous cell cancer. Cancers most commonly treated include salivary gland carcinomas and esthesioneuroblastomas.

WHAT IS THE ROLE OF PALLIATIVE CHEMOTHERAPY FOR RECURRENT OR METASTATIC HEAD AND NECK CANCER?

We do not presently have the means to cure either recurrent or metastatic squamous head and neck cancer with chemotherapy. The goal of chemotherapy in these patients is palliation. In the small proportion who achieve a complete response there appears to be some prolongation of life. The proper use of chemotherapy in patients with recurrent or metastatic cancer requires that the care team keep the limitations and goals of chemotherapy clearly in focus. The benefits of chemotherapy must be continually weighed against the risks and toxicities that are encountered. If the treatment is without a net palliative benefit, therapy should be discontinued. In most patients with metastatic head and neck cancer or with recurrent tumor that is not potentially curable with surgery or radiotherapy, a trial of chemotherapy is indicated. A decision for a palliative attempt must take into consideration the various contraindications to chemotherapy such as severe malnutrition, renal or hepatic failure, unresolved infection, and inability of the patient to comply with the regimen.

Almost all currently used chemotherapy programs for squamous cell head and neck cancer include methotrexate, cisplatin, or both. Several of the more prominent multidrug regimens are listed in Table 8–2. Treatment results such as response rates and survivals are purposely omitted from Table 8–2 since the studies that are quoted are uncontrolled and represent varying patient populations. The main value of these studies is to establish general efficacy and toxicity for the regimens. Several subsequent randomized protocols have com-

TABLE 8–2.—CHEMOTHERAPY REGIMENS FOR RECURRENT SQUAMOUS HEAD AND NECK CANCERS

STUDY, YEAR	CHEMOTHERAPY REGIMEN	
	Regimens Containing Cisplatin (DDP)	
Vogl and Kaplan,[8] 1979	**MBD:**	3-week cycles
	Methotrexate	40 mg/m^2 IM, days 1, 15
	Bleomycin	10 units IM, days 1, 8, 15
	Cisplatin (DDP)	50 mg/m^2 IV, day 4
Amer et al.,[12] 1980	**COB:**	3-week cycles
	Cisplatin (DDP)	100 mg/m^2 IV, day 1
	Vincristine (Oncovin)	1 mg IV, days 1, 5
	Bleomycin	30 units/24 hr IV infusion × 4 days (d 2–5)
Perry et al.,[13] 1982	**VBP:**	3-week cycles
	Vinblastine	4 mg/m^2 IV, day 1
	Bleomycin	15 units IM, days 1–7
	Cisplatin (DDP)	60 mg/m^2 IV, day 8
Kish et al.,[14] 1984	**DF:**	3-week cycles
	Cisplatin (DDP)	100 mg/m^2 IV, day 1
	5-FU	1,000 mg/m^2/24 hr/IV infusion × 4 days (d 1–4)
	Regimens Not Including Cisplatin (DDP)	
Cortes et al.,[15] 1981	**Bleo-CMF:**	3-week cycles
	Bleomycin	15 units/24 hr IV infusion, days 1–3
	Cyclophosphamide	500 mg IV, day 5
	Methotrexate	50 mg IV, day 5
	5-FU	500 mg IV, day 5
Pitman et al.,[16] 1983	**MTX/5-FU:**	1-week cycles
	Methotrexate	250 mg/m^2 IV, day 1 (followed at 24 hr by leucovorin, 10 mg/m^2 IV, then 10 mg/m^2 PO q. 6h × 5)
	5-FU	600 mg/m^2 IV, day 1 (1 hr after MTX)

pared alternative regimens for the treatment of advanced squamous cell head and neck cancer (Tables 8–3 and 8–4). It is these prospective, controlled studies that are emphasized in this discussion.

Methotrexate, 40 mg/m^2 IV weekly (with dose escalations as tolerated to weekly doses as high as 60 mg/m^2 IV), represents the current standard of palliative single agent chemotherapy for squamous head and neck cancer. Response rates of 25%–35% are consistently obtained with relatively mild toxicity. However, complete responses are infrequent and the response duration is usually only 3–4 months. A randomized study showed that cisplatin (50 mg/m^2 IV on days 1 and 8 of each 28-day cycle) was comparably effective but less well tolerated than methotrexate. The cisplatin produced more nausea, vomiting, and anorexia.[18] Other single-agent regimens utilizing bleomycin, hydroxyurea, vinca alkyloids, or 5-FU appear considerably less effective than methotrexate, although controlled comparisons have not been reported.

In order to improve response rates and to delay the emergence of resistance, many combined active drug regimens have been developed (see Table 8–2). Theoretically, the use of multiple active drugs in a single treatment regimen should attack different malignant cell components at different phases of the cell replication cycle. It is hoped this would counter the problem imposed by tumor heterogeneity when multiple cell populations within a given carcinoma have varying sensitivity profiles to chemotherapeutic agents. The regimens in Table 8–2 are generally reported to produce response rates of 40%–55% in patients with recurrent disease (but no prior chemotherapy). Previously untreated patients with advanced regional disease have 70%–90% response rates with the same regimens. While these results of pilot studies are encouraging, the regimens must be tested against less toxic single-agent therapy in randomized prospective trials before they can be accepted as clearly superior. Five studies outlined in Tables 8–3 and 8–4 performed this type of controlled comparison.

An Eastern Cooperative Oncology Group (ECOG) study compared weekly standard-dose methotrexate to higher-dose methotrexate with leucovorin rescue with

TABLE 8–3.—RANDOMIZED COMPARISONS OF ALTERNATIVE CHEMOTHERAPY REGIMENS FOR THE TREATMENT OF RECURRENT SQUAMOUS HEAD AND NECK CANCER

			RESPONSE (%)		MEDIAN DURATION (MO.)	
STUDY	REGIMEN	N*	CR	CR + PR	Response	Survival
Hong et al.[18]	Methotrexate, 40 mg/m^2 IV weekly (escalate to max. 60 mg/m^2)	17	0	24	2.8	6.1
	vs.					
	Cisplatin, 50 mg/m^2 IV d 1, 8, q4w	21	5	29	3.1	6.3
Jacobs et al.[19]	Cisplatin, 80 mg/m^2 IV 24-hr infusion q3w	40	8	18	7.6	6.3
	vs.					
	Cisplatin, 80 mg/m^2 IV 24-hr infusion q3w Methotrexate, 250 mg/m^2 IV 30-min infusion prior to cisplatin; followed at 24 hr with leucovorin	39	15	33	4.4	6.9
Vogl et al.[20]	Methotrexate, 40 mg/m^2 IV weekly (escalate to max. 60 mg/m^2)	83	8	35	5.0	5.3
	vs.					
	Methotrexate, 40 mg/m^2 IM d 1, 15 Bleomycin, 10 units IM d 1, 8, 15 Cisplatin, 50 mg/m^2 IV d 4 } q3w	80	16	48	5.8	5.9
Williams et al.[21]	Methotrexate, 45 mg/m^2 IV weekly (escalate to max. 60 mg/m^2)	68	. . .	16	4.7	6.4
	vs.					
	Cisplatin, 60 mg/m^2 IV, d 1 Vinblastine, 0.1 mg/kg IV, d 1, 15 Bleomycin, 15 units IV, d 1, 8, 15, 22 } q4w	66	. . .	20	3.6	5.1
Drelichman et al.[22]	Methotrexate, 40 mg/m^2 IV weekly	24	8	33	. . .	5.3
	vs.					
	Cisplatin, 100 mg/m^2 IV d 1 Vincristine, 1 mg IV d 1, 5 Bleomycin, 30 units IV 24-hr infusion × 4 d (d 2–5) } q3w	27	11	41	. . .	3.8

*N, number of evaluable patients.

TABLE 8–4.—RANDOMIZED PROTOCOLS ADDRESSING QUESTIONS OF DOSE AND SCHEDULE IN THE CHEMOTHERAPY OF SQUAMOUS HEAD AND NECK CANCER

STUDY	REGIMEN	N*	RESPONSE (%) CR	RESPONSE (%) CR + PR	MEDIAN RESPONSE DURATION (MO.)
DeConti and Schoenfeld[6]	Methotrexate, 40 mg/m^2 IV qw (escalate to toxicity)	77	8	27	3.5
	vs.				
	Methotrexate, 240 mg/m^2 IV q2w + leucovorin† at 42 hr	74	3	26	1.4
	vs.				
	Methotrexate, 240 mg/m^2 IV q2w + leucovorin† at 42 hr Cyclophosphamide, 0.5 gm/m^2 IV immediately before each MTX Ara-C, 300 mg/m^2 IV over 15 min after each MTX	71	3	20	1.6
Browman et al.[17]	Methotrexate, 200 mg/m^2 IV + leucovorin‡ at 24 hr, d 1, 8 5-FU, 600 mg/m^2 IV just before MTX, q3w *(simultaneous)*	42	12	62	. . .
	vs.				
	Methotrexate, 200 mg/m^2 IV + leucovorin‡ at 24 hr, d 1, 8 5-FU, 600 mg/m^2 IV 1 hour after MTX, q3w *(sequential)*	37	5	38	. . .
Coates et al.[23]	Methotrexate, 250 mg/m^2 IV + leucovorin§ at 24 hr 5-FU, 600 mg/m^2 IV 1 hr after MTX } Each week	35	11	51	. . .
	vs.				
	5-FU, 600 mg/m^2 IV Methotrexate, 250 mg/m^2 IV 1 hr after 5-FU + leucovorin§ at 24 hr Each week	35	6	40	. . .
Kish et al.[11]	Cisplatin, 100 mg/m^2 IV day 1 5-FU, 1,000 mg/m^2 24-hr IV infusion × 4 days, (d 1–4) } q3w	17	24	76	. . .
	vs.				
	Cisplatin, 100 mg/m^2 IV day 1 5-FU, 600 mg/m^2 IV bolus day 1 and day 8 } q3w	20	15	20	. . .

*N, number of evaluable patients.
†Leucovorin, 25 mg PO q6h × 8, starting 42 hours after MTX.
‡Leucovorin, 10 mg/m^2 PO q6h × 6, starting 24 hours after MTX.
§Leucovorin, 15 mg PO q6h × 8, starting 24 hours after MTX.

or without added cyclophosphamide plus Ara-C[6]). That study found no advantage for either the high-dose methotrexate alone or the combination regimen (see Table 8–4). When a similar high dose of methotrexate was added to cisplatin it did not significantly improve either the response rate ($P = 0.11$) or survival over that obtained with cisplatin alone. However, there was a trend toward an increased CR rate with the 2-drug regimen.[19]

Combinations of vincristine or vinblastine with bleomycin and cisplatin were originally reported to yield response rates approaching 50% in recurrent disease.[12, 13] Two randomized trials have compared COB or a vinblastine, cisplatin, bleomycin combination standard weekly methotrexate. These studies failed to show any increased efficacy for the combination regimens (see Table 8–3).[21, 22]

Only the recent ECOG study reported by Vogl and co-workers appears to demonstrate modest benefit for the combination regimen over methotrexate alone.[20] In that 163 patient study, patients treated with weekly methotrexate had a 35% response rate (8% CR) compared with 48% responses (16% CR) for patients treated with a methotrexate, bleomycin, platinum (MBD) regimen ($P = .04$) (see Table 8–3). The median duration of CR was nearly 8 months and was similar for the two therapies, as was average survival time. The degree of toxicity was similar between the 2 arms except for the frequency of cisplatin-induced vomiting. It would appear that the MBD regimen is more likely than methotrexate alone to provide several months of palliation to patients with recurrent or metastatic squamous head and neck cancer. MBD is a reasonable combination drug choice for patients who have adequate renal function, who can tolerate the cisplatin hydration, and who are not overly troubled by the cisplatin-induced nausea and vomiting. Earlier results with longer follow-up suggest that patients who achieve CR may have some survival benefit as well.[8, 24]

Two other regimens that have not yet undergone randomized comparison to standard therapy do have some unique properties that merit discussion. The sequential administration of methotrexate followed by 5-FU appears to be synergistic based on studies utilizing *in vitro* and in vivo animal tumor models. A treatment program based on this sequence was reported by Pitman and co-workers to yield a 65% response rate in 23 patients with recurrent head and neck cancer.[16] Their results were corroborated by a second group using the same regimen.[25] In addition to its possible pharmacologic significance, the methotrexate/5-FU regimen is of interest because it achieved exceptional response rates without employing cisplatin. However, two recently reported randomized studies cast doubt on the clinical significance of the sequential administration of the 2 agents (see Table 8–4). In one study patients were randomized to receive 5-FU simultaneously with methotrexate or to receive 5-FU 1 hour after methotrexate as in the Pitman regimen.[17] With 79 evaluable patients the response rate was actually higher with the simultaneous administration schedule than in the sequential one ($P < .06$). The trend was similar in patients with or without prior therapy. In a second study similar response rates and survivals resulted whether the methotrexate preceded or followed the 5-FU by 1 hour.[23] However, the response rates in both studies were higher than those usually obtained with methotrexate alone. These results suggest that further investigation of the methotrexate, 5-FU combination might be worthwhile.

The combination of high dose cisplatin coupled with 4- or 5-day IV infusion of 5-FU appears more promising.[14] In a preliminary uncontrolled study of this regimen in 30 patients with recurrent disease, 27% obtained CR while the total response rate (CR + PR) was 90%. The rarity of severe myelotoxicity and absence of severe nephrotoxicity was striking. When cisplatin plus infusion 5-FU was compared to cisplatin plus bolus 5-FU the results strikingly favored the infusion regimen (see Table 8–4).[11] Cisplatin/5-FU has never been compared to a standard regimen in a randomized trial. Therefore, an ECOG study has been proposed to compare cisplatin/5-FU to the MBD regimen.[8]

At the present time MBD or cisplatin/5-FU appear to represent effective and well tolerated palliative therapy for recurrent squamous head and neck cancer. Weekly IV methotrexate is a reasonable compromise offering palliation to about 30% of patients. No current palliative regimen has been demonstrated to consistently improve survival but further studies with the cisplatin/5-FU regimen are awaited.

WHAT CHEMOTHERAPY IS AVAILABLE FOR NONSQUAMOUS CELL CANCERS OF THE HEAD AND NECK?

Chemotherapy is actively used for palliative treatment of nonsquamous head and neck cancer. However, because of the relative rarity of these tumors, data are sparse. Undifferentiated head and neck carcinoma and lymphoepithelioma are two variants of squamous cell cancer that can be expected to respond to chemotherapy regimens designed for squamous cell cancer. Lymphoepithelioma is a nasopharyngeal carcinoma with a lymphoid stroma that sometimes appears in its cervical metatases. In one study four of seven patients with lymphoepithelioma treated with the COB or the cisplatin/5-FU regimen (see Table 8–2) showed an objective response that generally exceeded 10 months.[26] In another study of 12 patients with previously untreated lymphoepithelioma treated with a combination of Adriamycin, bleomycin, vinblastine, and dacarbazine (ABVD), 33% had a complete response and another 33% had a partial response.[27]

In a group of 13 patients with advanced salivary gland cancers who received a moderate dose program consisting of 3-weekly cycles in which cyclophosphamide, 450 mg/m^2, and Adriamycin, 45 mg/m^2, were administered on the first day of each week, five patients showed objective responses. The series included patients with adenoid cystic carcinoma, acinic cell tumor, malignant mixed tumor, and adenocarcinoma.[28] The regimen was ineffective in three patients with mucoepidermoid carcinoma, but two of three patients with mucoepidermoid cancer subsequently responded when treated with a combination of methotrexate, bleomycin, and cisplatin. In two other series a complete or partial response was achieved in 13 of 21 patients with various nonsquamous head and neck cancers with regimens containing cyclophosphamide, Adriamycin, and cisplatin.[29, 30] All but two patients in those series had adenocarcinoma, acinic cell carcinoma, adenoid cystic carcinoma, or malignant mixed tumor of the parotid.

Esthesioneuroblastoma is a rare tumor that arises from the olfactory epithelium of the nasal vault. A recent review demonstrated that 8 of 13 patients treated with chemotherapy have responded.[31] A regimen including treatment cycles of cyclophosphamide, 600–1,000 mg/m^2, and vincristine, 2 mg, produced responses of 1 or more years in three patients. The only other durable response was achieved with cyclophosphamide, vincristine, dacarbazine, and Adriamycin.

HOW DO MULTIMODAL PROGRAMS UTILIZE CHEMOTHERAPY FOR SQUAMOUS HEAD AND NECK CANCER?

The main strategies for combining chemotherapy with other treatment modes were discussed earlier (see Table 8–1). It should be reemphasized that even though these approaches are promising, they are still experimental. They should only be employed as part of a research protocol and with the formal, signed informed consent of the patient. Furthermore, their current applications must be limited to selected patients with stage III or IV disease. Based on current data, multimodal chemotherapy should not be given to patients with stage I or II disease.

"PRETREATMENT" CHEMOTHERAPY TO REDUCE TUMOR BULK

This treatment approach, sometimes termed neoadjuvant therapy, has had considerable popularity in recent years for the treatment of regionally advanced squamous head and neck cancer without distant metastases. Regimens such as COB, MBD, DF (see Table 8–2), or a combination of high-dose cisplatin followed by bleomycin infusion are administered for two or three cycles, followed by definitive regional therapy. This can consist of surgery, surgery with postoperative radiotherapy, or radiotherapy alone, depending on the postchemotherapy resectability of the lesion. A dramatic reduction in tumor size is regularly obtained with the chemotherapy that is used in all of these programs. Response rates to the initial chemotherapy regimens range from 70% to 90% in most reports. For many patients, the tumor is converted from clearly unresectable disease to potentially resectable cancers. The surgery is generally well tolerated.[10, 32–35] Unfortunately, as further follow-up has become available for most of these studies, the survival benefits and cure rates appear disappointingly modest, despite the impressive early response rates. For example, in a study of 24 patients treated by Vogl and co-workers with MBD chemotherapy prior to regional treatment, the initial response rate was 77%, but only two patients survived beyond 30 months.[34] Patient compliance can be a substantial problem. Al-Sarraf and co-workers were able to achieve a 55% complete response rate after three cycles of the highly effective DF regimen (see Table 8–2). Approximately half of these patients refused the subsequent planned surgery.[35] Thus, dramatic tumor reduction produces a mirage of cure that lures many patients away from accepting the arduous but necessary surgical or radiotherapeutic step. The prognosis for long-term disease control in these patients is very poor.

Recently a major National Cancer Institute–sponsored multi-institutional study of adjuvant therapy in advanced resectable stage III and IV squamous cancer of the oral cavity, hypopharynx, and larynx was reported. This study included 462 patients who were randomized to one of three groups: standard therapy, induction chemotherapy followed by standard therapy, or induction chemotherapy followed by standard therapy followed by maintenance chemotherapy (Table 8–5).[36] The response rate to the one cycle of induction chemotherapy was 37%. Unfortunately, the 2-year survival was virtually identical for the three regimens, ranging from 56% to 59%. Similarly, there were no significant differences in 2-year disease-free survival. Thus, the major controlled study of neoadjuvant therapy to date reports no survival or disease control benefits. It is conceivable that more aggressive regimens such as multiple cycles of DF chemotherapy will prove more effective in neoadjuvant treatment. To date, no definitive studies to support or reject this hypothesis have been reported. Therefore, despite its initial attractiveness, neoadjuvant therapy cannot yet be recommended as a standard treatment approach to head and neck squamous cell cancer.

CHEMOTHERAPY ADMINISTERED SIMULTANEOUSLY WITH RADIOTHERAPY AS A RADIOSENSITIZER

Irradiation treatment of locally advanced unresectable head and neck squamous carcinoma usually fails because of regional persistence of the cancer. Despite intensive radiotherapy, long-term regional disease control is achieved in less than one third of these patients, and 5-year survivals seldom exceed 15%. In an attempt to improve the effectiveness of radiotherapy in these advanced regional lesions, several different chemotherapy agents have been combined with irradiation. A very large randomized trial of methotrexate combined with radiotherapy versus radiotherapy alone was reported by Fazekas and co-workers.[37] There was no significant survival benefit observed for patients who received simultaneous methotrexate and radiation. The toxicity, particularly mucositis, was increased in this group. Bleomycin has been combined with radiation therapy but does not produce consistently better results than radiation therapy alone. Again, there is an increase in the incidence and severity of mucositis. Hydroxyurea has also been administered with radiation therapy. It has produced conflicting results but no consistent benefit in controlled trials. In one intriguing study 136 patients were randomized to receive radiation therapy alone or radiation therapy with 5-FU. This study, initiated in 1961, utilized a 5-FU regimen of 10 mg/kg/day for the first 3 days of radiation therapy, 5 mg/kg on day 4, and then 5 mg/kg 3 days a week until the end of radiation therapy unless severe local toxicity developed.[38] A 5-year survival of 35% was found in the radiation + 5-FU group, compared with a 15% 5-year survival in those patients who received radiation therapy alone. This result was statistically significant and was attributable to a treatment advantage that was most striking in patients presenting with oral cavity lesions.

In a recent ECOG study[39] cisplatin was administered weekly for the duration of a 7,000-rad course of radiation therapy. The dose of cisplatin was 10 mg/m^2/week in 4 patients, 20 mg/m^2/week in 18 patients, and 30 mg/m^2/week in 13 patients. All patients had stage III or IV unresectable head and neck cancer without distant metastases. Twenty-four of the 35 patients had lymph node involvement, and 16 had T_4 lesions. Eighty-six percent of these patients achieved a complete response on this regimen. Approximately two thirds of all patients have achieved long-term local-regional disease control. Because of this promising pilot study in a group with an unfavorable prognosis, a randomized study of radiotherapy alone versus radiotherapy plus cisplatin has been instituted by the ECOG.

POSTOPERATIVE ADJUVANT CHEMOTHERAPY

As surgical or radiotherapeutic approaches for stage III and IV head and neck cancer have improved local control, the problem of treatment failure due to *distant* metastases has increased. At least 30% of patients with regional control of advanced head and neck cancer ultimately die of distant spread. Since many head and neck cancers respond to chemotherapy, the concept of posttreatment adjuvant chemotherapy is attractive. Can adjuvant chemotherapy cure metastatic deposits of tumor cells while they are still microscopic and clinically undetectable? Unfortunately there are scanty published data from controlled studies to allow one to evaluate this important issue. The major *controlled* study addressing this issue has been the multi-institutional adjuvant study outlined in Table 8–5. Thus far this important and well-conducted study has only been preliminarily reported. It is already clear that the results do not show any survival advantage for those patients who received postoperative maintenance chemotherapy. Further detailed reports from that study will be of interest. An intergroup study to be done by several cooperative groups randomizes patients to three cycles of DF chemotherapy to be administered postoperatively versus no postoperative chemotherapy. This regimen would appear likely to be more active than the chemotherapy administered in the previous multi-institutional trial (see Table 8–5) and could give the concept of adjuvant chemotherapy a more convincing test. At present, however, there is no proved role for adjuvant chemotherapy in head and neck cancer.

REGIONAL CHEMOTHERAPY

Intra-arterial chemotherapy for advanced head and neck cancer has been attempted. The technical difficulties of such treatment approaches are substantial. Severe toxicity and complications have been encountered. Thus far, no clearcut regional disease control or survival advantage has been demonstrated.

SUMMARY

Chemotherapy has a major role in the palliative treatment of advanced recurrent or metastatic head and neck squamous cell cancer. This tumor is moderately sensitive to present-day chemotherapy. Impressive and

TABLE 8–5.—ADJUVANT CHEMOTHERAPY FOR RESECTABLE STAGE III AND IV HEAD AND NECK SQUAMOUS CARCINOMAS: SCHEMA FOR THE NCI-SPONSORED MULTI-INSTITUTIONAL TRIAL*

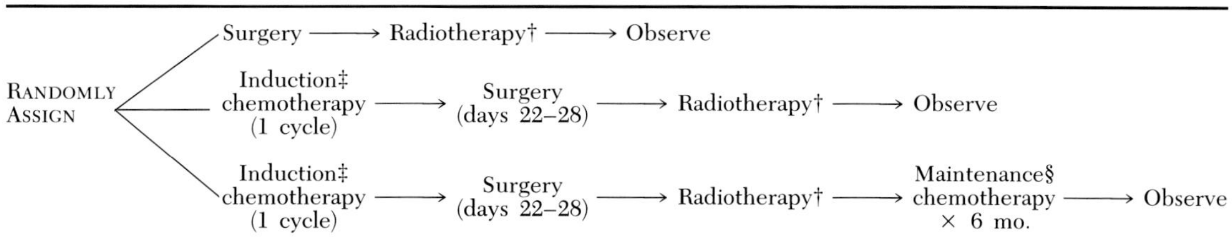

*From Baker et al.[36] Reproduced by permission.
†Radiotherapy given 4–10 weeks after surgery.
‡Induction chemotherapy: cisplatin, 100 mg/m^2 IV bolus on day 1; bleomycin, 15 mg/m^2 IV bolus on day 3, followed by 15 mg/m^2/day for 5 days, continuous infusion on days 3–7.
§Maintenance chemotherapy: cisplatin, 80 mg/m^2 as 24-hour IV infusion, every month for 6 months, starting 4 weeks after radiotherapy.

clinically useful tumor reduction can be obtained in approximately half the patients and can afford 6 months or more of clinical improvement for many afflicted individuals. The use of chemotherapy combined with other treatment modalities is more controversial. Adjuvant chemotherapy is tantalizingly promising and certainly worthy of considerable continued investigation. Unfortunately, it does not yet have a proved role for the treatment of squamous head and neck cancer. Several well-controlled and innovative clinical trials are in progress. In the future, one should be prepared to continuously reassess this question in light of new developments and the results of these systematically and prospectively controlled studies.

Acknowledgment

Work was supported in part by research grant No. CA20365 from the National Institutes of Health.

REFERENCES

1. Skipper H.E., Schnabel F.M., Wilcox W.S.: Experimental evaluation of potential anticancer agents: XII: On the criteria and kinetics associated with "curability" of experimental leukemia. *Cancer Chemother. Rep.* 35:1–111, 1964.
2. DeVita V.T. Jr.: The relationship between tumor mass and resistance to chemotherapy: Implications for surgical adjuvant treatment of cancer. *Cancer* 51:1209–1220, 1983.
3. Jacobs C., Wolf G.T., Makuch R.W., et al.: Adjuvant chemotherapy for head and neck squamous carcinomas. *Proc. Am. Soc. Clin. Oncol.* 3:182, 1984.
4. Bertino J.R., Boston B., Capizzi R.L.: The role of chemotherapy in the management of head and neck cancer: A review. *Cancer* 36:752–758, 1975.
5. Griswold D.P. Jr.: The potential for murine tumor models in surgical adjuvant chemotherapy. *Cancer Chemother. Rep.* 5:187–204, 1975.
6. DeConti R.C., Schoenfeld D.: A randomized prospective comparison of intermittent methotrexate, methotrexate with leucovorin and a methotrexate combination in head and neck cancer. *Cancer* 48:1061–1072, 1981.
7. Vogler W.R., Jacobs J., Moffitt S., et al.: Methotrexate therapy with or without citrovorum factor in carcinoma of the head and neck, breast and colon. *Cancer Clin. Trials* 2:227–236, 1979.
8. Vogl S.E., Kaplan B.H.: Chemotherapy of advanced head and neck cancer with methotrexate, bleomycin, and cis-diamminedichloroplatinum II in an effective outpatient schedule. *Cancer* 44:26–31, 1979
9. Skeel R.T.: Antineoplastic drugs: Classification and clinically useful agents, in Skeel R.T. (ed.): *Manual of Cancer Chemotherapy.* Boston, Little, Brown & Co., 1982, p. 44–45.
10. Decker D.A., Drelichman A., Jacobs J., et al.: Adjuvant chemotherapy with cis-diamminedichloroplatinum II and 120-hour 5-fluorouracil in stage III and IV squamous cell carcinoma of the head and neck. *Cancer* 51:1353–1355, 1983.
11. Kish J., Ensley J., Weaver A., et al.: Superior response rate with 96 hour 5-fluorouracil infusion vs 5-FU bolus combined with cis-platinum in a randomized trial for recurrent and advanced squamous head and neck cancer. *Proc. Am. Soc. Clin. Oncol.* 3:179, 1984.
12. Amer M.H., Izbicki R.M., Vaitkevicius V.K., et al.: Combination chemotherapy with diamminedichloroplatinum, Oncovin, and bleomycin (COB) in advanced head and neck cancer. *Cancer* 45:217–223, 1980.
13. Perry D.J., Weltz M.D., Brown A.W., et al.: Vinblastine, bleomycin and cisplatin for recurrent or metastatic squamous cell carcinoma of the head and neck. *Cancer* 50:2257–2260, 1982.
14. Kish J.A., Weaver A., Jacobs J., et al.: Cisplatin and 5-fluorouracil infusion in patients with recurrent and disseminated epidermoid cancer of the head and neck. *Cancer* 53:1819–1824, 1984.
15. Cortes E.P., Kalra J., Amin V.C., et al.: Chemotherapy for head and neck cancer relapsing after radiotherapy. *Cancer* 47:1966–1970, 1981.
16. Pitman S.W., Kowal C.D., Bertino J.R.: Methotrexate and 5-fluorouracil in sequence in squamous head and neck cancer. *Semin. Oncol.* 10(suppl. 2):15–19, 1983.
17. Browman G.P., Archibald S.D., Young J.E.M., et al.: Prospective randomized trial of one hour sequential versus simultaneous methotrexate plus 5-fluorouracil in advanced and recurrent squamous cell head and neck cancer. *J. Clin. Oncol.* 1:787–792, 1983.
18. Hong W.K., Schaefer S., Issell B., et al.: A prospective randomized trial of methotrexate versus cisplatin in the treatment of recurrent squamous cell carcinoma of the head and neck. *Cancer* 52:206–210, 1983.
19. Jacobs C., Meyers F., Hendrickson C., et al.: A randomized phase III study of cisplatin with or without methotrexate for recurrent squamous cell carcinoma of the head and neck. *Cancer* 52:1563–1569, 1983.
20. Vogl S.E., Schoenfeld D.A., Kaplan B.H., et al.: A randomized prospective comparison of methotrexate with a combination of methotrexate, bleomycin and cis-platinum in head and neck cancer. *Cancer* (in press).
21. Williams S.D., Einhorn L.H., Velez-Garcia E., et al.: Chemotherapy of head and neck cancer: Comparison of cisplatin + vinblastine + bleomycin (PVB) versus methotrexate (MTX). *Proc. Am. Soc. Clin. Oncol.* 1:202, 1982.
22. Drelichman A., Cummings G., Al-Sarraf M.: A randomized trial of the combination of cis-platinum, Oncovin and bleomycin (COB) versus methotrexate in patients with advanced squamous cell carcinoma of the head and neck. *Cancer* 52:399–403, 1983.
23. Coates A.S., Tattersall M.H.N., Swanson C., et al.: Combination therapy with methotrexate and 5-fluorouracil: A prospective randomized clinical trial of order of administration. *J. Clin. Oncol.* 2:756–761, 1984.
24. Chiuten D., Vogl S.E., Kaplan B.H., et al.: Effective outpatient combination chemotherapy of advanced head and neck cancer. *Surg. Gynecol. Obstet.* 151:659–662, 1980.

25. Ringborg U., Ewert G., Kinnman J., et al.: Methotrexate and 5-fluorouracil in head and neck cancer. *Semin. Oncol.* 10(suppl. 2): 20–22, 1983.
26. Decker D.A., Drelichman A., Al-Sarraf M., et al.: Chemotherapy for nasopharyngeal carcinoma: A ten-year experience. *Cancer* 52:602–605, 1983.
27. Galligioni E., Carbone A., Tirelli U., et al.: Combined chemotherapy with doxorubicin, bleomycin, vinblastine, dacarbazine and radiotherapy for advanced lymphoepithelioma. *Cancer Treat. Rep.* 66:1207–1210, 1982.
28. Posner M.R., Ervin T.J., Weichselbaum R.R., et al.: Chemotherapy of advanced salivary gland neoplasms. *Cancer* 50:2261–2264, 1982.
29. Creagan E.T., Woods J.E., Schutt A.J., et al.: Cyclophosphamide, adriamycin and cisdiamminedichloroplatinum (II) in the treatment of advanced nonsquamous cell head and neck cancer. *Cancer* 52:2007–2010, 1983.
30. Alberts D.S., Manning M.R., Coulthard S.W., et al.: Adriamycin/cis-platinum/cyclophosphamide combination chemotherapy for advanced carcinoma of the parotid gland. *Cancer* 47:645–648, 1981.
31. Wade F.M., Smith R.E., Johns M.E.: Response of esthesioneuroblastomas to chemotherapy: Report of 5 cases and review of the literature. *Cancer* 53:1036–1041, 1984.
32. Hong W.K., Shapshay S.M., Bhutani R., et al.: Induction chemotherapy in advanced squamous head and neck carcinoma with high-dose cis-platinum and bleomycin infusion. *Cancer* 44:19–25, 1977.
33. Witter R., Heller K., Randolph V., et al.: *cis*-Dichlorodiammineplatinum(II)-based chemotherapy as initial treatment of advanced head and neck cancer. *Cancer Treat. Rep.* 63:1533–1538, 1979.
34. Vogl S.E., Lerner H., Kaplan B.H., et al.: Failure of effective initial chemotherapy to modify the course of stage IV (M_O) Squamous cancer of the head and neck. *Cancer* 50:840–844, 1982.
35. Al-Sarraf M., Kish J., Ensley J., et al.: Induction cisplatinum and 5-fluorouracil infusion before surgery and/or radiotherapy in patients with locally advanced head and neck cancer: Progress report. *Proc. Am. Assoc. Cancer Res.* 25:196, 1984.
36. Baker S.R., Makuch R.W., Wolf G.T.: Preoperative cisplatin and bleomycin therapy in head and neck squamous carcinoma. *Arch. Otolaryngol.* 107:683–689, 1981.
37. Fazekas J.T., Sommer C., Kramer S.: Adjuvant intravenous methotrexate or definitive radiotherapy alone for advanced squamous cancers of the oral cavity, oropharynx, supraglottic larynx or hypopharynx. *Int. J. Radiat. Oncol. Biol. Phys.* 6:533–541, 1980.
38. Lo T.C.M., Wiley A., Ansfield F.J., et al.: Combined radiation therapy and 5-fluorouracil for advanced squamous cell carcinoma of the oral cavity and oropharynx: A randomized study. *AJR* 126:229–235, 1976.
39. Haselow R.E., Adams G.S., Oken M.M., et al.: Cisplatinum with radiation therapy for locally advanced unresectable head and neck cancer. *Proc. Am. Soc. Clin. Oncol.* 2:160, 1983.

9 / Cervical Lymphatics: Decisions and Variations in Managing Existing or Potential Cervical Lymph Node Metastases

DONALD G. MCQUARRIE, M.D., PH.D. / GEORGE L. ADAMS, M.D. / YASHODA RAO, M.D.

WHY IS CONTROL OF METASTATIC CERVICAL LYMPH NODE DISEASE CRUCIAL IN ACHIEVING CURE OF HEAD AND NECK CANCERS?

FREQUENT UNCONTROLLED cervical node metastases produced most of the failures which were seen in the early efforts to treat head and neck squamous cell cancers.[1] Studies of head and neck cancer deaths show that approximately 25% of uncured patients have recurrence at the primary site. About 50% succumb to invasion and compression from uncontrolled lymphatic or soft tissue spread in the neck. About 25% die with distant metastases.

Typical data comparing site, tumor size, and frequency of metastases are given in Table 9–1. There are three obvious points; some sites metastasize earlier and more frequently; as a squamous cell cancer grows, the likelihood of node metastases increases; and many patients will die of cancer if neck node metastases are ignored.

Crile's pioneering surgical efforts were directed to neck node control.[8] In those patients with proved node metastases, he found that 9 of 12 (75%) in whom his "block" dissection had been done survived for 3 years, compared to 9 of 48 patients (19%) in whom lesser procedures had been done. (Some of the "cured" patients had thyroid cancer.) By the midperiod of therapy (1920–1940), neck dissection was usually done as a second-stage procedure after the primary lesion appeared to be controlled by surgery or radiation. Finally, from 1940 on, composite resections were done as the primary procedure.[9–11] The excellent survival results in Kremen's early series (1956) and the 70% overall 5-year survival (98% NED survival for node negative and 48% NED survival for node positive) in Kremen's 1967 report illustrates the better results achieved with aggressive composite, in-continuity surgical procedures.[12, 13]

For all head and neck sites, survival rates are diminished as the number of nodes containing metastases increases. For example, the data of De La Pava and Pickren, reported in 1967, demonstrated a 74% 3-year survival for composite laryngeal resections with no involved nodes, 60% with one involved node, 25% with two, 28% with three, and less than 12% with more than four nodes positive.[14]

In the final analysis, the neck nodes must be considered in any treatment plan. The mortality from elective neck irradiation and/or neck dissection as an isolated procedure is small (<< 1% in most contemporary series). Disabilities from treatment are not severe if the spinal accessory nerve can be preserved. For the purposes of this chapter, the frequency and lethality of squamous cell cancer make it *the* prominent pathologic entity in disease of the neck lymphatics. As is discussed in chapters 19, 22, and 24, cancer of the thyroid, connective tissue tumors, and melanoma poses special problems.

WHY IS THERE EARLY FREQUENT INVASION OF LYMPHATICS BY SQUAMOUS CELL CANCERS?

In the 7-week human embryo there are five large lymphatic sinuses. The two most prominent are the jugular sacs, which are located lateral to the jugular vein. These sacs begin to proliferate, forming a rich network of channels through the neck and arms. By gestational age 3 months, there are budding segments of channels that form nodular masses. The nodular areas are subsequently populated with lymphocytes. By adulthood, an average unilateral cervical lymphadenectomy that is cleared and carefully studied will yield an average of 50 nodes (20–80 nodes in 88% of cases).[14] After 30 years of age, the number of obtainable lymph nodes decreases.

Primitive lymphatic precursors condense in the pharyngeal region and contribute to the components of Waldeyer's ring. In these areas, even small oropharyngeal cancers have easy access to dense lymphatic channels and the intrinsic ring of tonsillar, adenoidal, and lingual lymphatics in the subepithelial position. The oropharynx differs from the skin because it does not have a dense subepithelial collagen (dermal) barrier between the surface and the numerous lymphat-

TABLE 9–1.—FREQUENCY OF CERVICAL LYMPH NODE METASTASES BY STAGE OF PRIMARY LESION

STUDY, YEAR	NO. OF CASES	SITE	FREQUENCY OF METASTASES TO CERVICAL LYMPHATICS (%)			
			T_1	T_2	T_3	T_4
Mendelson et al.,[2] 1977	667	Alveolar ridge	16	23	13	
		Floor of mouth	26	35	32	
		Tongue	18	33	60	
DeSanto et al.,[3] 1977	265	Supraglottic	39	34	46	71
Razack et al.,[4] 1978	164	Epiglottis	32	50	50	62
Razack et al.,[5] 1978	97	Piriform Sinus	83	93	90	
Joyce and McQuarrie,[6] 1976	178	Oral	30	63	70	62
Wurman et al.,[7] 1975		Lip	5	52	73	

ic channels. The true vocal cords differ because they have no easily detectable subepithelial lymphatic channels (see Chap. 16). Within a centimeter, the hypopharynx and the subglottic area have rich lymphatics.

The frequent forced movements of chewing, swallowing, and speaking probably help propel tumor emboli and lymph. Chewing and deglutition can generate pressures of 50–100 mm Hg. It is not surprising that lymph node metastases are common. If viable cells lodge in the peripheral sinuses of the lymph nodes, they may grow. They then appear to extend by concentric growth. In some cases growth is exuberant and the tumor may break through the capsule into surrounding tissue. Nodes larger than 3 cm usually have broken through the node capsule.

The real question is, why are metastases not universal?—especially when studies such as those by Sandberg and Moore[15] and Watne et al.[16] show how frequently malignant cells can be recovered from the blood without subsequent systemic metastases being seen. Their studies were done on blood samples, but one must assume that lymphoid invasion is equally common. Because of local tissue nutritive factors, tumor cell age, host immunity, or unknown factors, only a few lymphogenous cancer emboli ever establish continued growth.

Some malignancies are not as predictable as squamous cell cancer. Melanomas may spread by both hematogenous and lymphatic routes. Conley observed that when melanomas of the scalp metastasize, the metastases are found in cervical nodes 70% of the time.[17] He also noted that the locus of melanoma spread is unpredictable. Treatment of lymph nodes with cervical mesodermal cancers is less clear cut. Soft tissue tumors spread by direct invasion as well as by hematogenous and lymphatic routes. Some sarcomas never involve regional lymphatics. Thyroid cancer is a special case and will be discussed in chapter 19.

WHAT ARE THE IMPORTANT NODE GROUPS IN THE NECK, AND HOW ARE THEY ARRANGED?

Rouviere in 1938 gave us an excellent description of the lymphatic anatomy of the neck.[18] His concepts seem valid when compared with contemporary clinical data and data obtained by lymphangiography and lymphangioscintigraphy.[19] Taillens suggested useful functional modifications of Rouviere's description.[19] The major groups are shown in Figure 9–1. The cervical nodes can be regarded as first-level target nodes and draining chains.

First-level nodes include (1) the high jugular nodes, which drain the rhinopharynx; (2) the subdigastric-jugular node(s), which drain the posterior mouth, posterior tongue, and tonsillar area; (3) the submandibular nodes, and (4) the submental nodes, which drain the anterior mouth, tongue, and gums. The cervical descending drainage nodes can be regarded as chains in general groups: (1) a jugular chain or triple chain (Taillens chain) on the anterior, posterior, and deep side of the internal jugular vein; (2) the spinal accessory chain; (3) the nuchal chain (shown but not labeled in Fig 9–1); (4) the transverse cervical chain; and (5) the scalene node group. Other significant lymph node groups are shown in Figure 9–2. The retropharyngeal nodes assume importance in nasal and sinus cancers. The nodes in the tracheoesophageal groove are involved in thyroid and hypopharyngeal cancers. There is wide individual variability in node location and lymphatic channel flow. Higher nodes may be bypassed.[20]

Knowledge of the general anatomy allows some insight into what epithelial area might have produced a cryptic metastasis, or which nodes might be involved for a particular primary. Table 9–2, modified from Ballantyne and Jackson,[21] gives some "good bets" as to where a primary lesion might be located when a cervical node is found to be enlarged or involved with cancer. The frequent involvement of first-line nodes high

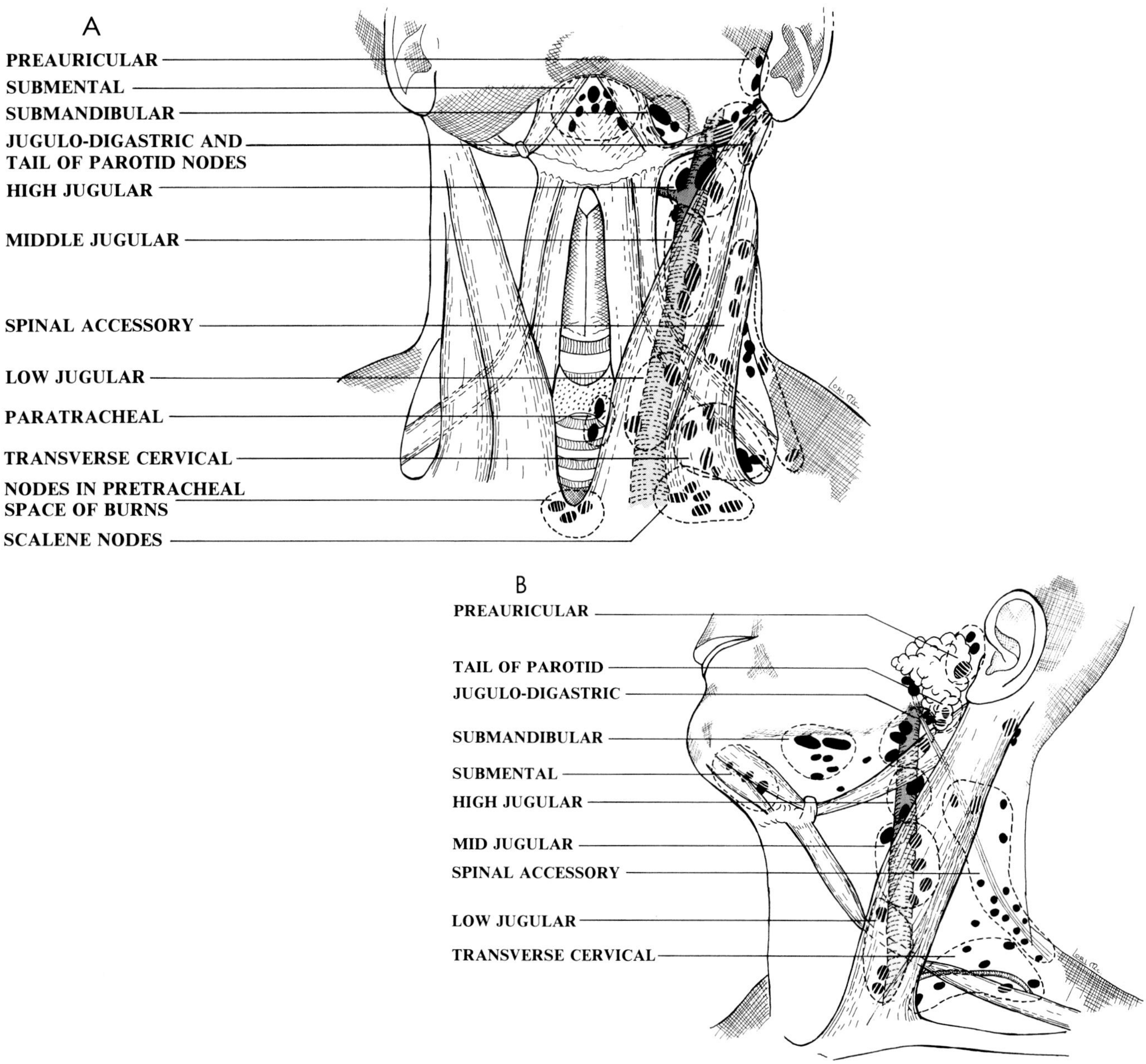

Fig 9–1.—A, major cervical lymph node groups with their approximate location in a frontal view. It should be understood that the node group divisions are quite arbitrary. The nodes are richly interconnected by a slightly directional network of interconnecting lymphatic channels. **B,** side view of the major cervical lymphatic groups. The close relation of the nodes to the superficially located spinal accessory nerve explains the frequency of trapezius muscle paralysis after node biopsy by an unskilled person.

in the jugular and subdigastric area suggests that effective treatment must reach these higher nodes and encompass them. Although discussions generally omit the preauricular nodes and nodes in the pterygoid space, they may be involved by metastases from pharyngeal, parotid, and auricular cancers. In addition, there are nodes in the paratracheal and tracheoesophageal grooves (see Fig 9–2) as well as in the pretracheal space of Burns (between the manubrium and the two layers of the deep cervical fascia; see Fig 1,A). These lower nodes are important thyroid metastatic sites.

HOW DO WE DETERMINE IF CERVICAL LYMPH NODES ARE LIKELY TO BE INVOLVED WITH CANCER?

Table 9–1 relates T staging to the probability of finding metastases in cervical lymph nodes. The probability

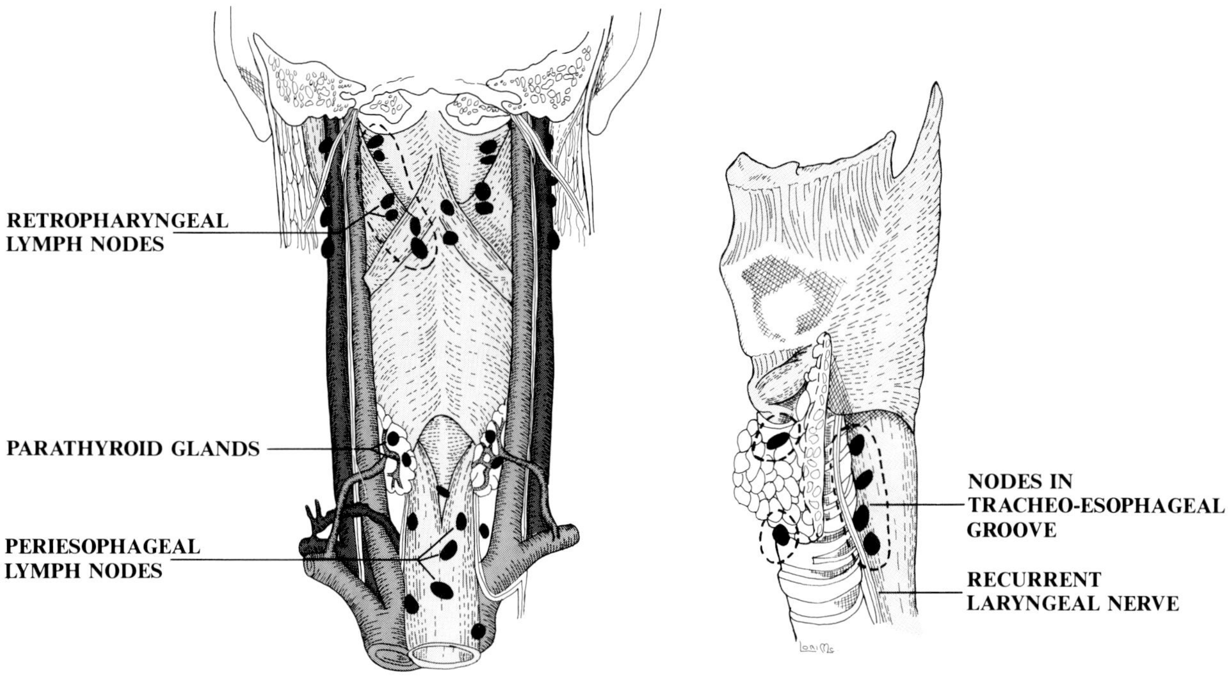

Fig 9–2.—*Left,* posterior view of the pharynx showing the deep retropharyngeal lymph nodes and the lower periesophageal lymph nodes. A left side view showing the nodes in the fat pad around the recurrent laryngeal nerve in the tracheoesophageal groove.

of node metastasis varies with *site* of the primary (5% for T_1 cancer of the lip, vs. 83% for a T_1 piriform sinus cancer) and *size* (when lip lesion grows to a T_3 size, the probability of lymph node metastasis jumps to 73%). *Clinical staging* is a useful guide to prognosis and therapy. Where nodes are large and obvious, clinical staging comes close to matching histologic staging. When metastases are small or located in nodes where fat and overlying tissue obscures findings, staging is reduced to inaccurate palpation and an educated guess. If the guess is wrong and an erroneous decision is made to withhold treatment of the neck, the patient's disease may progress from N_1 to N_3 before detection. In some series this is related to a decrease in 5-year survival of

TABLE 9–2.—PROBABLE LOCATION OF PRIMARY TUMOR ASSOCIATED WITH LYMPH NODE METASTASES

Preauricular (parotid)	Ear, scalp, skin
External maxillary	Lip, nose, skin
Submental	Lip, skin, anterior oral cavity
Submaxillary triangle	Submaxillary gland, oral cavity, skin lip, paranasal sinus
External jugular	Parotid, skin, ear
Suboccipital	Scalp, postauricular skin
Jugulodigastric	Oral cavity, oropharynx, paranasal sinus, nasopharynx, hypopharynx, larynx, parotid
Midjugular	Hypopharynx, larynx, thyroid, oral cavity, oropharynx
Lower jugular	Thyroid, larynx, cervical esophagus
Upper posterior cervical triangle	Nasopharynx occasionally, paranasal sinus, oropharynx, skin, scalp; a metastatic mass high in the neck extending beneath the sternocleidomastoid muscle into the posterior triangle of the neck almost always represents spread from a nasopharyngeal cancer
Prelaryngeal	Larynx, thyroid
Lower supraclavicular	Primary cancer below the clavicles—breast, lung, stomach, pancreas, colon, ovary, cervix, uterus, testis, bladder
Tracheoesophageal	Thyroid, esophagus
Retropharyngeal	Nasopharynx, skin of nose, paranasal sinus
Pterygoid	Buccal mucosal, tonsillar, pharyngeal

as much as 50%. *An erroneous no-treatment decision produces excess deaths in node-positive patients by avoiding low-risk therapy or operations.*

The aversion of some clinicians to treating the neck surgically really comes down to two issues: the functional loss of the trapezius muscle when the spinal accessory nerve is sacrificed, and the change in neck contour (without loss of essential function) when the sternocleidomastoid muscle is taken. The radical neck dissection may have been an impressive tour-de-force in 1908, but it is far from "radical" in the present surgical world. A better term is cervical lymphadenectomy. As the chapter progresses, we will see that the adenectomy has a number of variations. For all variations, mortality is 1% or less. If an eleventh nerve–sparing operation is done, morbidity is minimal. Similar to surgery, elective neck irradiation has a mild morbidity. Early mucosal inflammation and late progressive vascular sclerosis occur. Elective neck irradiation avoids initial tissue loss. The early mortality risk is nil.

In deciding on whether to treat the neck and how to treat it, we must know how well the palpate-and-guess evaluation of nodes compares with actual histologic findings. Table 9–3 gives data comparing palpation-derived clinical staging with actual histology. Other authors have noted a higher false negative rate, in the 20%–30% range,[12, 26] and a false positive rate of 15%–30%.[27] Why should false positives occur at all? Open tumor surfaces with infection, periodontitis, and tooth extractions can all induce benign lymphoid hyperplasia, which can enlarge and firm up a cervical lymph node or two.

Sensitivity and *specificity* are clearer terms for stating diagnostic reliability. Sensitivity denotes the ability of a test or examination to detect proved disease. Specificity denotes the ability of a test or examination to exclude another diagnosis. The two terms are defined and related graphically in Figure 9–3, in which data of three experienced examiners are plotted. The darkly shaded area represents the probable zone of accuracy of good to very good examiners. Other authors' data suggest that the area of error is larger than that shown. The final decision to treat the neck must be made on the basis of (1) the location of the primary, (2) the size of the primary lesion, and (3) previous experience with similar cases in similar locations. Histology of the biopsy specimen may help in an unusual case of a verrucous cancer (less likely to metastasize) or a highly anaplastic piriform sinus cancer (likely to metastasize early). If the nodes are palpable, one should treat the neck and accept the few false positives. If no nodes are palpable and past experience with cancers of similar location, size, and histology suggests that the probability of metastasis exceeds 5%–10%, then one should strongly consider treating the neck. Whether standard lymphadenectomy, a modified lymphadenectomy, or elective neck irradiation is chosen will depend largely on the stage and manner of treatment of the primary cancer. Untreated necks require frequent careful examination.

WHAT DECISION PROBLEMS ARE CAUSED BY POTENTIAL CONTRALATERAL OR BILATERAL LYMPH NODE SPREAD?

Contralateral spread occurs with cancers that approach the midline floor of the mouth, tongue, or the posterior oropharynx. A bulky tumor may not be strictly assignable to one side or the other. There is no firm barrier to lymph flow across the midline, especially if propelled by asymmetric masticatory and swallowing pressures. Table 9–4 summarizes some data on the incidence of contralateral metastases. These studies show that large T_2-T_3 deeply invasive, centrally located lesions of the lip and floor of the mouth as well as cancers of the posterior tongue and pharyngeal arch *do* have a significant (25% of cases) rate of metastasis to the contralateral neck. In making treatment decisions for these specific patients, one should (1) assign a higher risk of contralateral spread to lesions near the midline, (2) extend a higher likelihood of contralateral involvement to larger lesions of the tonsil, posterior tongue, epiglottis, and hypopharynx, (3) know that T_3 lesions are more likely to have crossover, (4) consider treating both sides of the neck in the initial plan for the high-crossover-rate lesions, (5) place incisions to accommodate treatment of

TABLE 9–3.—COMPARISON OF CLINICAL STAGING WITH HISTOLOGIC FINDINGS IN NECK DISSECTIONS

		% DISTRIBUTION TO EACH CATEGORY			
STUDY, YEAR	NO. OF CASES	Clin. Neg., Path. Pos. (False Negative)	Clin. Neg., Path. (True Negative)	Clin. Pos., Path. Pos. (True Positive)	Clin. Pos., Path. Neg. (False Positive)
Beahrs and Barber,[22] 1962	615	8	15	73	4
Mendelson et al.,[23] 1976	340	20	. . .	. . .	. . .
Sako et al.,[24] 1964	235	14	38	34	13
Spiro and Strong,[25] 1973	699	15	41	44	0

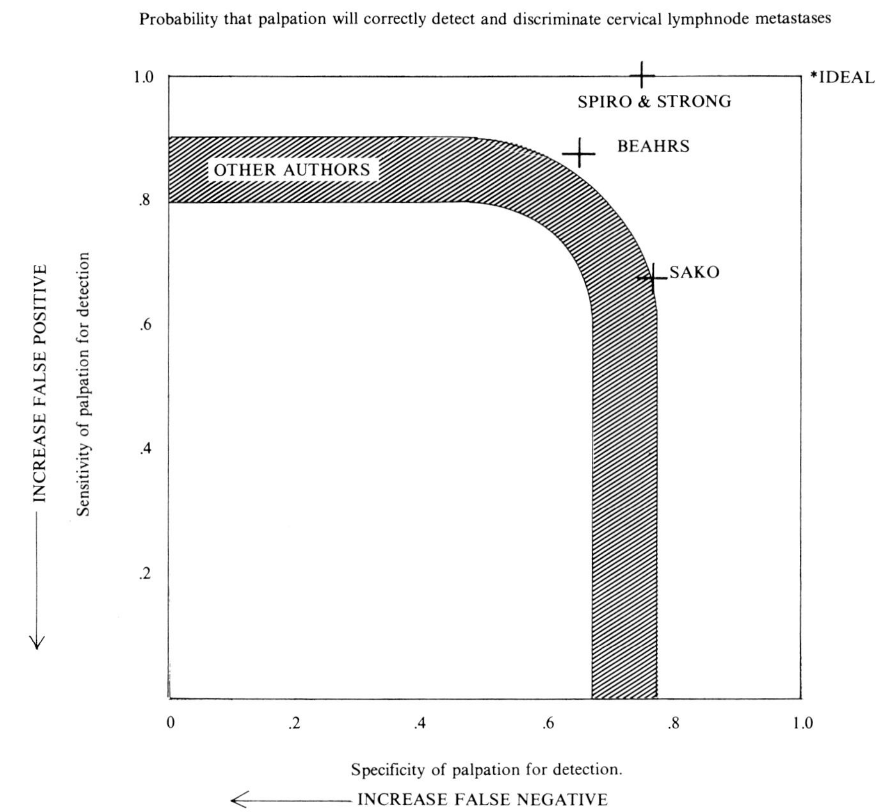

SENSITIVITY - SPECIFICITY

a = Has Disease, test positive

b = Has Disease, test negative

Sensitivity = $\frac{a}{a+b}$ = Ability to detect disease

c = Disease not present, test negative

d = Disease not present, test positive

Specificity = $\frac{c}{c+d}$ = ability to exclude disease

Fig 9–3.—Analysis of specificity and sensitivity of palpation examination of the neck in the detection of metastases.

both sides of the neck, (6) follow-up both sides of the neck rigorously, and (7) know that a contralateral mass is likely a metastasis.

At present, bilateral neck dissection has a low enough risk to warrant applications when indicated. In 17 selected patients with stage T_3 oral lesions and bilaterally positive nodes in whom we did simultaneous bilateral neck dissections, the 5-year tumor-free survival was 65% (data extended 2 years from time of report).[30] We have had no deaths in many additional bilateral neck dissections. Other authors have reported minimal operative mortality for bilateral lymphadenectomy.[2, 31, 32] Techniques and management are discussed later in the chapter.

IN CENTRALLY LOCATED ANTERIOR ORAL LESIONS WHERE METASTASES ARE PROBABLE, WHY NOT DO AN ELECTIVE LYMPHADENECTOMY ON THE DOMINANT SIDE AND A SUPRAHYOID DISSECTION ON THE CONTRALATERAL SIDE AS A STAGING PROCEDURE? IF THE SUPRAHYOID SIDE IS POSITIVE, SHOULD ONE DO A COMPLETE LYMPHADENECTOMY?

A suprahyoid dissection taking the anterior belly of the diagastric and geniohyoid muscles gives good anatomical access to the floor of the mouth. It is *not* useful as a staging procedure to determine if downstream

TABLE 9–4.—INVOLVEMENT OF CONTRALATERAL NECK NODES: INITIAL PATHOLOGIC FINDINGS AND SUBSEQUENT DEVELOPMENT OF NODE METASTASES

STUDY, YEAR	TUMOR LOCATION	NO. OF TOTAL CASES	% WITH CONTRALATERAL METASTASES
McQuarrie et al., 1982	Floor of mouth	99	35*†
McQuarrie et al., 1982	Ant. ⅔ of tongue	50	10
Healy et al.,[27] 1976	Palatine arch	130	13
DeSanto et al.,[3] 1977	Supraglottic	267	18*
Fletcher and Lindberg,[28] 1966	Palate and tonsillar fossa	88	24
Feind and Cole,[29] 1969	Lip	12	25
	Floor of mouth	53	17
	Ant. ⅓ of tongue	21	19
	Mid. ⅓ of tongue	80	4
	Post. ⅓ of tongue	24	25
	Epiglottis	25	28
	Hypopharynx	50	10
	Larynx	96	5
	Palate	12	10

*Combines results of bilateral neck dissection and nodes treated in subsequent procedures.
†40% of tumors were at (within 0.5 cm) or crossing midline.

nodes are involved. This statement is derived from our experience with the last 99 floor of the mouth cancers we treated. A contralateral suprahyoid dissection was done in 52 of the 99 cases (53%). An additional 10 patients (10%) underwent simultaneous bilateral neck dissection. Of the 52 patients in whom a suprahyoid dissection was performed, six had positive nodes, and a second lymphadenectomy or elective neck irradiation was done on that admission; eight (15%) of the node-negative patients in whom a suprahyoid dissection was done subsequently developed deep jugular node metastases on the side where the suprahyoid dissection was done. Only two of these eight patients lived 5 years following salvage procedures. Our experience parallels that of Chu and Strawitz[33] and others.[34, 35] Hidden in our small group is a second lesson. You cannot count on patients to return on schedule for follow-up. Four of our patients knew they had masses and knew that the mass was likely a recurrence. They failed to return for appointments until the cancer registry contacted them.

In summary, if the contralateral neck is palpably negative, but the intelligent estimate of involved nodes exceeds 10%–15% (pick your own cutoff point), there should be strong consideration of an eleventh nerve–sparing simultaneous lymphadenectomy on the contralateral side if the primary and ipsilateral neck are treated surgically. If radiation is the primary therapy, both sides of the neck are staged N_O, and a subsequent lymphadenectomy is not contemplated, then both sides of the neck should receive full therapeutic radiation doses.

WHY TREAT CERVICAL LYMPH NODES ON SUSPICION OF INVOLVEMENT? WHAT IS THE PRICE OF WAITING UNTIL NODES ARE PALPABLE?

Immediately there is a decision error by not detecting involved nodes (see Table 9–3). Deep nodes may progress from N_1 to N_3 status before detection. Some patients do not return for scheduled follow-up. In our patient population, approximately 20% refuse and actively avoid follow-up unless extraordinary efforts are made to trace them via a tumor registry. Salvage procedures after nodes are detected on follow-up palpation are less likely to cure the cancer. Marshall and Edgerton described ten patients with lip cancer who were observed and in whom cervical node metastases subsequently developed. Despite treatment, seven died, even though the primary was controlled.[36] In a large series of 340 patients with tongue cancer, Mendelson et al. found 32 patients who did not have neck dissections but were observed until nodes appeared. Palpable cervical lymph nodes developed in these 32 in the follow-up period. Although they would be expected to have a 50%–60% 5-year survival if they had had an elective node dissection, delay in this group resulted in ten (31%) surviving for 5 years.[23] Other authors have noted a poor survival rate with delayed treatment of cervical nodes that are detected by palpation during follow-up.[37]

WHAT EFFECTIVE TREATMENTS ARE AVAILABLE FOR CONTROL OF EXISTING OR SUSPECTED CERVICAL LYMPH NODE METASTASES?

Several general features are common to most squamous cell cancers. At present, surgery and irradiation are the only two therapies that have a chance of curing neck node metastases from squamous cell cancer. There are different ways to employ these two treatments, alone and in combination. Table 9–5 shows a matrix of 27 possible choices for treatment. If we tried to stratify these decisions by four stages of primary tumor disease, there would be 108 possible treatment groups. At this level of detail, carefully drawn randomized studies testing all possibilities for comparable cancer stages would take centuries to produce evaluable data. Fortunately, accumulated experience has reduced broad differences in some selections for some stages of disease to minimal decision differences. The perspicacious reader can think of specific examples in which one therapy or combination may be a desirable or an undesirable option. In the final analysis, decisions are adjusted for a particular stage at each site, as discussed in the appropriate chapters. Figure 9–4 outlines a general approach. The flowchart is just a beginning algorithm for managing the neck nodes in most oropharyngeal lesions. Treatment of the neck must be coordinated with treatment of the primary lesion.

WHAT ARE THE GUIDELINES FOR STAGING NECK NODES?

Cervical node classification is helpful. The following regional node classification is applicable to all head and neck cancers. In clinical evaluation, the actual size of the nodal mass should be measured and allowance should be made for intervening soft tissues. Masses over 3 cm in diameter do not always represent single nodes, but may be confluent nodes or tumor in soft tissues of the neck.

Clinical staging is good for initial planning. As more information becomes available from operative staging or from a careful pathologic study, further decision-making and ultimate results analysis should be based on the data with higher precision, i.e., pathologic staging. There are three stages of clinically positive nodes: N_1, N_2, and N_3.

The use of subgroups a, b, and c is not required, but is recommended. Midline nodes are considered as homolateral nodes.

N_X—Nodes cannot be assessed.

N_0—No clinically positive node.

N_1—Single clinically positive homolateral node 3 cm or less in diameter.

TABLE 9–5.—MATRIX OF POSSIBLE OPTIONS TO BE CONSIDERED IN TREATING EXISTING OR POTENTIAL NECK NODE METASTASES*

SURGICAL PROCEDURES PROPOSED \ IRRADIATION TREATMENT PROPOSED	Elective Neck Irradiation	Preop. Low-Dose Irradiation	Preop. High-Dose Irradiation	Postop. Irradiation	No Irradiation
Classic lymphadenectomy	S	a	b		R
Lymphadenectomy that spares spinal accessory n. XI	S	a	b		R
Lymphadenectomy that spares n. XI and internal jugular v.	S	a			R
Lymphadenectomy that spares n. XI, IJ, v., and SCM m.	S	a			R
Suprahyoid and/or local node excision	Rare				R
No surgery					

*S, subsequent surgical salvage of radiation failure; *a*, studies to date show minimum effectiveness; *b*, current studies use in combination with chemotherapy; R, radiation treatment of surgical failure.

N_2—Single clinically positive homolateral node more than 3 but less than 6 cm in diameter, or multiple clinically positive homolateral nodes, none more than 6 cm in diameter.

N_{2a}—Single clinically positive homolateral node more than 3 cm but less than 6 cm in diameter.

N_{2b}—Multiple clinically positive homolateral nodes, none more than 6 cm in diameter.

N_3—Massive homolateral node(s), bilateral nodes, or contralateral node(s).

N_{3a}—Clinically positive homolateral node(s), one more than 6 cm in diameter.

N_{3b}—Bilateral clinically positive nodes (in this situation, each side of the neck should be staged separately; that is, N_{3b}: right, N_{2a}; left, N_1).

N_{3c}—Contralateral clinically positive node(s) only.

WHAT THERAPEUTIC SELECTIONS CAN BE MADE IN TREATING CERVICAL NODES?

In selecting therapeutic options, the major objective of cancer cure should be paramount. One should not get lost in illogical pursuit of some trendy technique. Some practical guidelines follow.

1. Some cosmetic loss and functional disability are more desirable than severe cosmetic loss and function disability followed by death. This means that a tissue-conserving procedure should not be done unless there is no degradation of 5-year survival.

2. The lymphadenectomy must be planned and altered to encompass the resection of the primary as well as the likely location of metastases.

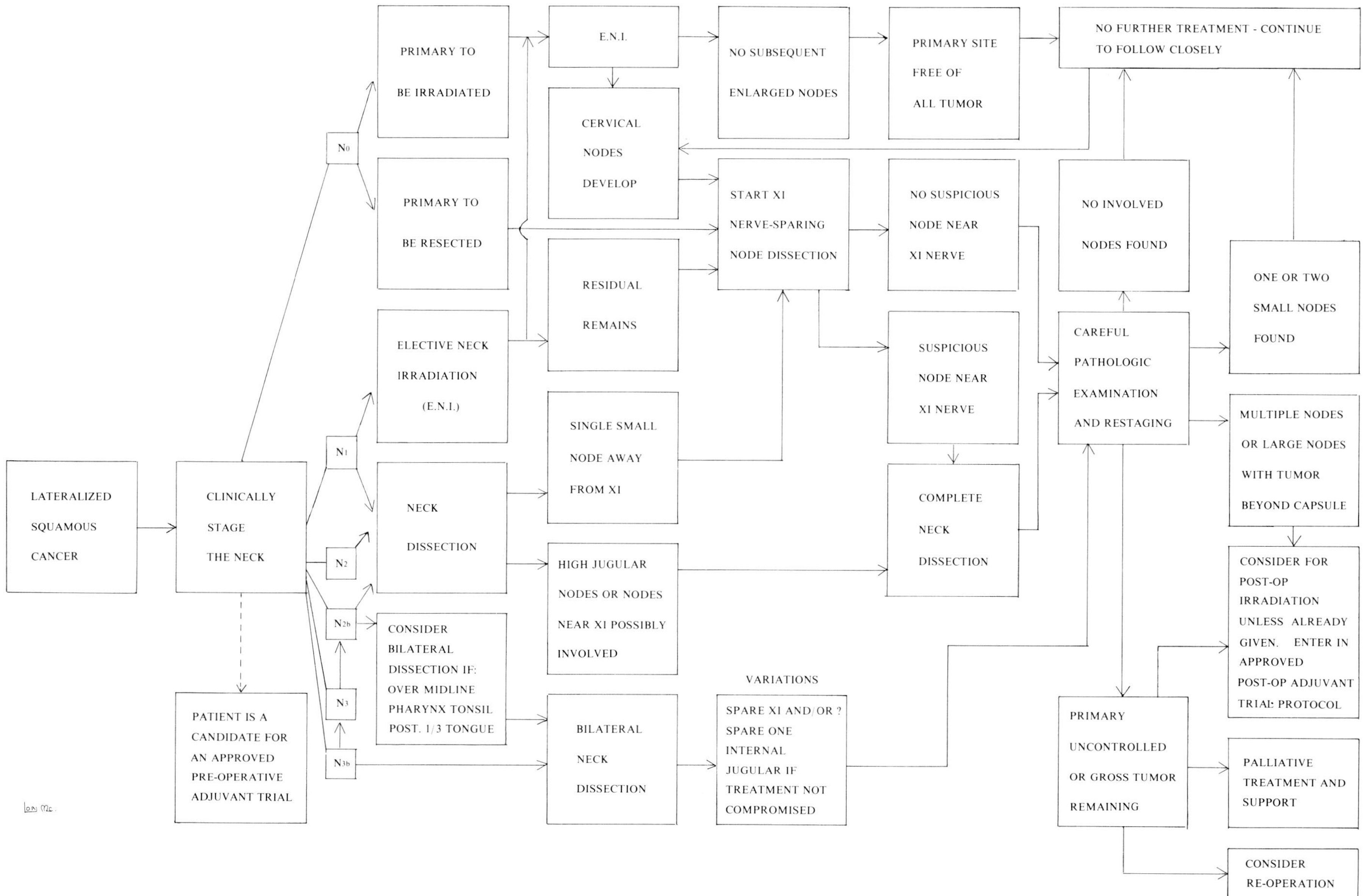

Fig 9–4.—Simplified flow chart of options for the treatment of potential or existing cervical lymph node metastases.

3. Loss of one internal jugular vein has no functional or detectable long-term physiologic effects. Loss of both veins may produce a transient increase in cerebral venous pressure which is easy to manage (see bilateral lymphadenectomy, below).[30] Conserving one vein in a bilateral dissection might ease postoperative care if no high jugular nodes are expected to be involved.

4. Loss of one sternocleidomastoid muscle in an adult is only a cosmetic contour loss, most noticeable in the suprasternal area.

5. Loss of the spinal accessory nerve is a significant disability. Abduction of the arm is impaired. Lifting is limited. Without rehabilitation and exercise in the immediate postoperative period, a frozen, painful shoulder will result.

6. If the sternocleidomastoid, digastric, and stylohyoid muscles are left intact, along with the internal jugular vein, then the more frequently involved upper jugulodigastric nodes are almost impossible to harvest without fragmentation. The conservative resections as advocated by Bocca and Pignataro[38] have their application to very specific clinical circumstances.

7. Unless the larynx is sacrificed, it is desirable to preserve the superior laryngeal nerve.

8. In selecting between irradiation and surgery, it should be remembered that irradiation also has a morbidity cost.[39] Early, there is some mucositis and stomatitis. Later, there will be xerostomia and complaints of "funny tastes." After 4–6 months there is a progressive decline in blood flow through the distributive arterioles. Decreased wound healing is noticeable at 6 months. Surgical procedures in irradiated tissues will have an increased likelihood of complications as time progresses after high-dose radiation.

9. The "wager" with elective neck node irradiation is that the net survivorship of irradiation and no further treatment plus irradiation with surgical salvage for any persisting disease produces as many survivors as surgery alone. The validity of this plan depends on irradiation of many N_0 patients, punctilious follow-up, and avoiding wide variation in treatment techniques between institutions.

10. In general, true N_0 and some N_1 disease is initially treated by neck irradiation when irradiation is used to treat the primary cancer site. With the exception of nasopharyngeal cancers, more *advanced* nodal disease is best treated by surgery. The problem in this decision is that many clinically staged N_0 patients are really N_1 or N_2. Leipzig and Hokanson[40] and Nahum[41] have pointed out the high frequency of positive ipsilateral nodes and contralateral nodes for tongue cancer in patients that are clinically staged N_0.

11. There is key question for which there is only anecdotal experience. What is the role of cervical irradiation in the postoperative period when pathologic examination of the specimen shows more than two or three positive nodes? We have offered our patients postoperative irradiation when the submitted specimen is pathologically staged N_2 or greater. This is done on the basis of favorable unpublished experience from friends in other centers. A poor data base.

HOW CAN RADIATION BE EMPLOYED TO CONTROL LYMPH NODE METASTASIS IN THE NECK?

Radiation treatment plays an important role in the control of neck metastases. The chapter on radiation therapy discusses the indications for the use of radiation therapy alone in subclinical neck metastases or in early stage neck metastases. The use of irradiation in an adjuvant manner (as preoperative or postoperative irradiation) in advanced disease is also discussed in detail elsewhere. Only the clinical approach to treating neck is discussed here.

Elective treatment of potential or existing neck metastases by irradiation depends on the location of the primary, the stage of the primary, and the definitive treatment of the primary tumor. If radiation is the sole treatment for the primary, then elective neck irradiation is usually a planned component of the therapy. Specifics depend on the anatomical location of the primary. Generally, elective neck irradiation is reserved for clinically N_0 or N_1 neck involvement.

In combined treatment, the primary tumor is surgically removed, along with unilateral or bilateral neck dissections. The adjuvant irradiation is given either preoperatively or postoperatively. In the case of preoperative irradiation, the primary tumor is included in the treatment field. A total dose of 5,000 rad is delivered over 5–6 weeks. Surgery is done about 4 weeks later. In postoperative radiation, the treatments are started 4–6 weeks following surgery and the whole tumor bed area is included in the primary beam. Total treatment dose would be 6,000 rad.

WHAT ARE SOME TECHNICAL FEATURES OF ELECTIVE NECK IRRADIATION?

Most often the patient is treated in a supine position. Different types of head immobilizers are used to make the daily treatment setups spatially reproducible. The primary target nodes along with first echelon of draining lymph node chains are included in the two parallel opposed lateral neck fields. The lower cervical and supraclavicular nodes are treated with a single anterior field. The junction between the lateral fields and the anterior supraclavicular field varies with the location of the primary. If the primary is in the oral cavity, oropharynx, or nasopharynx, the junction is at the thyroid notch (Fig 9–5). If the primary is in the larynx or hypopharynx, the junction is brought as low as possible (usually 2 cm below the thyrocricoid notch) to include the entire larynx and hypopharynx in the lateral neck field (Fig 9–6).

The upper margin of the lateral neck field extends up to the zygomatic arch to include high cervical, preauricular, and posterior pharyngeal wall nodes. For oral cavity lesions, the anterior margin extends to cover the entire mouth (including the submental and submandibular lymph nodes). The lips, including the corners of the mouth, are shielded to prevent painful mucositis. For the remaining lesions, it is sufficient to extend the

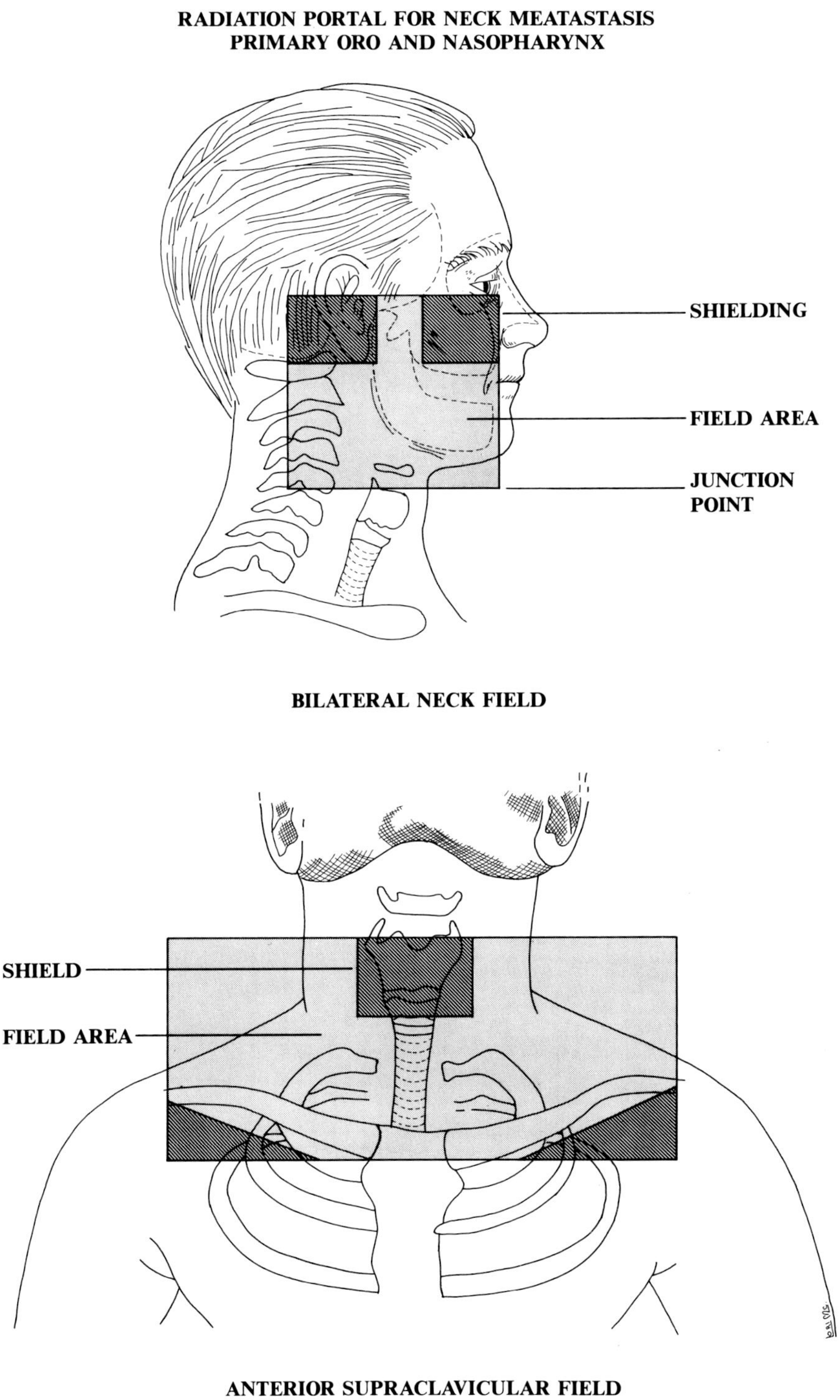

Fig 9–5.—Radiation field for elective neck irradiation with an oropharyngeal primary.

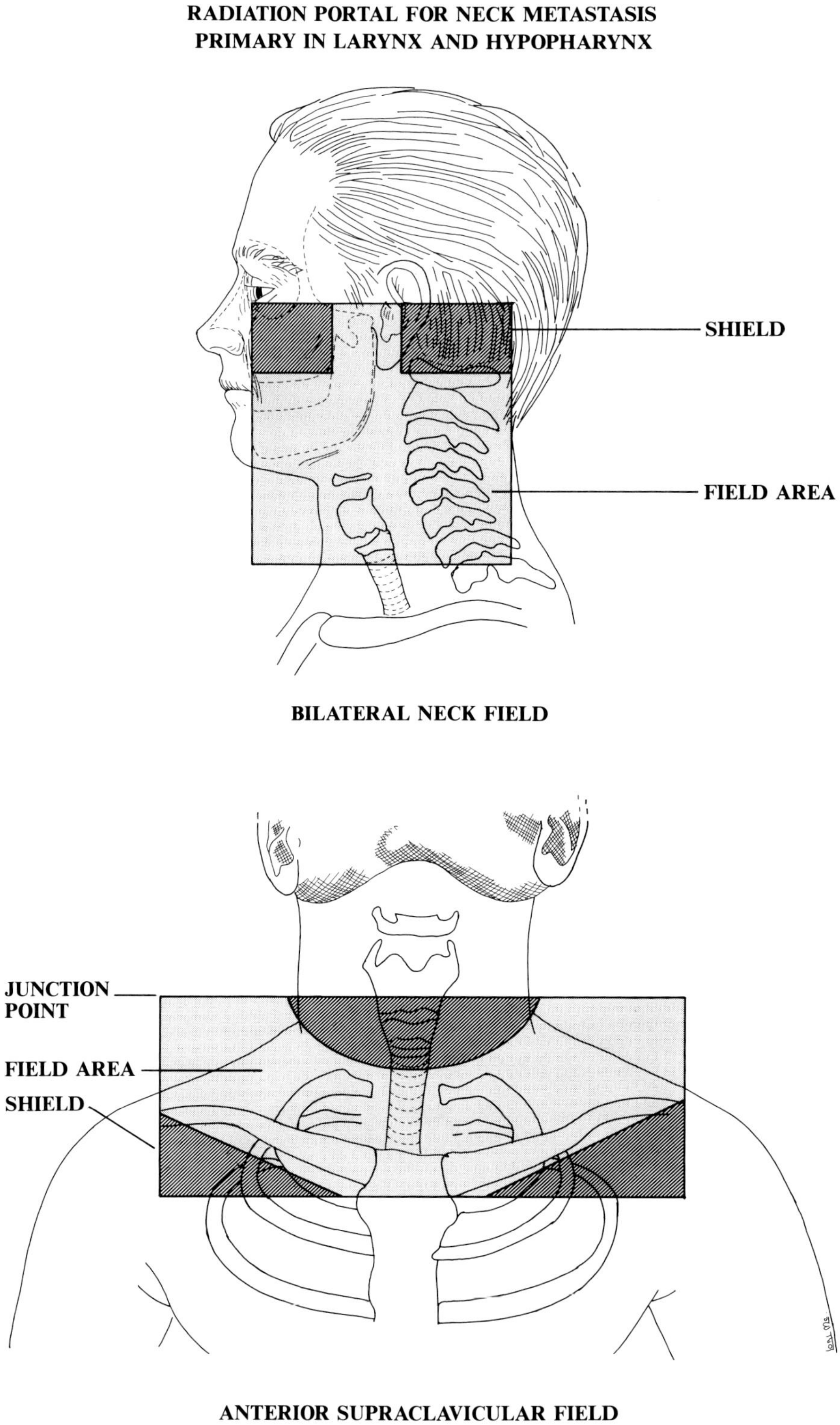

Fig 9–6.—Radiation field for elective neck irradiation with a laryngeal or hypopharyngeal primary.

anterior margin up to the lateral orbital ridge, thereby reducing the area of oral mucositis. Lesions that arise in the base of the tongue, posterior tonsillar pillar, and posterior pharyngeal wall have a higher incidence of occult metastasis in the posterior cervical chain; the posterior border of the field is designed to cover these areas adequately. In such cases, the treatment portal doses are adjusted to come off the spinal cord at 4,500 rad. The external auditory canals, the mastoids, and appropriate parts of the oral cavity are blocked with lead shields, depending on the site and extent of the tumor.

An anterior supraclavicular field includes lower cervical and supraclavicular nodes bilaterally and extends to the sternal notch. The infraclavicular areas are shielded (see Figs 9–5 and 9–6). In oral and oropharyngeal lesions in which the larynx is free of disease, the larynx is shielded with a small block (see Fig 9–5). In a majority of cases both supraclavicular areas are treated except in cases such as early lesions of tonsillar fossa, buccal mucosa, or retromolar trigone, where the incidence of contralateral supraclavicular metastases is very low.

If surgery is done subsequent to elective neck irradiation, it is important to remember the approximate location of fields and shielded areas. Planning of incisions, the use of flaps, and operative strategies must take into account the doses delivered and the time since irradiation.

WHAT ARE THE KEY STRATEGIES IN DOING A CERVICAL LYMPHADENECTOMY?

The procedure was originally discussed and illustrated by Crile in 1906.[8] Later refinements came from Brown and McDowell in 1944,[42] from Ward et al. in 1959,[9] and from Beahrs et al. in 1955 and 1977.[43, 44] Dr. Beahrs' updated description of the surgical anatomy of neck dissection is commended to the reader.[44] Hayes Martin's method was done in color by the noted illustrator F. Netter.[11] Bakamjian illustrated the use of the McFee incision.[45] Ballantyne illustrated and contrasted a standard cervical lymphadenectomy and one that preserves the spinal accessory nerve, the internal jugular vein, and the sternocleidomastoid muscle.[22] His approach is much more straightforward than Bocca's.[38]

A key problem in planning therapy is the variability in types of lymphadenectomy. This chapter is detailed in order to discuss the several common variations. The most practical and most frequent variation on the classic lymphadenectomy entails preservation of the spinal accessory nerve. Roy and Beahrs[46] successfully saved the spinal accessory nerve in 89 of 208 patients who underwent a total of 250 neck dissections. Forty-seven of the 89 were node negative. Forty-two were node positive. Except in two patients, the involved node(s) was far from the spinal accessory chain. There was no detectable degradation of cure rate *if* a very careful surgeon with a massive experience makes the patient selection and the judgment. Others have also been very selective and preserved trapezius muscle function with other technical modifications.[22, 47–50] The modifications are discussed in detail later. We will begin with the standard lymphadenectomy.

Whether one does the "classic" lymphadenectomy or one of its many variants, the surgical tactics are the same.

1. Remove the cover—skin and platysma.
2. Delineate the margins.
3. Remove the block of tissue. This can be done from bottom to top, back to front or front to back. Dissect the specimen of node-containing tissue from the pretracheal fascia. Preserve essential structures.
4. As you approach the area of the primary, plan to surround the site with adequate deep margins.
5. If a combined procedure is not planned, detach the specimen superiorly, preserving the lingual nerve.

This is a simple plan, but it will receive needed illustration later. The standard operation aims to remove the major lymph node chains shown in Figure 9–1, except the posterior auricular and occipital group. Embryologically, the rich reticular nets of lymph channels and nodes develop in juxtaposition to the venous structures. Most of the node-bearing tissues are enveloped between the deep and superficial leaves of the investing (deep) cervical fascia. The area to be resected in the lower neck is shown in cross section in Figure 9–7 at two levels.

HOW DO YOU CHOOSE A SKIN AND SUBCUTANEOUS INCISION FOR THE FLAPS?

The incision should give adequate exposure for the procedure in the neck and extend naturally into any incisions required to treat the primary cancer. Some of the incisions that have been proposed are shown in Figure 9–8. Version *A* is useful for a general dissection of the neck. The incision shown in *G* is good for an in-continuity laryngectomy, where 10% or more of patients may need a simultaneous bilateral or second neck dissection. The classic double Y, shown in diagram *B*, presents flap survival problems by cutting across blood supply at the base. Adequate medial exposure can be obtained by extending a vertical limb several centimeters below the clavicle, as in diagram *D*. If marginal necrosis of a flap occurs, it almost always involves the posterior flap. Because of this, we prefer designs with longer anterior and shorter posterior flaps. The three-corner junctions in some flap designs are most vulnerable to necrosis. The carotid bulb should never lie directly under a trifurcated junction! The trifurcation in diagrams *D* and *H* should be more posterior, as in *A*. An irreverent rule is: "God hates sharp corners! If you make them he will round them off with necrosis." The variations of the "hockey stick" incisions are quite ulititarian for discontinuous or pull-through excisions (diagrams *E* and *F*).

In dissecting the medial lower portion of the flap, the tissue around the tracheotomy site should not be disturbed so that there will not be a postoperative communication under the flap to the tracheostomy site. If there is potential communication, as in diagrams *E* and

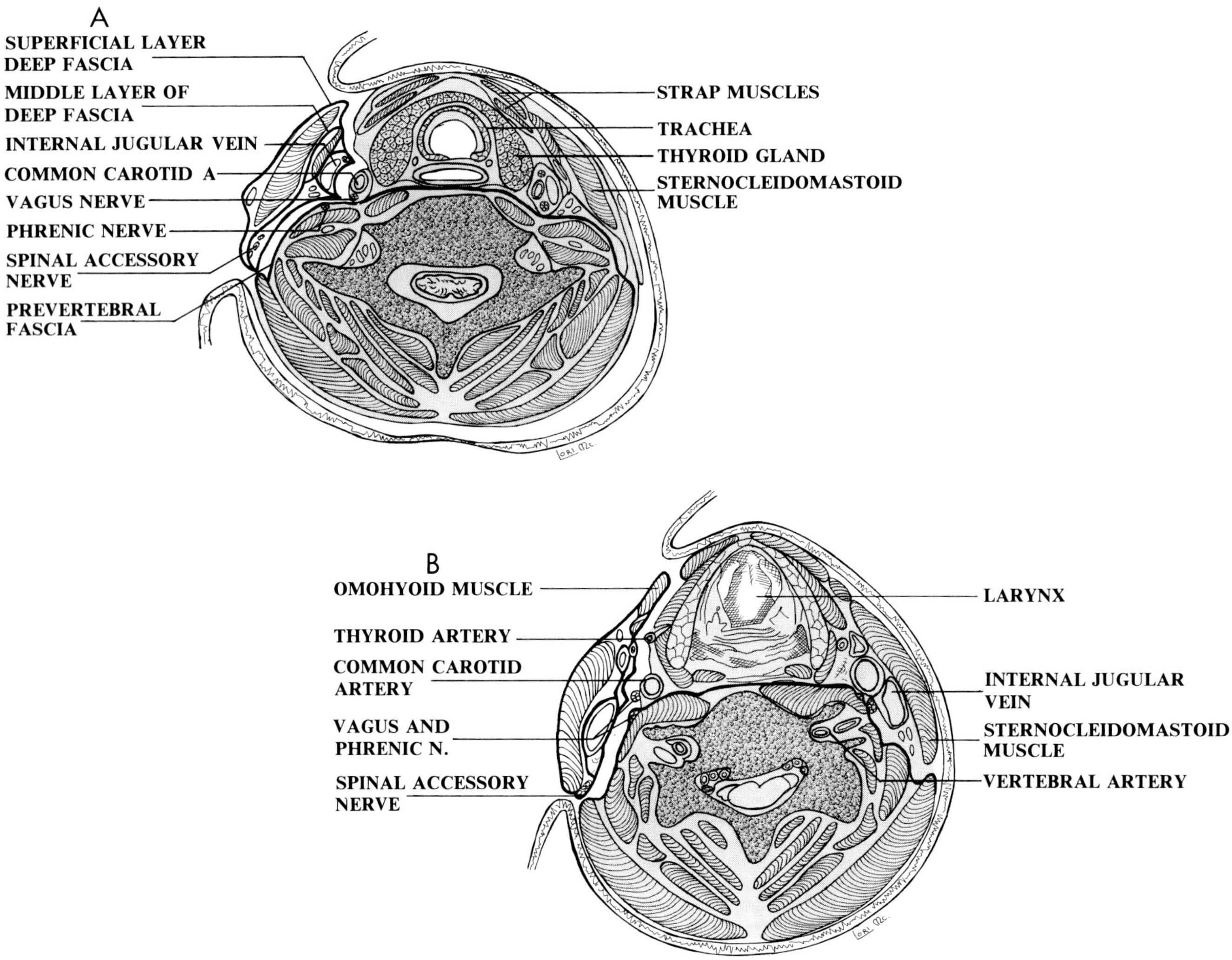

Fig 9–7.—A, Cross-sectional view of the neck at the thyroid isthmus; the block of tissue between the leaves of the deep cervical fascia is being dissected from the prevertebral fascia. **B,** cross-sectional view of the neck at the level of the larynx showing the plane of dissection. It is relatively easy to carry the dissection from back to front and incorporate the strap muscles and thyroid in an extended laryngeal resection.

F, the routes from the tracheostomy site to the lateral neck should be sutured securely.

Maintaining a viable flap requires care throughout the procedure. Too much compressive force is generated if a slippery flap is gripped with fingers or a sponge. Repeated pinching produces ecchymosis, thrombosis, and tissue injury. Flaps are handled only with skin hooks or stay sutures. They are kept moist and unkinked.

The final reconstructive maneuvers must be anticipated at the start of the operation and the design of any needed transfer flaps must be incorporated into the incisions (see Chap. 6). In general, we retain the platysma on the superficial flap. If large tumors invade near the platysma and skin, the full thickness is excised with a broad margin (> 2 cm). The area is then resurfaced with a planned full-thickness pedicle flap if direct closure would be under tension.

HOW CAN FLAP NECROSIS BE AVOIDED IN A HEAVILY IRRADIATED NECK?

When 5,000 rad or more have been given to the neck, there are blood flow changes. By 6 months, the subdermal vascular plexus is reduced by progressive proliferative sclerosis. The crucial perivascular multipotential fibroblastic stem cells are reduced or partially inactivated. Wound healing is impaired. By 2 years, blood supply is markedly reduced. Fibroblastic activity is barely present. Survival and healing of flaps is tenuous. For dissections late after heavy irradiation, the double transverse incision described by McFee is pre-

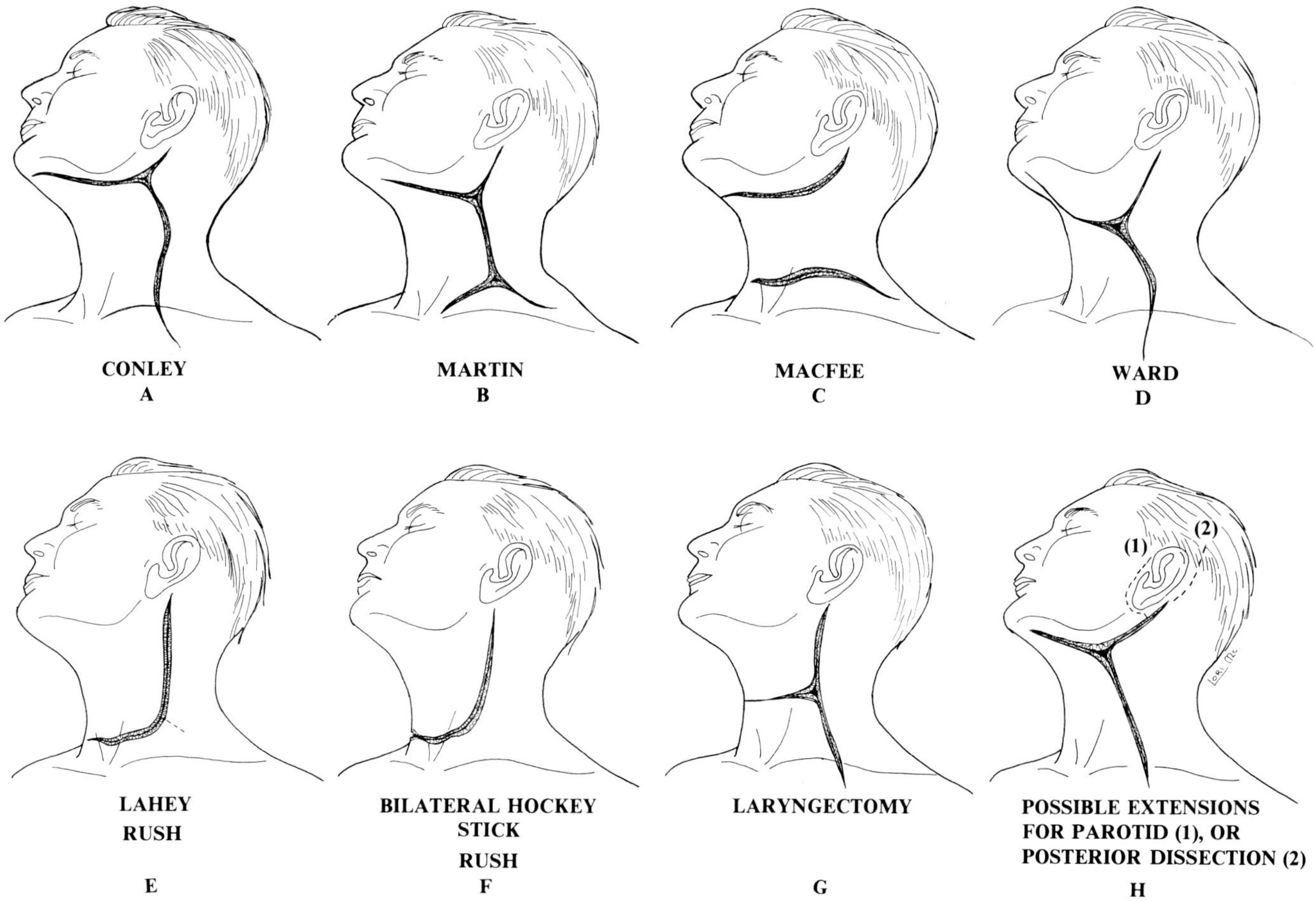

Fig 9–8.—Various incisions used for cervical lymphadenectomy.

ferred (see Fig 9–8, *C′*). For a McFee incision, flaps are handled with minimal tension, using a soft 1 inch penrose to loop and retract the middle flap. There are occasional patients with severe tissue damage from radiation treatment given years previously. When such a patient has a new primary needing surgical resection, resurfacing with a vascularized pedicle is planned. With the contemporary assortment of flaps that can transfer good viable neck coverage, there is little excuse to have a carotid exposed unless there is massive loss of oropharyngeal closure.

THERE ARE SEVERAL WAYS OF REMOVING THE BLOCK OF NODE-CONTAINING TISSUE. WHICH IS BEST?

Figure 9–9 shows the neck after the flaps have been raised. At this time, the superficial layer of the cervical fascia is exposed. The marginal mandibular nerve has been identified and preserved. The cervical lymphadenectomy can now be done back to front or bottom to top. There may be occasions when a large cervical node or the location of the primary makes one or the other method preferable. In either approach, it is an anatomical dissection. It should be done in an orderly and tidy manner. Hemostasis must be precise. Gentle blunt dissection can help develop the deep plane on the prevertebral fascia. The other tissues are sharply divided. All vessels over 1 mm are ligated. Large and significant veins are tied *and* suture ligated. Large veins will slip loose from a single simple ligature. For our illustrations we chose the left side of the neck for consistency. The lower portion of the borders are marked out first. The trapezius is followed down posteriorly, as shown in Figure 9–10. If the spinal accessory nerve is to be preserved, it is found as discussed below. The tissues are dissected clean of the trapezius border down to the clavicle.

The lower border is outlined by dividing the lower end of the sternocleidomastoid muscle. The deep investing fascia is incised above the clavicle between the lateral edge of the jugular and omohyoid. The omohyoid muscle is divided. Traction and elevation of the cut anterior stump of the omohyoid with a clamp will

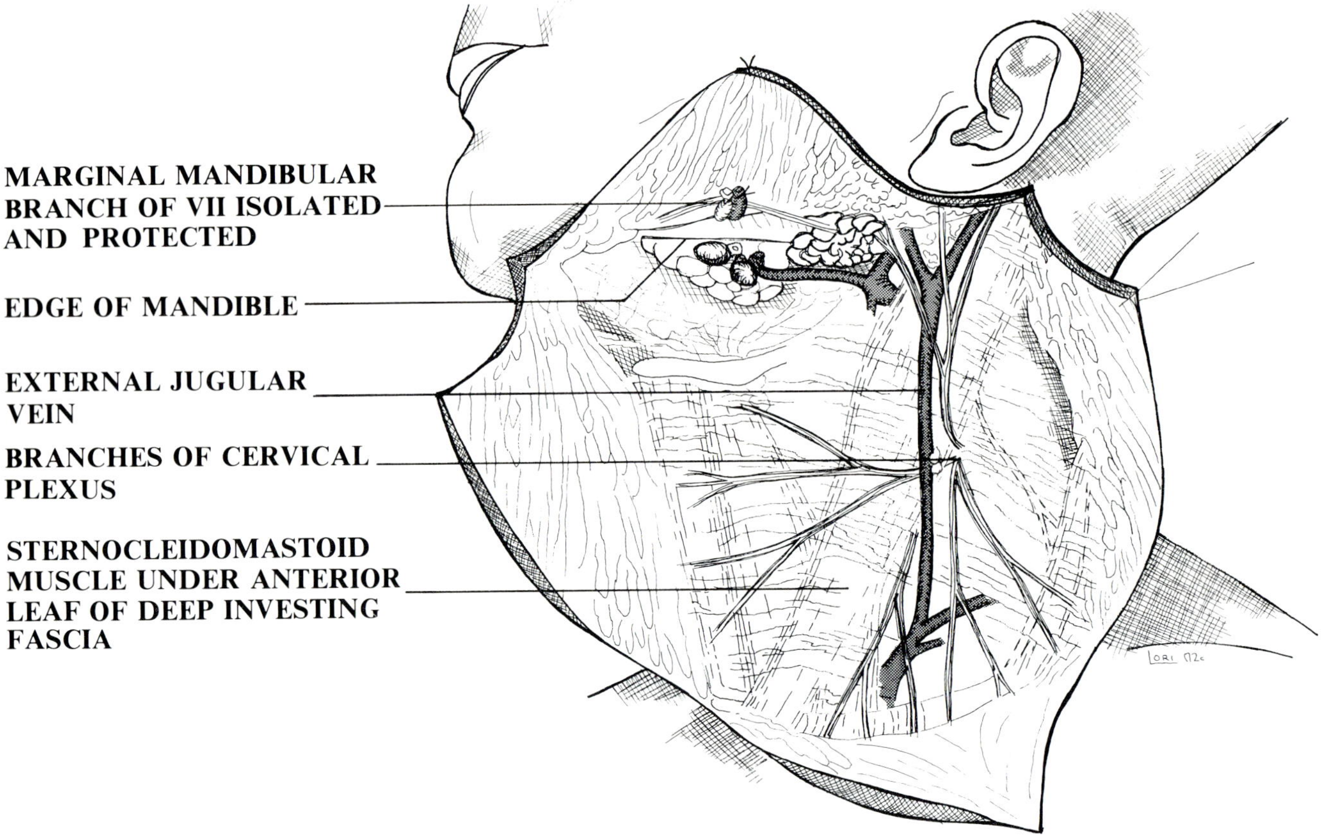

Fig 9–9.—Standard cervical lymphadenectomy. Flaps have been raised deep to the platysma. The marginal mandibular branch of the facial nerve has been identified and freed and is held upward by looping the ligated facial vessels upward.

make the area for the fascial incision line along its anterior border easy to see and easy to dissect up to the hyoid (Fig 9–11).

To raise the block of tissue with the internal jugular it is necessary to divide the internal jugular vein after opening the carotid sheath anteriorly. The jugular vein is dissected in a subadventitial plane, as in any vascular procedure. The vein can be rolled side to side so that its walls can be dissected free under direct vision. The vein is ligated in continuity and secured with suture ligatures on both ends. At this point the scalene fat is swept upward by some blunt dissection and the phrenic nerve, brachial plexus, carotid artery, and vagus nerve are identified. Dissection of the carotid sheath is done as shown in Figure 9–12. The tissues can be pulled superolaterally after the sheath of the carotid has been incised (Fig 9–12,A). This allows nodes in the retrocarotid position to be collected in the specimen (Fig 9–12,B). As the dissection progresses superiorly, the thin leaf of fascia should be left covering the phrenic nerve. This nice areolar plane can be cleanly dissected to the origins of the cervical nerves with one sweep of the finger. The transverse cervical vessels are divided (Fig 9–13).

An easy way to manage the posterior triangle is shown in Figure 9–11. Dissection is made on the scalenes laterally from the front to meet the previous posterior border incision. This creates a tunnel under the fat pad. A finger or Penrose drain can be used to lift the specimen and dissect it toward the axilla. With upward traction the fat pad can be divided in the front. The firmer deep tissue is vascular and should be divided between clamps.

If going from bottom to top in dissection, the dissection should be kept as a convex horizontal plane. The good assistant keeps the specimen lifted at an angle of 90° to 110° to the dissection plane while the surgeon exerts mild countertraction (Fig 9–14, A). The tyro tends to work deeper and deeper in a dissected tunnel, as in Figure 9–14, B.

Pulling the specimen straight cephalad obscures the dissection angle (Fig 9–14, C).

At the level of the cervical plexus the sensory nerve branches traverse the specimen from deep to superficial and tether it down. The dissection is carried superiorly, as shown in Figure 9–13. The supraclavicular, auricular, and occipital branches of the cervical plexus are cut about 1.5 cm out to avoid any possible damage to the

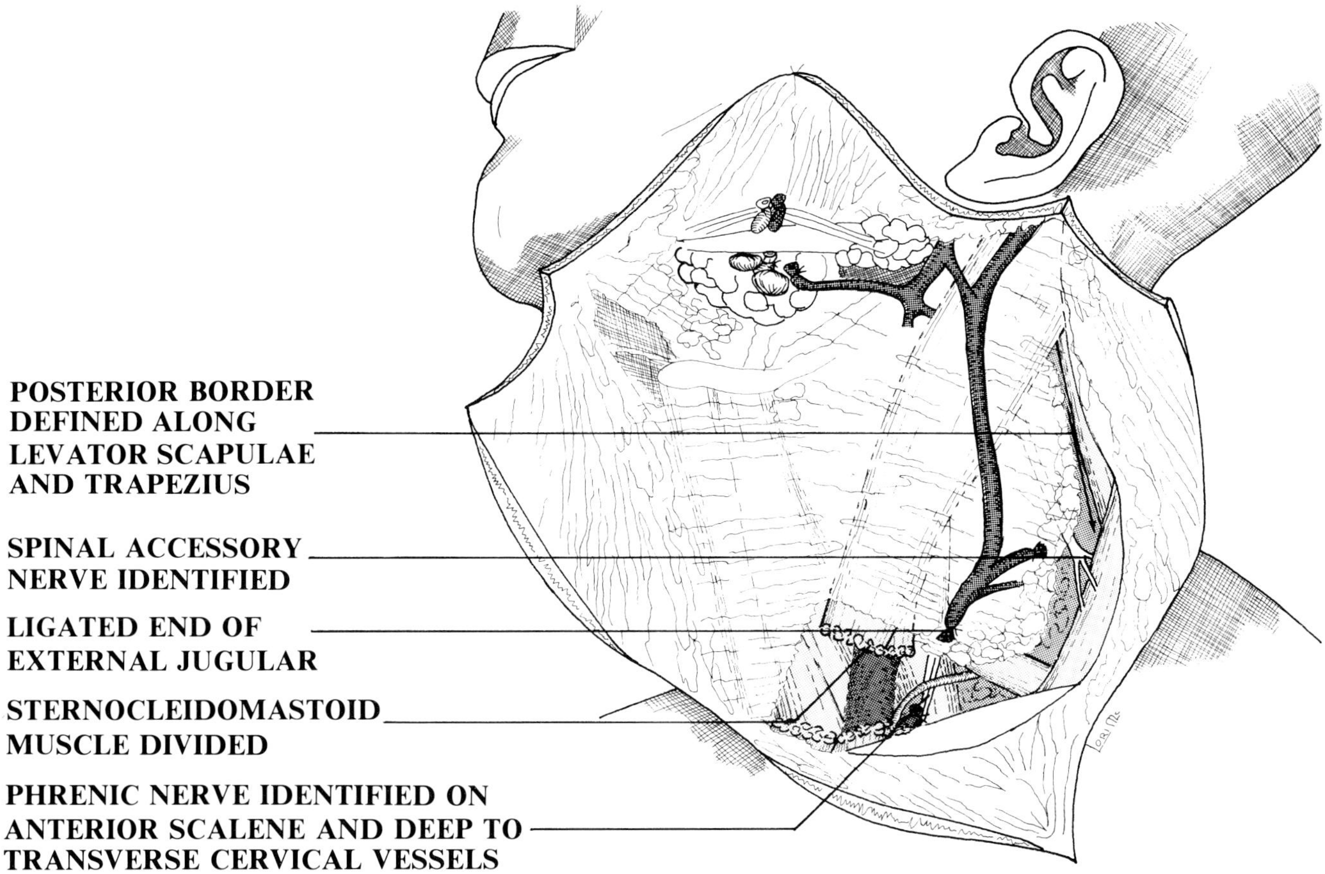

Fig 9–10.—Standard cervical lymphadenectomy. The posterior border is defined along the levator scapulae and trapezius muscles. If the spinal accessory nerve is to be preserved, it must be identified at this time. The lower border is defined by division of the sternocleidomastoid muscle. The anterior and middle leaves of the deep cervical fascia are divided centrally, exposing the carotid sheath, the omohyoid muscle. The scalene fat pad is swept upward, exposing the transverse cervical artery and phrenic nerve.

phrenic nerve. The dissection is continued superiorly. The omohyoid is detached superiorly. Posteriorly, the sternocleidomastoid is sharply freed along the mastoid process. There are useful technical principles that aid dissection for this phase of the operation (see Fig 9–14).

To avoid stimulating the carotid sinus vasodilatory-bradycardic reflex, the carotid bulb is injected subadventitially with 1% xylocaine using a fine 25-gauge needle. The hypoglossal nerve is identified at or slightly above the carotid bulb. There is a small plexus of thin-walled veins from the pharynx and/or thyroid. A moment of careful dissection, isolation, and ligature in-continuity (with added suture ligature) is less time-consuming than tidying up after tearing a thin-walled vein. With cranial nerve XII used as a guide to depth, the dissection is carried anteriorly and superiorly. The tail of the parotid gland and the posterior facial vein are sectioned at or below the level of the marginal branch of the seventh nerve. The completed "classic" neck dissection is shown in Figure 9–15. The classic operation preserves the posterior belly of the digastric and the stylohyoid muscles. The question is whether you want to remove the higher jugular nodes cleanly and with a better superior margin. It is difficult to have a clean high dissection at this point without exposing the upper jugular area by dividing the stylohyoid and posterior belly of the digastric muscle. An attempt to remove the higher medial jugular nodes without removing the internal jugular vein produces fragmentation of the jugulodigastric lymphatics which are frequently involved. Table 9–6 gives the frequency of involvement of the higher jugular nodes. Even the larynx has a significant frequency of upper jugular nodal involvement.

If the jugular nodes are involved and the posterior mandible is to be sectioned, then ligation and division of the internal jugular can wait until after sectioning the mandible. Then it is ligated nearer the base of the skull, with the higher jugulodigastric nodes cleanly encompassed in the specimen (Fig 9–16).

If a combined operation is planned, the deep border of the specimen is freed under the mandible and the submaxillary gland. The anterior facial artery is divided

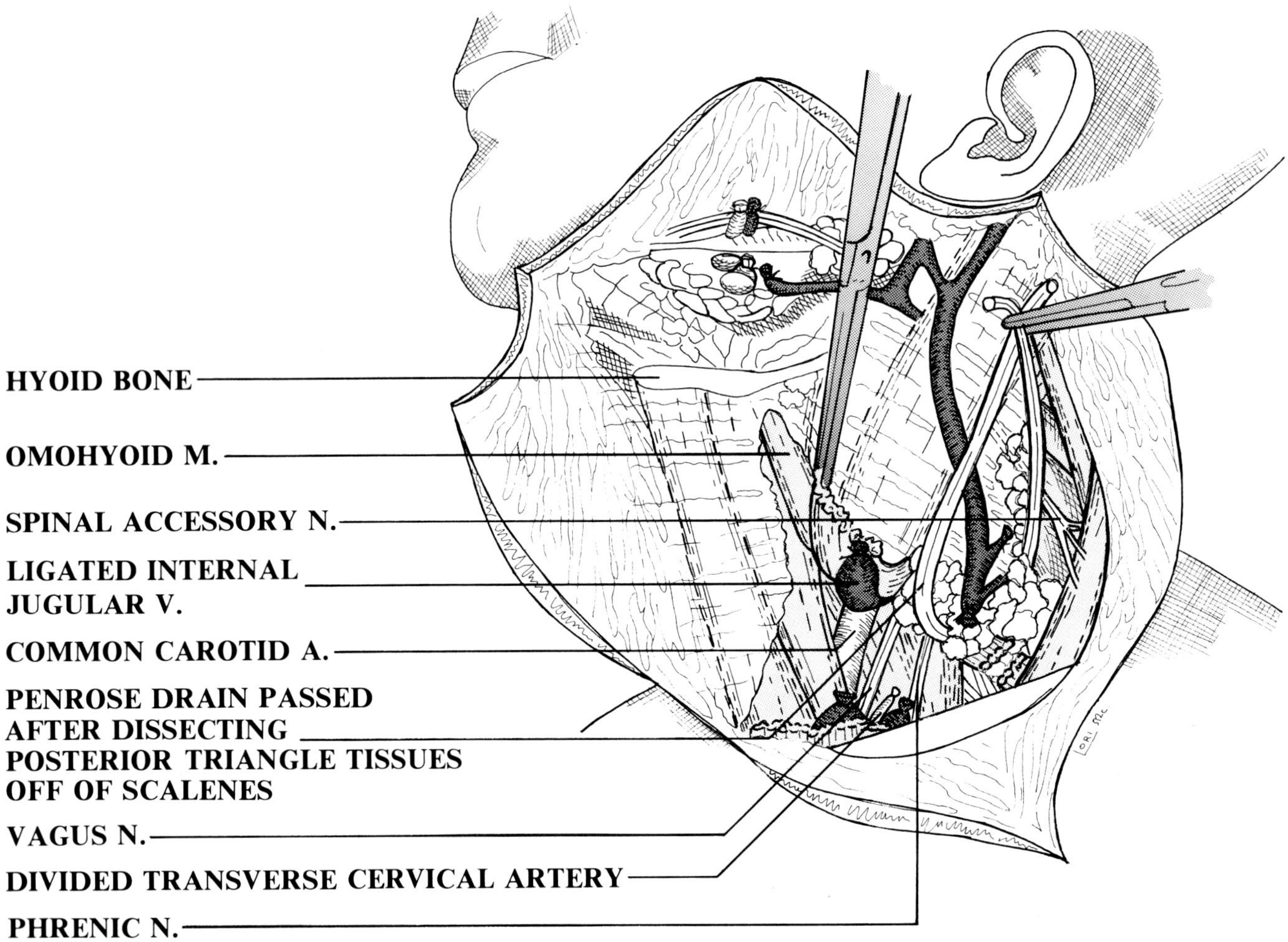

Fig 9–11.—The omohyoid muscle is divided. It is followed anteriorly to the hyoid to mark the anterior border. The internal jugular vein is divided. To free the posterior triangle tissue, a plane is created deep to the block of specimen on the scalenes to join the lower incision and the posterior border. A Penrose drain is passed underneath and used to retract the tissues for further dissection toward the axilla. The tissues are pulled up and divided at an arbitrary point.

at its origin. The specimen is freed anteriorly or posteriorly until it is attached only to the area to be resected.

If no composite operation is planned, the upper border is cleaned from the submental space and freed of the mandible, and the specimen and submaxillary gland are pulled downward. The chordatympany branch of nerve VII which travels with the lingual nerve ("secretory control" to the submaxillary gland) is sectioned, with care taken that the lingual nerve, now pulled down to a V, is not injured. The submaxillary duct is dissected along nerve XII under the geniohyoid, then divided and ligated. This completes classic neck dissection (see Fig 9–15). Bakamjian et al.[45] have illustrated the dissection, carried in an inferior-posterior to superior-anterior sweep. They also show how to do the operation using the parallel McFee incisions. The important idea is that cervical lymphadenectomy can be approached from several points if anatomical principles are understood. The procedure has a number of variations.

In dissection of the neck lymph nodes there are three common variations: preservation of nerve XI (as shown

TABLE 9–6.—DISTRIBUTION (%) OF CERVICAL METASTASES IN 393 NECK DISSECTIONS*

	SITE OF PRIMARY CANCER	
LOCATION	Oropharynx, thyroid, and major Salivary Glands	Larynx
Submaxillary triangle	71	42
Upper third of jugular	43	62
Middle third of jugular	29	52
Lower third of jugular	15	14
Posterior triangle	14	12
Lowest node	2	4

*Summarized from De La Pava and Pickren.[14]

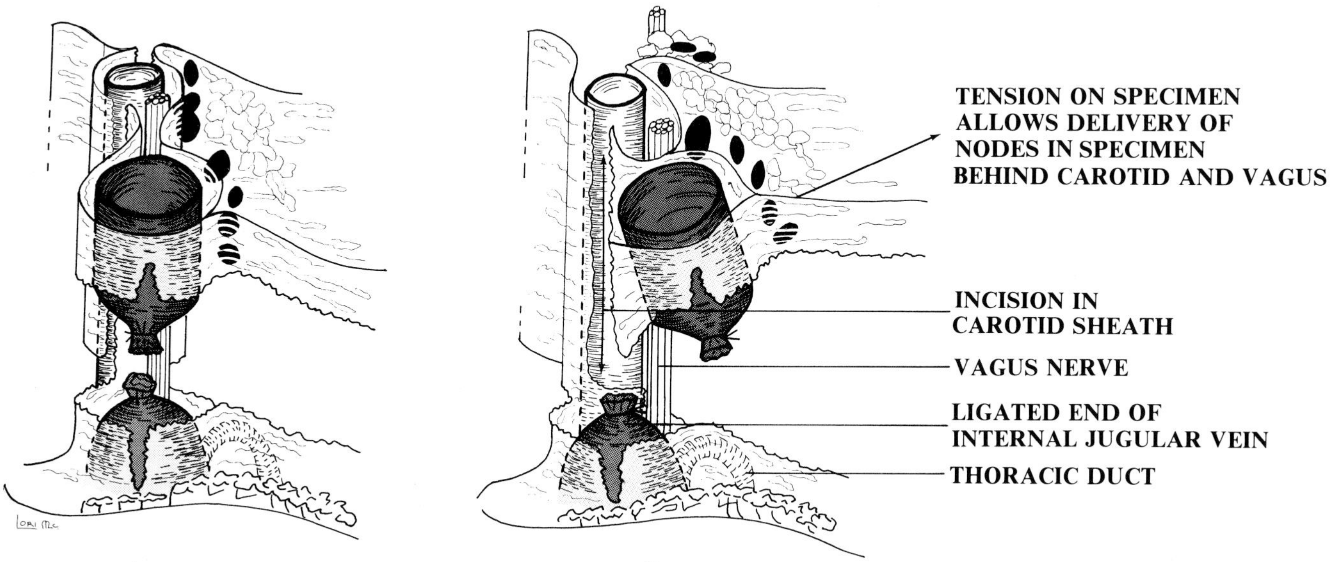

Fig 9–12.—Clearing the node-containing tissue from the carotid sheath. The nodes are most frequently found in the perivascular soft tissue. The carotid sheath is formed by the divided encircling layers of the middle leaf of the deep cervical fascia. In **A** the carotid sheath has been incised vertically on the anterior border. In **B** the tissues are retracted laterally. The vagus is freed in a similar way. Finally, the posterior part of the sheath is incised, with care taken to free the tissue behind the carotid and spare the cervical sympathetic chain.

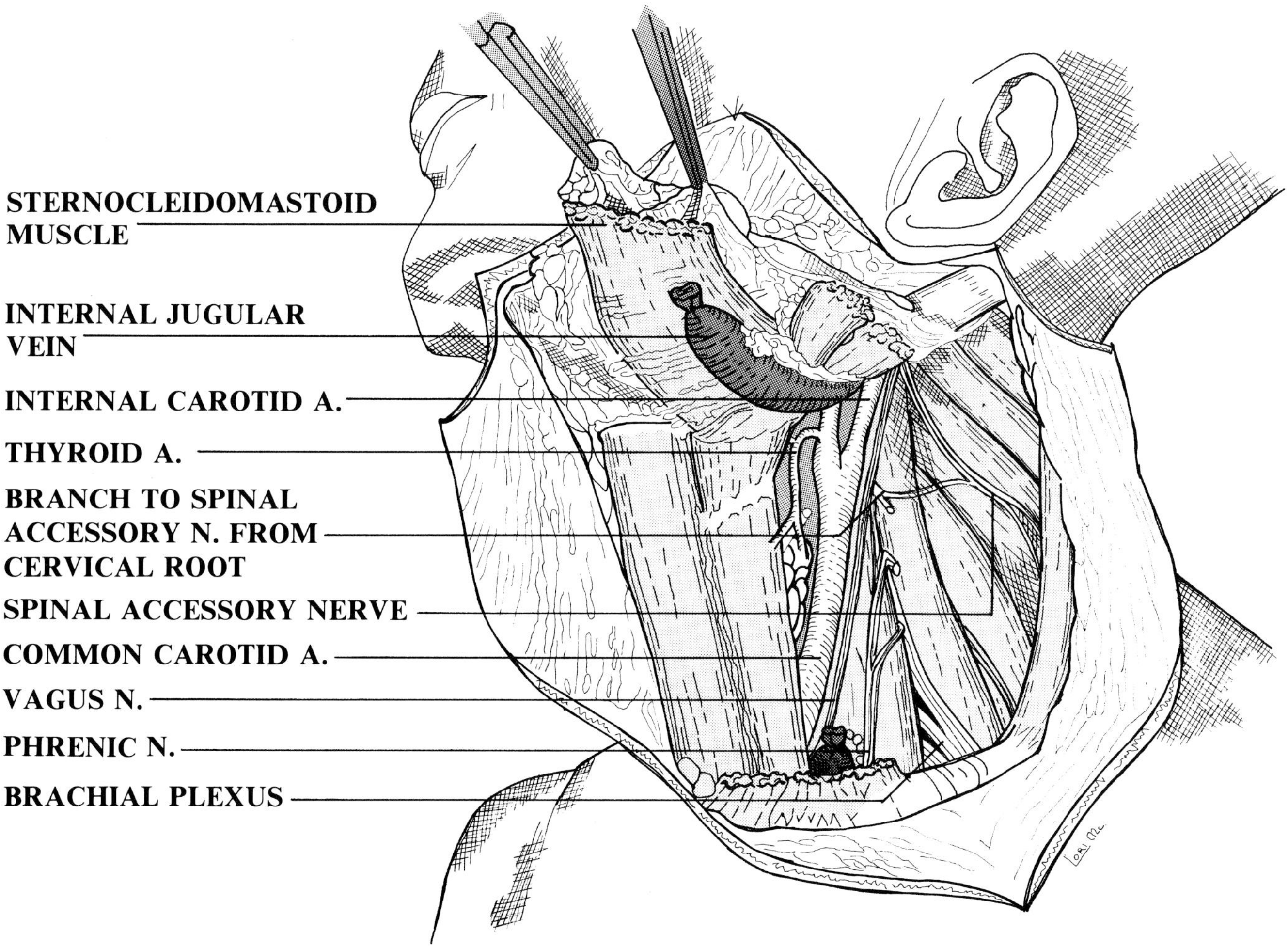

Fig 9–13.—Standard cervical lymphadenectomy. In this illustration the spinal accessory nerve is shown being preserved to illustrate the small contributing branch from the cervical plexus which may preserve some trapezius function if the eleventh nerve is divided superiorly. Failure to remember that the cervical sensory nerves traverse the specimen may perplex a neophyte during a neck dissection and bring progress to a halt.

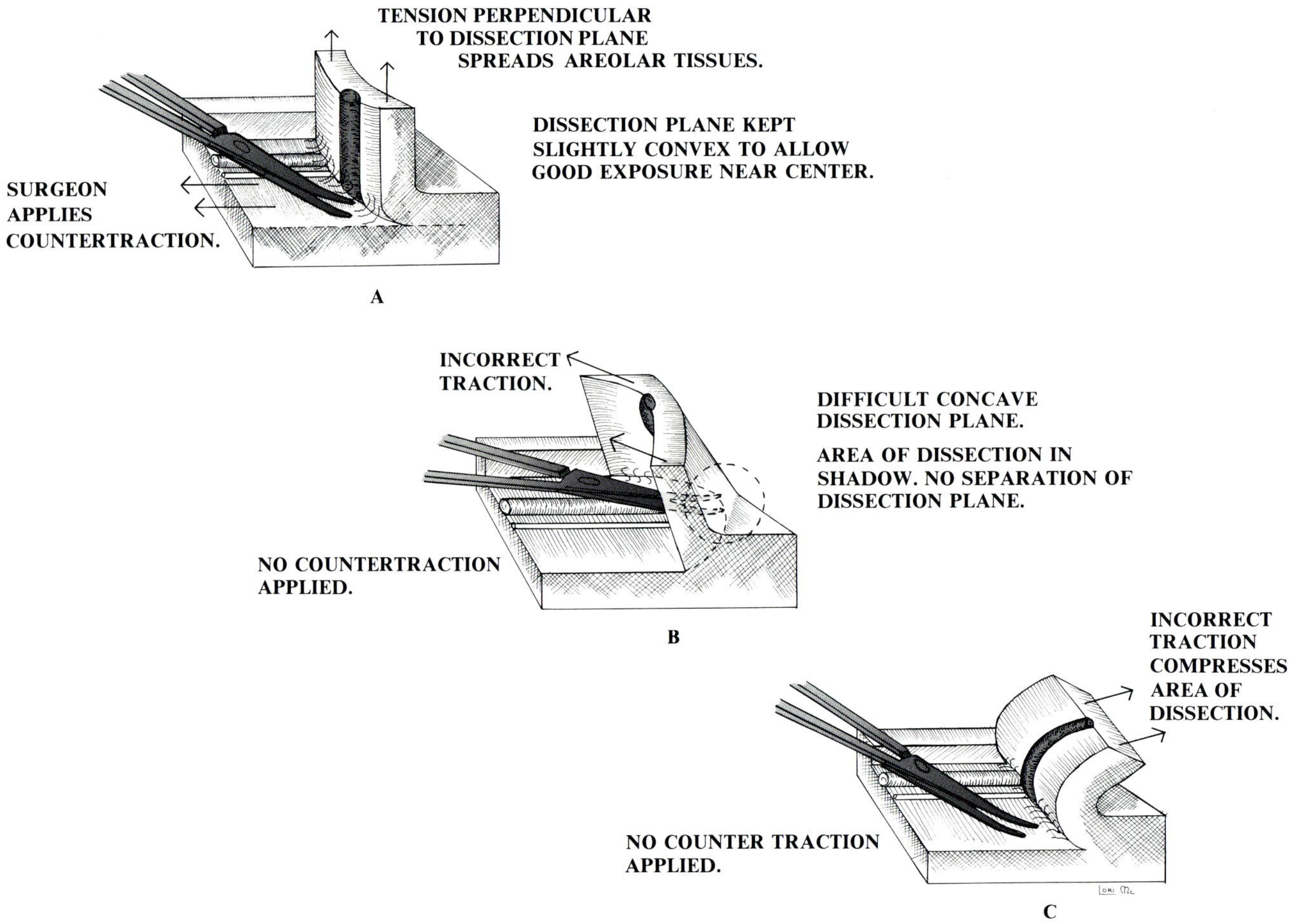

Fig 9–14.—Useful and difficult approaches to dissection of the cervical lymphatics. **A,** useful approach. The assistant applies tension perpendicular to the plane of dissection while the surgeon applies countertraction with a free hand. The dissection plane is kept in the open at all times. Do not make cuts at the bottom of a deep, dark, surgical abyss, especially in anatomically scenic areas, as shown in **B.** If your assistant is lazy and you don't provide countertraction, dissection is difficult, as shown in **C.**

in Fig 9–13), preservation of the digastric and stylohyoid (see Fig 9–15), and preservation of neither (see Fig 9–16).

HOW DO YOU IDENTIFY THE ACCESSORY NERVE DURING A FUNCTIONAL NECK DISSECTION?

As noted before, the spinal accessory nerve can be preserved in highly selected cases, clinical N_0 cases (perhaps N_1 if the node is far away from nerve XI). In order to preserve the nerve, it is identified in the early dissection of the posterior border (see Figs 9–10 and 9–13).

The spinal accessory or eleventh cranial nerve exits the skull from the jugular foramen. It supplies both the sternocleidomastoid and trapezius muscles. In two thirds of cases, the nerve lies lateral to the jugular vein, but in one third it may lie deep to the vein. It passes downward and posteriorly approximately 2 inches below the mastoid process and, along with the occipital artery, passes deep to or through the sternocleidomastoid muscle. It is most easily recognized as it exits from behind or from the substance of the sternocleidomastoid muscle to enter the posterior triangle of the neck. This point of exit is usually 2 cm above where the greater auricular nerve surfaces before it passes along the anterior lateral aspect of the sternocleidomastoid muscle. This is known as Erb's point. The accessory nerve is the only motor nerve that lies superficial to the deep cervical fascia of the posterior triangle of the neck. Approximately 1–2 inches above the clavicle the nerve passes beneath the inferior border of the trapezius muscle. The lesser occipital nerve exits from behind the sternocleidomastoid muscle at approximately the same level as the accessory nerve. It passes *upward* and

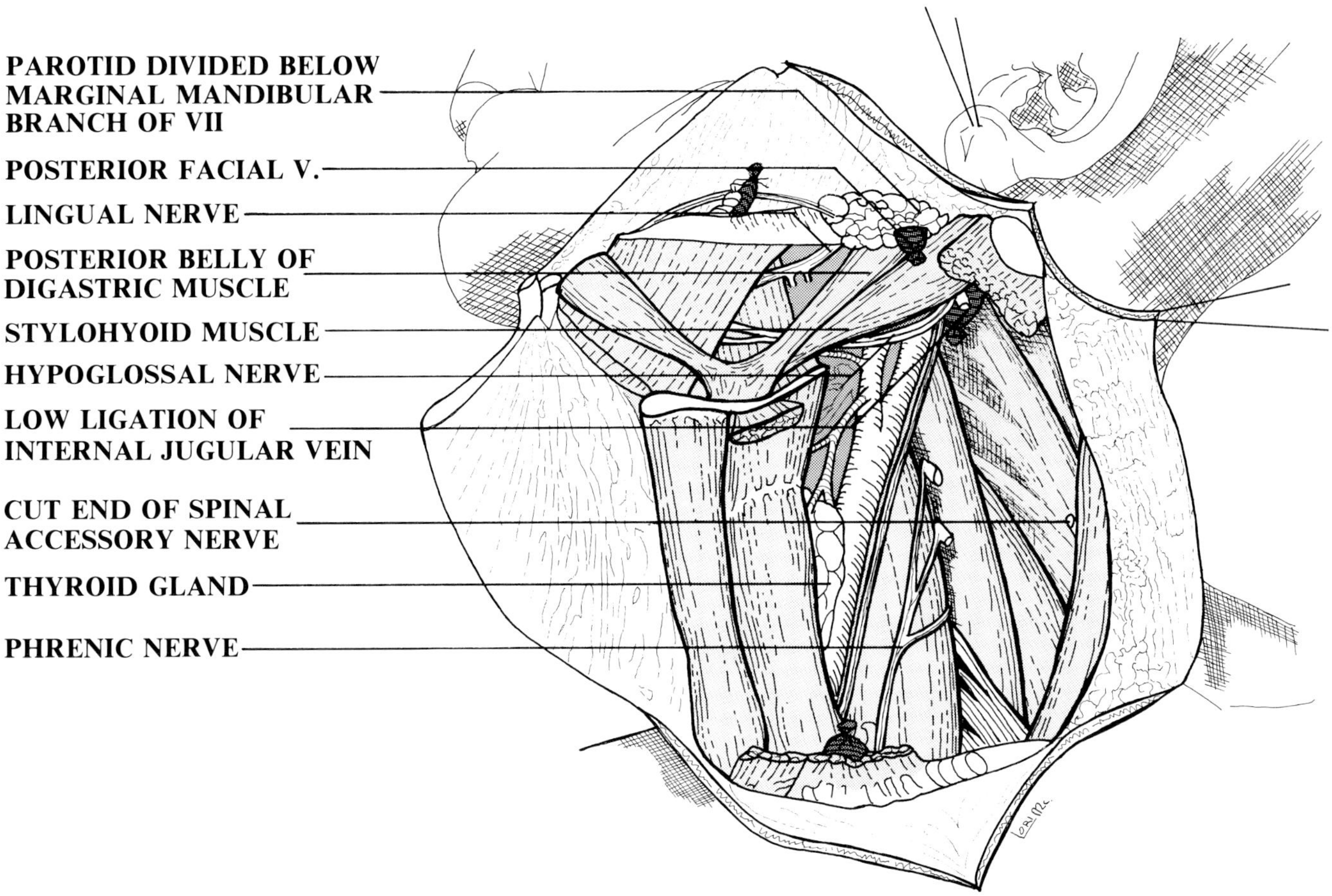

Fig 9–15.—Standard cervical lymphadenectomy. The upper portion of the jugular vein has been suture ligated and the spinal accessory nerve sectioned. The tissues have been swept from the posterior belly of the digastric. Not shown is the division of the facial artery near the external carotid. The submaxillary gland is removed, the duct is dividied, and the submental triangle is cleared, completing the dissection.

posteriorly, and where it reaches the occipital artery is the posterior-superior limit of the neck dissection.

There is a connection between cranial nerve XI and the third ramus of the cervical plexus. Even if nerve XI must be sacrificed above this point, some trapezius function will remain if this connection is preserved (see Fig 9–13). If any suspicious nodes are around the nerve, it should be sacrificed.

WHEN CAN THE SPINAL ACCESSORY NERVE BE PRESERVED?

We agree with the guidelines of Roy and Beahrs[46] which were introduced earlier. They preserve the spinal accessory when (1) the neck is staged N_0 and suspicious nodes are not encountered along the nerve or in the high jugular chain; (2) when there is a single node (N_1) well away from the course of the spinal accessory chain; and (3) in many thyroid cancers. To this might be added: (4) in the N_0 neck in a laryngectomy for a larger invasive cancer. The careful selection of patients is critical. Other authors have used the same general indications with no detectable degradation of cure rate.[47–51] It is interesting to note that an eleventh nerve–sparing procedure is used by the advocates of the procedure in no more than 30% of their major resections with lymphadenectomy. They are selective! Schuller et al. found minimal differences in patients' discomfort, appearance, or ability to return to work when radical neck dissection and modified neck dissection were compared in 243 study patients.[51b] We differ with Schuller and have found that trapezius function is nearly normal if nerve dissection of XI is gentle and undue traction is not placed on the nerve.

When the nerve must be sacrificed, Ballantyne and Guinn[52] have used an interposed free graft of greater auricular nerve. They reported function in 35 of 44 such nerve grafts. They reserve a section of the greater auricular nerve for this purpose. Previous irradiation pre-

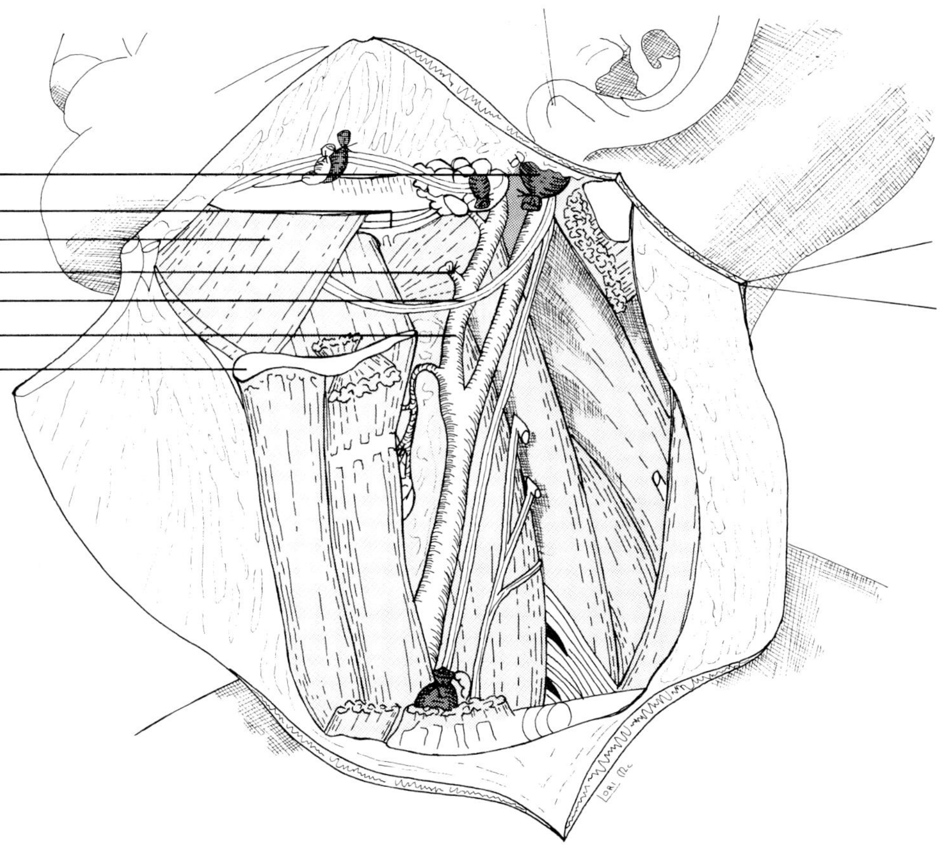

Fig 9–16.—A modification of the standard cervical lymphadenectomy with the digastric and stylohyoid muscles removed to give better access to the higher jugular nodes. This maneuver does sacrifice some lateral support of the larynx.

vents successful maintenance of the graft. There has not been a general adoption of free-nerving grafting.

ARE THERE VARIATIONS OF CERVICAL LYMPHADENECTOMY THAT CONSERVE MORE STRUCTURES THAN JUST THE SPINAL ACCESSORY NERVE?

In the past few years, several authors have written about operations that remove the major portion of the cervical lymphatics while preserving the spinal accessory nerve, the sternocleidomastoid muscle, the digastric and stylohyoid muscles, and the internal jugular vein. There is a tendency to perform a new procedure indiscriminantly just because it is new. The so-called conservation neck dissections do have a role in managing selected head and neck cancer patients. Some diseases such as early papillary carcinoma of the thyroid were probably overtreated in the past with a "classic" cervical lymphadenectomy. As we have pointed out, there are variations in cervical lymphadenectomy that enlarge the limits of the node removal. Conversely, there are indications for a conservation dissection. Ballantyne, who described one method of conservation lymphadenectomy, cautioned: "One should not press the indications for doing a modified neck dissection."[53] Methods of performing a modified dissection have been illustrated and discussed by Bocca[38, 54] and Ballantyne.[21, 51, 53]

WHAT IS THE RATIONALE FOR MODIFIED CONSERVATION NECK DISSECTION?

There are three reasons cited to justify a modification of the standard neck dissection. First, the lymph nodes of the neck lie within specific aponeurotic planes, which can be carefully dissected with preservation of underlying muscle and other important structures. Second, tumors of specific sites are known to metastasize primarily to certain areas. For example, laryngeal cancers seldom metastasize to the submental or submandibular nodes or to the spinal accessory chain of nodes. However, isolated cases of single metastases to these areas have been reported. Third, in a neck in which there are no clinically palpable nodes, the majority of potentially involved nodes can be removed and studied by

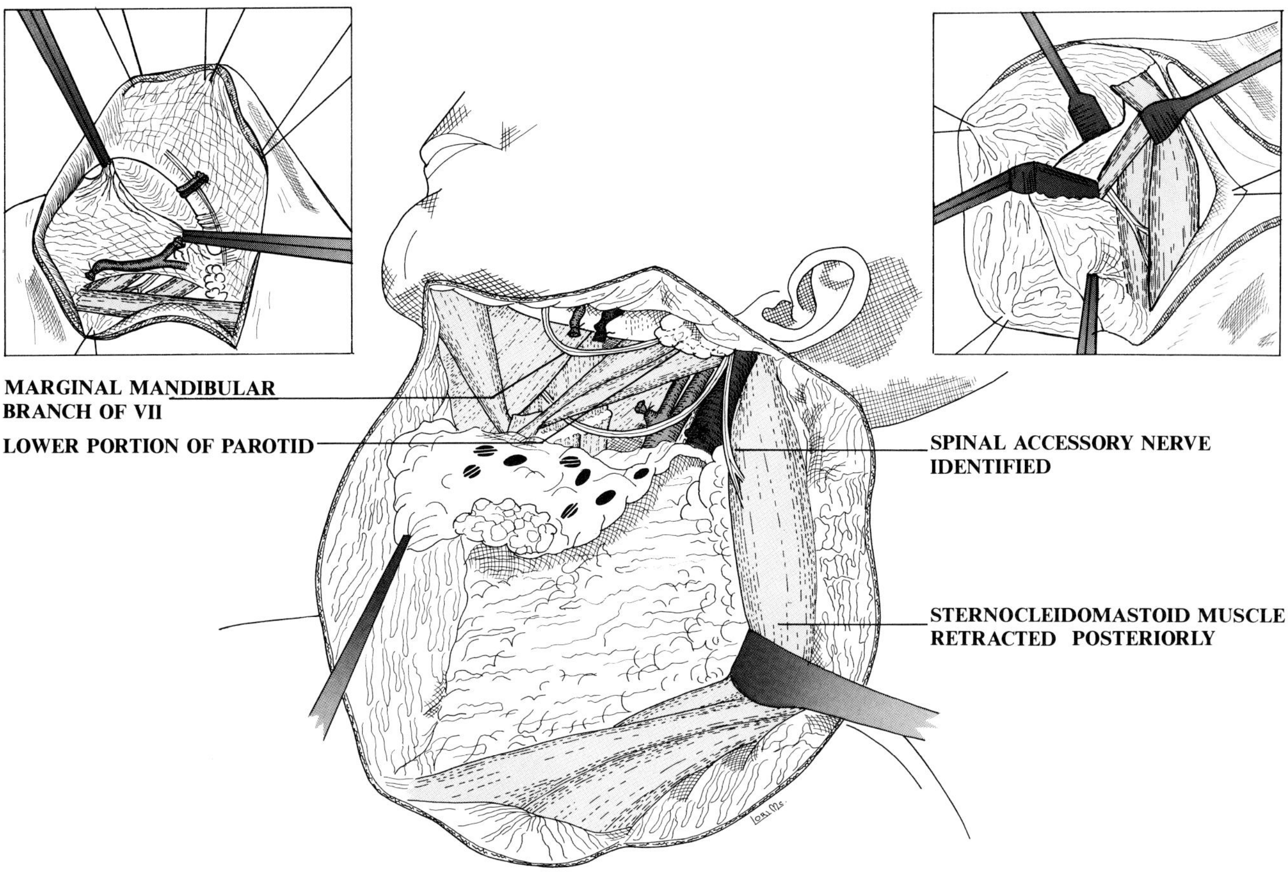

Fig 9–17.—Preservation neck dissection. Skin flaps are developed as for other dissection. The upper margin, near the mandible, is dissected as for a standard procedure *(left inset)*. The tissue and fascia over the digastric are cleared *(right inset)*. The spinal accessory nerve is identified and the branches to the sternocleidomastoid are preserved. The jugular vein is identified along with the carotid, vagus, and hypoglossal nerve. The submaxillary gland is dissected downward.

the pathologist. If positive nodes are found and tumor is extending out of the nodal capsule, postoperative irradiation is used by advocates, a questionably effective practice.

WHAT ARE THE INDICATIONS FOR MODIFIED CONSERVATION NECK DISSECTION?

There are no absolute indications for this procedure. Some general guidelines include the following:

1. A clinically negative neck in which there is a high risk of microscopic spread (a high risk is defined as at least 15%–25% likelihood that there are occult positive nodes).
2. The presence of N_1 cervical node disease in which the palpable node is not a high jugular node or in the spinal accessory group of lymph nodes.
3. In well-differentiated forms of thyroid carcinoma.
4. When a bilateral neck dissection is being performed and it is desirable to retain at least one jugular vein and one spinal accessory nerve.

WHEN IS A MODIFIED CONSERVATION NECK DISSECTION CONTRAINDICATED?

1. In the presence of N_2 or N_3 disease.
2. In lesions where there is a high probability that upper jugular nodes are involved.
3. In the presence of clinically positive nodes after a course of irradiation.
4. In the presence of malignant melanoma with clinically positive nodes.
5. Finally, it is not an operative procedure to perform when it compromises treatment of the primary lesion in a combined oropharyngeal resection.

Bocca et al. reported 30 years' experience with supraglottic laryngectomy and bilateral modified neck dissection for N_0, N_{1A}, and N_{1B} necks.[54] In Bocca's experience, 13% of N_0 and N_{1A} necks revealed metastatic cancer. He prefers simultaneous bilateral modified neck dissection and supraglottic laryngectomy to preoperative radiation therapy. This allows histologic examina-

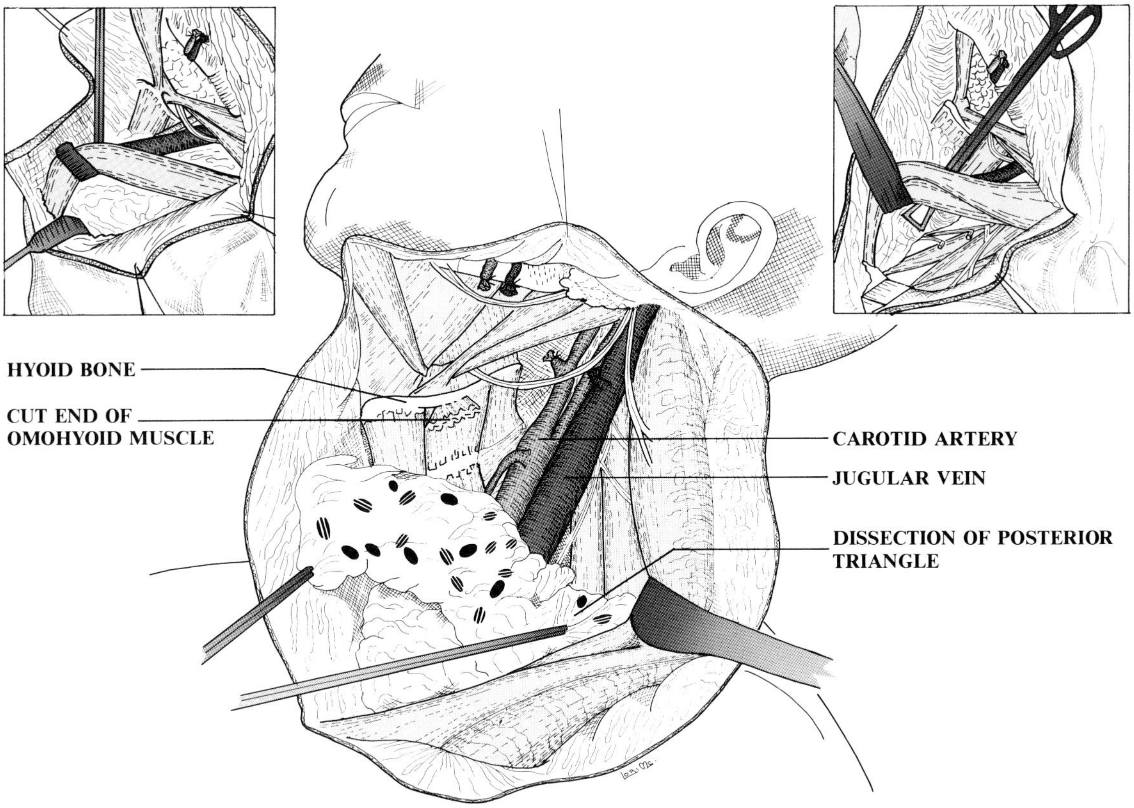

Fig 9–18.—Preservation neck dissection. Dissection is continued along the posterior border. Ballantyne removes as much posterior triangle tissue as can be obtained by posterior retraction on the sternocleidomastoid muscle. Bocca begins this posterior part of the dissection by pulling the sternocleidomastoid anteriorly *(left inset)* and then completing the dissection by passing the tissues under the sternocleidomastoid muscle *(right inset)*.

tion of the cervical lymph node tissue, and if there is evidence of "capsular rupture," Bocca recommends giving postoperative radiation therapy.

HOW DO YOU PERFORM A PRESERVATION NECK DISSECTION (THE BOCCA NECK PROCEDURE)?

Bocca and Pignataro[38] and Ballantyne and Jackson[21] have described and illustrated the procedure. The principal steps, as Ballantyne does the procedure, are shown in Figures 9–17 to 9–19. The insets to these figures show Bocca's variations. Basically, the spinal accessory nerve, sternocleidomastoid muscle, and internal jugular vein are identified and preserved. The areolar tissue is freed superiorly and along the usual posterior border (see Fig 9–17, *insets*). The digastric muscle is stripped of its fascia (*right upper inset,* Fig 9–17). The sternocleidomastoid muscle is retracted and lifted up while the spinal accessory nerve that innervates it is preserved. The specimen is dissected back to front. Bocca lifts the sternocleidomastoid up and passes the specimen from the posterior triangle under the muscle (see Fig 9–18, *insets*). Ballantyne removes as much areolar node-containing tissue from the posterior triangle of the neck as can be delivered from beneath the sternocleidomastoid when it is retracted posteriorly (see Fig 9–18). Finally, the specimen is cleared from the vessels, sparing the internal jugular vein (see Fig 9–19). The specimen can be pedicled on the strap muscle for in-continuity resection with the thyroid or the laryngeal structures (see Fig 9–19, *inset*). For thyroid carcinoma, Marchetta et al.[50] use a third variation in which the lower sternocleidomastoid muscle is detached and dissected upward. They then resect the node-containing block, preserving nerve XI and the jugular vein. At the conclusion, they reattach the sternocleidomastoid muscle.

HOW DO YOU MANAGE A SIMULTANEOUS BILATERAL NECK DISSECTION?

For many years, surgeons avoided simultaneous bilateral neck dissections because of early reports of lethal CNS complications. Sugarbaker and Wiley showed that there was some transient (24–48 hours) increase in ce-

nodes in carcinoma of the tongue. *Head Neck Surg.* 5:3–9, 1982.
41. Nahum A.M.: Head and neck cancer: Management of early lesions, editorial. *Head Neck Surg.* 5:1, 1982.
42. Brown J.B., McDowell F.: Neck dissections for metastatic carcinoma. *Surg. Gynecol. Obstet.* 79:115–124, 1944.
43. Beahrs O.H., Gassel J.D., Hollingshead W.H.: Technique and surgical anatomy of radical neck dissection. *Am. J. Surg.* 90:490–516, 1955.
44. Beahrs O.H.: Surgical anatomy and technique of radical neck dissection. *Surg. Clin. North Am.* 57:663–700, 1971.
45. Bakamjiam V.Y., Miller S.E., Poole A.G.: A technique for radical dissection of the neck. *Surg. Gynecol. Obstet.* 144:419–424, 1977.
46. Roy P.H., Beahrs O.H.: Spinal accessory nerve in radical neck dissection. *Am. J. Surg.* 118:800–804, 1969.
47. Weitz J.W., Weitz S.L., Mc Elhinney A.J.: A technique for preservation of spinal accessory nerve function in radical neck dissection. *Head Neck Surg.* 5:75–78, 1982.
48. Marchetta F.C., Sako K.: Modified neck dissection for carcinoma of the thyroid gland. *Surg. Gynecol. Obstet.* 119:551–558, 1964.
49. Carenfelt C., Eliasson K.: Cervical metastases following radical neck dissection that preserved the spinal accessory nerve. *Head Neck Surg.* 2:181–184, 1980.
50. Marchetta F.C., Sako K., Matsura H.: Modified neck dissection for carcinoma of the thyroid gland. *Am. J. Surg.* 120:452–454, 1970.
51. Jesse R.H., Ballantyne A.J., Larson D.: Radical or modified neck dissection: A therapeutic dilemma. *Am. J. Surg.* 136:516–519, 1978.
51b. Schuller D.E., et al.: Analysis of disability resulting from treatment including radical neck dissection or modified radical neck dissection. *Head Neck Surg.* 6:551–558, 1983.
52. Ballantyne A.J., Guinn G.A.: Reduction of shoulder disability after neck dissection. *Am. J. Surg.* 112:662–665, 1966.
53. Ballantyne A.: Selecting the proper type of neck dissection. Surgical Rounds 6(9):84–89, 1983.
54. Bocca E., Pignataro O., Oldini C.: Supraglottic laryngectomy: 30 years of experience. *Ann. Otol. Rhinol. Laryngol.* 92:14–18, 1983.
55. Sugarbaker E.D., Wiley H.M.: Intracranial pressure studies incident to resection of the internal jugular veins. *Cancer* 4:242, 1951.
56. Loeb M., McQuarrie D.G.: Management of simultaneous bilateral neck dissection. *Surg. Gynecol. Obstet.* 127:1322–1323, 1968.
57. McQuarrie D.G., Mayberg M., Ferguson M., et al.: Reduction of free water clearance with cephalic venous hypertension. *Arch. Surg.* 113:573–580, 1978.
58. Kennedy J.T., Krause C.J., Loevy S.: The importance of tumor attachment to the carotid artery. *Arch. Otolaryngol.* 103:70–73, 1977.
59. Ehrenfeld W.K., Stoney R.J., Wylie E.: Relation of carotid stump pressure to safety of carotid artery ligation. *Surgery* 93:299–305, 1983.
60. McCready R.A., Hyde G.L., Bivens B.A., et al.: Radiation-induced arterial injuries. *Surgery* 93:306–312, 1983.
61. Djalilian M., Weiland L.H., Devine K., et al.: Significance of jugular vein invasion by metastatic carcinoma in radical neck dissection. *Am. J. Surg.* 126:566–569, 1973.
62. Wander J.V., Chandhuri P.K.: Dissection of the posterior part of the neck. *Surg. Gynecol. Obstet.* 143:97–100, 1976.

10 / Interdisciplinary Care and Management: Planning for the Patient's Informed Involvement

DONALD G. MCQUARRIE, M.D., PH.D.

THE CHAPTERS to this point have presented some common aspects of head and neck cancer that are fundamental to treatment and management decisions. When these are combined with the site- and tumor-specific information that will be provided in subsequent chapters, detailed clinical plans can be made. In actual clinical practice, it is frequently necessary to ask the patient for permission to proceed when there is only a suspicion of malignancy, or without an absolute plan. It is necessary to make tentative treatment plans with several options. This chapter introduces a general management framework that can be used in sharing information with the patient and the patient's family. The planning must have the latitude to accommodate unexpected findings and changes in the patient's condition. Informed consent is required.

WHO SHOULD BE IN CHARGE OF PRODUCING A TREATMENT PLAN AND COORDINATING CLINICAL CARE FOR THE PATIENT?

Most patients try to identify one professional who is in charge of their care. They wish to relate to an individual, not a committee. Some *one* physician must assume this role, particularly if the patient has some sense that he or she does or may have a life-threatening cancer. The physician in charge has the responsibility of identifying special patient needs. He must organize appropriate resources from other specialties and disciplines. The primary physician and primary ward nursing staff are helped when there is an easy and cooperative interspecialty exchange. Each patient's care plan can be put together by means of formal (rounds and conferences) or informal contacts. The composition of the care team will reflect the specific needs of the patient—one might call it "creative ad hocery." Achieving a "cure" or maximal control of the cancer is paramount. Function, cosmesis, a patient's emotional state, and rehabilitative potential can only deteriorate with uncontrolled disease.

When patients see multiple health care professionals, they wish to have one anchor person who serves as *their* doctor and interprets the often bewildering currents of care. Make sure one such person is identified and available.

WHO IS INVOLVED IN CARE FOR A HEAD AND NECK CANCER PATIENT?

Figure 10–1 presents a comprehensive framework for a care and management program. The more detailed algorithms provided in other chapters can be inserted to augment the details of care. This way of presenting a management program emphasizes three points. First, effective care requires intellectual and individualized input from the many disciplines noted along the top of the flow chart. Second, rehabilitation must be built into the initial planning phases. If rehabilitation is not adequately considered, procedures may be undertaken that prevent the later use of some rehabilitative techniques. Third, it is essential to communicate to the patient that the plan for his care extends far beyond a simple ablation of the malignancy. In his Grant Ward memorial address, the late Dr. Robert Chambers reported on a comprehensive head and neck cancer rehabilitation center at John Hopkins University.[1] He stressed the primary purposes as "(1) The best possible care for the head and neck cancer patient, utilizing a team approach; (2) preoperative and postoperative education, treatment, and counseling; and (3) total rehabilitation of the patient encompassing emotional, mental, physical, social and vocational aspects." Most medical centers with lower case loads must attempt to match the same functions with a more impromptu organization.

The plan shown in Figure 10–1 does not emphasize adequately the key role of nursing personnel. They must support and help inform the patient in the preoperative, perioperative, and postoperative phases. They must project a positive attitude and interest to produce favorable patient responses.

HOW DO WE GO WRONG WITH PLANS FOR TREATMENT AND REHABILITATION OF HEAD AND NECK CANCER?

When a patient thought to have a head and neck cancer is seen, the physician's judgment must be evaluated for common errors. Two experienced surgeons, Dr. John Loré and Dr. Donald Shedd, summarized 19 major points of error:[2]

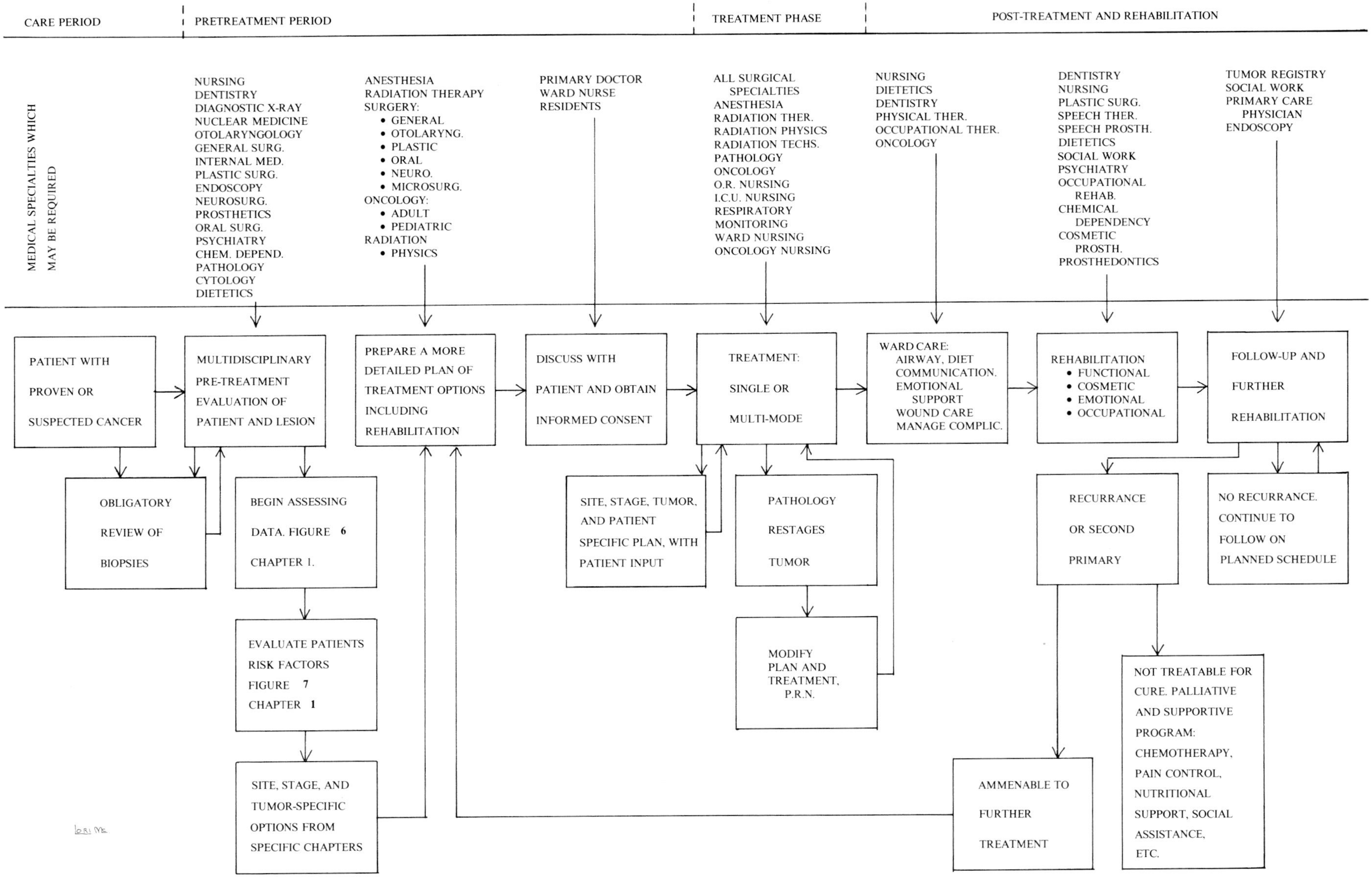

Fig 10–1.—Comprehensive approach to the care and management of a patient with head and neck cancer.

Sound clinical management, as collectively developed over years of accumulated experience, is sometimes better expressed in negative rather than positive terms — what should not be done, or pitfalls to avoid.

The following are stated in terms of *unsound* practices:

1. Open biopsy of a lump in the neck before performing a complete head and neck and general physical examinations.
2. Inadequate *incisional* biopsy of an oral cavity lesion.
3. Inadequate *excisional* biopsy of a suspicious oral cavity lesion.
4. Failure to review previous histopathology slides.
5. Permitting a single histopathologic benign diagnosis to override a clinical diagnosis of carcinoma. Repeat biopsies may be needed.
6. Biopsy of the larynx, hypopharynx, nasopharynx, esophagus, or trachea prior to radiologic studies, when such studies are indicated to aid in the evaluation of the extent of disease.
7. Lack of multidisciplinary approach, where indicated.
8. Tailoring the scope of surgical resection to the ability of the surgeon rather than to the objective requirements imposed by the lesion.
9. Compromise of the ablative phase of surgery in order to accommodate limited reconstructive skills.
10. Compromise of surgical margins because radiation therapy or chemotherapy was or is to be given. Conversely, giving less than an adequate tumor dose of radiation therapy with the intent of resorting to surgical excision of any residual disease.
11. Performing the right operation on the wrong patient. Some patients may not tolerate a technically feasible operation.
12. Assessing the degree of success or failure of radiation therapy on the basis of the response of the lesion during or immediately on completion of treatment.
13. Failure to realize the implications of the "condemned mucosa" or multiple primary syndrome.
14. Failure to perform a complete general physical examination, as well as a complete head and neck examination.
15. Prolonged watch-and-wait attitude in the face of an asymptomatic mass.
16. Inadequate search for an occult primary.
17. Abandonment of the patient with neck metastasis from an undetectable primary.
18. Enucleation of tumors of the major salivary glands and thyroid gland.
19. Treating a patient with a head and neck lesion with antibiotics for an extended period of time without a biopsy.

WHAT DO WE NEED TO TELL THE PATIENT ABOUT HIS HEAD AND NECK CANCER AND THE TREATMENT PLANS?

Dr. Hayes Martin proposed good and humane suggestions for discussing therapeutic options with patients:[3]

> "Experience proves that if the surgeon (therapist) firmly believes in the soundness of his recommendations and if he gives due consideration to the sensibilities of the patient, he will have few refusals of even the most extensive operation (treatment). While it is obvious that some person in the family should be apprised of the facts, no matter how grim, the patient may well be approached more gently, carefully avoiding such cruel and careless terms as take out your larynx, remove your eye, or cut off your breast.
>
> Expressions like these, and blunt references to cancer, which are so often associated in the lay mind with desperate connotations of hopelessness, suffering, and death, may well result in panic, causing the patient to run for cover to anyone (sometimes even charlatans) who may offer what appears to be a less drastic solution to the problem.
>
> Many patients can face danger with less fear if they are spared the exact specifications of the risk. In certain cases they will accept with confidence total laryngectomy or radical resection of the maxilla if they are sustained by the surgeon's promise that he will do his best to save the larynx, or the eye, or other important structure. This statement is, of course, the truth, for he always would save what he could.

Since the early 1960s, when this was written, there has been a drastic change in legal and societal attitudes toward involving patients in the therapeutic decision process. Casual patient aquiescence will not prevent agonizing, post facto unscientific litigation. The contemporary patient usually wants to participate in decision-making. Informed consent is the order of the day. The wide spectrum of treatment options for head and neck cancer is producing an increasing number of lawsuits. Many are based on failure to obtain informed consent or lack of timely diagnosis. It is doubtful whether patient understanding, memory retention, or bent of mind allows a truly informed consent, but the responsible physician has a clear duty to present alternatives, plans, risks, and benefits to patients. You must work to retain a humane gentility in carrying out the requirements of informed consent. It is difficult but not impossible.

WHAT CONSTITUTES INFORMED CONSENT?

Any person treating head and neck cancer should be familiar with the minimum criteria.

In the classic case of *Schloendoff v. Society of New York Hospital*, 211 NY 125, 105 NE 92, 93 (1914), the courts held that:

> Every human being of adult years and sound mind has a right to determine what shall be done with his own body, and a surgeon who performs an operation without his patient's consent commits an assault for which he is liable in damages.

There are two recognized forms of consent: express consent and implied consent. *Express consent* is given in words, which may be spoken or written. The practical problems involved in proving an effective oral consent are substantial. Always strive to get a specifically detailed written consent. *Implied consent* arises by reasonable inference from the conduct of the patient. Its underlying basis is that the patient's actions demonstrate his acceptance of the procedure. This assumes that his action is voluntary and that the patient has actual or apparent knowledge of what is to transpire. In actual practice this may be sufficient for minor procedures, like venipuncture. However, it would be difficult to show that a nonprofessional patient understood the risks and problems of complex cancer care. For treatment of head and neck cancer, written consent with adequate documentation specific to the procedure(s) and the patient is a must.

Extension of Consent

As a general rule, the patient's consent is limited to those procedures contemplated when consent is given. Additional modified consent is needed for additional procedures to remedy conditions discovered during performance of the contemplated procedure. The physician should try to obtain formal consent which covers as many contingent problems as possible. The requirement for additional permission is subject to two major exceptions. The first exception applies when the context of the permission indicates that the patient consented to treatment for the general purpose of remedying a *condition* rather than limiting consent to a particular therapeutic procedure. The background facts and documentation are important. The courts have not paid much attention to a routine carte blanche on a preprinted consent form. In treating a head and neck cancer, or the possibility of cancer, permission and documentation should show that the patient agrees to treating the malignant disease and to making all necessary efforts to achieve cure. It is better if possible variations are specifically discussed. There should be no specific prohibitions against removal of tissues or against any specific procedures (see below). If the consent of a patient is directed to one specific procedure, there may be an implied prohibition of any other procedure. For example, courts usually require specific consent when a body part is to be removed and will not readily accept implied consent to significant tissue removal. *The courts have been reluctant to recognize implied consent where the procedure alters reproductive capacity, removes a breast, removes an eye, or produces significant cosmetic deformity.* Presumably this would extend to laryngectomy, removal of a mandible, removal of an ear, and so forth. For head and neck cancer, nothing replaces good informed consent and permission for adequate therapeutic options in achieving the best chance of cure.

The second exception in a cancer operation the patient cannot be consulted in midprocedure. There may not be a spouse or someone who can give consent on the patient's behalf. In a much quoted case, *Kennedy v. Parrot,* the court fashioned the following rule:

> In short, where an internal operation is indicated, a surgeon may lawfully perform, *and it is his duty to perform,* such operation as good surgery demands, even when it means an extension of the operation further than was originally contemplated, and for so doing he is not to be held in damages for an unauthorized operation.

This particular opinion held because no organ was removed and reproductive capacity was not impaired. The extension of the procedure was minor, permission had been granted to have a condition remedied, and the procedure did not materially increase the risk to the patient. If there is an unforeseen necessity to alter or extend procedures beyond that covered by the permission form, the surgeon should get adequate, additional broad consultation in the operating room and have the consultants document their concurrence with the changes.

A patient may express limits of consent. For head and neck cancer treatment, if a patient expressly prohibits a specific medical or surgical procedure, the surgeon cannot claim implied consent. If a patient has expressly prohibited extension of a procedure to include orbital exenteration or laryngectomy, the surgeon may *not* extend the procedure to these areas without the patient's consent. The courts have a strong regard for a patient's stated wishes, even when those wishes conflict with the exercise of sound medical judgment. Prior restraints of this nature should be taken seriously. Where medical judgment dictates the possibility of certain procedures, special efforts should be made to convince the patient to withdraw any such obstacles prior to surgery, regardless of how trivial or unlikely to occur they may seem.

The patient must also be informed as to the exact identities and status of the surgeons who will be performing the procedure. Where an educational program or other special factors make substitution of practitioners desirable, the patient's knowledgeable agreement to the substitution should be carefully documented.

Informed Consent

Cases have been won on the basis of negligent nondisclosure. It is important to know that *formal consent* and *informed consent* are very different terms. The mere act of signing a consent form is construed by most courts as evidence of the fact that some type of discussion was held with the patient about the contemplated procedure. A related but separate question revolves around the information given by the physician to the patient about the procedure. The courts have held that the physician must disclose enough information to allow the patient to make an informed decision about the surgery.

The standards of disclosure are as follows:

1. The *reasonable physician* standard requires that the information communicated to the patient be similar to that given by other physicians in similar circum-

stances. A minority of states currently recognize this standard.

2. The *reasonable patient* standard requires that the physician give the amount of information which a reasonable patient in similar circumstances would need to make an informed decision. This view is held by the majority of states.

3. One state Supreme Court has held that a physician can be held liable for negligent nondisclosure if he fails to disclose the risks or alternatives to a proposed course of treatment when "a reasonable person in what the physician knows or should have known to be the patient's position would likely attach significance to that risk or alternative in formulating his decision to consent to treatment." Similar rulings have been made in other states.

4. *For a plaintiff to be successful in a case based on informed consent, he must first establish that the physician breached his duty to the patient, that there was damage, and that the damage was caused by the procedure. More specifically, a plaintiff must establish a duty on the part of the physician to know of a risk or alternative treatment program. He must also show a duty to disclose the risk or alternative treatment plan by evidence establishing what a reasonable person would likely consider significant. He would use knowledge of that risk or alternative to formulate his decision to consent to treatment.* The objective test is whether a reasonable person in the plaintiff's position would have refused treatment had he been informed of the risks. If the plaintiff successfully sustains the burden of proof on the breach of duty and causation, he must also prove that the undisclosed risk produced harm.

The key elements of informed consent are:

1. Patient is competent (over age 18 with unimpaired mental capacity).
2. Consent is voluntary.
3. Sufficient information is given about the following:
   The nature of the procedure.
   Probable consequences (desirable and undesirable results that will probably occur).
   Possible material risks that may occur.
   Alternatives, with their probable consequences.
   Problems in recuperation and/or rehabilitation.
4. The information is understood by the patient.

Situations which may not require informed consent:

1. *Risks generally known.*—When a relatively minor risk is also inherent in a procedure and is common knowledge to a reasonable patient, then the risk need not be disclosed. Thus, in the case of blood transfusion, the 0.13% chance of hepatitis did not have to be disclosed, according to a federal court in Tennessee.

2. *Patient asks not to be told.*—If the patient has the right to know the procedure's nature, risks, and alternatives, then the patient has the right to waive the right.

3. *Emergency.*—An emergency is a condition which constitutes an immediate danger to the life or health of the patient and which precludes taking time to obtain consent from the patient or next of kin. If an emergency tracheotomy is needed to restore an airway, do not debate the niceties of informed consent. Do it. If time permits, a reasonable effort should be made to obtain a consent. The record should show this effort.

4. *Therapeutic privilege.*—When in the physician's opinion disclosure would complicate or hinder treatment, cause psychological harm, or upset the patient so much as to render him unable to make a decision, then consent need not be obtained from the patient. *The fact that disclosure might create anxiety in a patient is not sufficient to warrant application of this exception.*

Before opting to treat a patient under the therapeutic privilege, a physician should obtain consultation with another physician to make an independent determination that there is a real basis to rely on this exception. He should document exactly what risks are being withheld from the patient's knowledge and why. The physician is then best advised to disclose those risks to the appropriate next of kin and to document that fact also.

An adequate documentation of consent includes:

1. Name of the physician(s) who will perform the procedure.

2. Name of the possible operations or procedures which may be done.

3. Approval to treat a particular condition and correct it.

4. Nature and purpose of the operation or procedure, and what is expected to be accomplished, in plain English.

5. Statement of general risks (e.g., death, paralysis, hemorrhage, and infection), and risks specific to this procedure, in plain English. Any tissues which must be removed should be stated, as should any permanent functional impairment.

6. Alternatives and their probable consequences which are discussed with the patient should be mentioned in plain English.

Some suggested guidelines for complying with consent requirements:

1. Understand the state consent laws, and the hospital's requirements for obtaining and documenting consent.

2. Discuss the proposed treatment or procedure with the patient, or with his legal guardian, preferrably with a witness present.

3. Obtain a consent form. We use the back of the

form to draw diagrams of procedures or to outline alternative programs.

4. *Document the consent discussion in a separate progress note or office chart. When the consent discussion is waived by the patient, or when the physician elects to forego it, the reasons should be documented.*

NOTE: This material is not intended as legal advice. Surgeons should discuss the contents of consent forms and review consent requirements with a qualified attorney. It is advisable to obtain hospital approval before changes are made in established policies and procedures.

How can a physician blend the good advice of Dr. Martin with the conflicting rigors of legal responsibility under informed consent?

We have been fairly successful in patient relations with a policy of full and honest sharing of information with the patients. The presentation of the therapy plan is balanced by discussing each problem created by treatment in the context of a parallel rehabilitation effort. If large tissue losses are needed to encompass a tumor, the patient is presented with the efforts for maximum primary reconstructive effort during the major resective operation. Future reconstructive options are sketched in general terms. If radiation xerostomia is anticipated, we discuss the posttreatment use of the synthetic salivas. Occasionally, if a patient is unusually anxious about a procedure that is minimally disfiguring, a photograph of a patient who has undergone a similar procedure is reassuring. Most larger communities have a laryngectomy support group who will be happy to send a rehabilitated patient of similar gender, age, and occupation to visit the patient and discuss speech rehabilitation. It is essential at this early stage to set an optimistic tone and help establish the patient's motivation to achieve his rehabilitation potential. He should meet the members of the care team.

Many times, the largest help to the patient is to give him the time and emotional support to work through the decision process at his own pace. The physician in charge should be available to answer initial questions and subsequent repeated questions. If a spouse or other family members are involved, the physician should schedule at least one leisurely session with them. It is amazing how the retelling of a medical team's advice, recommendations, and plans can be distorted. The family should know the risks, the plans, and the rehabilitation effort which is planned. From day to day, the powerful forces of denial will alter the patient's perceptions of what is going on.

Through the years, you learn to volunteer answers to many unasked questions.

Q. What is the risk to my life of the treatment?

A. Minimal risk to your life!

Q. Will I look like some of the patients I see on the ward, like Mr. ______?

A. Some of the patients on the ward have far-advanced cancers. Your treatment will be entirely different. Mr. ______ has never had a cancer; he is being reconstructed after a severe shotgun injury to the face.

Q. Will I loose my voice? (when the operation will never be near the larynx).

A. No, your voicebox will work just fine. You may have trouble forming some sounds (if the mouth or pharynx is involved). When you first wake up, the temporary tracheostomy will keep you from talking for 10 days or so unless you put your finger over the end to let air go through your voicebox.

Q. What happens to me if the treatment doesn't cure the cancer?

A. There are other effective treatments we can employ in an attempt to salvage failure from one type of therapy, and sometimes this does produce a cure. If not, there are other steps we can take to achieve additional periods of useful comfortable living. We'll be here to help you.

Q. Why did I get this (squamous cell oropharyngeal) cancer?

A. In almost every instance (of squamous cancer) the cancer can be related to the use of tobacco in one form or other. Alcohol use aggravates the problem. If you are to avoid a new cancer, you must stop using tobacco and alcohol. We will help you find a program to help you.

Q. Will people be repelled by my appearance?

A. There are many people with war injuries or accidental injuries who have more deformity than the treatment will produce. After a short time, close friends no longer notice. Many steps can be taken to change or mask the deformity. Most strangers are quite understanding. When you are up and around after your operation, we'll have you go into different areas of the hospital where visitors are and you will see that there are very few problems. Those you encounter, we will help you with.

In general, you should anticipate the unexpressed fears of the patient and provide answers or a "leading" opportunity to bring hidden questions and issues into rational discussion.

REFERENCES

1. Chambers R.G.: The Grant E. Ward Memorial Lecture: Total rehabilitation of the patient with head and neck cancer. *Am. J. Surg.* 142:431–433, 1981.

2. Loré J.M., Shedd D.P.: Common departures from sound management, in Hamner J.E. III (ed.): *Management Guidelines for Head and Neck Cancer,* NIH publication No. 80–2037. Washington, D.C., U.S. Department of Health, Education and Welfare, September 1979, pp. 7–31.
3. Martin H.: Radical neck dissection. *Ciba Clin. Symp.* 13(4):103–116, 1961.

11 / Perioperative Adjunctive Care in Head and Neck Cancer Surgery

James T. Lee, Jr., M.D., Ph.D. / Graeme A. Browne, B.Sc., M.Sc., B.D.S., F.R.C.D.

I. Perioperative Prophylactic Antibiotics

James T. Lee, Jr., M.D., Ph.D.

WHAT ARE THE KEY ELEMENTS IN PREVENTING WOUND INFECTION?

A PATIENT'S smooth recovery from a potentially curative operation for head and neck cancer can be ruined by a wound infection. Extra morbidity, discomfort, expense, and even death can be the consequences. Emphasis on this iatrogenic complication should always rest squarely on *prevention*. Wound infection requires antecedent wound contamination. All elective surgical wounds probably become contaminated to some degree during the operation, yet many heal without infection after suture closure. The outcome hinges on the interplay of factors characteristic of both the patient and the bacterial pathogens. In head and neck surgery, intraoperative contamination may be slight and of no consequence (e.g., during a thyroidectomy) or may be serious and essentially continuous in the early postoperative recovery period (e.g., following floor of mouth tumor resection with node dissection). If local and systemic host defenses swiftly eliminate the bacteria from previously sterile planes, there will be minimal impact on orderly healing, infection will not occur, and local inflammation will be of appropriate intensity and duration. In contrast, if bacterial challenge is overwhelming from the onset, if the challenge is unchecked in wound depths postoperatively, if host defenses are suboptimal (e.g., in diabetic, malnourished, or steroid-dependent patients), or if local factors (e.g., technically imperfect closure, dead space, hematoma, or prior radiation therapy) mitigate the delivery or crisp expression of host defenses, then wound contamination may progress unchecked to invasive soft tissue infection with stimulation of inflammation beyond levels customarily associated with normal repair. These undesired circumstances define wound infection; healing will be delayed until the infection resolves.

In the dynamic contamination-infection sequence just described, a surgeon has limited opportunities to sense trouble and tip the balance in favor of natural processes whose aggregate purpose is rapid, early destruction of all bacteria, clearance of their toxic products, and restoration of a wound repair sequence leading to healing. Wound infection in modern head and neck surgical practice can often be prevented or held to very low rates by attention to the many facets of aseptic surgical technique and thoughtful exploitation of various adjunctive maneuvers. Surgical antibiotic prophylaxis, defined as the administration of antibiotics *before* the onset of intraoperative bacterial contamination to prevent subsequent bacterial growth and invasive infection, is an adjunct whose value has been established in general surgery by laboratory[1, 2] and clinical studies.[3–5] It is important to distinguish this use of antibiotics from therapeutic applications, in which antibiotics are prescribed, often for prolonged time periods, to treat established and clinically obvious infections, which may or may not be culture proved at the time therapy begins. Antibiotic prophylaxis is therefore a *presumptive* intervention calculated specifically to kill bacteria that will lodge in a sterile wound during the discrete time period between skin incision and wound closure.[6, 7] The timing of the dose(s) and accurate preoperative prediction of the most likely contaminants are the determinants of success, which may be dramatic. The proper place of antibiotics in the armamentarium has not always been clear, and the surgical literature contains thousands of pages devoted to debate, discussion, and disagreement over this point. A few studies[8–12] pertain specifically to head and neck surgical procedures in which correctly designed trials have often shown a benefit of antibiotics. Much of the adverse criticism of past antibiotic use by surgeons was correctly directed at clearly inappropriate use of drugs in ways that produced, at best, no benefit, and at worst, patient hazards from allergic reactions, side effects, or infections by hospital organisms.[3, 13–15] Modern antibiotics are very safe and provide attractive risk-benefit ratios if used with discretion in head and neck cancer surgery. The most pertinent factors in justifying their use is classification of an operation's wound infection potential.

ARE ANTIBIOTICS INDICATED IN "CLEAN" HEAD AND NECK SURGERY?

In "clean" head and neck operations, where a dissection into the oropharynx, nasopharynx, or hypopharynx is not required, the potentially infecting bacteria are, predictably, the patient's skin flora or those from the hospital environment. Data from several studies confirm that *Staphylococcus* is the most frequent offender.[16–18] Proper skin decontamination before draping and strict aseptic operating room deportment are time-tested and effective prophylactic measures here, and many surgeons routinely realize wound infection rates of 1% or less. Clean case perioperative antibiotic use is *not* recommended. It has been impossible, in reliable studies,[8–10, 12, 18] to detect any impact of antibiotics on clean wound infection rates in head and neck surgery, which supports the arguments that antibiotic use in clean cases is superfluous,[3] dangerous,[3, 19] or economically irresponsible[13] and insidiously encourages a relaxed attitude toward other aspects of wound toilet.[14] Clinical experience must influence preoperative choices when patients scheduled for clean surgery might have an increased chance of wound infection. It has been suggested that prior irradiation of the neck area[20] may be adverse; malignancy, severe malnutrition, and diabetes are cited[7, 18] as generally inimical. Pending a randomized study that addresses exactly the question of whether clean cases in head and neck cancer surgery should ever be "covered" with prophylactic antibiotics, surgeons can only individualize preoperative decisions about their use. We follow the guidelines in Table 11–1, recognizing that the risk and cost of a few antibiotic doses are minimal.

WHY ARE ANTIBIOTICS NECESSARY IN "CLEAN-CONTAMINATED" CASES?

"Clean-contaminated" operations have been defined as procedures in which the respiratory, alimentary, or genitourinary tract is entered without unusual complications, or which produce wounds that are mechanically drained.[18] Routine antibiotic prophylaxis has not always been used by some surgeons in these types of operations, but composite head and neck cancer operations, those in which neck dissection and/or flap mobilization accompanies mucosal penetration of the oral cavity, are definitely exceptional. It is impossible to sterilize the oropharyngeal cavity, and there is always a significant risk of wound infection by the rich mixed flora of this cavity; *these infections can be disastrous.* An important characteristic of the reconstructed tissues in the early postoperative period cannot be overemphasized: continued bathing of fresh, sometimes tenuous mucosal suture lines with large inocula of live, pathogenic bacteria, with real potential for a trapped collection of these bacteria (with or without drains!) in a functionally closed space. Furthermore, the very patients who require these extensive operations are often in a poor-risk category at the outset, with poor general health and/or malnutrition.[21] It is our position that the omission of antibiotic coverage in clean-contaminated head and neck cases is an egregious mistake that will guarantee a prohibitive wound infection rate.

TABLE 11–1.—SUMMARY OF RECOMMENDATIONS FOR PERIOPERATIVE ANTIBIOTIC USE IN CLEAN AND CLEAN-CONTAMINATED HEAD AND NECK CANCER OPERATIONS

CATEGORY	ANTIBIOTIC	DOSE PATTERN
Clean case (e.g., thyroid surgery, radical neck dissection)	None	None
Clean case exception	Cefazolin*	1 gm IV at the induction of anesthesia; repeat q8h for total of 24 hr
Clean-contaminated case (e.g., composite resection for laryngeal cancer)	Cefazolin†	1 gm IV at the induction of anesthesia; repeat q8h for total of 72 hr‡

*In patients with definite penicillin allergy, substitute erythromycin, 500 mg IV, at the induction of anesthesia, then 500 mg IV q6h thereafter for a total dose period of 24 hours.

†In patients with definite penicillin allergy, substitution of tetracycline, chloroamphenicol, or aminoglycosides may be required, depending on sensitivity patterns of gram-negative aerobes in a given hospital; consultation with an infectious disease specialist is recommended.

‡Extension of dose period or empirical change to other antibiotic(s) may be indicated, based on wound examination, culture results, or clinical assessment. Extension is desirable in cases where exposed bone surfaces or prosthetic materials are contaminated.

HOW IS A PROPHYLACTIC ANTIBIOTIC CHOSEN?

The coverage spectrum of a "perfect" prophylactic antibiotic regimen would encompass only the bacterial populations encountered during the operation. There is no such drug or combination of drugs. In attempts to hone the accuracy of preoperative predictions of wound infection pathogens and provide data germane to more specific antibiotic selection, several workers have discovered that assiduous cultures of skin and oral flora before surgery are notoriously unreliable guides to subsequent wound infection isolates.[8, 17] Yoder and Silva have shown that even meticulous postoperative cultures of suction drain effluents will not provide better than coin-toss accuracy (47% vs. 50%) in forecasting which patients will have a wound infection after clean-contaminated head and neck operations.[22] In view of the uncertainties, selection of the prophylactic agent must be guided by literature reports and an updated awareness of microbiology laboratory sensitivity patterns for wound isolates in a particular surgeon's practice. Bacteriologic data from several investigations[8, 9, 17, 18] confirm the high frequency of mixed infections with aerobes (e.g., *Staphylococcus, Streptococcus, E. coli, Proteus, Klebsiella,* and *Pseudomonas sp.*) and numerous anaerobes, including fusiforms, *Actinomyces*, streptococci, and the *Bacteroides* species indigenous to the mouth. Colonization of the oral cavity with hospital-acquired gram-negative bacilli, often resistant to multiple antibiotics, is a frequent finding in chronically ill patients[19] and many head and neck cancer patients.

Is there a "best compromise" antibiotic for prophylactic use? Penicillin has excellent activity against many normal flora of the mouth, including the anaerobes, and will also kill many of the gram-positive skin flora.[4] However, many *Staphylococcus* strains and numerous gram-negative rods are not sensitive to this cheap, otherwise suitable drug. Recent investigations have addressed this problem. Some groups[9, 11] have employed penicillin derivatives (e.g., ampicillin, cloxacillin, carbenicillin), two-drug combinations, or single broad-spectrum agents[8, 12] to fill perceived penicillin coverage gaps. Cefazolin, a first-generation cephalosporin, is attractive. This drug is safe, cheap in short courses, has useful pharmacokinetic properties in man, and has a spectrum covering the gram-positive organisms, including *Staphylococcus*, many gram-negative aerobes, and the normal oral anaerobes.[23] *Pseudomonas* and some *Klebsiella* species are not sensitive to cefazolin. In the rare patient with a definite history of anaphylaxis or other severe and immediate allergic reaction to penicillin, any of the cephalosporins would be contraindicated.

What can the surgeon do when faced with this problem? Available literature is of little help. Coverage of both gram-negative bacilli and oral anaerobes must be provided and some improvisation is required. Our suggestions are outlined in Table 11–1. There is little disagreement that a prophylactic antibiotic will be maximally effective if given parenterally just before skin incision to guarantee bactericidal levels of drug in the tissues at the time of contamination,[3] but there is no consensus about the acceptable duration of coverage. Arbitrary definitions range from zero (i.e., just a preoperative dose) to 24 hours to even 3 days.[13] In clean-contaminated cases, clinical judgment may dictate that "prophylaxis" be continued for some days post-operatively as "therapy." This shift in tactics must be accompanied by two realizations: (1) every potential adverse effect of the drug (e.g., cost, superinfection, skin rash) will be directly proportional to the duration of its use, and (2) the process that one is attempting to "treat" may involve organisms that are not sensitive to the antibiotic. The most realistic approach is one that finds the surgeon focusing not on semantics but on the appearance of the wound and the patient's progress.

Five clinical studies (Table 11–2) have shown clear benefit of antibiotic prophylaxis in clean-contaminated head/neck cancer surgery. Robinson noted a 64% infection rate after laryngectomy without antibiotics but reduced the rate threefold by simply dusting the wound with an antibiotic mixture before closure.[11] A systemic route of administration probably provides a more dependable penetration of wound tissues.[3] Becker and Parell found that 29 placebo-treated patients undergoing clean-contaminated operations had an 87% infection rate;[8] this alarming statistic was reduced to 38% in 32 patients treated with perioperative cefazolin, and these workers argued that salivary contamination of the wound postoperatively was a likely cause of the high infection rate in the treated group and proposed that a period of therapy with the drug was one solution. Seagle et al. studied 34 patients and found a 70% wound infection rate without antibiotic use but an infection rate of 24% when perioperative cefazolin was given.[12] Dor and Klastersky used a double-drug regimen to broaden coverage in a study of 80 patients who received placebo or systemic ampicillin/cloxacillin.[9] The placebo group infection rate of 41% was bested by a treatment group infection rate of 20%. Finally, in the ultimate example of spectrum broadening, recent studies by Johnson et al. have substantiated the need for broad-spectrum coverage and provided the first results of third-generation cephalosporin prophylaxis in head and neck surgery.[24, 25] These new drugs offer the theoretical advantages of β-lactamase resistance and very broad coverage that includes many anaerobes, the common skin organisms, and an impressive assortment of

TABLE 11–2.—EFFICACY OF PROPHYLACTIC ANTIBIOTICS IN CLEAN-CONTAMINATED HEAD AND NECK CANCER OPERATIONS

STUDY	ANTIBIOTIC(S)	WOUND INFECTION RATES Treated	Placebo
Dor and Klastersky[9]	Ampicillin and cloxacillin by mouth or NG tube, 250 mg q6h for 5 days, started 24 hr preoperatively	20% (8/39)	41% (17/41)
Robinson[11]	2 gm 50% ampicillin/carbenicillin powder mixture; wound dusted before closure performed	23% (3/13)	64% (7/11)
Becker and Parell[8]	Cefazolin, 1 gm IV or IM 2 hr preop.; 500 mg q6h for total of 4 doses	38% (12/32)	87% (20/23)
Seagle et al.[12]	Cefazolin, 1 gm IV 12 hrs preop.; 1 gm q6h for total of 4 doses	24% (4/17)	70% (12/17)
Johnson et al.[24]	Cefotaxime or cefoperazone, 2 gm IV starting 1 hr preop; q6h for total of 4 doses	10% (7/71)	78% (7/9)

gram-negative aerobes. Newer multiple-drug combinations can match the third-generation drugs' impressive efficacy. Johnson et al. showed an improved wound infection rate (4%–7%) when clindamycin and gentamicin combined were compared to cefazolin alone (20%–33%) in clean-contaminated patients.[24] No benefits were realized by extension of dosing from 24 hours to 5 days. In a separate study, they additionally blindly randomized patients to receive placebo, cefotaxime, or cefaperazone before surgery. The wound infection rate was 10% in the combined antibiotic groups, but the nine placebo recipients had to be identified early in the study after seven serious infections (78%), including several systemic sepsis episodes.[25, 26] The patients receiving these two drugs had no detected side effects and the series is being extended. If the claimed infection rates are further verified in independent studies, a new era of improved infection control in head and neck cancer surgery may be at hand; alternatively, this optimism may ultimately be dampened by the occurrence of wound sepsis secondary to resistant organisms.

Taken together, the five quoted studies demonstrate an averaged infection rate of 20% in clean-contaminated head and neck operations when antibiotics have been used, a placebo group averaged infection rate of well over 65%, and no admitted instances of antibiotic complications. Two conclusions are in order: human studies research committees should no longer allow placebo groups in studies of head and neck surgical antibiotics, and prophylactic antibiotic use is mandatory in clean-contaminated cases.

REFERENCES

1. Alexander J.W., Altemeier W.A.: Penicillin prophylaxis of experimental staphylococcal wound infections. *Surg. Gynecol. Obstet.* 120:243–254, 1965.
2. Miles A.A., Miles E.M., Burke J.H.: The value and duration of defense reactions of the skin in primary lodgement of bacteria. *Br. J. Exp. Pathol.* 38:79–96, 1957.
3. Hunt T.K., Alexander J.W., Burke J.F., et al.: Antibiotics in surgery. *Arch. Surg.* 110:148–155, 1975.
4. Kisch A.L.: Principles of antimicrobial therapy of head and neck infections. *Surg. Clin. North Am.* 9:751–769, 1976.
5. Polk H.C. Jr., Lopez-Mayor J.F.: Postoperative wound infection: A prospective study of determinant factors and prevention. *Surgery* 66:97–103, 1969.
6. Darrell J.H.: Antibiotics in the prevention of postoperative infection, in Mathiew A., Burke J. (eds.): *Infection and the Perioperative Period.* New York, Grune & Stratton, 1982, pp. 119–135.
7. Ketcham A.S., Block J.H., Crawford D.T., et al.: The role of prophylactic antibiotic therapy in control of staphylococcal infections following cancer surgery. *Surg. Gynecol. Obstet.* 114:345–352, 1962.
8. Becker G.D., Parell G.J.: Cefazolin prophylaxis in head and neck cancer surgery. *Ann. Otol.* 88:183–186, 1979.
9. Dor P., Klastersky J.: Prophylactic antibiotics in oral, pharyngeal, and laryngeal surgery for cancer: a double-blind study. *Laryngoscope* 83:1992–1998, 1973.
10. Eschelman L.T., Schleuning A.J., Brummett R.E.: Prophylactic antibiotics in otolaryngologic surgery: A double-blind study. *Trans. Am. Acad. Ophthalmol. Otol.* 75:387–394, 1971.
11. Robinson J.M.P.: Wound infection following laryngec-

tomy: The effect of topical ampicillin and carbenicillin. *J. Laryngol. Otol.* 90:415–425, 1976.

12. Seagle M.B., Duberstein L.E., Gross C.W., et al.: Efficacy of cefazolin as a prophylactic antibiotic in head and neck surgery. *Otolaryngology* 86:568–572, 1978.
13. Crossley K., and Gardner L.C.: Antimicrobial prophylaxis in surgical patients. *JAMA* 245:722–726, 1981.
14. Strong M.S.: Wound infection in otolaryngologic surgery and the inexpediency of antibiotic prophylaxis. *Laryngoscope* 73:165–184, 1963.
15. Weiner J.P., Gibson G., Munster A.M.: Use of prophylactic antibiotics in surgical procedures: Peer review guidelines as a method for quality assurance. *Arch. Surg.* 139:348–351, 1980.
16. Beahrs O.H.: Complications of surgery of the head and neck. *Surg. Clin. North Am.* 57:823–829, 1977.
17. Becker G.D., Parell G.J., Busch D., et al.: Anaerobic and aerobic bacteriology in head and neck cancer surgery. *Otolaryngology* 84:592–602, 1977.
18. Dipiro J.T., Bivins B.A., Record K.E., et al.: The prophylactic use of antimicrobials in surgery. *Curr. Probl. Surg.* 20:76–132, 1983.
19. Johanson W.G., Pierce A.K., Sanford J.P.: Changing pharyngeal bacterial flora of hospitalized patients. *N. Engl. J. Med.* 281:1137–1140, 1969.
20. Ketcham A.S., Hoye R.C., Chrètien P.B., et al.: Irradiation twenty-four hours preoperatively. *Am. J. Surg.* 118:691–697, 1969.
21. Fairbanks D.N.: Antimicrobial prophylaxis in otolaryngologic surgery. *Laryngoscope* 89:490–492, 1979.
22. Yoder M.G., Silva J.: Anaerobic isolates in Hemovac lines. *Laryngoscope* 87:63–71, 1977.
23. Thompson R.L., Wright A.J.: Cephalosporin antibiotics. *Mayo Clin. Proc.* 58:79–87, 1983.
24. Johnson J.T., Myers E.N., Thearle P.B., et al.: Antimicrobial prophylaxis for contaminated head and neck surgery. *Laryngoscope* 94:46–51, 1984.
25. Johnson J.T., Yu V.L., Meyer E.N., et al.: Efficacy of two third-generation cephalosporins in prophylaxis for head and neck surgery: A prospective, randomized, double-blind trial. *Arch. Otolaryngol.* 110:224–227, 1984.
26. Thearle P.B.: Personal communication.

II. Perioperative Nutritional Considerations

JAMES T. LEE, JR., M.D., PH.D.

WHEN IS MALNUTRITION ADVERSE IN HEAD AND NECK CANCER SURGERY?

THE STRATEGIC LOCATION of all head/neck cancers near the "front end" of the alimentary tract obligates a thoughtful surgeon to plan a systematic approach for patient nutrition in both the preoperative and postoperative periods. A simplifying strategy in such an approach is the recognition that many patients will not need specialized biochemcial testing, hyperalimentation, or close monitoring of calorie or protein economies. Although any head and neck tumor is, in principle, capable of major and ultimately complete interference with eating, many individuals with serious malignant diseases of the head and neck enter the hospital without detectable nutrition problems. It is hardly a coincidence that such patients are frequently those undergoing operations for earlier stage cancers that have not yet compromised eating mechanics. The required operations seldom cause significant delay in resumption of eating postoperatively either because of the limits or because of the site of dissection (e.g., excision of a small lip cancer, thyroid lobectomy, or parotidectomy), and perioperative fluid and diet orders are rudimentary. It is a happy circumstance to identify patients in this category, which may include the majority of cases in some practices. At the other extreme is a small but significant fraction of patients with preoperative malnourishment ranging from worrisome to catastrophic, determined for the most part by the extent to which large, encroaching neoplasms have disturbed ingestion, chewing, and swallowing of adequate, balanced meals. The anatomical position, shape, and size of the cancer are major variables. Possible causal mechanisms include anorexia, painful mastication, abnormal taste or smell functions, and dysphagia. When radiation or chemotherapy is employed as an adjunct to surgery, oral pain, xerostomia, or nausea and vomiting may hamper oral intake. The evolution of resultant nutritional damage and its aggregate systemic consequences in a particular patient is further modulated by the delay before the patient contacts the health care system and by the impact of long-standing, adverse dietary patterns secondary to poverty, past alcoholism, poor dental health, or coincident medical disorders.

Apart from simple mechanical interference with chewing and swallowing, systemic effects of neoplastic tissue are of more than academic concern. Cancer cachexia[1] has been a puzzle for years, and abnormalities in glucose metabolism, amino acid metabolism, and gluconeogenesis have been demonstrated in animals and suspected in man when various types of tumors are present.[2] A traditional notion is that malignant tissue can engender negative energy balance merely by competing for vital nutrients. This "tumor glucose trap" concept may partly explain the putatively increased metabolic rates and corresponding increased nutritional needs in patients with some types of cancer. Recently, the increasing sophistication of technology in the rapidly growing medical nutrition industry, a legitimate and lingering concern about possible tumor growth promotion in cachectic cancer victims receiving "artificial feeding," and the recognition that cancer patients often seem to have lost homeostatic control mechanisms that would otherwise limit protein wasting have combined to stimulate interest in biochemical probes of the unexplained quirks of energy and protein metabolism in human cancer. Burt et al.[2] found that forearm tissue glucose uptake and lactate release in patients with *localized* distal esophageal cancer could not be explained by weight loss alone but required a dual mechanism: both the obligate nutrient consumption by tumor (the "trap") and a curious overstimulation of peripheral tissue energy metabolism, perhaps mediated by tumor-derived, hormone-like substances. Amino acid fluxes did not differ in cancer patients and normal control patients.

Regardless of ultimate mechanistic conclusions, the clinical consequence of disordered, ineffective energy and protein metabolism in cancer patients can be that nutritional needs substantially exceeding basal levels are unfulfilled, often for many days before proper medical intervention. Head and neck cancer patients are uniquely at risk because local tumor effects increasingly compound initially moderate malnutrition, with a spiraling course toward a definite nutritional crisis: striking weight loss secondary to negative energy balance, muscle wasting, and probably immune system dysfunction from depressed synthesis of essential proteins and catabolism of both the central visceral and peripheral muscle nitrogen sources, with deranged serum chemistries confirming advanced whole body effects. The implications of major surgery for such a patient are disturbing, and surgical efforts to cure a large head or neck cancer with a conscionable risk-benefit ratio may take on some characteristics of a high-wire act.

Secure healing of a complex, bacterially contaminated wound following radical head and neck cancer surgery is the primary issue. Various wound infection risk factors have been mentioned previously. It is almost a cliché that primary healing in clean surgical wounds has biologic priority and will proceed in the face of relatively severe prior malnourishment, but years of surgical experience confirm that malnutrition definitely interferes with recovery from serious surgical complications, especially nosocomial infectious complications. Infected wound repair as well as the function of local and systemic host defenses,[3, 4] specific and nonspecific, can suffer, with increased morbidity or even mortality resulting. The potential scenario is evident: calorie and protein requirements during infection and postsurgical stress increase significantly above basal levels,[5] patients with preoperative nutritional deficits are ill equipped to handle the additional metabolic requirements of a complicated postoperative course, and the complication itself may prevent adequate food intake. It is a serious error to overlook reversible perioperative factors that may increase substantially the probability of this calamity. Postoperative nutritional details also deserve organized diligence. Some of the iatrogenic aspects of head and neck cancer surgery are unavoidable. For example, radical operations for large oropharyngeal cancers always interfere temporarily (sometimes permanently) with the ability to eat regular foods. It is clear that attention to nutrition is important, not only in assuring that such patients are ready for operation but also in the immediately postoperative NPO phase when critical mucosal suture lines must achieve watertight healing beneath soft tissue flaps undisturbed by potentially disruptive stresses imposed by chewing or swallowing food. Equally important is the subsequent hospital convalescence period when some patients must literally learn to eat again. A team approach by the ward dietician, surgeon, and nurse is crucial here. Other types of iatrogenic nutritional damage are possible before the surgeon becomes involved. If weeks of radiation or chemotherapy precede salvage surgery for large, advanced cancers, patients with even modest initial nutritional deficits will lose substantial ground on every preoperative day unless an effective feeding strategy is devised and enforced. As in other general aspects of good surgical care, this insidious problem must be anticipated and contingency plans activated when appropriate. The axiom that malnutrition is much easier to prevent than to repair should be remembered.

In summary, the bulk and location of a head and neck tumor can be major determinants of the preoperative nutritional status and can influence directly the permissible scope and safety of an operation. In general, larger neglected tumors will be associated with more significant nutritional damage and will require more extensive radical operations with higher inherent risks. All dangerously malnourished patients must therefore be identified, even though the best available knowledge may force the use of approximation techniques that are insensitive, imperfect, or incomplete.

WHAT ARE THE ELEMENTS OF A NUTRITIONAL EVALUATION?

Conscientious preoperative preparation of each patient includes an expeditious nutritional status evaluation by the surgeon and the ward dietician or nutritionist who cooperatively integrate data from the patient interview, physical examination, and clinical laboratory tests. This evaluation ought to be viewed as an investment in patient safety but need not be elaborate or expensive. It should be shaped from the outset by three technical points that relate to the likelihood of complications and the projected eating disturbance in the postoperative period: (1) What operation is required? (2) What is its wound infection risk category? (3) What is a likely duration of the postoperative NPO period, assuming a smooth, uncomplicated recovery? A delayed operation date and an empirical course of nutritional support must be considered if the preoperative evaluation suggests that a patient presents an unacceptable nutritional risk. Alternatively, if no warning flags are found, the operation can be scheduled and attention centered on planning routine perioperative parenteral fluid needs with an expectation of a smooth transition back to regular eating a few days after surgery. The neuroendocrine responses to general anesthesia and surgery have been exhaustively studied, and it is clear that even a week of semistarvation in the face of a typically mild catabolism and negative nitrogen balance is tolerated perfectly well by patients receiving parenteral glucose for "protein-sparing" after uncomplicated elective surgery of far greater magnitude than many head and neck cases.[6]

Unlike organ-specific functional tests applicable to the cardiopulmonary or renal systems, the determination and subsequent relationship to surgical outcome of preoperative nutritional status is often inexact and may be an educated guess. Developments in the growing field of nutritional assessment must always be analyzed carefully. The interplay of general medical health, nutritional history and immune system function is complex and may never be amenable to strict analytic elucidation, but it has been the subject of a confusing literature. Certain aspects of the problem have been termed "an intellectual quagmire."[7] The waters have been muddied by the fact that several well-publicized studies have proved to be badly designed, technically flawed, or vague,[8–16] and by the realization that nutritional evaluation and the therapies prescribed in response to it can add an expensive increment to a hospital bill.

Despite enthusiasm for methods of deceptively variable complexity wherein multiple laboratory tests and anthropometric variables are merged in mathematical functions to quantify "nutritional state," many schemes, both simple and esoteric, have proved reliable only for post hoc epidemiologic categorization of patients. Companion data in the field of head and neck surgery per se are scarce, so that one must improvise with useful concepts and experiences from general surgery work, recognizing that currently available methods cannot infallibly predict operative complications related to nutritional deprivation. Prognostic nutritional stratification, a method developed recently by Mullen et al.[11, 12] through regression analysis of data from a large series of general surgical patients, has recently been applied for the first time in head and neck cancer surgery. In Mullen's technique values for the preoperative serum albumin level, serum transferrin level, triceps skin fold thickness, and a score from a battery of delayed cutaneous hypersensitivity tests are combined in a linear equation to give a prognostic nutritional index (PNI) used for predicting major complications. Mullen has realized rather impressive success for his four-variable linear equation.[12]

Hooley and co-workers applied this technique in 29 high-risk patients undergoing head and neck cancer surgery[13] and noted preoperative PNI values ranging from −22% to 30%. Six of seven patients experiencing serious postoperative complications had PNI values greater than 20%, but all patients who suffered minor complications had PNI values less than 20%. It was suggested that the method may guide the prediction of which patients need a period of preoperative nutritional support.

Mullen's approach has been simplified by Rainey-Macdonald et al.,[14] who questioned the technical ease, precision, and general availability of skin tests and athropometric measurements in routine hospital settings. They showed that a simple two-variable discriminant function, using serum albumin (Alb) and serum transferrin (Tf) values in the following relationship:

$$F = 1.20 \text{ Alb} + 0.013 \text{ Tf} - 6.43$$

provided an equally useful correlative function for 55 surgical patients (including nine head and neck cancer patients) studied prospectively. The mean albumin value for 33 patients surviving without major complications was 3.51 ± 0.58 gm/100 ml, but it was 2.66 ± 0.53 gm/100 ml for 22 patients who died or experienced a major complication. An albumin level below 3.0 gm/100 ml separated correctly 84% of the patients into outcome groups; this single variable had a predictive accuracy of 76% (sensitivity of 86% and specificity of 82%). When a lower limit serum transferrin level of 175 or less was included as a second factor of discrimination, 91% of the patients were correctly classified. In the resultant function, *F* greater than zero correlated with good outcomes and negative *F* values "predicted" serious morbidity or mortality after surgery with 88% accuracy, as did the Mullen method used with the same patients. It was concluded that hypersensitivity skin test results and triceps skin fold data are redundant. Pending refinements in current methods of preoperative assessment, the Rainey-Macdonald equation seems a reasonable adjunctive yardstick for subgrouping head and neck cancer patients facing high-risk operations and might be most useful when combined with clinically based patient management decisions. A truly prospective trial of screening techniques in stratified head and neck cancer patients, with surgical outcome as the bottom line, will be a welcome advance.

A skillful physical examination and an appropriately elicited history have an important, possibly singular role[15] in nutritional assessment and can yield reliable clues to preoperative nutritional deterioration (Table 11–3). It is important to seek specific information about weight loss, eating difficulty, diet habits, medication use (e.g., chronic steroids), and a history of diabetes. An experienced clinical dietician is invaluable for this task. Regardless of mechanism (swallowing problems, chewing problems, or anorexia) "eating difficulty" is considered here to mean inability to consume a daily requirement of calories, protein, and water. The patient must always be queried closely about his or her usual weight, and a history of unintended weight loss should be clarified as to both the extent and rate of the loss. Unless a patient is intentionally restricting food intake, weight loss is abnormal and solid evidence that total caloric intake has been repeatedly exceeded by net metabolic requirements. The problem of choosing a "normal" weight is well known. Should it be usual weight, ideal weight for height from epidemiologic data, or do classic rules of thumb give a reliable basis for evaluation?[16–18] A value of 7%–10% of usual weight is probably an acceptable and practical estimate of a clinically significant weight loss threshold. The surgeon should conduct the usual complete physical examination with a special awareness of the obvious signs of major nutritional damage (loose clothing, muscle wasting, edema). Of more than minor significance is the opportunity to determine if a patient's nutritional story is explained by his type of cancer. A clinically consistent picture that makes sense must be constructed. For example, one might consider it highly difficult to rationalize a 15-pound weight loss and anorexia in a patient admitted to the ward for excision of a 1.5 × 1.0-cm lip cancer! The possibilities of other malignancies or wasting diseases in the head and neck cancer population must always be kept in mind and appropriate screening tests (e.g., chest x-ray, guiac stool testing) employed. Suggested routine laboratory work is also listed in Table 11–3 and includes basic tests ordered on surgical inpatients in many hospitals. A serum albumin value at the time of admission can be useful if the patient is not dehydrated or overhydrated,[19] but only if the evaluation personnel keep in mind some albumin interpretation problems. Clinically significant visceral protein loss can exist but be unrevealed by a normal value as a consequence of the long albumin serum half-life,[20] but a clearly decreased albumin value (e.g., < 3.0 gm/100 ml) in a patient with significant weight loss and eating difficulty is a warning of possible major protein-calorie malnutrition[21] if overhydration, proteinuria, major liver disease, or, rarely, a protein-wasting enteropathy are excluded by standard methods. The serum level of transferrin, a protein with much shorter half-life, is ostensibly coupled more closely with changes in visceral protein status.[21] This variable can be measured directly[22] or estimated from the total iron-binding ca-

TABLE 11–3.—PREOPERATIVE NUTRITIONAL EVALUATION: KEY POINTS

PATIENT INTERVIEW
Weight loss
Eating difficulty
Dietary habits
Alcoholism
Diabetes
Medications
PHYSICAL EXAMINATION
Weight and height
Obvious cachexia
Loose clothing
Muscle wasting
Ascites/edema
Lesion fits picture
LABORATORY DATA
Complete blood cell count
Serum albumin*
Serum transferrin*
Liver function tests*
Urinary analysis
Fasting serum glucose

*Optional data for obviously minor cases

pacity,[23] a cheap test available in most hospitals. Significant anemia can accompany malnutrition and cause misleading transferrin levels;[21] a complete blood cell count allows assessment of this and also provides guidance for corrective red blood cell transfusions preoperatively.

CASE MANAGEMENT PHILOSOPHY: TWO PATTERNS

Clean category head and neck cancer operations carry a very low risk of wound failure or infection, almost never stimulate extraordinary stress hormone responses in the postoperative period, rarely involve extensive dissection requiring complicated flap coverage of a wound, and usually delay resumption of regular eating for 1–3 days. For these reasons, it is very unlikely that nutritional status will have much impact on the surgical outcome unless a patient is catastrophically malnourished. Table 11–4 summarizes a conservative approach to patients facing clean category head and neck cancer operations. Rarely, when combined findings strongly suggest a type IB status, two options will be open: (1) verify that there is no cryptic etiology for the malnutrition, then operate, with enteral nutrition being started as soon after anesthetic recovery as possible to check further deterioration; or (2) delay operation while further investigating and improving patient status (see discussion of type II patients below). Seasoned head and neck cancer surgeons almost always make the correct choice on the basis of one skill: clinical judgment.

Type II head and neck cancer patients face major extirpative operations that will involve dissection within the oropharyngeal cavity and reconstruction with tissue flaps. They must be evaluated and prepared cautiously. Table 11–5 summarizes our approach, in which an effort is made to segregate patients who could benefit from a 7- to 10-day period of empirical preoperative nutritional replenishment. The fiscal price of this tactic must be balanced against the emotional and physical price a patient will pay during an unwelcome postoperative complication plus the dollar expense of its morbidity. With DRG implementation at hand, such decisions will become more frequent but no less inexact and frustrating for surgeons. For all patients meeting type IIA criteria, critical malnutrition is improbable even if there has been eating difficulty, and operations can proceed when other preparations are complete. However, every type IIA patient should receive enteral nutrition through the nasogastric tube as soon as gastrointestinal tract function resumes postoperatively. The object is to supply at least the ongoing calorie and nitrogen needs and to blunt consecutive losses during NPO periods of unpredictable length. In type IIB patients, arbitrary and vigorous preoperative nutritional support is prudent, especially if the Rainey-Macdonald index and the clinician's interpretation of the patient in light of his past experience suggest a high-risk postoperative course. Enteral feeding should be used if a tube can be passed, but total parenteral nutrition (TPN) is somewhat more reliably brought up to an adequate total calorie level in a short period of time, and this modality should be used without hesitation if there are problems with maintaining an adequate enteral rate.

The rationale for preoperative "nutritional repair" must be fully understood. A currently unsolved vital problem in the field of surgical nutrition is the differentiation of patients who will benefit from *preoperative* TPN or enteral feeding from those in whom it will not

TABLE 11–4.—PERIOPERATIVE NUTRITION: CLEAN CASES

DEFINITION OF "CLEAN" CASE
Oropharyngeal cavity not entered in conjunction with neck dissection
No mucosal suture lines covered by soft tissue flaps

TYPICAL CASES
Thyroidectomy, parathyroidectomy, parotidectomy, neck node dissection, soft tissue cancer of face, neck, or lips; minor intraoral biopsies; partial glossectomy without node dissection

CATEGORY IA CHARACTERISTICS
Weight loss insignificant
No eating difficulty
Serum albumin above 2.9

CATEGORY IB CHARACTERISTICS
History of eating difficulty *and* either significant weight loss *or* albumin below 3.0

PERIOPERATIVE NUTRITION
IA: IV fluids until taking food
IB: Delay needed to confirm malnutrition, etiology? Postoperative enteral feeding at 30–35 kcal/kg if not eating at 48 hours

TABLE 11–5.—PERIOPERATIVE NUTRITION: CLEAN-CONTAMINATED CASES

DEFINITION OF "CLEAN-CONTAMINATED" CASE
Oropharyngeal cavity entered and mucosal suture line covered by soft tissue flap reconstruction

TYPICAL CASES
Radical laryngectomy, floor of mouth tumor resections, composite resections of all types

CATEGORY IIA CHARACTERISTICS
Insignificant weight loss *and* serum albumin above 3.0 *and* serum transferrin above 190 with/without eating difficulty

CATEGORY IIB CHARACTERISTICS
Any IIA criteria failure

PERIOPERATIVE NUTRITION
IIA: Standard perioperative IV fluids; start enteral feeding as soon as possible postoperatively and continue at *maximal tolerable rate* until full oral diet can be resumed
IIB: Rainey-Macdonald index; for preoperative albumin below 2.6 gm/100 ml consider albumin infusions daily; delay surgery for 7–10 days, feeding at 30–35 kcal/kg; nitrogen balance review on day 7; postoperative enteral feeding at *maximum rate* until eating; TPN may be indicated

change outcome; this issue is entirely separate from the question of whether the methods can sustain life normally (they obviously can and are enormously effective). It is naive to suppose that a starved patient could be returned to normal nutritional status with 1 week of *any* therapy, but there is suggestive evidence from a few general surgical studies that at least 1 week of intensive nutritional support (such as TPN) is the minimum acceptable period. Enteral alimentation should accomplish the same result if given at isocaloric and isonitrogenous levels.[24] Mullen et al. discovered from retrospective investigations of patients who received preoperative TPN that patients with lower PNI values tended to cluster in a subpopulation that benefited from TPN, in contrast to patients who did not receive a course of TPN before operation.[25] This work has been criticized because it did not involve a randomized, prospective design. Muller, Brenner, and co-workers[26] randomly chose 66 cancer patients for an arbitary 10-day course of preoperative TPN and found a clear reduction in complications relative to 59 prospectively chosen control patients. It is interesting that nutritional evaluation was not performed or used as the basis for therapy in a single patient.

Excepting research techniques used in a few centers to estimate, for example, the lean body cell mass,[27] there are no simple analytical methods that can sense a patient's early response to short courses of nutritional therapy. A malnourished patient will have met metabolic demands prior to hospitalization by consumption of his adipose tissue and both central visceral and muscle proteins, and the extracellular fluid expansion that results during this catabolic state is mixed with lean body mass decreases, making weight changes during a period of brisk refeeding undecipherable. Furthermore, sequential serum albumin levels[28, 29] and probably transferrin levels[30] are unpredictably sensitive to short-term therapy. Burt et al.[30] showed that 2 weeks of TPN therapy in cancer patients stimulated whole body protein synthesis and decreased skeletal muscle catabolism, as measured by elaborate radiotracer studies and 3-methylhistidine excretion, but such measurements are not a simple affair, and questions can be raised about the meaning of 3-methylhistidine excretion data in patients being refed. Serial nitrogen balance studies can detect cessation of net catabolism and show that net nitrogen flux has turned inward, suggesting anabolism, but cannot necessarily calibrate progress along a tissue repair trajectory. Nitrogen balance data may be a risky basis for navigation while stressed or starving patients are aggressively refed.[31, 32] Nonetheless, Kudsk and Sheldon[33] have argued that a simple nitrogen balance remains the best measure of dynamic changes during nutritional therapy. This 24-hour tally of nitrogen intake and loss[31] is inexpensive to perform. It requires a 24-hour urine collection, an accurate log of total nitrogen ingested or infused (simple with TPN or enteral feeding), small corrections for nonurinary nitrogen losses, and estimates[33] of nonurea urine nitrogen. It may not be unreasonable to use the attainment of at least a small positive balance as a hopeful sign in the type IIB patient after 7–10 days of preoperative feeding.[34] An alternative is to await expectantly an early diuretic response to repair feeding, said to be a beneficial sign in recent work by Kinney's group.[28] Until clarifying positions are reported, decisions regarding preoperative nutritional preparation in type IIB cases will require a shrewd mix of intuition, soft biochemical data, guessing, and luck.

After successful postoperative recovery, and if there is no evidence of wound infection, dehiscence, or early fistula, all specialized nutritional methods can be tapered as the patient becomes ready and able to eat. The surgeon and dietician should tailor diet orders to the particular patient (e.g., mechanically soft diet for the initial solid food in a patient with partial glossectomy). It is always helpful for the dietician to actively follow type II cancer patients after surgery not only to ensure adequate inputs during the enteral feeding phase, but also to confirm that patients actually consume full calorie and protein rations after all nourishment is being taken orally. A current practice in many hospitals is a discharge review with the dietician or ward nurse, at which time any special diet needs at home can be outlined with the patient and family members. Concern for proper nutrition should continue in long term follow-up. Patient reports of good appetite, no insurmountable mechanical problems with eating, and the return of stable body weight are all welcome markers of a successful alimentary rehabilitation.

WHAT ARE THE PATIENT'S NUTRITIONAL REQUIREMENTS?

Energy intake requirements are ongoing and are determined by many factors, including body size, age, sex, presence of infection or other stresses, and the degree of physical activity.[5, 35] Resting requirements can be indirectly derived from calculations, nomograms, or rules of thumb.[35, 36] Estimates are suitable for successfully managing all head and neck cancer patients. Published guidelines[37] suggest daily maintenances of 25–30 kcal/kg for most hospitalized patients, with increases to 35–40 kcal/kg for patients with malnutrition or mild stress. Spanier and Shizgal[38] have carefully studied critically ill, stressed patients and recommend 46 kcal/kg for this hypermetabolic subset. For illustration, by these recommendations a 160-lb patient would require approximately 2,100, 2,800, or 3,400 kcal/day, respectively. The corresponding protein requirements are also determined by many factors. In particular, the net utilization of protein intake is a function of the nonprotein calorie level,[35] so that the calorie-nitrogen ratio of any nutritional mixture, regardless of the route of administration, is a key specification. As a first approximation, we approach type II cancer patients who require preoperative repair and postoperative feeding via enteral or parenteral nutrition by targeting minimal energy needs at 30 kcal/kg at a nonprotein calorie-nitrogen ratio of approximately 150. In major septic complications, we aim for levels approaching 40–45 kcal/kg while vigorously controlling the infection with antibiotics and/or surgical drainage.

All head and neck cancer patients, whether or not they are experiencing eating difficulty, should receive *at least* 25 kcal/kg of basal needs by the simplest and cheapest route available during preoperative workup periods. Type IIB patients thought to be nutritionally threatened to the extent that scheduled surgery is ill advised must be considered for arbitrary repair feeding and "pushed" to receive increased requirements by multiple meals and flavored supplemental liquids if they can swallow, by enteral tube feedings if they cannot, or even by TPN if necessary and clinically indicated, and as soon postoperatively (usually as enteral feeding) as is practical and safe. One exception, supported by years of clinical success, is the use of IV glucose and electrolytes in routine (e.g., type IA) cases. This standard postoperative technique, which can always supply 100% of water and electrolyte needs but only about 25% of calorie needs and none of the nitrogen needs, is a low-risk gamble that a clinician will almost always win because of the low stress level following an uncomplicated clean case, the quick recovery of eating ability, and the body's capacity to tolerate and repair a mild protein loss. In any other setting, formal provision of daily calorie/nitrogen needs cannot be justifiably avoided.

WHAT NUTRITIONAL METHODS ARE AVAILABLE?

Three inpatient nutritional methods (regular meals, enteral alimentation, and TPN) can supply required water, protein, calorie, and mineral needs. A detailed recital of vitamin requirements will not be attempted here. An excellent summary has been compiled by Jeppsson and Gimmon.[39] We routinely provide a daily supplement capsule to other than type IA patients to exceed all of the B complex and vitamin C requirements if the patient is taking oral nutrition. Otherwise we rely on enteral feeding to provide these substances. For our patients on TPN we infuse 1,000 mg of vitamin C IV and one dose of an IV multivitamin mixture (MVI-12, Armour) each 24 hours. Patients on TPN or enteral nutrition need exogenous vitamin K, and this is given weekly unless oral feeding has resumed. When a patient's thirst mechanisms and appetite are intact, minimal mechanical problems exist with ingestion of food or with function of the gastrointestinal tract, and there are no medical indications for witholding feedings, the preferred nutritional method is a series of regular meals served in a palatable fashion at proper temperatures. This method is the province of the hospital dietician who (1) ensures that the meals provide a balance of adequate portions that include healthy mixtures of fat, carbohydrate, proteins, and vitamins; (2) verifies that the diet is consistent with the medical orders and overall treatment objectives; (3) documents, when necessary, actual calorie and nitrogen intakes; (4) alerts the surgical team to problems encountered in meeting nutrition goals; and (5) teaches good nutrition habits to patients and their families. Through knowledge of food composition and the capabilities of the hospital kitchen or pharmacy as well as ongoing awareness of advances in medical nutrition, a dietician can often improvise a number of tricks such as feedings of between-meal supplements [chilled Isocal (Mead-Johnson) or Ensure (Ross)] and alterations of food consistency, frequency, or taste that ensure proper nourishment. If any patient cannot or will not eat enough food to satisfy ongoing nutritional needs, this must be promptly noted and other techniques pressed into service without delay. Enteral alimentation, in which nutrients, water, vitamins, or oral medications are infused by tube into the stomach or the proximal small intestine via nasogastric or pharyngostomy tubes, has been part of the head and neck cancer surgeon's armamentarium for many years. Improved understanding of basic gastrointestinal physiology, new and more comfortable feeding tubes, choices of formulas for practically every conceivable clinical contingency, and the clear demonstration that enteral alimentation is safe, economical, and effective have provided solid support for the axiom, "if the gut works, use it." Every head and neck cancer surgeon should be familiar with enteral alimentation and exploit it fully. Encyclopedic review of the method is beyond the scope of this chapter; excellent books and articles[40–42] should be consulted. Briefly, the surgeon and dietician need to choose an appropriate formula, select a practical and comfortable tube, and devise nursing orders that guarantee safe delivery of the mixture at a rate that meets targeted calorie/nitrogen needs.

HOW IS ENTERAL ALIMENTATION USED?

An almost bewildering assortment of tube feeding preparations is commercially available. They differ in cost, content, and type of protein, calorie source, mineral content, osmolality, nonprotein calorie/nitrogen ratio, and caloric density, but are nutritionally complete in the context of even a 3- to 4-week course and provide, with few exceptions, essential trace minerals and vitamins except for vitamin K. An important advantage of almost all commercial preparations over blenderized hospital food is their low viscosity, which obviates problems of tube plugging and allows use of more comfortable, small-diameter tubes.[43, 44] A 24-hour-a-day infusion is preferred when nursing attention is adequate. The method is contraindicated in patients who are not alert or have no gag reflex. We have had excellent results with an isotonic mixture (Isocal) that provides 1,000 kcal and 34 gm of protein per liter at full strength and contains no lactose. Many other choices are available, and these alternatives have been exhaustively tabulated by Matarese.[45]

The cheapest, most comfortable tube should be used for preoperative enteral alimentation. Any of the newer, flexible tubes with weighted tips can be used, and we have found these especially handy in patients undergoing postoperative radiation therapy. A plain radiograph should always be obtained to ensure proper placement in the stomach.

The provision of an enteral feeding route in the postoperative patient deserves comment. All patients with a complex wound reconstruction (type II) have traditionally had nasogastric tubes passed distally at the time of surgery to allow gastric decompression and to prevent vomiting during the early postoperative ileus period. Although larger (18 French) tubes seem to be frequently used in adults for this purpose (a habit developed on general surgery wards?) a smaller tube should be considered (14 French sump nasogastric tube) since it can easily handle swallowed air and gastric juice outputs, yet can simply be taken off suction when ileus resolution indicates that the gastrointestinal tract is functioning and ready to receive feeding, then used for comfortable enteral feeding. Solutions can be gravity dripped or pumped into the gut.

The orders for administration of enteral feeding should be carefully planned and reviewed with the nursing staff. In most large practices detailed protocols are followed routinely. Many potential tolerance problems can be avoided by a strictly followed schedule in which both formula strength (i.e., osmolality) and feeding rate are advanced. If an isotonic mixture is dripped into the stomach (our preference), it is often possible to start with slow (25–30 ml/hour) rates of the full strength solution and advance hourly flow stepwise over a controlled 24 to 48 hour period. In many patients, it should be possible to secure a tolerated rate of infusion that will give 24-hour total loads near 2,400 kcal. When warranted, higher calorie/nitrogen input per unit volume is possible using concentrated mixtures (1.5 or 2.0 kcal/ml), but some well-known strategies for gradually approaching tolerance to any of the hypertonic mixes will be necessary.[41, 42]

Responsible, systematic patient monitoring during enteral alimentation is critical. Mechanical problems such as aspiration or vomiting must be absolutely prevented by upright positioning of the patient and nursing vigilance. Diarrhea suggests incomplete absorption secondary to high infusion rates; solutions include addition of psyllium, kaolin, or narcotics to slow transit time.[46, 47] Numerous potential metabolic problems are known[48, 49] and the clinician must be on guard for them. When enteral alimentation is used for repair feeding of severely depleted patients in negative nitrogen balance, hypophosphatemia can develop; many of the commercial mixtures are adequate for maintenance requirements but modification is necessary when used for preoperative repair. Water balance, electrolyte levels, and tolerance of the glucose load must all be followed closely, just as in a TPN patient. Daily body weights and regular, appropriate laboratory studies are essential. (See discussion of complications in chapter 27.)

In summary, most patients on a head and neck cancer ward can be managed well using enteral technique. However, if exigencies of any sort preclude delivery of needed calorie/nitrogen requirements by the oral or enteral routes, TPN must be employed. The two clinical settings most likely to require this shift in strategy are (1) a gravely malnourished preoperative IIB patient in whom it is impossible to adequately elevate the enteral rate to repair levels, and (2) any postoperative patient with a catastrophic complication that elevates metabolic requirements and mandates heroic support.

HOW IS TPN USED IN HEAD AND NECK CANCER SURGERY?

Clinical application of hyperosmolar central venous nutrition (TPN) has occurred over the past two decades, and this powerful adjunct has been ranked alongside general anesthesia, antisepsis, and antibiotics as a pivotal development in modern surgery.[50] Many surgeons use TPN, and the technology is available even in small community hospitals.

Several caveats are in order: TPN is much more expensive than enteral alimentation, has potentially more serious, although rare, iatrogenic complications than enteral technique, demands assiduous monitoring attention by surgical and nursing team members and 24-hour-a-day cooperation of a knowledgeable pharmacy staff and clinical laboratory, and has been shown by Sako and co-workers[51] in a randomized trial to provide no benefits postoperatively over conventional enteral feeding methods in head and neck cancer surgery. For these reasons, TPN should never be prescribed casually but kept in abeyance as an elective tool for special circumstances where there is proved success of its use.[52, 53] Though risks of TPN are low in the hands of an experienced team, informed consent discussions with patients may be prudent. A brief description of TPN follows, but a number of excellent sources[54–57] are required reading for any physician who plans to use the technique.

The initiation of TPN is never an emergency and is contraindicated in patients who are not hemodynamically stable. We routinely use a mixture containing 2.75% amino acids and 20% dextrose, which will supply 792 calories and 27.5 gm of protein per liter at a nonprotein calorie/nitrogen ratio of 148. At an infusion rate of 150 cc/hour, this solution provides 2,850 calories and 99 gm of protein per day. There are other possible dextrose/amino acid combinations that provide higher or lower nonprotein calorie/nitrogen ratios.[5] Special TPN mixtures are available for patients with hepatic insufficiency, renal failure, or high stress levels.[5, 56] Metering devices that control the rate, monitor the stream for air bubbles, and signal the nurse by audible alarm for untoward events such as catheter plugging or disconnection are standard equipment. The TPN method gives a clinician absolute, 24-hour-a-day control of the patient's metabolic fueling, and thus can be used for either maintenance nutrition under circumstances that grossly elevate calorie/nitrogen requirements (e.g., severe sepsis) or for intensive feeding to repair past nutritional deficits. An obvious limitation can be a patient's inability to tolerate water loads near 4 L/day (renal or cardiac insufficiency must be absent or under control).

The mechanical complications of TPN comprise all misadventures that can accompany placement of a subclavian vein catheter. Every conceivable mistake has been reported, with pneumothorax being the most common. Serious and fatal bleeding has also followed damage to the subclavian vein or artery, and air embolism, cardiac perforation, and cardiac tamponade are all rare but grave possibilities. Catheter placement must therefore be viewed strictly as a surgical procedure, to be performed only by a skilled and cautious doctor under ideal conditions of good light, absolute sterile technique, proper patient positioning, and adequate assistance. Head and neck surgeons should choose the side of subclavian vein cannulation with an eye toward planned operative fields and required flap sites when TPN is used preoperatively. A postoperative decision to use TPN may find the surgeon faced with operative wounds that preclude subclavian catheterization; a "long arm" central venous line placed from either antecubital fossa can be used. Rosen, Latto, and Ng[59] have provided an excellent compendium of catheterization techniques. A small sterile bandage is placed at the skin puncture site and a chest x-ray film is used to rule out pneumothorax and verify proper catheter position in the superior vena cava before beginning infusion of TPN.

When administration of TPN begins, metabolic complications of the method, some of which can be dramatic and fatal, must be clearly anticipated by monitoring. The consequences of the sustained hypertonic glucose load can include osmotic diuresis with hyperosmolar coma secondary to severe dehydration. The urine and blood glucose levels must be regularly followed to detect this problem at its onset so that infusion rates can be adjusted accordingly. Subcutaneous or IV insulin administration may be needed under a variety of common circumstances, including stress states, in the overtly or subclinical diabetic patient, or in the patient on steroids. A sudden reduction in the TPN infusion rate, with or without insulin administration, can precipitate severe and lethal hypoglycemia. A senior nurse with proved experience in managing TPN must be available on the ward 24 hours a day to oversee orderly and safe infusion. Numerous other metabolic problems can result, including serious imbalances of potassium, calcium, magnesium, and phosphorus metabolism and acid/base disturbances. Essential fatty acid deficiency can develop after a variable period of TPN, and many clinicians routinely administer 500 ml of commercially available 10% fat emulsion (e.g., Intralipid) twice weekly as prophylaxis.[60] This maneuver also increases the total caloric input by 550 kcal on infusion days. It is unclear whether a fraction of daily TPN calorie needs should *always* be provided by fat, and debate is unsettled about the correct carbohydrate-fat ratio when fat is used. Cerra[5] has outlined the various approaches. The variation of TPN called peripheral parenteral nutrition, in which peripheral veins are used for infusing daily mixtures of 10% dextrose, amino acids, and lipid emulsion, involves a number of compromises. In our judgment it offers no advantages over enteral alimentation technique in head and neck surgery and we do not currently use it.

Special TPN flowsheets posted in the patient's room are common practice; we use this method routinely and strongly encourage it. On these large "scoreboards" the daily weights, vital signs, fluid input/output records, and myriad laboratory values can be serially entered for viewing on rounds. The initial goal in early TPN administration is a gradual, smooth increase in the rate of delivery up to target levels over a day or two, without taxing unnecessarily the patient's homeostatic mechanisms. A long-term goal is the sterility of the patient's "lifeline," and a potentially grave complication is that of line infection. The TPN mixture is an excellent culture medium for many pathogens and the catheter itself is a chronic foreign body positioned in a tract linking the outside world and the central circulation. It is hardly surprising that early use of TPN was accompanied by alarming reports of both bacterial and fungal sepsis. A number of simple lessons have been learned. We consider TPN lines sacrosanct and never use them for blood sampling or any other IV infusion. The skin dressing over the site of entry should be applied with sterile technique at the time of catheter placement and changed thereafter on a 48-hour basis by a trained nurse following a rigid protocol. When fresh bags of TPN mixture must be connected to the line, sterile precautions are observed. At the earliest suspicion of sepsis in any TPN patient, the possibility of line infection must be entertained and ruled out if possible. If there are any doubts, the surgeon should remove or change the catheter.

In summary, TPN can be a powerful adjunct in head and neck surgical therapy when patients are not able to eat or cannot be maintained by a preferred enteral technique. TPN can be safely used for as long as necessary after a catastrophic complication to support vital body processes but should be tapered slowly and discontinued at the first indication that either of the two less complex, safer, and cheapter routes is available.

REFERENCES

1. Dempsey D.T., Feurer I.D., Knox L.S., et al.: Energy expenditure in malnourished gastrointestinal cancer patients. *Cancer* 53:1265–1273, 1984.
2. Burt M.E., Aoki T.T., Gorschboth C.M., et al.: Peripheral tissue metabolism in cancer-bearing man. *Ann. Surg.* 198:685–691, 1984.
3. Fischer J.E. (ed.): *Relevance of Nutrition to Sepsis: Report of the Third Ross Conference on Medical Research.* Columbus, Ohio, Ross Laboratories, 1982.
4. Alexander J.W., Stinnett J.D.: Changes in immunologic function, in Fischer J.E. (ed.): *Surgical Nutrition.* Boston, Little Brown & Co., 1983, pp. 535–549.
5. Cerra F.B. (ed.): *Pocket Manual of Surgical Nutrition.* St. Louis, C.V. Mosby Co., 1984, pp. 59–85.
6. Moore F.D.: Surgical care and metabolic management of the postoperative patient, in Winters R., Greene H. (eds.): *Nutritional Support of the Seriously Ill Patient.* New York, Academic Press, 1983.
7. Meguid M.M., Twomey P., Buzby G., et al.: Nutrition in the cancer patient. *Contemp. Surg.* 23:85–111, 1983.
8. McLaren D.S., Meguid M.M.: Nutritional assessment at the crossroads. *JPEN* 7:575–579, 1983.
9. Moore F.D.: Delayed scientific hypersensitivity. *JPEN* 6:1–2, 1982.
10. Twomey P., Ziegler D., Rombeau J.: Utility of skin testing in nutritional assessment: A critical review. *JPEN* 6:50–58, 1982.
11. Mullen J.L., Gertner M.H., Buzby G., et al.: Implications of malnutrition in the surgical patient. *Arch. Surg.* 114:121–125, 1979.
12. Buzby G., Mullen J.L., Matthews D.C., et al.: Prognostic nutritional index in gastrointestinal surgery. *Am. J. Surg.* 139:160–167, 1980.
13. Hooley R., Levine H., Flores T.C., et al.: Predicting postoperative head and neck complications using nutritional assessment. *Arch. Otolaryngol.* 109:83–85, 1983.
14. Rainey-Macdonald C.G., Holliday R.L., Wells G., et al.: Validity of a two-variable nutritional index for use in selecting candidates for nutritional support. *JPEN* 7:15–20, 1983.
15. Baker J.P., Detsky A.S., Wesson D.E., et al.: Nutritional assessment: A comparison of clinical judgment and objective measurements. *N. Engl. J. Med.* 306:969–972, 1982.
16. Clouse R.E.: Practical use of body weight in nutritional therapy. *Clin. Consult. Nutr. Suppl.* 3:2–5, 1983.
17. Blackburn G.L., Thornton P.A.: Nutritional assessment of the hospitalized patient. *Med. Clin. North Am.* 63:1103–1115, 1979.
18. Silberman H., Eisenberg D. (eds.): *Parenteral and Enteral Nutrition for the Hospitalized Patient.* New York, Appleton-Century Crofts, 1982, pp. 20–24.
19. Forse R.A., Shizgal H.M.: Serum albumin and nutritional status. *JPEN* 4:450–454, 1980.
20. Wright R.A.: Nutritional assessment. *JAMA* 244:559–560, 1980.
21. Grant J.P., Custer P.B., Thurlow J.: Current techniques of nutritional assessment. *Surg. Clin. North Am.* 61:437–463, 1981.
22. Tsung S.H., Rosenthal W.A., Milewski, K.A.: Immunological measurement of transferrin compared with chemical measurements of total iron-binding capacity. *Clin. Chem.* 21:1063–1066, 1975.
23. Markowitz J., Fairbanks V.F.: Transferrin assay and total iron-binding capacity. *Mayo Clin. Proc.* 58:827–828, 1983.
24. Heymsfield S.B., Bethel R.A., Ansley J.D., et al.: Enteral hyperalimentation: An alternative to central venous hyperalimentation. *Ann. Intern. Med.* 90:63–71, 1979.
25. Mullen J.L., Buzby G.P., Matthews D.C., et al.: Reduction of operative morbidity and mortality by combined preoperative and postoperative nutritional support. *Ann. Surg.* 192:604–613, 1980.
26. Muller J.M., Brenner U., Dienst C., et al.: Preoperative parenteral feeding in patients with gastrointestinal carcinoma. *Lancet* 1:68–71, 1982.
27. Shizgal H.M.: Body composition and nutritional support. *Surg. Clin. North Am.* 61:729–741, 1981.
28. Starker P.M., Lasala P.A., Askanazi J., et al.: The response to TPN: A form of nutritional assessment. *Ann. Surg.* 198:720–724, 1983.
29. Starker P.M., Gump F.E., Askanazi J., et al.: Serum albumin levels as an index of nutritional support. *Surgery* 91:194–199, 1982.
30. Burt M.E., Stein T.P., Schwade J.G., et al.: Whole-body protein metabolism in cancer-bearing patients. *Cancer* 53:1246–1252, 1984.

31. Heymsfield S.B., Tochilin N., McManus C.B., et al.: Nitrogen balance. *Clin. Consult. Nutr. Suppl.* 4:6–10, 1984.
32. Bistrian B.R.: A simple technique to estimate severity of stress. *Surg. Gynecol. Obstet.* 148:675–678, 1979.
33. Kudsk K.A., Sheldon G.F.: Nutritional assessment, in Fischer J. (ed.): *Surgical Nutrition.* Boston, Little, Brown & Co., 1983, pp. 407–420.
34. Mackenzie T.A., Blackburn G.L., Flatt J.P.: Clinical assessment of nutritional status using nitrogen balance. *Fed. Proc.* 33:683, 1974.
35. Silberman H., Eisenberg D. (eds.): *Parenteral and Enteral Nutrition for the Hospitalized Patient.* New York, Appleton-Century-Crofts, 1982, pp. 52–64.
36. Rainey-Macdonald C.G., Holliday R.L., Wells G.A.: Nomograms for predicting resting energy expenditure of hospitalized patients. *JPEN* 6:59–60, 1982.
37. Jeejeebhoy K.N.: Total parenteral nutrition. *Ann. R. Coll. Phys. Surg. Can.* 9:287–300, 1976.
38. Spanier A.H., Shizgal H.M.: Caloric requirements of the critically ill patient receiving intravenous hyperalimentation. *Am. J. Surg.* 133:99–104, 1977.
39. Jeppsson B., Gimmon Z.: Vitamins, in Fischer J. (ed.): *Surgical Nutrition.* Boston, Little, Brown & Co., 1983, pp. 241–281.
40. McArdle A.H., Palmason A.R.T., Morency I., et al.: A rationale for enteral feeding as the preferable route for hyperalimentation. *Surgery* 90:616–623, 1981.
41. Freeman J.B., Fairfull-Smith R.J.: Current concepts of enteral feeding. *Adv. Surg.* 16:75–112, 1983.
42. Taylor K.B., Anthony L.E. (eds.): *Parenteral and Enteral Nutrition for the Hospitalized Patient.* New York, McGraw-Hill Book Co., 1983, pp. 78–114.
43. Dobbie R.P., Hoffmeister J.A.: Continuous pump-tube enteric hyperalimentation. *Surg. Gynecol. Obstet.* 143:273–276, 1976.
44. Cobb L.M., Cartmill A.M., Barry M., et al.: A tube for enteral nutrition of patients with aphagopraxia and patients with ventilator assistance. *Surg. Gynecol. Obstet.* 155:81–84, 1982.
45. Matarese L.E.: Enteral alimentation, in Fischer J. (ed.): *Surgical Nutrition.* Boston, Little, Brown & Co., 1983, pp. 727–739.
46. Kaminski M.V., Sailesh M.D., Gray D.S.: Prolonged enteral nutritional support. *Clin. Consult. Nutr. Suppl.* 3:6–8, 1983.
47. Frank H.A., Green L.C.: Successful use of a bulk laxative to control the diarrhea of tube feeding. *Scand. J. Plast. Reconstr. Surg.* 13:193–194, (1979).
48. Cataldi-Betcher E.L., Seltzer M.H., Slocum E.A., et al.: Complications occurring during enteral nutrition support: A prospective study. *JPEN* 7:546–552, 1983.
49. Vanlandinghamn S., Simpson S., Daniel P., et al.: Metabolic abnormalities in patients supported with enteral tube feeding. *JPEN* 5:322–324, 1981.
50. Stevens J.C.: Surgical nutrition: The fourth coming. *JAMA* 239:192, 1978.
51. Sako K., Lore J.M., Kaufman S., et al.: Parenteral hyperalimentation in surgical patients with head and neck cancer: A randomized study. *J. Surg. Oncol.* 16:391–401, 1981.
52. Ruberg R.L., Dudrick S.J.: Intravenous hyperalimentation in head and neck tumour surgery: Indications and precautions. *Br. J. Plast. Surg.* 30:151–153, 1977.
53. Copeland E.J., MacFadyen B.V., MacComb W.S., et al.: Intravenous hyperalimentation in patients with head and neck cancer. *Cancer* 35:606–611, 1975.
54. Fischer J.E.: Nutritional support in the seriously ill patient. *Curr. Probl. Surg.* 17:469–531, 1980.
55. Goodgame J.T.: A critical assessment of the indications for total parenteral nutrition. *Surg. Gynecol. Obstet.* 151:433–441, 1980.
56. Fischer J.E., Freund H.R.: Central hyperalimentation, in Fischer J.E. (ed.): *Surgical Nutrition.* Boston, Little, Brown & Co., 1983, pp. 663–702.
57. Brennan M.F.: Total parenteral nutrition in the cancer patient. *N. Engl. J. Med.* 305:375–382, 1981.
58. Wagman L.D., Burt M.E., Brennan M.F.: The impact of total parenteral nutrition on liver function tests in patients with cancer. *Cancer* 49:1249–1257, 1982.
59. Rosen M., Latto I.P., Ng W.S. (eds.): *Handbook of Percutaneous Central Venous Catheterisation.* London, W.B. Saunders Co., Ltd., 1981.
60. Goodgame J.T., Lowry S.F., Brennan M.F.: Essential fatty acid deficiency in total parenteral nutrition: Time course of development and suggestions for therapy. *Surgery* 84:271–277, 1978.

III. Management of Dentition for Surgical and Irradiation Therapy

GRAEME A. BROWNE, B.SC., M.SC., B.D.S., F.R.C.D.

THE MANAGEMENT of dentition for oropharyngeal surgery is relatively simple when there will be no irradiation treatment. The major objectives are to preserve good dentition and to reduce the oral bacterial contamination. Restorable healthy teeth outside the area of resection are preserved because they are useful as structural anchors for subsequent reconstruction. The major decisions to be made are outlined in the algorithm shown in Figure 11–1.

Much more controversy surrounds the management of dentition when irradiation is to be used as either the principal treatment or as a preoperative or postoperative adjunct. In order to make appropriate decisions, it is necessary to understand how irradiation will affect the periodontal tissues, oral mucosa, salivary gland function, and bone.

Tumoricidal doses of radiation injure both neoplastic and contiguous nonneoplastic tissues. Mitotically active cells with short cell cycle times are radiosensitive and undergo rapid necrosis. Long-term cell injury may be clinically apparent in nonneoplastic tissues whose cells have been in the G_0 phase of the cell cycle or in cells where a prolonged interphase of mitosis occurs due to a protracted G_1 phase. Actin, a constituent of the cell cytosol, together with the microtubules and microfilaments that form the cytoskeleton, are believed to be altered by ionizing radiation. This alteration substantially contributes to the postulated malfunctioning of the transport of intracellular organelles. The damage results in breaches of intercellular barrier integrity and reduces regenerative cell repair. The barrier between cells is required for integrity of the periodontal membrane. Tumoricidal doses of irradiation delivered to nonneoplastic oral tissue will, in time, produce some degree of irreversible degenerative changes that may precipate postirradiation sequelae.

WHAT ARE THE EFFECTS OF IRRADIATION ON PERIODONTAL TISSUES?

The anatomical barrier between the external environment of the oral cavity and the "internal milieu" of tissues is the crevicular attachment apparatus of the periodontium. In the edentulous patient, the interface is the mucoperiosteum of the alveolar processes and the palate of the maxilla. Under normal physiologic conditions the epithelial attachment actively transports tissue fluid in and around the cells and into the oral cavity, providing cellular and humoral protection to this zone. The gingival crevice anatomy facilitates the interchange of ions and larger molecules (including some immunoglobins) via the intercellular gap junctions or nexi. The periodontium has a brief cell cycle time that makes this zone particularly susceptible to the effects of ionizing radiation. Interruption of normal mitotic activity in the gingiva, whether it is caused by physical, chemical, or irradiation injury, will result in periodontal disease. The periodontal degeneration is accompanied by a profound change in the bacterial microenvironment. Typically, periodontal disease creates a host environment for a mixed flora of microaerophilic, facultative, and obligative anerobic organisms. Associated with these bacteria are proteolytic enzymes, leukocidins, endotoxins, and exotoxins. Individually or collectively, the bacterial actions depress normal periodontal cytodynamics and accelerate gingival necrosis. Periodontal injury permits local invasion by the oral flora to the subjacent alveolar bone by direct infiltration, or possibly by systemic spread from episodic bacteremias.

Two major radiobiologic effects on the periodontal tissue are (1) *direct cell death,* with an approximate 30%–40% reduction in viable cell counts, and (2) *indirect cellular effect* from radiation, which accounts for 60%–70% of ultimate cell injury. This effect does not occur immediately but may be observed following one or more mitotic cycles.

WHAT ARE THE EFFECTS OF RADIATION THERAPY ON NORMAL SALIVARY GLANDS?

The paired major salivary glands supply between 1,000 and 1,500 ml of saliva to the oral cavity and oropharynx during waking hours. Approximately 80%–90% of the daily production is the result of gustatory and masticatory stimuli associated with eating. The parotid and submandibular glands are located paraorally,

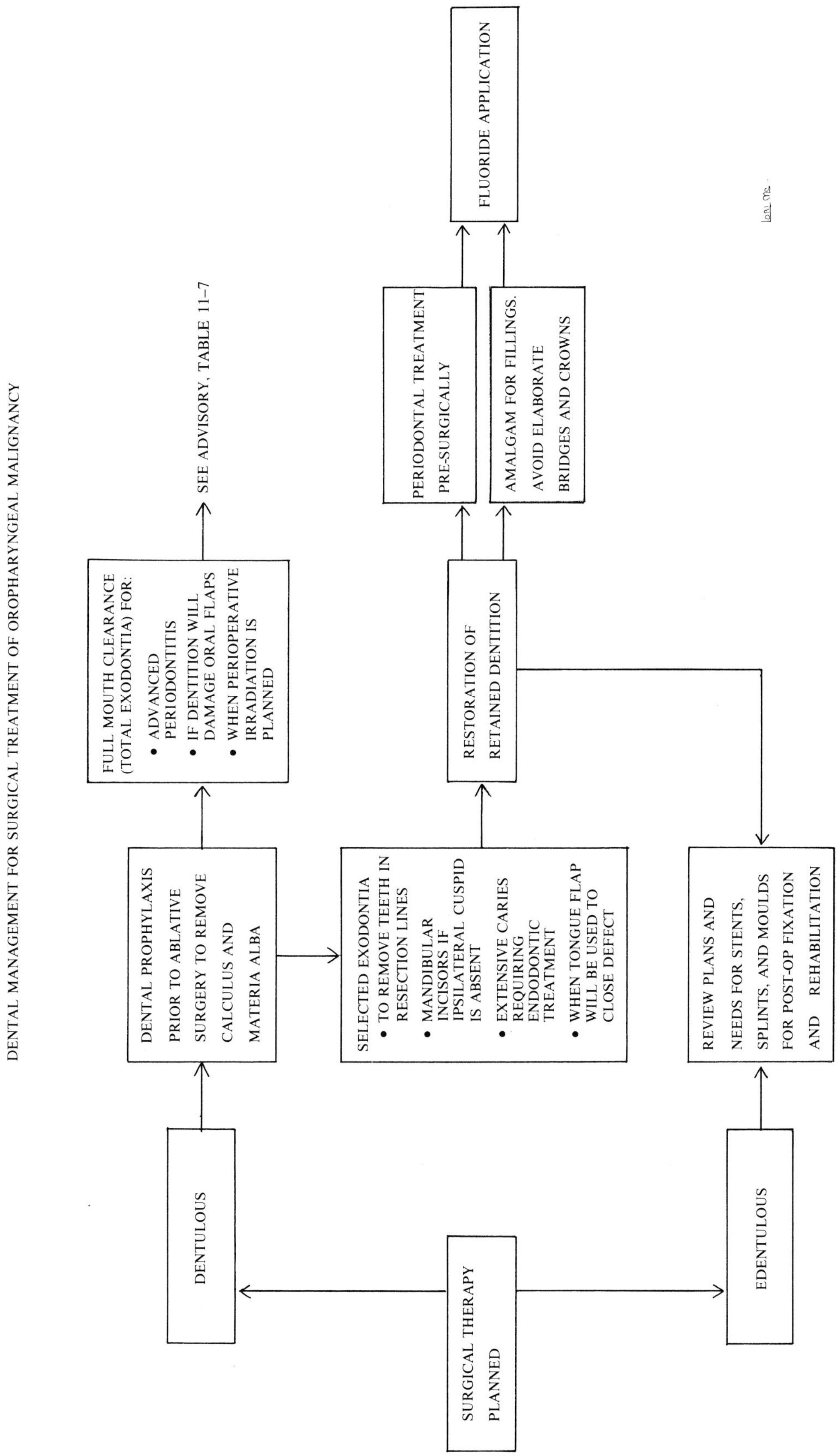

Fig 11–1.—Major decisions that must be made about dentition if treatment entails surgery.

while the sublingual glands are located submucosally in the floor of the mouth. The entrance of the respective salivary ducts into the mouth is constant except for the sublingual gland, which shows great variability as it enters via the ducts of Rivinus (opening along the plica sublingualis) and Bartholin's duct (which opens directly into the submandibular duct in 10%–50% of cases). In addition to the major salivary glands, numerous accessory salivary glands are distributed throughout the oral cavity within the investing mucosa. These glands are seen on the posterolateral aspect of the hard palate and the buccal and labial mucosa.

Saliva is isosmolar when it is initially secreted by an acinar cell. Then, selective reabsorption of sodium and excretion of potassium occurs, producing a fluid that is hypotonic with respect to plasma. Saliva is composed of three principal types: serous, seromucous, and mucous saliva. Typically, the parotid gland produces a serous saliva. The submandibular gland produces a nearly equal mixture of serous and mucous saliva. The sublingual gland, although composed of a histologic admixture of serous demilunes and goblet mucus-secreting acini, produces a preponderance of mucous saliva. Radiation will change the proportions of each type.

The volume of serous saliva that is produced varies according to the individual's state of wakefulness and the state of hydration. Volume decreases with dehydration and with advancing age.

Systemic disease can be reflected in salivary gland function and should be recognized during preirradiation assessment of salivary gland activity. For example, patients with diabetes, alcoholism, or collagen disease disorders show a diminished flow associated with glandular fibrosis. We may often overlook the concomitant effects of drug management of allergies and the assorted minor and major psychiatric disorders that have significant parasympatholytic effects. Frequently, these agents induce profound (oral) xerostomia.

The principal putative effect of ionizing radiation on the salivary glands is to quantitatively and qualitatively alter the quantity and physical properties of saliva. This change in function may be temporary, lasting several weeks to many months, or it may be permanent. Postirradiation salivary gland function has a direct relationship to (1) the location of the irradiation ports, (2) the individual dose and its frequency, (3) the cumulative amount of radiation given, (4) the preexisting health of the salivary glands, (5) the health of the periodontium, (6) the presence of dentition, (7) functional oral habits (gum chewing, etc.), (8) consumption of alcohol, and (9) the continued use of tobacco products, including smoking or the use of chewing tobacco.

An early predictor of the susceptibility of salivary serous acini to subsequent therapeutic doses of irradiation is the production of saliva with markedly higher viscosity. Xerostomia and viscid saliva may be encountered in the more sensitive glands following delivery of as little as 460 rad. Uniform glandular response is observed when 1,500 rad have been targeted through the salivary glands. Postirradiation salivary viscidosis precedes symptomatic mucositis.

WHAT IS THE PROPOSED MECHANISM OF RADIATION-INDUCED XEROSTOMIA?

The striated ducts are responsible for active transport of electrolytes and water. Autonomic nervous system parasympathetic activity induces acinar secretion. This activity is impeded by sympathetic nervous stimulation. In a histologic examination of salivary adenomeres, the subbasalar vascular rete are prominent during secretion, reflecting the active transport function of salivary excretion. Few studies on the impact of irradiation to salivary glands have been undertaken because of difficulties in obtaining postirradiation saliva samples when xerostomia is present. In addition, there is a lack of histologic material to correlate with salivary sample analysis. Thus, a cogent explanation will contain only inferences about water transport, electrolyte secretion, and intra-ductal absorption. About 75% of patients receiving radiation treatments have an immediate xerostomia followed by some *improvement in flow rate* of saliva over a period of 6 months to 2 years following radiation treatment. Qualitatively, the viscosity remains consistently higher than that noted prior to radiation therapy, even 2–3 years following the completion of therapy.

The clinical usefulness of the salivary gland function index lies in being able to predict which patients will show an unremitting xerostomia. It therefore enables the clinician to offer an opinion on (1) the probability of retaining natural dentition without significant radiation-induced dental caries and associated periodontal disease, and (2) the probable duration of a period that will elapse before the patient may safely wear prosthodontic appliances following radiotherapy.

Two major features of salivary function are clinically evaluated before radiation: the total salivary gland capacity after stimulation, a measure of the combined output of the major and minor glands; and the viscosity of the secretion.

A rapid clinical assessment of salivary function can be made by having the patient chew on dental wax for a few minutes to stimulate glandular secretion. Measurement of the volume collected after a standard interval provides a working estimate of total secretory function.

Viscosity can be clinically evaluated by lifting the pooled saliva from the floor of the mouth or the buccal vestibule with a tongue blade. Normal pooled saliva, which represents an admixture of serous, seromucous, and mucous saliva, can usually maintain a vertical salivary web to a distance of 5 cm. Viscous salivary webs which exceed 15 cm prior to radiation portend a poor glandular response to salivary stimulation after radiotherapy (Table 11–6). Patients with low total volumes and high viscosity will have a poor prognosis for avoiding progressive caries. If the patient is edentulous, low volume and high viscosity portend an extended delay for resumption of salivary secretory function. Poor salivary rebound following radiation therapy precludes the successful use of a dental prosthesis. In the dentulous patient it implies that retained natural dentition will have an exceedingly poor prognosis. Thus, the salivary web index, together with stimulated flow rates, is useful in selecting those patients for whom preradiation therapy dental extractions are indicated. Better advice can be given to these patients about the probability of being able to tolerate a dental prosthesis during the late postirradiation period.

WHAT IS THE ROLE OF SECRETORY IGA IN SALIVA?

There are plasma cells interspersed within the connective tissue of salivary adenomeres that secrete IgA, which combines with a proteinaceous secretory piece. This complex molecule, S-IgA, is resistant to enzymatic degradation and probably reflects a defense mechanism to any retrograde intraductal passage of pathogens. Normally, increased levels of S-IgA are identifiable in salivary samples obtained from bacterial parotitis. Following a tumoricidal course of radiotherapy to the oropharynx, the plasma cells in the interlobular connective tissue fail to produce an elevated S-IgA.[1] In the absence of suppression, one would expect a retrograde migration of microflora into the salivary ducts and acini to stimulate IgA production as flow rates decline. We failed to find an elevated IgA level. The patients in our study had severe advanced periodontitis and radiation-induced dental caries and would be expected to have had high oral bacterial counts.[1]

The relationship between saliva and serum agglutination titers in postirradiation patients shows a significant inverse relationship between S-IgA depression, dental caries, and lower agglutination titers to *S. mutans*, *S. sanguis*, and *L. fermenti*.[2, 3]

TABLE 11–6.—TWO SIMPLE TESTS TO EVALUATE SALIVARY FUNCTION

1. Stimulated total salivary gland capacity (5 minutes):	
Normal	25 ml
Hyposecretor	< 15 ml
Hypersecretor	> 35 ml
2. Clinical assessment and guide to significant viscosity changes:	
Maximum length of viscous salivary web:	
Normal	5 cm
Viscous	15 cm

WHAT ARE THE ULTIMATE EFFECTS OF IRRADIATION CHANGES ON THE DENTITION?

Characteristically, the dental caries that are secondary to ionizing irradiation commences at the cervical margin of the tooth. This area coincides with the cementoenamel junction (CEJ). The CEJ is usually above the level of the gingiva. When the CEJ is above the gum margin, it is susceptible to the tenacious levans and dextrans produced by *S. mutans*, which provides a low pH medium for dental demineralization. Interproximal dental areas are the primary sites affected. Clinically, one observes progressive buccal and labial extension of the demineralization until eventually the teeth have ring-bark circumferential caries, pathognomonic for radiation exposure.

The clinical effects of irradiation to the dentition are primarily due to the changes that occur in the periodontal tissues and the salivary glands. The changes are not due to any direct alteration of the tooth structure by irradiation. Attempts at dental restoration are uniformily unsatisfactory because of progressive caries. Continued loss of tooth tissue from the margins of the restoration does lead to the loss of mechanical retention of most of the restorative materials. The fillings are dislodged from the tooth. Amalgam has superior physical properties when compared to other composite restorative materials. It provides the mainstay of the management of radiation-induced dental caries. Teeth that are affected by circumferential caries are prone to frequent spontaneous amputations, usually without antecedent pulpitis. The absence of pulpitis is due to fibrosis and neural destruction secondary to the chronic effects of radiation.

Occasionally periapical inflammation occurs. The intramedullary alveolar bone is vulnerable to infection. Systemic transport of antibiotics must penetrate into areas of poor vascularity in order to achieve therapeutic levels in the locality of a periapical infection. Tissue antibiotic levels are probably not as high as desired.

Management of periapical inflammation is best undertaken by conservative endodontic therapy as opposed to dental extraction. Osteoradionecrosis may follow an isolated extraction in an irradiated mandible. Any endodontic management must emphasize that the intraradicular biomechanical preparation must not extend beyond the confines of the root. Care must be taken not to extrude the pulpal debris into or beyond the periodontal ligament. Doing so will likely precipitate an acute apical abscess.

Root canal obturation appears to be most successful with silver points rather than gutta percha points. The reason for this is speculative. It is thought that the silver oxides that form about the silver points are more bacteriostatic than the leachable root canal sealants used with both gutta percha and silver points. A significant disadvantage with silver points is that they are not biodegradable. Therefore, inadvertent extrusion beyond the root apex will precipitate a localized osteitis. For this reason, accurate apical preparation is critical to the overall success of root canal therapy for teeth that have been retained for dental and prosthetic management of selected radiation patients.

The unwary practitioner or occasional dental clinician may make optimistic treatment plans and make zealous efforts in head and neck irradiation patients to preserve teeth, particularly in younger patients. This ideal frequently becomes a long-term clinical albatross when the associated problems of osteoradionecrosis emerge. Preirradiation evaluation of patients should be undertaken with the following risk criteria:

MAJOR CRITERIA

1. Ports and dosage are transoral and the planned dose to the teeth in question will exceed 3,000 rad.
2. No useful purpose is served by retention of the teeth/tooth.
3. Dental function will be limited to a few months, rather than have the teeth remain indefinitely, e.g., preoperative irradiation is given before a large segment of tooth-bearing mandible or maxilla is resected.
4. Advanced periodontal disease (is this a monoradicular tooth or a multiradicular tooth?).
5. Significant previous dental problems for that tooth, for example, deep restoration, crown, etc.
6. The therapy is not palliative.
7. Low salivary flow of higher viscosity.

MINOR CRITERIA

1. The patient will not be cooperative in a complex care program.
2. Minimal dental caries is present.
3. No previous regular dental care in the setting of generalized horizontal alveolar bone loss.
4. Logistic difficulties for follow-up for dental prophylaxis and topical fluoride therapy.

One major criterion determines the need to perform preradiation edentulation, and two or more minor criteria strongly suggest that dental extractions are indicated as an integral part of the preirradiation or presurgical management and for the subsequent care for the patient. Figure 11–2 summarizes some of the major decision points for patients who will be irradiated.

CAN MAXILLARY TEETH BE RETAINED IN RADIATION PATIENTS WHEN MANDIBULAR EDENTULATION HAS BEEN PLANNED OR IS PRESENT?

The mechanical trauma to an edentulous mandible from opposing natural teeth will eventually precipitate either direct or indirect injury of the mandibular alveolar mucoperiosteum. This is a particular problem for patients who have had or will undergo radiation therapy to the jaws. Loading forces to a dental prosthesis by natural dentition exceeds the loading force that is generated by an opposing dental prosthesis. In addition, the oral flora in the dentulous patient is markedly different from that in the edentulous patient. In the dentate mouth the bacteria are typically obligative and faculatative anaerobic organisms, together with the microaerophilic and acidophilic organisms. The change in milieu of the edentulous mouth favors saprophyte overgrowth by *Candida albicans*. There are significant reductions in numbers of peptostreptococci, fusiform bacilli, and *Bacteroides melanogenicus*. If teeth are retained in the postirradiated oral cavity where nasopharyngeal organisms can flourish in the mouth, then patients with xerostomia will have a high bacterial acidogenic oral flora, with the predictable result of severe dental caries and accelerated periodontal injury.

Proponents of dental maintenance claim satisfactory dental preservation with regular topical fluoride therapy, administered daily by the patient, either in a custom dental arch tray that fits over the maxillary and mandibular teeth or by toothbrush application after regular oral hygiene has been completed. Interspersed at regular intervals of 2–4 weeks are clinical follow-up examinations and prophylaxis and fluoride applications. Clearly, any change in patient compliance or ability to carry out meticulous oral hygiene will quickly produce rapid deterioration of retained dentition.

IS TOPICAL FLUORIDE EFFECTIVE IN ALLOWING PRESERVATION OF TEETH IN THE IRRADIATED PATIENT?

Stannous fluoride 1.4% causes less direct gingival injury than does sodium fluoride when correctly applied. It also has less of an emetic effect than sodium fluoride. If the topical fluoride is to be incorporated into the superficial crystal lattice of tooth hydroxyapatite, then it must not be diluted or displaced by other active ions. In our clinic, even with meticulous dental care, radiation-induced caries becomes evident in the long term (3+ years). This unfortunate demise of well-nurtured teeth has also been documented elsewhere[3, 4] in a longitudinal study which noted the microbial population

DENTAL MANAGEMENT FOR IRRADIATION THERAPY OF OROPHARYNGEAL MALIGNANCY

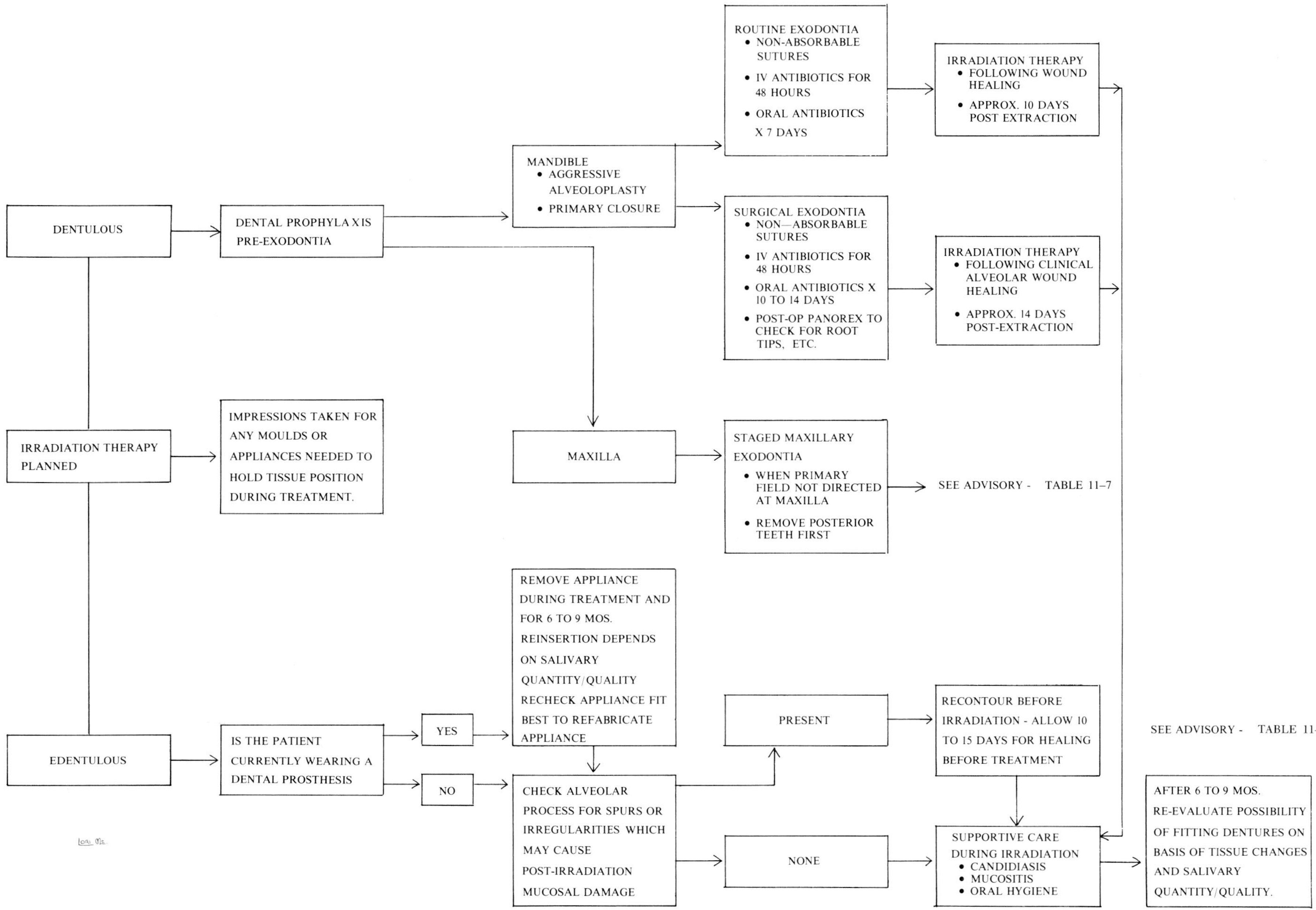

Fig 11–2.—More complex decisions about dentition are required if treatment entails irradiation or irradiation plus surgery.

shifts following radiation therapy. Dental caries occurred following alterations in the microflora, irrespective of the type of topical fluoride applied. Of 36 patients, 23 developed an average of 17.9 caries/patient within 30 months following irradiation, despite careful fluoride treatment and use.[3]

The large bulk of patients with oral cancers do not have impeccable dentition with healthy periodontium. They rarely display a reliable willingness to maintain excellent oral hygiene and follow a complex program with fluoride. The ability to retain teeth requires young patients with impeccable dentition and a ready willingness to participate in a lifelong compulsive ritual.

Any discussion of the preservaton of teeth with effective irradiation treatment must conclude that teeth that are directly in a high-dose field are usually expendable in the overall assessment of patient well-being. No matter how noble the motives for preservation of teeth, the initial hopes of the clinician usually undergo an entropic shift as the clinical condition continues to shuffle downhill to osteoradionecrosis.

WHAT IS THE CLINICAL PATTERN OBSERVED WITH IRRADIATION OF THE ORAL MUCOSA?

Radiation mucositis is painful, debilitating, and emotionally taxing during the course of treatment. The onset and severity vary considerably among patients. The clinical degree of mucositis has a direct relationship to the degree of oral xerostomia. Its time of onset is related to the rate of the absorbed dose of radiation. Twice-daily radiation treatment protocols produce a more intense mucositis that develops earlier in the therapy. The patients have more difficulty adjusting to the discomfort. Once-daily treatments do not cause as frequent disruptions of treatment scheduling as twice-daily protocols.

When the clinician sees radiation mucositis, it is an intensely erythematous, edematous, and often ulcerative mucosal state. All areas of the mouth and oropharynx may be simultaneously involved. A partial xerostomia coexists with the mucositis. Salivary changes usually precede mucositis by approximately 7–10 days. Saliva is typically frothy, with an apparent loss of the anticipated spinnbarkeit. Desquamated epithelium, usually mechanically removed by tongue and cheek movements or irrigated away, now lies over the mucosa, adding to its water-logged appearance and the opalescence of the scant pool of saliva that may be seen in the mouth. The commissures of the mouth are cheilotic, with some evidence of small hemorrhages. The exquisitely tender mouth is examined only with difficulty. When a florid mucositis is present, swallowing, speaking, and chewing are painful and avoided by the patient. Oral hygiene is usually abandoned by both the patient and the dentist due to the intensity of the discomfort. Frequently the oral cavity and oropharynx are overgrown by *C. albicans,* thus aggravating the condition.

HOW DO YOU MANAGE RADIATION MUCOSITIS?

Symptomatic management of radiation mucositis is principally dependent on maintaining a moist mucosa. This may be done by having the patient refrain from using commercial mouth rinses, which often contain 14%–18% alcohol. Alcohol in these preparations (as well as in alcoholic beverages) adds to mucosal dessication. Artificial saliva should be used instead of mouthwashes. It is available as Oralube to federal health care facilities, and is commercially available as Xerolube. These moistening agents provide a lubricating medium that is palatable and therapeutically beneficial. The formulation of both of these saliva substitutes permits oral ingestion without concern for cardiovascular, renal, or hepatic toxity or fluid overload. Patients should be vigorously discouraged from using candies to stimulate salivary flow and from drinking sweet carbonated beverages, since the sugar will facilitate rampant dental caries, particularly in patients with xerostomia.

Diphenhydramine, when held in the mouth in contact with the mucositis for 3–5 minutes, will provide symptomatic relief of the mucositis-related pain. This antihistamine may augment xerostomia if it is ingested. As the mucositis progresses in severity, milk of magnesia may be applied to the mucosa. It should be used in 10- to 15-ml volumes after oral hygiene has been completed. It is applied directly to the inflamed mucosal surfaces. The high pH of milk of magnesia neutralizes the oral acid that is present in radiation mucositis. In addition, the surface retention of the dense suspension of milk of magnesia confers a long-lasting protective covering to the mucosa. If significant discomfort persists after the use of these agents, then topical xylocaine 10% or diclonine hydrochloride 0.5% may be tried. Rapid absorption of these agents will occur through the ulcerated and hyperemic mucosa. Therefore, these topical anesthetics should be used sparingly to avoid specific systemic drug-induced toxicities. The goal is to achieve symptomatic relief of the discomfort of mucositis in order to enable the patient to eat and maintain adequate total caloric intake.

Candida infections should be managed with systemic antifungal agents. Mycelia may lie protected beneath accumulating organic debris. Consequently, the more deeply placed *Candida* organisms will not be affected by topical pharmaceuticals. Treatment for oral fungal infections should continue beyond the observed clinical resolution for a minimum of 14 days. Oral candidiasis is often associated with gastrointestinal tract involvement. In women, the urogenital area may become secondarily infected and require management. Acute radiation mucositis usually resolves about 8–12 weeks following the last dose of radiation. Chronic saprophytic overgrowth may persist indefinitely.

WHAT ARE THE CHRONIC CHANGES TO THE ORAL MUCOSA FOLLOWING RADIATION THERAPY?

Over 12–24 months the oral mucosa develops a pallor and increased firmness associated with a loss of resiliency. Distensibility of the buccal tissues diminishes, and the tongue and floor of the mouth become more stiff and take on a shiny, bald appearance.

A close examination of the buccal mucosa and the mucosa of the sulcus areas will reveal a paucity of blood vessels; there is no longer a well-defined junction between the formerly richly vascular free mucogingival connection to the gingiva. Those vessels that are present are telangiectatic capillary collaterals formed as small arterioles are obliterated. For comparison, pressure on these areas in the nonirradiated patient will be followed quickly by rapid vascular refilling with a transient rebound hyperemia. In an irradiated patient, palpation produces local pallor with no subsequent rebound hyperemia. Qualitatively, irradiated tissue does not possess the resiliency of healthy tissue and may feel "boggy" or firm, depending on the stage of local lymphedema.

Heavily irradiated oral mucosa has minimal healing response to such "minor" surgical manipulations as dental extractions or to prosthodontic trauma. Loss of mucosal coverage may lead to osteomyelitis or osteoradionecrosis. The mandible has more than ten times the incidence of osteoradionecrosis than does the maxilla. The difference in incidence is thought to be due to the bony architecture and its regional blood supply.

WHAT ARE THE EFFECTS OF RADIATION ON MANDIBULAR AND MAXILLARY BONE?

The viability of bone requires an adequate blood supply. It is generally assumed that the mandible derives its vascular requirements from the inferior dental artery. The mandible is actually dependent on its muscle attachments for about 75% of its blood supply. This is a critical concept when the incidence of postirradiation morbidity is considered. Many studies fail to identify patients who have had major soft tissue and muscle resection with treatment of a primary carcinoma or neck dissection, both of which may significantly reduce the vascular perfusion of the target bone.

Modern irradiation sources and precise treatment planning are the best way to prevent bone damage. Not all irradiated patients get clinically significant osteoradionecrosis. The declining incidence and the management of the problem are discussed in chapter 27.

Radiation directly damages osteoblasts and osteoclasts in long bones; the critical level is stated to be 3,000 rad. No specific data have been analyzed for the mandible; however, it may reasonably be assumed that the 3,000-rad range will probably have a similar effect on mandibular osteoblasts and osteoclasts. Bone death will occur at 5,000 rad for adult tissue. Juvenile bone is more susceptible to ionizing radiation because of its inherently higher rate of cell turnover. Growth centers are arrested in children at less than 3,000 rad.

In the undissected irradiated mandible, progressive vascular intraluminal obliteration affects all exposed vessels, but more importantly, the distributive capillaries undergo the more significant flow changes due to a greater relative cross-sectional area reduction. With vascular ischemia, normal osteoblastic and osteoclastic activity will decline. Definable changes can be seen in the bony trabecular pattern of cancellous bone when viewed on an intraoral periapical film. These changes of ischemia and decreased bone growth kinetics are helpful in assessing the degree of effect of radiation in the region under examination. Trabecular augmentation is an initial change and contrasts markedly with the local marrow spaces. Progressive radiopacity of the marrow spaces occurs. The area under examination may therefore erroneously be interpreted as a radiographic artifact rather than as exhibiting changes in the ratio of inorganic salt to organic matrix that occur with radiation exposure of bone.

Osteoradionecrosis of the jaws is due to vascular ischemia of bone marrow following radiation. It usually occurs in conjunction with a mixed secondary infection following a disruption in the overlying mucoperiosteum. Osteomyelitis is an infection of bone marrow arising from an odontogenic infection, trauma, or hematogenous spread of microorganisms. The radiographic appearance and clinical signs and symptoms may be similar. Uninfected areas of demineralization may be present. Correct diagnosis of the bone infection is important. It does not rely solely on a history of exposure to irradiation. Radiograms provide static information of past physiologic or pathologic events. For bony changes to be detected, 50% or more of the inorganic matrix

TABLE 11–7.—PRACTICAL ADVICE AND SUGGESTIONS FOR DECISIONS ABOUT DENTITION

1. If maxillary natural teeth are allowed to function against an edentulous irradiated mandible with or without a prosthetic appliance in place, then the stronger maxillary forces will cause mandibular erosion.
2. Maxillary teeth should not be left where they will erode and abrade a flap closure.
3. If radiation is planned for a patient who has previously had some form of marginal mandibulectomy, any remaining teeth should be extracted prior to irradiation to avoid fracture from irradiation changes and function overload on the weakened mandible, which may produce pathologic fractures.
4. Postirradiation dental treatment and extractions require special conservative management.
   (a) Endodontic therapy must avoid extra-apical instrumentation.
   (b) Topical fluoride is used regularly to decrease the rate of dental demineralization of any retained teeth.
   (c) Any dental surgery should be limited to single tooth extractions and mucoperiosteal flaps should be avoided.
   (d) Avoid using local anesthetics containing vasoconstrictors.
   They are unnecessary because the blood flow is already low.
   Prolonged vasoconstriction can cause local tissue necrosis.
   (e) Remove extensive bridge construction to improve oral hygiene.
   (f) Support mobile teeth by interproximal bonding or with an intracoronal splint.
5. A mandible that has been partially resected or had blood supply reduced by dissection or irradiation will have a reduced transport rate for antibiotics.
6. Patients for full-dose chemotherapy require about the same care during active therapy that a radiation patient does. Severe periodontal disease requires dental extractions. Restoration of debilitated but restorable dentition must be completed before active therapy is initiated.
7. In general, younger patients with periodontitis have much less likelihood of maintaining dentition than do older patients with a similar stage of periodontitis.
8. Patients with parafunctional oral movements (i.e., dyskinesias, tics, tardive (drug-induced) or acquired behavioral dyskinesias) should not wear dentures during chemotherapy, to avoid mucosal injury.

must be affected. Utilization of radionuclide imaging will assist the clinician in determining the relative degree of vascularity to the area in question. A photopenic focus implies vascular ischemia. Combining both modalities will offer the clinician optimal information to facilitate differentiating between osteomyelitis and osteoradionecrosis.

The reader is referred to chapter 27 for a discussion of the management of osteoradionecrosis and osteomyelitis. Some practical recommendations on the management of patients who are to undergo irradiation and/or surgical dissection are listed in Table 11–7.

REFERENCES

1. Browne G.A.: Unpublished data.
2. O'Neill P.A., Brown L.R., Dreizen S., et al.: Immunoglobulin class of agglutinins to microorganisms in post-irradiation cancer patients. *J. Dent. Res.* 60:1639–1647, 1981.
3. Brown L.R., O'Neill P.A., Dreizen S., et al.: Relationship between saliva and serum agglutination titers and post-irradiation caries activity in cancer patients. *J. Dent. Res.* 60:10–18, 1981.
4. Brown L.R., Dreizen S., Handler S., et al.: Effect of radiation-induced xerostomia on human oral microflora. *J. Dent. Res.* 54:740–750, 1975.

12 / Cancer of the Lip

ALAN R. SHONS, M.D., Ph.D. / BARRY H. J. PRESS, M.D.

CARCINOMA OF THE LIP is a common and easily accessible malignancy of the head and neck. Early visual detection of lip tumors usually leads to prompt treatment at an early stage. Thus, the prognosis is better than for other head and neck cancers. Carcinoma of the lip is 20 times more frequent in the lower lip than in the upper lip.[1, 2] Carcinoma of the lip occurs most commonly in patients aged 50–70 years, and the male-female ratio is approximately 20:1.[2] Squamous cell carcinoma accounts for approximately 97% of lip cancers and basal cell cancer for 3%.[3] Lip cancer, like skin cancer in other areas, occurs most commonly in fair-skinned persons with extensive sun exposure.

HOW ARE LIP CANCERS CLASSIFIED?

Several different classification systems for carcinoma of the lip have been used by various authors in reporting results. In some centers, the TNM staging system for the oral cavity including the lip has not been applied because of a perceived difference in prognosis of lip cancer as compared to oral cavity cancer. A large study of our experience by Wurman et al.[4] suggests that lip cancer staged as T_2 and T_3 by the TNM system for oral cancer has a metastatic rate comparable to oral cavity cancer (Table 12–1).[5] Broders' classification is recommended for histologic tumor grading by cell differentiation.[6, 7] Chapter 4 discusses the prognostic significance of this classificatory system.

The prognosis for cure of lip cancer varies with the extent of the disease and the degree of cellular differentiation at the time of initial examination. T_1 N_0 M_0 or T_2 N_0 M_0 lesions involving only the lower lip have cure rates of approximately 90%. Similar cure rates have been achieved with either surgery or radiation in several large series of patients with early lip cancers. In a series of 2,066 patients treated by radiation, an 86% 5-year determinate survival was noted.[2] An 82% 5-year determinate survival was reported in a series of 835 patients treated surgically.[8]

Cure rates decrease as the size of the primary increases. Ward and Hendrick, in a surgical series, reported a 5-year cure rate of 95% for lesions less than 1 cm. The cure rate decreased to 41% for lesions more than 3 cm in diameter.[9] Cure rates decrease as histologic differentiation decreases. A 5-year cure rate of 71.6% for grade I and 46.9% for grade III carcinomas was reported in a series of 563 patients treated primarily by surgery.[10] The two variables of size and grade may be related, since higher grades of anaplasia are found in larger lip cancers.

Achievement of cure of lip cancer in patients with metastases to the neck is difficult. The 5-year absolute survival in patients with lip primaries who present with neck metastases is reported to range from 35.9% to 55.5%.[1, 10–12] Lower survival rates are found in patients with fixed cervical nodes or mandibular invasion. Similarly, lower survival rates are found in patients in whom primary treatment failed.

HOW DO YOU DIAGNOSE AND MANAGE THE MINIMAL LIP LESION?

The alert examiner is the best detection device. The most common presentation of lip carcinoma is a nonhealing ulcer with rolled and indurated margins; this is easily recognized as carcinoma. However, the cancer may also present in other less typical forms which may resemble either benign, hyperkeratotic changes or actinic chelitis-type lesions. Gross areas of leukoplakia may encompass histologic changes ranging from hyperkeratosis to invasive carcinoma. Leukoplakia of the lip is best managed by lip shave, which constitutes both treatment and diagnosis. An elliptical incision is outlined to include the area of surface change. The outer margin of the ellipse is normally placed slightly outside

TABLE 12–1.—STAGING OF CARCINOMA OF THE LIP*

T_0	No evidence of primary tumor.
T_{IS}	Carcinoma in situ.
T_1	Greatest diameter of primary tumor 2 cm or less.
T_2	Greatest diameter of primary tumor more than 2 cm but not more than 4 cm.
T_3	Greatest diameter of primary tumor more than 4 cm.
T_4	Tumor more than 4 cm in diameter with deep invasion of bone and muscle.

*From Beahrs and Heyers.[5] Reproduced by permission.

the vermillion border. To prevent distortion of the lip, the ellipse should be oriented symmetrically, even if this means sacrifice of some normal mucosa. After the elliptical excision has been completed, the mucosa of the lip is undermined to the buccal sulcus and then advanced into the defect.

Biopsy of localized suspicious lesions should entail an elliptical incision to encompass all of a portion of the lesion as well as adjacent normal tissues. The biopsy specimen should be of sufficient depth to allow evaluation of invasiveness (see Chap. 4). Alternatively, a small skin punch biopsy may be used. Both methods can be performed under local anesthesia.

When the diagnosis of lip cancer has been made with certainty, the minimal lesion (1–1½ cm) can be treated by radiation or operative therapy with similar cure rates of 80%–90%. Surgical therapy has several advantages. They include immediate eradication of disease, absence of effect on adjacent normal tissue, one-stage excision and reconstruction, and the opportunity to examine pathologically the specimen. For invasive cancer, a simple wedge excision and primary closure are performed (Fig 12–1). A gross margin of at least 0.5 cm of normal-appearing tissue beyond the recognized limits of the tumor is advised. Frozen section examination is done to confirm tumor-free margins. Wedge excision or a variant can be used for lesions which require resection of up to one third of the vermillion. For more extensive excisions some type of cheiloplasty is necessary as an adjunct to lip reconstruction.

ARE UPPER LIP CANCERS DIFFERENT THAN LOWER LIP CANCERS?

Approximately 90%–95% of all squamous cell carcinomas of the lip occur on the lower lip. The rare upper lip lesions may have a worse prognosis because routes of nodal metastasis are more diverse and may include the parotid, preauricular, and facial nodes as well as the various cervical and submandibular lymph node groups. Danish investigators have recently reported substantial differences in the various epidemiological characteristics of upper and lower lip cancer, suggesting that the two are indeed separate entities.[13, 14] Metastases are more likely to be found at the initial examination of a patient with upper lip cancers than lower lip cancers. The higher rate of metastasis is reflected in a lower 5-year survival rate of approximately 50%.[2, 15]

In 1%–2% of cases, both lips or the commissure are involved. The prognosis for lesions of the commissure is not as good as for carcinomas located elsewhere on the lips. Recurrence is common. Commissural cancers behave more like those that involve the mucous membrane of the buccal area and have similar cure rates.

WHAT IS THE ROLE OF NECK DISSECTION IN THE TREATMENT OF CERVICAL METASTASES FROM LIP CANCER?

Lip cancer does cause death. In most instances uncontrolled disease is associated with metastatic cancer spread to lymph nodes of the neck. These few deaths occur in a large cohort of patients where the majority of lip cancers are well differentiated and diagnosed at an early stage before metastases occur. The management of the larger advanced cancer or the poorly differentiated cancer presents a special challenge.

The incidence of nodal metastases from lip cancers varies considerably in different reports. The aggregate number of patients who develop cervical metastases from cancer of the lip is low, less than 10% in most series (Table 12–2). Most often recommendations for cervical node treatment vary with the personal experience of the reporting group. There is a general agree-

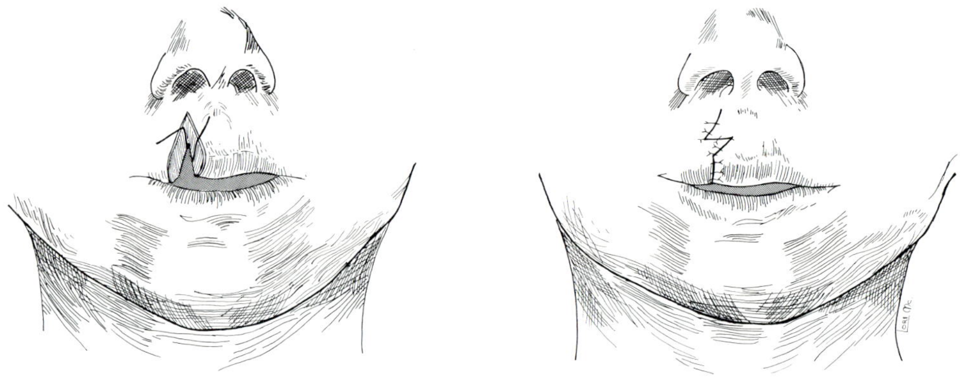

A B

Fig 12–1.—The more demanding wedge excision of the upper lip is illustrated to show a procedure to minimize the linear scar. **A,** a defect following wedge excision of a lip lesion can be closed with a Z-plasty to prevent linear contracture and vermillion border distortion. Secure approximation of the os orbiculare muscle must be achieved in the repair to allow satisfactory postoperative lip function. **B,** the flaps are interdigitated and the repair is completed. The same type of repair can be performed on the lower lip.

TABLE 12–2.—INCIDENCE OF NODE METASTASIS IN PATIENTS WITHOUT METASTASES ON ADMISSION

STUDY, YEAR	NO. OF PTS.	% WITH SUBSEQUENT METASTASES
Jorgensen et al.,[12] 1973	869	5.2
Gladstone and Kerr,[17] 1958	498	7.8
Regato et al.,[18] 1959	519	9.1

ment that the incidence of cervical node involvement depends on two major factors, the size of the primary lesion and the degree of cellular differentiation. Ashley et al.[16] noted an incidence of lymphatic involvement in 2% of patients with primary lesions less than 1 cm, in 7% of patients with lesions 1–2 cm, and in 18% of patients with lesions larger than 2 cm. Wurman et al.[4] reported a 52% incidence of metastasis from primaries 2–4 cm in the largest dimension. There was a 73% incidence of metastasis from primaries larger than 4 cm in size.

Routine full prophylactic neck dissection is not advocated for all cases of lip cancer. The usual justification for not including elective treatment of the neck *with* treatment of the primary lip cancer is that the cure rate for *therapeutic* neck dissection for subsequently confirmed occult metastases compares favorably with the results of *elective* radical neck dissection. The findings of Marshall and Edgerton sharply question the above assumption.[19] Seven of their patients developed cervical metastases after initial treatment of lip cancer and underwent subsequent therapeutic radical neck dissection. All seven died of metastatic disease. It is apparent that tumor spread in the upper anterior cervical nodes, while not common, is a major factor in mortality from this disease. In our series, patients with T_2 and T_3 cancers had a significant incidence of lymph node metastases. Thus, if there is to be improvement in the curative results in patients with advanced lip cancers, it is necessary to anticipate node metastases in large lip cancers, detect recurrence earlier, and excise enlarged nodes before there is penetration of the lymph node capsule by tumor.

Marshall and Edgerton recommend aggressive treatment, including bilateral suprahyoid neck dissection, if there is (1) a primary lesion greater than 1.5 cm in diameter, (2) cancer of the commissure or upper lip, (3) recurrent cancer, (4) poorly differentiated cancer, (5) palpable cervical adenopathy, or (6) an unreliable patient likely not to return for regular follow-up examination. If tumor is found in these suprahyoid specimens, a full radical neck dissection is performed on the side of the node involvement. The inherent problems with suprahyoid dissections are discussed in chapter 9.

Because about 50% of patients with pathologically positive nodes in the suprahyoid region will also have tumor in the jugular nodes, and because metastases may also bypass the suprahyoid nodes, suprahyoid dissection fails as the *only* therapeutic procedure and as a predictive maneuver. Where suspicion of node metastases is confirmed or high (i.e., a larger tumor > 2 cm or a 1.5 cm lesion of high grade, grade III or grade IV), we prefer an eleventh-nerve-sparing neck dissection. The techniques are discussed in chapter 9.

WHAT ARE THE OPTIONS IN RADIATION THERAPY

Radiotherapeutic treatment of lip cancer may consist of interstitial, contact, or external beam therapy. Contact and interstitial applications of radium have now largely been supplanted by external radiotherapy, which is more versatile, controllable, and can penetrate to a greater depth. While low voltage x-irradiation (100 kV) has produced satisfactory results for small, shallow lesions, higher energy is preferable for tumors greater than 1.5 cm in diameter. Total doses of 3,000–6,000 rad are delivered in daily fractions over a 4 to 6-week period. More recently, electron beam irradiation (7–18 MeV) has been used with advantage. Additional depth of penetration is achieved, while 80%–100% of delivered energy is still present to a depth of 2–3 cm. There is a rapid fall-off in dose beyond these depths. Thus, the mandible receives very little radiation with electron beam therapy. Regardless of the method of delivering radiation therapy, care must be taken to protect the adjacent uninvolved tissue by proper shielding. This will confine the sequelae of mucositis and radiodermatitis to a restricted area. After radiation therapy, permanent hypersensitivity to thermal and actinic stimuli is present. For patients having occupations associated with sun exposure, the local skin change remains a disadvantage of irradiation therapy. Late local changes include cutaneous depigmentation and atrophy of the lip musculature in the irradiated field.

The place of prophylactic neck irradiation of the patient with cancer of the lip has not been prospectively studied. It may be chosen for the treatment of unreliable patients with clinically negative (N_0) necks. For obvious metastatic nodes, therapeutic neck irradiation has proved to be less successful than operative extirpation.

WHAT ARE THE SURGICAL OPTIONS FOR RESECTING AND RECONSTRUCTING LARGE LIP CANCERS?

Repair by excision and primary closure will produce a satisfactory result when less than one third of the lip must be resected (see Fig 12–1). Larger defects require additional tissue from another location for reconstruction. The operations for lip reconstruction may be classified in order of preference, as follows: (1) those which are limited to the remaining lip segments, (2) those which borrow from the opposite lip, (3) those which utilize adjacent cheek tissue, and (4) those which employ distant flaps. Local flap reconstruction is preferable because of close facial skin color and texture match, as well as the availability of mucous membrane. The best technique which borrows tissue from the opposite lip is the lip switch, Abbe or Estlander flap. The Abbe technique is used for defects medial to the oral commissure in both upper and lower lip (Fig 12–2). The width of the Abbe flap should be one-half the width of the resected segment so that the two lips are reduced proportionately with flap transposition. The pedicle should be made as narrow as possible to facilitate rotation. Special care must be taken to avoid injury to the labial artery. With meticulous dissection the flap can be created as an island flap pedicled only on the vessels. After there is good healing, the pedicle of the Abbe flap can be divided in 2 weeks. If the division of the Abbe flap pedicle is done by performing an associated inset by the technique illustrated in Figure 12–3, then satisfactory lip contour will result.

Lesions near the oral commissure can be treated by the Estlander modification of the Abbe procedure (Fig 12–4). This technique does not involve a cross-lip pedicle. It does require a second-stage reconstruction of the commissure. The technique of commissure reconstruction that is illustrated in Figure 12–5 is the procedure of choice.

WHAT PROCEDURES CAN BE USED WHEN MOST OF THE LIP IS EXCISED?

Resection of large lip cancers will produce large defects that will constitute a near-total loss of the upper or lower lip. A more extensive lip reconstruction must use some type of lateral advancement flap incorporating the mobilized tissue of the cheek. The Gillies fan technique may be used for large central defects of either the upper or lower lip (Fig 12–6). Mucosal lining can be obtained by mobilization of the remaining oral mucosa.

Another technique is the Camille-Bernard operation, which employs lateral advancement flaps. Medial rotation of soft tissue is facilitated by the excision of Burow's triangle (Fig 12–7). Oral mucosa on the inside of Burow's triangle is preserved and used to restore the vermillion border (Figs 12–7,B and C). The lower lip

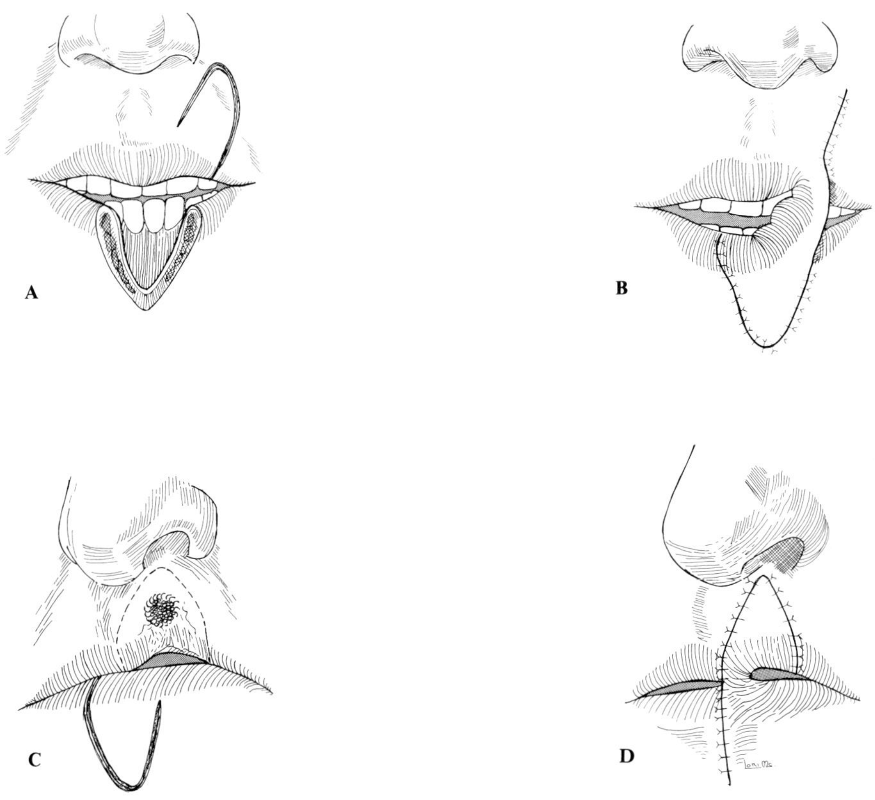

Fig 12–2.—The Abbe lip-switch technique. **A** and **B,** the technique employed for a lower lip defect. **C** and **D,** the technique employed for an upper lip defect. Full-thickness flaps are designed one-half the width of the original defect. The narrow pedicle is created to facilitate rotation to the donor site for reconstruction. The pedicle is divided and inset at 10–14 days, as shown in Figure 12–3.

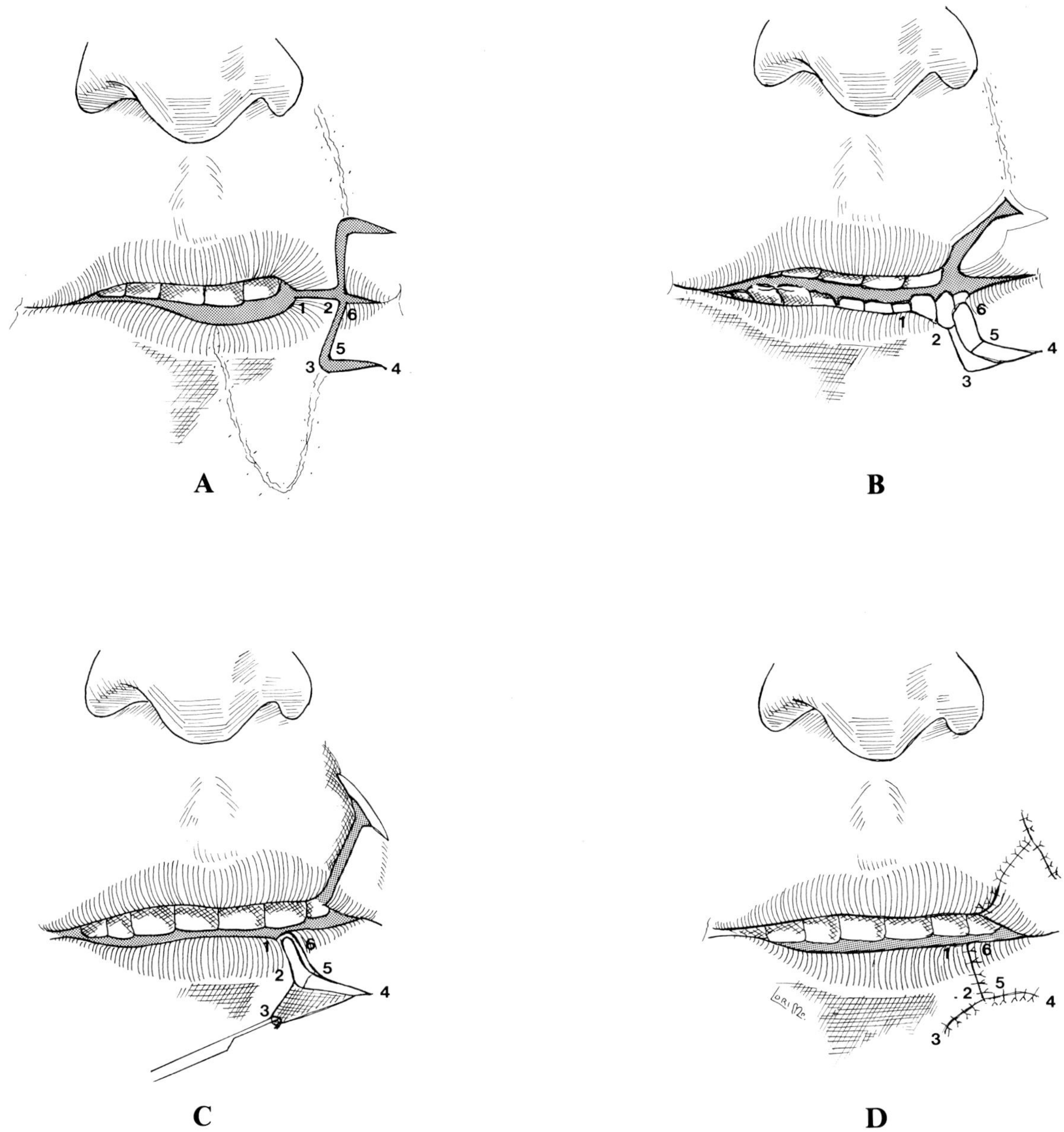

Fig 12–3.—Division of the Abbe pedicle by the technique of May. **A,** the previous line of closure *(2–3)* is opened for a distance of 1 cm. One-centimeter lateral incisions are made *(3–4).* **B,** the incisions are made and the flaps created. **C,** Z-plasty transposition of the flaps while tension is maintained at *3.* **D,** closure completed with vermillion edge aligned.

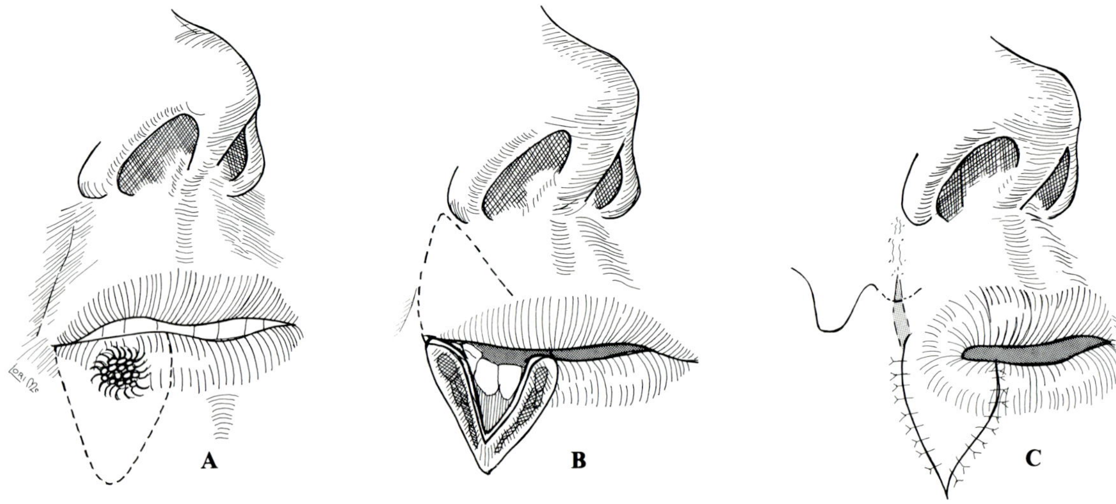

Fig 12–4.—The Estlander technique for lateral lip defects. **A,** the excision extends to the oral commissure. **B,** the flap is outlined with a medial labial artery pedicle. **C,** the flap is transposed, with a round commissure as a result.

cheek flaps cannot be advanced medially unless there is wide undermining along the lateral mandible (see Fig 12–7,B). The main complaints of patients undergoing lip reconstruction are drooling, poor speech intelligibility, cracking and fissuring, lack of sensibility, and inadequacy of stomal size. While many lip reconstructions may have an acceptable appearance in repose, the functional result with attempted animation of the face may not be as satisfactory because most reconstructive methods either partially or totally denervate the flaps. A more pleasing functional result can be obtained in the reconstruction of large lip defects by using the Karapandzic principle, which consists of mobilizing *arterialized innervated* flaps of skin and os obiculare muscle from the surrounding network of suspensory muscles. These flaps are utilized to form a new and smaller oral sphincter (Fig 12–8).[20] When the neural integrity and anatomical position of the os obiculare sphincter mechanism are preserved, there are the salutary results of good oral continence, sphincter function, and symmetric lip movement. The resultant microstomia created by this operation does not cause a functional problem.

Finally, in very large lip defects lacking appropriate adjacent flap tissue, a distant flap must be considered. The deltopectoral flap is perhaps most commonly used for lower lip reconstruction, while the temporally based forehead flap may be used for upper lip reconstruction. Both of these flaps must be lined with skin grafts, or, as an alternative, the deltopectoral flap may be turned

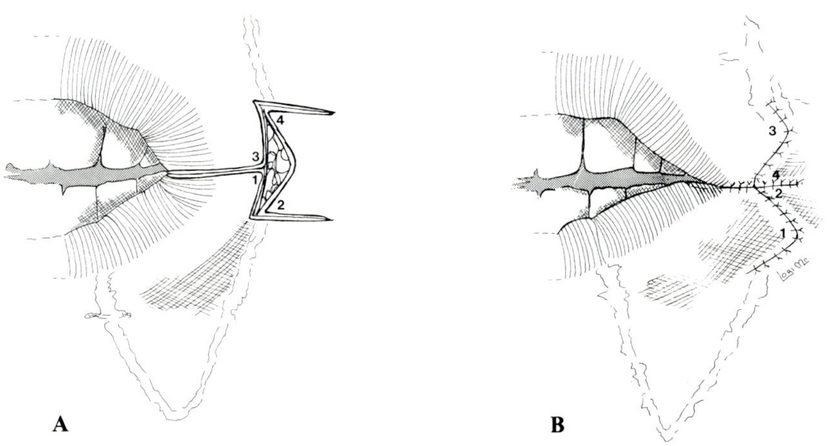

Fig 12–5.—Double Z-plasty technique of May for the correction of a round commissure following the Estlander reconstruction. **A,** the previous incision is opened lateral to the commissure for a distance of 2 cm *(2–4).* Superior and inferior 1-cm lateral extensions are incised. **B,** double Z-plasty flaps are transposed as shown and the repair is completed.

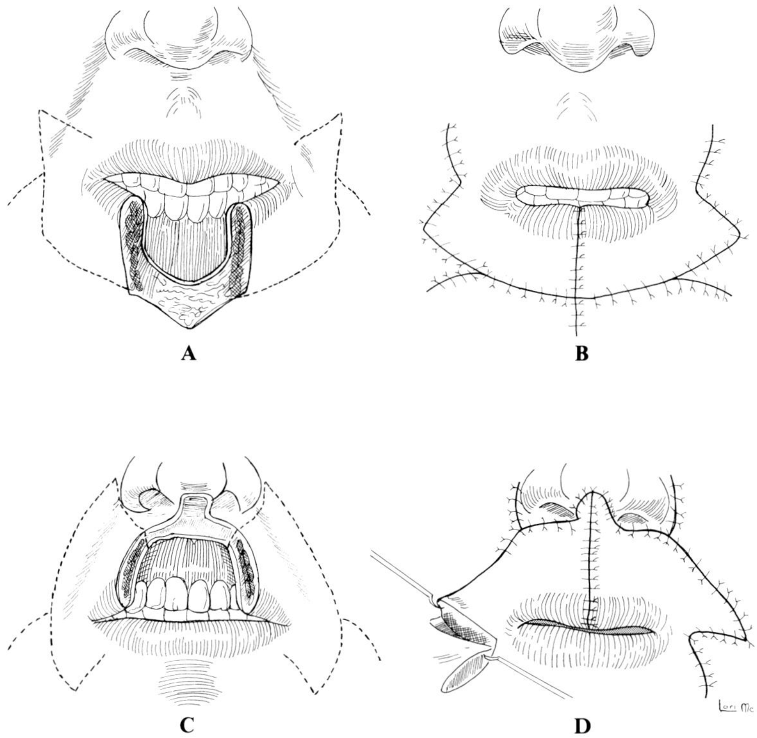

Fig 12–6.—The Gillies fan flap technique. **A** and **B,** the technique is applied to a large central lower lip defect. **C** and **D,** the technique is applied to a large central upper lip defect. The lateral defects are closed by transposition flaps.

on itself to supply the inner lining of the reconstructed lip. Such distant flap reconstructions are cosmetically and functionally less satisfactory than local transposition flap reconstruction.

Wound care following surgical resection of lip carcinoma should include skin suture removal between days 4 and 7 postoperatively unless the patient has been previously irradiated. Postoperative feeding should be restricted to a liquid diet for the first 48 hours, followed by a soft diet for 4–5 days. If the patient wears dentures, do not let him or her attempt to insert them for at least 3–4 weeks. Of course, patients with pedicle flaps crossing the oral stoma must be maintained on a liquid diet until division of the pedicle takes place.

Common technical problems include misalignment of the vermillion, microstomia, and ectropion. Ectropion and disruption of the vermillion can be minimized by tension-free suture lines and careful approximation of the vermillion border. Microstomia can be prevented by the liberal use of local and regional flaps. If a pa-

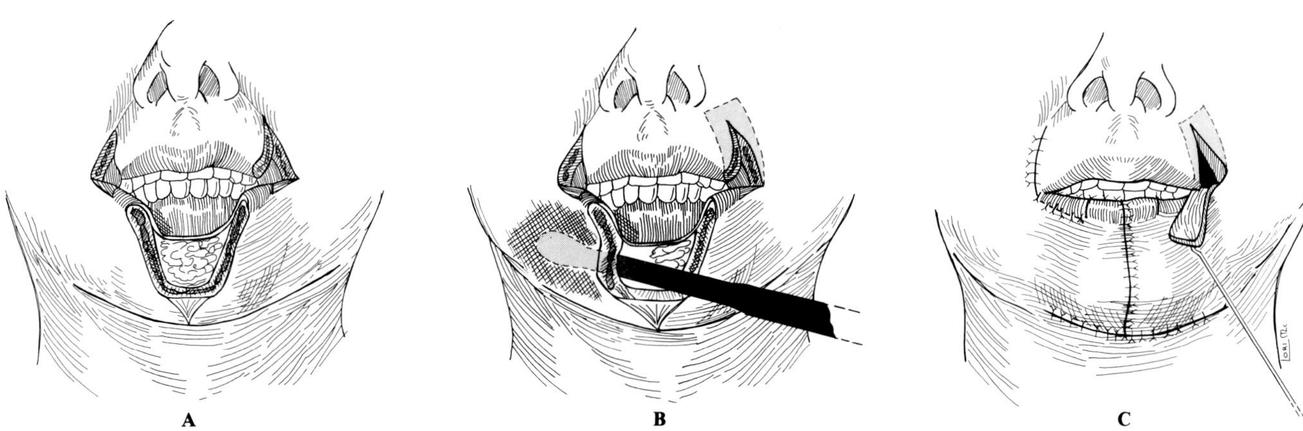

Fig 12–7.—Camille-Bernard procedure. **A,** Burow's triangles are outlined laterally, with the apex of the triangle oriented in the nasolabial fold. **B,** extensive lateral mobilization of the cheek is required to free the flap off the underlying mandible to allow for medial advancement of the cheek flaps. The flaps of preserved mucosa are indicated by *dotted lines.* **C,** the closure is completed by bringing downward the mucosal flaps that underlie Burow's triangle. The mucosal flap is based inferiorly, brought down, and adjusted to restore the vermillion border.

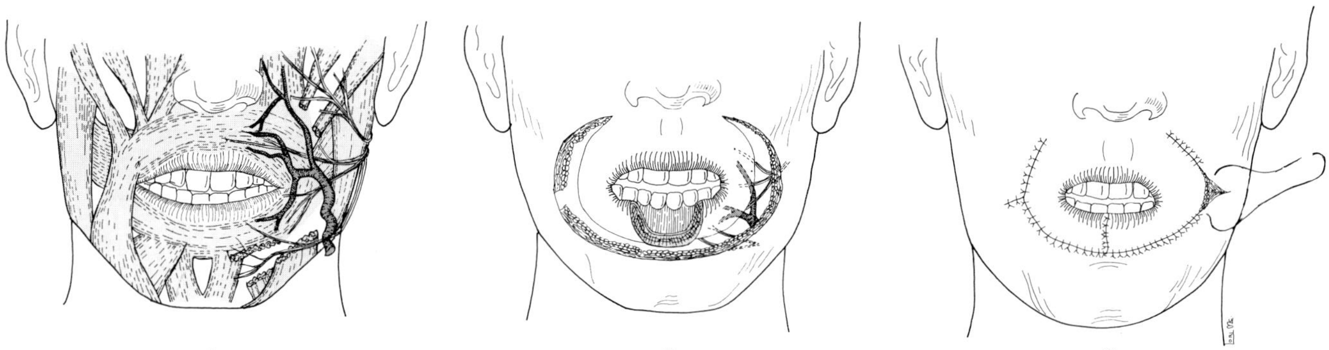

A B C

Fig 12–8.—The Karapandzic lip reconstruction. **A,** perioral anatomy illustrating facial nerve innervation of the os obiculare muscle. **B,** the dissection, nearly completed, involves division of the suspensory musculature with preservation of innervated os obiculare muscle and overlying skin. **C,** medial mobilization of lip flaps with closure of lateral defect employing a Y-V technique.

tient's speech is intelligible and drooling is controlled, microstomia is not a major problem and is generally well tolerated. Distortion of the commissure is a frequent occurrence with lip-switch flaps as well as lateral advancement flaps. Commissuroplasty as a secondary procedure can improve the appearance of the reconstructed commissures. Patients should also be cautioned to avoid smoking and sun exposure postoperatively.

REFERENCES

1. MacKay E.N., Seller A.H.: A statistical review of carcinoma of the lip. *Can. Med. Assoc. J.* 90:670, 1964.
2. Molnar L., Ronay P., Tapolesanyi L.: Carcinoma of the lip: Analysis of the material of 25 years. *Oncology* 29:101, 1974.
3. Stoddard T.G.: Conference on cancer of the lip. *Can. Med. Assoc. J.* 90:666, 1964.
4. Wurman L.H., Adams G.L., Meyerhoff W.L.: Carcinoma of the lip. *Am. J. Surg.* 130:470, 1975.
5. Beahrs O.H., Heyers M.H. (eds.): *Manual for Staging of Cancer.* Philadelphia, J.B. Lippincott Co., 1983, p. 25.
6. Broders A.C.: Squamous cell epithelioma of the lip. *JAMA* 74:656, 1920.
7. Broders A.C.: Carcinoma. *Arch. Pathol.* 2:376, 1926.
8. Bernier J.L., Clark M.L.: Squamous cell carcinoma of the lip: A critical, statistical and morphological analysis of 835 cases. *Milit. Surg.* 109:379, 1951.
9. Ward G.E., Hendrick J.W.: Results of treatment of carcinoma of the lip. *Surgery* 27:321, 1950.
10. Cross J.E., Guralnick E., Daland E.M.: Carcinoma of the lip: A review of 563 case records of carcinoma of the lip at the Pondville Hospital. *Surg. Gynecol. Obstet.* 87:153, 1948.
11. Jorgensen K., Elbrond O., Anderson A.P.: Carcinoma of the lip. *Acta Otolaryngol.* 75:312, 1973.
12. Jorgensen K., Elbrond O., Anderson A.P.: Carcinoma of the lip: A series of 869 cases. *Acta Radiol.* 12:177, 1973.
13. Lindquist C., Teppo L.: Is upper lip cancer "true" lip cancer? *J. Cancer Res. Clin. Oncol.* 97:187, 1980.
14. Lee E.S., Wilson J.S.P.: Cancer of the lip. *Proc. R. Soc. Med.* 63:685, 1970.
15. Schreiner B.F., Christy C.J.: Results of irradiation treatment of cancer of the lip: Analysis of 36 cases from 1926–1936. *Radiology* 39:293, 1942.
16. Ashley F.L., McConnell D.V., Machida R., et al.: Carcinoma of the lip. *Am. J. Surg.* 110:549, 1965.
17. Gladstone W.S., Kerr H.D.: Epidermoid carcinoma of the lower lip: Results of radiation therapy of the local lesions. *AJR* 79:101, 1958.
18. Del Regato J.A., Sala J.M.: The treatment of carcinoma of the lip. *Radiology* 73:839, 1959.
19. Marshall K.A., Edgerton M.T.: Indications for neck dissection in carcinomas of the lip. *Am. J. Surg.* 133:216, 1977.
20. Jabaley M.E., Clement R.C., Orcutt T.W.: Myocutaneous flaps in lip reconstruction: Applications of the Karapandzic principle. *Plast. Reconstr. Surg.* 59(5):680, 1977.

13 / Oral Cancer

DONALD G. MCQUARRIE, M.D., PH.D.

THE BOUNDARIES of the oral cavity include all of the structures anterior to the tonsillar pillars and the circumvalate papillae of the tongue. The discussion in this chapter will exclude the lips (covered in Chap. 12). The areas and boundaries of the oral cavity are defined in Table 13–1. There are cancers that obviously straddle one or more of the anatomical divisions of the oral cavity. Consequently, assignment of location may be quite arbitrary. Modest-sized cancers may extend through the oral cavity into the oropharynx. The division between the oral cavity and the oropharynx is conceptually useful because for oral cancer, detection and treatment is easier, there is a wider range of therapeutic options, and surgical margins can be larger. As might be expected, patients with oral cavity cancers generally have a better aggregate survival rate than patients with oropharyngeal cancers. A T_1N_O oral cancer should have a high rate of cure with minimal disability or deformity.

NINETY-SEVEN PERCENT OF ORAL PRIMARY CANCERS ARE SQUAMOUS CELL CANCERS

Squamous cell cancer causes characteristic irregularity and ulceration of the mucosal surface. The rare adenocarcinoma (1%–3%) arises in a minor salivary gland. It has normal intact overlying mucosa until late in its course, when the mucosa may degenerate and ulcerate. Adenocarcinomas are generally painless and regular in outline.

WHICH AREAS OF THE ORAL CAVITY ARE MOST FREQUENTLY INVOLVED WITH CANCER?

Chapter 2, on diagnosis, called attention to the particular areas of oral vulnerability. These areas are identified by the shaded areas of Figure 13–1. The vulnerable areas probably are made so by a higher concentration of carcinogenic exposure and by failure to

TABLE 13–1.—DEFINITION OF ANATOMICAL LIMITS OF ORAL CAVITY*

The oral cavity extends from the lips anteriorly to but not including the soft palate and posteriorly to the base of the tongue. It is divided into specific subsites, as defined below.

Buccal mucosa.—All the membrane lining the inner surface of the cheek and lips from the line of contact of the opposing lips to the line of attachment of mucosa of the alveolar ridge (upper and lower) and the pterygomandibular raphe.

Lower alveolar ridge.—The alveolar process of the mandible and its covering mucosa (lower gingiva), which extends from the line of attachment of mucosa in the buccal gutter to the line of free mucosa of the floor of the mouth. Posteriorly it extends to the ascending ramus of the mandible.

Upper alveolar ridge.—The alveolar process of the maxilla and its covering mucosa (upper gingiva), which extends from the line of attachment of mucosa in the upper gingival buccal gutter to the junction of the hard palate. Its posterior margin is the upper end of the pterygopalatine arch.

Retromolar gingiva (trigone).—The attached mucosa overlying the ascending ramus of the mandible from the level of the posterior surface of the last molar tooth to the apex superiorly, adjacent to the tuberosity of the maxilla.

Floor of mouth.—A semilunar space over the myelohyoid and hyoglossus extending from the inner surface of the lower alveolar ridge to the undersurface of the tongue. Its posterior boundary is the base of the anterior pillar of the tonsil. It is divided into two sides by the frenulum of the tongue and contains the ostia of the submaxillary and lingual salivary glands.

Hard palate.—The semilunar area between the upper alveolar ridges and the mucous membrane covering the palatine process of the maxillary palatine bones. It extends from the inner surface of the superior alveolar ridge to the posterior edge of the palatine bone.

Anterior two thirds of tongue.—A freely mobile portion of the tongue which extends anteriorly from the line of circumvallate papillae to the undersurface of the tongue at the junction of the floor of the mouth. It is composed of four areas: (1) tip, (2) lateral borders, (3) dorsum, and (4) undersurface (nonvillous surface of the tongue).

*Based on AJC clinical staging system.

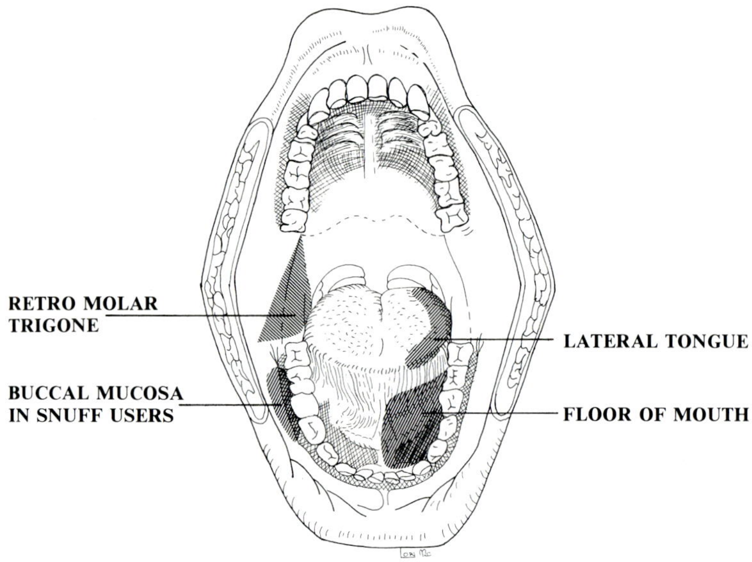

Fig 13–1.—Areas of vulnerability to oral cancer. *Shading* indicates sites of most frequent cancer occurrence. Note the absence of cancers in the upper tongue and upper portions of the oral mucosa.

clean the carcinogens from mucosal surfaces. If one observes the mouth of heavy tobacco users, the accumulation of tobacco residue may be correlated with the areas involved: the puddle in the anterior floor of the mouth, tongue irritation in pipe smokers, buccal mucosal or floor of the mouth leukoplakia in tobacco chewers or snuff users, and tar collection, with the dental plaque keeping a reservoir of carcinogens in constant contact with gingiva and lateral tongue.

DO DIFFERENT LOCATIONS WITHIN THE ORAL CAVITY HAVE A DIFFERENT PROGNOSIS WITH SIMILARLY STAGED SQUAMOUS CELL CANCERS?

Table 13–2 gives some selected survival statistics drawn from different centers at different times. There are important features of an aggregate group like oral cancer patients. No one site in the oral cavity differs greatly in the proportion of 5-year survivors. Most series show a deterioration of survival when larger cancers extend posteriorly into the oropharynx. Many oral cancer series do include more patients with cancer of the tongue and floor of the mouth *detected* at an earlier stage.[7] The most important feature of Table 13–2 is that patients with early node-negative cancers (stages I and II) can have a much better 5-year survival than patients with advanced cancers. The second major lesson, not shown by tabular data, is that curative treatment of early oral cancers produces very little deformity or functional loss. At all sites amenable to both radiation (with surgical salvage) and surgical therapy, there is minimal difference in 5-year survival for stage I and II disease. Planned combined therapy does not yield any striking improvement when applied to early oral cancers.

After an oral cancer is diagnosed and carefully staged by the criteria given in Table 13–3, decision-making then focuses on methods of treatment. The discussion in this chapter begins by considering smaller early cancers and progresses to the treatment of advanced cancers. Rigid anatomical boundaries are not stressed, so that some general decision-making concepts can be emphasized.

WHAT ARE THE MAJOR TREATMENT OPTIONS FOR A SMALLER LOCALIZED ORAL CANCER STAGED AS T_1 OR T_2?

The spectrum of options may include:

1. Local ablation of the cancer with cryotherapy, cautery, or laser.
2. Wide local intraoral excision.
   - No treatment of cervical lymph nodes.
   - Discontinuous conservation lymphadenectomy.
   - Elective neck irradiation.
3. Irradiation of the primary with teletherapy, with or without implanted radiation boost.
   - Elective or therapeutic neck irradiation may be added.
   - Add surgical salvage if irradiation fails.
   - Surgical cervical lymphadenectomy.
4. Wide excision of cancer in-continuity with cervical lymphadenectomy.
   - As a pull-through procedure.
   - With cheek flap exposure.
   - With temporary section of the mandible for exposure.

TABLE 13–2.—DETERMINATE SURVIVAL AFTER TREATMENT OF SQUAMOUS CELL ORAL CANCERS WITH DIFFERENT SITES OF ORIGIN

		% 5-YEAR SURVIVAL BY STAGE			
SITE AND TREATMENT*	STUDY, YEAR	I	II	III	IV
Floor of mouth					
Mixed	Ildstad et al.,[1] 1983	62	60	30	10
Rad.	Mendenhall et al.,[2] 1983	100†	100†	58	0
Surg.	Mendelson et al.,[6] 1977	81	67	44	
Surg.	Harrold,[8] 1971	69	49	24	7
Rad. and Surg.	Fayos and Lampe,[10] 1972	71	58	12	
Tongue					
Rad.	Mendenhall et al.,[2] 1983	100†	71	35	50†
Surg.	Kremen,[3] 1967	94	94	48	
Mixed	Leipzig and Hokanson,[4] 1982	70	65	30	10
Surg.	Mendelson et al.,[6] 1977	85	61	54	
Rad.	Fu et al.,[9] 1976	43	41	15	5
Rad. and Surg.	Fayos and Lampe,[10] 1972	64	32	6	
Rad. and Surg.	Holm et al.,[11] 1983	77	69	13	
Alveolar ridge					
Surg.	Mendelson et al.,[6] 1977	83	80	68	
Rad. and Surg. Salv.	Fayos and Lampe,[10] 1972	33	37	38	
All oral cavity					
Surg.	Joyce and McQuarrie,[5] 1976	74	67	38	38
Mixed	Shaw et al.,[7] 1976	70	55	50	24

*All radiation series include surgical salvage of radiation failures.
†Fewer than six patients in group.

With marginal resection of the mandible.
Resection of a mandible segment.
With primary bone repair.
With delayed repair.
With no repair.

5. Combined resection with any of the above plus oral resurfacing.
   Local flaps—tongue, mucosa.
   Cervical or forehead flaps.
   Myocutaneous flap.
   Free microvascular graft.
6. Add consideration of preoperative or postoperative adjunctive irradiation, particularly if pathologic staging shows advanced metastases.
7. Adjunctive chemotherapy with planned approved protocols only (usually reserved for more advanced cancers).

On an active head and neck cancer service, there are specific instances in which one may consider each of these modes alone, or a combination of modes. The therapy is tailored to the particular stage of the cancer given in Table 13–3 as well as specific tumor location, tumor size, the likelihood of involved cervical nodes, and the size of palpably suspicious nodes. In addition, particular tumor characteristics are critically important for decision purposes. Is the cancer exophytic, superficial, moderately infiltrating, deeply infiltrating, or ulcerating? Does the cancer extend to or overlie bone, cause gross erosion of bone, produce radiographically evident erosion of bone? Potential involvement of neighboring structures must be noted. The patient's complicating diseases are found and characterized. Thus, one may start objective treatment planning using the tools listed in chapter 5. Occupational requirements

TABLE 13–3.—STAGING OF ORAL CANCER: TNM CLASSIFICATION

Primary tumor (T)	
T_X	Tumor that cannot be assessed by rules.
T_0	No evidence of primary tumor.
T_{IS}	Carcinoma in situ.
T_1	Tumor 2 cm or less in greatest diameter.
T_2	Tumor more than 2 cm but not more than 4 cm in greatest diameter.
T_3	Tumor more than 4 cm in greatest diameter.
T_4	Massive tumor more than 4 cm in diameter with deep invasion to involve antrum, pterygoid muscles, base of tongue, or skin of neck.

Nodal involvement (N). See staging guidelines in Chapter 9.

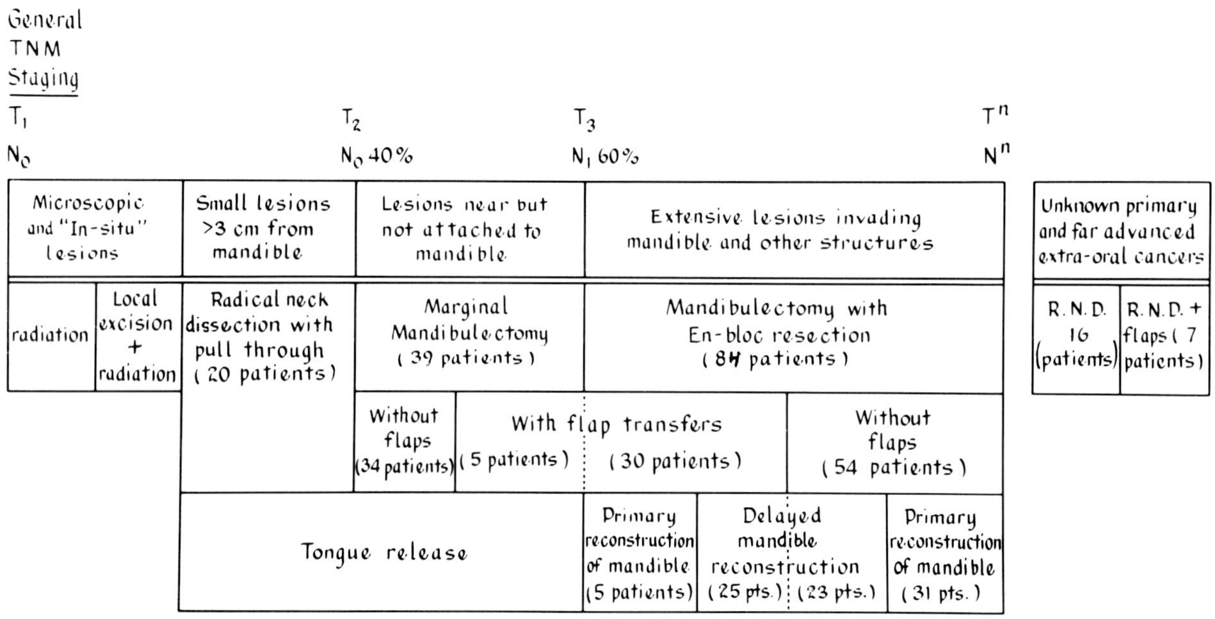

Fig 13–2.—The spectrum of treatments we used in caring for 166 consecutive oral cancer patients. It emphasizes the mixture of options and the increased complexity of treatment as the cancers become larger, involve contiguous tissues, and have more metastases to cervical lymph nodes. (Joyce L., McQuarrie, D.G.[5] Reproduced by permission.)

or emotional attitudes (of the patient) may weigh heavily in the ultimate treatment choice.

The priorities are still the following: (1) Cure the primary cancer! (2) Treat potential or proved cervical metastases. (3) Preserve or maximize oral function. (4) Make cosmetic restoration. Almost always, the treatment must trade some disability for a chance to cure the lethal disease. One must match the spectrum of disease against a spectrum of therapy. Figure 13–2 lists some of the variations we employed in a series reported in 1976.[5] This clearly expresses the need for an eclectic repertoire of therapy. That series (166 patients) did not include patients with in situ cancers and a few very small T_1 lesions treated by irradiation. Advances since 1976 have increased the options for reconstruction. Today, we would avoid delayed reconstruction in favor of primary reconstruction.

When Can You Use Local Excision as the Sole Treatment of a Small Superficial Oral Squamous Cell Cancer?

Local excision is applicable only where there is a very low likelihood of cervical metastases and when the patient's condition or adamant attitudes prevent more certain methods of eliminating the squamous cancer. The decision problem is best exemplified when there is a complete excisional biopsy of a minimal T_{IS} or superficial T_1 lesion with very skimpy margins in a very sick elderly person. The most important procedure is to have the surgeon review the microscopy slides with the pathologist. Verbal and written miscommunications are thus avoided. (The problems of biopsy are discussed in Chap. 4.) If the epithelial changes in the specimen are all in situ, then it is the surgeon's responsibility to be certain that there are no residual or adjacent lesions. In a younger person or an unreliable person, a wider excision must be done for an in situ lesion if any margin, particularly the deep margin, is close (< 1.0 cm) or questionable. A careful search is made for invasive characteristics in the biopsy specimen and any reexcised tissue. If even minimal (1–2 mm) invasion is found, there must be wide local ablation. If deeply invasive components are found (> 2–4 mm), we regard it as a more advanced T_1 lesion and treat the neck lymph nodes by lymphadenectomy or elective neck irradiation.

For local excision to be considered, the cancer must be thin, minimally invasive, and located to allow good peripheral and deep margins. The patient must be reliable to impeccable follow-up. For consideration of local excision, dissection should not extend into the neck, where it may impair the ability to do a subsequent thorough lymphadenectomy. In reviewing "localized" excisions, remember that experienced surgeons take a wide swath around the tumor (Figs 13–3 and 13–4). In a series of 126 floor of the mouth cancers, Marks and co-workers found only five which they felt were suitable for limited local excision.[12] Spiro and Strong treated 185 of 563 (33%) favorably situated cancers of the tongue by partial glossectomy alone.[13] It must be noted

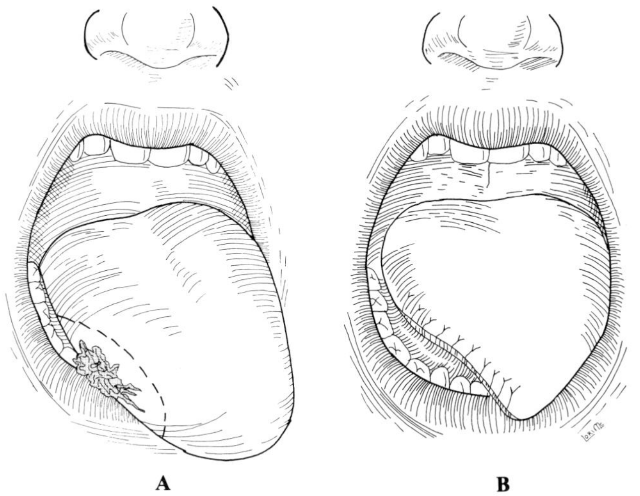

Fig 13–3.—Inadequate excision of an invasive cancer of the tongue.

that there were local recurrences (8% in T_1, 18% in T_2 cancers). Thirty-eight percent of the 185 patients developed cervical lymph nodes requiring treatment. The aggregate 5-year survival of patients with locally excised lesions was 62%. In a subsequent publication, the same group found increased survival (in the larger T_1T_2 cancers) when neck dissection was done before cervical lymph nodes became apparent.[14] Marks and co-workers achieved 91% "ultimate control" by local excision for a smaller group of superficial minimally invasive tongue cancers.[15] The Roswell Park group reviewed their experience with 50 patients treated by local excision.[16] After a 5-year follow-up, "one out of every three patients developed recurrent disease and one out of every four patients died of cancer." They concluded, and we concur, that small "localized" cancers are not to be treated as a trivial problem. Local treatment must be contrasted to the better results—in the 85% range—reported in other published series of wide excisions when treatment of cervical nodes is added.[3, 6] If the local treatment fails, a more deforming radical salvage attempt is required to achieve a cure.

When Can Cryotherapy Be Used for Early Oral Cancers?

Small superficial cancers can be destroyed with cryonecrosis as well as local excision. Local excision has the definite advantage of permitting microscopic examination of the tissues to confirm the initial diagnosis and the complete removal of the lesion.

Cryotherapy was originally introduced by Cooper in 1961.[17] Gage has been a pioneering advocate for the *judicious* use of cryosurgery in selected oral cancer patients.[18–21] Neel et al. have demonstrated that repetitive freezing (at least three times) to $-30°$ C to $-40°$ C is required to assure tumor cell death.[22, 23] Cryosurgery can be used to ablate oral dysplasia. Advocates of cryosurgery still reserve its use in oral cancer to very high risk patients who are clinically node negative. We have found the technique of particular use when there is a severe clotting disorder, there is a need for contin-

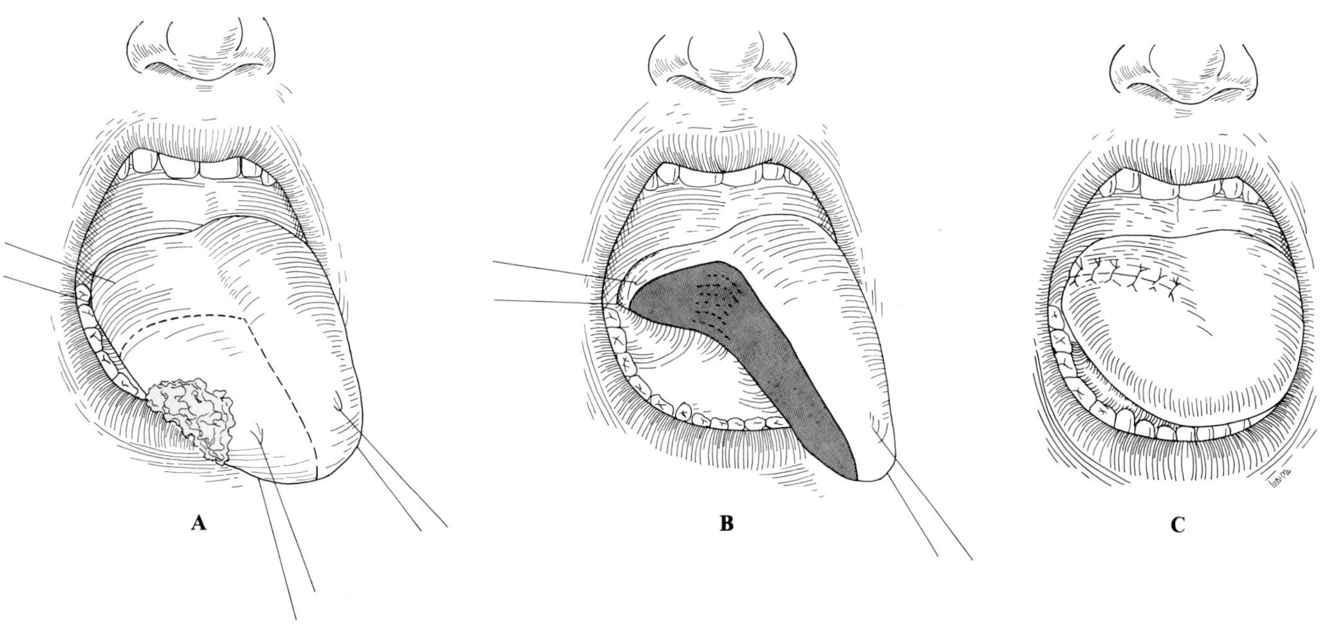

Fig 13–4.—The dimensions of an adequate excision of a smaller invasive cancer of the tongue. Because of the pliancy of the tongue tissues, the deep portion of a tongue cancer will have a much different border when the tongue is extended than when it is contracted inward. The error is to make the deep margin too shallow, resulting in frequent local recurrence. With minimal extension, this type of resection can be made contiguously with a cervical node dissection. The procedure becomes a pull-through operation.

uing anticoagulation, the patient is recovering from a myocardial infarct, or the patient has a short life expectancy from some other disease.

Cryosurgery needs either a light general anesthetic, in an uncooperative patient, or good local anesthetic, in a cooperative patient. The area to be frozen must be insulated from the surrounding tissues. Styrofoam cups broken into appropriate-sized pieces are useful and cheap insulation. The basic objective is to freeze the tissue in situ two or three times. Other general recommendations are: (1) Use an implanted thermocouple control to ensure freezing at adequate depth. (2) Use liquid nitrogen systems for oral cancers. (3) Maintain good tissue contact with the cryogenic probe. (4) Freeze as quickly as possible by using the equipment as cold as possible. (5) Thaw slowly. (6) Overlap the frozen areas. (7) Repeat the freezing at least once, preferably twice after the first freezing thaws. (8) Include a margin of normal tissue.[24] Cryosurgery produces no posttreatment pain. The areas are allowed to heal by secondary intention after necrosis.

Gage found he could control T_1N_0 disease in 21 of 21 highly selected patients.[18] Nineteen patients lived 5 years without recurrence; two died of other causes.

In conclusion, there is a highly selective role for cryosurgical treatment in oral cancer: in debilitated patients in whom there is little likelihood of cervical node spread. Does local cautery have any use for local tumor control? No! It is a painful, barbaric means of local tissue destruction. Laser surgery is discussed at the end of the chapter.

How Do You Decide Between Irradiation Therapy and Surgery in Early Invasive Oral Cancer?

Early detection is the key to cure for oral cancer. Unfortunately, only 20%–25% of oral cancers are detected in an early T_1 stage. Shedd[25] and Mashberg et al.[26] have reconfirmed the areas of high cancer risk in the mouth (see Fig 13–1). The *very early* cancers are quantitatively distributed in the mouth as shown in Table 13–4. In the table, note the absence of early cancers on the alveolar ridge. This suggests that the alveolus is usually involved secondarily.

TABLE 13–4.—DISTRIBUTION OF 222 EARLY ASYMPTOMATIC CANCERS AT VARIOUS SITES WITHIN THE ORAL CAVITY*

SITE	% OF ORAL CANCERS
Floor of mouth	45.5
Oral tongue	16.5
Soft palate	13.5
Anterior pillar	10.0
Lip	6.7
Lingual aspect retromolar trigone	5.4
Alveolar ridge	1.3
Buccal mucosa	1.0
Hard palate	0.5

*Summarized from Mashberg and Meyers.[28]

The white thickening of leukoplakia is easily recognized, but it is the reddish erythroplakic area that is the most common presentation of an early cancer. In Mashberg's first study of 207 oral cancers, 33% were erythematous, 4.9% were white, while 60% were mixed with a red predominance.[27] In a subsequent extended report of 222 early lesions, $T_1N_0M_0$, Mashberg and Meyers found that 20% were in situ and 80% were invasive, with small nests of cells penetrating below the basement membrane.[28] Forty-two percent of these cancers were less than 1 cm in greatest dimension. About 15% will have positive cervical nodes. These early, thin, T_1 cancers are distinctly different from a T_1 cancer that is deeply invasive, ulcerated, and grossly 1.5 × 1.8 × 1.8 cm in size. Even though the latter cancer is also staged as a T_1 lesion, it is a more vicious malignancy. Despite the frequent absence of palpable nodes, the invasive T_1 cancer has been microscopically node positive in 56% of our patient population. When considering T_1 lesions, it is well for the surgeon to adjust his decision-making to the specific characteristics of the cancer.

Almost all of the early thin small cancers without metastases can be cured by irradiation *or* surgery. There are two reservations. Follow-up must be reliable, and surgical salvage must be effectively applied if radiation therapy fails. There is very little cosmetic or functional loss to the patient by either therapy. Because of the close parity between treatments, both groups of therapists find it satisfying to successfully treat such patients. In a larger cancer center, spirited discussions may occur. Table 13–5 summarizes data from several irradiation series, and Table 13–6 summarizes data from surgical series. Some of the variation in results could well be due to the different proportions of *early* (i.e., small, thin) T_1 lesions included in different series.

Most, but not all, radiotherapists recommend that a T_1 cancer directly on bone is best treated by surgical removal. If a good, aggressive, curative irradiation dose is delivered, ulceration and/or bone damage may result (see the discussion of osteoradionecrosis in Chap. 27). From Table 13–4 it may be ascertained that less than 8%–10% of early cancers are directly on bone. Many other floor of the mouth lesions are near enough to the mandible to pose some problems. Many large centers recommend that surgical excision be the mainstay for floor of the mouth cancers.[6, 12] This is to avoid radiation complications. This leaves 60%–70% of oral cancers as a decision problem.

If we use the example of a 60-year old white male salesman with a T_1N_0 invasive tongue cancer, we can make the life expectancy decision calculations we made

TABLE 13–5.—5-YEAR TUMOR-FREE SURVIVAL AFTER RADIATION TREATMENT OF T_1N_O (STAGE I) ORAL CANCERS, BY LOCATION

	% 5-YEAR SURVIVAL BY ORAL SITE					
STUDY, YEAR	All Sites	Tongue	Buccal Mucosa	Gingiva	Floor of Mouth	Palate
Ash,[29] 1962		67.5	78	55	73	83
Easson,[30] 1963		60				
Hirata et al.[31]* 1975	67					
Patterson et al.,[32]† 1950			82			
Lampe,[33]† 1955			53	33		
Fu et al.,[9, 34] 1976		43			82	
Marks et al.,[15] 1981		88				
Chu[35]					98	
Ildstad et al.,[1] 1983					58	

*Results show a definite improvement of survival between orthovoltage period (1947–1963) and supervoltage period (1964–1970, 80%) survival.
†Older series (1950).

in chapter 4. The example can be complicated by the history of a myocardial infarction 18 months previously, with angina pectoris, no congestive failure. The coronary angiogram shows moderately diffuse left and right coronary disease with a nearly occlusive distal right coronary contricting lesion. How should we treat the cancer? We may use an age-corrected 5-year N.E.D. cancer survival estimate of 80% for irradiation and 85% for surgery (a surgeon has to be allowed a little bias) from Tables 13–5 and 13–6, and estimate his uncorrected 5-year mortality from heart disease at 30% (data in Chap. 5). Then, with a 2% operative mortality and a 10% reduction in quality of life from long-term disability from surgical resection and a 0.1-year convalescence, and using the equations given in chapter 5,

$$LE_{Surg.} = \left[\frac{1}{.0581 + .0325 + .0131} \times (.98) \times (.90)^*\right] - 0.1 = 8.41 \text{ years}$$

If irradiation takes 5–6 weeks (0.1 year) with some convalescence, then:

$$LE_{Rad.} = \left[\frac{1}{0.581 + .0446 + .0131} \times (1.0) \times (1.0)^*\right] - 0.1 = 8.53 \text{ years}$$

The decision between treatments is virtually a toss-up. It becomes obvious that the critical difference is really a function of the patient's and the doctor's estimate of the quality of life reduction by long-term disability (LTD, marked by an asterisk in the above calculations), which may include speech changes or some cosmetic differences. The additional factor to consider is the percentage of irradiated patients who may need surgical salvage later with the full surgical risk. The amount of risk from the heart disease does not sway the decision much (2% operative mortality). This risk is offset by some of the late radiation morbidity with xero-

TABLE 13–6.—5-YEAR TUMOR-FREE SURVIVAL AFTER SURGICAL TREATMENT OF EARLY ORAL CANCERS T_1N_O (STAGE I)

	% 5-YEAR SURVIVAL BY ORAL SITE					
STUDY, YEAR	All Sites	Tongue	Buccal Mucosa	Gingiva	Floor of Mouth	Palate
Kremen,[3]* 1967		95				
Hirata et al.,[31] 1975	96					
Mendelson et al.,[6]		85		83	81	
Marks et al.,[15] 1981		91				
Shons et al.,[36] 1985					72	
Ildstad et al.,[1] 1983					63	
McQuarrie et al.,[38] 1985†		82				
Shah et al.,[7] 1976	70					
Barton,[37]*1977					89	
Spiro and Strong,[13] 1971		85				

*Includes some T_2N_O patients.
†Series overlaps with cases in Shons A. R. et al.[36]

stomia and poor tissue healing. There is a growing recognition that tumoricidal irradiation dosages may produce a 10%–50% frequency of difficult and even late lethal complications.[12, 39–42] These complications can include carotid artery necrosis, carotid artery occlusive disease, and other late tissue loss. The decisions for therapy are frequently based on the patient's unwillingness to accept one therapy or the other. There are strong emotional components in patient's decisions. Many women totally reject a surgical option. A growing number of patients have an irrational fear of irradiation of any type. For a patient who is unreliable to follow-up, we strongly urge surgical therapy.

In summary, either treatment may be used as the primary therapy for early cancers. Cures are accomplished by *full-dose* irradiation or *full surgical margins* in the therapy. Makeshift and comprised "hope it works" treatments will not yield the 80%–90% 5-year cure rate that should be expected. For *invasive* oral squamous cell cancers, the probability of lymph node involvement is too high to ignore, and the physician should not aovid treating the neck nodes with low-risk techniques (see Chap. 9). The neck should be treated by elective neck dissection or modified lymphadenectomy even though it is clinically stage N_0. The appropriate dissection is done for N_1, N_2, or N_3 disease. It is conceptually better to resect the primary and cervical nodes in continuity, but the neck dissection can be discontinuous if oral excision is adequately wide. If the primary is irradiated, an N_0 neck should also be treated as outlined in chapter 9 and as advocated by Jesse and Fletcher.[43] They used 4,500–5,000 rad delivered over 4½–5 weeks.

What Are the Decision Options in the Larger, More Invasive T_1 and T_2 Oral Cancers?

Unfortunately, the early lesions described by Mashberg and Meyers[28] made up only 10% of their series and a maximum of 25%–30% of other reported oral cancer series. The larger, more aggresive nodular, ulcerated, or deeply invasive cancer poses a therapeutic challenge. At least one third to one half of patients with a deeply invading oral cancer will have cervical node metastases palpable on admission. The cervical nodes must be included in the treatment. It is in the T_1 (large) and T_2 cancers that surgery and irradiation are said to *compete*. The absolute therapeutic dichotomy is not good for selecting a decision path. Surgery and irradiation are *complementary* to each other. Each has specific advantages with early and late consequences. Some of these are listed in Table 13–7. With T_1, T_2, N_0, or N_1 cancers, a 5-year actuarial survival should approach or exceed 55%, even for stage III disease.[44]

It is true that larger invasive cancers pose greater agonies in the decision-making process. In the aggregate group, adequate extensive surgery for T_1 or T_2 lesions will result in as many long-term survivors as irradiation, and frequently more. It is equally true that cosmetic and functional loss with surgical therapy increases directly with tumor size. In direct parallel, radiation is less able to achieve a cure without surgical salvage, i.e., a postirradiation operation with wider margins, a higher risk, and more extensive surgery than would have been required if surgery had been the initial treatment. As we shall see shortly, the results of radiation and surgical salvage are about equivalent to the results of surgery alone. There are patients in whom the avoidance of any cosmetic change and/or oral soft tissue loss is critical to employment and daily function. In this case, *the surgeon* would strongly recommend irradiation as first therapy. For this patient, the chance of avoiding soft tissue resection may be worth the uncertainty, time, and expense of potentially double therapy. In contrast, there are larger oral cancers near bone, or in totally unreliable patients. In this instance, *the radiation therapist* would strongly recommend surgery. Other patients with large involved nodes will require neck dissection for management. The surgery in the neck will approach the primary and hence will make an in-continuity dissection of the primary the most desirable option. In this case, the management of the primary is best included with the lymphadenectomy. As cancers increase in size (large T_2 or T_3), the end results seem to favor surgical resection. The question of preoperative and postoperative adjunctive irradiation was discussed in chapter 7. The rational for cervical lymph node removal or ablation is covered in chapters 7 and 8.

Figure 13–5 is a decision diagram which gives some beginning structure to the complexity of our questions. The diagonal division in the large box indicates that there are varying proportions of patients who will be selected for surgery or irradiation as the initial mode of treatment. A number of questions need further examination.

The two most important decision factors for type of treatment have been patient reliability to follow-up and the patient's perceptions of the long-term morbidity because of fear of appearance change or because of occupational requirements for impeccable speech.

We studied our own nonrandomized retrospective experience with cancer of the anterior two thirds of the tongue as illustrative of decision problems wherein surgery or irradiation can be applied without a question of proximity to bone or major vessels.[45] We asked four questions of our data. (1) Does irradiation therapy spare a significant proportion of patients from the tissue loss of surgery? (2) Does prior irradiation reduce local or

TABLE 13–7.—CONSIDERATIONS FOR SELECTING IRRADIATION OR SURGERY FOR TREATMENT OF T_1 (LARGER) OR T_2, N_0 OR N_1 ORAL CANCERS

IRRADIATION	SURGERY
Advantages	
No immediate soft tissue loss if successful; speech and oral function good.	Immediate direct ablation of tumor with ability to immediately confirm margins with frozen sections.
No anesthetic or surgical risk.	Reconstruction can be part of resective procedure.
Margins can be covered.	Removes draining lymphatic nodes.
May control some cervical lymphatic micrometastases.	No changes in healing abilities of tissues.
Disadvantages	
Requires patient reliable for follow-up.	Loss of oral function (speech, swallowing difficulty) with soft tissue loss, depending on resection location and extent.
Failures have fewer options for surgical salvage or late reconstruction. Some patients will have the complications and problems of both modes of treatment.	Variable but predictable cosmetic changes, depending on resection location and extent.
Cannot use radiation later for 2d primary in adjacent area.	Potential loss of spinal accessory nerve function.
Xerostomia, dental complications, acute mucositis.	Some cervical sensory loss.
"Dental delay" of 2–3 weeks in treatment unless patient is edentulous.	Risk of infection.
Osteoradionecrosis of mandible (low frequency at lower doses).	External scars and some change of appearance.
Impaired tissue healing after 1–2 years.	Small but real surgical mortality.
Vascular sclerosis (late); ? hypothyroidism.	
Tissue stiffness and muscular atrophy (late).	
Emaciated patient will not maintain nutrition during and after treatment.	
Reasons for Selection of Treatment Mode	
Strong patient aversion to surgical disabilities.	Tumor near bone.
Survival after irradiation and surgical salvage is about equal to surgery only. Some patients do not need operation (see text).	Patient not reliable for follow-up.
Extremely elderly patient with severe end-stage disease with complications.	Younger patient in whom late complications of irradiation should be avoided.
Occupational requirements for speech and unblemished appearance.	Patient occupational requirements for early return to work.
	Strong patient aversion to irradiation treatment.

cervical recurrence rates in patients who subsequently require salvage surgery? (3) Are surgical options altered by previous irradiation? (4) Are the survival results of irradiation plus aggressive surgical salvage as good as those of surgical treatment alone? The answers for our population were no, no, yes, and, for the big question, yes. There is a big caveat in our study. The patients were *not* randomly allocated between groups. In our study the cases of 53 consecutive patients with oral tongue cancer were retrospectively reviewed. All T_1 cancers were invasive and beyond the very early superficial stage (this is important in comparison to the other reported series). After pathologic staging of the groups, they were similar, with equivalent and typical distribution of tumor stages between 28 irradiated patients (Fig 13–6,*A*) and 25 patients treated by surgery (Fig 13–6,*B*). The determinate survival was calculated by the life table method. Eighty-two percent (23/28) of the primary irradiation patients ultimately had surgical treatment after histologically proved failure. Of the five patients not operated on, three had advanced stage IV disease. Treatment in these patients should be considered as palliative attempts only. Two irradiated patients with T_1 lesions were 5-year tumor-free survivors. In the surgical survivors, irradiation was added to the therapy of five patients who were pathologically staged N_2.

In the patients undergoing surgical salvage, tumor invasion plus the effects of irradiation made it inadvisable to attempt a marginal mandibulectomy in most lesions recurring near the mandible. The results of recurrence and survival are shown in Table 13–8. Irradiation followed by surgery was associated with more, not less, neck recurrence. In the end, the determinate 5-year survival was exactly the same for the two groups. Our provincial experience without a large number of early T_1 cancers would lead to the conclusion that only a limited fraction of patients with larger oral cancers will be able to avoid tissue loss because of successful irradiation treatment. These successes are bought at the price of a larger group of patients who have the late effects and complications of both modes of treatment. The need for

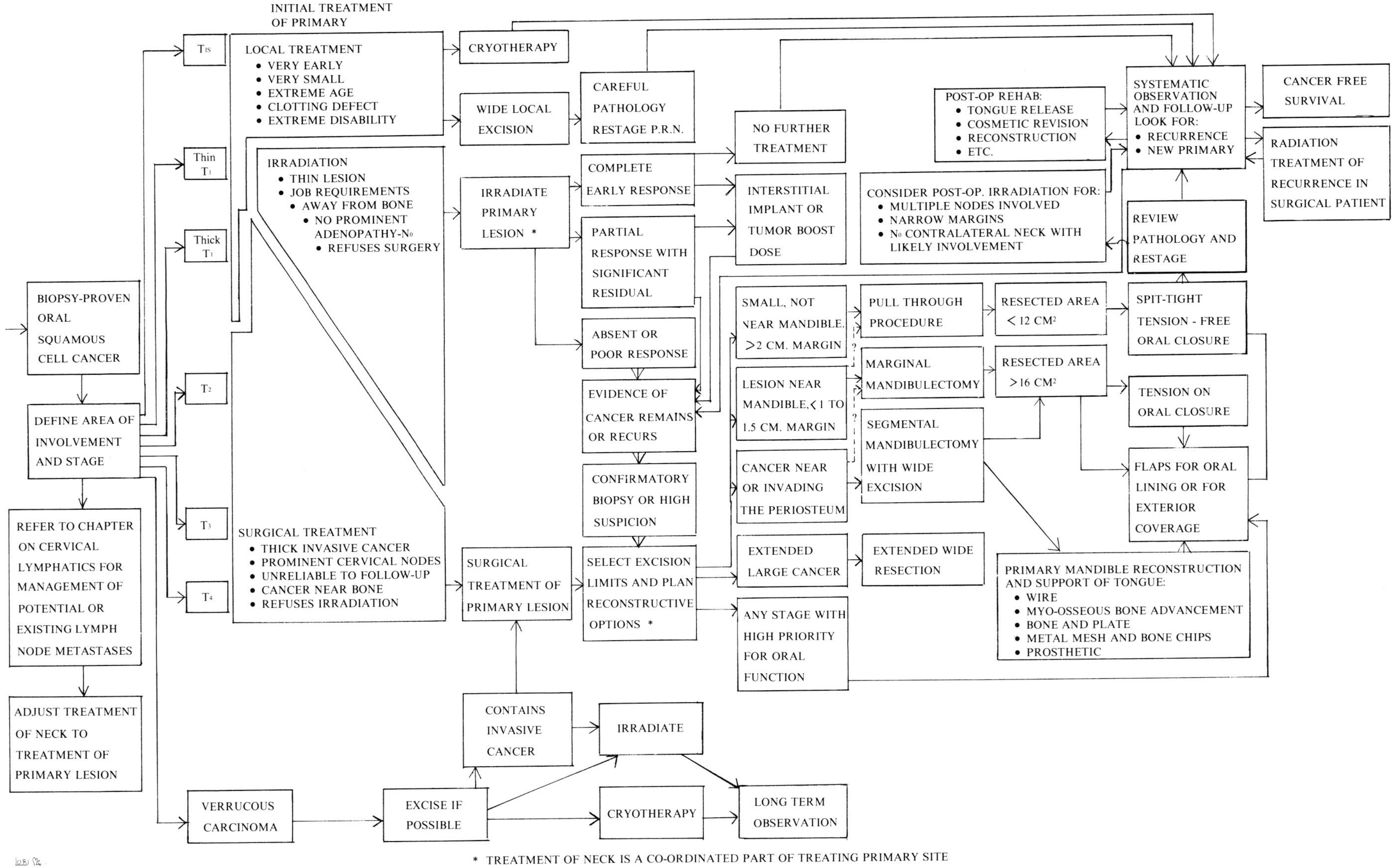

Fig 13–5.—Decision diagram outlining some of the general decision paths for the treatment of oral cancer. Knowledge of the tumor stage and an estimate of cervical node status is required; the patient's characteristics and preferences must also be taken into account. These factors are important in early decision-making for selection of therapy.

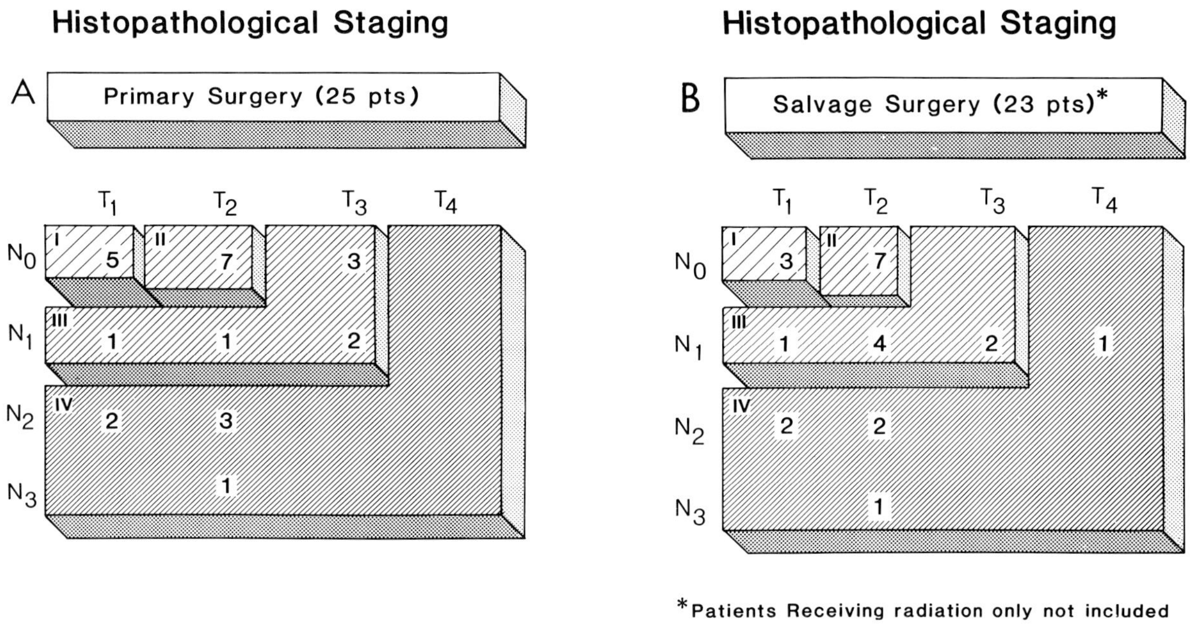

Fig 13–6.—A, histopathologic stage distribution of patients with tongue cancer initially treated by irradiation. Of the 28 patients 23 subsequently required surgical salvage. If all 28 patients were included, there would most likely be two additional T_1 patients, for a total of five. Three additional patients received only palliative irradiation for T_4N_2 disease. **B,** histopathologic stage distribution of patients treated primarily by surgery. Elective postoperative irradiation was given to the five N_2 patients. The results in patients included in **A** and **B** are given in Table 13–8. (From Shons A.R., et al.[36] Reproduced by permission.)

surgical salvage in our series is higher than the results cited in the literature (see following discussion). These conclusions may have to be modified for the future with newer radiotherapy techniques. Many of our patients were treated before good treatment simulators and linear accelerators were available.

HOW OFTEN IS SURGICAL SALVAGE REQUIRED IN IRRADIATED PATIENTS WITH ORAL CANCERS?

Table 13–9 lists some of the available data on the percentage of surgical salvage attempts required after irradiation. The data vary most in patients with T_1 cancers, reflecting the differing mix of early T_1 and larger invasive T_1 cancers in different centers. For stage II (T_2N_o) and stage III (T_1N_1, T_2N_1, T_3, and T_3N_1) oral cancers, a significant proportion of patients (estimated range, 33%–70%) required surgical treatment after irradiation. The proportion requiring salvage attempts increased with primary tumor size. Hirata et al. concluded that more patients were treated with radiotherapy, but better control was obtained with surgery for each stage of the disease in the entire period of study (1964–1970).[31] In the classic 1961 Janeway Lecture by Ash, reporting on 1,944 cases of oral cancer treated by irradiation, the patients were divided into early and late cases.[29] Initial "control" was 51% in the early cases and 26% in the late cases. Subsequent surgical treatment "controlled" 49% of the early uncontrolled cases and 30% of the late cases which recurred or persisted. The final actual aggregate 5-year survival of the 1,944 patients was 33%. Since these earlier reports, both irradiation and surgical techniques have improved. In patients with advanced disease and in those with positive cervical nodes, surgery has a distinct edge

TABLE 13–8 —RECURRENCE AND SURVIVAL IN PREVIOUSLY IRRADIATED AND PRIMARY SURGICAL PATIENTS WITH ANTERIOR TONGUE INVOLVEMENT

TREATMENT GROUP	N	LOCAL RECURRENCE AT 2 YR (%)	NECK RECURRENCE AT 5 YR (%)	SYSTEMIC METASTASES AT 5 YR (%)	DETERMINATE SURVIVAL 5 YR(%)
Primary surgery	25	5.5	36.7	16.0	55.5*
Irradiation failures	23	10.0	74.8	13.0	55.2†

*Five of 25 patients received planned postoperative irradiation (N_2).
†This number would be slightly higher if the 2/25 radiation successes were included.

TABLE 13–9.—% OF PATIENTS REQUIRING SURGICAL SALVAGE ATTEMPT AFTER IRRADIATION THERAPY FAILED TO CONTROL ORAL CANCER (LIP EXCLUDED)

		% OF PTS. REQUIRING SURGICAL SALVAGE ATTEMPT, BY STAGE				
STUDY, YEAR	SITE	All Stages	I	II	III	IV
Mullholland et al.,[45] 1984	Tongue		60	100	100*	
Leipzeg and Hokanson,[4] 1982	Tongue		100†	83	77	
Hirata et al.,[31] 1975	All sites	49				
Mendenhall et al.,[2] 1982	Oral tongue		13	57	50	
	Floor of mouth	32				
Vermund and Gollin,[46] 1973	Tongue		33 I and II		45 III and IV	
Marks et al.,[12] 1983	Floor of mouth	44				

*Irradiation used largely for palliative purposes before patient accepted surgery.
†Small number of T_1N_0 patients.

in achieving long-term survival. The more recent results are summarized in Tables 13–2, 13–9, 13–10, and 13–11.

What Are the Criteria for Deciding That Surgical Resection Is Needed After Irradiation Treatment?

There are no hard and fast rules for managing patients who do not show durable complete irradiation response. In general, the following groups are seen: (1) early failures with minimal response or continued growth; (2) those who respond partially but in whom there is a significant neoplastic residual; and (3) those who have initial ablation of the gross tumor with subsequent reappearance 9 months to more than a year later. For these last patients, it is frequently difficult to distinguish scirrhous invasive tumor from postirradiation fibrosis. There should be histologic confirmation of persisting malignancy.

Local and cervical node cancer may recur in 10%–15% of irradiated patients well beyond the magic 2-year period semantically used as the "total control" index in some published series. This accounts for the continuing decline in accurate actuarial survival slopes, so that 2-year "control" is a far different number from disease-free 5-year survival. Several simple points are essential to secure good patient survival. A persisting or new palpable node in the neck of an irradiation-treated patient is cancer so often that other diagnoses should not be

TABLE 13–10.—RECURRENCE RATES AND SURVIVAL FOLLOWING SURGICAL THERAPY FOR TONGUE CANCER

STUDY, YEAR	ANATOMICAL SITE	N	TUMOR STATUS	STAGE	LOCAL RECURRENCE (%)	CERVICAL RECURRENCE (%)	5-YR SURVIVAL (%)
Marchetta and Sako,[44] 1975	Tongue	72		III			56%
Lam et al.,[47] 1980	Tongue	56					50.6 overall
Spiro and Strong,[13] 1971	Anterior tongue	185	T_1		8		61.1 overall
			T_2		14		
			T_3		30		
Spiro and Strong,[48] 1974*	Anterior tongue	314	T_1				69.2
			T_2				52.7
			T_3				36.6
Shah et al.,[7] 1976	Anterior tongue	191		I			83
				II			63
				III			37
				IV			11
Whitehurst and Drovlias,[49] 1977	Anterior tongue	137	T_1		9.8	15.9	67.1
			T_2		14.3	42.9	25.0
			T_3		23.1	42.9	42.9
White and Byers,[50] 1980	Tongue	152	T_1		7.3	17.1	
			T_2		3.8	19.2	
			T_3		21.4	28.5	
Johnson et al.,[51] 1980	Anterior tongue	28	T_1		10.7	35.7	
Razack et al.,[52] 1982	Tongue	206		I			64
				II			62
				III			44
				IV			11

*May have overlap of cases with the series above.

TABLE 13–11.—RECURRENCE RATES AND SURVIVAL FOLLOWING RADIATION THERAPY FOR TONGUE CANCER

STUDY, YEAR	ANATOMICAL SITE	N	TUMOR STATUS	STAGING	LOCAL RECURRENCE (%)	CERVICAL RECURRENCE (%)	5-YEAR SURVIVAL (%)
Gilbert et al.,[53] 1975	Anterior tongue	56	T_1		9		73
			T_2		38		37
			T_3		64		19
Fletcher and Jesse,[54] 1977	Anterior tongue	Not stated	T_1				98
			T_2				91
			T_3				81
			T_4				32
Johnson et al.,[55] 1980	Anterior tongue	12	T_1		25	33.3	
De Croix and Ghossein,[56] 1981	Anterior tongue	682	T_1		14		80
			T_2		22		56
			T_3		29		25
Razack et al.,[52] 1982	Tongue	73		I			16
				II			38
				III			21
				IV			0

considered even in wishful thinking. The person observing the patient should be willing and able to biopsy questionable lesions. If resection is necessary, the optimum curative attempt is usually larger, not smaller, than a planned early operation would have been.

WHERE DOES SURGICAL TREATMENT FAIL IN THE LARGER ORAL CANCERS?

If we ignore our treatment successes and analyze our failures, we get a clearer idea as to where to concentrate future effort. In our own review of 99 consecutive patients with floor of the mouth cancers, 94 were available for follow-up. The operations used are listed in Figure 13–7. Figure 13–8 shows recurrence rates in the primary site. Patients that had pull-through (floor of mouth excision only) procedures had a higher percentage of local recurrence. Figure 13–9 shows the data for recurrences in the neck. The data from our experience (see Fig 13–9) and the data of others (reviewed in Chap. 9) show that the suprahyoid node dissection neither harvests involved nodes, nor does it predict the need for additional lymphadenectomy. At a minimum, a spinal accessory nerve–conserving procedure is needed to harvest nonpalpable but involved contralateral high jugular nodes.

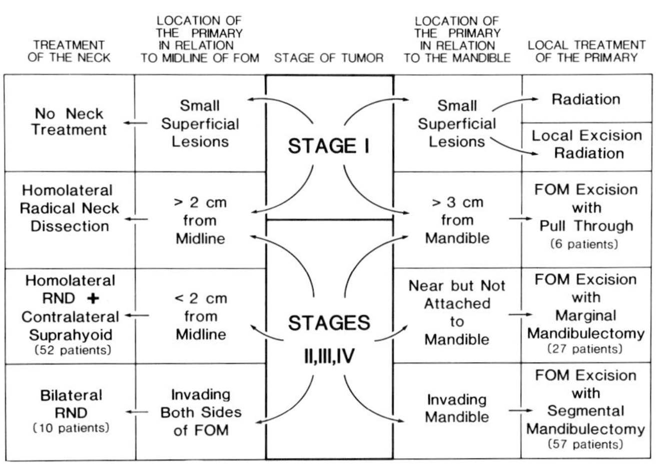

Fig 13–7.—The decision scheme we used in treating a series of patients with floor of the mouth cancer, and the number of patients treated by each scheme relative to treatment of the primary site and treatment of the neck lymphatics. The numbers in the boxes indicate the number out of 99 treated in each way. At present the treatment of the neck nodes in patients with a large midline cancer would include a homolateral radical neck dissection and a contralateral conservation neck dissection rather than the suprahyoid dissection that was done in 52 patients (third box in first column). (From Shons A.R., et al.[36] Reproduced by permission.)

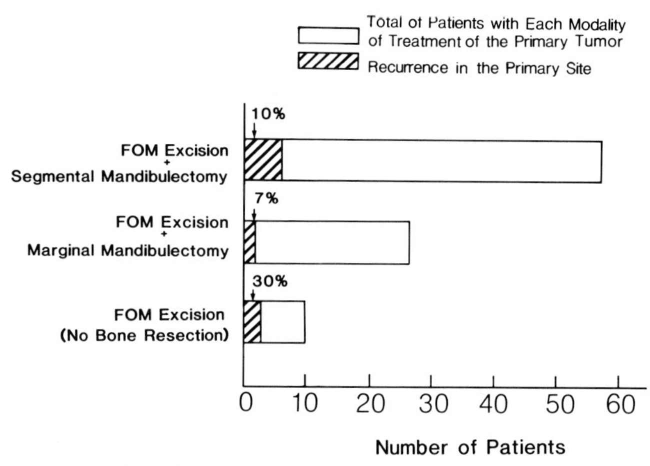

Fig 13–8.—The frequency of local recurrence with types of resection of the primary. One would expect the third group to have the most favorable outcome, since these patients required no bone resection. Nevertheless, they had the highest percentage rate of recurrence (3/10 = 30%). Usually there was a strong desire to save dentition in a "favorable" lesion. One should be circumspect about compromising margins in the "favorable" lesions. Two of the recurrences were salvaged with secondary surgery. (From Shons A.R. et al.[36] Reproduced by permission.)

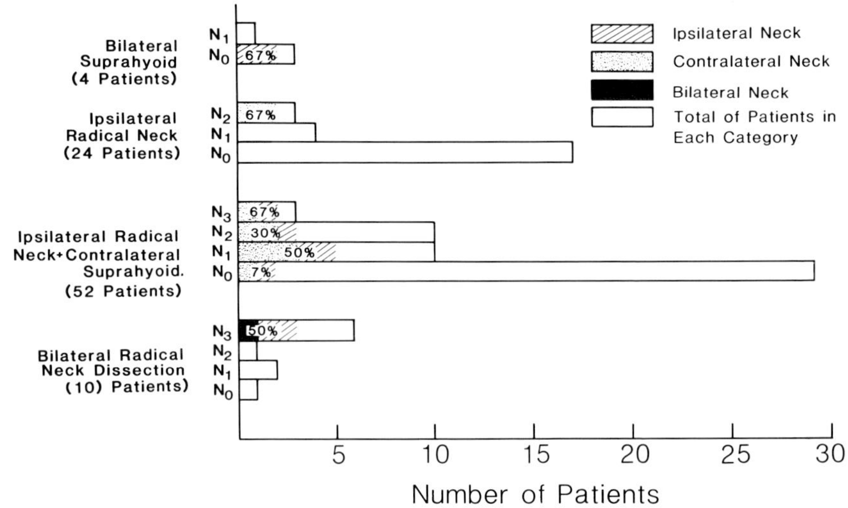

Fig 13–9.—Sites of recurrence in the neck. In the top group and the third group down, it can be seen that recurrence after a suprahyoid dissection was frequent. A suprahyoid dissection is not a good operation for therapy or for predicting other nodal involvement. (From Shons A.R. et al.[36] Reproduced by permission.)

Crossover or bilateral metastases are a major source of recurrence. Contralateral cervical node recurrences have a high salvage rate if an operation is done early.

The data from Figure 13–8 suggest that we frequently underestimated the need for wider margin in the T_2 lesion. There were fewer recurrences in patients in whom cervical flap transfers were planned and used, implying that margins were more freely extended, with the consequent result that there were fewer local recurrences, even in patients with massive cancers. Local recurrence really means that inadequate initial resection margins were taken, or, much less likely, some local wound seeding occurred. The determinate survival of patients with floor of the mouth cancers by stage is shown in Figure 13–10.

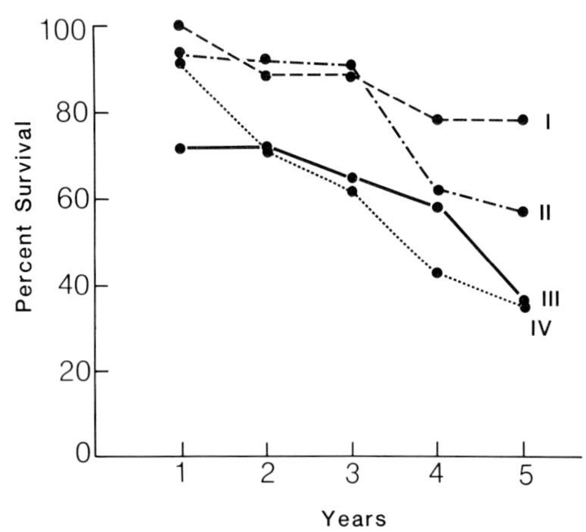

Fig 13–10.—The age-corrected determinate survival of patients with floor of the mouth cancers, by stage. Note that about 33% of stage IV oral cancers can be cured for a 5-year period by surgery. (From Shons A.R. et al.[36] Reproduced by permission.)

Shah and co-workers studied the causes of treatment failure in 334 of 704 oral cancer patients.[7] In their series, women had a higher recurrence rate than men (is this due to smaller margins to preserve appearance?). Increasing tumor depth and higher stages were associated with more recurrence. Extracapsular extension from invaded cervical nodes resulted in more frequent neck recurrences. Positive or questionable resection margins were deadly (78%), despite additional radiation therapy. Invasion of soft tissues of the face and neck was associated with a 69% recurrence rate.

Some suggestions for prevention of recurrence of oral cancer after surgery are as follows:

1. Uncompromising wide excision of the primary cancer is essential. Oral cancers usually allow technical achievement of adequate margins.
2. Radiation cannot be counted on to correct inadequate surgical excision.
3. A suprahyoid dissection is a means to gain access to the floor of the mouth. It is not effective in removing involved cervical nodes, nor is it a good staging procedure.
4. Contralateral cervical node spread is a common problem (10%–20%) (see Chap. 9). Any node that appears in the contralateral neck should be assumed to be metastatic cancer.
5. Ipsilateral neck recurrence is associated with soft tissue invasion and extracapsular extension of lymph node metastases. Give large nodes (> 2–3 cm) as wide a margin as possible. A "conservation" neck dissection is contraindicated in the face of large nodes or multiple nodes.
6. Surgical margins tend to be wider when planned full-thickness flaps are available for reconstruction.

WHAT IS THE PLACE OF PRIMARY RECONSTRUCTIVE PROCEDURES IN ORAL CANCER?

Chapter 6 outlined and illustrated the spectrum of techniques available for oral reconstruction after ablative surgery. *Reconstruction must be a planned component of the larger ablative operation.*

It is difficult to quantify improvement in appearance and function, but most experienced surgeons know the disaster of no oral reconstruction. Our previous review[5] showed that one can incorporate primary reconstructive techniques successfully into the initial treatment without compromising the resectability of the entire tumor mass. The functional and partial cosmetic improvement is apparent when compared to the old unreconstructed "commando" procedures.

Our experiences with reconstructive techniques lead us to several general observations:

1. Primary reconstruction is technically easier and less time-consuming than later secondary reconstructive techniques, such as a tube-pedicle transfer. Stranc, Labandter, and Roy[57] summarized their experience with 196 tube-pedicle transfers. They found that a tube pedicle reconstruction took 3–12 months (average, 5.8 months) to complete. Completion involved three to ten operations (average of six). A primary local flap or myocutaneous flap transfer will obviate reopening the surgical area. The use of this flap for oropharyngeal closure is illustrated for this chapter and for the oropharynx in chapter 14. We and others have advocated primary repair where possible in tumor patients[58–60] and in those with traumatic facial injuries. Many surgeons now reliably transfer free composite full-thickness pedicles with microvascular surgical anastomosis of the flap blood supply to vessels in the recipient area. This can be used when local adjacent tissues are not usable.

2. You can plan and accomplish replacement of oral lining by using a selection of chest flaps, cervical flaps, skin grafts,[61] or forehead flaps. The additional oral lining adds motility to the tongue and mouth, which facilitates speech and swallowing.

3. We agree with Mendelson et al.[6] and Hoopes[62] that "mandibular *resection* is never performed solely for the purpose of facilitating either wound exposure or closure." Many patients with tumor abutting but not invading the mandible can be managed effectively by marginal mandibular resection[63] without sacrificing the contour and support of oral structures which the mandible provides. Figure 13–11 shows some of the many possible variations.

4. When the mandible must be sacrificed, there are several effective means that allow primary reconstruction (Fig 13–12). Other methods are described and illustrated in chapter 6. When no other means are available, we have effectively used a simple silicon rubber wire prosthesis. This device avoids most of the early problems of erosion when an unpadded single wire is used for support. To date it has been used in 40 patients, with more than 75% of the patients retaining the prosthesis. The local myo-osseous advancement of the lower remaining portions of the horizontal ramus (illustrated in Chap. 6) has led us to use bone advancement, where possible, in preference to a prosthesis. In larger spans, a myo-osseous flap or osteomyocutaneous flap of some sort is required to achieve prolonged success. Maisel and Adams recently studied the improved reconstruction and time and cost savings of the myo-osseous technique in four patients.[64] If a long span of bone is to maintain both structure and calcification, it must bring its own blood supply with it. All mandible replacement requires effective fixation as well as adequate oral and external full-thickness soft tissue coverage.

5. Having a repertoire of reconstructive techniques allows the surgeon to perform a wider cancer excision and achieve a higher rate of planned reconstruction.

IS ANY THERAPY EFFECTIVE IN STAGE IV ORAL CANCERS?

Occasionally one encounters statements such as the following from Million et al.:[65] "There are anecdotal cases in which patients with advanced stage IV disease have been cured. However, the cure rate for some advanced lesions may be estimated at 1%–2% at best. The question then becomes, is it rational to put 100 patients through major therapy with a treatment-related mortality rate of 5%–10% and a high morbidity to cure one or two patients?" Even though there is a disclaimer about "advanced stage IV," the tendency is to carry this nihilistic thinking to all stage IV disease. The roman numeral stage designation of classification has many flaws. They are most severe in stage IV. Remember that stage IV disease contains any N_2 and N_3 and all T_4 cancers. Many T_1, T_2, T_3, N_2, or N_3 patients are quite curable. Some large exophytic T_4 lesions are node negative or N_1 when studied pathologically. Data from our oral cancer series showed the following determinate 5-year survival without evidence of disease: T_2N_2 and T_2N_3, 66%; T_4N_1 and T_4N_2, 36% (see the results for stage IV floor of the mouth cancers shown in Fig 13–10). There should be no discouragement unless histologically positive nodes extend to the clavicle, the tumor is fixed to the paraspinous muscles or transverse processes, or the upper end of the internal carotid is not free. Computerized axial tomography has proved invaluable in determining resectability.

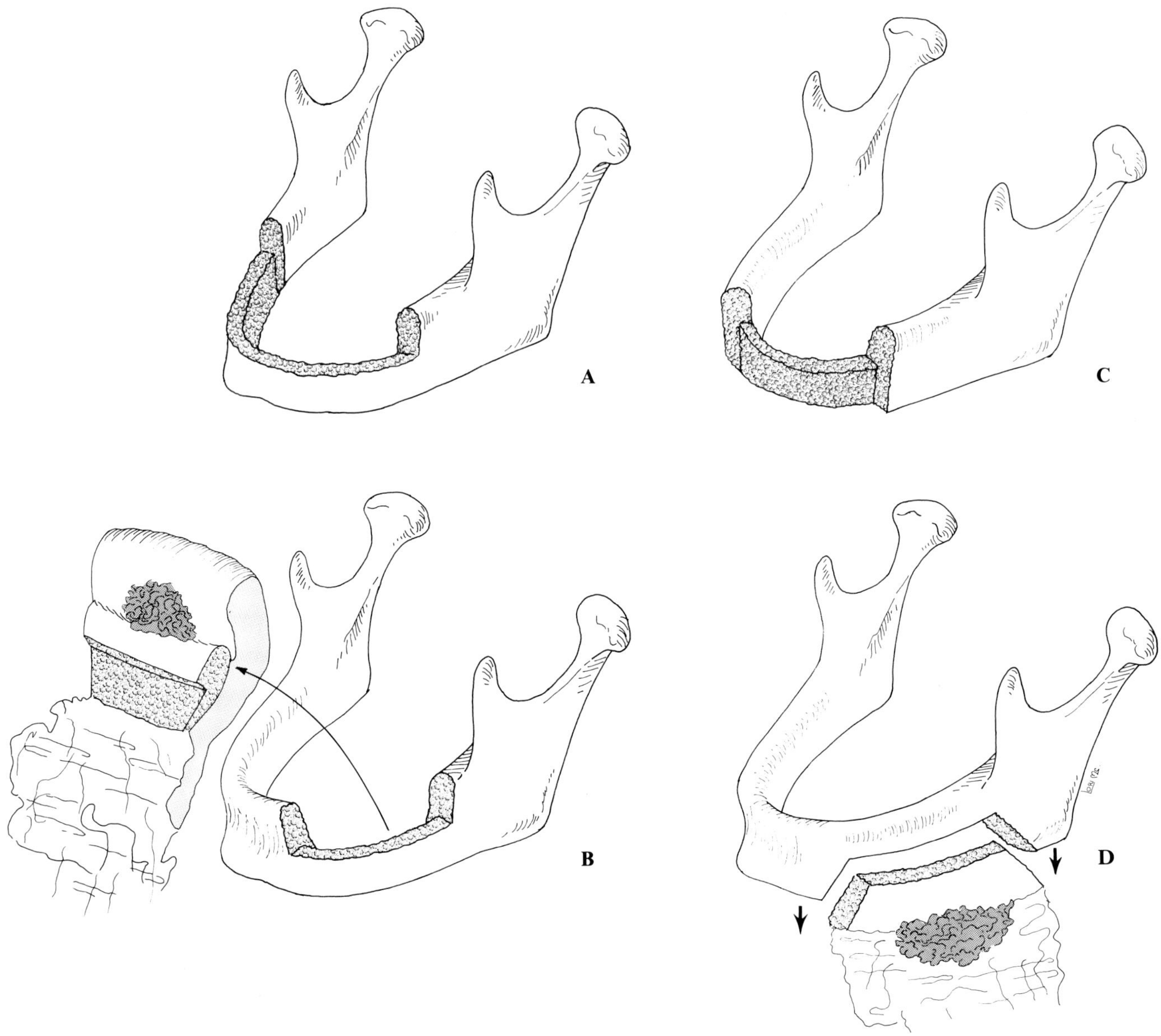

Fig 13–11.—Four variations of marginal resection of the mandible where tumor is very close to or immediately abutting the mandible. **A,** the usual amount of mandible resected for a moderate-sized midline floor of the mouth cancer. **B,** a lateral resection for a lesion involving the alveolus. **C,** resection useful for larger lip cancers growing near the mandible. **D,** large submandibular nodes may be fixed to the lower edge of the mandible, requiring bone resection.

If Adequate Surgical Margins Are the Key to Successful Cure of Larger Oral Cancers, How Do You Achieve These Margins?

The first problem is deciding on a measurable dimension to substitute for the term adequate margin. Histologically, tumor strands frequently extend along tissue planes a centimeter or so from the visible or palpable edges, particularly in the musculature of the tongue. A 2- to 3-cm gross margin is what more cognizant surgeons recommend. The residents have accused the author of using a "rule of thumb," the width of a pudgy thumb (2.57 cm). Margins in the mobile portions of the mouth can be deceptive when retraction distorts or stretches tissues. Margins should be plotted in the undeformed, unretracted state. There should be a mental construction of a deep margin in the resective tactic which will give a 2- to 3-cm deep margin. Where the tumor approaches, encases, or invades a nerve, such as the lingual or inferior alveolar nerve, one should resect the nerve as far proximally as possible. This has a better chance of capturing perineural extension.

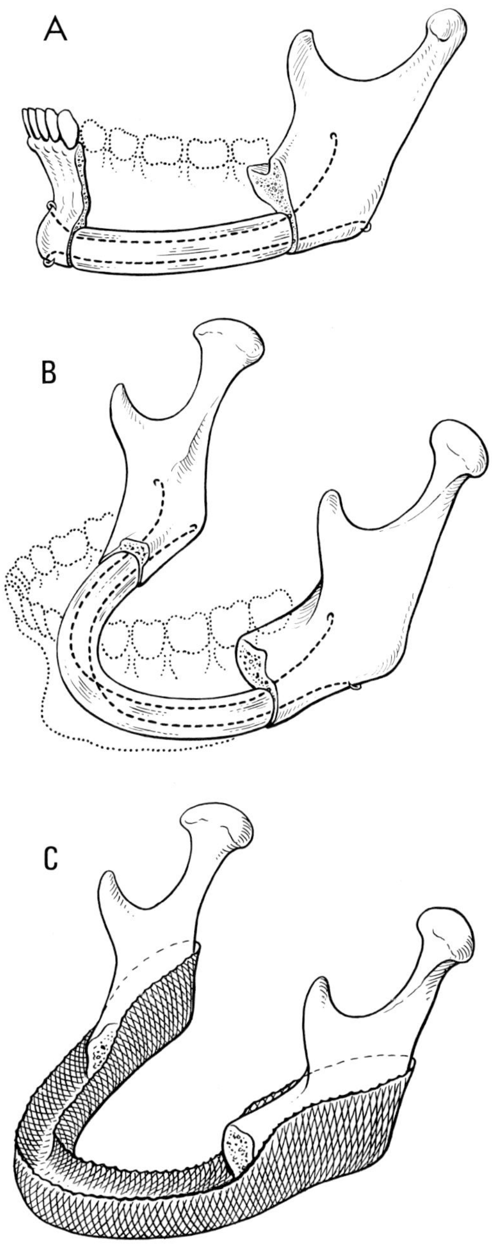

Fig 13–12.—When bone advancement is not possible or where other bone replacement is not feasible, a simple prosthesis made from a silicone rubber block with inserted Kirchner wires can be used as a support. It can be used in a lateral position **(A)** or as replacement for the whole arch **(B).** This is a secondary procedure. More desirable options are discussed in chapter 6 **(C).** If there is no oral contamination a dacron-urethane or Vitallium mesh tray can be used to hold cancellous bone chips. Trying to fill a large span, as illustrated, is quite unreliable for long-term firm bone mineralization.

Several guides for each area are discussed and illustrated.

TONGUE

For the usual T_2 middle third of the tongue lesion, a pull-through hemiglossectomy can be done, as described by Kremen in 1951.[66] The tongue is easily divided down its midline to a point well behind the tumor. This can be done transorally and with a "hockey stick" neck incision for the lymphadenectomy. The primary lesion is freed laterally from the mandible by the transoral route. The tongue is divided down the midline. The final resection is performed in the neck after "pulling" the specimen beneath the mandible and sectioning tongue muscle transversely in the posterior portion. The transoral resection is a little more awkward than dividing the lip and developing cheek flaps, but it will leave the front of the face unscarred. The tongue is then closed to the gingiva. A tongue release may be done 3 months later. For massive tongue cancers, exposure and resection may require division of the lip, cheek flaps, and/or some sort of mandible resection (see illustrations in Chap. 14). Some authors divide the mandible at the symphysis or at the canine tooth to gain exposure, wiring the ends at closure. This type of exposure is most applicable to more posterior oropharyngeal lesions, which frequently require mandible resection.

LESIONS OF TONGUE, FLOOR OF THE MOUTH, AND ALVEOLAR RIDGE INVOLVING THE MANDIBLE

The right hand side of Figure 13–5 gives a reasonable scheme of management. If voluntary movement of the tongue by the patient reveals a 2- to 3-cm gross margin between the edge of the cancer and the lingual gingiva, then the entire mandible and dentition can be retained. Before the 1960s there was a commonly held armchair opinion that the oral cavity lymphatics drained via mandibular periosteal lymph channels. This was used as a justification for routine segmental mandibulectomy in many cases where the tumor was at some distance from bone. Marchetta et al. studied 80 resected, serially sectioned specimens.[67] The periosteal lymphatics did *not* contain cancer cells unless there was direct contiguous invasion by tumor. This study and the availability of high-speed cutting drills made marginal mandibulectomy a rational option which was easy to perform. When cancer approaches but does not attach to or invade bone, we perform a marginal mandibulectomy with one of the variations shown in Figure 13–11. Figure 13–13 shows the extent of resection for a floor of the mouth cancer, well away from the mandible (see Fig 13–13,A). The more extensive cancer requires mar-

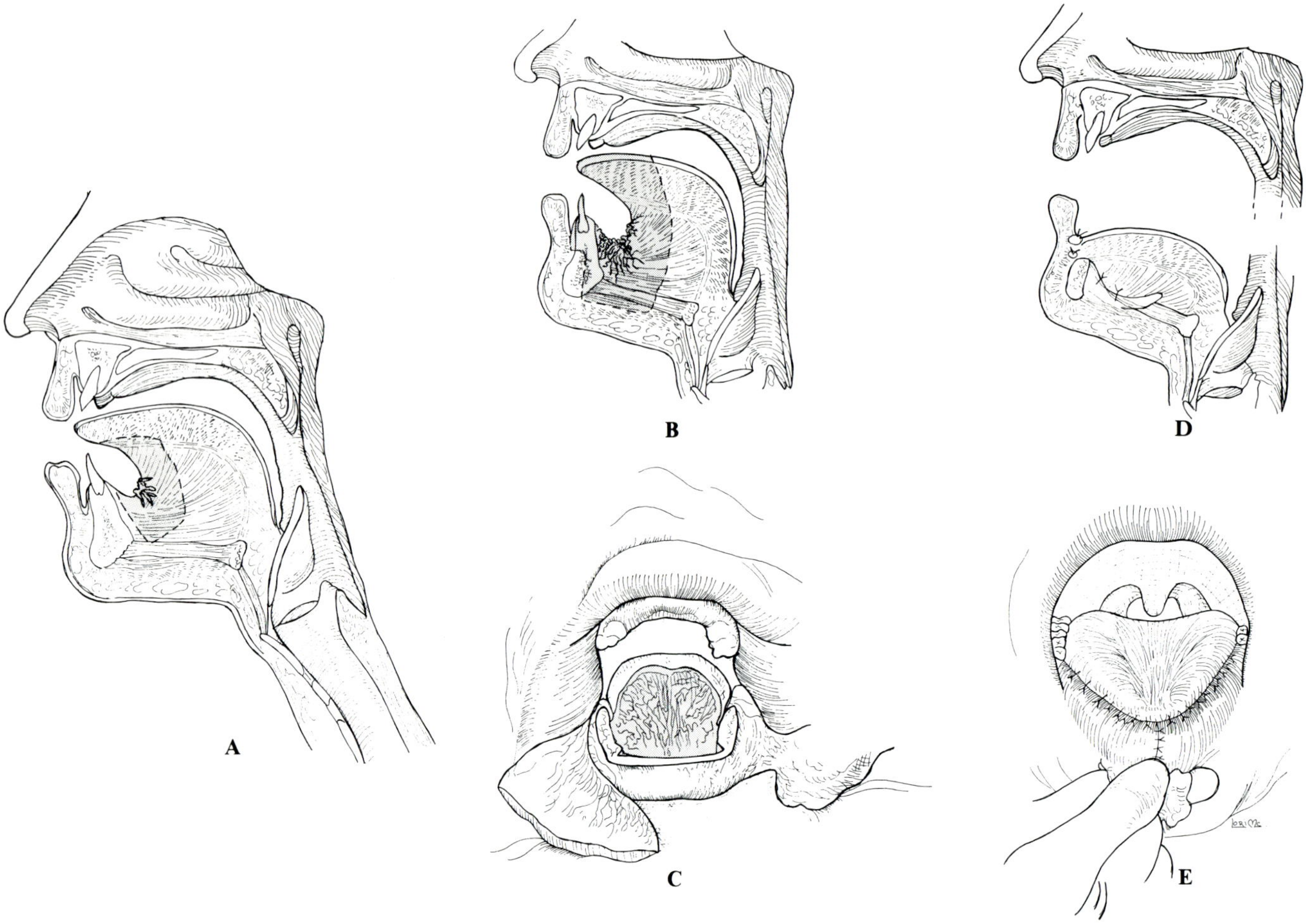

Fig 13–13.—**A,** resection for a small cancer away from the mandible. Note the sizable and deep margin. **B,** the more extensive floor of the mouth cancer near the mandible requires a marginal mandibulectomy. The specimen is usually removed in continuity with the cervical lymphatics, leaving the defect shown in **C.** Oral closure is shown in **D** and **E.**

ginal mandibulectomy (see Figs 13–13,B and C). Usually this is contiguous specimen with the lymphadenectomy. Figs 13–13,D and E show the method of closure. A tongue release at 3 months may improve oral function. If there is radiographic evidence of bone invasion, we strive for 2- to 3-cm lateral bone margins. If there is deep invasion near the inferior alveolar nerve, we section the vertical ramus above the entry foramen of the nerve. If the entire anterior mandibular arch is resected, some provision must be made to replace the supportive component of the arch. Failure to provide support allows the remaining tongue musculature to collapse and attach to the hyoid (Fig 13–14). Late reconstruction is then virtually impossible. Overzealous anterior fixation of the tongue prevents adequate swallowing (see Fig 13–14,D).

DEEPER STRUCTURES OF THE MOUTH

Excision of the floor of the mouth and underside of the tongue requires the surgeon to develop a cone of surrounding tissue beginning just above the hyoid (see Fig 13–13,B). We usually include the digastric, the geniohyoid, some of the hyoglossus, the styloglossus, and as much intrinsic tongue muscle as necessary. The distance from the hyoid to the underside of the tongue is small. Place the middle finger of the right hand on the floor of the mouth and the thumb on the hyoid. The short distance will surprise you.

It is possible to adapt the resection of involved tongue to whatever is needed to achieve adequate margins. Cancers do not respect the borders of a "standard" resection. A midline division of the tongue is simple and relatively avascular. Larger tumors may require additional diagonal or extended transverse resections.

RETROMOLAR TRIGONE

A few small lesions ($<$ 1–1.5 cm, superficial) may be excised with a tissue-bone block and closed primarily. The neck is then treated by ENI or a discontinuous

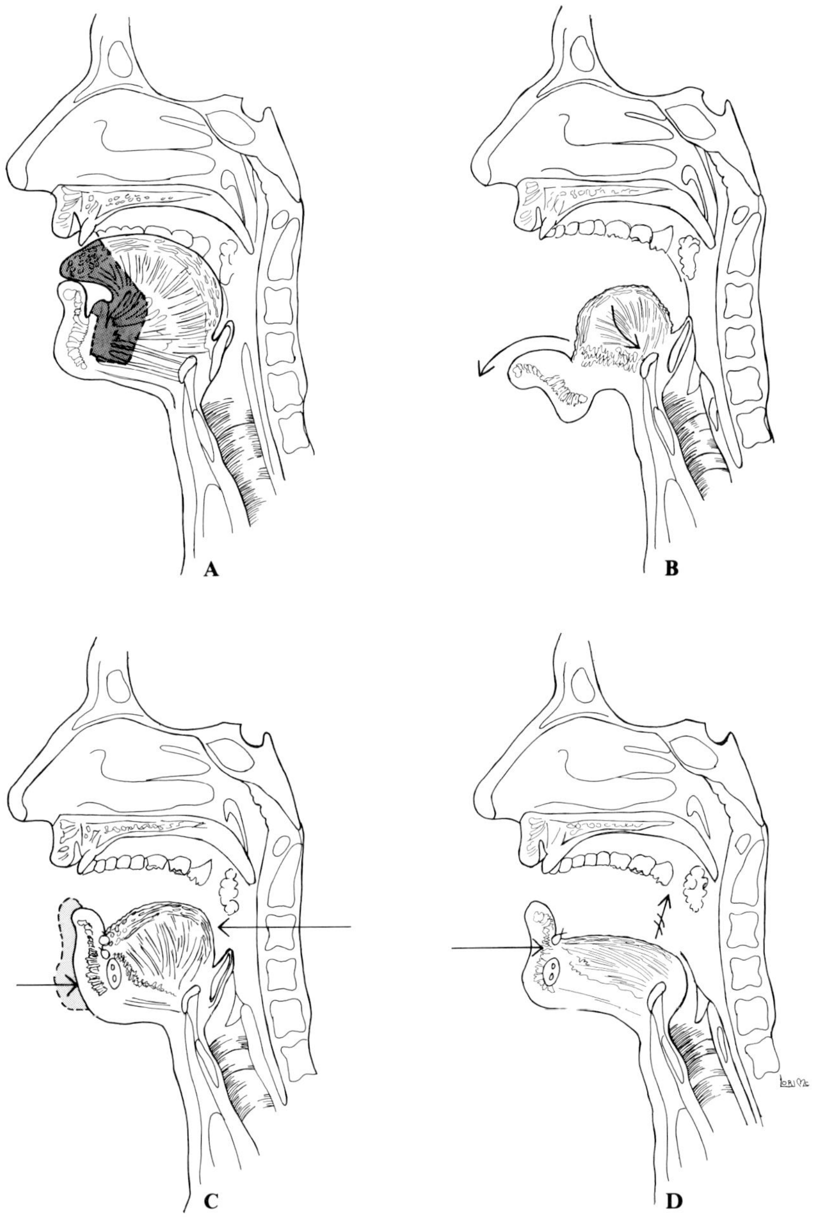

Fig 13–14.—A, resection leaving a strut of mandible will preserve support of the tongue on closure. **B,** if no support is provided, the tongue heals and contracts down to the hyoid. Contraction of the tongue on swallowing pushes oral contents forward. **C,** if a significant amount of tongue is taken with the mandibular arch, it may be necessary to recess the mandible on reconstruction to avoid excessive tension on the tongue and allow it to contract and raise the posterior portion on swallowing. **D,** if the tongue is pulled tightly forward in closure, the tongue cannot be raised for effective swallowing. A slight overbite as created in **C** is better than an inability to swallow.

lymphadenectomy. With larger retromolar trigone cancers, a more extensive resection is planned which incorporates the local elements of the lymphatic ring of Waldeyer, i.e., the tonsil and adjacent lingual tonsil (see illustrations in Chap. 14.) Pterygoid space recurrences have been encountered. Therefore it is desirable to completely remove involved bone, much of the muscle and the deep facial lymphatics in the pterygoid space, the tonsil, and contiguous tongue and lingual tonsillar tissue. If necessary, the resection can include tonsil, soft palate, maxillary tubosity, the buccinator muscle and buccinator fat pads, and associated lymph nodes. An occasional involved node is harvested in the pterygoid or buccinator tissue. One cannot be sure this translates to increased survival. Eilber and Zarem have used and illustrated pterygoid resection in 14 patients.[68] In 12 cases the cancers were not squamous cell cancers.

LESIONS OF THE HARD PALATE

A Ferguson maxillectomy incision is used and the involved segment removed, as is done for a maxillectomy. With larger cancers, it may be hard to distinguish between maxillary antrum or oral origin. Basically, the resection is a maxillectomy. The techniques and guidelines are covered in chapter 17. Neck dissection is discontinuous by necessity.

Is There a Valid Indication for a Total Glossectomy? Is a Laryngectomy Always Required?

Selected patients may tolerate a total glossectomy with adequate reconstruction.[69, 70] Aspiration may force a subsequent laryngectomy. This subject is discussed in chapter 14 and in articles by Effron et al.[71] and Harrold.[72]

When are Flaps Required in Oral Closure After Resecting Larger Oral Cancers?

A hemiglossectomy or resection of the anterior floor of the mouth (with or without marginal mandibulectomy) can be closed without difficulty by pulling the tongue laterally or forward, using some of the intrinsic redundancy of oral lining membranes (see Fig 13–14). This does tether the tongue and produces a marked functional deficit. When there is a limited amount of tongue remaining, it is necessary to support the tongue farther back if one is replacing anterior mandible (see Fig 13–14,C). If pulled too far forward it may heal but it cannot function for speech or swallowing (see Fig 13–14,D). Some minimal improvement can be realized with a tongue release. If distinct speech is a major occupational requirement, if more than 12–16 sq cm of mucosal or tongue surface is to be resected, or if the lateral oropharynx must be widely resected, it is prudent to plan on full-thickness flaps for additional oral lining. A tongue flap can only be used to close small defects (6–10 cm^2) in adjacent areas. This type of flap aggravates impaired oral function. Larger defects require cervical, Bakamjian flaps[73] (Fig 13–15), forehead flaps, or a myocutaneous flap.

An oral closure under *any* tension will break down. If there is tension on frail mucosa, the closure may fail as early as 24 hours. Larger retromolar trigone resections are virtually impossible to close primarily without fixing the tongue in the rear of the mouth and converting the faucial arch to a tight stenosis. This closure under tension produces a precarious oral suture line which is prone to frequent orocutaneous fistulas. An ap-

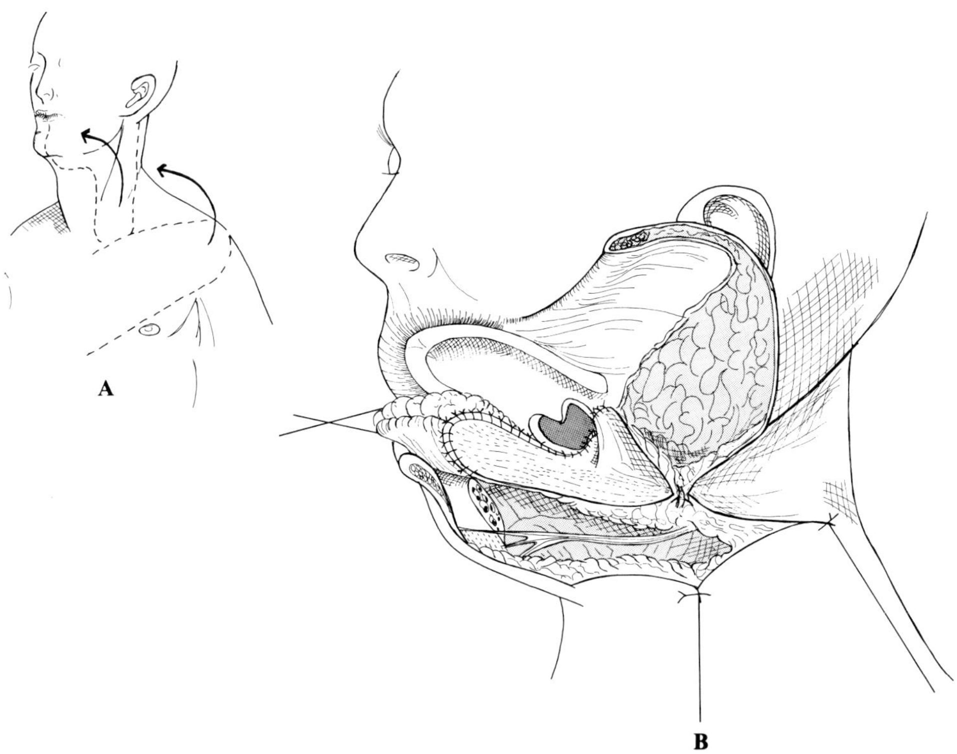

Fig 13–15.—Cervical and pectoral flaps used for oral reconstruction. *Inset* shows the general design of the two flaps. The cervical flap incorporates the platysma. It is tubed "skin-side-in" for a short distance and then folded outward for oral lining. The cheek flap then covers the non-epithelialized surface. Careful attention must be paid to achieve good closure at all "three-sided" junctions of flap and mucosa. The deltopectoral flap is brought up to cover the lateral neck. The deltopectoral flap donor site is covered with split-thickness skin.

propriate flap which is placed in an irradiated host field must bring a good blood supply with it if healing is to be reliable, i.e., a cervicle flap cannot be used if it has an irradiated base. The flap must be custom-designed for each patient. The common error is to plan the flap too small. Make the flap 20% bigger than the defect. Frequently we use the utilitarian Bakamjian flaps with variations in unirradiated patients.[58] They are reliable up to 3–5 months after irradiation if a preliminary "delay" procedure is done. After that time, a well-vascularized pectoral myocutaneous flap becomes the preferred method for irradiated fields (see Chap. 14). We agree with Conley[74] that we should first think of simpler methods and shift regional tissues where possible and not use more spectacular tissues transfers with compulsive enthusiasm and increased risk unless they are absolutely required.[74]

IS PREOPERATIVE IRRADIATION OF VALUE IN IMPROVING ORAL CANCER SURVIVAL?

The use of irradiation was discussed in chapter 7. In general, the combined modalities of treatment are only considered for larger stage III and IV cancers. A definitive answer is not available for oral cancer in particular. Condict Moore et al. summarized observations up to 1972 with a question:[75] "Why is this combination of treatment so irresistible, yet so hard to prove it of patient benefit?" Combined treatment became popular by the middle to late 1960s when a number of authors had reported effects in laryngeal cancer after short follow-ups using historical controls for comparison. In 1967 the Memorial Hospital group reported results of preoperative irradiation before neck dissection in a nonrandomized group of oral cancer patients. The small difference in cervical recurrence rates in the irradiated patients was tantalizing rather than overwhelming.[76] Cady did a comprehensive review of laboratory results and clinical experiences with preoperative irradiation at all sites reported in the literature from 1914 to 1968.[77] He concluded that for head and neck cancer, there *may* be some small beneficial effect. For preoperative irradiation in general, he cautioned that "the potential benefit to be realized may be modest in terms of overall survival." In 1968, the Memorial Hospital group published a prospective nonrandomized trial of low-dose preoperative cervical irradiation. Again, there were slightly fewer node recurrences. Unfortunately, there was no proportionate increase in 3-year survivors.[78] A higher (5,000-rad) preoperative treatment was tried in a mixed group of 45 patients by Sanfilippo et al.:[79] there was a hint of increased control, but no evaluable survival data. Moore et al.[75] paired irradiated patients and historical control patients by similar characteristics. They felt that irradiation had some benefit, largely confined to the group thought to be staged N_1. Two randomized prospective studies show no significant difference in survival in a group made up largely of patients with oral cancers[80] or supraglottic cancers.[81] The Radiation Therapy Oncology group has found no difference in survival following preoperative (5,000 rad) and postoperative (6,000 rad) therapy when combined with surgery in a mixed group of randomly allocated head and neck cancer patients.[82] Data are extended to 40 months. Marchetta and Sako reasoned that "if the increment of [survival] improvement is not greater than 5 percent, preoperative irradiation is not warranted since about 56 percent of patients with squamous cell carcinoma of the intraoral cavity, stage III, would receive unnecessary irradiation."[44]

Combination preoperative chemoradiotherapy is currently being evaluated in independent studies[83–84] and as planned protocols. We can also expect tests of particle therapy, hypoxic cell sensitizers, and hyperthermia.[85] Some of these studies are discussed in chapter 8.

At this time one may conclude that if preoperative irradiation has any salutary effect in prolonging life in *oral* cancer patients, the effect is minimal and confined to small subgroups of patients with early node involvement. Because of the significant increment in mortality and morbidity with higher dose or multidrug chemotherapy with irradiation, the combined adjuvant use should be confined to the context of participation in approved randomized prospective clinical trials.

IS RADIATION SALVAGE OF SURGICAL FAILURES EFFECTIVE?

Very rarely will irradiation control or cure a bulky recurrence after surgical failure. Repeat surgery has a low yield but is still the best opportunity. Radiation therapy for recurrences can reduce bulk and control local pain from bone invasion. Irradiation for surgical failure is palliative at best.

IS VERRUCOUS CARCINOMA OF THE MOUTH DIFFERENT FROM THE USUAL ORAL SQUAMOUS CELL CANCER?

It is difficult to fit verrucous carcinoma into the discussion so far. The problem presents itself to a clinician who finds a floridly exuberant whitish lesion when he examines the mouth of an elderly patient, typically 75–85 years old. It may be velvety or irregular and warty on its surface. The differential diagnosis includes exophytic squamous cell cancer, verrucous carcinoma, benign verrucous hyperplasia (?), and proliferative papillomatous leukoplakia. The beautiful gross and histologic illustrations of Burkhardt and Maerker[86] show the various lesions in color. Any of these lesions may be surrounded by wide areas of leukoplakia. An adequate biopsy specimen should be obtained which includes the edge of the lesion and a decent section from the deep margin. The diagnosis of verrucous hyperplasia of the oral mucosa should not give a sense of complacency. Shear and Pindborg reviewed 68 cases from Copenhagen and Johannesburg, a real north-south sample.[87] Twenty of the 68 lesions (29%) were called verrucous carcinomas, 7 (10%) were associated with invasive squamous carcinoma; and 45 (66%) were associated with epithelial dysplasia. Obviously there were overlaps in this spectrum of groupings. The distinction between verrucous hyperplasia and verrucous carcinoma is fuzzy and somewhat dependent on the size of the sample submitted to pathology. The pathology of reported clinical series has been reviewed.[88] The conclusion is that verrucous cancer fits somewhere between nonverrucous squamous cell cancer and the hyperplasias such as leukoplakia. The term verrucous hyperplasia is probably semantically and clinically confusing. The *absence* of a carcinoma cannot be assured until the entire lesion is removed and microscopically examined. Verrucous carcinoma is also known as Ackerman's tumor, after his nonoriginal description in 1948.[89] Verrucous "epithelioma" was clearly illustrated and sensibly discussed by Butlin in 1885.[90] Verrucous carcinoma represents less than 2% of oral cancers. It occurs in patients over 50 years old in 95% of cases. The verrucous cancers are located in the buccal mucosa (43%), gingiva (30%), tongue and floor of the mouth (9%), palate (7%), and other sites.[90] Histologically confirmed cervical metastases occur in less than 2% of all cases in the oral cavity. These have occurred following irradiation. Postirradiation anaplastic transformation is a minimal risk (4%–10%) shibboleth. McDonald et al. reviewed the best way to treat the lesions.[91] They found 193 patients with adequate follow-up. Of these, 53 (27.5%) were treated by irradiation, and 22 (41.5%) of those patients that received irradiation were apparently "cured." Anaplastic malignant growth followed irradiation in 7.5% of these 53 cases. Of the 138 patients (67%) treated surgically, 74% were cured and 26% experienced recurrence. Local excision, when technically possible, appears to be the best treatment. Neck dissection is unnecessary unless there are palpable nodes or invasive squamous cell cancer is found in the deeper sections. Gage suggested that it is conceptually valid to treat them by cryosurgery, although he does not identify specific numbers of verrucous carcinoma cases.[92, 93] The lesions we have seen cover a wide area and drape over the mandible. Because of diagnostic problems, it would be desirable to have the whole lesion excised and carefully examined for its pathology. If that is inordinately risky for the patient, or difficult because of site, radiation and cryotherapy are good second and third choices. Cervical lymphadenectomy would be reserved for cases with detectable cervical nodes or a clearly invasive component to the verrucous cancer.

IS THERE A SPECIFIC USE FOR LASERS IN TREATING ORAL CANCER?

Lasers are both trendy and very expensive. For ablation and excision of any superficial lesion, a CO_2 laser will provide another means of destroying cell structure with heat. The advantage of the laser is that the system can focus the effective area to a fine point. It does seal off vessels of 0.5 mm or smaller, but it can punch an exciting defect if used near large vessels. There is a low level of postoperative pain. Laser use is limited to areas where the beam can be directly focused. Carruth has emphasized that margins still must be maintained.[94] He has used the laser in lieu of a knife to remove a larger segment of tongue containing cancer.[95] The exact indications for use and comparative effectiveness are "still very much *sub judice*."[94]

REFERENCES

1. Ildstad S.T., Bigelow M.E., Remensmyder J.P.: Intraoral cancer at the Massachusetts General Hospital. *Ann. Surg.* 197:34–41, 1983.
2. Mendenhall W.M., VanCise W.S., Bova F.J. et al.: Analysis of time dose factors in squamous cell carcinoma of the oral tongue and floor of mouth treated by radiation therapy alone. *Int. J. Radiat. Oncol. Biol. Phys.* 7(8):1005–1010, 1981.
3. Kremen A.J.: Surgical management of cancer of the tongue. *Surg. Clin. North Am.* 47:1125–1129, 1967.
4. Leipzig B., Hokanson J.A.: Treatment of cervical lymph nodes in carcinoma of the tongue. *Head Neck Surg.* 5:3–9, 1982.
5. Joyce L., McQuarrie D.G.: Application of contemporary reconstructive techniques in head and neck surgery for anterior oral-facial cancers. *Surgery* 80:373–378, 1976.
6. Mendelson B.C., Hodgkinson D.J., Woods J.E.: Cancer of the oral cavity. *Surg. Clin. North Am.* 57:585–596, 1977.
7. Shah J.P., Cendon R.A., Farr H.W., et al.: Carcinoma of the oral cavity: Factors affecting treatment failure at the primary site and the neck. *Am. J. Surg.* 132:504–507, 1976.
8. Harrold C.C.: Management of cancer of the floor of the mouth. *Am. J. Surg.* 122:487–493, 1971.
9. Fu K.K., Ray J.W., Chan E.K., et al.: External and interstitial radiation therapy of carcinoma of the oral tongue. *AJR* 126:107–115, 1976.
10. Fayos J.V., Lampe I.: Treatment of squamous cell carcinoma of the oral cavity. *Am. J. Surg.* 124:493–500, 1972.
11. Holm L.E., Lundquist P.G., Silfversward C., et al.: Combined preoperative radiotherapy and surgery in the

treatment of carcinoma of the anterior two-thirds of the tongue. *Laryngoscope* 93:792–796, 1983.
12. Marks J.E., Lee F., Smith P.G., et al.: Floor of mouth cancer: Patient selection and treatment results. *Laryngoscope* 93:475–480, 1983.
13. Spiro R.H., Strong E.W.: Epidermoid carcinoma of the mobile tongue: Treatment by partial glossectomy alone. *Am. J. Surg.* 122:707–710, 1971.
14. Spiro R.H., Strong E.W.: Epidermoid carcinoma of the oral cavity and oropharynx: Elective vs. therapeutic radical neck dissection as treatment. *Arch. Surg.* 107:382–384, 1973.
15. Marks J.E., Lee F., Freeman R.B.: Carcinoma of the oral tongue: A study of patient selection and treatment results. *Laryngoscope* 91:1548–1559, 1981.
16. Marchetta F.C., Sako K., Razack M.S.: Management of "localized" oral cancer. *Am. J. Surg.* 134:448–449, 1977.
17. Cooper I.S., Lee A. St. J.: Cryothalamectomy-hypothermia coagulation. *J. Am. Geriatr. Soc.* 9:714–718, 1961.
18. Gage A.A.: Five-year survival following cryosurgery for oral cancer. *Arch. Surg.* 111:990–994, 1976.
19. Gage A.A.: Experimental cryogenic injury of the palate: Observations pertinent to cryosurgical destruction of tumors. *Cryobiology* 13:415–425, 1978.
20. Gage A.A.: Current issues in cryosurgery. *Cryobiology* 19:219–222, 1982.
21. Gongloff R.K., Samit A.M., Greene G.W., et al.: Cryosurgical management of benign and dysplastic intraoral lesions. *J. Oral Surg.* 38:671–676, 1980.
22. Neel H.B. III, Farrell K.H., Payne W.S.: Cryosurgery of respiratory structures: I. Cryonecrosis of trachea and bronchus. *Laryngoscope* 83:1062–1071, 1973.
23. Neel H.B. III, Ketcham A.S., Hammond W.G.: Requirements for successful cryogenic surgery for cancer. *Arch. Surg.* 101:43–48, 1971.
24. Carpenter R.J. III, Snyder G.G. III: Cryosurgery: Theory and application to head and neck neoplasia. *Head Neck Surg.* 2:129–141, 1979.
25. Shedd D.P.: Clinical characteristics of early oral cancer. *JAMA* 215:955, 1971.
26. Mashberg A., Morrissey J.B., Garfinkel L.: A study of the appearance of early asymptomatic squamous cell carcinoma. *Cancer* 32:1436, 1973.
27. Mashberg A.: Erythroplasia vs. leukoplakia in the diagnosis of early asymptomatic oral squamous carcinoma. *N. Engl. J. Med.* 297:109–110, 1977.
28. Mashberg A., Meyers H.: Anatomic site and size of 222 early asymptomatic oral squamous cell carcinomas. *Cancer* 37:2149–2153, 1976.
29. Ash C.L.: Oral cancer: A 25-year study. The Janeway Lecture. *AJR* 87:417, 1962.
30. Easson E.: Radiotherapy in oral cancer, 1932–1962. *Br. Dent. J.* 115:239, 1963.
31. Hirata R.M., Jacques D.A., Chambers R.G., et al.: Carcinoma of the oral cavity: An analysis of 478 cases. *Ann. Surg.* 182:98–103, 1975.
32. Patterson R., Tod M., Russel M.: *The Results of Radium and X-Ray Therapy in Malignant Diseases.* Edinburgh, E. & S. Livingston, 1950.
33. Lampe I.: Radiation therapy of cancer of the buccal mucosa and lower gingiva. *AJR* 73:628–635, 1955.
34. Fu K.K., Lichter A., Galante M.: Carcinoma of the floor of the mouth: An analysis of treatment results and the sites and cases of failures. *Int. J. Radiat. Oncol. Biol. Phys.* 1:829, 1976.
35. Chu A., Fletcher G.H.: Incidence and causes of failure to control by irradiation the primary lesions in squamous cell carcinomas of the anterior two-thirds of the tongue and floor of the mouth. *AJR* 117:502–508, 1973.
36. Shons A.R., Magallanes F., McQuarrie D.G.: The results of aggressive regional surgery in the treatment of floor of the mouth cancer. *Surgery* 96:29–33, 1984.
37. Barton R.T., Ucmakli A.: Treatment of squamous cell carcinoma of the floor of the mouth. *Surg. Gynecol. Obstet.* 145:21–27, 1977.
38. McQuarrie D.G., Shons A.R., Magallanes F.: The results of aggressive regional surgery and immediate reconstruction in oral cancer. Unpublished data.
39. MacComb W.S.: Necrosis in treatment of intra-oral cancer by radiation therapy. *AJR* 87:431–440, 1962.
40. McCready R.A., Hyde G.L., Bivins B.A., et al.: Radiation-induced arterial injuries. *Surgery* 93:306–312. 1983.
41. Levinson S.A., Close M.B., Eherenfeld W.K., et al.: Carotid artery occlusive disease following external cervical irradiation. *Arch. Surg.* 107:395–397, 1973.
42. Larson D.L., Lindberg R.D., Lane E., et al.: Major complications of radiotherapy in cancer of the oral cavity and oropharynx: A 10-year retrospective study. *Am. J. Surg.* 146:531–536, 1983.
43. Jesse R.H., Fletcher G.H.: Treatment of the neck in patients with squamous cell carcinoma of the head and neck. *Cancer* 39:868–872, 1977.
44. Marchetta F.C., Sako K.: Pre-operative irradiation for squamous cell carcinoma of the head and neck: Does it improve 5 year survival or control figures? *Am. J. Surg.* 130:487–488, 1975.
45. Mulholland M.W., Magallanes F., Press B.H.J., et al.: Aggressive surgical therapy after radiation failure in treatment of cancer of the oral tongue. *Arch. Surg.* 119:394–399, 1984.
46. Vermund H., Gollin F.E.: Role of radiotherapy in the treatment of cancer of the tongue. *Cancer* 32:333–345, 1973.
47. Lam K.H., Wong J., Lim S.T., et al.: Surgical treatment of cervical lymph nodes in carcinoma of the tongue. *Aust. NZ J. Surg.* 50:37–41, 1980.
48. Spiro R.H., Strong E.W.: Surgical treatment of cancer of the tongue. *Surg. Clin. North Am.* 54:759–765, 1974.
49. Whitehurst J.O., Drovlias C.A.: Surgical treatment of squamous cell carcinoma of the oral tongue: Factors influencing survival. *Arch. Otolaryngol.* 103:212–215, 1977.
50. White D., Byers R.M.: What is the preferred initial method of treatment for squamous carcinoma of the tongue? *Am. J. Surg.* 140:553–555, 1980.
51. Johnson J.T., Leipzig B., Cummings C.W.: Management of T_1 carcinoma of the anterior aspect of the tongue. *Arch. Otolaryngol.* 106:249–251, 1980.
52. Razack M.S., Sako K., Patel J.K.: The role of initial mo-

dality in treatment of squamous cell carcinoma of the tongue. *J. Surg. Oncol.* 19:136–138, 1982.
53. Gilbert E.W., Goffinet D.R., Bagshaw M.A.: Carcinoma of the oral tongue and floor of the mouth: Fifteen years' experience with linear accelerator therapy. *Cancer* 35:1517–1524, 1975.
54. Fletcher G.H., Jesse R.H.: The place of irradiation in the management of the primary lesion in head and neck cancers. *Cancer* 39:862–867, 1977.
55. Johnson J.T., Leipzig B., Cummings C.W.: Management of T_1 carcinoma of the anterior aspect of the tongue. *Arch. Otolaryngol.* 106:249–251, 1980.
56. De Croix Y., Ghossein N.A.: Experience of the Curie Institute in treatment of cancer of the mobile tongue: Treatment, policies, and result. *Cancer* 47:496–502, 1981.
57. Stranc M.F., Labandter H., and Roy A.: A review of 196 tubed pedicles. *Br. J. Plast. Surg.* 28:54, 1975.
58. Shons A.R., McQuarrie D.G.: Cervical-pectoral flaps in the treatment of advanced oral cancer. *J. Surg. Oncol.* 7:213–218, 1975.
59. Spira M., Gerow F.J., Hardy S.B.: Subcutaneous pedicle flaps on the face. *Br. J. Plast. Surg.* 27:258, 1974.
60. McQuarrie D.G.: Immediate functional restoration of the mandible after surgical treatment of advanced oral cancer. *Arch. Surg.* 102:447–452, 1971.
61. Rush B.F. Jr., Swaminathan A., Knightly J.J.: Use of split thickness grafts in the repair of excisions of the oropharynx, base of tongue and larynx. *Am. J. Surg.* 128:553, 1974.
62. Hoopes J.E.: The forehead flap in intraoral reconstruction, in Anderson R., Hoopes J.E. (eds.): *Symposium on Malignancies of the Head and Neck.* St. Louis, C.V. Mosby Co., 1975, vol. 2, pp. 193–195.
63. Flynn M.E., Moore C.: Marginal resection of the mandible in the management of squamous cancer of the floor of the mouth. *Am. J. Surg.* 128:490, 1974.
64. Maisel R.H., Adams E.L.: Osteomyocutaneous reconstruction of the oral cavity. *Arch. Otolaryngol.* 109:731–734, 1983.
65. Million R.R., Cassisi N.J., Wittes R.E.: Cancer in the head and neck, in DaVita V.T., (ed.): *Cancer: Principles and Practice of Oncology.* Philadelphia, J.B. Lippincott Co., 1982, chap. 13.
66. Kremen A.J.: Cancer of the tongue: A surgical technique for a primary combined en bloc resection of the tongue, floor of the mouth and cervical lymphatics. *Surgery* 30:227, 1951.
67. Marchetta F.C., Sako K., Murphy B.: The periosteum of the mandible and intra-oral carcinoma. *Am. J. Surg.* 122:711–713, 1971.
68. Eilber F.R., Zarem H.A.: Pterygoid dissections for extensive cancer: An old concept revisited. *Plast. Reconstr. Surg.* 59:545–550, 1977.
69. Razack M.S., Sako K., Bakamjian V.Y., et al.: Total glossectomy. *Am. J. Surg.* 146:509–511, 1983.
70. Krespi Y.P., Sisson G.A.: Reconstruction after total or subtotal glossectomy. *Am. J. Surg.* 146:455–491, 1983.
71. Effron M.Z., Johnson J.T., Myers E.N., et al.: Advanced carcinoma of the tongue: Management of total glossectomy without laryngectomy. *Arch. Otolaryngol.* 107:694–697, 1981.
72. Harrold C.C.: Surgical treatment of cancer of the base of the tongue. *Am. J. Surg.* 114;493–498, 1967.
73. Bakamjian V., Littlewood M.: Cervical skin flaps for intraoral and pharyngeal repair following cancer surgery. *Br. J. Plast. Surg.* 17:191–210, 1964.
74. Conley J.: Hayes Martin Lecture: Changes in head and neck surgery. *Am. J. Surg.* 146:425–428, 1983.
75. Moore C., Mullins F., Scott R.M.: Pre-operative irradiation in cancer of the head and neck. *Am. J. Surg.* 124;555–558, 1972.
76. Catlin D., Strong E.W.: Pre-operative irradiation for neck dissection. *Surg. Clin. North Am.* 47:1131–1137, 1967.
77. Cady B.: Pre-operative radiation. *Surg. Gynecol. Obstet.* 126:851–865, 1091–1105, 1968.
78. Strong E.W.: Pre-operative radiation and radical neck dissection. *Surg. Clin. North Am.* 49:271–276, 1969.
79. Sanfilippo L.J., Sherman P., Steichen F.M.: Treatment of advanced cancer of head and neck with intensive preoperative irradiation and radical surgery. *Am. J. Surg.* 118:701–707, 1969.
80. Lawrence W., Tery J.J., Rogers C., et al.: Pre-operative irradiation for head and neck cancer: A prospective study. *Cancer* 33:318–323, 1973.
81. Snow J.B., Kramer S., Marcial V.A., et al.: Lowry L.D.: Evaluation of randomized preoperative and postoperative radiation therapy for supraglottic carcinoma. *Ann. Otol.* 87:686–691, 1978.
82. Snow J.B., Belber R.D., Kramer S., et al.: Randomized pre-operative and postoperative radiation therapy for patients with carcinoma of the head and neck: Preliminary report. *Laryngoscope* 90:930–945, 1980.
83. Pearlman N.W., Meyers A.D., Johnson F.B., et al.: Preoperative chemo-radiotherapy in advanced head and neck cancer. *Head Neck Surg.* 5:10–14, 1982.
84. Cruy A.B., McInnis W.D., Aust J.B.: Triple drug intra-arterial infusion combined with x-ray therapy and surgery for head and neck cancer. *Am. J. Surg.* 128:573–579, 1974.
85. Segren S.L.: Recent advances in radiation therapy of head and neck cancer. *Head Neck Surg.* 4:227–232, 1982.
86. Burkhardt A., Maerker R.: *A Colour Atlas of Oral Cancers.* Chicago, Year Book Medical Publishers, Inc., 1981.
87. Shear M., Pindborg J.J.: Verrucous hyperplasia of the oral mucosa. *Cancer* 46:1855–1862, 1980.
88. Batsakis J.G., Hybels R., Crissman J.D., et al.: The pathology of head and neck tumors: Verrucous carcinoma. *Head Neck Surg.* 5:29–38, 1982.
89. Ackerman L.V.: Verrucous carcinoma of the oral cavity. *Surgery* 23:670–678, 1948.
90. Butlin H.T.: *Diseases of the Tongue* London, Cassell & Co., 1885, pp. 126–190, 291.
91. McDonald J.S., Crissman J.D., Gluckman J.L.: Verrucous carcinoma of the oral cavity. *Head Neck Surg.* 5:22–28, 1982.

92. Gage A.: Indication, techniques and results of cryosurgery for dysplastic and neoplastic oral diseases, in *Proceedings of the IV World Congress of Cryosurgery*, September 1980.
93. Gongloff R.K., Samit A.M., Greene G.W., et al.: Cryosurgical management of benign and dysplastic intraoral lesions. *J. Oral Surg.* 38:671–676, 1980.
94. Carruth J.A.S.: The role of lasers in otolaryngology. *World J. Surg.* 7:719–724, 1983.
95. Carruth J.A.S.: Resection of the tongue with the carbon dioxide laser. *J. Laryngol. Otol.* 96:529–532, 1982.

14 / Cancer of the Oropharynx

George L. Adams, M.D.

Malignant tumors of the oral cavity and pharynx account for nearly 50% of malignancies of the upper aerodigestive tract. The National Cancer Institute estimates that 27,000 new cases occur per year, with a 2:1 male preponderance. These tumors often reach considerable size before they are recognized. Cancers in the oropharynx frequently involve nodes on either or both sides of the neck. The long-term use of tobacco products is the principal cause of oropharyngeal and tonsillar squamous cell cancer. Later in this chapter, we will discuss the oropharynx and tonsillar areas separately because there are some differences in therapeutic management.

An unfortunate number of patients come for care with advanced lesions. Tumors commonly reach sizes of 2 and 3 cm without symptoms. A dull ache or a mild sore throat is usually the initial symptom and may be present for several months. Referred otalgia to the ipsilateral ear occurs because sensory divisions of the glossopharyngeal nerve supply this area. The pain radiates directly to the ear, as it does following a tonsillectomy. The key to diagnosis is careful examination with adequate illumination, looking for any area of ulceration or asymmetry between the sides of the oropharynx. More so than in any other in the examination of the head and neck, palpation of the area with one's fingers is necessary. A better examination is obtained when a topical anesthetic agent such as 10% xylocaine or cetacaine is applied to an area which is markedly tender or ulcerated. Any lesion in a patient who is a tobacco user will require an immediate biopsy.

WHAT ARE THE AREAS OF THE OROPHARYNX, AND WHERE DO THE CANCERS OCCUR?

The oropharynx begins at the anterior tonsillar pillar of faucial arch. The retromolar trigone is a distinct area posterior to the molar tooth, overlying the alveolus of the mandible and the ascending ramus. With the mouth closed, a triangular region is formed. With the mouth open, this area spreads out and becomes a continuous region from the posterior aspect of the molar tooth up along the anterior or faucial arch. The arch then blends with the uvula. The tonsil fills the space between the anterior and posterior tonsillar pillars. It is peculiarly nonsensitive to pain from early malignancy, which perhaps explains why tumors in the tonsil can reach such a large size without symptoms. Figure 14–1 shows a large cancer.

The posterior tonsillar pillar or posterior arch is a less common site for the development of malignancy. The region behind the posterior tonsillar pillar blends with the posterior oropharyngeal wall. Tumors are less common in this region than in the tonsillar area or region of the anterior pillar. Because of their location, they can directly extend into the underlying cervical spine. These tumors are noted for their propensity to develop multiple ulcerations, with areas of normal-appearing mucosa between several distinct lesions. What actually occurs is submucosal extension between the tumorous sites. The entire area between two or three specific ulcerations must be assumed to contain cancer.

The superior boundary of the oropharyngeal area is the soft palate, and above this is the nasopharynx. The inferior boundary is the entrance to the hypopharynx, which begins at the glossopharyngeal fold, a fold of tissue extending from the attachment of the epiglottis to the lateral pharyngeal wall. The anterior limit is the posterior third, or base, of the tongue. This includes the region posterior to the circumvallate papillae that lies approximately at the level of the anterior tonsillar pillar and extends inferiorly to the region of the epiglottis. A band of tissue in the midline connects the midportion of the epiglottis with the base of the tongue and is known as the glossoepiglottic fold. Small depressions on each side of this band are known as valleculae.

It is in the region of the posterior or base of the tongue that palpation plays an essential role in early detection and diagnosis of malignancy. Any patient with otalgia and a normal-appearing tympanic membrane and a history suspicious for malignancy requires direct palpation of this region, no matter how uncomfortable it is for the patient. The multiple folds of tissue at the base of the tongue that make up the lingual tonsil fill this portion of the posterior tongue. The bulk and irregularity of normal and malignant tissues makes it difficult to detect an early malignancy by indirect mirror laryngoscopy.

WHERE DO THESE MALIGNANCIES SPREAD?

Tumors arising on the anterior tonsillar pillar or tonsil tend to invade inferiorly into the base of the tongue.

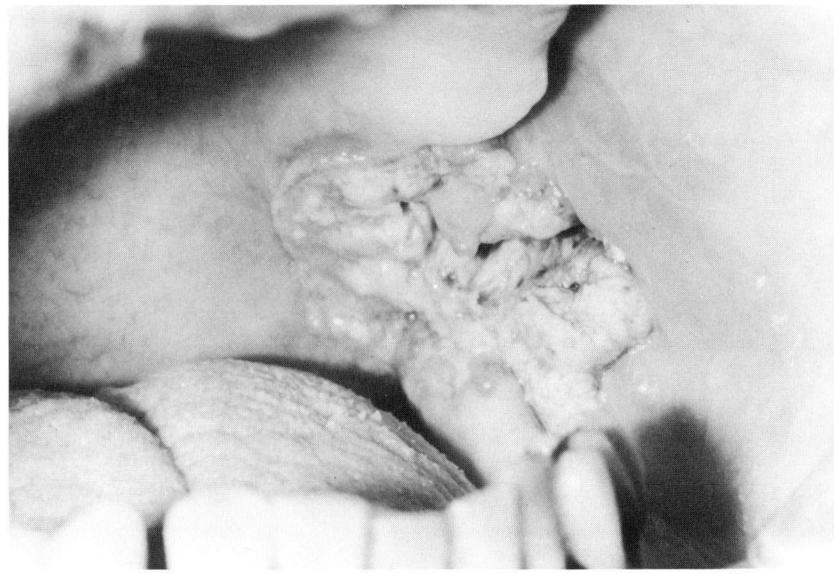

Fig 14–1.—An ulcerative squamous cell carcinoma fills the area of the retromolar triangle on the patient's left.

They fill the gutter space between the tongue and the tonsil. By using either two tongue blades or careful manual palpation, the examiner will find this depression to be filled by a tender or ulcerating lesion. Once the tumor has extended into the base of the tongue, it can grow rapidly toward the midline of the tongue or more deeply into the root of the tongue. At this point the patient exhibits the "hot potato" voice, and swallowing is disturbed or painful. Tumors can extend superiorly along the anterior tonsillar pillar toward the uvula. In advanced cases, the tumor actually extends across the midline to involve the opposite tonsillar pillar.

Malignant tumors arising in the base of the tongue tend to grow anteriorly throughout the tongue. The muscular tongue appears to have no boundary limiting the extension of tumor. Trapped anteriorly by the hyoid bone, the tongue then is pushed upward and outward. In such a situation, a laryngoscope introduced in an anesthetized patient cannot compress the tongue forward, making the larynx difficult to visualize. Bleeding can occur and an emergency tracheostomy becomes absolutely essential.

Tumors on the posterior pharyngeal wall tend to grow superiorly and inferiorly, the ulcerations skipping areas of normal mucosa. When they grow posteriorly, they develop fixation to the cervical spine. Clinical evaluation then requires not only delineating the extent of the disease, but determining the mobility of the tumor against the posterior spine.

WHAT CANCER TYPES INVOLVE THE OROPHARYNX?

More than 90% of malignant tumors in the oropharynx are squamous cell or epidermoid carcinoma. Tumors consisting of lymphocytic aggregates of tissue have been referred to as lymphoepitheliomas. In actuality they should be considered high-grade squamous cell carcinomas. Transitional cell carcinoma is another name given to squamous cell carcinoma which is similar to that seen in the bladder. It occurs in the nasopharynx and oropharyngeal region. For practical purposes it should be considered to be like other forms of squamous cell carcinoma. Adenocarcinoma occurs in the minor salivary glands but is rare in the oropharynx.

The greatest diagnostic confusion occurs with lymphoma, generally of the histiocytic form. The tonsil and base of the tongue can be a primary site of such malignancy, particularly in young individuals. A unilaterally enlarged tonsil in a young individual should be considered a malignancy until excisional biopsy in the form of a tonsillectomy is performed. A lymphoma can present as a large ulcerating tumor with cervical adenopathy, often with multiple lymph nodes. The treatment of lymphoma is so different from that of squamous cell carcinoma that it is essential that large, adequate biopsy specimens be obtained when lymphoma is a possibility. Lymphoma is generally seen in a patient of a younger age with no associated history of heavy drinking or smoking (Figs 14–2 and 14–3).

As in other areas, squamous cell malignancies in the region of the tonsil and base of the tongue have been divided into grades 1 through 4, with grade 4 being the least differentiated and grade 1 being the most differentiated. Clinically, the well-differentiated tumors are less likely to metastasize, but other factors such as the duration of the tumor and its stage also determine the likelihood of metastasis. In 80% of cases, the jugulodigastric or jugulocarotid lymph node is the involved node. The relationship of clinical to pathologic nodes in

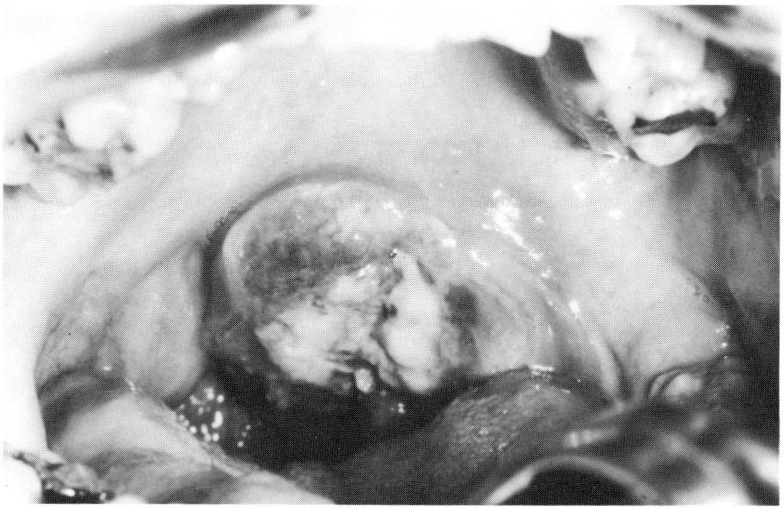

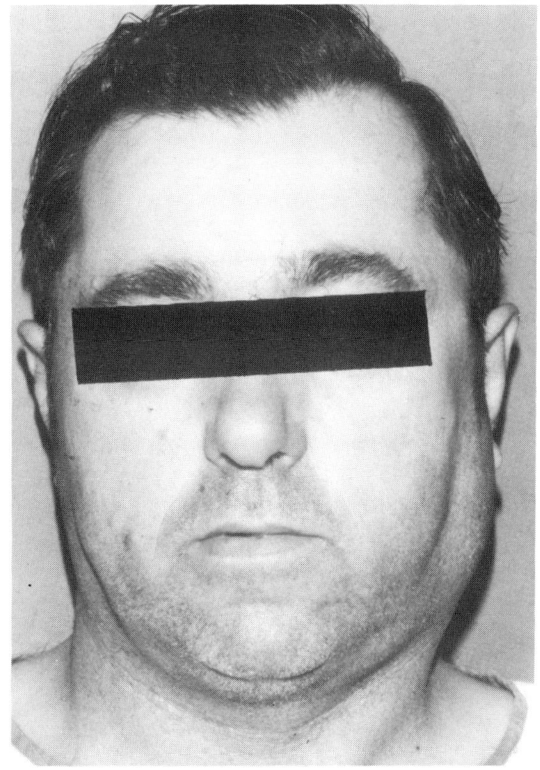

Fig 14–2.—The multiple cervicle lymph nodes in this younger patient suggested the possibility of a lymphoma.
Fig 14–3.—Same patient as in Figure 14–2. A generous biopsy showed an ulcerating lymphoma of the left tonsillar area.

709 cases of previously untreated carcinoma was studied by Cachene. He found that 20% of patients thought to have N_{1a} nodes had no metastases on pathologic examination (false positives). The study also demonstrated that 50%–60% of patients had capsular rupture of the cervical metastases, a factor considered by many to represent a poor prognosis.[1]

For each of these regions, the TNM system of classification of staging and of reporting of end results is presented in Table 14–1. Unfortunately, there is no factor in this system for deep infiltration. Thus, a thin T_3 lesion may have significant spread along the anterior tonsillar pillar toward the uvula and down toward the base of the tongue, yet clinically it appears that such a tumor will respond well to therapeutic irradiation. A smaller tumor deeply infiltrating into the base of the tongue may be staged as T_2 and survival will not be expected to be as good. An earlier system of classification divided the T system according to number of sites involved; thus, if the tongue and tonsil were involved, this would be a more advanced T stage. The American Joint Commission on Cancer currently prefers to use the size of the tumor for comparison of results.

What Unique Factors Affect Decision-Making in the Management of Oropharyngeal Cancer?

Malignancies of the oropharynx have the highest associated incidence of second primary malignancies. This incidence reaches as high as 37% in the series described by Jesse and Sugarbaker: 54 of 144 patients with carcinoma of the oropharynx.[2] In our own series, reported in 1971, the highest incidence of second primary malignancies was associated with carcinoma of the base of the tongue. There was an incidence of 20% (10/50) in patients who survived more than 2 years. The problem in collecting the data was the question of whether a second primary developed in the lung or whether it represented a pulmonary metastasis.

Other series have demonstrated that between 50% and 75% of second malignancies which do develop will develop in this same organ complex. Because of these statistics, it has become common practice to perform panendoscopy, or endoscopic evaluation of the entire

TABLE 14–1.—TNM STAGING FOR CARCINOMA OF THE OROPHARYNX AND BASE OF TONGUE

T_{IS}	Carcinoma in situ
T_1	Tumor 2 cm or less in greatest diameter
T_2	Tumor more than 2 cm but not more than 4 cm in greatest diameter
T_3	Tumor more than 4 cm in greatest diameter
T_4	Massive tumor more than 4 cm in diameter with invasion of bone, soft tissues of neck, or root (deep musculature) of neck, or root (deep musculature) of tongue

The development of trismus is suggestive of invasion of the pterygoid muscle and is considered T_4 in our series.

upper aerodigestive tract. Even if it is apparent that the tumor involves only the tonsillar region or base of tongue, direct laryngoscopy with evaluation of the larynx, hypopharynx, pharynx, esophagus, and nasopharynx is performed under general anesthesia. The physician is looking for a second primary malignancy. While synchronous tumors may occur in only 1%–3% of patients, they so drastically change the approach to the malignancy that it is considered worthwhile to search for them. In our experience, bronchoscopy for a second primary malignancy is not warranted if there are no symptoms and if a chest x-ray film is normal.

A second important factor contributing to decision-making in the management of oropharyngeal cancer is the poor general nutritional status of many of these patients. There is a high incidence of alcoholism, cirrhosis of the liver, esophagitis with varices, and generally poor nutritional status in patients with oropharyngeal carcinoma. Patients who continue to drink in spite of or during their treatment make their management excessively difficult.

A third factor is the high incidence of early and bilateral metastatic carcinoma. Carcinomas arising in the soft palate have a 15% incidence of bilateral metastasis. Tumors of the base of the tongue similarly have an early propensity to bilateral metastasis. Carcinoma of the base of the tongue, except for the earliest T_1 lesions, is assumed to have cervical metastases at the time of presentation. In most series, 80% of tumors of the base of the tongue have positive cervical metastases at the time of recognition. The incidence of contralateral metastasis is considered to be in the range of 15% (see discussion in Chap. 9).

A fourth factor is that surgical resections will interfere greatly with the patient's ability to swallow and to handle secretions. Consideration must be given to protecting the upper airway at the time of such resections. Prolonged use of a cuffed tracheotomy tube postsurgically will solve some of the lesser problems. When an extensive amount of tissue is resected, it is essential to bring in nonirradiated tissue in the form of a forehead flap or myocutaneous chest flap so as not to create a funnel that pours the oral secretions directly into the larynx.

For resections of the base of the tongue, total glossectomy/laryngectomy must be done in the majority of cases. Large tumors will involve the hypoglossal nerve or lingual artery. When both are removed in a total glossectomy and the flap is brought into position, there is no longer a base of the tongue with which to propel food away from the open larynx. Supraglottic laryngectomy leaves the upper airway even more vulnerable to chronic aspiration. In selected cases in which a small portion or a remnant of tongue base can be preserved and an adequate flap is available, it is possible to save the larynx. Preservation of the larynx can be considered only in a cooperative, nonalcoholic patient with good pulmonary function.

CARCINOMA OF THE TONSIL

What Malignant Tumors Involve the Tonsillar Area?

The tonsillar area is the most common site of oropharyngeal malignancies. Tumors of this region are grouped together, for in the case of advanced tumor, it is impossible to discern whether the tumor began in the faucial arch and extended into the tonsil, or vice versa. The enlarging tumor soon encroaches on the soft palate or crosses the lingual sulcus to invade the base of the tongue. Some physicians still insist on distinguishing the sites of origin of these tumors. They believe that tumors originating on the faucial arch are more likely to extend into the base of the tongue and are more aggressive. In large tumors, radiation therapists try to determine the exact site of origin by recording the region of tumor last to respond to the radiation. Several groups believe that tumors originating in true tonsillar tissue have a higher rate of response to therapeutic irradiation. Therefore, they treat such malignancies with therapeutic irradiation, reserving surgery for persistence.

Since the Tonsil is Composed of Functioning Lymphoid Tissue, Can There be Metastasis to the Tonsil?

The tonsil itself can also be the site of metastatic disease. Tumors that commonly metastasize to the tonsil include squamous cell carcinoma of the lung and carcinoma of the breast. Other tumors reported include seminoma, hypernephroma, and adenocarcinoma from the stomach or pancreas. Malignant melanoma has also been reported to metastasize to the tonsil. Bilateral metastatic disease has been seen with both malignant melanoma and breast carcinoma.

What is the Management of Carcinomas of the Tonsillar Area?

There are five approaches to the management of epidermoid carcinoma of the tonsillar area.[3–14] These include:

1. Primary therapeutic irradiation, including the site of the primary and the neck.
2. Surgery only: a composite resection which includes removal of the tonsillar region and a segment of the mandible, and in-continuity radical neck dissection.
3. A full course of therapeutic irradiation to the primary, with a moderate dose to the neck, followed by a radical neck dissection.
4. Either preoperative or postoperative therapeutic

irradiation, usually a dose of 4,000–5,000 rad. If radiation is given preoperatively, then there is a delay of 4–6 weeks before a composite resection is performed. The extent of the resection is determined before the effects of the therapeutic irradiation are seen and is not altered by the response to radiation.

5. An approach utilizing an investigational protocol in which a combination of radiation, surgery, and chemotherapeutic agents is employed. The agents most frequently selected in this situation include cisplatin, methotrexate, bleomycin, and 5-fluorouracil. The combination and sequence of the irradiation and chemotherapy in relation to the surgery depend on the specific investigational protocol.

APPROACH 1—THERAPEUTIC IRRADIATION ONLY

WHAT ARE THE REASONS FOR PRIMARY IRRADIATION? Arguments in favor of therapeutic irradiation include: (1) Cosmetic as well as functional preservation of the mechanism for swallowing. (2) Irradiation can be administered to the ipsilateral and contralateral aspects of the neck. Irradiation has been demonstrated to be effective in controlling disease in N_0 necks. (3) Failure to respond to therapeutic irradiation, or recurrence in the region, can be treated by surgical resection.

WHY NOT IRRADIATE ALL MALIGNANCIES OF THE TONSILLAR AREA? Early T_1 tonsillar carcinomas do respond well to irradiation, and most centers prefer this method. The exceptions would include (1) a patient in whom radiation is being reserved for the development of another primary in a patient with a demonstrated propensity for multiple malignancies, (2) an uncooperative alcoholic, and (3) an elderly patient who would not tolerate irradiation well.

Most tonsillar carcinomas are T_3 in size at the time of presentation. Cervical metastases are present in at least 50% of such patients. While irradiation might effectively control the primary site, it is less effective in controlling clinical cervical metastases. When an initial response to irradiation is followed by recurrence, the surgery required is attended by multiple complications. Dehiscence of the wound, oropharyngeal fistula, and carotid blowout are among the possible complications. In our study, the survival rate in patients with recurrent carcinoma treated in this manner was 20%. Even though a successful operative procedure could be performed, recurrence regionally or in a distant area was the rule.

APPROACH 2—SURGERY ONLY

The surgical cure rate for advanced carcinoma of the tonsillar area remains about 35%–50% in most studies. Surgery alone is utilized in patients who have already had therapeutic irradiation to the head and neck for another carcinoma. There are very few surgeons who advocate only surgery for advanced malignancies with clinical cervical metastases.

APPROACH 3—IRRADIATION TO PRIMARY, FOLLOWED BY RADICAL NECK DISSECTION

If the rate of cure were acceptably high, irradiation to the primary followed by a radical neck dissection for cervical metastases would represent a reasonable approach to the management of this cancer. Functional results would remain excellent, and morbidity is minimal for a neck dissection alone without entrance into the pharynx. This method is currently utilized by few centers because of the statistics on survival (poor). The main opportunity to use this approach is in patients with a small primary malignancy and a large N_2 cervical metastasis.

APPROACH 4—PREOPERATIVE OR POSTOPERATIVE IRRADIATION

There are strong proponents of preoperative therapeutic irradiation in the management of carcinoma of the tonsil. They believe that combining the two modalities should improve the overall statistics for survival. Indeed, for $T_3N_0N_1/N_2$ carcinomas, the series studied demonstrate approximately 70% 5-year survivals. Preoperative therapeutic irradiation requires tattooing of the extent of the initial lesion. Radiation of 4,000–5,000 rad, depending on the specific protocol, is administered to the tonsillar area and to the neck. A composite resection is performed in 4–6 weeks, after the mucositis has resolved and the patient's nutritional status has improved. Advocates of preoperative irradiation feel that the oxygenation and blood supply to the tumor prior to any surgery in the area permit a greater effect from the irradiation. Lymphatics are sealed to prevent distant spread, and the tumor mass itself is decreased in size prior to surgical manipulation.

Proponents of postoperative irradiation feel that the tumor mass can be better encompassed at surgery, as the margins will be more distinct. Operating in a nonirradiated field should be easier and the incidence of severe complications reduced. A larger dose of postoperative therapeutic irradiation can be administered, usually about 6,000 rad. Irradiation must, however, include the entire field of the neck dissection, including all margins of the resection in both the neck and the site of the primary.

Opponents of combined radiation and surgery point to the lack of controlled studies demonstrating that the combined modalities offer better survival than either modality alone. Prospective studies compare preoperative versus postoperative irradiation and generally show that the results are approximately the same. Claims of improved results with preoperative therapeutic irradiation and/or with protocols combining therapies almost always compare the results in patients so treated with the results in historical controls. The utilization of therapeutic irradiation preoperatively precludes its use later, should there be a second primary or a recurrence.

APPROACH 5—A COMBINATION OF CHEMOTHERAPY, RADIATION, AND SURGERY

There are currently several prospective trials combining one investigational use of chemotherapy with radiation or surgery, or both. The chemotherapeutic agents may be administered prior to surgery or as an adjuvant in the postoperative period. The initial rate of response to the preoperative chemotherapy has been excellent, in the range of 60%–70% partial response, with a few (10%–15%) complete remissions. However, the statistics for 5-year survival in this group of patients have not shown significant improvement. Such prospective randomized trials still play an important role in future investigational areas, trying to improve these statistics for survival.

Extremely large carcinomas of the tonsil are treated in all medical centers by a full course of therapeutic irradiation. Recently, combinations of chemotherapy during, before, or after therapeutic radiation have also been utilized. For a period of 2–6 months a patient has decreased pain, decreased mass in the pharynx, and improved swallowing. Survival from inoperable carcinoma of the tonsil treated by therapeutic irradiation remains less than 10%.

With This Variety of Treatment Modalities, Which Is the Best Treatment for a Given Patient?

If one excludes investigational protocols, the literature suggests that there are currently two primary means of treating carcinoma of the tonsillar area. These are a full course of therapeutic irradiation, with surgery reserved for persistent disease or recurrence, known as surgical salvage; and combined preoperative or postoperative therapeutic irradiation with a composite resection. The reasons for preoperative or postoperative therapeutic irradiation have previously been mentioned. The decision as to which method to use remains unresolved because of a lack of prospective, randomized studies. Virtually all studies to answer this question are retrospective.

The tumor that gives rise to the most discussion is the T_3, a relatively large tumor that is still amenable to surgical resection. Most T_4 tumors are associated with trismus or other features that make them inoperable, and they therefore fall into the category for therapeutic irradiation only. Early T_1 and T_2 tumors have a satisfactory cure rate with irradiation alone. The only argument that can be used to avoid irradiation in such cases is the possibility, based on the patient's history and habits, that he or she is likely to develop a second primary for which irradiation might be the preferred treatment.

WHAT ARE THE ARGUMENTS FOR AND AGAINST PREOPERATIVE RADIATION?

Using irradiation with surgical salvage, Horwitz and Boles[13] had an overall survival rate of 46%. Irradiation alone, studied by Fayos and Lampe, gave an overall cure rate of 39.8%.[14] When looking at all such studies, it is important to determine the initial staging of the majority of the tumors. Rabuzzi et al., reporting statistics from New York, revealed a 66% overall 5-year survival for patients with T_3 carcinoma of the tonsillar area treated by combined preoperative irradiation and therapy.[11] Again, this was a nonrandomized study. Schumrick and Quenelle in 1976 presented similar results: an overall survival rate of approximately 65% in patients treated with preoperative radiation.[12]

A Minnesota study reported a 75% 2-year survival in patients with T_3 carcinomas treated by combined therapy.[15] Of those patients who received radiation only, 22% later developed distant metastases precluding any surgical resection. The 2-year survival from T_3 cancers treated by therapeutic irradiation alone was 27%, compared with a 75% 2-year survival with combined therapy. The absolute survival rate with preoperative irradiation in Maltz's study was 56% overall, with an 80% 5-year survival following preoperative irradiation for T_1 lesions and only a 33% 5-year-survival in patients with a T_3 lesion.[15a]

A nonrandomized study reported by Perez et al. in 1976 revealed that preoperative irradiation provided no better survival than irradiation with surgical salvage.[10] Pathologic examination of the specimens in that study revealed that the 3-year cure was 90% if there was no tumor in the pathologic specimen. If there were two to three positive nodes after preoperative irradiation, the survival rate fell to 25%. Perez et al. utilized only 2,000–3,000 rad preoperatively in this study. The overall survival rate for patients with T_3N_0 lesions given combined therapy was 42.8%, and with radiation alone, 45.4%.[10] Fleming's study in 1976 yielded two interesting findings: patients with poorly differentiated or undifferentiated carcinoma of the tonsil, regardless of treatment, had a 20% 5-year survival, and 21.5% of the patients developed a second primary malignancy in the period of study.[15b]

In studies comparing preoperative and postoperative

therapeutic irradiation, no statistical difference has been noted for carcinoma of the tonsillar area. This is not true for carcinoma of the supraglottic or piriform sinus area, where postoperative therapeutic irradiation appears to be more effective than preoperative irradiation. Thus, there is currently a greater tendency to give radiation postoperatively. This permits the surgeon to have a better evaluation of the extent of disease at the time of surgery, thus reducing the surgically positive margins. The marked effectiveness of preoperative irradiation, particularly at the site of the primary lesion, may tempt the surgeon to excise less tissue than would have been excised initially without the preoperative irradiation. It is essential that all tumors in the tonsillar region treated with preoperative irradiation be adequately tatooed, and that margins of tissue for pathologic evaluation be taken from the patient, rather than from the specimen.

In summary, therapeutic irradiation alone is utilized for smaller carcinomas of the tonsillar area or for larger tumors that spread superficially but do not appear to be deeply invasive, and when no nodes in the neck are palpated clinically. Combined therapy, either with preoperative or postoperative therapeutic irradiation, is used primarily for T_3 tumors. It is also used for T_4 tumors when they remain operable. Combined therapy is recommended when there are palpable, clinically positive nodes. It is used for larger and more invasive tumors or when there is evidence of tumor extending into the mandible. In a true composite resection, a segment of the mandible is removed and generally not reconstructed at the time of surgery. There are no statistics to establish whether preoperative or postoperative irradiation is more effective. Selected data from several key studies are summarized in Table 14–2 with 2-, 3-, and 5-year survival statistics.

COMPOSITE RESECTION

The standard surgical approach for malignant tumors of the tonsillar area involves a composite resection. This includes a standard radical neck dissection, resection of a segment of mandible, generally from the midbody to high on the mandibular ramus, in continuity with wide resection of the tumor from the area of the soft palate to the base of the tongue, including the anterior and posterior tonsillar pillars.

PART 1: PREPARATION.—The first phase of the operative procedure includes preparation for general anesthesia. Orotracheal intubation is utilized and a Foley catheter is inserted. Sufficiently large intravenous lines are established as well as a central line in a debilitated patient. The entire neck, including across to the opposite side as well as the face, is prepared. Depending on the specific case and the desires of the surgeon, a tracheostomy can be performed now or at the end of the operative procedure. A personal preference is to perform the tracheostomy at the start, to exclude endotracheal tubes from the operative field. A spiral wound tube is utilized and sutured in position so that it cannot slip into the right mainstem bronchus.

PART 2: NECK DISSECTION.—A standard neck dissection on the ipsilateral side is performed (Fig 14–4). In almost all cases of carcinoma of the tonsil in which surgery is required, a neck dissection is a standard part of the procedure, even when no clinically palpable nodes are present. This is based on the high incidence of histologically proved pathologic lymph nodes even in clinically negative necks. The incision utilized is shown in Figure 14–4. Variations in this incision include an extension to the opposite submandibular region or elevation so that the lip need not be split. In a debilitated patient, it is preferable not to swing the incision around the chin but to split the chin immediately down the midline. This should be done especially if the mandible will be taken more anteriorly than the submental foramen. Now the standard neck dissection is performed, including resection of the submandibular triangle and its contents, with the pedicle of the specimen attached to the region of the angle of the mandible. The jugular vein is ligated as high as is feasible and the tail of the parotid gland is included in the resection. Our preference is to remove the digastric muscle as well, as this allows an even further resection of this triangle, which is the site of the earliest and most frequent nodal disease.

PART 3: RESECTION OF THE MANDIBLE.—If a lip-splitting incision is utilized, the intraoral portion of the incision is extended posteriorly, leaving at least 2 cm of healthy normal mucosa attached to the buccal alveolar surface. This will permit closure later. With this wide exposure, it is possible to determine the site at which the mandible will be resected. Periosteum is elevated from this area, and utilizing either a Gigli saw or an oscillating right-angled drill, the operator resects the mandible anteriorly. Determination of the posterior mandibular cut on the ramus is dependent on the extent of the tumor (Fig 14–5). In large tumors with bony invasion we disarticulate the mandible from the condylar fossa. The condyle is removed by remaining in the subperiosteal plane to avoid extensive hemorrhage from the pterygoid veins. This posterior cut is more easily made with a Gigli saw.

PART 4: RESECTION OF THE PRIMARY.—The surgeon now has maximal exposure of the primary malignancy (Fig 14–6). A previously tattooed lesion can be resected

TABLE 14–2.—RESULTS OF TREATMENT OF CARCINOMA OF THE TONSIL

STUDY, YEAR, INSTITUTION	NO. OF PTS.	LENGTH OF FOLLOW-UP*	RESULTS	
Givens et al.,[16] 1981 (Univ. of Virginia)	104	. . .	*Overall 5-year survival:*	38%
			Stage I	93%
			Stage II	57%
			Stage III	27%
			Stage IV	17%
			By nodal disease:	
			N_0	70%
			N_1	27%
			N_2	23%
			N_3	0%
			Surgery	87%
			Radiation	27%
			Combined	32%
Shrewsbury et al.,[15] 1981 (Univ. of Minn.)	96	2 yr	*Overall 2-year survival:*	48%
			Radiation:	
			T_1	7/9
			T_2	5/10
			T_3	4/27
			T_4	0/10
			Combined:	
			T_1	5/5
			T_2	9/11
			T_3	16/21
			T_4	1/3
			By Nodal Disease:	
			N_0	63%
			N_1	49%
			N_2	33%
			N_3	17%
Perez et al.,[10] 1976 (Washington Univ., St. Louis)	98	3 yr	Radiation:	
			$T_{1,2}N_0$	16/21
			$T_{1,2}N_{1,2}$	4/9
			$T_3N_{0,1,2}$	10/22
			$T_{1,2,3}N_3$	4/16
			Combined:	11/17
			$T_{1,2}N_0$	11/22
			$T_{1,2}N_{1,2}$	18/42
			$T_3N_{0,1,2}$	3/9
			$T_{1,2,3}N_3$	
			Surgical salvage of irradiation failures:	3/10
Rebuzzi et al.,[11] 1982 (Upstate Medical Center, Syracruse, NY)	58	. . .	All treated with combined therapy;	62%
			overall survival:	68%
			$T_{1,2}$	64%
			$T_{3,4}$	67%
			Stage II	82%
			Stage III	55%
			Stage IV	
Shumrick and Quenell,[12] 1979 (Univ. of Cincinnati)	80	2 yr	All treated with combined therapy; *overall survival:*	58%
			T_1	5/5
			T_2N_0	4/10
			T_2N_1	3/6
			T_3N_0	10/12
			T_3N_1	11/21
			T_3N_2	1/4

*For purposes of determining survival statistics.

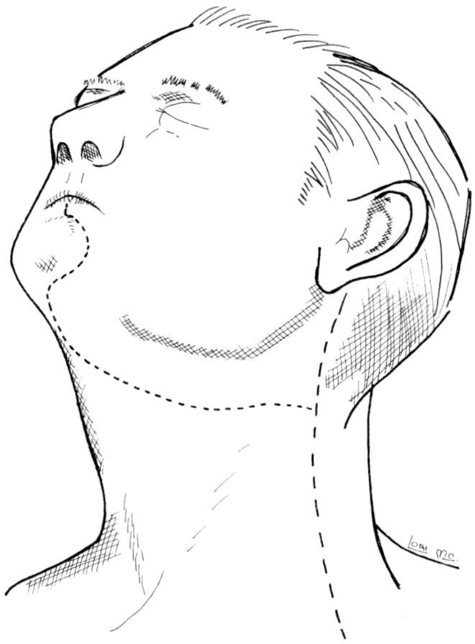

Fig 14–4.—Preferred incision for a composite resection. Note the following aspects: there is gentle curvature around chin; the incision is made two to three fingerbreadths below the mandible; the transverse incision meets the posterior incision at a right angle; the incision crosses the carotid artery at only one point.

just outside the area of the tattooing (Fig 14–7). Resection can be performed with a cutting cautery or scissors. One hand is held on the specimen to help in establishing its depth. This is particularly essential if there is evidence of extension into the lingual area.

Part V: Closure.—When a segment of mandible has been resected and not primarily reconstructed, in most cases it is now possible to perform primary closure at the site of the tonsillar resection. In larger tumors this will not be possible without severely compromising the patient's later ability to swallow. Even though a closure can be performed, the patient is left not only with poor speech but also with either a very limited oral opening or a configuration that causes regurgitation into the nose and nasopharynx. To prevent this problem, there are a number of methods to close the defect.

These techniques include the follwing:

1. A myocutaneous flap can be made from the pectoralis major, with skin from the chest wall brought into the defect. This technique has the advantage of simultaneously providing coverage of the carotid artery with the muscle pedicle sutured to protect the carotid artery (Figs 14–8 through 14–10). It is probably the most popular and most effective way to close a large defect.

2. A forehead flap, while easier to construct, has the drawback of requiring a second operation in 5–6 weeks to replace the nonused flap and skin graft the forehead. It creates a definite cosmetic deformity to the frontal area. When a forehead flap is selected, either the zy-

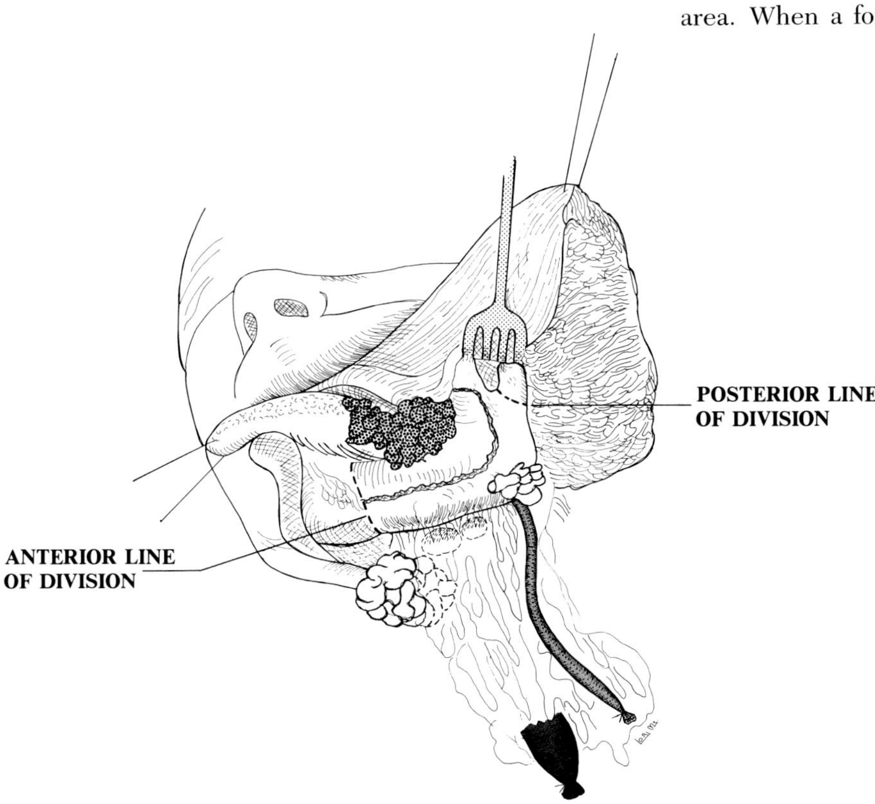

Fig 14–5.—Composite resection. A neck dissection has been completed. The contents of the neck are pedicled along the mandibular body and angle. The cheek flap is elevated posteriorly. The Gigli saw or an air-driven oscillating saw are used to divide the mandible. Anterior and posterior divisions vary on the site of the primary, but are usually in the midbody and ascending ramus.

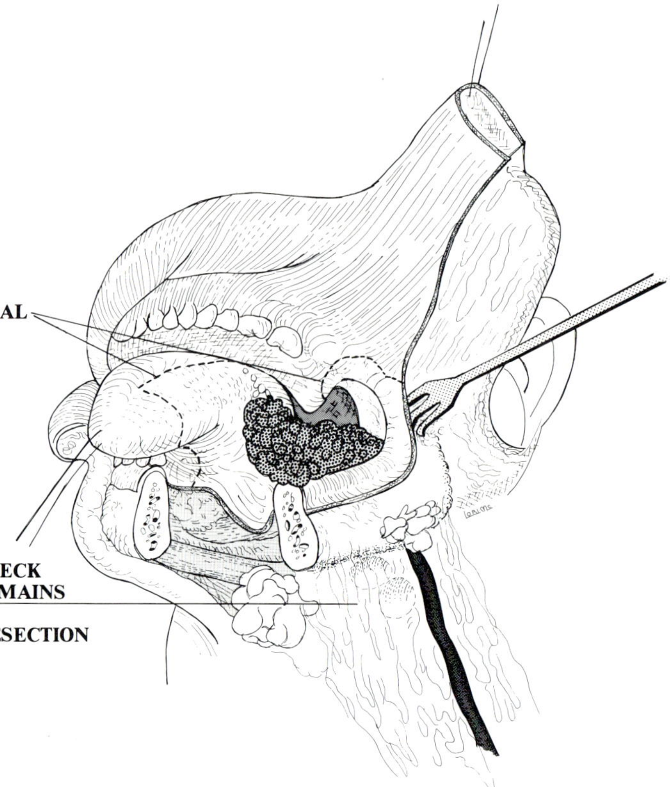

Fig 14–6.—Composite resection. Adequate exposure permits resection of the primary. A minimum of 2 cm of surrounding normal tissue is mandatory. Cutting electrocautery reduces the bleeding.

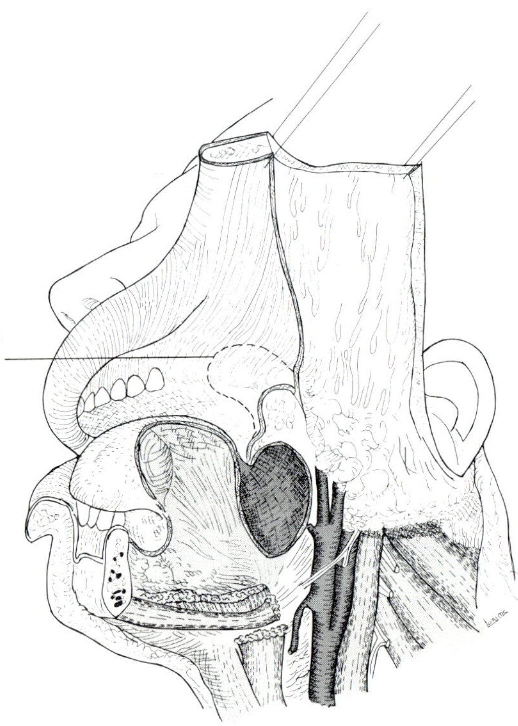

Fig 14–7.—Composite resection: Completion of resection. Specimen includes the tonsillar area, portion of base of the tongue, the posterior belly of the digastric muscle, the mandibular segment with the attached portion of masseter muscle, and contents of submandibular triangle. The exposed carotid artery is protected with a muscle flap or dermal graft.

gomatic arch is removed or the flap is placed lateral to the zygoma. In this situation there is also a possibility of injury to the buccal division of the facial nerve (see Chap. 6).

The advantage of the forehead flap is its excellent blood supply, the ease of operative procedure, and the fact that the flap is very effective in replacing tissue loss when the resection has been large or particularly high, including a large area of the soft palate or posterior lateral pharynx. It is also considerably thinner than the myocutaneous flap, which brings a large amount of bulk into the region. The forehead flap is used by us at this time only in more debilitated patients or those with significant vascular disease, in whom it is thought that a pectoralis major flap may not be effective. When the flap is used, the forehead is dressed with bacitracin ointment smeared on Telfa and is allowed to granulate. When the forehead flap is taken down, in 5–6 weeks, significant granulation tissue should have filled in the defect. It is leveled to the edges of the skin and a split-thickness skin graft is applied. The defect in the cheek is closed after removing the flap by closing the deep layers with chromic suture and the skin with a 5–0 nylon. The procedure is generally done 5 weeks after the original operation. The tracheotomy tube is left in place for this additional anesthetic procedure.

3. Split-thickness skin graft of the oropharynx. This technique utilizes a large split-thickness skin graft sutured to the margins of the defect. An antibiotic oint-

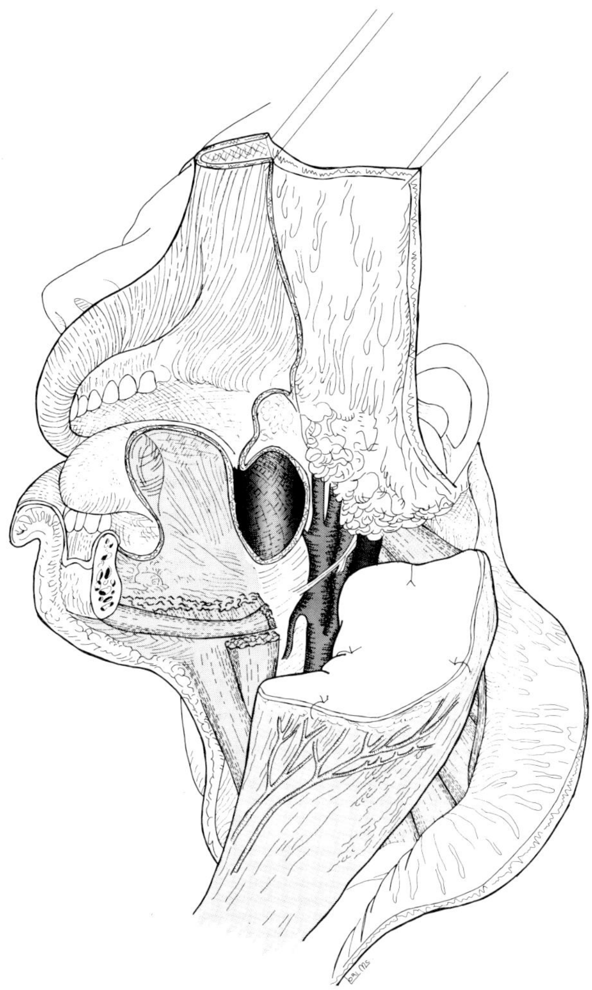

Fig 14–8.—Composite resection. A pectoralis major myocutaneous flap is developed and tunneled into position. The skin paddle ranges from 2 × 4 to 3 × 5 inches. Closure of the defect and carotid artery protection are provided by the flap.

ment–impregnated gauze is used to create a large bolus stent, which is then sutured into position. A watertight closure with suture is essential to prevent leakage. This technique is used in patients with teeth, who can then be maintained in interdental fixation for a period of 3 weeks before the gauze bolus is removed. This creates the least cosmetic deformity and has been used without drawback even in patients who have received preoperative irradiation.

4. The Bakamjian flap technique, illustrated in chapter 13.

When reconstruction of the tonsillar area is completed, the wound is closed in at least three layers, the deep layers and muscle and mucosa closed first and the vermilion border appropriately realigned. Two large Hemovac or other similar drains are inserted into the neck and brought out posteriorly. No external dressing is applied. The skin is closed with chromic suture in a subcutaneous area and a 4–0 nylon skin suture. Recently, a stapler has been used to close the skin in nonirradiated patients.

The spiral wound tracheostomy tube is replaced with a No. 6 or 8 cuffed tracheotomy tube which is sutured in place. This avoids accidental decannulation in the first 24 hours and prevents flap ischemia from compression by the tracheotomy tie across the skin wound. A nasogastric tube is placed for suction the first 24 hours, and then left in place as a feeding tube. Postoperative feedings through the nasogastric tube begin on the second postoperative day. The Hemovac drains are removed when the drainage is less than 50 cc, or in 3–4 days. The prophylactic antibiotics are maintained until 24 hours after the Hemovac drains are removed. Depending on the extent of the operative procedure, the patient is allowed to take oral fluids or a semisoft diet on the tenth postoperative day. In patients with teeth it is important to initiate good oral hygiene as early as the third postoperative day. This includes brushing the teeth as well as use of a saline or peroxide mouth rinse.

CARCINOMA OF THE BASE OF THE TONGUE

The base of the tongue has arbitrarily been defined as that region of the tongue posterior to the circumvallate papillae. It extends from the region of the anterior tonsillar pillar posteriorly to the vallecula, a small bilateral symmetric valley-like area associated with the base of the epiglottis. The base-of-tongue surface includes the lingual tonsil. While the median raphe of the tongue divides the entire tongue into two sides, it does not serve as a barrier for tumors developing in the posterior tongue. Thus, tumors originating on one side may rapidly extend to the other, posteriorly toward the epiglottis, or deeply toward the root of the tongue.

In most series, cancer of the base of the tongue accounts for approximately 30% of all carcinomas of the tongue. It is more common in men, with a male-female ratio of 3:1, but more recent studies show an increasing incidence in women. In studies of patients under the age of 30, cancer of the anterior two thirds of the tongue outnumbers cancer of the posterior tongue by 9:1.[16a]

What Are the Signs and Symptoms of Cancer of the Base of the Tongue?

The most common presenting symptom is a chronic sore throat. The patient usually has a history of tobacco and alcohol use. Also, he or she may exhibit poor oral hygiene with a "black hairy" tongue. Larger tumors cause fixation of the base of the tongue, creating the "hot potato" voice. This voice quality results from pooling of saliva in the area and the patient's efforts to swallow the saliva rapidly before talking so that he does not

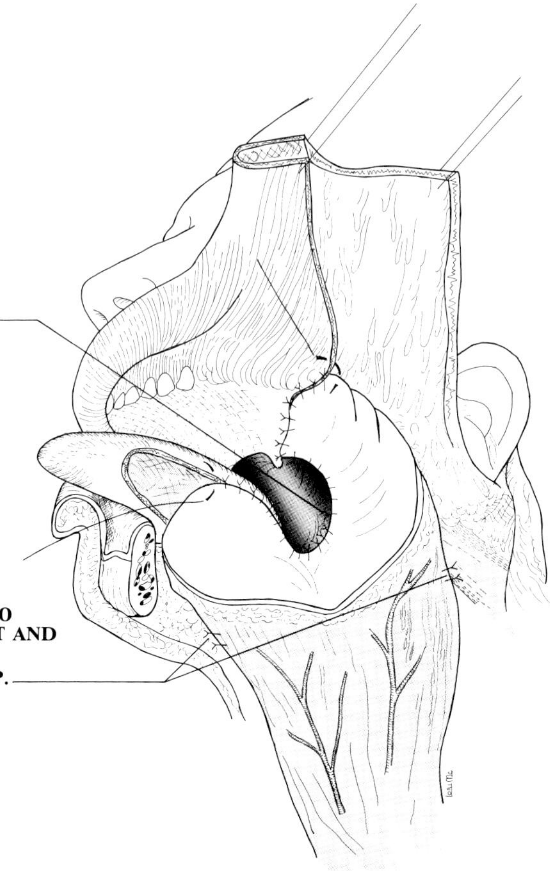

Fig 14–9.—Composite resection. The composite flap is sutured into position and support is provided to prevent the skin being separated by the downward pull of the muscle.

aspirate it. A mass in the neck, usually an enlarged jugulodigastric node, is often the presenting complaint. There can be referred otalgia to the ipsilateral ear and yet no tumor may be apparent on initial examination. In such situations, careful mirror examination of the tongue must be followed by careful palpation of the base of the tongue. Any area of ulceration or area of explicit tenderness requires direct laryngoscopy with biopsy. In fact, a mass in the neck without an apparent primary source is suspicious of carcinoma of the base of the tongue, and biopsies of this region should be performed in all cases of "unknown" primary tumors.

There are eight major points to consider in the management of carcinoma of the base of the tongue:

1. It is difficult to diagnose clinically, which often results in a delay in proper diagnosis.
2. There is a high incidence of early metastatic disease.
3. There is a high incidence of bilateral cervical metastases.
4. There is a high incidence of poorly differentiated tumors.
5. There is a high incidence of second primary malignancies developing in these patients, and a higher incidence of synchronous primaries.

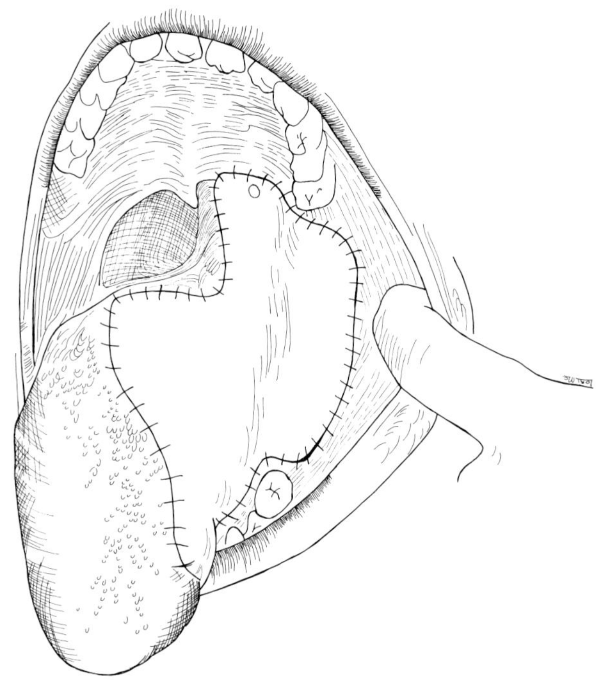

Fig 14–10.—Composite resection. After the flap is sutured into position, the cheek flap is replaced. Two large Hemovac drains are placed in the neck on each side of the muscle flap, and two separate drains are placed in the chest wall.

6. Surgical resection creates greater disability than does surgery for lesions in the anterior tongue, with marked effects on swallowing and speaking and interference with laryngeal function.

7. Total glossectomy with total laryngectomy may be required, even when the larynx is free of evidence of carcinoma.

8. Primary closure and preservation of the larynx frequently are not possible, necessitating use of regional and local flaps.

Each of these major points will be discussed.

DELAY IN DIAGNOSIS

Large series report an average delay of 4½–6 months from the time the patient complains of a constant sore throat until the diagnosis is made. The referred otalgia may mislead the physician and divert attention to neuralgia and ear disease. Tumors developing deep within the crypts of the tongue can be difficult to see on mirror examination and impossible to see on tongue blade examination. Careful palpation remains the key. The tongue may have to be topically anesthesized to permit such an examination. A carcinoma of the anterior tongue is recognized far sooner by both the patient and the physician because of its pain and ulcerating appearance. The diagnosis is even more difficult when the tumor develops beneath intact mucosa.

HIGH INCIDENCE OF EARLY METASTASIS

Carcinoma of all regions of the tongue has a very high incidence of early metastasis.[17] Patients in many series with T_2 and T_3 tumors of the posterior third of the tongue have a 50%–80% incidence of metastatic disease detectable on palpation on initial examination. Patients with no palpable cervical disease have a 30%–34% incidence of positive pathologically proved cervical metastases at the time of neck dissection.

HIGH INCIDENCE OF BILATERAL CERVICAL METASTASIS

The incidence is so high that specific management is directed to the opposite side of the neck as well. This requires treatment by either surgery or radiation therapy, depending on the protocol of the institution. Another exception to the rule regarding most carcinomas of the head and neck is the appearance of a contralateral node with no apparent ipsilateral cervical metastasis. However, pathologic examination of the specimen from the neck will reveal the presence of ipsilateral nodes.

HIGHER INCIDENCE OF POORLY DIFFERENTIATED TUMORS

Whether there is a higher incidence of poorly differentiated tumors depends on the studies. Studies at the Mayo Clinic[18] and at New York Memorial Hospital[19] found that the incidence of poorly differentiated tumors in the base of the tongue was no significantly higher when compared to the cancers of the anterior two thirds. On the other hand, the Stanford group found that approximately 70% of their patients had moderately or poorly differentiated tumors of the base of the tongue. The Stanford group also reported a better survival rate in patients with well-differentiated tumors.

HIGH INCIDENCE OF SECOND PRIMARIES

Perhaps more so than any other primary site of malignancy, cancer of the base of the tongue has the highest incidence of second primary malignancies.[20] These occur either within the 5-year follow-up since the time of diagnosis and treatment or as a synchronous primary. Therefore panendoscopic evaluation of all patients with cancer of the base of the tongue is encouraged before a treatment plan is determined. Also, when considering the use of radiation therapy, one must recognize that these patients may develop a second primary malignancy that may require irradiation.

GREATER DISABILITY FOLLOWING SURGERY FOR CANCER OF THE BASE OF THE TONGUE

Any glossectomy of the anterior two thirds of the tongue results in some change in voice, but generally no significant disability in the mechanism for swallowing. It is the base of the tongue that propels food past the larynx and prevents aspiration. Resection of the hypoglossal nerve or base of the tongue greatly diminishes this capacity. It also greatly affects speaking if the hypoglossal nerve and a portion of the base of the tongue are resected. However, the greatest problem with aspiration results when efforts are made to preserve the larynx. Resection of the supraglottic larynx, because of a concern for infiltration into the epiglottis and preepiglottic space, often results in a larynx unable to protect the airway. The larynx becomes incompetent if the superior laryngeal nerve on either or both sides is removed with the resection. The patient cannot withstand the resulting aspiration pneumonia.[21]

OPERATIVE PROCEDURE FOR CARCINOMA OF THE BASE OF THE TONGUE

In many ways, resection of cancer of the base of the tongue is similar to the composite resection described earlier in this chapter for carcinoma of the tonsillar area. The following discussion points out the special considerations in resecting a cancer at the base of the tongue.

NECK DISSECTION.—Because of the high incidence of metastatic tumor, virtually all patients with carcinoma of the base of the tongue undergo either a therapeutic or a prophylactic neck dissection. Not only is this helpful for removing the cervical metastatic disease, but it provides improved access to the area. Because of the high incidence of high jugulodigastric positive nodes, we do not make an effort to preserve the accessory nerve in this dissection, nor is the neck dissection modified on the ipsilateral side. When simultaneous neck dissections or a delayed second-stage neck dissection is performed on the contralateral side, this dissection is modified to preserve the jugular vein and accessory nerve if there were no clinically palpable nodes and if radiation therapy will be utilized postoperatively.

MANDIBULECTOMY OR MANDIBULOTOMY.—Access to the area is improved by splitting the mandible just anterior to the angle. When this is done and the mandible is preserved, it is referred to as a mandibular osteotomy. It provides excellent access to the base of the tongue for limited tumors, those 2–4 cm in size. It also facilitates closure, which will be described later. However, if a tumor extends toward the mandible or toward the tonsillar fossa, this segment of mandible must be removed in the form of a partial mandibulectomy. A mandibulotomy is performed by making a stepwise incision to allow rewiring of the mandible, similar to that performed for mandibular fracture through this area. We have experienced an increased incidence of osteoradionecrosis in patients who have had this procedure followed by irradiation. Thus, we recommend that a period of at least 6 weeks elapse before the planned postoperative radiation therapy is begun. We do not perform an osteotomy in patients who have had prior high-dose therapeutic irradiation.

WHY ISN'T PRIMARY CLOSURE POSSIBLE? Primary closure in tonsillar and anterior lesions of the tongue is facilitated by resection of a portion of the mandible, if that segment is not reconstructed. In tumors of the base of the tongue, resection of the portion of the mandible does not permit an easier closure. In such situations, the larynx is pulled upward and the remaining tongue pulled posteriorly. This further distorts the passage for swallowing and leads to increased aspiration. Thus, with any sizable primary malignancy in this area, either a setback type of procedure, myocutaneous flap, or forehead flap reconstruction is required. The pectoralis major myocutaneous flap has become the workhorse for reconstruction of the tongue. This is one of the most useful flaps to fill in the defect created when a large segment of tongue is removed. Conley has even proposed innervating the myocutaneous flap with the hypoglossal nerve to obtain some function in the tongue. This, of course, is in the presence of a total glossectomy.

RESECTION OF THE PRIMARY.—Tumors limited to the posterior one third of the tongue and not extending past the circumvallate papillae can be approached in several ways. If a tongue flap reconstruction is planned, efforts are made to preserve both the hypoglossal nerve and the lingual artery. Preoperative evaluation should have established whether the supraglottic larynx must be resected at the same time, for this definitely modifies the approach. In such cases, the incisions used are similar to those utilized in supraglottic laryngectomy with resection of the superiormost portion of the thyroid cartilage and epiglottis to permit removal of the pre-epiglottic space.

This approach applies to tumors which arise in the vallecula. Tumors not extending into the vallecula but arising more anteriorly, yet still posterior to the circumvallate papillae, can be approached by the osteotomy method. After resection, a lingual flap is used to repair the defect, with preservation of the epiglottis and pre-epiglottic space. Larger tumors extending across the midline or those where the vascular pedicle and hypoglossal nerve must be sacrificed will require use of a pectoralis major flap in reconstruction. Tumors extending into the area of the circumvallate papillae cannot be repaired by the lingual setback or regional lingual flaps, and require a pectoralis major flap or forehead flap for reconstruction.

Currently the pectoralis major myocutaneous flap is the preferred method. This is required because there is not sufficient anterior tongue remaining to allow an adequate margin of resection and reconstruction. Closure is performed so as not to distort the larynx and create a chute that would allow food to pass directly into the upper airway. Every effort is made to preserve superior laryngeal nerves. Postoperative care and management are similar to that for oropharyngeal carcinomas, and feeding is usually initiated on the 14th postoperative day.

What Tongue Flap Procedures Are Used for Local Reconstruction?

The lingual setback tongue flap for carcinoma of the base of the tongue as described by Schechter et al. is the preferred reconstructive method when posssible.[22] Unfortunately, some tumors are so large that this setback procedure cannot be safely used without compromising the margins of resection. However, Schechter et al. have used it for tumors involving up to 90% of the base of the tongue. More generally, it is used for tumors 2–4 cm in size and those not extending across the midline. It has three advantages: (1) it provides the best functional reconstruction, (2) it requires less operative time, and (3) it maintains bulk, as the innervated flap does not atrophy.

The procedure requires preservation of the hypoglossal nerve and lingual artery. The lateral pharyngotomy and mandibulotomy approach is utilized. After resection of the specimen, the anterior two thirds of the tongue is split down the midline to the hyoid bone. The anterior ipsilateral two thirds is then pulled posteriorly and sutured in place to perform the reconstruction. This reconstruction cannot be used when tumor extends into the area of the circumvallate papillae. It is preferable to use this when the hypoglossal nerve can be preserved, but if that is not possible, the flap can still be used. The vascular pedicle or lingual artery, however, must be preserved.

When Is a Laryngectomy Necessary?

There are two reasons for removing the larynx: (1) direct invasion by tumor, and (2) prevention of chronic, permanent aspiration. In large series, approximately 40% of patients with cancer of the base of the tongue require a simultaneous laryngectomy. In the series from New York Memorial Hospital, 42% of 204 patients treated surgically required laryngectomy. Seventy percent of these had direct invasion of the larynx. This implies that 30% (25) of the larynges were removed for large cancers (greater than half of the base of the tongue), where preservation would have left a larynx that could not prevent aspiration. Even though the larynx can be preserved for speaking, it can not effectively prevent the pouring of saliva directly into the trachea.

Specific indications for removal of the larynx for a cancer of the base of tongue when it is clinically not involved by cancer include: (1) when it is not feasible to perform an extended supraglottic laryngectomy so as to remove the pre-epiglottic space, and (2) there is extensive cancer involving more than 75% of the base of the tongue and the hypoglossal and superior laryngeal nerves cannot be preserved.

Ogura and Biller have described the basis for extending a supraglottic laryngectomy for resecting carcinoma of the vallecular area.[23] The tumor cannot extend to the circumvallate papillae or onto the lateral pharyngeal wall. The pre-epiglottic space must be resected en bloc and an ipsilateral radical neck dissection performed. For limited and especially vallecular tumors, this may be an effective method, especially for unilateral tumors or when at least one superior laryngeal nerve can be preserved.

More bulky tumors are best approached through a lateral mandibulotomy and require resection of 75%–90% of the base of the tongue with an in-continuity neck dissection. If the superior laryngeal nerve and at least one hypoglossal nerve can be preserved, the larynx can be saved.

Laryngectomy as part of the initial procedure should be considered when any one of the following conditions obtains: (1) both superior laryngeal nerves are resected, (2) both hypoglossal nerves are resected, (3) more than 90% of the base of the tongue is resected and mandibulectomy and radical neck dissection are also carried out, (4) there is direct extension into the pre-epiglottic space (base of the tongue will be fixed and hyoid bone forward), (5) an elderly person undergoes this extensive procedure who will not tolerate any degree of aspiration, or (6) a large tumor extends significantly onto the lateral pharyngeal wall. Total glossectomy becomes necessary when there is insufficient functional tongue left to obtain a 2-cm margin surrounding the tumor.[24, 25] This includes tumors extending to over 90% of the base of the tongue or well anterior to the circumvallate papillae into the middle third of the tongue. This anterior extension of tumor necessitates resection of the hypoglossal and lingual nerves.

Preservation of the mandible by mandibulotomy and flap reconstruction preserves the larynx and maintains a greater degree of function than did older techniques. However, specific limitations have been established as to when this technique can be safely applied.

What Is the Preferred Treatment for Cancer of the Base of the Tongue?

In few areas of surgery for cancer of the head and neck is there such a diversification of methods and opinions. Management of all aspects of cancers of the base of the tongue is controversial, with strong advocates for primary irradiation with surgical salvage[26] and for surgical resection combined with irradiation.[27] Overall statistics on survival from large series vary from 10% to 55%. Results in a selected group of larger studies are shown in Table 14–3. Of utmost importance to survival statistics are the stage of the primary and the presence of cervical metastases at presentation. Clearly, patients with early carcinomas with no clinical cervical metastasis will do as well as patients with lesions of the anterior tongue, and are often treated similarly. Larger lesions are subject to both diversity of opinion on treatment modality and a certain amount of philosophy as to the quality of life provided to a patient with a total laryngectomy, partial mandibulectomy, and bilateral radical neck dissection.

Even such large resections as are often performed can provide palliation to the patient suffering from fixation of the tongue, chronic aspiration, and continuous pain from an ulcerating tumor. Radiation likewise can be palliative for large bulky tumors, and the use of irid-

TABLE 14–3.—RESULTS OF TREATMENT OF CANCER OF THE BASE OF THE TONGUE

STUDY, YEAR, INSTITUTION	NO. OF PTS.	LENGTH OF FOLLOW-UP*	PROCEDURE AND RESULTS	
Ogura and Biller,[23] 1969 (St. Louis)	30	3 yr	Extended supraglottic laryngectomy:	
			Survival:	
			No nodes	67%
			Nodes	27%
Harrold,[28] 1967 (NY Memorial)	252	5 yr	*Survival overall:*	
			Radiation (56 pts.)	13%
			Surgery (182 pts.)	25%
			Survival with nodes:	
			Overall	15%
			Unilateral	17.5%
			Bilateral	9%
Riley et al.,[29] 1983 (Stanford)	119	5 yr	Radiation (97 pts.):	
			T_1	41%
			T_2	38%
			T_3	5%
			T_4	12%
			Combined therapy: survival no different from that for radiation therapy. Local control by combined therapy, 78%; by radiation, 47%.	
Thawley et al.,[26] 1983 (St. Louis)	101	5 yr	Combined therapy, preoperative radiation (3,000 rad in 3 wk):	
			T_1	57%
			T_2	72%
			T_3	30%
			T_4	22%
			Local control:	
			Stage I	100%
			Stage II	75%
			Stage III	67%
			Stage IV	40%
Schleuning and Summers,[30] 1972 (Univ. of Oregon)	84	. . .	Radiation:	
			Stage I 1/1 recurred, not salvaged	
			Stage II 2/3 recurred, 1/2 salvaged	
			Stage III N_0 5/5 recurred, 1 salvaged (surgery)	
			N_1 15/16 recurred, 3/15 salvaged	
			Surgery:	
			Stage I 1/1 salvaged	
			Stage II 2/2 recurred, 0/2 salvaged	
			Stage III N_0 2/3 recurred, none salvaged	
			N_1 1/1 recurred, not salvaged	
Parsons et al.,[27] 1983 (Univ. of Florida) (provide most complete data)	95	. . .	Radiation alone (65 pts.):	
			T_1N_0	2/2
			T_1N_1	1/1
			T_1N_2	0/2
			T_2N_0	2/2
			T_2N_1	2/3
			T_2N_{2a}	1/3
			T_2N_{2b}	2/2
			T_2N_{3a}	1/2
			T_2N_{3b}	0/4
			T_3N_0	1/3
			T_3N_1	2/5
			T_3N_{2a}	0/0
			T_3N_{2b}	1/4
			T_3N_{3a}	2/3
			T_3N_{3b}	2/6
			T_4N_0	1/2
			T_4N_1	0/1
			T_4N_{2a}	0/3
			T_4N_{2b}	0/4
			T_4N_{3a}	0/2
			T_4N_{3b}	1/10

TABLE 14–3.—RESULTS OF TREATMENT OF CANCER OF THE BASE OF THE TONGUE *(cont.)*

STUDY, YEAR, INSTITUTION	NO. OF PTS.	LENGTH OF FOLLOW-UP*	PROCEDURE AND RESULTS	
			Combined therapy (6 pts.):	
			Better results with postoperative radiation.	
			Radiation failure: 36.	
			11 treated by surgery; 2 pts. survived 2 yr.	
Whicker et al.,[18] 1972 (Mayo Clinic)	102	5	*Survival by treatment:*	
	Primary tumor size:		Planned preop. radiation	3/15
	25%, T_1		Surgical salvage after radiation	3/11
	55%, T_2		Radiation salvage after surgery	1/22
	22%, $T_{3,4}$		Planned postop. radiation	2/8
			Survival by stage:	
			Stages I and II	55%
			Stages III and IV	35%
			Survival by nodes:	
			No nodes	50%
			Positive nodes	35%
Strong,[19] 1979 (N.Y. Memorial)	84		*Survival by stage:*	
			Stage I	1/1
			Stage II	7/11
			Stage III	18/49
			Stage IV	5/23

*For purposes of determining survival statistics.

ium 192 implants has added another dimension. Chemotherapy is given for palliation, for distant metastases, and in prospective combined protocols. It has not added to survival, but by reducing bulk and ulceration, it has helped alleviate pain in our patients.

Guidelines for management of carcinoma of the base of the tongue are listed in Table 14–4. These guidelines are based on the statistics given in Table 14–3.

Treatment Summary

Preferred treatment for T_1 and small T_2 tumors without evidence of nodal disease is radiation therapy. For

TABLE 14–4.—GUIDELINES FOR TREATMENT OF CARCINOMA OF THE BASE OF THE TONGUE

SIZE AT PRESENTATION	TREATMENT
Early lesions	
T_1N_0, vallecula	Radiation therapy or extended supraglottic laryngectomy (radiation if no suggestion of invasion of pre-epiglottic space)
T_1, posterior tongue	Radiation therapy to primary and both sides of the neck
T_2N_0	Radiation therapy to primary and both sides of the neck; lesions clearly to one side are treated surgically with prophylactic neck dissection
T_2N_1	Surgery, including ipsilateral neck dissection; postoperative radiation therapy to primary and both sides of the neck
	In selected cases, full-course irradiation to primary and neck, ipsilateral neck dissection
Larger lesions	
T_3N_0	Radiation therapy to both sides of the neck and primary, either preoperatively postoperatively; recently postoperatively favored; resection of primary and ipsilateral neck dissection
$T_3N_1N_2$	Same as above; possible simultaneous bilateral neck dissection, preserving contralateral jugular vein
$T_4N_0N_1$	90% glossectomy, ipsilateral neck dissection, postoperative radiation therapy; may require total glossectomy and laryngectomy
T_4N_2	Preoperative radiation therapy and probable total glossectomy and total laryngectomy; simultaneous bilateral neck dissection preserving contralateral jugular vein; or staged neck dissection; most of these patients receive palliative full-course radiation

OROPHARYNGEAL CANCER

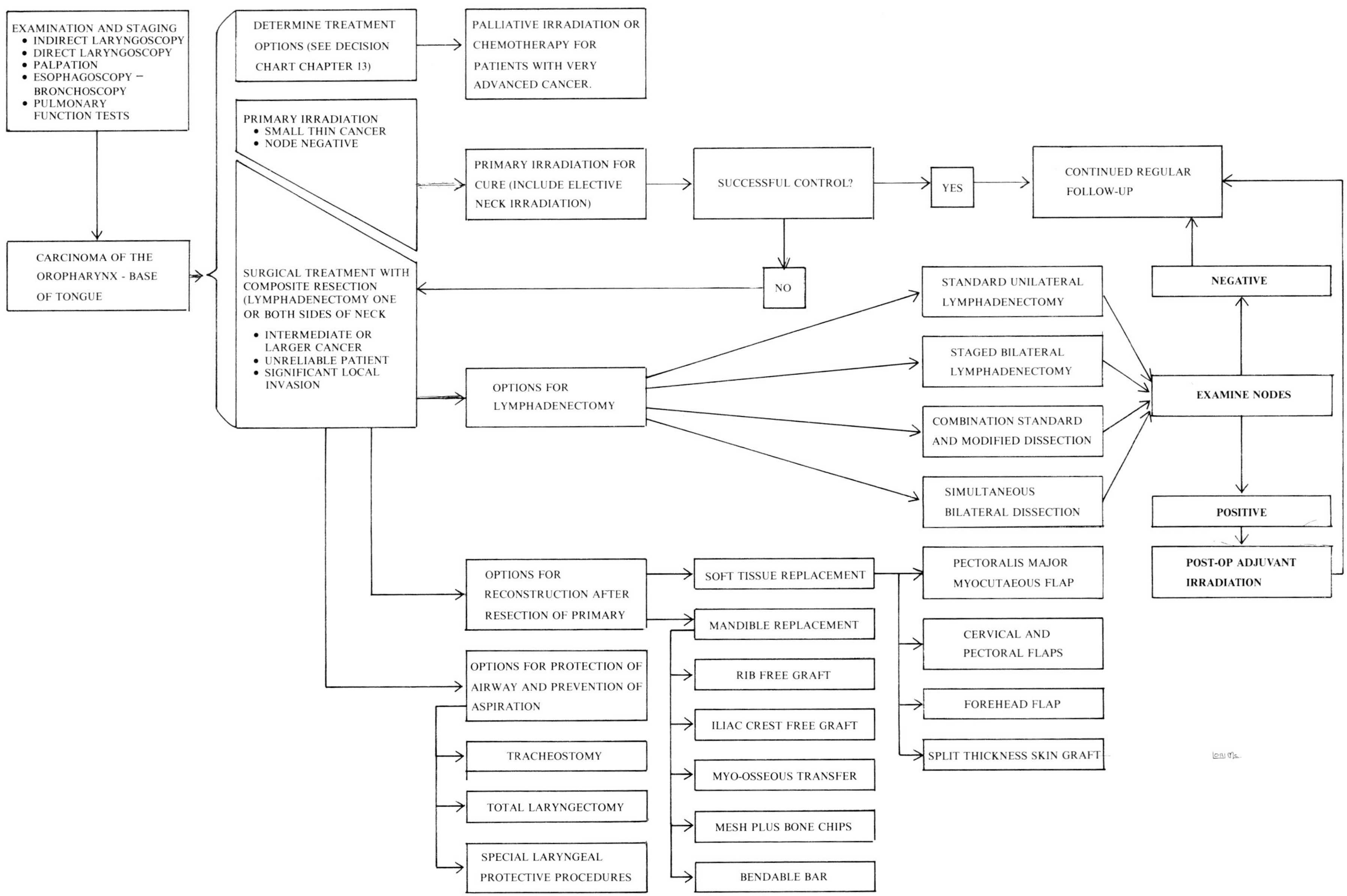

Fig 14–11.—Schema for management of oropharyngeal cancer. Diagram summarizes the surgical options for management of lymph nodes, soft tissue replacement, mandible replacement, and protection of the airway.

larger T_2, all T_3, and T_4 tumors, the preferred treatment is combined radiation therapy and a composite resection, when feasible. Even though combined therapy has not provided a longer survival, it has definitely decreased the incidence of local recurrence. Very large T_4 tumors or those with N_{2a} or N_{2b} disease are treated with preoperative radiation therapy followed by resection. Patients whose tumors fail to show a significant response to preoperative radiation therapy are carried to a full course of irradiation for palliation, and surgery is not attempted. Some of the surgical options are shown in Figure 14–11.

Results of Treatment

Interpretation of results for treatment of tumors of the base of the tongue requires stage-by-stage comparison. It is not representative of the results of the primary treatment modality to give overall 5-year cure rates or measures of local control. Clearly, treatment of the site of the primary fails in 60% of patients. Eighty percent of patients at some time in the course of the disease develop cervical metastases. In most series, 75% of patients have palpable metastases at presentation and 20% have bilateral cervical disease. Comparison of results prior to 1960 also is not indicated. Prior to that time, irradiation alone was the most common treatment modality, and as surgical techniques have improved to provide better margins and better functional results, radiation therapy has likewise improved.

REFERENCES

1. Johnson J.T., Barnes E.L., Myers E.N., et al.: The extracapsular spread of tumors in cervical node metastasis. *Arch. Otolaryngol.* 107:725–729, 1981.
2. Jesse R.H., Sugarbaker E.V.: Squamous cell carcinoma of the oropharynx: Why we fail. *Am. J. Surg.* 132:435–438, 1876.
2. Wang C.C.: Management and prognosis of squamous cell carcinoma of the tonsillar region. *Radiology* 104:667–671, 1972.
4. Allen G.W., Hemenway W.G.: Carcinoma of the tonsil: Surgical treatment. *Laryngoscope* 70:246–257, 1960.
5. Andrews P.E., Sprinkle P.M.: Carcinoma of the tonsil: A comparison of two treatment modalities. *South. Med. J.* 65:982–984, 1972.
6. Terz J.J., Farr H.W.: Carcinoma of the tonsillar fossa. *Surg. Gynecol. Obstet.* 125:581–590, 1967.
7. Hamberger A.D., Fletcher G.H.,, Guillamondequi O.M., et al.: Advanced squamous cell carcinoma of the oral cavity and oropharynx treated with irradiation and surgery. *Radiology* 119:433–438, 1976.
8. Calamel P.M., Hoffmeister F.S.: Carcinoma of the tonsil. *Am. J. Surg.* 114:582–585, 1967.
9. Barrs D.M., DeSanto L.W., O'Fallon W.M.: Squamous cell carcinoma of the tonsil and tongue base region. *Arch. Otolaryngol.* 105:479–485, 1979.
10. Perez C.A., Lee F.A., Ackerman L.V., et al.: Nonrandomized comparison of preoperative irradiation and surgery versus irradiation alone in the management of carcinoma of the tonsil. *AJR* 126:248–260, 1976.
11. Rabuzzi D.D., Mickler A.S., Chung C.T., et al.: Treatment results of combined high-dose preoperative radiotherapy and surgery for oropharyngeal cancer. *Laryngoscope* 92:989–992, 1982.
12. Shumrick D.A., Quenelle D.J.: Malignant disease of the tonsillar region, retromolar trigone, and buccal mucosa. *Otolaryngol. Clin. North Am.* 12:115–124, 1979.
13. Horwitz M.R., Boles R.: Carcinoma of the tonsillar region. *Trans. Am. Acad. Ophthalmol. Otolaryngol.* 78:ORL-368-ORL-377, 1974.
14. Fayos J.V., Lampe I.: Radiation therapy of carcinoma of the tonsillar region. *AJR* 111:85–94, 1971.
15. Shrewsbury D., Adams G.L., Duvall A.J., et al.: Carcinoma of the tonsillar area: A comparison of irradiation compared to preoperative irradiation and surgery. *Otolaryngol. Head Neck Surg.* 89:979–985, 1981.

15a. Matz R., Shumrick D.A., Aron B.S., et al.: Carcinoma of the tonsil: Results of combined treatment. *Laryngoscope* 84:2172–2180, 1974.

15b. Fleming P.M., Matz G.J., Powell W.J., et al.: Carcinoma of the tonsil. *Surg. Clin. N.A.* 56:125–136, 1976.

16. Givens C.D., Johns M.E., Cantrell R.W.: Carcinoma of the tonsil. *Arch. Otolaryngol.* 107:730–734, 1981.

16a. Newman A.N., Rice D.H., Ossoff R.H., et al.: Carcinoma of the tongue in persons younger than 30 years of age. *Arch. Otolaryngol.* 109:302–304, 1983.

17. Leyszig B., Hobanson J.A.: Treatment of cervical lymph nodes in carcinoma of the tongue. *Head Neck Surg.* 5:3–9, 1982.
18. Whicker J.H., Desanto L.W., Devine K.D.: Surgical treatment of squamous cell carcinoma of the base of the tongue. *Laryngoscope* 82:1853–1860, 1972.
19. Strong E.W.: Carcinoma of the tongue. *Otolaryngol. Clin. North Am.* 12:107–114, 1979.
20. Odette J., Szymowski R.T., Nichols R.D.: Multiple head and neck malignancies. *Trans. Am. Acad. Ophthalmol. Otolaryngol.* 84:805–813, 1977.
21. Harrison D.F.N.: The questionable value of total glossectomy. *Head Neck Surg.* 6:632–638, 1983.
22. Schechter G.L., Sly D.E., Roper A.L., et al.: Set-back tongue flap for carcinoma of the tongue base. *Arch. Otolaryngol* 106:668–674, 1980.
23. Ogura J.H., Biller H.F.: Conservation surgery in cancer of the head and neck. *Otolaryngol. Clin. North Am.* 641–665, 1969.
24. Biller H.F., Lawson W., Baek S.: Total glossectomy: A technique of reconstruction eliminating laryngectomy. *Arch. Otolaryngol.* 109:69–73, 1983.
25. Sessions D.G., Stallings J.O., Brownson R.J., et al.: Total glossectomy for advanced carcinoma of the base of the tongue. *Laryngoscope* 83:39–50, 1973.
26. Thawley S.E., Simpson J.R., Perez C.A., et al.: Preoperative irradiation and surgery for carcinoma of the base of the tongue. *Ann. Otol. Rhinol. Laryngol.* 92:485–490, 1983.

27. Parsons J.T., Million R.R., Cassisi N.J.: Carcinoma of the base of the tongue: Results of radical irradiation with surgery reserved for irradiation failure. *Laryngoscope* 92:689–696, 1982.
28. Harrold C.C.: Surgical treatment of cancer of the base of the tongue. *Am. J. Surg.* 114:493–497, 1967.
29. Riley R.W., Fee W.E.. Goffinet D., et al.: Squamous cell carcinoma of the base of the tongue. *Otolaryngol. Head Neck Surg.* 91:143–150, 1983.
30. Schleuning A.J., Summers G.W.: Carcinoma of the tongue: Review of 220 cases. *Laryngoscope* 82:1446–1454, 1972.

15 / Nasopharyngeal Carcinoma

Yashoda Rao, M.D. / Seymour Levitt, M.D.

Cancer of the nasopharynx is one of the most challenging malignant tumors of the head and neck region. Although it occurs worldwide, the highest incidence is found in people of southern Chinese origin living in Southeast Asian countries.[1] A high risk is maintained among first-generation Chinese immigrants to countries like Australia and the United States. However, recent epidemiologic studies have shown a decline in the incidence of nasopharyngeal carcinomas in Chinese immigrants of second and subsequent generations living in California.[2, 3]

WHAT ARE THE ETIOLOGIC FACTORS ASSOCIATED WITH NASOPHARYNGEAL CANCER?

The etiologic hypotheses for induction of nasopharyngeal carcinoma have been well summarized by John H. C. Ho.[4] Three factors are thought to be involved: (1) the constant association of Epstein-Barr virus (EBV)—ubiquitous with nasopharyngeal carcinoma, independent of geography—acting as a carcinogen; (2) a high incidence of nasopharyngeal carcinoma in Chinese, suggesting genetically determined susceptibility; and (3) an environmental factor, which may vary from one population group to another, such as the habit of eating salted preserved fish and the deficiency of vitamin C in the diet in young southern Chinese boat people.

Recent studies have suggested that some vegetable products may activate dormant EBV. One of the more active products in vitro was derived from the croton plant, common in southern China.

WHAT IS THE EFFECT OF AGE AND SEX ON THE INCIDENCE OF NASOPHARYNGEAL CARCINOMA?

The incidence by age and sex of nasopharyngeal carcinoma varies between the Chinese and non-Chinese population. The highest incidence is found in the third and fourth decades of life in Chinese, while in non-Chinese groups the incidence is highest in the fifth and sixth decades of life. There is a high incidence of nasopharyngeal carcinoma among Chinese men, with a male to female ratio of 3:1, compared to a 2:1 male-female ratio in non-Chinese populations.[5, 6]

In children, rhabdomyosarcoma is the most commonly encountered malignancy in the nasopharynx, while carcinoma drops down to the second common cancer of the nasopharynx. In children, nasopharyngeal carcinoma accounts for about 30% of all malignancies in this site, whereas in adults, 85% of the tumors are carcinomas.[7, 8] (See Chapter 24, part II.)

HOW DOES THE ANATOMY OF THE NASOPHARYNX INFLUENCE THE CLINICAL PRESENTATION AND LOCAL SPREAD OF NASOPHARYNGEAL CARCINOMA?

The nasopharynx is an open cavity situated below the base of the skull and behind the nasal cavity. The posterior wall is formed by posterior pharyngeal wall at the level of the first two cervical vertebral bodies. Anteriorly it opens into the posterior nares. The soft palate forms the inferior wall, where the nasopharynx communicates with oropharynx. The medial end of the eustachian tubes opens into the lateral wall of the nasopharynx and is bounded by thc fossa of Rosenmüller, which is the lateral recess lying above and behind the medial end of the eustachian tubes. The complexity of the adjacent anatomical structures of the nasopharynx is important in understanding and diagnosing the local extension of tumors (Fig 15–1). When the tumor invades the base of the skull, it can extend directly into the middle cranial fossa, through the cranial foramina, with involvement of cranial nerves III, IV, V, and VI. Similarly, the tumor can invade the retroparotid space laterally, or metastasize into the lymph nodes in the periparotid area with entrapment of cranial nerves IX, X, XI, and XII, along with the internal carotid artery, internal jugular vein, and cervical sympathetic chain. Anteriorly, the tumor can spread into the nasal cavity and grow through the cribriform plate into the anterior cranial fossa to involve the optic and ophthalmic division of the trigeminal nerves. Cranial nerve VI is commonly involved, affecting the lateral rectus muscle. Anteriorly, the cancer can also extend into the posterior maxillary antrum and posterior orbit. Inferiorly, the tumor may spread submucosally along the posterior pharyngeal wall into the prevertebral muscles and cervical vertebral bodies.

The soft tissue of the nasopharynx forms part of

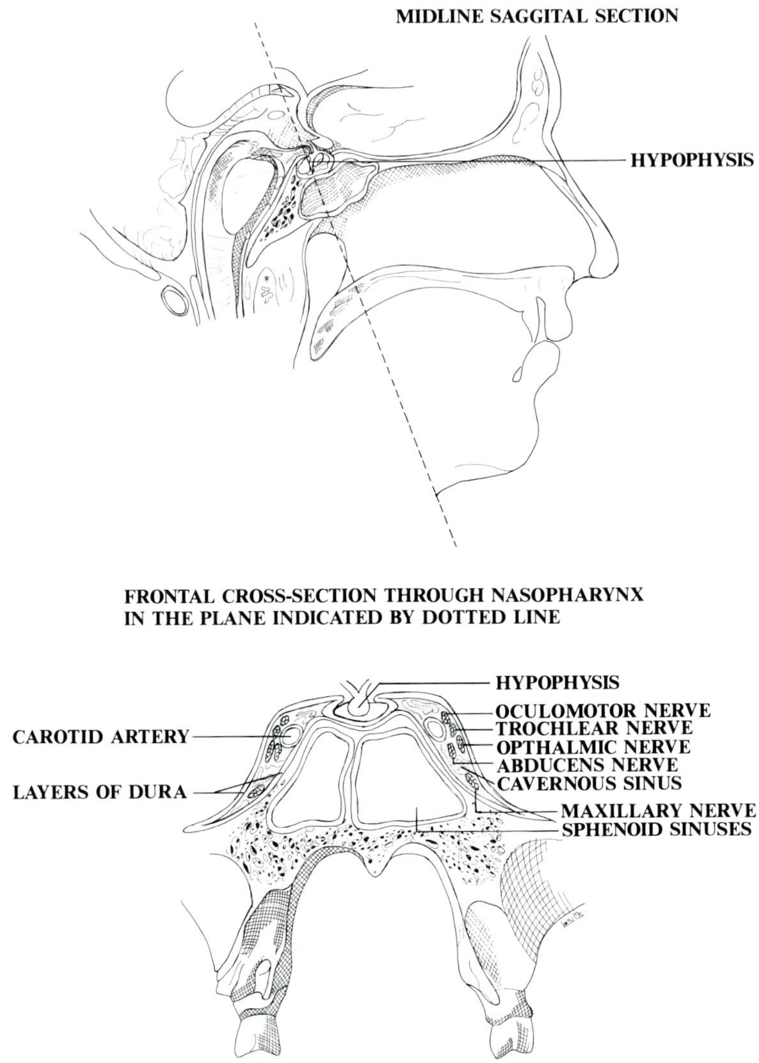

Fig 15–1.—Anatomical cross-sections of the nasopharynx: sagittal section, and frontal section along the line indicated in the sagittal section. Note the relationship of the nerves in the lateral wall of the cavernous sinus and their close proximity to the nasopharynx and the sphenoid sinus.

Waldeyer's ring and has abundant lymphoid stroma in the submucosa. The ease of access to rich lymphatic channels is probably responsible for the high incidence of cervical lymph node metastases in nasopharyngeal carcinoma. Well-differentiated squamous cell carcinomas have about a 70% incidence of node metastases, whereas high-grade or undifferentiated carcinomas or lymphoepitheliomas have over a 90% incidence of node metastases. The first echelon of lymph nodes to be involved by a nasopharyngeal cancer comprises the high upper cervical (which lie deep to the sternomastoid muscle at its insertion), posterior spinal accessory, jugulodigastric, and retropharyngeal nodes. Inferior spinal accessory, lower cervical, and supraclavicular nodes are affected in the second stage of metastatic spread in the neck. (See Chapter 2 and Chapter 9.)

The nasopharynx is a midline structure. Therefore, it is not surprising to find a high rate of bilateral neck node metastases. Clinically detectable bilateral node metastases are seen in 20%–30% of cases.

Early lesions of the nasopharynx produce very few symptoms. Because of the high incidence of neck node metastases, 40%–50% of patients see a physician with the sole complaint of an asymptomatic mass in the neck (see discussion on Unknown Primary in Chap. 25). If the tumor has its origin in the lateral nasopharyngeal wall, blockage of the eustachian tube can cause fullness in the ear, pain referred to the ear or the mastoid, and hearing impairment. Unexplained unilateral serous otitis media in an adult requires examination and biopsy of the nasopharynx. Depending on the degree of anterior spread of the cancer, the patient may present with nasal obstruction or epistaxis. Invasion of the posterior orbit may cause proptosis. Sore throat and swallowing discomfort secondary to spread of the disease to the tonsillar bed or oropharynx is encountered late in some cases. A variety of syndromes showing single or collective involvement of cranial nerves is seen in patients with advanced disease. Intracranial extension of tumor takes place through the cranial foramina. Involvement of the petrous apex and cavernous sinus causes palsies of cranial nerves II through VI, with appropriate visual disturbances. The extension of tumor through the lateral pharyngeal wall into the retroparotid space causes symptoms referable to sensation in the ear, vocal cord weakness, and palsy of the trapezius. When the cervical sympathetic chain is affected, Horner's syndrome results. Spread of the disease into prevertebral muscles and cervical vertebrae can cause severe pain on movement of the head. About 15%–25% of patients have cranial nerve involvement at the time of initial presentation. The most common cranial nerves involved are V and VI, followed by IX and X.

WHAT ARE THE APPROPRIATE DIAGNOSTIC PROCEDURES FOR STAGING NASOPHARYNGEAL CARCINOMAS?

The American Joint Committee staging system for nasopharyngeal carcinoma is based on the anatomical location and local spread of tumor in the nasopharynx.[9] The nasopharynx is divided into two sites—the posterior superior wall, or "vault," and the lateral wall.

PRIMARY TUMOR: T STAGE

T_{IS}—Carcinoma in situ.

T_1—Tumor confined to one site of the nasopharynx or no tumor visible (positive biopsy only).

T_2—Tumor involving two sites (both posterior superior and lateral walls).

T_3—Extension of tumor into nasal cavity or oropharynx.

T_4—Tumor invasion of skull or cranial nerve involvement, or both.

Node staging is the same as is outlined in chapter 9.

Physical examination of the head and neck region, including a thorough neurologic examination (of cranial nerves), is essential to the initial workup. The nasopharynx is poorly seen on routine examination. Direct endoscopic visualization of nasopharynx and biopsy of the lesion are the only definitive way of establishing the diagnosis of nasopharyngeal carcinoma. Indirect examination of the nasopharynx by mirror is of limited value and requires good patient cooperation. A flexible fiberoptic nasopharyngoscope and camera equipment are available for direct visualization of the nasopharynx. These visual tools help to define the extent of local involvement.[10] Often the patient presents with metastatic disease in the neck without a visible primary lesion in the nasopharynx. The presence of a high jugular node mass or of posterior cervical node metastases should make one suspect an occult primary harbored in the nasopharynx. Directed biopsies of normal appearing tissue in this area are both justified and useful. Radiographic studies of the base of the skull (submentovertical views, CT scan, or tomogram of the base of the skull) are helpful in establishing the extent of the tumor in this area (see Chap. 3). These studies, particularly the CT scan, will define any evidence of destruction of the pterygoid plates, foramen lacerum, foramen ovale, foramen spinosum, or foramen jugulare. Information regarding tumor extension into the ethmoid and sphenoid sinus can be obtained by sinus x-rays and refined by CT. With the availability of newer CT scanners with the ability to do frontal and sagittal reconstructions, CT examination is the procedure of choice. CT scans are helpful in clinical decision-making for previously diagnosed nasopharyngeal carcinoma where information concerning the extent of the disease is necessary to plan radiation therapy. In such cases, CT scans can show deep spread of tumor beyond the mucosal surface, intracranial extension of the tumor, invasion of the paranasal sinuses or orbit, bone involvement in the region of the base of the skull, and lymph node metastases in the neck.[11–13] The most common areas of distant metastases are bone, lung, and liver. A routine chest x-ray film, liver function tests, and bone scans are helpful in ruling out distant metastases.

WHAT ARE THE DIFFERENT HISTOLOGIC VARIANTS OF NASOPHARYNGEAL CARCINOMA?

The most common malignant tumors of the nasopharynx are of epithelial origin. The posterior wall of the nasopharynx is lined by squamous epithelium, whereas the roof and lateral walls have stratified ciliated columnar epithelium with mucous and serous secreting glands. Squamous cell carcinoma constitutes 85% of all malignant tumors of the nasopharynx. Well to moderately differentiated squamous cell carcinoma, poorly differentiated squamous cell carcinoma, undifferentiated carcinoma, and lymphoepithelioma (lymphocytic infiltration among the tumor cells) are the four structural variants of squamous cell carcinomas. Lymphomas constitute 10% of the remaining tumors, and the rest (5%) consist of rare tumors like plasmacytomas, adenocarcinomas, and sarcomas.

WHAT IS THE ROLE OF SURGERY IN NASOPHARYNGEAL CARCINOMA?

In nasopharyngeal carcinomas, both the primary disease and the neck node metastases are unsuitable for surgical excision. The anatomical location of the nasopharynx and the direct spread of the cancer to adjacent structures such as the base of the skull, the orbit, and the prevertebral space make surgical resection of the primary disease impossible. Similarly, radical neck dissection is often not desirable or effective because of involvement of high cervical nodes (close to the base of the skull) and retropharyngeal nodes, and the frequent presence of extensive bilateral neck node metastases. Hence, the role of surgery in the treatment of nasopharyngeal carcinoma is limited to biopsy of the primary lesion for histologic diagnosis and to removal of the residual disease in the neck nodes following radiation, when the primary is proved by biopsy to be under control.

WHAT ARE THE DIFFERENT FACTORS TO CONSIDER BEFORE PLANNING RADIATION TREATMENT FOR NASOPHARYNGEAL CARCINOMA?

Radiation therapy is the primary treatment modality for most cases of nasopharyngeal carcinoma. However, there are certain situations when definitive radiation is not indicated or when modification of the treatment is necessary. Figure 15–2 is a useful guide in making decisions regarding radiation treatment for nasopharyngeal carcinoma.

Squamous cell carcinoma and its variants, such as lymphoepithelioma, or undifferentiated carcinoma, account for over 85% of cases of nasopharyngeal carcinoma. As shown in Figure 15–2, they are treated by irradiation, with the lymphoepitheliomas treated on occasion with slightly lower doses. Lymphomas and other uncommon tumors need individual treatment planning and will not be discussed in this chapter.

Once a diagnosis of squamous cell carcinoma is made, the next step is to establish the stage of the disease and to exclude distant metastases. If the disease is limited to the head and neck region, minor variations in field size and in the total dose are necessary, depending on the T and N stages of the disease and the histologic variation.

Most nasopharyngeal carcinomas are poorly differentiated tumors with a high incidence of node metastases. Nasopharyngeal carcinoma has a great propensity for local spread. Because of these factors, for any given T stage of the disease, a large radiation field encompassing the following anatomical structures is needed: (1) the nasopharynx, (2) the base of the skull, to include cranial foramina and sphenoid and cavernous sinuses, (3) posterior ethmoid sinus, posterior orbit, posterior maxillary antrum, and posterior nasal cavity, and (4) the oropharynx and retropharyngeal nodes. When there is evidence of spread of the disease into base of the skull, the superior border of the radiation field should include the entire pituitary fossa, suprasellar region, base of the brain, and floor of the middle and anterior cranial fossae.

It has been shown that elective irradiation of uninvolved neck (N_0) to 4,500–5,000 rad reduces the probability of appearance of neck metastases at a later date.[14] Therefore, given the high incidence of neck node metastases in nasopharyngeal carcinoma, prophylactic irradiation of both sides of the neck in patients clinically staged N_0 is recommended. To achieve better control of clinically involved nodes, a higher dose of radiation (6,000–7,000 rad) is needed to achieve better local control.

For a full course of radiation, a cobalt 60 or 4- or 6-MeV linear accelerator is used to deliver an adequate dose to the primary and the neck nodes. Parallel opposed lateral fields are used to treat the primary and the upper neck nodes up to 4,500 rad. At this point the treatment field is reduced to exclude the spinal cord. Clinically positive posterior neck nodes should be boosted with electrons or a small tangential photon beam (avoiding the spinal cord). The lower neck is treated through a single anterior field to 5,000 rad, with a shield over the larynx. Treatment setup becomes more complicated when an anterior facial field is used to deliver an adequate dose in cases of anterior extension of the tumor into the nasal cavity. Because of the large volume of tissue that is treated, 175–180 rad/day is better tolerated than higher daily doses.

Several authors believe there is a definite difference in radiosensitivity between squamous cell carcinomas and lymphoepitheliomas.[15, 16] Local failures are rare with 6,000–6,500 rad for lymphoepitheliomas, where squamous cell carcinomas require 6,500–7,500 rad (depending on the T stage of the disease) for local control of the disease.

HOW EFFECTIVE IS RADIATION FOR TREATMENT OF NASOPHARYNGEAL CARCINOMA?

There are several prognostic factors that dictate the results of radiation treatments. The most important of them are the T and N stages of the disease. To a certain degree, age, sex, histologic subtype, and technical precision of the radiation treatment may also influence the results. Because nasopharyngeal carcinoma is a rare tumor and most commonly seen in certain restricted geographic locations, just a few authors have accumulated large enough experience to make definitive conclusions about treatment results. Tables 15–1, 15–2, and 15–3, give 5-year disease-free survival of patients with nasopharyngeal carcinoma treated by radiation. The second most important prognostic factor (after stage) appears to be the histologic subtype of the cancer, at least in the early stage of the disease. As seen in Table 15–4, patients with lymphoepitheliomas show better survival

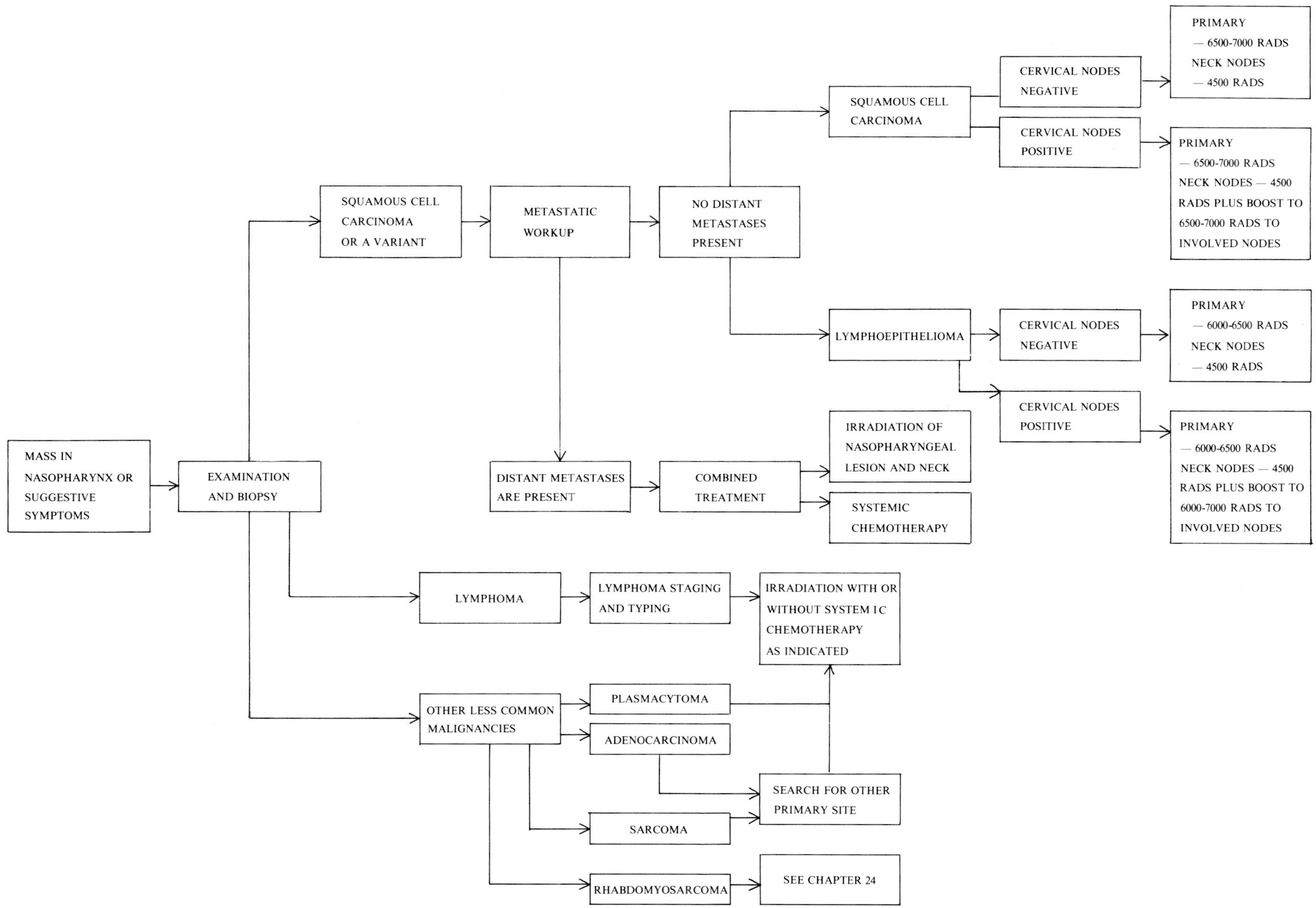

Fig 15–2.—Decisions for treatment of nasopharyngeal carcinoma.

TABLE 15–1.—5-YEAR DISEASE-FREE SURVIVAL (%) BY STAGE OF DISEASE

STUDY, YEAR	STAGE I	STAGE II	STAGE III	STAGE IV
Hsu and Tu,[19] 1983	81	75	48	20
Huang,[17] 1980	65	46	23	0
Ho,[4] 1978	68	50	28	7

TABLE 15–2.—5-YEAR DISEASE-FREE SURVIVAL (%) OF TREATED NASOPHARYNGEAL CANCER, BY T STAGE

STUDY, YEAR	T_1	T_2	T_3	T_4
Wang,[20] 1983	60	48	27	29
Hoppe et al.[21] 1976	76	63	55	0
Dickson,[5] 1981	33	41	14	8

following radiation treatments than do patients with squamous cell carcinomas or undifferentiated carcinomas. Younger patients (less than 40 years old) have better prognosis than older patients, and females have a slight survival advantage over males.[4, 16–18]

Because of the aggressive nature of nasopharyngeal carcinoma and its rich lymphatic supply, advanced local and regional disease is common. In many other head and neck squamous cancers, far-advanced node disease is a sure harbinger of therapeutic failure. In contrast, aggressive radiation treatment for advanced node stages of nasopharyngeal carcinoma is often fruitful. Disease-free survivals ranging from 15% to 30% have been reported when these advanced local carcinomas (without apparent dissemination beyond the head and neck region) have been treated with radiation.[24–27] One may speculate why irradiation of some of these advanced cancers of the nasopharynx is successful when irradiation of advanced node-positive cancers arising in other oropharyngeal sites clearly is not, or not to the same degree.

Unlike other head and neck cancers, late recurrence is not uncommon in nasopharyngeal carcinoma. Long-delayed recurrence is mainly seen with lymphoepitheliomas. Local persistence or recurrence of tumor in the nasopharynx and base of skull is the primary cause of failure following irradiation. Neck disease alone or distant metastases alone do not represent more than 20% of the treatment failures. The most common site of distant metastases is bone. Metastasis to lung and liver is seen in squamous cell carcinomas. The frequency of distant metastasis is more related to the increased N stage of the disease than to the T stage. Up to 50% of patients with N_2 or N_3 disease in the neck develop distant metastases. For these patients, the only hope for improved survival is to add an effective systemic therapy.

TABLE 15–3.—5-YEAR DISEASE-FREE SURVIVAL (%) OF TREATED NASOPHARYNGEAL CANCER BY N STAGE

STUDY, YEAR	N_0	N_1	N_2	N_3
Wang,[20] 1983	60	42	42	21
Hoppe et al.,[21] 1976	78	70	42	39
Dickson,[5] 1981	37	32	29	13

TABLE 15–4.—5-YEAR DISEASE-FREE SURVIVAL (%) BY HISTOLOGIC TYPE

STUDY, YEAR	SQUAMOUS	LYMPHOEPITHELIOMA	UNDIFFERENTIATED
Dickson,[5] 1981	22	52	42
Wang,[22] 1983	25	70	41
Hoppe et al.,[16] 1978	47	58	43
Mesic et al.,[23] 1981	44	68	15

Table 15–5 shows the ultimate sites of cancer spread in ten patients at the University of Minnesota who were carefully studied shortly before death (four patients) or were autopsied after dying from nasopharyngeal carcinoma (six patients). Over half of the patients had hepatic metastases. All but three patients had extensive systemic metastases. Effective control of nasopharyngeal carcinoma will require some means to treat the systemic spread.

Retreatment of recurrent disease in the nasopharynx and base of the skull is often palliative and occasionally curative. External radiation alone to a dose of 4,000–6,000 rad or a combination of external radiation to 3,000 rad and interstitial implant or intracavitary radium is often useful.[28, 29] The reirradiation of 108 patients with local recurrence in the absence of coexisting distant metastases has resulted in 21% 2-year and 5% 5-year survivals in one series reported by Hsu and Tu.[19]

WHAT ARE THE SIDE EFFECTS AND COMPLICATIONS RELATED TO RADIATION TREATMENT OF NASOPHARYNGEAL CARCINOMA?

The usual side effects of radiation treatment include anorexia, fatigue, radiation dermatitis in the treatment field, and mucositis of the oropharynx leading to odynophagia. These symptoms subside 4–6 weeks following completion of radiation treatment. The most common persistent side effect of radiation is xerostomia because of inclusion of salivary glands in the treatment fields. A pretreatment dental checkup is helpful in preventing radiation-related dental problems, which may lead to osteoradionecrosis of the mandible or maxilla. Hoarseness, dyspnea due to persistent edema of the larynx, trismus secondary to radiation of the temporomandibular joint, subcutaneous fibrosis of both sides of the neck, cataract formation, and keratoconjunctivitis (if eyes are

TABLE 15–5.—TERMINAL FINDINGS IN TEN PATIENTS DYING FROM MALIGNANT TUMORS OF THE NASOPHARYNX

PT.	TUMOR TYPE	AREAS OF SPREAD
1	Malignant lymphoma	Heart, liver, L. kidney, lung*
2	Undifferentiated carcinoma	Sphenoid, dura, L. temporal lobe*
3	Undifferentiated carcinoma	Liver (70%–80%) (exploratory lap.), chest x-ray negative
4	Undifferentiated carcinoma	Lungs, liver*
5	Squamous cell carcinoma	Posterior fossa, pituitary*
6	Squamous cell carcinoma	Lung, liver, bone marrow, lymph nodes*
7	Squamous cell carcinoma	Sella, clivus, petrous ridge, base of skull (x-ray)
8	Squamous cell carcinoma	Hemorrhage—erosion of tumor, R. int. carotid artery
9	Squamous cell carcinoma	Heart, lungs, liver, spleen, kidneys, pancreas, esophagus, adrenals, mesentery*
10	Embryonal cell rhabdomyosarcoma	Clivus (x-ray), lung (x-ray)

Areas of spread determined by autopsy* (6 patients), x-ray findings (3 patients), and exploratory laparotomy (1 patient).
Note: five patients had hepatic involvement when they died.

included in the radiation fields) are some of the late and persistent complications of radiation. The most severe complication of radiation is damage to the brain stem and cervical spinal cord. Ballantyne reported the causes of the 6% late mortality attributable to radiation treatment of nasopharyngeal cancer at M. D. Anderson Hospital.[30] Transverse myelitis occurred in 8 of 218 treated patients in that series. In three the complication was not fatal. With meticulous modern treatment techniques, this dread complication should be infrequent (see chap. 27).

REFERENCES

1. Ho J.H.C.: Nasopharyngeal carcinoma. *Adv. Cancer Res.* 15:57–92, 1972.
2. Buell P.: The effect of migration on the risk of nasopharyngeal carcinoma among Chinese. *Cancer Res.* 34:1189–1194, 1974.
3. Zippin C., et al.: Studies on heredity and environment in cancer of the nasopharynx. *JNCI* 29:483–490, 1962.
4. Ho J.H.C.: An epidemiological and clinical study of nasopharyngeal carcinoma. *Int. J. Radiat. Oncol. Biol. Phys.* 4:183–193, 1978.
5. Dickson R.I.: Nasopharyngeal carcinoma: An evaluation of 209 patients. *Laryngoscope* 91:333–354, 1981.
6. Laing D.: Nasopharyngeal carcinoma. *Otol. Clin. North Am.* 71:703–725, 1968.
7. Jereb B., Huvos A.D., Steinberg P., et al.: Nasopharyngeal carcinoma in children: Review of 16 cases. *Int. J. Radiat. Oncol. Biol. Phys.* 6:487–491, 1980.
8. Jaffe B.F., Jaffe N.: Head and neck tumors in children. *Pediatrics* 51:731–740, 1973.
9. American Joint Committee for Cancer Staging and End Result Reporting: *Manual for Staging Cancer,* ed. 2. Philadelphia, J.B. Lippincott Co., 1983.
10. Chiang T.C., Jund P.E.: The nasopharyngoscope and camera examination of the primary carcinoma of the nasopharynx. *Cancer* 40:2353–2364, 1977.
11. Maneuso A.A., Bohman L., Hanafee W., et al.: Computed tomography of nasopharynx: Normal and variants of normal. *Radiology* 137:113–121, 1980.
12. Sliver J.A., Mawad M.E., Hilal S.K., et al.: Computed tomography of the nasopharynx and related spaces. *Radiology* 147:725–731, 1983.
13. Elie G., Vazel P., Renand-Salis J.L., et al.: CT of primary malignant tumor of the nasopharynx: Computerized tomography. *J. Radiol.* 4:235–241, 1980.
14. Fletcher G.M.: Elective irradiation of subclinical disease in cancer of the head and neck. *Cancer* 29:1450–1454, 1972.
15. Chen K.Y., Fletcher G.H.: Malignant tumors of the nasopharynx. *Radiology* 99:165–172, 1971.
16. Hoppe R.T., Williams J., Warnke R., et al.: Carcinoma of the nasopharynx: The significance of histology. *Int. J. Radiat. Oncol. Biol. Phys.* 4:199–205, 1978.
17. Huang S.C.: Nasopharyngeal cancer: A review of 1605 patients treated radically with cobalt 60. *Int. J. Radiat. Oncol. Biol. Phys.* 6:401–407, 1980.
18. Meyer J.E., Wang C.C.: Carcinoma of the nasopharynx. *Radiology* 100:385–388, 1971.
19. Hsu Mow-Ming, Tu Shih-Mien: Nasopharyngeal carcinoma of Taiwan: Clinical manifestation and results of therapy. *Cancer* 52:362–368, 1983.
20. Wang C.C.: *Radiation Therapy for Head and Neck Neoplasms.* Littleton, Mass., Wright/PSG Publishing Company, Inc., 1983, p. 208.
21. Hoppe R.T., Goffinet D.R., Bagshaw M.A.: Carcinoma of the nasopharynx. *Cancer* 37:2605–2612, 1976.
22. Wang C.C.: *Radiation Therapy for Head and Neck Neoplasms.* Littleton, Mass., Wright/PSG Publishing Company, Inc., 1983, p. 210.
23. Mesic J.B., Fletcher G.H., Goepfert H.: Megavoltage irradiation of epithelial tumors of the nasopharynx. *Int. J. Radiat. Oncol. Biol. Phys.* 7:477–453, 1981.

24. Cooper J.S., Rowe J.D., Newell J.: Regional stage IV carcinoma of the nasopharynx treated by aggressive radiotherapy. *Int. J. Radiat. Oncol. Biol. Phys.* 9:1737–1745, 1983.
25. Amornmarn R., Prempree T., Sewchand W., et al.: Radiation management of advanced nasopharyngeal cancer. *Cancer* 52:802–807, 1983.
26. Petrovich Z., Cox J.D., Roswit B., et al.: Advanced carcinoma of the nasopharynx. *Radiology* 144:905–908, 1982.
27. Bedwinek J.M., Perez C.A., Keys D.J.: Analysis of failure after definitive irradiation for epidermoid carcinoma of the nasopharynx. *Cancer* 45:2725–2729, 1980.
28. Wang C.C., Schulz M.D.: Management of locally recurrent carcinoma of the nasopharynx. *Radiology* 86:900–903, 1966.
29. McNeese M.D., Fletcher G.H.: Retreatment of recurrent nasopharyngeal carcinoma. *Radiology* 138:191–193, 1981.
30. Ballantyne A.J.: Late sequellae of radiation therapy in cancer of the head and neck with particular reference to the nasopharynx. *Am. J. Surg.* 130:433–436, 1975.

16 / Carcinoma of the Larynx and Laryngopharynx

ROBERT H. MAISEL, M.D.

HISTORY AND TREATMENT OF LARYNGEAL CANCER

FOR MANY YEARS carcinoma of the larynx was recognized only in its late stages. Effective treatment, however, required earlier diagnosis. The recognition of earlier and treatable phases of the carcinoma was pioneered by Manuel Garcia, a Spanish singing teacher, who was able to perform indirect examination of the larynx with dental mirrors, employing reflected sunlight as the light source. He reported his results to the Royal Society of London in 1855. Subsequent to this, the science of laryngology developed in Europe. Both infectious disease and neoplastic growths of the larynx could be studied. Early treatments entailed the use of cautery and biopsy excision for laryngeal neoplasia. The first recognized laryngectomy for treatment of a large carcinoma was reported by Bilroth in 1873. The operation, performed on a patient with a subglottic vocal cord carcinoma, represents a milestone in our treatment of laryngeal cancer.

The most famous case of laryngeal carcinoma, and one with the greatest impact on world history, was that of Emperor Fredrick III of Germany.[1] This case was mentioned in chapter 1.

Babe Ruth was another famous person who suffered from laryngeal carcinoma. He died of laryngeal cancer on Aug. 16, 1948, after his active career as an American sports hero was complete.

Little significant progress occurred in the treatment of carcinoma of the larynx from the turn of the century until the 1930s, when radiation therapy of laryngeal cancer was introduced and produced some success. Because of skin and soft tissue injury due to poor penetration of the x-ray beam, the morbidity from treatment in the 1930s and 1940s was striking. Little progress was made during the decade. The introduction of endotracheal anesthesia, the wider use of good tracheostomy tubes, early antibiotics, and improved techniques in blood transfusion allowed additional advances in the treatment of carcinoma of the larynx in the period following World War II. At the same time, radiation therapy techniques were improved by using higher energy particles to deliver the radiation beam. Superficial skin damage was limited, while tissue destruction at the site of carcinoma was improved. Fletcher, working with many co-workers at the M. D. Anderson Hospital, spearheaded this technique of radiation.[2]

Alonso in South America and Ogura and Som in the United States began to recognize that partial laryngectomy was possible and effective. Their work was built on the experimental work of Pressman, who demonstrated the compartmentalization of the larynx that determined the pattern of lymphatic spread of carcinoma.[3, 4] The predictability of extension was the scientific foundation for partial laryngectomy.

The two-stage supraglottic laryngectomy of Alonso was modified by Ogura and Mallen[5] and by Som[6] into a single-stage partial laryngectomy to preserve the voice in patients with supraglottic cancer. The operation was performed by others and recognized to be equal in its survival characteristics to the debilitating total laryngectomy.

In the 1960s, Powers, Holtz, Ogura, and others[7] began careful studies on what is now considered low-dose preoperative radiation therapy in combination with surgery. Their careful work in a large series of patients led to acceptance of high-dose preoperative radiation therapy and the alternative technique of high-dose postoperative radiation therapy for carcinoma of the larynx and pharynx. Chemotherapy has not had much of an impact on primary treatment of carcinoma of the larynx except for very specialized cell types.

When therapy is correctly selected, good survival can be achieved by vertical hemilaryngectomy, horizontal (supraglottic) laryngectomy, and radiation therapy for cure. Despite these important improvements of therapy in the 1950s and 1960s, there were still many patients with large tumors that required total laryngectomy, leaving them aphonic. Restoring a communicative voice to patients who had a total laryngectomy required the major interest of people like Asai,[8] Komorn et al.,[9] and Singer and Blom.[10]

WHAT STRUCTURES MAKE UP THE LARYNX AND HYPOPHARYNX?

Figure 16–1 illustrates the general structure of the area. The particular structures and anatomical limits are defined below (based on the American Joint Commission clinical staging system).

Larynx

The *anterior limit* is composed of the anterior or lingual surface of the suprahyoid epiglottis, the thyrohyoid membrane, the anterior commissure, and the anterior

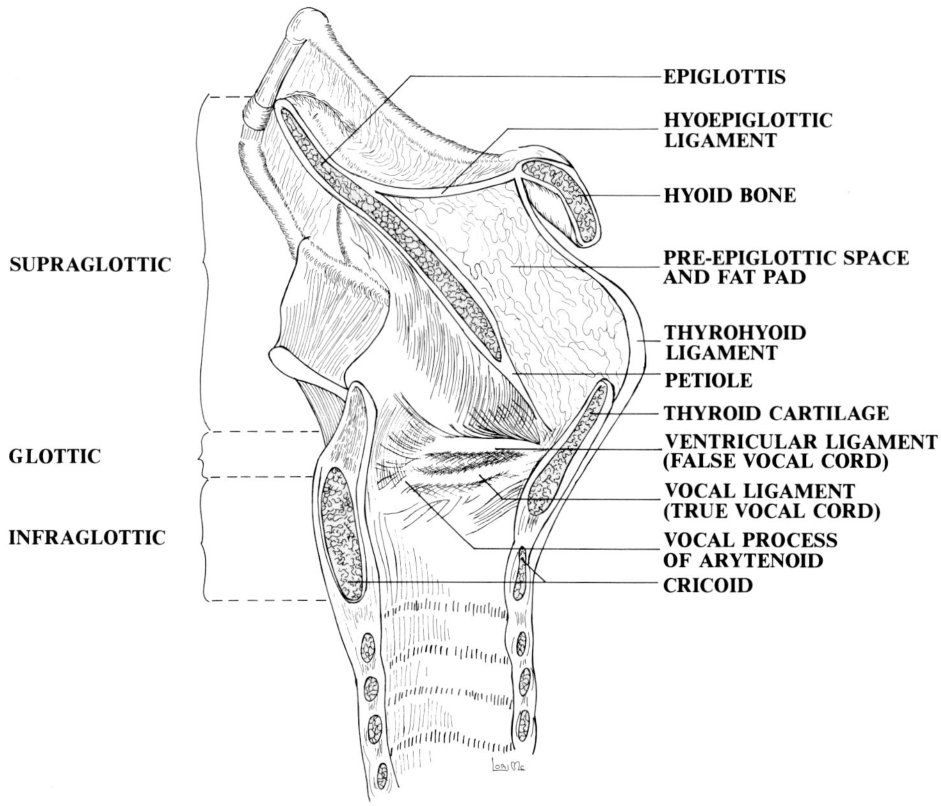

Fig 16–1.—Anatomy of the larynx.

wall of the subglottic region, which is composed of the thyroid cartilage, the cricothyroid membrane, and the anterior arch of the cricoid cartilage.

The *posterior and lateral limits* include the aryepiglottic folds, the arytenoid region, the interarytenoid space, and the posterior surface of the subglottic space, represented by the mucous membrane covering the cricoid cartilage.

The *superolateral limits* are the tip and the lateral border of the epiglottis.

The *inferior limits* are determined by a plane passing through the inferior edge of the cricoid cartilage.

Sites within the supraglottic region (superior to horizontal plane passing through the apex of the ventricles) include the epiglottis (both its lingual and laryngeal aspects), aryepiglottic folds, arytenoids, and ventricular bands (i.e., false cords).

Sites within the glottic region (horizontal plane of the apex of the ventricles to a point 1 cm below this plane) include the true vocal cords and the anterior and posterior glottic commissures.

Subglottic region (inferior border of glottis to inferior border of cricoid cartilage).

Hypopharynx

The hypopharynx is that portion of the pharynx that extends from the plane of the hyoid bone superiorly to the plane of the lower border of the cricoid cartilage inferiorly (Fig 16–2). It is partitioned into three distinct sites: the *piriform sinuses*, the *postcricoid area* (the posterior surface of the larynx, extending from the posterior limit of the arytenoid cartilage and its connecting folds to the inferior limit of the cricoid cartilage and bounded laterally by the piriform sinuses), and the *posterior and lateral pharyngeal walls* (the lateral walls appearing quite distinct above the level of the piriform sinuses).

It is useful to try to define tumor extent as precisely as possible. We will see that effective decision-making and communication depend on a good definition of tumor location. The larynx and hypopharynx are defined separately, but the actual distances are small and the areas contiguous, so it is useful to combine the discussion of both areas.

HOW COMMON IS LARYNGEAL CARCINOMA?

If particular sites are not grouped, carcinoma of the larynx is the most common tumor of the *upper* aerodigestive system (see Chap. 1). Its incidence approximates 10% that of lung cancer, and there are 10,000 new cases of laryngeal carcinoma each year, including the cancers of the intrinsic and extrinsic larynx. This comes close to half the cancers of the head and neck

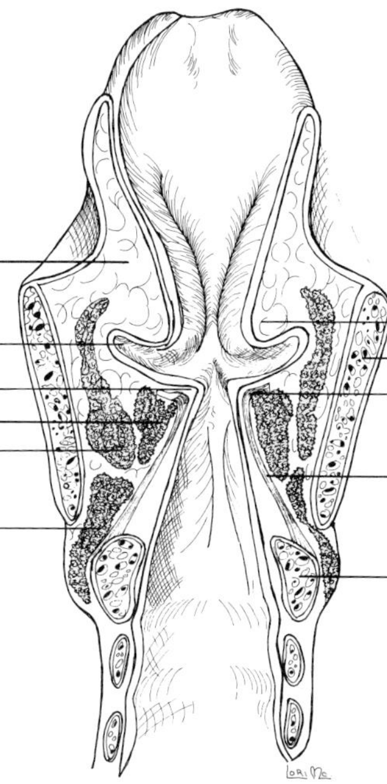

Fig 16–2.—Anatomy of the larynx.

when the skin and thyroid gland cancers are excluded. In the past, there was a 9:1 male-female ratio. Recent studies show a closing gender gap. The peak incidence of carcinoma of the larynx is between the ages of 50 and 70. Carcinoma of the larynx is very unusual under the age of 35. In the United States, the etiology appears to relate to smoking of cigarettes. Alcohol does not appear to be a causal factor.

DIAGNOSTIC MANEUVERS

What Symptoms and Findings Are Present in Laryngeal and Hypopharyngeal Cancer?

The commonest and earliest symptom of laryngeal carcinoma is hoarseness. A high index of suspicion is necessary in the examining physician, particularly if the patient is a smoker. Patients with supraglottic and hypopharyngeal carcinomas usually present with a "hot potato voice" or the more usual hoarseness. The patient may complain of pain or dysphagia, and the first sign of tumor may be a neck mass. Occasionally, patients with hypopharyngeal cancer will complain of hemoptysis, ipsilateral otalgia, a persistent cough, or the sensation of a lump in the throat. Other symptoms that frequently occur are dysphagia, odynophagia, hemoptysis, and airway obstruction (in patients with large tumors). Throat pain is unusual in the small glottic tumor, but can occur when there is invasion of the adjacent structures. Whenever the suspicion of cancer is entertained, a good indirect examination of the entire larynx and hypopharynx must be achieved. When the symptoms are ignored or the tumor is in a location that allows the patient to delay seeking medical help, the opportunity for cure as well as for preservation of organ function is reduced.

The most frequent site of origin for laryngeal carcinoma is on the true vocal cord. The most frequent location on the vocal cord is the free edge on the superior surface of the membranous true vocal cord. According to English,[11] 50% of laryngeal tumors occur on the vocal cord, and 75% of these originate on the anterior half of the cord. Glottic tumors are occasionally seen at the anterior commissure or posteriorly on the arytenoid, but usually only as an extension of a tumor originating on the mobile vocal cord. Indirect laryngoscopy is the mainstay of early diagnosis. Topical anesthesia of the area or mild sedation can be used to help examination in the office. The newer flexible fiberoptic instruments which are passed transnasally allow patients with a violent cough and gag reflex to be examined more easily in the office and reduce the need for general anesthesia to conduct a first examination. The fiberoptic scopes do have a limited sharpness of image.

The gross pathology of all carcinomas of the larynx is usually easy to recognize on mirror examination as an exfoliating or keratotic and friable-appearing lesion. In larger lesions, mobility of the larynx is impaired. Chronic granulatomous disease of the larynx can occasionally mimic malignant patterns, although a granuloma usually occurs on the posterior aspect of the vocal cord. Because of these alternative possibilities, histologic confirmation of carcinoma is mandatory before one begins treatment of the suspected laryngeal carcinoma patient.

Occasionally a node in the neck is the presenting symptom. The neck must be carefully examined in all patients and the normal structures palpated. Lymph node metastases from carcinoma of the larynx are to the anterior jugular nodes. When a single node is present, it is in the midjugular group of these anterior nodes. The nodes are palpable and abnormal clinically when they are 2 cm in size. Most nodes are nontender, firm, not fixed to the soft tissue, and relatively easy to recognize if the examiner makes a careful search. Nodes may be less easy to palpate in the fat or muscular neck until the patient is completely relaxed. When the patient is under general anesthesia for endoscopy, it provides another opportunity to palpate the neck and discover enlarged nodes. Occasionally lymph nodes as large as 2 cm are not recognized on the preoperative examination or on the examination under anesthesia and become apparent during the course of neck dissection and/or laryngeal surgery.

Patients with supraglottic and hypopharyngeal lesions may be more difficult to examine. If the lesion is favorably placed for examination, the appearance of the lesion is characteristic. The patient must be carefully examined by indirect mirror techniques not only to be sure the suspected lesion is not ignored, but also to be certain that a second small lesion adjacent to it is not missed. None of the laryngeal-hypopharyngeal cancers can be seen using only an examining tongue blade and a direct light source. Indirect examination using mirrors or more extensive direct examination is necessary. It is possible that an office examination will disclose only the edema of the mucosa when the patient has symptoms of throat pain or hoarseness. Edema of either the arytenoids or the piriform sinus requires direct laryngoscopy. This will usually show the ulcerated, friable lesion deep to the bulging folds of the edematous mucosa.

What Preoperative Diagnostic Radiographic Studies Are Useful in Evaluating Laryngeal and Hypopharyngeal Cancers?

Soft tissue technique regular x-ray examination, tomography, contrast laryngography, xeroradiography, and computerized axial tomography have all been used. General applications were discussed in chapter 3. The radiographic evaluation of the larynx requires a diagnostic radiology expert with a particular interest in the task. The best early radiographic technique was laryngography, originally described by Holtz et al. in St. Louis.[12] This technique allows reasonably good examination of both piriform sinuses, and the valleculae, as well as the entire endolarynx. It allows a reasonable estimation of vocal cord size and shows whether or not there is subglottic extension of tumor. The technique is moderately difficult since it requires a slow drip of oily Dionosol or similar contrast material onto the cords (topically anesthetized) of awake patients. Routine neck films are then taken with the patient in different stages of phonation.

Laryngography still has a place, particularly for the patient with a piriform sinus lesion in whom radiographic evaluation of the base of the piriform sinus is necessary before planning surgery. The laryngogram is valuable in cases where either vocal cord mobility or the integrity of the laryngeal ventricle is questioned. Laryngography has been largely supplanted by tomography because it takes less time and is less difficult to perform. Tomography does not define the folds of the larynx nearly as well as laryngography since no contrast material is applied to the mucosal tissues.

Laryngeal tomography is a noncontrast technique that allows the air shadow to be evaluated next to the soft tissue mass of the larynx. The primary value of tomography is to assess vocal cord paralysis and to evaluate the subglottic angle. It is not very helpful in recognizing tumor bulk. Whereas correctly performed tomography may demonstrate cartilaginous invasion, plain soft tissue radiographs will often yield the same information. Xeroradiography of the larynx is a little-used technique that has some value in defining large soft tissue shadows and detecting foreign bodies in the airway.

These earlier techniques have been replaced for most purposes by the CT scan of the larynx, our best present-day technique for detecting cartilage invasion and estimating soft tissue bulk.[13–15] In conjunction with endoscopy, the CT scan gives the best pretreatment map of the location of a tumor and the depth of invasion, both within the soft tissues of the larynx and extralaryngeally. CT is of primary value to the decisions of the surgeon when defining cartilage invasion by carcinoma. The radiologist often can measure cartilage invasion accurately using this technique and can contribute to decisions on partial surgery. Surgical exploration will, on occasion, show that the CT scan was incorrect. The surgeon must always reserve the opportunity to disregard "soft" x-ray findings and do a procedure based on prior clinical experience with similar cancers.

CT scanning is important to define the depth of invasion into the soft tissues of the neck. The CT scan should *not become a required routine* pretreatment examination since the diagnosis of carcinoma is suspected on laryngoscopy and confirmed by biopsy, and the treatment is largely planned on the basis of the information gained from direct examination of the primary tumor and from palpation of the neck for possible positive lymph nodes. With an accurate evaluation, one can then use statistics from similarly staged patients and past experience as a guide to making decisions on surgery or radiation.

Finally, a chest radiograph is needed, but metastatic bone surveys as well as CT scans of the head, chest, and body are not commonly indicated. Patients with laryngeal carcinoma that has not spread outside the larynx to the neck occasionally have lung metastases (< 3%), but only in very unusual circumstances do such tumors metastasize to distant sites in the liver, brain, or bone. Simultaneous lung cancer can occur and will often be discovered by routine chest radiography.

What Is the Role of Direct Laryngoscopy?

Patients who have had complete evaluation by indirect examination and by radiographic study must then be considered by the physician for endoscopy under anesthesia. If one is going to dismiss a suspicion of cancer, it is necessary to prove that cancer is not present. Direct laryngoscopy is done in virtually all patients who have a suspicious lesion or persistent symptoms that require careful examination and/or biopsy. It is only by direct laryngoscopy that a satisfactory biopsy specimen may be obtained.

How Are Direct Laryngoscopy and Biopsy Conducted?

If the patient can tolerate safely a general anesthetic, this is the preferred mechanism of patient control during direct laryngoscopy. A small endotracheal tube (6.0–6.5 mm internal diameter) is passed. The surgeon must be in the room to help, in case the laryngeal tumor interferes with the opportunity to control the airway. After intubation has been completed and relaxation achieved, the lighted laryngoscope is introduced.

Endoscopy for laryngeal carcinoma requires experience and a delicate hand as well as the willingness to take substantial pieces of tissue for biopsy. While the flexible fiberoptic instruments as well as the mirror examination permit a reasonable and dynamic view of the endolarynx in most patients, a suspicious lesion requires direct laryngoscopy with a hard instrument that can move tissues out of the way. General anesthesia allows the physician a much better view and permits him to palpate, push, and biopsy any areas of interest or suspicion. The anterior commissure laryngoscopes of Dedo and Jako are both quite adequate for this purpose and introduce enough light for good visualizaiton of all aspects of the larynx (Fig 16–3). In selected cases, they may be used in conjunction with the operating microscope. The area of the tumor should be the last part of the larynx to be examined since the tissue is more friable. If any bleeding is induced, it will obscure visibility in the rest of the larynx.

In general, the extrinsic larynx should be examined first in patients with an endolaryngeal tumor. The piriform sinuses are examined and opened to the apex with the lighted laryngoscope. The arytenoids are then examined and palpated to ensure mobility of the cricoarytenoid joint. Similarly, the vallecula and base of the tongue must be examined on entry or withdrawal of the laryngoscope by placing the scope between the epiglottis and the tongue. This ensures that a small carcinoma has not been ignored either as a presenting lesion or as a second simultaneous primary cancer. The endolarynx

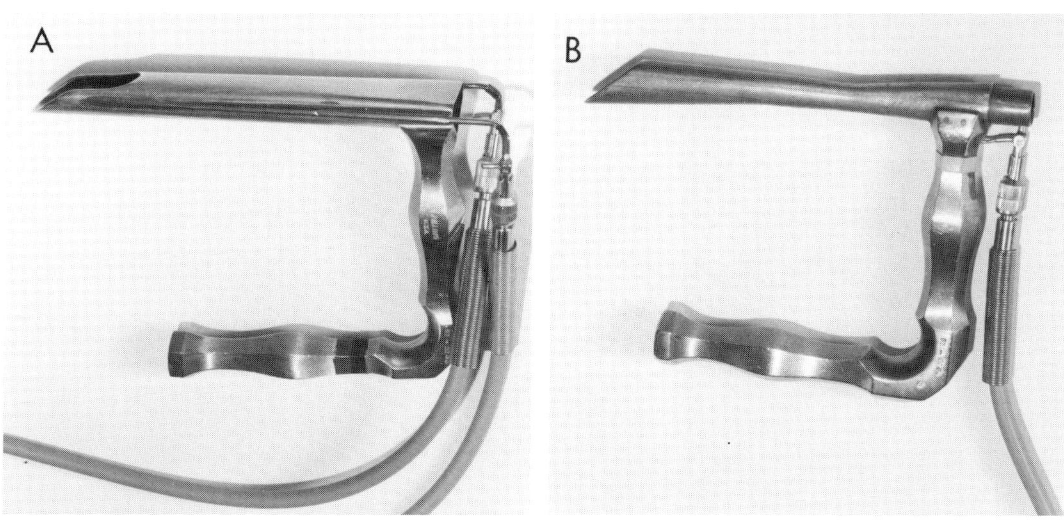

Fig 16–3.—Laryngoscopes used in endoscopy. The Jako laryngoscope *(left)* was among the first to allow careful well-lighted laryngoscopy with particular attention to the endolarynx. The Dedo laryngoscope *(right)* is a modification of the Jako scope and has a smaller tip. This allows better visibility of the anterior commissure and allows one to see the small (in the female) endolarynx more easily. Both scopes are equally good for examining the hypopharynx and postcricoid area.

is examined next. The anterior commissure *must* be clearly seen in all cases. The ventricle of the larynx must be opened to visualization using the blade of the laryngoscope, to ensure that what is apparently a glottic tumor is not concealing transglottic extension through the ventricle.

Deep biopsy specimens of suspected laryngeal carcinoma are taken so that the presence or absence of invasive characteristics of the neoplasm can be evaluated by the pathologist. If insufficient biopsy samples are submitted, the pathologist can only diagnose the tissue as malignant; he cannot judge the depth of invasion. Good biopsy technique will eliminate the need for repeating the procedure.

At the conclusion of the examination a map of the relationship of the tumor to the larynx (Fig 16–4) is drawn. It is good discipline to do this when writing the postoperative orders. The drawing produces a map of the direct laryngoscopic findings, the extent of the tumor, and the site of any biopsies. The drawing is added to a second appropriately labeled drawing that was made earlier during the office examination. Together, they reflect the observer's interpretations on both indirect and direct laryngoscopy. These visualizations are the surgeon's map for tumor staging and for the planning of treatment or resection.

The drawings are ultimately matched to the findings in the surgical specimen. Many such comparisons will help enlarge the surgeon's judgmental experience and are a method of checking the accuracy of both indirect and direct laryngoscopy. As such, they are an important self-teaching tool as well as an important part of the record to be shared with the pathologist in searching for clear surgical margins and with the radiation therapist during consultation about radiation therapy, either for definitive or adjuvant treatment.

When Are Bronchoscopy and Esophagoscopy Indicated?

It is our present recommendation that all patients who have a carcinoma of the head and neck undergo upper airway endoscopy to include not only laryngoscopy, as described above, but also esophagoscopy to the gastric introitus.[16, 17] When pulmonary symptoms are present or if the chest x-ray film is abnormal, bronchoscopy is done. These studies can be done with one anesthetic if there are no contraindications to extending the anesthetic. There is one important warning. If the patient is to undergo bronchoscopy, the upper airway carcinoma to be evaluated must not present any risk of obstructing or compromising the airway during or after the procedure. Bronchoscopy creates some risk of losing control of the airway in a patient with a large obstructing lesion. In our experience, bronchoscopy has not been rewarding in patients who have a normal chest x-ray film and no chest symptoms. In a series of 534 patients in whom we routinely used bronchoscopy, all carcinomas noted on bronchoscopy were found in patients who had an abnormal chest x-ray film. Therefore, we are more judicious in deciding when to include bronchoscopy. Several recent reports are in conflict about the value of positive bronchial washings with negative bronchoscopy examination and negative lung radiographs, and we presently do not depend on bronchial washings. We do search for a lung primary by CT scan if the cytology is positive, but the laryngeal tumor is the more likely site of the exfoliated cells.

Esophagoscopy is a low-risk procedure because the airway is controlled by an endotracheal tube. We have discovered four otherwise unrecognized and asymptomatic carcinomas of the esophagus in patients with simultaneous upper aerodigestive system carcinoma and a negative barium swallow.

HOW DO YOU CLASSIFY AN ABNORMAL LARYNGEAL BIOPSY SPECIMEN?

The diagnosis of laryngeal carcinoma requires a successful representative biopsy specimen of the lesion as well as effective communication with the pathologist who must interpret the microscopic pattern of the biopsy sample. It is important to give the pathologist a gross description of the lesion along with the adequate sample of the abnormal tissue. Whenever possible, a full stripping of the vocal cord under direct laryngoscopy is the best specimen for the pathologist to examine. Small-bite biopsies of abnormal tissue that do not include the full thickness of mucosa makes it impossible for the pathologist to recognize invasive cancer. Multifocal areas of carcinoma are common in the larynx and hypopharynx. It is wise to sample questionable areas adjacent to the obvious tumor. The biopsy information will help in making treatment decisions.

Carcinoma of the larynx is classified by its cell of origin. The single most frequent carcinoma is squamous cell carcinoma. Within the spectrum of epidermoid abnormalities, there are five general diagnoses the pathologist must consider: hyperkeratosis, hyperkeratosis with atypia, carcinoma in situ, superficially invasive carcinoma, and invasive carcinoma. Since there are different implications for the treatment of each category, the pathologist should define the particular characteristics of the lesion. All of these lesions may clinically present as only a white vocal cord or as erythroplakia. The vocal cord will often look swollen, which accounts for the patient's frequent complaint of a voice change or obvious hoarseness.

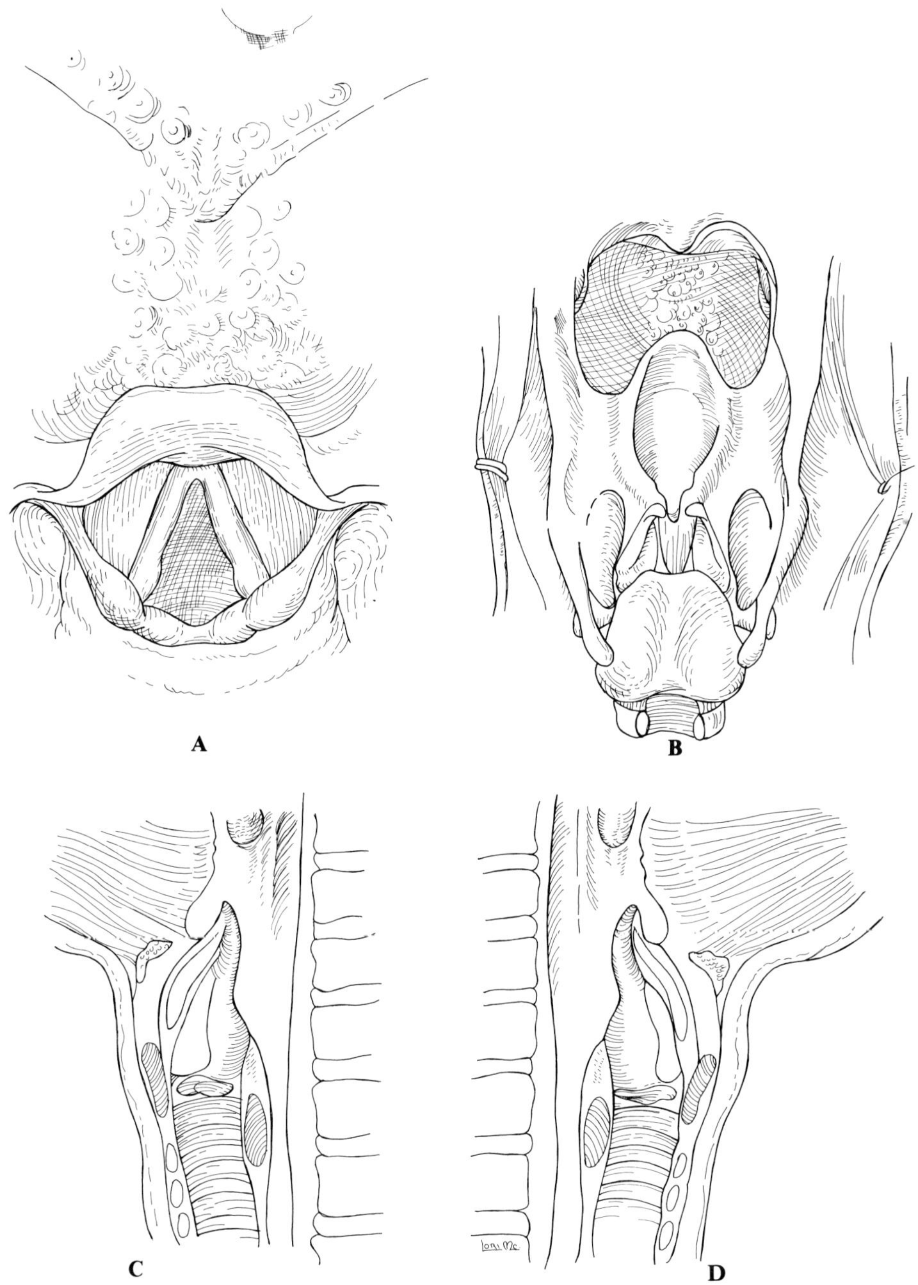

Fig 16–4.—Drawing of larynx for indirect laryngoscopy and direct endoscopy mapping of cancer. The location of tumor as recognized on indirect laryngeal drawing is penciled in. A similar and hand-labeled drawing of the tumor is made after direct laryngoscopy. These are used as a teaching aid; the tumor as it is drawn is compared to the surgical specimen.

Epidermoid Cancers

Hyperkeratosis.—Hyperkeratosis of the vocal cord is a histologic diagnosis used to describe an abnormally thick layer of keratin in a true vocal cord. It is imperative that the examining pathologist be aware of the normal depth of the vocal cord squamous layer to recognize what qualifies as hyperkeratosis. The biopsy specimen should show a good strip of lining showing normal underlying basement membrane to determine whether satisfactory stripping of all the abnormal tissue has been accomplished. Hyperkeratosis does not imply a precancerous lesion. However, hyperkeratosis with any atypia requires more careful observation and repeat stripping whenever the mucosa becomes suspicious again. Since most of these patients do continue to smoke, an invasive laryngeal carcinoma is likely to be detected on some subsequent examination. Patients with hyperkeratosis are followed up regularly for the rest of their lives and reexamined and biopsied as necessary under anesthesia in the operating room. Should the presenting symptom recur in an interval between examinations, the patient is obviously invited back to the office for reexamination.

HYPERKERATOSIS WITH ATYPIA.—The next diagnosis, hyperkeratosis with atypia, is more ominous. In such a biopsy specimen, there will be parakeratosis, or the presence of mature ghost cells closer to the basement membrane than would be normally expected. There is dyskeratosis with variable degrees of disorientation and proliferation of epithelial cells. This atypical pattern blends on its more benign side with pure hyperkeratosis and on its more malignant end with carcinoma in situ.[18]

CARCINOMA IN SITU.—In the larynx, carcinoma in situ may be considered as intraepithelial carcinoma. In such circumstances cytologic abnormalities exceeding dysplasia are present. The architecture is disrupted. As is true of carcinoma in situ in other sites, the diagnosis of carcinoma in situ in the larynx often is based on a biopsy specimen taken from an area adjacent to an invasive carcinoma. The clinical findings must be correlated with the pathology in light of this possibility. A second biopsy is probably needed if any gross mucosal lesion remains. More substantial tissue samples should be taken.

SUPERFICIAL CARCINOMA.—Superficial carcinoma should be treated.[19] Superficial carcinoma is beyond carcinoma in situ. It is diagnosed when shallow or early invasion extends below the basement membrane level. Some surgeons have been quite successful at adequate stripping of the vocal cord, with stripping repeated several months later to prove no more carcinoma is present. Radiation therapy has been also successful but probably represents overtreatment. At present, it appears that stripping can be repeated until the lesion recurs frequently or becomes more aggressive microscopically and therefore suggests the need for radiation therapy or surgery.[20] Laser techniques also can be used for the accurate removal of confirmed superficial carcinoma.

INVASIVE CARCINOMA.—The diagnosis of invasive carcinoma requires treatment in all cases. The criteria for deciding between radiation therapy or various types of surgery is individual and is discussed later.

Nonepidermoid Cancers

Not all cancers found on hypopharyngeal or laryngeal biopsy are epidermoid. The other cell types are briefly considered below.

PSEUDOSARCOMA.—Pseudosarcoma is a pathologic diagnosis made on rare occasions in patients with laryngeal carcinoma. At the University of Minnesota, our pathologist recognized six cases of pseudosarcoma out of 350 laryngeal malignancies.[21] A seventh case was recognized on slide review 8 years after treatment. Four of the patients had a pedunculated smooth mass. In three cases the mass was described as exophytic and more like the usual appearance of squamous carcinoma.

Histologically, pseudosarcoma is composed of areas of invasive squamous cell carcinoma extending through a stroma which has a sarcomatous appearance. It probably represents a malignant morphological variant of squamous cell carcinoma, in which the stomal cells are spindle-shaped epithelioid cells. It appears that these spindle cells possess independent metastatic capability, and therefore we now call these tumors *spindle cell carcinomas*.

Evidence of squamous differentiation as well as characteristics of invasiveness do not have prognostic value. In our experience as well as experience reported in the literature, metastases presage a bad prognosis.[22] Primary radiation therapy may be considered in selected cases. In general, we usually recommend surgical treatment. The usual pattern of metastasis and survival appears to parallel that of laryngeal squamous cell carcinoma, and therefore treatment should be comparable to that for similarly located staged squamous cell carcinoma of the larynx.

VERRUCOUS CARCINOMA.—Verrucous carcinoma is an unusual variant of laryngeal carcinoma. It represents 1%–2% of carcinomas. It is recognized both by its exophytic velvety appearance and by the absence of the conventional histologic features of invasive neoplasia.[23] Microscopically, it may resemble extensive hyperkeratosis, so the pathologist needs to know the gross clinical presentation and its resemblance to carcinoma. The age and sex distribution of patients with this lesion are similar to those of patients with squamous cell carcinoma. This lesion is relatively slowly growing and has a pushing margin rather than an infiltrating, submucosal, finger-like pattern.

It is generally accepted that verrucous carcinoma is not managed successfully by radiotherapy or cryotherapy. This lesion has developed into an anaplastic or sarcoma-like lesion after irradiation or cryotherapy in a sufficient number of cases that surgical treatment is favored. Conservation surgery can be employed for selected cases. Verrucous carcinomas of the larynx have not been reported to metastasize to cervical nodes; therefore, elective neck dissection is not warranted.

SMALL CELL CARCINOMA.—Small cell carcinoma was rarely described in the past. More recently it is being identified with more frequency as pathologists have refined their diagnostic criteria. Since the lungs and larynx share a common embryologic origin from primitive foregut, the neuroectodermal oat cell carcinoma must be considered in laryngeal cancer patients when the histologic and cytologic characteristics are present. If electron microscopy demonstrates neurosecretory granules and the biopsy suggests oat cell carcinoma, laryngectomy is not done immediately.

The treatment of such patients with chemotherapy may be the best therapeutic choice since the disease has a rapid systemic dissemination (which may represent multicentric origin). If the primary tumor remains after chemotherapy, radiation therapy or surgery can be added. This tumor is the one exception where an extensive metastatic workup is done before treating laryngeal cancer.

Head as well as body CT scanning is done before treatment is initiated for a laryngeal small cell tumor. When the tumor is treated by resection alone, the prognosis is grim. However, the occasional cases in the literature treated with chemotherapy have shown some suggestion of prolonged survival compared to previous treatment modalities.[24]

ADENOCARCINOMA.—Adenocarcinoma of the larynx is rare, accounting for less than 1% of all laryngeal malignancies.[25] Most institutional series, therefore, are very small, and the nine patients described by Sessions et al. represent a very large series.[26] The adenocarcinoma seems to arise in subglottic and supraglottic locations since there are very few salivary glands at the glottic level. Sessions feels that the adenocarcinoma is a highly lethal disease. The adenocystic variety appears to follow the persistent invasive pattern seen in both major and minor salivary glands with frequent recurrence and an ultimately poor prognosis. Because of slow growth, survivors may function well for 10–15 years. Based on his experience and a literature review, Sessions believes that radical surgery for laryngeal adenocarcinoma does not decrease the recurrence rate or prolong survival time. Therefore, it is recommended that wide local excision or conservation modes of surgery be undertaken whenever feasible. Neck dissection is not indicated unless palpable nodes are detected. The possibility that the adenocarcinoma represents a metastatic lesion to the larynx must be considered and discussed with the pathologist. A review of organ systems likely to be the site of a primary, such as breast, kidney, and gastrointestinal tract, must be undertaken before extirpative surgery is performed. An isolated pulmonary metastasis does not contraindicate aggressive treatment of the primary lesion since adenocystic carcinoma occasionally will lie dormant in a metastastic site for many years before requiring further attention.

WHAT ARE THE CHARACTERISTICS OF SPREAD OF LARYNGEAL AND HYPOPHARYNGEAL CANCERS?

To effectively stage and plan treatment for an epidermoid carcinoma involving the larynx, one must understand the biologic behavior of tumors in this unique area. The structure of the larynx and the somewhat different pattern of squamous cancer growth result in a functional "compartmentalization" in the larynx. Many intrinsic laryngeal lesions have a pushing margin, in contrast to hypopharyngeal lesions, which usually invade submucosally. The compartmentalization of the larynx (Pressman)[3] and the different patterns of tumor growth and extension determine survival and are reflected in tumor staging criteria. The predictable behavior is the keystone to conservation surgical techniques in laryngeal carcinoma (Fig 16–5).

Glottic carcinomas that arise on the free edge of the vocal cord usually spread along the vocal cord and involve the submucosal space of Reinke before they breach this compartment. Tumor growth occurs along this plane before extending across the ventricle to the supraglottis or before reaching more than 10 mm subglottically. By the time either of these advanced extensions has occurred, the lymphatic channels have generally been penetrated. With extension, the risk of metastasis to the neck nodes is substantially increased.

Once fixation of the deep structures of the intrinsic laryngeal muscles and arytenoid cartilage has occurred, the risk of invasion into the thyroid cartilage and to the neck has significantly increased, as has the likelihood of death from cancer. A tumor that originates at (or extends to) the anterior commissure is more likely to penetrate the thyroid cartilage since the anterior commissural ligament of Boyle is a weak point in the cartilaginous barrier to tumor spread. These biologic growth characteristics underlie the TNM system of laryngeal tumor classification. It should be noted, for example, that T_3 tumors represent laryngeal fixation, not gross tumor size. Fixation can occur with a relatively small tumor and is important in prognosis.

Ultimately, laryngeal carcinomas spread through lymphatic channels. Distant metastatic lesions from laryngeal carcinoma are unusual in the early stages. In the late stages, the patients who ultimately die of laryngeal cancer do have distant metastases that are a major contributing cause of death.[27–29]

The subglottic tumors spread earlier than glottic cancers because subglottic lesions can penetrate the cricothyroid membrane. This membrane, in contrast to thyroid or cricoid cartilage does not present a barrier of internal perichondrium, cartilage, and external perichondrium before tumor cells can reach the soft tissues of the neck. It is because of this early penetrating extension that partial surgery is less successful and rarely undertaken for tumors that originate in the subglottic location.

Supraglottic tumors, which usually form on the epiglottis or false vocal cord, spread within the supraglottic compartment before extending transglottically. They penetrate through the epiglottis to the pre-epiglottic

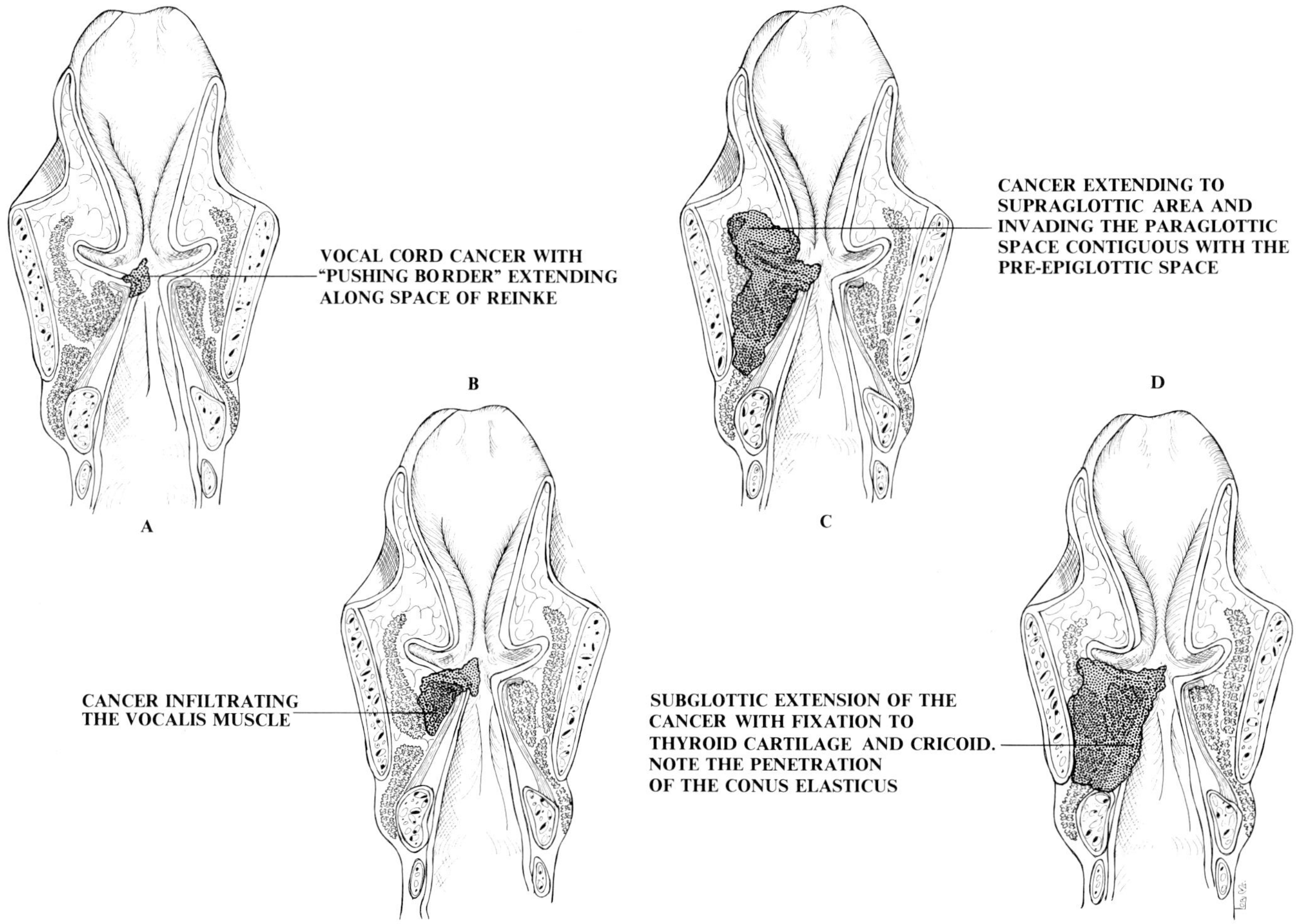

Fig 16–5.—Biology and patterns of invasion of laryngeal/hypopharyngeal cancer.

space before metastasizing more widely in the soft tissues. It is the nature of this predictable pattern of extension that allows partial surgery but anatomically limits the tissues that can be preserved. For example, supraglottic laryngectomy requires the excision of the hyoid bone and the superior half of the thyroid cartilage in conjunction with the laryngeal lumen to ensure adequate margins around the pre-epiglottic space.

HOW ARE LARYNGEAL AND HYPOPHARYNGEAL CARCINOMAS STAGED?

Because of the anatomical characteristics of the complex laryngeal mechanism and the biologic behavior of laryngeal epidermoid cancer, this area has a different basis for staging than other areas of the head and neck. Staging criteria are not based on size of the primary cancer for the T component of TNM staging. The staging of laryngeal cancer is shown in Table 16–1. The nodal staging criteria are the same as for other squamous cell cancers.

Hypopharyngeal cancer staging is also outlined in Table 16–1. Again, the proximity of such lesions to the structures of the pharyngolarynx and the frequent laryngeal involvement guide the staging.

WHAT TREATMENTS ARE AVAILABLE FOR CARCINOMA OF THE LARYNX?

The previous sections outlined how the various cancers are characterized and classified. There were hints of treatment modalities. Before treatment planning is discussed, it is appropriate to summarize the broad categories of treatment options. They are as follows:

- Radiation therapy
  - Primary site only
  - Primary site and cervical lymphatics
- Repeated local stripping of mucosa by endolaryngeal route
- Endolaryngeal laser excision
- Surgery
  - Frontolateral hemilaryngectomy
  - Extended frontolateral hemilaryngectomy with muscle flap reconstruction

TABLE 16–1.—TNM CLASSIFICATION OF CARCINOMA OF THE LARYNX AND LARYNGOPHARYNX

PRIMARY TUMOR (T)	
T_x	Minimum requirements to assess the primary tumor cannot be met
T_0	No evidence of primary tumor
Supraglottis	
T_{IS}	Carcinoma in situ
T_1	Tumor confined to site of origin with normal mobility
T_2	Tumor involves adjacent supraglottic site(s) or glottis, without fixation
T_3	Tumor limited to larynx with fixation or extension to involve postcricoid area, medial wall of piriform sinus, or pre-epiglottic space
T_4	Massive tumor extending beyond the larynx to involve oropharynx, soft tissues of neck, or destruction of thyroid cartilage
Glottis	
T_{IS}	Carcinoma in situ
T_1	Tumor confined to vocal cord(s) with normal mobility (including involvement of anterior or posterior commissures)
T_2	Supraglottic or subglottic extension of tumor with normal or impaired cord mobility
T_3	Tumor confined to the larynx with cord fixation
T_4	Massive tumor with thyroid cartilage destruction or extension beyond the confines of the larynx, or both
Subglottis	
T_{IS}	Carcinoma in situ
T_1	Tumor confined to the subglottic region
T_2	Tumor extension to vocal cords with normal or impaired cord mobility
T_3	Tumor confined to larynx with cord fixation
T_4	Massive tumor with cartilage destruction or extension beyond the confines of the larynx, or both

Anterior commissurectomy with keel
Subtotal laryngectomy with reconstruction
Supraglottic (horizontal) laryngectomy
Partial laryngopharyngectomy
Total laryngectomy
Total laryngopharyngectomy

The use of irradiation is discussed below in the detailed treatment of various stages. Endolaryngeal resection is done for small carcinomas limited to the free edge of the true vocal cord or to the epiglottis. Suspension laryngoscopy is used. The epiglottis can be resected with appropriately designed instruments that will reach through the metal tube. With the use of the operating microscope, microdissection of a small lesion of the true vocal cord is possible. Repeated vocal cord stripping may be sufficient treatment for *very small* microinvasive tumors on the free edge of the vocal cord.

This technique is extended by using the CO_2 laser and has allowed small lesions to be vaporized and removed.[30] Laser surgery is not magic. It is just another controlled method of removing tissue using microlaryngeal cutting or laser techniques.

Endolaryngeal cordectomy and epiglottectomy are possible. In selected *very small* lesions; local excision may be the treatment of choice. It is mandatory in such circumstances to ensure that the actual surgical margins are clear, since this microsurgery approaches within 2 mm of the border between normal tissue and tumor. This close margin is usually successful in carcinoma of the intrinsic larynx because the tumor has a pushing behavior rather than a tendency to be deeply infiltrating. As a result of this clinical characteristic, it is possible to achieve gross margins on endolaryngeal tumors of 2–3 mm and still be successful in curing the patient. Such a small margin would be totally unsatisfactory for resecting hypopharyngeal or oral cavity carcinomas, where the gross margin may be 5–15 mm from the microscopic free edge.

Glottic carcinoma is detected early because of symptoms of hoarseness. Most of the tumors discovered are at a T_1 (60%) or T_2 (25%) stage when first recognized. The options for treatment include surgical resection and radiation therapy.[31] For tumors that are isolated to one side of the larynx and that originate on the mobile vocal cord, a hemilaryngectomy offers a good opportunity for both cure and rehabilitation. Vertical hemilaryngectomy is 90%–95% successful as the sole treatment for eradication of clinical stage T_1 cancer of the mobile vocal cord.[32] A vertical hemilaryngectomy will encompass the internal perichondrium and cartilage and excise sufficiently wide margins around all of the tumor (Fig 16–6). Early glottic cancers almost never metastasize to the neck nodes. Therefore, vertical hemilaryngectomy need not include a neck dissection unless a palpable node is noted. An in-continuity hemilaryngectomy with radical neck dissection is kept as an option. The limited lymphatic drainage from the vocal cord is thought to be the reason for the paucity of lymph node metastases in vocal cord cancers detected early. Only if the cancer penetrates through cartilage or invades the rich lymphatic channels in the supraglottis and subglottis does it then spread to the neck nodes.

Small-port x-ray therapy is the alternative to limited laryngeal surgery.[33, 34] This mode is usually quite successful for small glottic cancers. In many centers irradiation is the preferred treatment for vocal cord carcinoma limited to the mobile vocal cord. The remaining voice is better. Not all patients are spared operative treatment. Salvage laryngeal surgery is required to bring the cure rate of irradiation to that of surgery alone.

Patient series reporting success with either radiotherapy or partial surgery must be carefully analyzed. The results of limited primary treatment are bolstered by subsequent salvage surgery. If this added effect is not accurately reported, the data will reflect spuriously optomistic results of irradiation.

TREATMENT OF T_1 VOCAL CORD CARCINOMA

Most T_1 vocal cord carcinomas are treated by radiation therapy. Approximately 10%–20% of carcinomas so

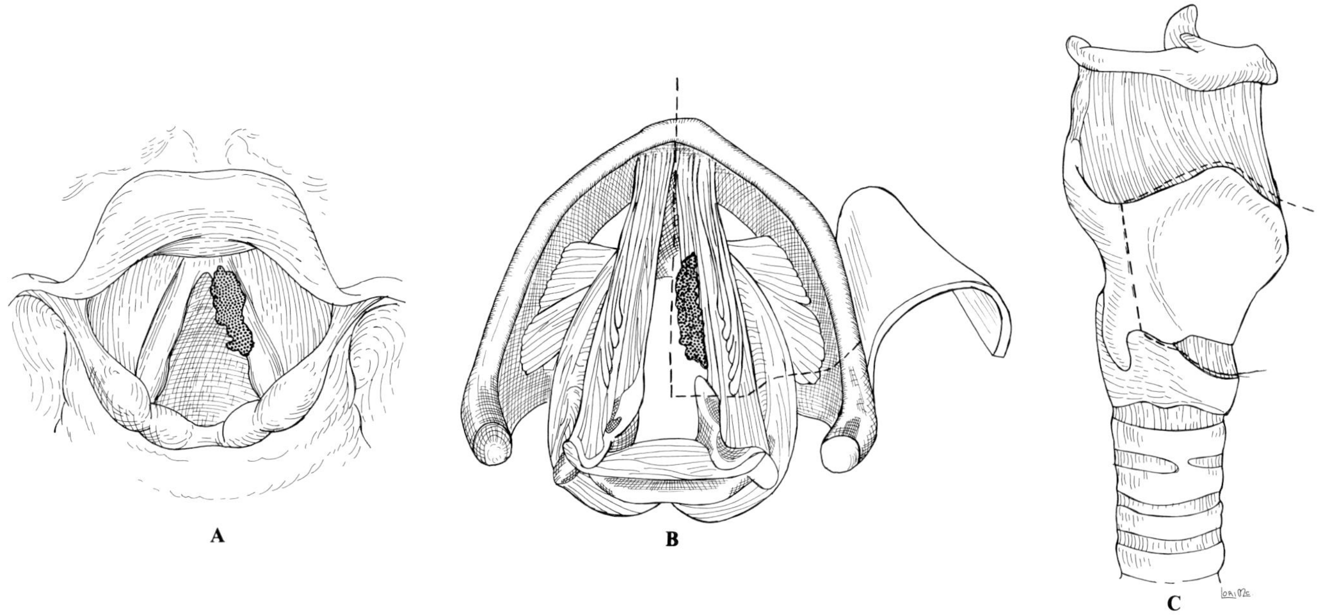

Fig 16–6.—Vertical hemilaryngectomy. **A,** true cord tumor located on a mobile cord is seen to be approaching the anterior commissure. **B** and **C,** the perichondrium is elevated and subsequently used for closure. Cartilage and mucosal cuts are made.

treated either fail to respond to irradiation or recur in the same location, a circumstance which is encountered by even the most skilled radiation therapist. Salvage surgery is then necessary. Where a T_1 lesion persists or recurs and has the same gross appearance as it originally did, a vertical hemilaryngectomy can be a safe tumor operation. The operating surgeon must have examined the patient before radiation therapy so that he is aware of the original margins of the tumor. To achieve a cure, these original margins must be excised even if the tumor is not as large as it was originally.

After radiation failure it is necessary to have wider margins around the tumor than would be necessary if the tumor had been initially treated by surgery alone. Radiation therapy changes the histologic and clinical pattern from a pushing, less invasive tumor of a true vocal cord to a more aggressive burrowing pattern.

The surgical margins are carefully checked on frozen sections. Occasionally the pathologist will report that the mucosal margins appear positive on permanent histologic section when the original gross examination had suggested that there were several millimeters of clear mucosa. The preparation of the microscopic slide may cause more contraction of the mucosal margins than shrinkage of the tumor, thus creating a false image that the tumor is crowding the edge of resection.[35] This is hypothesized to explain the evidence that the cure rate of T_1 lesions with positive and negative margins is virtually the same.

Not all T_1 lesions should be treated by irradiation as a "first therapy." Unreliable patients and selected patients, such as those under 40 years of age, should have hemilaryngectomy as the preferred treatment for mobile vocal cord lesions. There is some long-term hazard of radiation-induced cancer. Some centers favor initial surgical treatment because of their excellent experience with cure and voice preservation. If excellent radiotherapy facilities are close at hand and the patient can tolerate 6–7 weeks of outpatient therapy, radiation is recommended for most mobile cord $T_1N_oM_o$ lesions. The surgeon must have correctly mapped the tumor and must not have underdiagnosed a cancer that is actually too large to expect a reliable cure from irradiation.

Often, when a T_1 vocal cord carcinoma recurs, it is too large or has invaded too widely or deeply to allow hemilaryngectomy. A wide-field laryngectomy is then performed and the patient rehabilitated, as described below.

A glottic lesion is defined to be no greater than 10 mm below the ventricle. Tumors with 12–15 mm of subglottic extension can be excised by removing the superior third of the cricoid plate. Further extension of this operation for larger subglottic extension risks destroying the function of the larynx in speaking and creates chronic aspiration.

A vertical hemilaryngectomy can be planned for tumors that recur after radiation if both the original and recurrent tumors are localized to the area where the lesion can be easily encompassed.

The frontolateral hemilaryngectomy is the appropriate operation for small recurrent tumors. The larynx is entered through cartilage cuts made on the posterior lamina of the ipsilateral thyroid cartilage and through a separate cut just to the contralateral side of the midline of the thyroid cartilage. Before the cartilage cuts are made, the external perichondrium is peeled back and preserved for use for closure of the anterior larynx. The true and false cords are excised, including the muscular process of the arytenoid cartilage. Mucosal closure and flap rotation are not needed.

The perichondrium is closed after the contralateral cord has been sutured to the midline anteriorly. The preserved strap muscles form the next layer of closure, and the skin incision is then approximated in layers. A pseudocord of scar tissue forms and opposes the mobile contralateral cord. A satisfactory but hoarse voice results. Swallowing is not impeded.[36, 37]

T_1 ANTERIOR COMMISSURE CANCER

The anterior commissure resection is used for horseshoe-shaped tumors of the anterior commissure that remain at the glottic level. Resection is often done with the insertion of a keel to prevent laryngeal stenosis due to webbing and foreshortening of the larynx (Fig 16–7). While more radiotherapists are adept in treating midline anterior laryngeal tumors than previously, the anterior commissure of the larynx is among the more difficult areas of the body in which small tumors may be successfully treated by radiation therapy. The constant movement of the front of the larynx with respiration during irradiation will occasionally alter the dose actually administered from the desired calculated radiation dose. The radiotherapist must place the machine firmly against the larynx, creating significant discomfort during the treatment, to ensure that an accurate and complete tumoricidal dose is administered.

Because of the poor cure rate achieved with radiation therapy for lesions of the anterior commissure, many surgeons recommend an anterior commissure hemilaryngectomy.[38] The anterior third of each vocal cord along with the corresponding section of thyroid cartilage is removed and the larynx is stented in the open position by a keel, which is preferable to an intraluminal stent since the keel restores the triangular appearance of the glottis and prevents foreshortening. The keel can be intraluminal and secured by translaryngeal wires tied in the lateral neck. This permits endoscopic removal without an external incision.[39, 40] The keel is removed, often under local anesthesia, 5–6 weeks postoperatively. The treatment is quite successful as a cancer operation and leaves the patient swallowing easily, albeit with a hoarse and often weaker voice. Such a voice is serviceable but unpredictable.

The usual hemilaryngectomy requires an epiglottoplasty suturing the petiole securely around the hyoid bone with a large 2–0 suture. Tucker et al.[41] and Schechter[42] have used the epiglottis in the repair of the anterior commissure and extended ventral lateral hemilaryngectomies. They find this technique to offer the best glottic aperture after such resection, with no significant aspiration. Their technique requires retraction of the epiglottis into the surgical defect after removing mucosa, fibrofatty tissue, and the suspensory ligaments on the anterior surface of the epiglottis. The flap is sutured in place with interrupted sutures that bring the mucosal edges into close approximation. Voice quality after this operation is variable and is a function of arytenoid mobility.

T_1 VOCAL CORD CARCINOMA WITH ARYTENOID INVASION

The extended frontolateral hemilaryngectomy, often with total arytenoidectomy on the involved side, offers a third opportunity to preserve the voice and remove a vocal cord carcinoma.[43] [This operation has been extended for use with reasonable success in more ad-

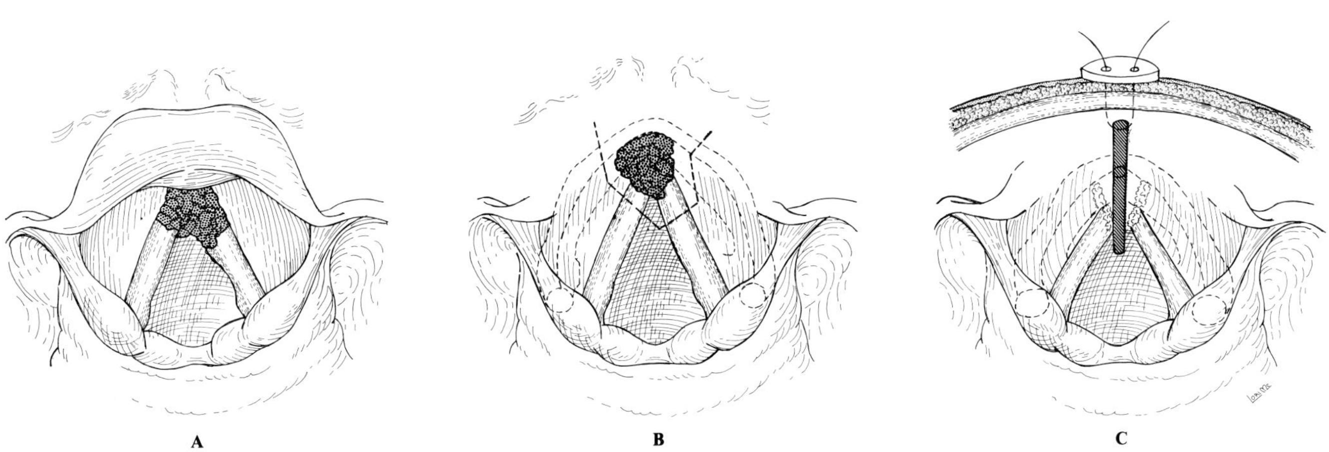

Fig 16–7.—Anterior commissure resection with insertion of keel.

vanced T_3 (fixed cord) carcinomas of the vocal cord.] The extended frontolateral hemilaryngectomy allows resection of up to one third of the opposite cord, along with total hemilaryngectomy to include resection of the body of the arytenoid. Strap muscle flaps (sternohyoid and sternothyroid) are necessary to reconstruct the posterior bulk removed with the arytenoid (Fig 16–8).[44] Some surgeons rotate mucosal flaps from the piriform sinus to allow earlier mucosal healing and prevent scarring. It is necessary to overcorrect the needed bulk on the arytenoid and to try to use the tendinous portion of the strap muscles with lysis of the ansa hypoglossi nerve to prevent motion of the muscle flap. Should the muscle flap remain overgenerous after a satisfactory duration of healing, endoscopic removal of the obstructing bulk can be achieved using CO_2 laser techniques.

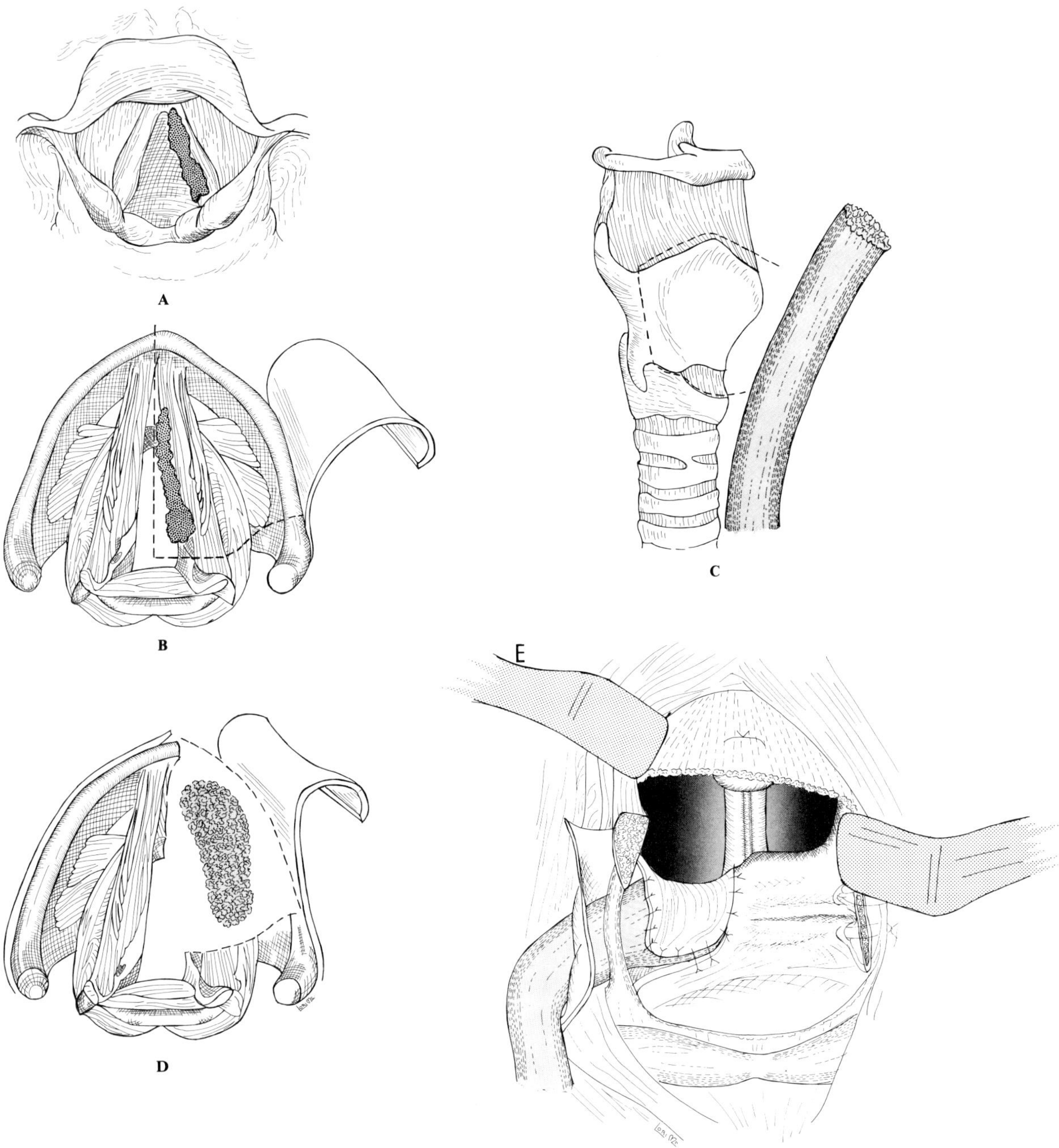

Fig 16–8.—Use of muscle flap in extended vertical hemilaryngectomy. **A,** tumor is located posteriorly and seen to involve the vocal process. **B,** tissue to be excised is outlined. **C,** strap muscle flap is prepared for insertion. **D,** bed for muscle flap. **E,** muscle flap is inserted through perichondrium.

OTHER FEATURES OF HEMILARYNGECTOMY

Can Hemilaryngectomy Be Extended to More Advanced Cancers of the Vocal Cord?

A technique introduced by Pearson et al. has permitted even wider resection of the larynx with primary reconstruction, with the objective of retaining both vocalization and swallowing despite a need for permanent tracheostomy.[45] In an effort to treat T_3 carcinoma of the larynx with surgery while preserving vocalization, Pearson has endeavored to preserve one side of the larynx along with the vascular supply and nerve supply from the recurrent laryngeal nerve. This surgical excision of a transglottic or glottic cancer with a fixed cord includes resection of the ipsilateral vertical hemilarynx, including the cricoid. The contralateral laryngeal mucosa is combined with the pyriform sinus flap to allow a tracheal hypopharyngeal phonotory shunt to be created. As a result of preserving the recurrent laryngeal nerve, this tube contracts on swallowing to prevent aspiration. A permanent tracheostoma is necessary, but, in selected cases with localized disease, this neoglottic technique has been quite successful. The extended hemilaryngectomy should be considered as an alternative to total laryngectomy. Other techniques of phonotory shunting have also been very successful and will be described later in this chapter.

What Are Some of the Complications of Hemilaryngectomies?

Vertical hemilaryngectomy is a procedure that has little operative or perioperative morbidity since the surgeon enters only the larynx, not the pharynx. Feeding is by nasogastric tube or esophagostomy tube for a period of 5–7 days. After that time, oral feedings can usually be resumed. A tracheostomy tube is left in place until the glottic airway is sufficient. It is then removed and the stoma allowed to close by secondary intention after the size of the tracheostomy tube has been reduced to a No. 5 Jackson tube or a comparable tube and this smaller tube has been plugged for a period of 24 hours. Occasionally patients aspirate after hemilaryngectomy because of either excess glottic aperture or an incompetent and inadequate cough reflex. Most patients do not have clinically important aspiration problems, as shown by barium swallow. The occasional debilitated patient with poor pulmonary reserve may have long-term problems after hemilaryngectomy, but this is much less frequent than after other forms of partial laryngectomy.

Failure to secure the epiglottis petiole to the hyoid bone with a suture can permit the epiglottis to obstruct the larynx both functionally and visually. Consequently, the airway is partially obstructed, and postoperative indirect mirror evaluation searching for tumor recurrence is difficult. This problem is presently treatable to some extent by laser surgery. Open reduction of the epiglottis may be necessary.

Surgery may leave the patient with an incompetent larynx. He aspirates food and saliva. Such patients also have a barely audible voice. Treatment of both problems must be offered. The incompetent larynx requires either a maintenance tracheostomy or open technique to increase the bulk of the residual pseudocord. Teflon injection rarely is successful in this circumstance since no thyroid cartilage lamina remains to buttress the injected Teflon and keep it where the surgeon injects it. Teflon injection is more successful after a horizontal hemilaryngectomy, as it is for patients with unilateral vocal cord paralysis.

Extension of the hemilaryngectomy indications by allowing resection of half the vertical dimension of the anterior aspect of the cricoid has allowed voice preservation and safe tumor resection in patients with subglottic extension. Resecting the cricoid, however, does increase the risk of chondritis and loss of the subglottic airway. It may also produce a prolonged period of aspiration. Reconstruction of the cricoid with autogenous cartilage from other parts of the body, including the opposite thyroid cartilage lamina, has been successful.[46]

On rare occasions the glottis remains edematous or overly bulky after the reconstruction. The patient is unable to be decannulated. Subglottic stenosis may occur due to surgery on the cricoid or from a tracheostomy placed either too high or complicated by excessive granulation tissue. These situations can be corrected using the CO_2 laser to excise the excess tissue. An occasional patient, however, requires a persistent tracheostomy to maintain an adequate airway.

Orocutaneous fistula occasionally occurs in the heavily irradiated patient when the two laminae of the thyroid cartilage fail to heal. Fistulization through the strap muscles occurs anteriorly. If secondary healing does not occur, rotation flaps can be used to close the fistula. The patient usually continues to swallow satisfactorily while healing, so morbidity from this complication is not major.

Chronic thyroid cartilage chondritis secondary to infection or radiation damage can contribute to persistent laryngeal edema. Treatment consists of long-term antibiotics and, if available, hyperbaric oxygen "diving" to try to reduce acute exacerbations.

Patients with persistent laryngeal edema must be suspected of having an occult tumor recurrence. Biopsy, while necessary, can exacerbate the chondritis. A nonfunctional, edematous, painful larynx may need to be excised to preserve swallowing, to isolate the lungs, and to remove the tissue to be sure no cancer remains.

How Successful Is Vertical Hemilaryngectomy?

The risk of local recurrence when the tumor is correctly assessed preoperatively is small. The cure rate for primary surgery should be 90%–95% for mobile cord tumors and about 80% for most T_2 lesions. The success rate falls approximately to 60% when this operation is used for small T_3 lesions. Kirchner and Som studied serially sectioned laryngeal specimens of T_3 cord cancers and concluded that with less than 10 mm of subglottic extension (anteriorly) and 5–6 mm extension posteriorly, hemilaryngectomy would be 60% successful in curing the tumor.[47] Total laryngectomy offers approximately the same cure rate. Large T_3 lesions are not effectively managed by partial surgery. It is mandatory, however, that the surgeon carefully select patients with T_3 lesions for such partial surgery. The unsophisticated surgeon should not attempt this operation. These lesions, with a fixed cord, can invade deeply. Statistically, surgery is clearly superior to radiation, by a margin of almost 3:1, in patients with T_3 cancers.[47, 48]

While reconstruction of the cricoid using fragments of thyroid cartilage has been successful,[46] we presently do not perform extended partial resections for subglottic tumors. We have elected total laryngectomy with immediate voice restoration techniques in their stead. An occasional patient with a small transglottic tumor (T_2) that barely comes to the false vocal cord is eligible for hemilaryngectomy rather than total resection. The patient must be prepared to accept a total laryngectomy when such surgery is contemplated, since deep invasion may be discovered in the operating room. Postoperative radiation therapy for invasive tumors is not necessary if the surgical margins are free of tumor and confirm the clinical impression.

When Is a Horizontal Hemilaryngectomy Indicated?

Supraglottic laryngectomy is indicated for a tumor limited to the supraglottic compartment of the larynx when there is no evidence of thyroid cartilage invasion. The pre-epiglottic space may be invaded by tumor and must be emcompassed by the operative procedure (Fig 16–9). The pulmonary reserve in such patients must be adequate to tolerate loss of the protection of the epiglottis and false vocal cords. All patients who have this operation will aspirate frequently in the early postoperative period and continue to do so in some minor degree. Those whose physiologic function is equivalent to

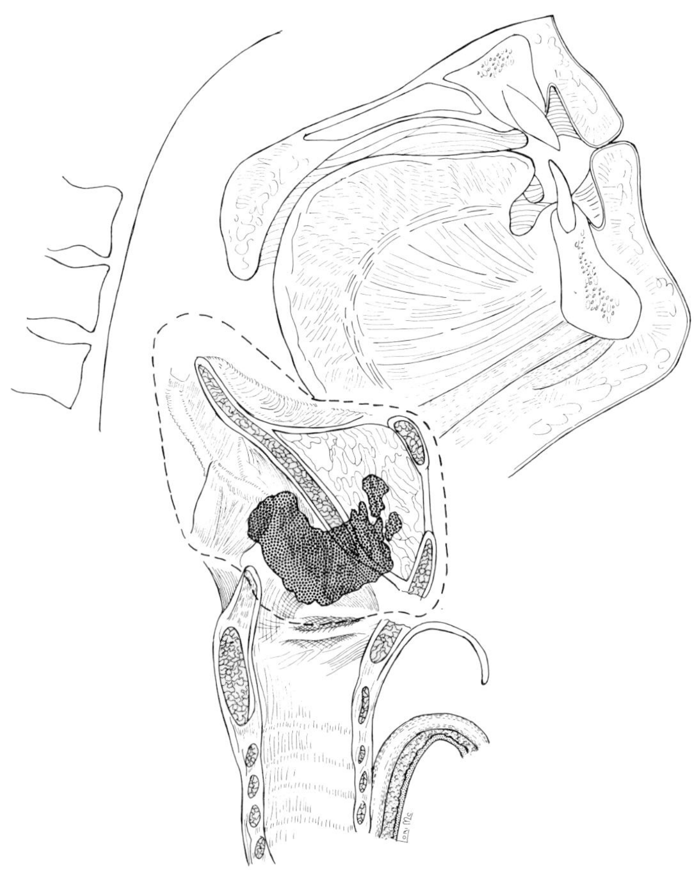

Fig 16–9.—Supraglottic cancer invading through the pre-epiglottic space.

that of someone over 65–70 years of age and who have chronic obstructive lung disease are at great risk of recurrent bouts of postoperative pneumonia. Careful selection must be done before considering partial surgery for supraglottic cancers. Supraglottic lesions have a substantial risk of being associated with occult metastases. Preoperative pulmonary function tests must be completed. We generally want at least 50% of predicted 1-second expiratory volume before recommending partial surgery in patients with supraglottic tumors. Simple clinical tests such as the ability to walk a flight of stairs without stopping will contribute to the preoperative evaluation (see the "treppen-sprechen" test, described in Chap. 5).

The pure subtotal supraglottic laryngectomy for epiglottic and false vocal cord lesions is standard and quite successful in obtaining local control of the disease (Fig 16–10).[49–54] Supraglottic cancers have a definitive probability that there are lymph node metastasis (Table 16–2) (up to 15%–33%), depending on the location of their primary lesion. For this reason radical neck dissection is usually done in conjunction with the supraglottic laryngectomy on the ipsilateral side.[55] A conservation neck dissection for N_0 necks is accepted by many people. Cranial nerve XI as well as the sternomastoid muscle may be preserved. Some physicians prefer radiation therapy to both sides of the neck as an alternative to lymphadenectomy in N_0 necks. The cure rate with partial surgery is equivalent to that with total laryngectomy and approximates 70% in T_1 and T_2 lesions of the supraglottis. Local recurrence is very rare if the surgical margins are secure. Jacobs et al.[56] found an 8.5% risk of local recurrence after supraglottic laryngectomy, with most failures found after treating lesions requiring extended subtotal supraglottic laryngectomy. Lesions of the epiglottis (which either perforate to the lingual surface or which flow over the lingual surface) and cancers that involve the vallecula (but are more than 1 cm from the circumvallate papillae) are amenable to an extended supraglottic laryngectomy in which the superior margin of resection goes through the base of the tongue. This procedure requires closure under greater tension and brings the base of the tongue and the laryngeal remnant closer together (Fig 16–11). As a result, aspiration is more likely and more severe. Since these tumors involve (at least partly) the oropharynx, the cure rate is lower and similar to that of oropharyngeal cancers.

The risk of wound breakdown and fistula formation is greater than after a horizontal hemilaryngectomy. After *extended* supraglottic laryngectomy, patients should be referred for radiotherapy consultation since their risk of local recurrence is much higher than that of patients who undergo simple supraglottic laryngectomy.

It appears to be useful to do a cricopharyngeal myotomy on a patient at the same time as the extended partial laryngectomy. We continue to recommend it. It is not clear whether a myotomy is necessary with a pure supraglottic laryngectomy.

In summary, the indications for a supraglottic laryngectomy include all T_1 and T_2 tumors involving the supraglottis. Tumors located inferior to the hyoid bone are more aggressive in invading the pre-epiglottic space and therefore are recommended for surgery. Suprahyoid supraglottic lesions may be more successfully treated with radiation therapy, and surgery is not always necessary for these tumors.

HOW IS A SUPRAGLOTTIC LARYNGECTOMY DONE?

The technique for supraglottic laryngectomy requires a horizontal cartilage cut across the thyroid cartilage after elevating and preserving the perichondrium (see Figs 16–10,A and B). In men, this is usually performed at the junction of the upper and middle thirds of the thyroid cartilage, and in women, at about 50% of the vertical height of the thyroid cartilage. The incision usually is made with a oscillating saw, as a transverse

TABLE 16–2.—INCIDENCE OF CERVICAL METASTASES IN 401 CASES TREATED BY TOTAL OR PARTIAL LARYNGECTOMY WITH NECK DISSECTION*

LOCATION	NO. OF CASES	INCIDENCE OF METASTASES (PALPABLE AND OCCULT)	INCIDENCE OF OCCULT METASTASES
Supraglottic			
Epiglottis	51	16/51 (31%)	7/42 (16%)
Epiglottis and false cord	63	35/63 (55%)	12/40 (30%)
Epiglottis, false and true cords	21	11/21 (53%)	5/15 (33%)
Piriform	111	84/111 (75%)	19/46 (41%)
Aryepiglottic fold	2	2/2 (100%)	. . .
Pharyngeal wall	6	5/6 (83%)	2/3 (66%)
Base of tongue	49	30/49 (61%)	6/25 (24%)
Transglottic (true and false cords only)	66	21/66 (31%)	7/52 (13%)
Glottic and subglottic	32	6/32 (18%)	2/28 (7%)

*From Ogura and Biller.[50] Reproduced by permission.

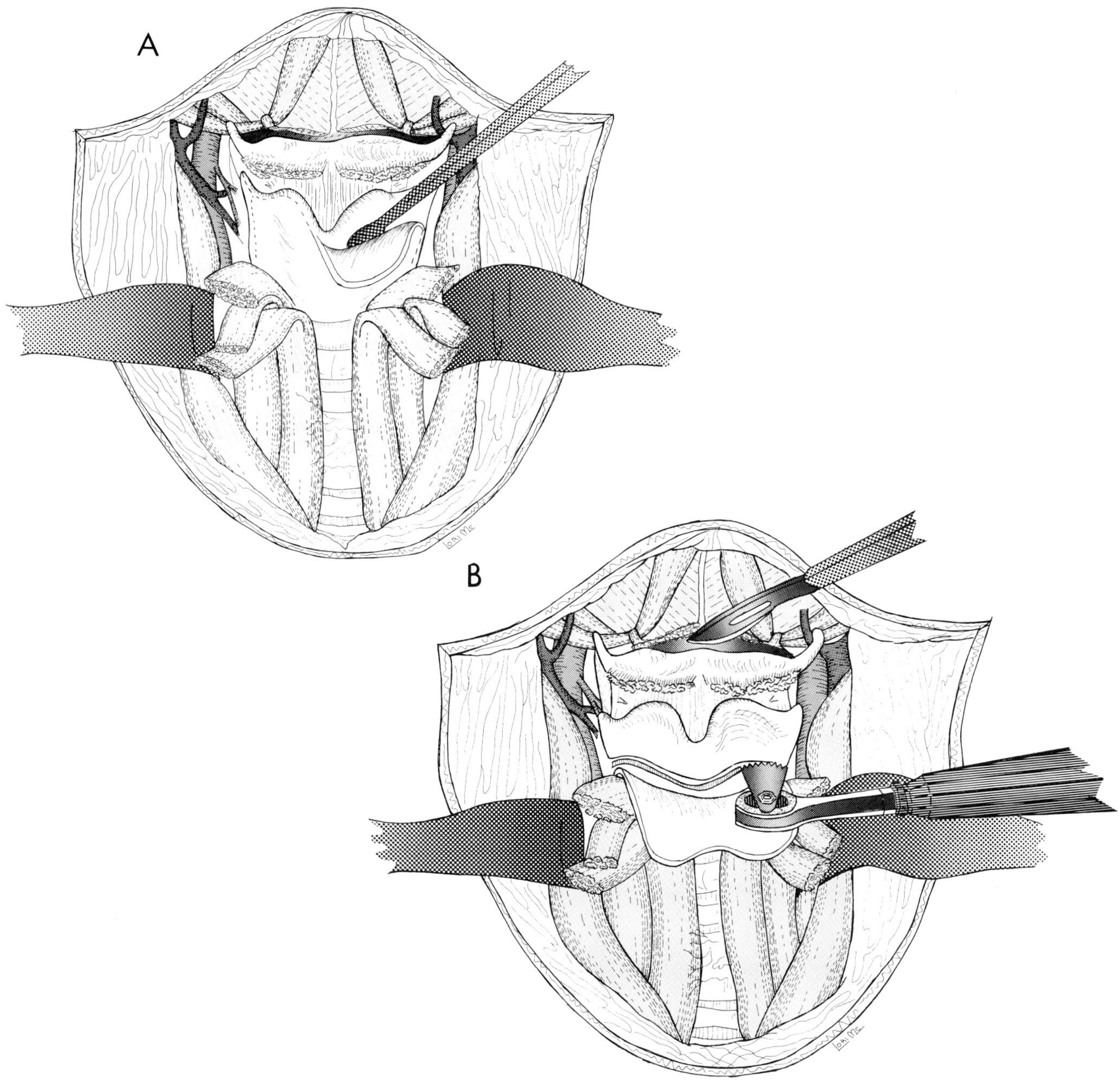

Fig 16–10.—Supraglottic laryngectomy. **A,** perichondrium is elevated off the thyroid cartilage. **B,** thyroid cartilage is incised with a saw. A knife is used to skeletonize hyoid bone and the greater cornua of thyroid cartilage. *(continued).*

incision, and the resected cartilage should include both superior cornu. The hyoid bone is skeletonized and is removed completely (see Fig 16–10,B). Some surgeons preserve the contralateral hyoid and superior cornu of the thyroid lamina and incorporate them into the closure. This is done to preserve the sensory function of the superior laryngeal nerve and reduce early aspiration problems. The suprahyoid muscles are stripped from the hyoid. This is necessary to be sure that the entire pre-epiglottic space is removed as a surgical block. The larynx is entered either in the vallecula or the contralateral piriform sinus, and good visualization of the tumor is achieved (see Fig 16–10,C). The epiglottis is grasped, and under direct vision the aryepiglottic folds are cut with a scissors, one blade placed internally in the ventricle of the larynx and the other placed externally through the thyroid cartilage cut. The cut is made on the less involved side and moving toward the mid-

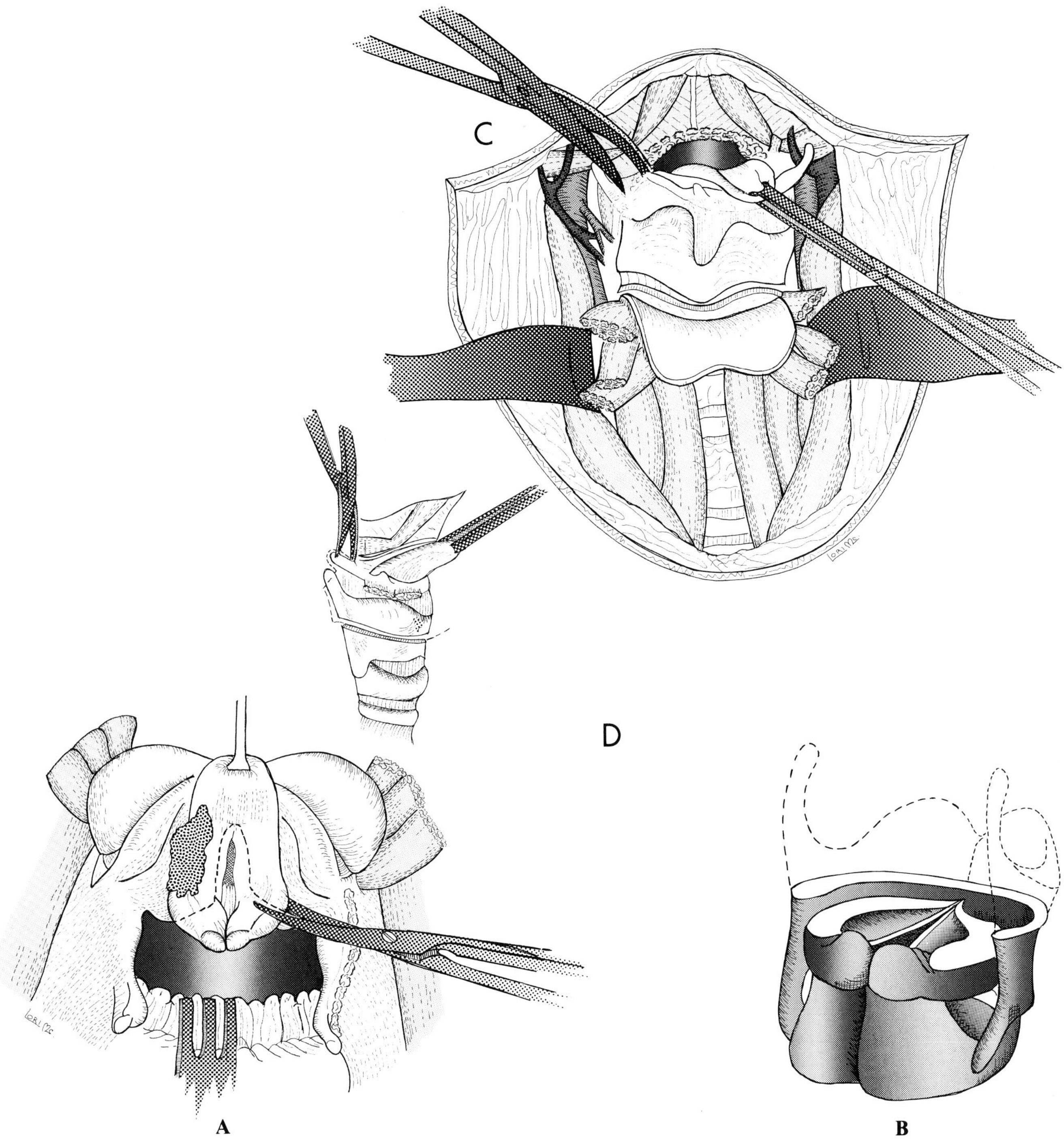

Fig 16–10 (cont.).—C, vallecula is entered. **D,** tumor and supraglottis are excised.

line; then the side with the bulk of the tumor is resected. In this way the larynx is opened like a book so that the most important page (involved side) may be under optimal visualization for resection. At the completion of this part of the procedure, both false vocal cords have been removed and the superior mucosal surface of the true vocal cords is left intact (see Fig 16–10,D). If there is then a clinical suspicion of cord involvement, a strip of the true vocal cord can be taken for frozen section to be sure margins are adequate. If necessary, the superior half of the true vocal cord can be removed to achieve satisfactory margins (see Fig 16–11,A). It is important to have bilateral mobile vocal cords to minimize the risk of aspiration. The wound is

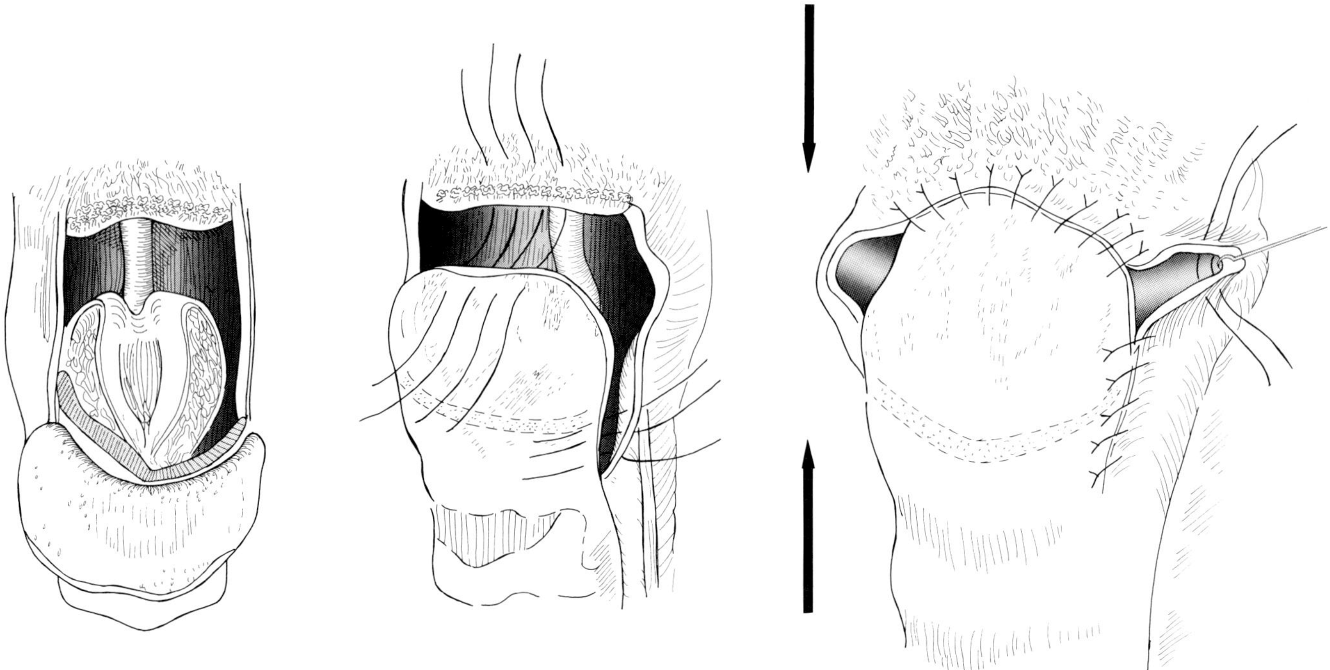

A B C

Fig 16–11.—Closure of supraglottic laryngectomy. **A,** resection completed. **B,** sutures placed from tongue base and from lateral pharyngeal wall to thyroid perichondrium. **C,** pharynx closed on itself (with sutures) to complete watertight closure.

closed by interrupted nonabsorbable sutures incorporating the perichondrium of the larynx and approximating it to the base of tongue musculature. The mucosa is not included in the suture since it will increase the tension of closure and the risk of suture line breakdown. These sutures are placed and then tied from the midline laterally, to decrease tension on the suture line. Two or three layers of strap muscle are approximated and the skin incision is closed in two layers (see Fig 16–11,B).

Alternative techniques of closure to ensure primary healing and avoid fistualization include placing the sutures through the thyroid cartilage directly, or using wire suspension sutures from the thyroid cartilage to lateral and anterior midline drill holes placed in the mandible.[57, 58] The techniques of laryngeal suspension have not improved swallowing as they were intended to do. Suspension wires are used only when the tension of closure is high and the risk of fistualization is increased.

Constant suction drainage is necessary when a radical neck dissection has been done. The suction drains are removed approximately 3–6 days postoperatively, usually when the drainage has decreased to below approximately 30 cc per 8-hour shift of observation.

If wound closure is unsatisfactory, then planned fistula formation is wiser and safer. The planned fistula avoids extensive flap necrosis and carotid artery exposure. A planned fistula should be created in the midline to keep salivary flow away from the carotid artery. The direct fistula can be kept clean with dressings and intermittent suction. At 2 weeks the fistula is usually well matured and can be closed by inversion of mucosa, with a secondary closure of skin drawn from local flaps in the neck.

Partial supraglottic laryngectomy requires that several important decisions be made by the surgeon and medical consultants. The patient must tolerate the expected complications as well as the occasional but anticipated complication of an orocutaneous fistula. The patient must be prepared to experience, and the physician to treat, minor episodes of aspiration pneumonia and possibly a major lobar pneumonia. Aspiration pneumonia can occur after the tracheostomy tube is removed, the glottic edema is reduced, and the patient begins to swallow actively.

A foldover laryngectomy can be done if the supraglottic tumor has spilled onto the true vocal cord. In such an operation, the true vocal cord is removed and the thyroid cartilage rolled over to create a submucosal support against which the opposite cord can close. One must be careful not to injure the ipsilateral recurrent laryngeal nerve or the arytenoid cartilage in such an operation since posterior glottic closure is dependent on their integrity. Failure to take such precautions will create an incompetent glottis and lead to recurrent aspiration pneumonia. Should it become obvious that the recurrent nerve has been cut or the arytenoid deliberately sacrificed in the course of tumor surgery, the ipsilateral vocal cord is sutured in the midline to the cricoid and a cricopharyngeal myotomy performed. Successful rehabilitation will then ensue.

Supraglottic laryngectomy represents a partial pharyngectomy as well as a partial laryngectomy; therefore, deglutition must be retaught after mucosal healing has been completed. This has usually occurred by 10–14 days and the edema of the remaining larynx has subsided. At this point, the tracheostomy tube is reduced in size and plugged, and after the patient has demonstrated a tolerance for 24 hours without dyspnea or stridor, the tracheostomy tube is removed and the stoma allowed to close by secondary intention over 2–3 days. Only after the stoma has closed is the patient begun on an oral diet. The nasogastric tube is removed, allowing the patient to swallow without the presence of a foreign body in the pharynx. The postoperative supraglottic laryngectomy patient is then taught to swallow against a closed glottis. The habit he must create requires inspiring fully before ingesting food. The food is then placed deeply in the mouth and the patient swallows repeatedly. When he has completed his swallow, the patient is encouraged to cough, expectorate, and spit out any food remaining in his mouth. By repeated efforts of this type under observation by a nurse or physician, the patient learns to control his aspiration. With time, pharyngeal muscles become adapted to better control of the food bolus. The type of food initially presented is important both in learning how to swallow and in reducing the risk of aspiration. Water is usually not easily tolerated, but liquids with carbonation, as well as custards, scrambled eggs, Jell-O, and ice cream, are tolerated well by many people. An experimental food tray must be assembled. The patient selects foods from this tray that he can easily ingest. Should one food be particularly well tolerated, ample quantities of this food are given as the entire meal. As the patient enlarges his menu, adequate caloric intake will occur. The dietitian is an important member to the rehabilitative team at this point. Careful intake and output records as well as daily weights are necessary during this period of learning to ensure that the patient is not becoming dehydrated and does not get into negative nitrogen balance.

WHEN IS A TOTAL LARYNGECTOMY REQUIRED?

Total laryngectomy is indicated for all intrinsic laryngeal tumors that require surgery but do not permit partial laryngectomy. While the Europeans and Canadians recommend radiotherapy as primary treatment for large T_3 and T_4 laryngeal tumors, most American writers describe the need for total laryngectomy under such circumstances. It is the feeling of the latter that unsuccessful radiotherapy presents many problems. Recurrent tumor may be very difficult to recognize until it has extended through the laryngeal cartilage into the soft tissues of the neck after radiotherapy as a result of the tissue swelling that obscures laryngeal visualization. Furthermore, the tumor often changes its behavior and becomes a vicious submucosal invading tumor rather than an exophytic mucosal tumor with pushing margins. For these reasons, as well as the availability of newer techniques that allow voice restoration, wide-field laryngectomy is the first choice for patients with large laryngeal lesions.

Patients under consideration for partial surgery may need conversion to laryngectomy in the operating room if the cancer has extended farther than expected preoperatively. Patients undergoing conversion laryngectomy in the operating room have a better statistical survival than the whole population of total laryngectomy patients.[59] Better survival results might be expected since the conversion group represents patients with smaller tumors. The risk of spreading tumor by exploratory laryngotomy appears unfounded.

Two other indications for total laryngectomy are radiation failure resulting in a large recurrent tumor, and debilitated respiratory physiology that does not allow the risk of partial surgery even though the lesion fits the criteria for partial surgery.

A wide-field laryngectomy is done in all the above circumstances. The pharynx is entered away from the tumor. Wide-field laryngectomy requires resection of the strap muscles overlying the larynx (Fig 16–12,A). For narrow-field laryngectomy, the larynx is delivered from the strap muscles, as is done for horizontal partial laryngectomy. The rationale for including the prelaryngeal strap muscles is to increase the block of potentially invaded tissue and to decrease the chance of inadequate resection of a T_4 tumor. Partial surgery is employed in limited T_1 through T_3 lesions and therefore should not be done if the tumor has crossed the cartilage (thyroid) and invaded the strap muscles. A measure of insurance is afforded by including the strap muscles in the block dissection in every total laryngectomy.

For large supraglottic lesions, the contralateral pyriform sinus or opposite vallecula is the site of surgical entry. For glottic tumors, the vallecula can be entered and the epiglottis immediately grasped to obtain exposure. The hyoid bone is usually skeletonized and excised so that a persisting nubbin of lesser cornu does not remain in the neck to be misdiagnosed as recurrent

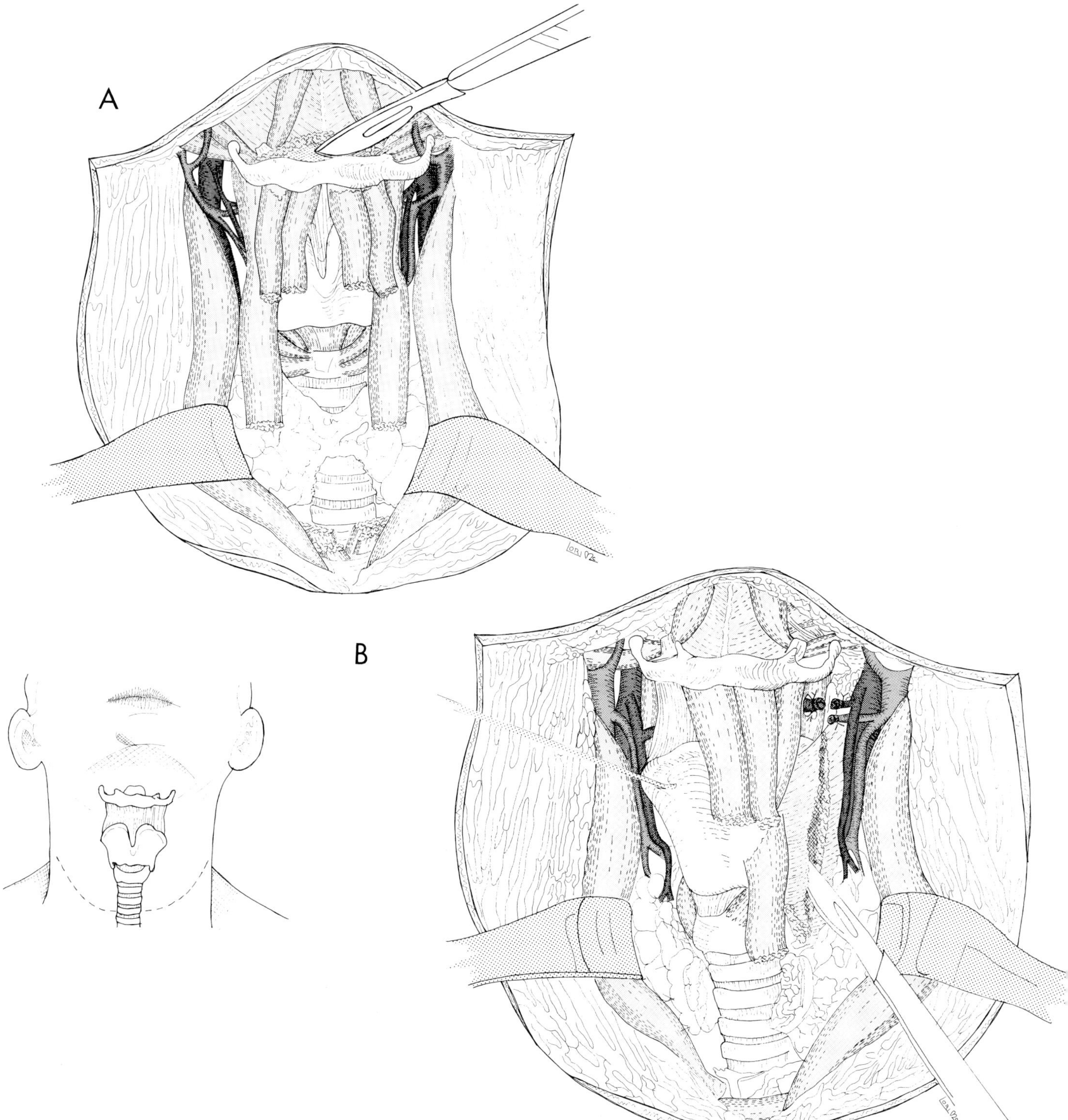

Fig 16–12.—Total laryngectomy. **A,** from above, the hyoid base is skeletonized and delivered and the strap muscles are cut. Skin incision is outlined against position of larynx and trachea. **B,** thyroid cartilage is delivered from the pharyngeal constrictors and the thyroid gland is elevated away from trachea. *(continued)*

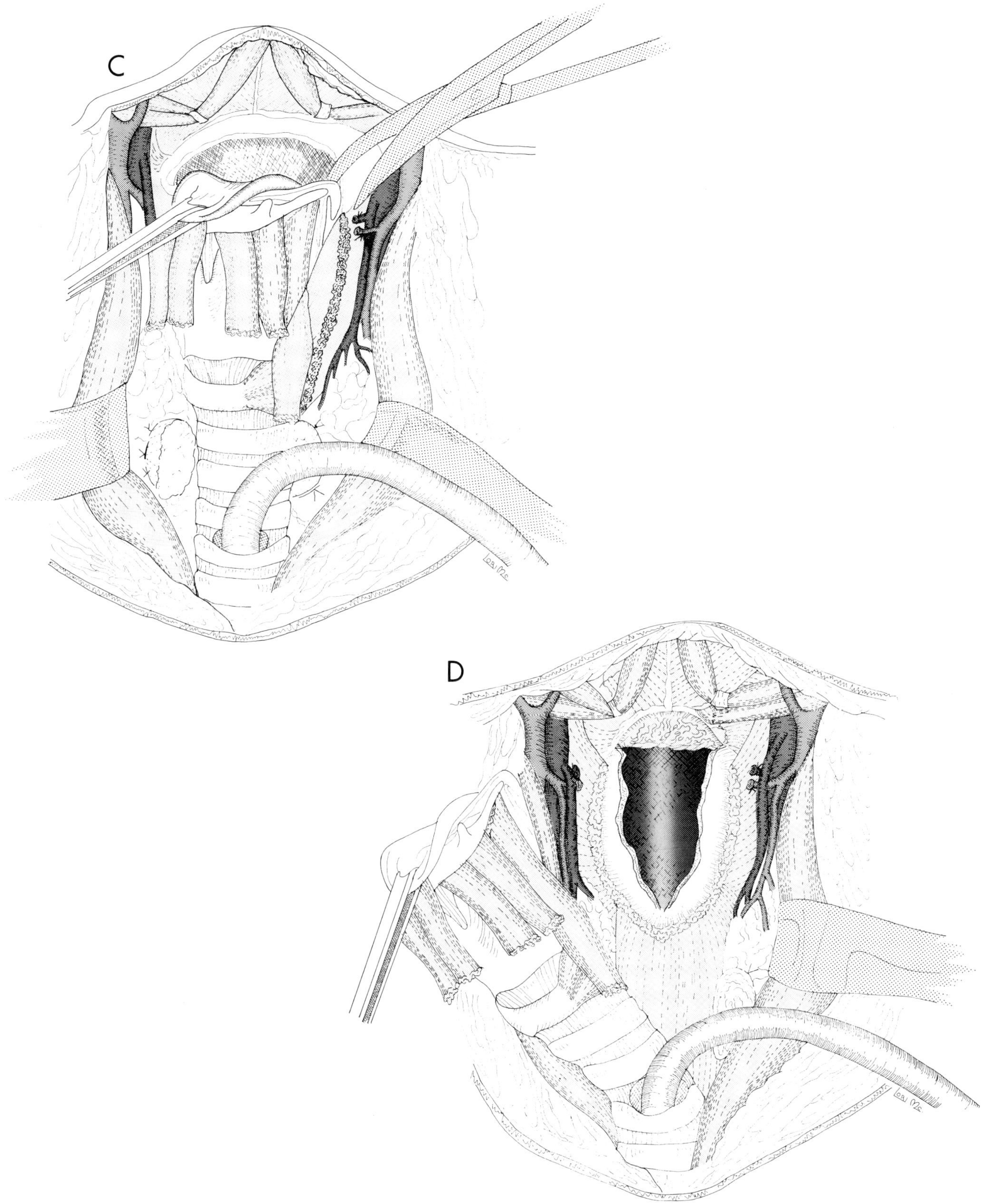

Fig 16–12 (cont.).—C, larynx is dissected from above and the tracheostoma created. **D,** larynx is delivered from pharynx—including the hyoid bone, thyroid and cricoid cartilage, and the first two tracheal rings.

tumor in a lymph node. The mucosal incisions are quickly connected and the tumor is well visualized before further excision is considered (Fig. 16–12,B and C).

An ipsilateral hemithyroidectomy may be necessary for glottic level tumors to minimize the risk of thyroid gland metastasis, which, while unusual, can occur. Thyroid gland resection is done, although the pathologic studies on glottic and subglottic tumors showed no thyroid gland invasion by squamous cell carcinoma in one series,[55] in contrast to the 10% risk of invasion cited in another report.[28] It is of note that in a study by Shafer et al.,[60] the risk of hypothyroidism after radiation therapy for carcinoma in the pharynx and larynx was 3%, but the incidence of hypothyroidism in patients given radiation as well as hemithyroidectomy was 50%. Vrabec and Heffron[61] as well as Murken and Duvall[62] have shown that the risk of hypothyroidism after combined therapy approaches 67%. Therefore, it is mandatory to monitor all such patients in the postoperative period. At 6 months after surgery they are fully evaluated for thyroid gland function.

We presently recommend that a total thyroidectomy be done only when there is identifiable gross invasion of the thyroid gland. Under such circumstances some parathyroid glands are studied by frozen section samples and preserved, if not invaded by squamous cell carcinoma. The remainder of the resection should include the cricoid cartilage and the second tracheal ring (Fig 16–12,D). If the tumor has a subglottic extension, frozen section study of the inferior margin of the trachea is necessary before closure is begun.

The total laryngectomy is closed by a running mucosal suture. Our preferred closure is in the shape of a T, with two or three layers of muscle closed over the mucosa before subcutaneous and skin layers are brought together (Fig 16–13). We no longer use a straight-line vertical closure because in our experience, this closure caused a higher incidence of postoperative stricture requiring dilation. Continuous suction drainage is used as after supraglottic laryngectomy. Vertical hemilaryngectomy wounds can often be allowed to drain open using Penrose drains or a Jackson-Pratt closed drainage system or small Hemovac.

The permanent tracheostoma is carefully created to prevent stenosis (see Fig 16–13). A midline ellipse of cervical skin and soft tissue is excised. Interrupted permanent sutures carefully secure the mucosa of the trachea to the skin of the neck. If the stoma is widely patent and the patient does not need respiratory support after surgery, a tracheostomy or laryngectomy tube is not necessary. Should there be a question of insufficient stomal size or the need for a cuffed stomal vent, a laryngectomy tube is placed and usually removed by the fifth to seventh day. Most patients have a sufficiently large stoma that there is no permanent need for a laryngectomy tube.

Radical neck dissection is a major component of the surgical treatment of carcinoma of the intrinsic and extrinsic larynx (see Chap. 9). All patients with palpable neck nodes undergo radical neck dissection. If fixation to the deep structures is suspected, we consider preoperative radiation therapy or induction chemotherapy to shrink the neck mass. If the neck mass shrinks, surgery is then carried out. While the prognosis is poor in patients with N_3 nodes, some patients have survived more than 2 years after such treatment, and therefore we continue to recommend it.

Full-course radiation for palpable nodes as a curative treatment is not advised. Elective neck dissection is performed in all patients in whom the statistical risk of occult metastasis to the neck nodes exceeds 15%. An alternative treatment for such occult metastases has been radiation therapy, but our preferred treatment is elective neck dissection, with consideration of postoperative radiation therapy to the neck as well as the site of the original primary tumor.

The data underlying our considerations are given in Table 16–2 and in general reflect the need for neck treatment with all large T_1 and all T_2 supraglottic lesions. It is of note that the risk of occult metastases is 30% in lesions involving the epiglottis and false vocal cord. Transglottic tumors have a risk of only 13%, and therefore the need for elective neck dissection is borderline in these circumstances. Larger transglottic tumors that infringe on the epiglottis suggest the need for treatment of the ipsilateral neck. All tumors with invasion of the lingual surface of the epiglottis, the base of the tongue, or the vallecula must be treated by ipsilateral radical neck dissection since the likelihood of occult nodes is 24%. Pharyngeal tumors similarly have a high risk of both palpable and occult metastasis. Piriform sinus carcinomas, as can be seen from Table 16–2, carry a 58% risk of palpable neck nodes, while 41% of those without palpable nodes have occult node metastases in the neck. Midline or bilateral lesions carry a similar risk of nodes in both necks, and therefore treatment must be considered carefully for these tumors. Bilateral neck dissection can be done with or without "conservation" modifications (outlined in Chap. 9). An alternate treatment recommendation is to do an ipsilateral neck dissection on the side of greatest disease. If occult metastases are found, radiation to the contralateral N_0 neck is an option. More lateral lesions such as piriform sinus and false vocal cord lesions are less likely to have contralateral metastases, although in some studies the risk has approached 20%.

In view of the aggressive and unpredictable nature of

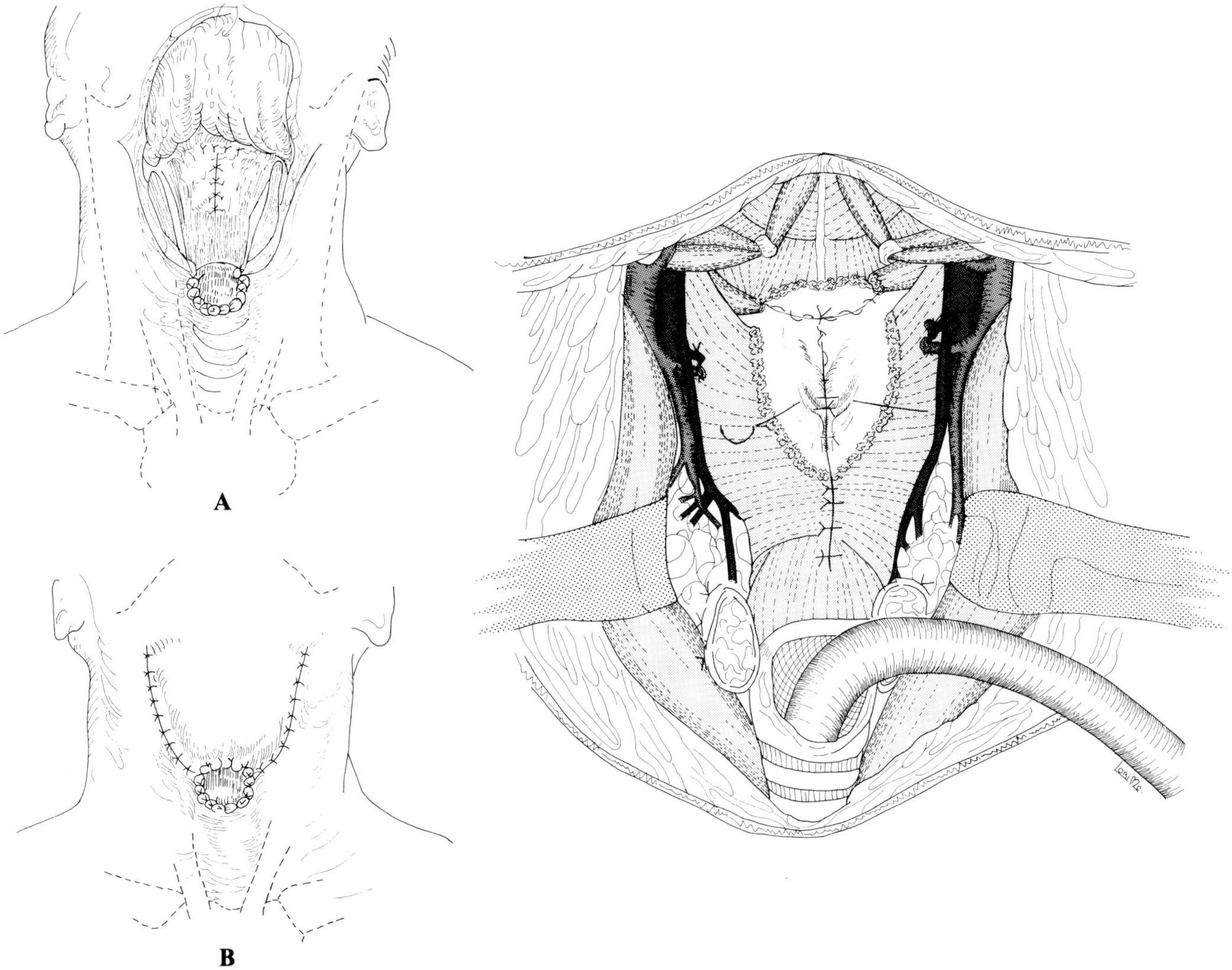

Fig 16–13.—Closure of total laryngectomy. First layer is closed in a T with running Connell suture. The submucosa is oversewn, and strap muscle remnants and the constrictor muscle make up the third layer.

cancers of the tongue base and hypopharyngeal tumors, radiation therapy includes both sides of the neck and the site of the primary if the primary lesion is treated by irradiation.

Most studies do not show an improved survival from combination therapy for intrinsic laryngeal lesions when compared to adequate surgery that includes resection of ipsilateral cervical lymph nodes.

HOW SHOULD RECURRENT LARYNGEAL CANCER BE MANAGED?

Local recurrence after total laryngectomy has a dire prognosis. The stomal margins are a frequent site of recurrence. Stomal recurrence also can occur at the location of the temporary tracheostoma after hemilaryngectomy and supraglottic laryngectomy. It has a less awesome prognosis in such circumstances. The incidence of recurrent cancer around the tracheostoma after a total laryngectomy is 5%–15%. Preoperative tracheostomy as well as microscopically positive inferior margins have been implicated in the higher range of incidence. Frozen section study of the inferior margin of the resection is needed for glottic tumors. However, the sampling at frozen section may not be complete enough, and permanent sections may reveal a positive margin.

In order to reduce the rate of stomal recurrences, several surgeons have recommended emergency laryngectomy within 48 hours after tracheostomy for an obstructing laryngeal tumor.[63] An alternative to tracheostomy presently is laser removal of the bulk of the endotracheal tumor. This allows time for planned treatment and eliminates the need for an unscheduled tracheostomy.

Sisson in 1962 was the first to describe wide operative removal for stomal recurrence. Patients with stomal recurrence superior to the tracheostoma have a better survival than patients with recurrence inferiorly. A 5-year survival of 17% has been reported in his series of 28 patients.[64] In a second report, 10 of 16 patients died of persistent carcinoma, with 25% of patients free of disease at 1 year.[65] This resection requires mobilization and resection of the trachea, followed by reimplantation of the trachea into the area of the manubrium. The clavicular heads and the manubrium are often removed. The soft tissue is replaced with deltopectoral or pectoralis major myocutaneous flaps. The extensive reconstruction as well as the mediastinal dissection produces significant postoperative complications and mortality. It is necessary to separate the trachea from the great vessels to minimize mediastinitis and to reduce tension on the trachea as it is inserted into the neck or chest skin. Careful selection of patients for this operation requires CT scan, mediastinoscopy, and exploratory surgery. The great vessels and the vertebral column must be clear of tumor. The pharynx or esophagus can be replaced if needed with intestinal interposition grafts. These challenging salvage attempts must be reserved for the very experienced surgical team, or the mortality of the operation will be overwhelming.

WHAT ARE THE INDICATIONS FOR COMBINATION TREATMENT FOR LARYNGEAL CARCINOMA?

Small glottic tumors and *small* suprahyoid supraglottic lesions merit treatment by x-irradiation alone. For the vigorous, healthy patient who can tolerate surgery, the decision on treatment for larger laryngeal carcinoma usually is in favor of surgery rather than irradiation as the sole treatment. Intermediate-sized tumors of the larynx often can be treated by surgery without the need for combination radiotherapy. Large lesions such as sizable T_3 and T_4 lesions of the intrinsic larynx carry such a high risk of local and regional spread that combination therapy is recommended in all such circumstances. In our judgment, all hypopharyngeal lesions should be treated with combination therapy because the invasive biologic behavior of hypopharyngeal lesions requires an aggressive treatment combination to achieve acceptable survival statistics.

WHEN DO YOU EMPLOY PARTIAL OR TOTAL LARYNGOPHARYNGECTOMY FOR HYPOPHARYNGEAL CANCERS?

Hypopharyngeal tumors are primarily defined as those located in the piriform sinus and usually on the anterior and medial wall of the sinus. Posterior hypopharyngeal tumors are also included in this group. Surgery is required for effective cure in all hypopharyngeal tumors. Radiation therapy for cure has a prognosis of half or less that of surgery alone or in combination with irradiation (Table 16–3). Cancer that is limited to the pyriform sinus and which does not extend to the apex of the sinus can be treated by partial laryngopharyngectomy, with preservation of the vocal cord anteriorly.[66] The operation is similar to a supraglottic laryngectomy except that the thyroid cartilage cuts are made toward the inferior cornu on the involved side. The arytenoid is usually severed and brought into the specimen, since the aryepiglottic fold is frequently involved. At the completion of the resection, the ipsilateral vocal cord is sutured with a sizable chromic suture to the posterior face of the cricoid cartilage in the midline. The patient is then awakened slightly during the operation and a cough reflex is elicited. Glottic closure must be complete at this time or the patient is likely to aspirate during the postoperative period, since he will have an immobile and lateralized vocal cord and no epiglottis. Therefore, the patient will have great difficulty in maintaining the glottis closed during swallowing. It is necessary to adjust the suture placement to give best closure for rehabilitation of deglutition to be successful. More mucosa is removed in this procedure than in a supraglottic laryngectomy, and the risk of postoperative fistula is increased. If the surgeon is concerned about the tension of the closure, a deliberate fistula should be created or a pectoralis muscle myocutaneous flap employed in the closure. Successful swallowing rehabilitation takes months and significant effort by the patient. Larger hypopharyngeal lesions such as T_3 and T_4 piriform lesions and posterior commissure lesions, which may be horseshoe shaped and come around to the esophageal introitus, require total laryngopharyngec-

TABLE 16–3.—THREE-YEAR SURVIVAL AFTER CONSERVATION SURGERY FOR LARYNGEAL TUMORS*

TREATMENT	NO. OF CASES	SURVIVAL (%)
Supraglottic tumors		
Supraglottic laryngectomy	119	67
Total laryngectomy	21	43
X-ray therapy	20	30
Total	160	
Pyriformsinus tumors		
Partial laryngectomy	85	59
Total laryngectomy	57	30
X-ray therapy	32	11
Total	175	
No Rx, nodal response rate: N_0	= 53%	
N_+	= 24%	

*From Ogura et al.: *Laryngoscope* 90:591–600, 1980. Reproduced by permission.

tomy. If large amounts of mucosa have not been removed, primary closure similar to that for a laryngectomy is carried out. Som has described a procedure for small postcricoid lesions in which the anterior larynx is preserved and used as replacement for the anterior hypopharynx (Figure 16–14).[67] A total laryngectomy is obviously required in such a procedure.

Posterior pharyngeal wall carcinomas are dangerous tumors. Their symptoms may be vague, and the visibility of the tumor to the physician will be limited. These tumors spread quickly down the prevertebral fascia to the retropharyngeal nodes, and because of their location, the cancer may metastasize to both sides of the neck. For these reasons, radiation therapy is added to the treatment of posterior pharyngeal cancers. Excision of this lesion is done through a suprahyoid approach (midline pharyngotomy with mucosal replacement either by split-thickness skin graft (for small lesions) or rotation flap (for moderate-sized lesions). The loss of pharyngeal musculature and its replacement by nonmoving tissue may temporarily inhibit swallowing, but all patients recover deglutition over the course of 1 year after surgery. Resection of larger lesions requires pectoralis major flap reconstruction of the hypopharynx.

The success of irradiation for posterior pharyngeal cancers is limited. The results of combination therapy appear to be better. It is of note that a posterior pharyngeal wall cancer is unusual. There were only six posterior pharyngeal wall lesions in a series of 401 larynx and pharynx cancers reported by Ogura and Biller.[50] Good statistical data on alternative treatment modalities are difficult to derive because all series are small in number.

Total laryngopharyngectomy is necessary for laryngeal tumors that extend out of the larynx as well as for hypopharyngeal tumors that extend across the midline. When such resection does not permit preservation of enough mucosa for primary closure, alternative methods of reconstruction are necessary.

High cervical esophageal lesions as well as postcricoid and pyriform lesions that extend to the cervical introitus also pose problems. Submucosal spread can go

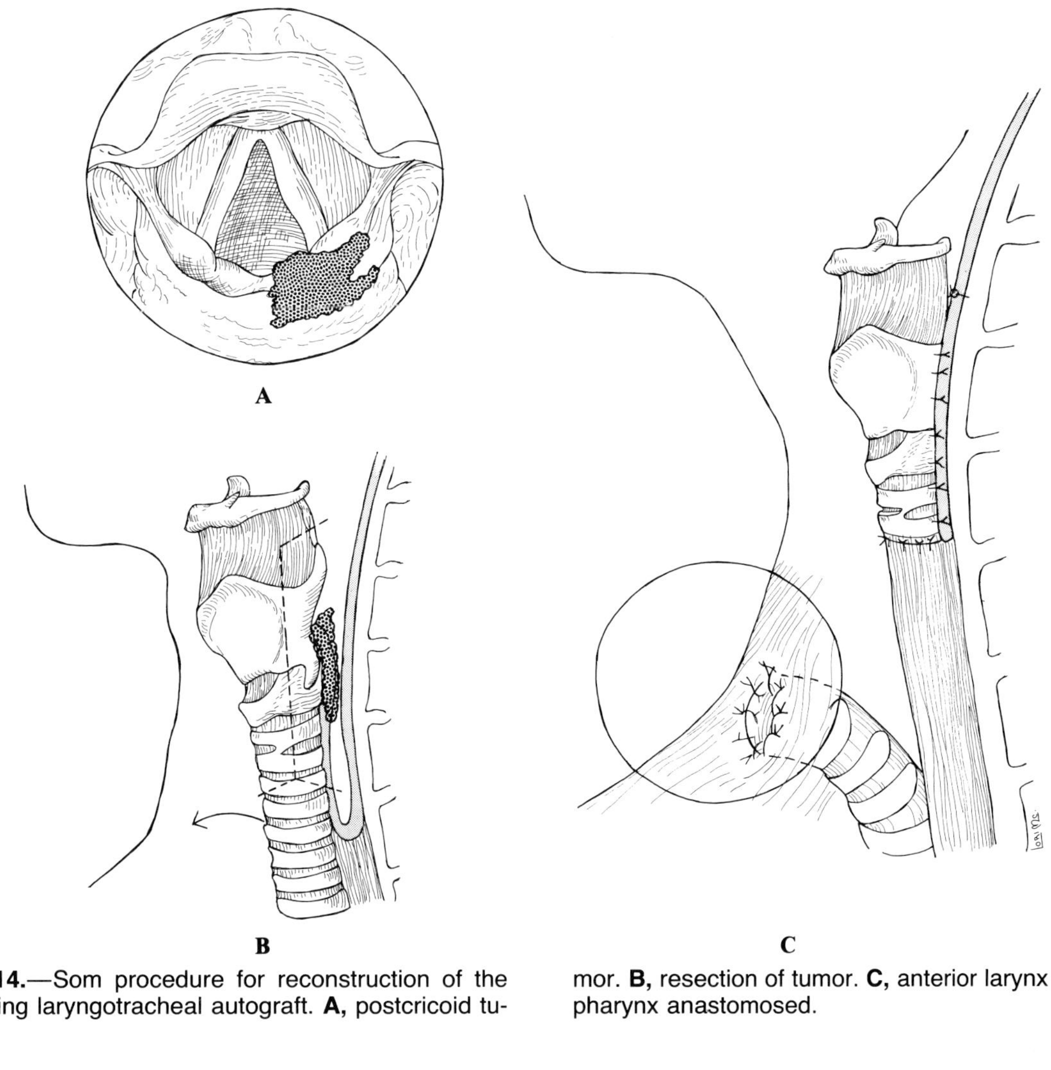

Fig 16–14.—Som procedure for reconstruction of the pharynx using laryngotracheal autograft. **A,** postcricoid tumor. **B,** resection of tumor. **C,** anterior larynx and posterior pharynx anastomosed.

down several centimeters. Similarly, these tumors have skip lesions where there is clear intervening mucosa and submucosa with a secondary tumor many centimeters distally.

Therefore, large hypopharygneal or pyriform sinus tumors that invade the larynx and extend down toward the esophageal introitus as well as laryngeal tumors that extend posteriorly through the cricoid plate require reconstruction with a neopharynx. Staged closures have been available since the mid-1950s, but because of the cost and duration of hospitalization that these multiple-stage procedures require, newer techniques have been explored.

Among the earlier techniques was the Wookey technique,[68] which entailed the creation of a posterior hypopharynx from the skin of the neck, with a rotation flap of lateral neck skin used to create an anterior tracheal wall. The remaining neck skin is then closed over the tube and swallowing can begin again. This technique works satisfactorily in the nonirradiated patient. Even under the best of circumstances, many stages are required. The operation is often unsuccessful because of scarring or breakdown of tissue if the patient has had radiation therapy.

The Bakamjian deltopectoral flap has been used successfully in reconstructing the hypopharynx.[69] The procedure is done in two to three stages and often results in stenosis. Colonic interposition grafts have worked satisfactorily and can be drawn in front of the sternum, although this creates both a functional and cosmetic deformity because the swallowing tube lies subcutaneously in the neck and chest.

The three techniques of pharyngeal reconstruction in current use are described in increasing order of preference. First, the pectoralis major muscle with the attendant chest skin can be used to resurface the hypopharynx after laryngectomy and to create a conduit for the passage of food from the mouth to the esophagus.[70] Tubing such a flap is difficult. One alternative is to use only the muscle of the flap and graft split-thickness skin on the muscle, rather than carrying the thick subdermal fat as well as the thick skin of the chest wall. In either case, it is suggested that a controlled fistula be created with secondary closure 10–14 days after the primary operation. This method represents the best of the skin-lined rotation flaps. The donor tissue is outside the portal of any preoperative irradiation. Because the complications are superficial and localized, this operation does not carry the risk of mortality and morbidity from peritonitis that the two following techniques do. Swallowing is not dynamic in this muscle-lined tube, and stenosis is more likely.

A second technique is total laryngoesophagectomy and replacement with a gastric tube. The procedure is performed through abdominal and cervical approaches. The esophagus is dissected free from the neck and abdomen and removed without a thoracotomy.[71] The stomach is brought up through the posterior mediastinum. The stomach carries its own vascular supply, but because of the long distance and the tension on vessels in the transfer, some surgeons recommend connecting the gastric vessels to those in the neck to augment the blood supply. One surgeon has verbally told us he has had better success by bringing up a gastric tube that is elongated because some of the proximal duodenum is carried with the greater curvature tube. The intact circumference of the duodenal bulb makes a better anastamosis to the pharynx. Some groups have reported excellent success with the operations that use the intact stomach or a greater curvature tube. Other groups have reported several serious complications. Those who favor the technique allow the patient to begin to swallow at 7 days. Acid regurgitation has occurred and must be dealt with subsequently. Bile stasis is another reported complication from this operation. It can be managed once the diagnosis is ascertained.

The third technique is to use a free graft of a loop of jejunum with its vascular arcade which is brought to the operative field, revascularized, and sutured proximally to the base of the tongue and distally to the esophagus.[72–75] This technique has been quite successful in our experience (Fig 16–15). The revascularization of the jejunal transplant works well with a microvascular anastomosis since the bowel vessels of 1.5 or 3.0 mm match up nicely with vessels found in the neck. Using large neck vessels (jugular vein and external carotid artery) for the anastomosis reduces the success rate because of the disparity in size and the risk of occlusion in the donor bowel vessels. The free bowel segment technique requires a two-team approach. A microvascular anastomosis increases the operative time. The intestinal segment can be visualized endoscopically and evaluated in the postoperative period. A failing vascular anastomosis can often be salvaged by revision of an area of vascular occlusion or congestion. In the successful case, the patient is permitted to eat at approximately 10–14 days. Swallowing is usually quite satisfactory.

Based on our experience, we presently recommend the free jejunal loop to patients who need total laryngopharyngectomy. We presently are not using the pectoralis major flaps for primary reconstruction.

IS IT BETTER TO USE PLANNED RADIATION THERAPY PREOPERATIVELY OR POSTOPERATIVELY FOR THE TREATMENT OF ADVANCED LARYNGEAL OR HYPOPHARYNGEAL CANCERS?

In the 1950s, when radiation therapy was combined with surgery in the treatment of cancer of the larynx,

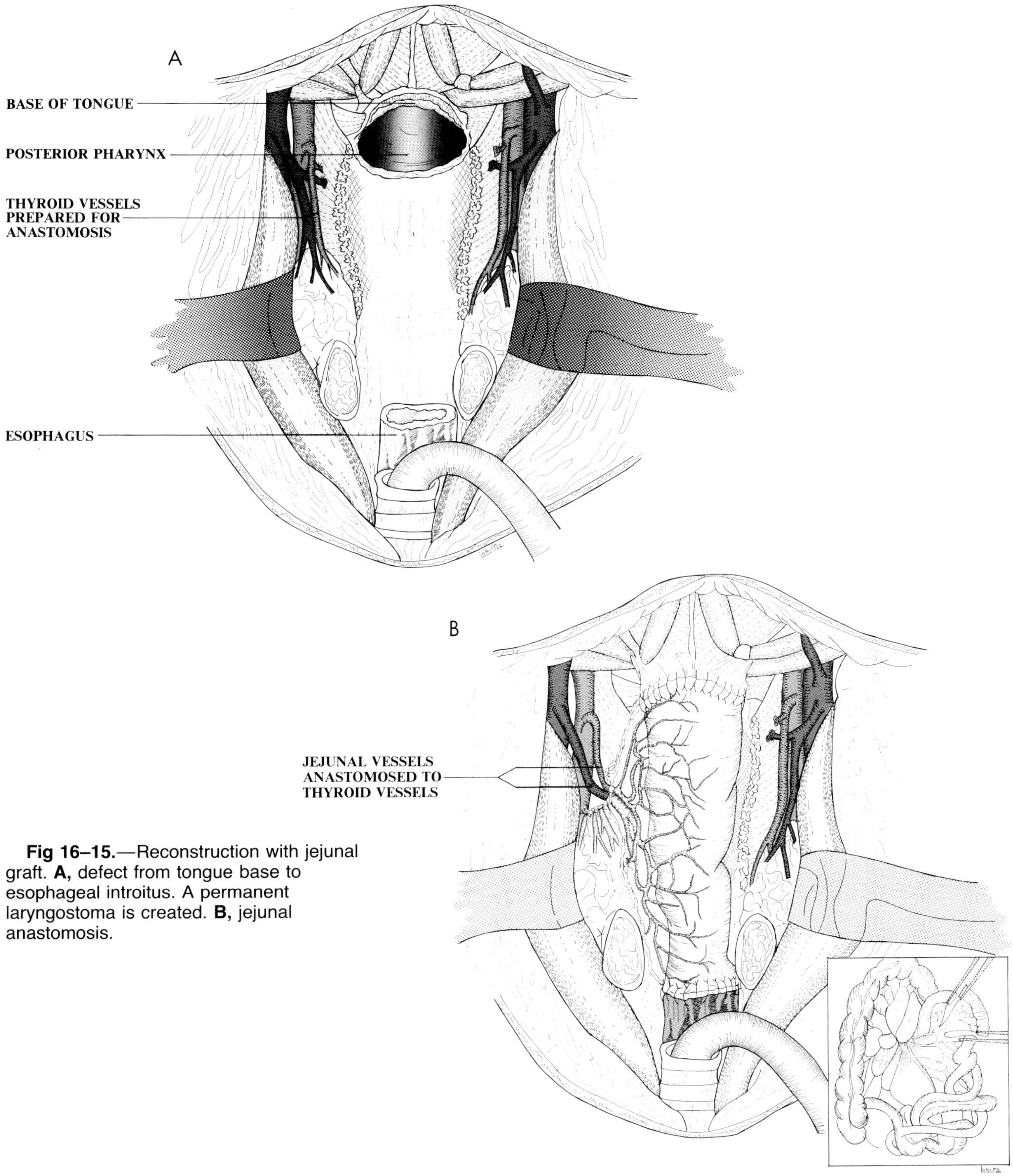

Fig 16–15.—Reconstruction with jejunal graft. **A,** defect from tongue base to esophageal introitus. A permanent laryngostoma is created. **B,** jejunal anastomosis.

attempts were made to balance the maximal dose against the increased risk of morbidity. The radiation therapist worked in conjunction with surgeons. The original protocol doses were of the order of 2,000–3,000 rad given over a period of 2–3 weeks. It was noted that high-dose preoperative irradiation at a level of approximately 5,000–6,000 rad given at a rate of 175–200 rad/day could be administered safely without significant acute morbidity during the treatment program and without skin breakdown (by using high-energy radiation). With the dose of 5,000–6,000 rad administered preoperatively, operating surgeons noted an increasing incidence of complications and an increasing severity of complications. Pharyngocutaneous fistulas were more difficult to close. The secretions often infected the tissues of the neck, occasionally destroying the skin flaps. Other soft tissues of the neck, including the adventitia and media of the carotid artery, were more vulnerable to necrosis, which risked carotid artery blowouts.

Postoperative irradiation was suggested as an alternative and has similarly met with good success. There are no results from controlled studies that show a curative advantage with postoperative irradiation. The choice between preoperative and postoperative irradiation, therefore, remains with the surgical and radiation therapy team. The advantages of preoperative irradiation are that the radiation therapy can be administered at a planned starting date and can be completed on schedule in almost all circumstances. Surgery can then be done after a usual waiting period of 5–6 weeks (1 week for every week of radiation therapy). Any complications from surgery do not delay adjunctive treatment since the preliminary treatment has been completed. The disadvantage of preoperative irradiation is the potential for increasing the number and severity of complications after surgery.

The advocates of postoperative radiation therapy point out the unirradiated tumor is unaltered, and therefore the gross margins of the tumor are more easily recognized by the surgeon and microscopic margins more accurately interpreted by pathologists. Complications in the unirradiated patient are less catastrophic. Fistulas and wound dehiscence are less frequent and usually less extensive. Healing after complications is more rapid.

The down-side risk is that complications of surgery must be cleared up before the radiation therapy can be administered. Since wound complications can require many weeks of rehabilitation, there may be a significant delay in initiating irradiation postoperatively. This may render the treatment sequential, not combinational, and lose the theoretical biologic advantage of using two modalities for the same disease.

HOW IS A PHARYNGOCUTANEOUS FISTULA MANAGED?

An occasional patient with a partial or total laryngectomy does not heal primarily despite careful surgical techniques. The risk of fistula formation is approximately 5%–15% after total laryngectomy and higher after laryngopharyngectomy because of the paucity of mucosa available for closure. For supraglottic laryngectomy, fistulas occur at the rate of 15%–20%. The risk is as high as 25% after partial laryngopharyngectomy.

As described above, the risk of fistula occurrence is not any greater in the irradiated patient. When a fistula occurs, the healing time is markedly prolonged. After a high dose of preoperative irradiation, or if surgery is carried out after irradiation (for cure) has failed, the fistula is likely to be larger and to destroy more of the skin flaps and local tissues of the neck. Early identification of the fistula is important. Edema of the skin flaps, persisting drainage through the Hemovac suction drains, and evidence of saliva or bubbles in the Hemovac drains are early and unequivocal clues to the presence of an impending or existing fistula. Once a diagnosis is definite, actions are aimed at minimizing the complications and trying to keep the fistula as small as possible so that secondary healing of the wound can occur. Should the fistula be delayed in onset and occur after oral feeding has begun, feeding is stopped. Accumulated infected oral secretions, usually contaminated with gram-positive bacteria, must be drained externally. Fistulas occur in the midline of the pharynx after total laryngectomy since this is the site of weakness of the T closure. After partial laryngectomy, fistulas occur laterally at the location of greatest tension in the closure.[76]

The external drainage point of a fistula should be controlled by the surgeon. Direct drainage makes the shortest fistula tract and allows packing of the wound to direct any secretions externally without continued undermining of the flap. A short tract also helps protect the carotid artery from being bathed by infected saliva. Several days are required for the lateral skin flaps to seal to the underlying tissues. During active treatment of a fistula, the patient should be given cephalosporin antibiotics IV or by nasogastric tube. Frequent wound cleaning and packing is also very important. The packs should include iodoform and often are soaked in Betadine. If *Pseudomonas* is a suspected organism, dilute acetic acid is also a valuable packing solution. As the wound begins to develop granulation tissue, the amount of packing is decreased daily. Most wounds will close spontaneously, and closure is accelerated by careful wound hygiene. If a fistula is large, the duration of debility can be decreased by rotating a pectoralis major myocutaneous flap or a deltopectoral flap into the wound once granulation has begun and the lateral flaps are sealed in place. Most fistulas will delay healing and the resumption of swallowing by 1–2 months. The patient, if reliable, need not be hospitalized during this period and can be cared for at home by either family or a trained nurse. The patient is observed in the office at weekly intervals to ensure that no weight loss is occurring. For patients who otherwise will need hospitalization, rotation of flaps to close such a fistula will save time and expense. The best treatment of fistulas is prevention. Careful wound closure technique with minimal tension is important. Preservation of as much normal mucosa as possible decreases tension on the closure. Perioperative antibiotics are necessary and are continued for a period of 5–10 days after surgery. There is no need for prolonged antibiotic administration once the wound has healed primarily. Antibiotics are superfluous after the fistula has begun to granulate.

While wound complications such as orocutaneous leaks will delay healing, they appear to have no relationship to the ultimate function of swallowing and speech over the long term. Stenosis of the hypopharynx after complications from total laryngectomy makes esophageal speech and voice shunting techniques much less successful. Similarly, swallowing is inhibited and may be limited to liquids and very soft foods. Repeated dilation with Maloney dilators in the office under local anesthesia is often sufficient to maintain a pharynx that is of adequate size to tolerate well-chewed semisolid foods. Rarely is secondary pharyngeal reconstruction necessary. However, bowel transplant with free jejunal grafts or large rotation skin flaps such as the pectoralis major myocutaneous flap are successful reconstructive techniques for the patient whose stricture prevents swallowing.

WHAT METHODS OF REHABILITATION ARE AVAILABLE AFTER LARYNGECTOMY?

The methods of rehabilitation after laryngectomy include (1) use of esophageal speech, (2) use of a prosthesis (Blom-Singer, or Panje), (3) surgical reconstruction of the sounding voice, or (4) use of an electromechanical device.

Speech restoration in the laryngectomy patient began many years ago. Speech therapists have been able to educate 30%–60% of all laryngectomy patients to use esophageal speech. Success depends on the psychosocial situation of the patient as well as on the amount of narrowing of the pharynx and esophagus due to surgery and subsequent irradiation. When successful, esophageal speech is intelligible. Some of the very best of the speakers are difficult to distinguish from the general population. They are able to speak in public. Useful voice extends to all functions that normal laryngeal speakers have.

Unfortunately, many patients do not do well with esophageal speech. They have increasing difficulty in periods of tension and anxiety. For these people electric vibrating devices have been used. These vibrate the neck and pharyngeal tissues and allow the lips and tongue to shape the vibrating air column into words. Most of these patients sound very similar to each other and the voice is quite mechanical and poorly modulated. To try to overcome these problems, surgeons have deliberately created fistulas in the neck to try to bring an air supply from the trachea into the mouth, as well as using external devices to bring a vibrating column of air from the trachea into the oral cavity. Most of these ideas have met with mixed success, at best.

In the 1960s, Asai in Japan proposed and performed a multistage operation to create a skin-lined flap from the laryngostoma to the base of the tongue.[8] This flap, which was created with the skin of the anterior neck, was occasionally successful but was often marred by wound breakdown, hair from the rotated skin obstructing the created stoma, and late stenosis. Komorn et al. developed a mucosa-lined tube to connect the proximal esophagus to the laryngostoma. This offered several advantages over the Asai technique.[9] It was a single-stage procedure that could be done at the time of laryngectomy. The lumen was stented by a plastic tube, and wound breakdown was unusual in the acute period. However, stenosis was frequent, since the plastic tube could not be left in place long term lest the patient aspirate through this pharyngotracheal fistula.

In the late 1970s Singer and Blom[10] and Panje,[77] working separately, revised the concept of the tracheal puncture. Their operations permitted, respectively, a puncture from the tracheostoma to the midline pharynx, and a perforation from the posterior tracheal wall to the esophagus. Through these small fistulas, both groups inserted a Silastic tube with a valve mechanism, invented independently, that would permit air under pressure to travel from the trachea to the pharynx but would not permit food or liquid to enter the trachea from the hypopharynx, either around the tube or through its lumen. The success rate with these procedures has been 75%–90% in several reports and the voice quality is quite good. The patient is able to speak to the full extent of his breathing capacity, and with a new valved tracheostoma cover, the patient can speak using either device without covering the tracheostoma with a finger (Fig 16–16).

This has been an interesting and exciting advance for the patient with a laryngectomy. These operations, which were originally proposed as secondary treatments for failures of esophageal speech, are now recommended by some to be done as part of the primary rehabilitation after laryngectomy. When the fistula is created at the resective operation it can be used for insertion of the nasogastric tube to drain the gastric contents during the acute postoperative convalescence, and it can be used to feed the patient until the mucosal suture line has healed. In general, we begin to feed laryngectomy patients on day 7 or 8 if they can control their secretions. Similarly, supraglottic laryngectomy patients are fed at 10–14 days postoperatively, after the tracheostomy tube has been plugged and usually not until it has actually been removed and the tracheostoma has begun to close. In the latter group of patients, the

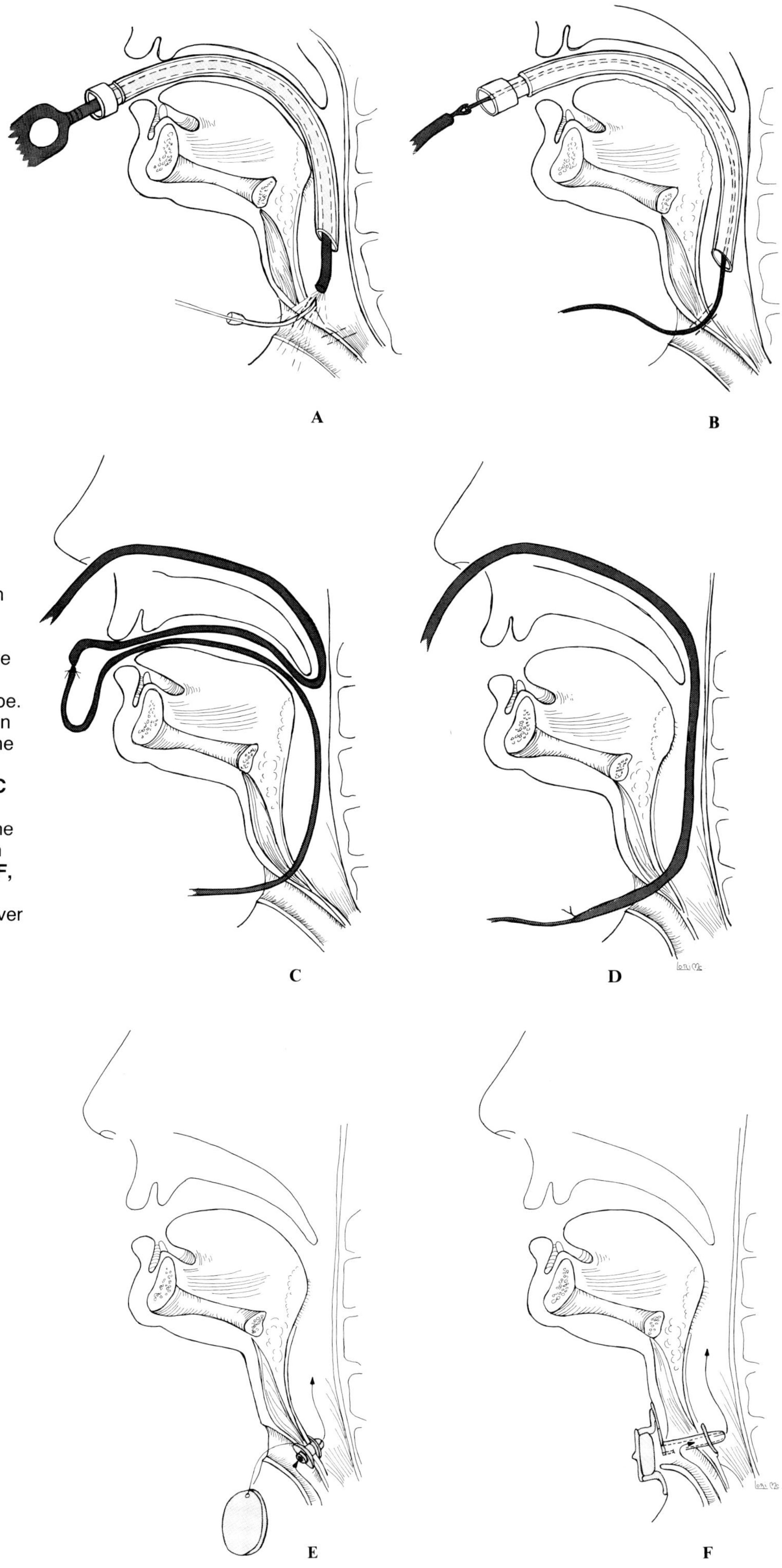

Fig 16–16.—Voice restoration procedures. **A,** 5 mm from the mucocutaneous junction, a 14-gauge needle is used to puncture the party wall in area transilluminated by the endoscope. **B,** a flexible endoscope has been used in the illustration to draw the thread and then the catheter through the pharynx and nose, **C** and **D.** Catheter is left in place 1 week after puncture to mature the tract. **E,** Panje-type prosthesis in place in posterior tracheal wall. **F,** Blom-Singer Duckbill voice prosthesis with valved stoma cover allows speech with both hands free.

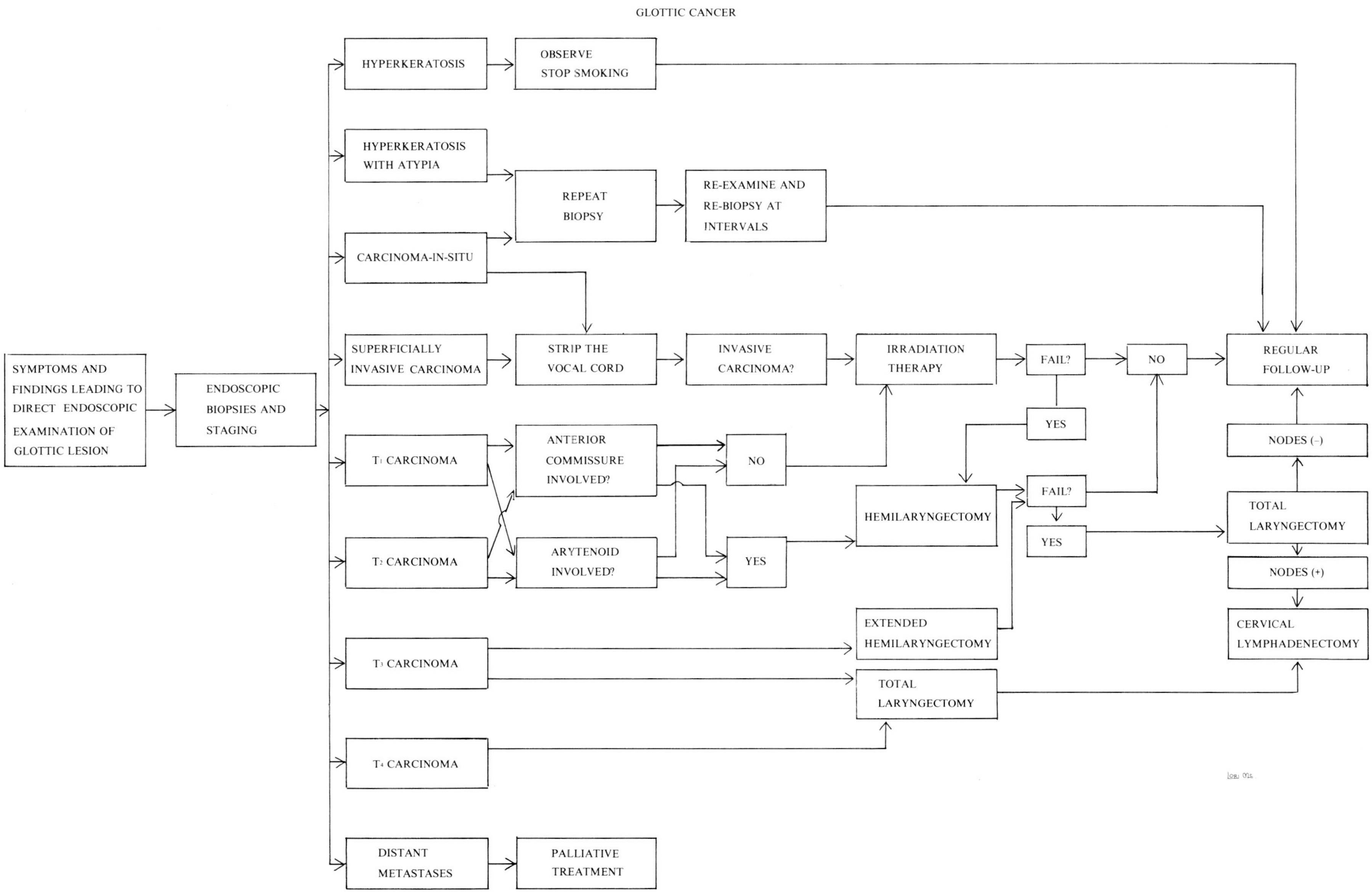

Fig 16–17.—Summary decision chart for management of laryngeal cancer.

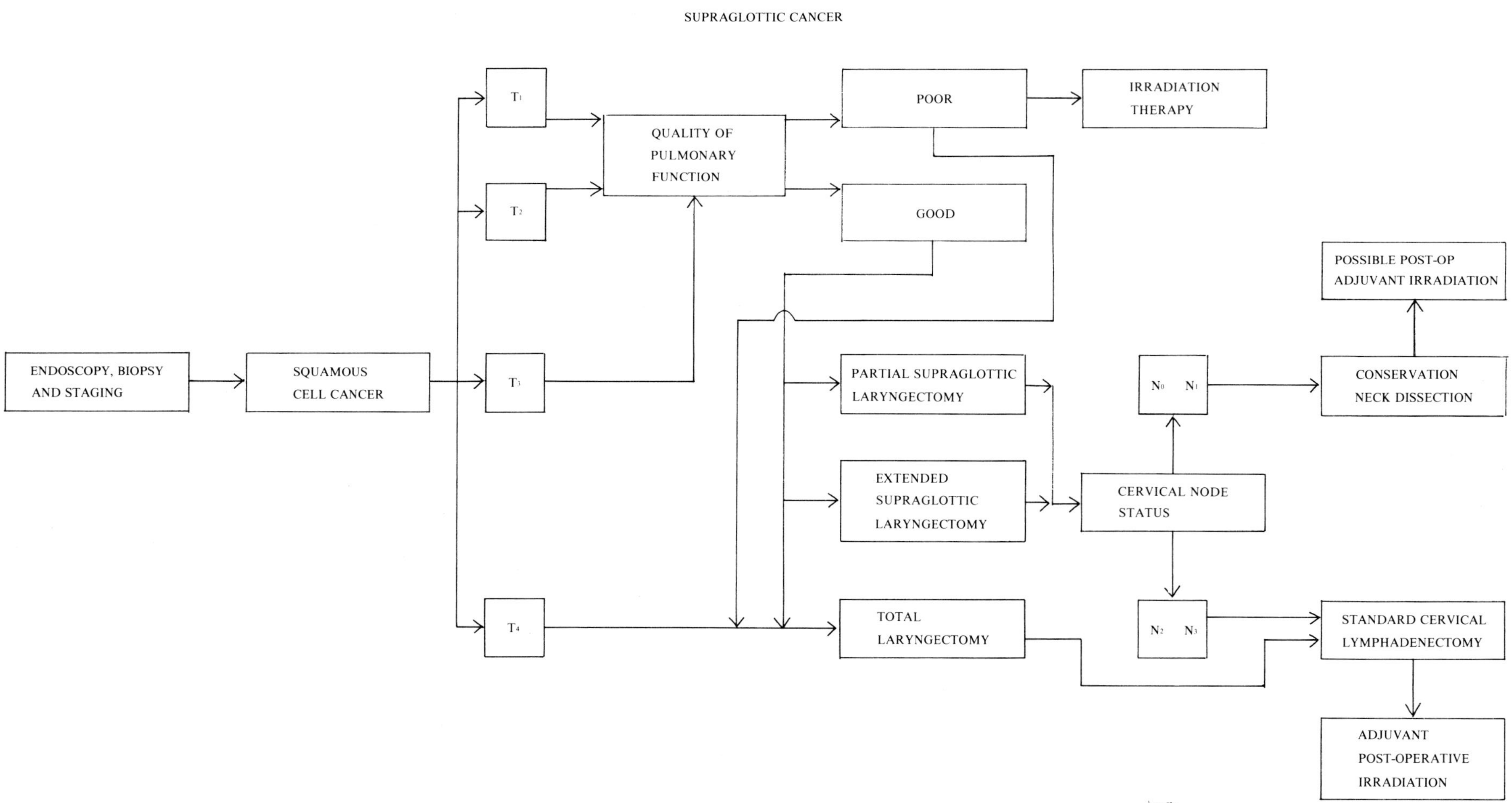

Fig 16–18.—Summary decision chart for management of hypopharyngeal cancer.

subglottic pressure is a necessary prerequisite for good swallowing.

One of the advantages of this immediate voice restoration technique is that it creates a fistula which may take the pressure off the suture line above it. In addition, it obviates placement of plastic nasogastric tube crossing the suture line and moving up and down with every swallow for the first 7–10 days. We have not yet studied whether these patients have fewer wound breakdowns, but they do experience a psychological boost when they are able to vocalize 2–3 weeks after surgery.

It is presently recommended that a cricopharyngeal myotomy to the posterior midline be done in all primary cases of voice reconstruction by the Blom-Singer technique. A myotomy is particularly important in patients who either fail to develop good esophageal speech or lack any voice. The Taub blow test may be considered in patients who are contemplating secondary surgery for voice restoration. Endoscopy and barium swallow are necessary to rule out stenosis above the entrance of the puncture into the pharynx.

Should complications from the fistula occur, removal of the plastic tube will usually permit cicatricial closure of the surgically created fistula. The counterpoint to this is that the patient must maintain the stoma with the plastic prosthesis in it most of the time, because in occasional patients the fenestra can close within 24–48 hours if not stented.

Decision charts for managing the patient with laryngeal and hypopharyngeal cancer are presented in Figures 16–17 and 16–18.

REFERENCES

1. Alberti P.W.: Historical development of laryngectomy: II. The evolution of laryngology and laryngectomy in the mid-ninteenth century. *Laryngoscope* 85:288, 1975.
2. Fletcher G.H., Klein R.: Dose-time-volume relationship in squamous cell carcinomas of the larynx. *Radiology* 82:1032–1042, 1964.
3. Pressman J.: Submucosal compartmentation of the larynx. *Ann. Rhinol. Otol.* 65:766, 1956.
4. Pressman J., Simon M., Monell C.: Anatomical studies related to the dissemination of cancer of the larynx. *Trans. Am. Acad. Ophthalmol. Otolaryngol.* 64:628, 1960.
5. Ogura J.H., Mallen R.W.: Partial laryngoesophagectomy for supraglottic and pharyngeal carcinoma. *Trans. Am. Acad. Ophthalmol. Otolaryngol.* 69:832, 1965.
6. Som M.L.: Conservation surgery for carcinoma of the supraglottis. *J. Laryngol. Otol.* 84:655, 1970.
7. Powers W.E., Holtz S., Ogura J., et al.: Contrast examination of larynx and pharynx: Accuracy and value in diagnosis. *AJR* 86:651–660, 1961.
8. Asai R.: Laryngoplasty after total laryngectomy. *Arch. Otolaryngol.* 95:114, 1972.
9. Komorn R.M., Weycer J.S., Sessions R.B., et al.: Vocal rehabilitation with a tracheo-esophageal shunt. *Arch. Otolaryngol.* 97:303, 1973.
10. Singer M.I., Blom E.D.: An endoscopic technique for restoration of voice after laryngectomy. *Ann. Otol. Rhinol. Laryngol.* 89:529, 1980.
11. English G.M.: Malignant neoplasms of the larynx, in English G.M. (ed.): *Otolaryngology: A Textbook.* Hagerstown, Md., Harper & Row, 1976, chap. 48.
12. Holtz S., et al.: Contrast examination of the larynx and pharynx: Glottic, infraglottic and transglottic tumors. *AJR* 89:10–28, 1963.
13. Nathan M.D., et al.: Diagnostic accuracy of xeroradiography: Assessment of extent of carcinoma of the larynx. *Trans. Ophthalmol. Otolaryngol.* 84:619–621, 1977.
14. Segal S.S., Aufterheide J.F., Aaronberg D.J., et al.: High resolution computer tomography in the staging of carcinoma of the larynx. *Laryngoscope* 91:292–300, 1981.
15. Mancuso A.A., Tamakawa Y., Hanafee W.N.: CT of the fixed vocal cord. *AJR* 135 (3):7529–7534, 1980.
16. Maisel R.H., Vermeersch H.: Panendoscopy for second primary tumors in head and neck cancer patients. *Ann. Otol. Rhinol. Laryngol.* 90 (5):460–464, 1981.
17. McGuirt W.F.: Panendoscopy as a screening examination for simultaneous primary tumors in head and neck cancer: A prospective sequential study and review of the literature. *Laryngoscope* 92:569–576, 1982.
18. Batsakis J.G.: *Tumors of the Head and Neck: Clinical and Pathological Considerations,* ed. 2. Baltimore, Williams & Wilkins Co., 1979, pp. 121–129.
19. McGavran M.H., Bauer W.C., Ogura J.H.: Isolated laryngeal keratosis: Its relation to carcinoma of the larynx based on the clinico-pathological study of 87 consecutive cases with long-term follow-up. *Laryngoscope* 70:932, 1960.
20. McGavran M.H., Stutsman M.D., Ogura J.H.: Superficially invasive epidermoid carcinoma of the true vocal cord, in Alberti P.W., Bryce D.P. (eds.): *Workshops From the Centennial Conference on Laryngeal Cancer.* New York, Appleton-Century-Crofts, 1976, p. 120.
21. Giordano A.M., Ewing S.L., Adams G.L., et al.: Laryngeal pseudosarcoma. *Laryngoscope* 93(6):735–740, 1983.
22. Lambert P.R., Ward P.H., Berci G.: Pseudosarcoma of the larynx. *Arch. Otolaryngol.* 106:700, 1980.
23. Biller H.F., Bergman J.A.: Verrucous carcinoma of the larynx. *Laryngoscope* 86:1698, 1975.
24. Posner M.R., Weichselbaum R.R., Carrol E. et al.: Small cell carcinomas of the larynx: Results of combined modality treatments. *Laryngoscope* 93:946–949, 1983.
25. Adams G.L., Duvall A.J.: Adenocarcinoma of the head and neck. *Arch. Otolaryngol.* 93:261, 1971.
26. Sessions D.G., Murray J.P., Bauer W.C., et al.: Adenocarcinoma of the larynx. *Can. J. Otolaryngol.* 4:293, 1975.
27. Ogura J.H., Bello J.A.: Laryngectomy and radical neck dissection for carcinoma of the larynx. *Laryngoscope* 62:1, 1952.
28. Ogura J.H.: Surgical pathology of cancer of the larynx. *Laryngoscope* 65:867, 1955.

29. Sessions D.G.: Surgical pathology of cancer of the larynx and hypopharynx. *Laryngoscope* 85:814, 1975.
30. Strong M.S.: Laser excision of carcinoma of the larynx. *Laryngoscope* 85:1286, 1975.
31. DeSanto L.W.: The options in early laryngeal carcinoma. *N. Engl. J. Med.* 306:910, 1982.
32. Biller H., Ogura J., Pratt L.: Hemilaryngectomy for T_2 glottic cancers. *Arch. Otolaryngol.* 93:238, 1971.
33. Perez C.A., Holtz S., Ogura J.H., et al.: Radiation therapy of early carcinoma of the true vocal cords. *Cancer* 21:764, 1968.
34. Wang C.C.: Treatment of glottic carcinoma by megavoltage radiation therapy and results. *Am. J. Roentgenol. Radium Ther. Nucl. Med.* 120:157, 1974.
35. Bauer W.C., Lesinski S.G., Ogura J.H.: The significance of positive margins in hemilaryngectomy specimens. *Laryngoscope* 85:1–13, 1975.
36. Ogura J.H., Sessions D.G., Spector G.J.: Analysis of surgical therapy for epidermoid carcinoma of the laryngeal glottis. *Laryngoscope* 85:1522, 1975.
37. Skolnik E.M., Martin L., Yee K.F., et al.: Radiation failures in cancer of the larynx. *Ann. Otol. Rhinol. Laryngol.* 84:804, 1975.
38. Sessions D.G., Ogura J.H, Fried M.P.: The anterior commissure in glottic carcinoma. *Laryngoscope* 85:1624, 1975.
39. Blitzer A., Pang M., Som M., et al.: Modification of the anterior commissure technique of partial laryngectomy. *Arch. Otolaryngol.* 106:503, 1980.
40. Som M.L., Silver C.E.: The anterior commissure technique. *Arch. Otolaryngol.* 87:42, 1968.
41. Tucker H., Wood B., Levine H., et al.: Glottic reconstruction after near-total laryngectomy. *Laryngoscope* 80:609, 1970.
42. Schechter G.L.: Epiglottic reconstruction and subtotal laryngectomy. *Laryngoscope* 93:729–734, 1983.
43. Lesinski S.G., Bauer W.C., Ogura J.H.: Hemilaryngectomy for T_3 (fixed cord) epidermoid carcinoma of the larynx. *Laryngoscope* 86:1563, 1976.
44. Quinn H.J.: A new technique for glottic reconstruction after partial laryngectomy. *Laryngoscope* 79:980, 1969.
45. Pearson B.W., Woods R.D., Hartman D.E.: Extended hemilaryngectomy for T_3 glottic carcinoma with preservation of speech and swallowing. *Laryngoscope* 90:1950, 1980.
46. Biller H.F., Som M.L.: Vertical partial laryngectomy for glottic carcinoma with posterior subglottic extension. *Ann. Otol. Rhinol. Laryngol.* 86:715, 1977.
47. Kirchner J., Som M.L.: Clinical significance of fixed vocal cord. *Laryngoscope* 81:1029, 1971.
48. Lawson W., Biller H.F.: Cancer of the larynx, in Suen J.Y., Myers E.N. (eds.): *Cancer of the Head and Neck.* New York, Churchill Livingstone, 1981, p. 459.
49. Ogura J.H., Marks J.E., Freeman R.B.: Results of conservation surgery for cancers of the supraglottis and pyriform sinus. *Laryngoscope* 90:591, 1980.
50. Ogura J.H., Biller H.F.: Partial and total laryngectomy in radical neck dissection, in English G.M. (ed.): *Otolaryngology.* Hagerstown, Md., Harper & Row, 1981, chap. 23.
51. Ogura J.H., Thawley S.E.: Conservation laryngeal surgery and radical neck dissection, in English G.M. (ed.): *Otolaryngology.* Hagerstown, Md., Harper & Row, 1981.
52. Nadol J.B.: Treatment of carcinoma of the epiglottis. *Ann. Otol.* 90:442, 1981.
53. Kirchner J., Som M.L.: Clinical and histological observations on supraglottic cancer. *Ann. Otol. Rhinol. Laryngol.* 80:638, 1971.
54. Som M.L.: Conservation surgery for carcinoma of the supraglottis. *J. Laryngol. Otolaryngol.* 84:655, 1970.
55. McGavran M.H., Bauer W.C., Ogura J.H.: Incidence of cervical lymph node metastases from epidermoid carcinoma of the larynx and their relationship to certain characteristics of the primary tumor. *Cancer* 14:55–66, 1961.
56. Jacobs J.R., Sessions D.G., Ogura J.H.: Recurrent carcinoma of the larynx and the hypopharynx. *Otolaryngol. Head Neck Surg.* 88:425, 1980.
57. Calcaterra T.: Laryngeal suspension after supraglottic laryngectomy. *Arch. Otolaryngol.* 102:716, 1976.
58. Goode R.: Laryngeal suspension in head and neck surgery. *Laryngoscope* 86:349, 1976.
59. Myers E.M., Ogura J.H.: Completion laryngectomy. *Ann. Otol.* 88:172–177, 1979.
60. Shafer R.B., Nuttal F.Q., Pollak K., et al.: Thyroid function after radiation and surgery for head and neck cancer. *Arch. Intern. Med.* 135 (6):843–846, 1975.
61. Vrabec D.P., Heffron T.J.: Hypothyroidism following treatment for head and neck cancer. *Ann. Otol. Rhinol. Laryngol.* 90:449, 1981.
62. Murken R.E., Duvall A.J.: Hypothyroidism following combined therapy in carcinoma of the laryngopharynx. *Laryngoscope* 82:1306, 1972.
63. Baluyot S.T., Shumrick D.A., Everts E.C.: Emergency laryngectomy. *Arch. Otolaryngol.* 94:414–417, 1971.
64. Sisson G.A., Bytell D.E., Becker S.P.: Mediastinal dissection—1976: Indications and newer techniques. *Laryngoscope* 87:751, 1976.
65. Schuller D.E., Hamaker R.C., Gluckman J.L.: Mediastinal dissection: A multi-institutional assessment. *Arch. Otolaryngol.* 107:715, 1981.
66. Kirchner J.A.: Pyriform sinus cancer: A clinical and laboratory study. *Ann. Otolaryngol.* 84:793, 1975.
67. Som M.L.: Laryngotracheal autograft for postcricoid carcinoma. *Ann. Otolaryngol.* 83:41, 1974.
68. Wookey H.: Surgical treatment of carcinoma of pharynx and upper esophagus. *Surg. Gynecol. Obstet.* 75:499–506, 1942.
69. Bakamjian V.Y.: A two-stage method for pharyngoesophageal reconstruction with a primary pectoral skin flap. *Plast. Reconstr. Surg.* 36:173–184, 1965.
70. Baek S., Lawson W., Biller H.F.: An analysis of 133 pectoralis major myocutaneous flaps. *Plast. Reconstr. Surg.* 69:460–467, 1982.
71. Schechter G.L., et al.: Combined treatment of advanced cancer of the laryngopharynx and cervical esophagus. *Laryngoscope* 92:11–15, 1982.
72. Flynn M.B., Acland R.D.: Free intestinal autografts for reconstruction following pharyngolaryngoesophagectomy. *Surg. Gynecol. Obstet.* 149:858, 1979.

73. Gluckman J.L., et al.: The free jejunal graft in head and neck reconstruction. *Laryngoscope* 91:1887–1894, 1981.
74. Grage T.B., Quick C.A.: The use of revascularized ileocolic autografts for primary repair after pharyngolaryngoesophagectomy. *Am. J. Surg.* 136:477–485, 1978.
75. McConnel F.M.S., Hester T.R. Jr., Nahai F., et al.: Free jejunal grafts for reconstruction of the pharynx and cervical esophagus. *Arch. Otolaryngol.* 107:476–481, 1981.
76. Kornblut A., Shumrick D.A.: Complications of head and neck surgery. *Arch. Otolaryngol.* 94:246–254, 1971.
77. Panje W.: Prosthetic voice rehabilitation following laryngectomy. The voice button. *Ann. Otol. Rhinol. Laryngol.* 90:116–120, 1981.

17 / Malignant Tumors of the Paranasal Sinuses and Nasal Cavity

George Adams, M.D.

Tumors arising in the nose and paranasal sinuses are uncommon. They appear to have no relationship to smoking, alcohol consumption, or other habits. However, there is a relationship to environmental factors. A higher incidence of cancer of the maxillary sinuses has been reported in workers in the chromium and nickel industries. Adenocarcinoma arising high in the vault of the nose has been reported in Wales among workers in the furniture industry, particularly those working with hard woods such as mahogany. Twenty years ago thorium was used as a contrast medium to outline the sinuses for specific x-ray studies. This was later found to excite the formation of a thorium-related malignancy of the maxillary sinus (Table 17–1).

The factor most commonly associated with malignancies of the nose and sinuses has been a longstanding history of chronic sinus disease. Therefore, the initial symptoms of malignancy and those of benign disease of the sinuses may be identical. A malignancy of the sinus can develop to large size or spread to adjacent sites before a correct diagnosis is made. In the early stages, routine radiographic studies of the sinus will not discriminate between malignancy and chronic inflammatory disease. In fact, by the time bony erosion is detected radiographically, the tumor is often far advanced. Early detection of malignancy of the sinus or nose requires a high suspicion of an underlying tumor when a patient fails to respond to customary medical management of a sinus problem. A basic scheme for the diagnosis and management of paranasal sinus cancer is shown in Figure 17–1.

HISTORICAL ASPECTS

The first wide resection for a malignancy of a maxillary sinus has been attributed to Richard Weissmann, surgeon to King Charles II. In 1671 he performed a radical resection on a 28-year-old man with a tumor causing decreased vision. In 1826 Lizzars formalized the operative procedure for resection of the upper jaw. He advised that the procedure be done quickly to avoid excessive hemorrhage and to reduce the suffering of the patient. The resection of the palatal tumor and the maxillectomy performed on President Grover Cleveland in 1893 were discussed in a previous chapter. This large sarcoma involved a portion of the soft palate and maxilla. A dentist at the same time made a prosthesis which was inserted immediately.[1]

TABLE 17–1.—Cancer of the Paranasal Sinuses: Suspected Etiologic Factors

Occupational risks
Nickel refining (squamous cell carcinoma)
Furniture workers, esp. hard woods (adenocarcinoma)
Chemical manufacturing
Radium dial-painters
Thorium dioxide (used as a contrast material)
Snuff (contains carcinogens)

In 1911 William Clark published a series of papers advocating the use of electrodissection and electrocauterization for cancers of the maxillary sinus.[2] Still, in 1917, the majority of patients seen at the Mayo Clinic with cancer of the upper jaw were no longer candidates for any type of operative procedure at the time of diagnosis.[3] Douglas Quick in 1929 advocated the combination of therapeutic x-irradiation, radium, and surgery in the management of maxillary malignancies.[4] Fifty percent of the patients he saw had already undergone a prolonged course of treatment, including local operative procedures, before the correct diagnosis was made. Seventy-three percent of the patients in his series had cervical metastases at the time of presentation. Again, this highlights the delay and difficulty of diagnosis in earlier periods.

Between 1930 and 1945, therapeutic irradiation became the preferred method of treatment of nasal sinus malignancies. Surgical resection failed to eradicate the tumor because the full extent of involvement could not be recognized prior to surgery.[5] Therefore resection of the maxilla frequently was inadequate, as a tumor could have extended through the posterior wall into the pterygomaxillary fossa or even the base of the skull. Frazell and Lewis in 1963 published data on 416 patients with carcinoma of the nose and paranasal sinuses.[6] They concluded that surgical resection was the preferred method of treatment. Tabb in 1959 again advocated surgical resection, but recommended postoperative therapeutic irradiation.[7]

In 1954 Smith, Klopp, and Williams were the first to present a series of patients with extensive disease involving the base of the skull.[8] They published their re-

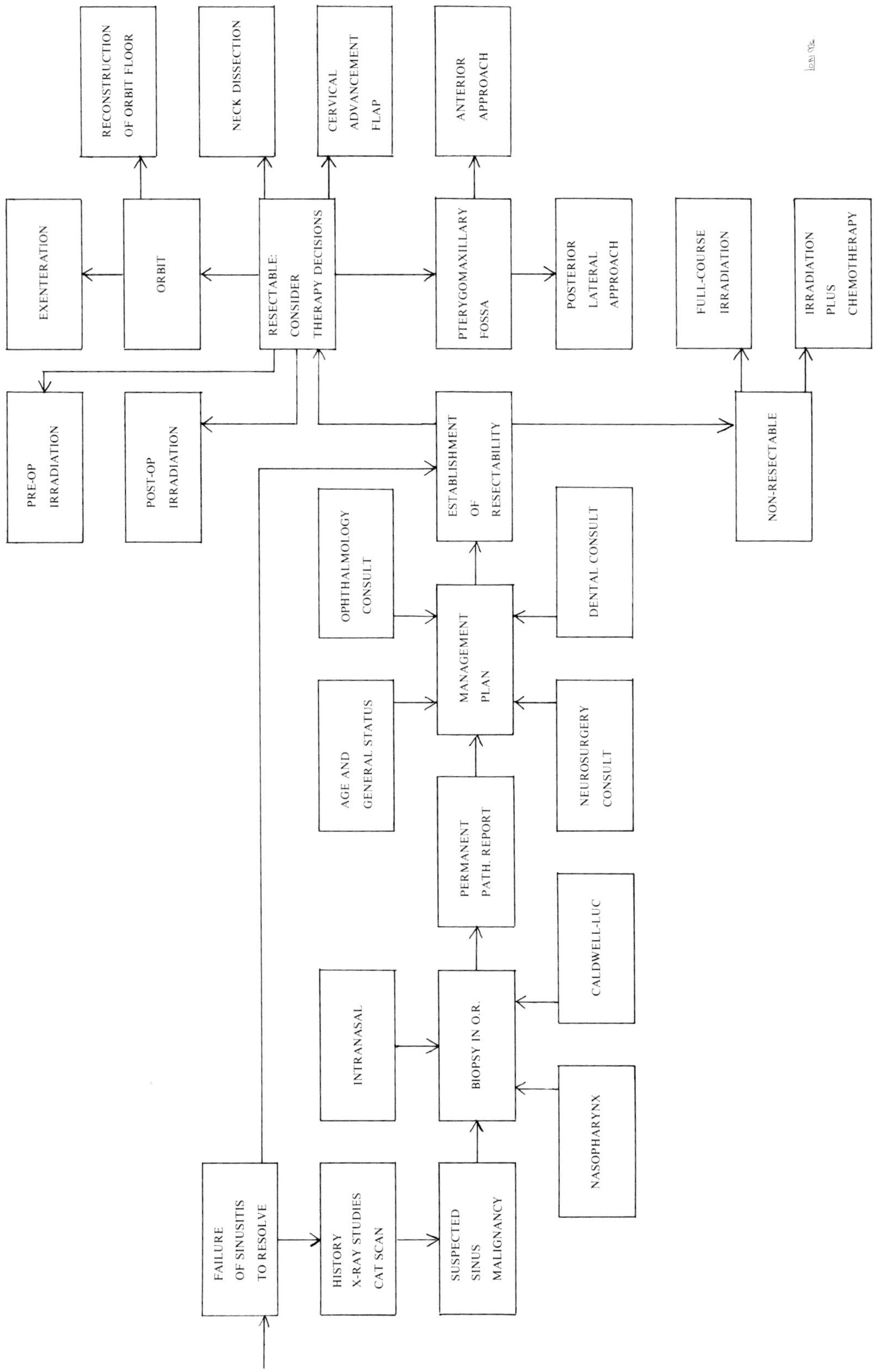

Fig 17–1.—Scheme for management of paranasal sinus cancer.

port of 19 cases in which a combined resection was performed, including the cribriform plate. A neurosurgeon would define the extent of the tumor intracranially. Then the combined procedure, which required dropping out the entire maxilla, ethmoid, and orbital contents from below, was performed. By 1966, this group had performed the operative procedure on 33 patients and had a 61% 3-year-survival with a 7% operative mortality.

PATHOLOGY

What Is the Most Common Type of Malignancy of the Nose and Paranasal Sinuses?

As in other areas of the head and neck, *squamous cell carcinoma* or *epidermoid carcinoma*[9–11] by far exceeds all other cell types as the most common form of malignancy. *Adenocarcinoma* is the second most common type of malignancy in adults.[12] The most common form of adenocarcinoma of the maxillary sinus is adenoidcystic carcinoma. Unlike its counterpart in the parotid or submandibular glands, adenoidcystic carcinoma occurring in the maxilla does not have a prolonged course. It aggressively extends posteriorly toward the base of the skull. Radiologic assessment will always underestimate the extent of the disease. Biopsy specimens should be obtained several centimeters from the site of the actual malignancy, as there can be submucosal as well as epineural extension of the disease.

Papillary adenocarcinoma occurs high in the vault of the nose. This is the type of malignancy described in furniture workers. It appears as a papillary lesion in the region of the superior turbinate or nasal vault. *Mucoepidermoid carcinoma* may arise in the salivary glands of the palate and extend directly upward (Figs 17–2 and 17–3). Most of these malignancies arise at the junction of the hard and soft palate and involve the maxilla by direct extension. *Adenoidcystic carcinoma* arising in a minor salivary gland in the palate may similarly extend upward into the maxilla.[13]

Squamous cell carcinoma is likewise the most common type of malignancy to arise primarily in the frontal sinus.[14] Nevertheless, cancer of the frontal sinus is extremely rare, and each published series includes only one or two such isolated cases, that is, cases in which the tumor did not extend upward from the maxilla and ethmoid area to involve the frontal complex. They may be associated with a prolonged history of chronic frontal sinusitis.

Malignant melanoma usually arises on the palate or nose and extends to involve the maxillary sinus.[15–17] This melanoma of the mucosal membrane is frequently difficult to diagnose, particularly if there is a lack of pigmentation. By the time of diagnosis, the disease has usually demonstrated extensive posterior erosion.

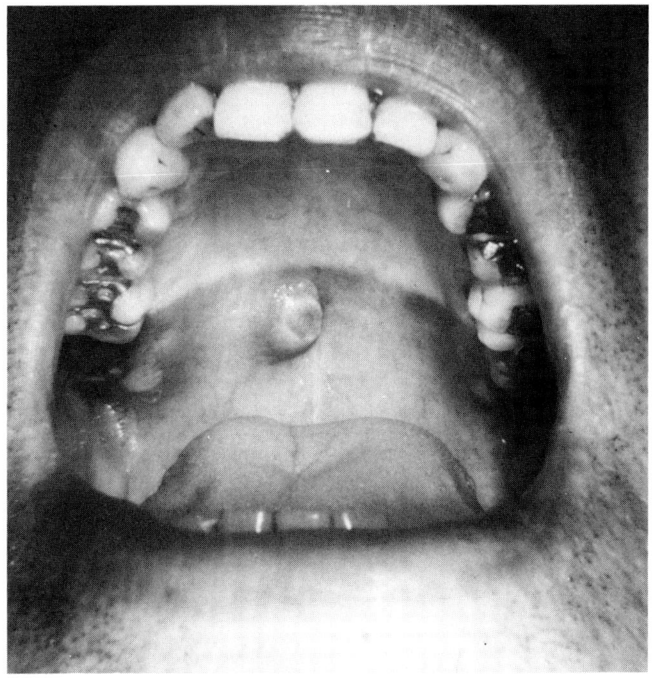

Fig 17–2.—Mucoepidermoid carcinoma, adenoidcystic carcinoma, malignant mixed tumor, and mixed tumor have this appearance. Note that the tumor is at the junction of the hard and soft palate and just off the midline. Compare with the torus in Figure 17–12. Partial maxillectomy is required.

Osteogenic sarcoma is the most common sarcoma of the maxilla and is treated with combined surgery and chemotherapy.[18] At times this malignancy has extended to adjacent areas, and radiation and chemotherapy are the only possible form of treatment.

Metastatic malignancies can also extend to the maxillary sinus. Any tumor that has a tendency to metastasize to bone would likely extend to the maxillary sinus. The most common such malignancy is renal cell carcinoma.

When Should You Suspect Malignancy of the Sinus, Nose, or Paranasal Sinus?

The initial symptoms of malignancy of the paranasal sinuses are almost identical to those of benign sinusitis. Some clues to differentiating these are as follows:

1. There is a lack of response to medical management.
2. There is frequently associated epistaxis.
3. Pain or swelling persists over the involved area.
4. Physical examination may reveal paresthesia of cranial nerve V.
5. There may be exophthalmos or other visual changes.
6. A denture may become ill-fitting.
7. Cranial nerve paralysis may develop.

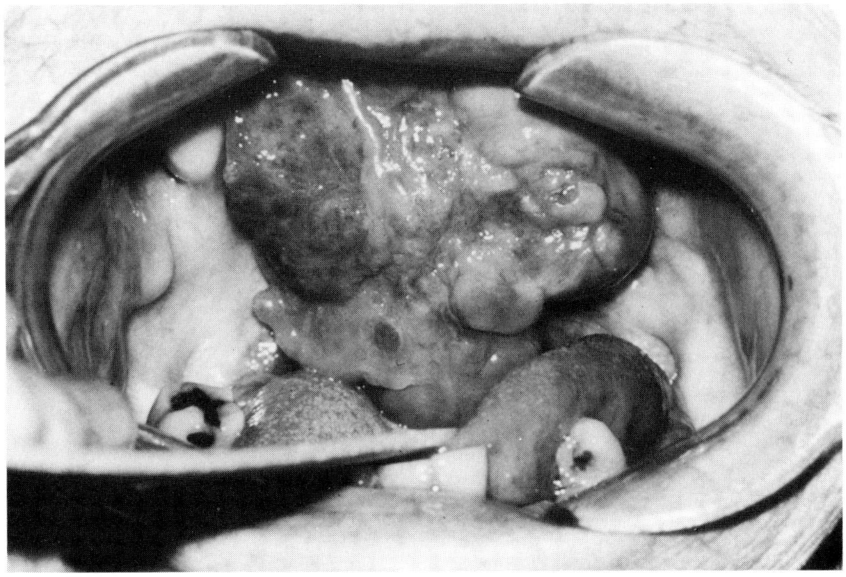

Fig 17–3.—Large fungating tumor involving the entire palate. Tumor has ulcerated because of its extensive size. Biopsy proved it to be a benign mixed tumor. Bilateral partial maxillectomy was required.

8. Persistent unilateral rhinorrhea may be present.
9. Radiologic evaluation may demonstrate bony erosion.
10. X-ray examination showing erosion of dental roots is highly suggestive of a tumor, although not necessarily one that is malignant.

Chronic benign disease generally does not cause resorption of maxillary roots. A persistently opacified maxillary sinus needs to be explored, if no explanation for the persistence is found.

HOW DO YOU ESTABLISH THAT THE PATIENT HAS NOT RESPONDED TO CUSTOMARY MEDICAL MANAGEMENT?

Acute sinusitis usually follows an upper respiratory tract infection or occurs in the patient with allergy problems. It is often bilateral or involves all sinuses, when it is referred to as pansinusitis. When there is persistent involvement of a single sinus, one must be suspicious that there is obstruction of the drainage of that sinus (Fig 17–4). Antibiotics, decongestants, or antihistamines are prescribed. Nasal topical decongestants may provide some relief and promote drainage when given for a short period of time, generally less than 5 days. After only 48 hours, the patient should receive some relief of the pain and headache associated with sinus disease.

Pain worsening on medical management requires either more intensive intravenous antibiotics or a drainage procedure. Most often it is the maxillary sinus that is involved, and an antral aspiration can be performed. Two popular techniques are aspiration in the canine fossa, directly above the canine tooth, and aspiration beneath the inferior turbinate. Direct puncture through the anterior wall of the maxillary sinus is easier. Xylocaine 2% with adrenaline 1:100,000 is injected. Then a sinus trocar is passed directly into the sinus. The fluid present in the sinus is aspirated and sent for culture and evaluation. Cytologic study can also be performed on this material, although interpretation is difficult because of the extensive amount of inflammatory cellular material present.

The initial antibiotic selected should cover the spectrum of *Pneumococcus*, *Streptococcus*, *Staphylococcus*, and *Hemophilus influenzae* organisms. Amoxicillin or ampicillin is currently a favorite drug for this purpose. In patients allergic to penicillin, one of the cephalosporins is preferred. Tetracycline and erythrocin are also effective for sinus disease. The aspirate should be sent to be cultured for identification of the responsible organism.

At the same time that the aspirate is obtained, normal saline can be flushed through the sinus. This not only washes the mucopurulence from the sinus, but may permit better function of the ciliary activity of the sinus, allowing it thereafter to cleanse itself. Radiographs obtained a few days after the irrigation may demonstrate persistence of a mass within the sinus. If there is still failure to respond and the sinus again fills with fluid, irrigation may again be performed.

A unilaterally opacified maxillary sinus that fails to respond to medical management and irrigation requires further exploration. Fungal infection, chronic hyperplastic sinusitis, and tumor are included in the differential diagnosis. It is always preferable to obtain a biopsy specimen for pathologic evaluation without actually entering the sinus. Therefore, a transnasal route is preferable. However, it is possible to miss the diagnosis of malignancy if only a nasal antrostomy is

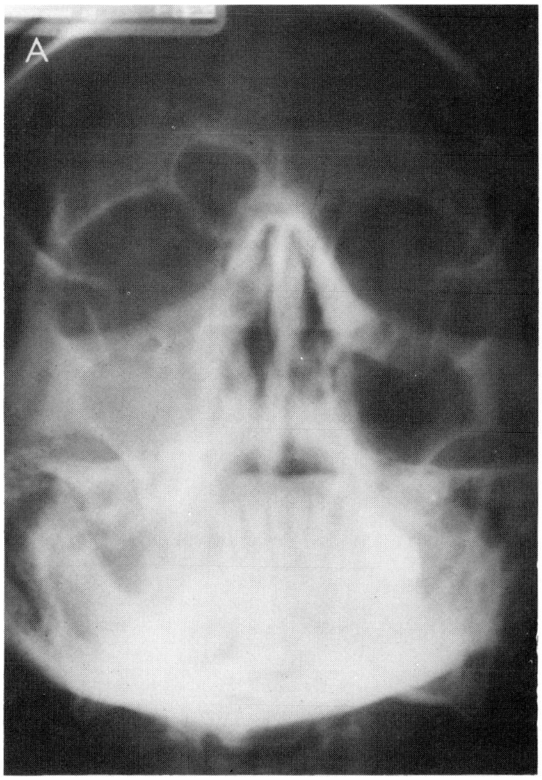

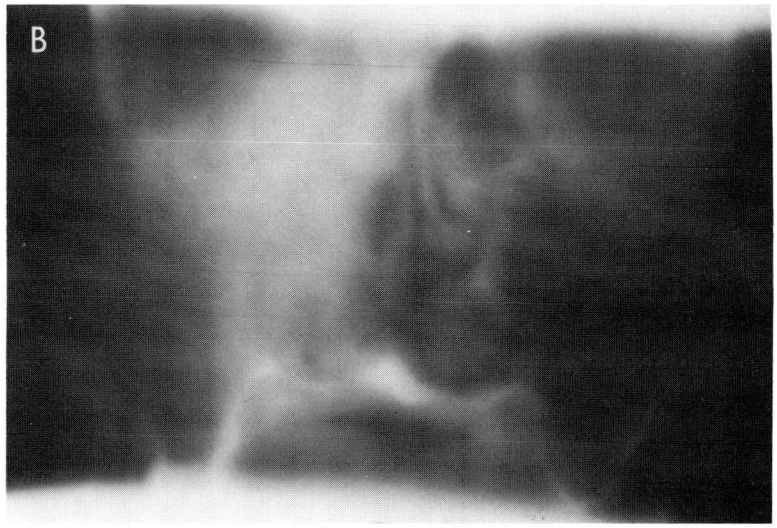

Fig 17–4.—A, x-ray of a patient with chronic sinusitis. A nasal antrostomy was performed in 1978. **B,** polytomograph obtained in 1983 showed extensive bone erosion. Biopsy by the Caldwell-Luc approach established the diagnosis of squamous cell carcinoma of the left maxillary sinus.

performed. If tissue obtained by this route reveals only chronic inflammation but tumor is suspected, a Caldwell-Luc approach is required.

The nasoantral window or nasoantrostomy involves removal of a 2 × 2 cm segment of bone beneath the inferior turbinate. While it is an excellent treatment for the management of chronic benign disease, it is not always helpful in diagnosing malignancy, because not all aspects of the sinus can be directly seen. In Europe, a special sinuscope has been devised to pass through this opening. It is a flexible fiberoptic type of scope that permits better evaluation of the maxillary sinus. If material obtained by transnasal antrostomy is not helpful, direct visualization is necessary.

The Caldwell-Luc operation provides a direct approach through the anterior wall of the maxillary sinus. Care is taken to remain sufficiently above the dental roots and to avoid permanent paresthesia of the face, which may occur from injury to the maxillary divisions of cranial nerve V. All abnormal tissue can be seen under direct vision through this approach and can be removed from the sinus and sent for pathologic examination. Material for culture is also obtained.

WHAT ARE THE SIGNS AND SYMPTOMS OF NASAL TUMORS?

Tumors arising high in the nasal vault or in the ethmoid area soon produce epistaxis or nasal obstruction. Unilateral nasal obstruction without an apparent cause requires x-ray study of the sinus. Some unusual nasal tumors may cause a decreased sense of smell, and later rhinorrhea. The nose can be decongested utilizing a ¼% Neosynephrin spray. Tumors of the ethmoid region will look like fleshy polyps. When palpated with the suction tip, they may be friable and bleed. For biopsy, cocaine pledgets can be packed into the area. After vasoconstriction is attained, biopsy can be performed directly through the nose, but the physician must be prepared to pack the nose, should extensive bleeding occur.

ARE THERE TUMORS OF THE SPHENOID SINUS?

The sphenoid sinus is the least likely site of a primary malignancy. It may be the site of metastasis from the prostate or breast. Tumors of the sphenoid sinus are best approached by the translabial/transnasal route, exposing the sphenoid sinus and pituitary gland, as is done in pituitary surgery. The area can only be cureted and the specimen sent for pathologic examination. Therapeutic irradiation is the mainstay of treatment. Malignancy of the sphenoid sinus is suspected when a lateral-view radiograph shows persistent opacification of the sinus and bony erosion. The sphenoid sinus is commonly involved with chronic sinusitis as part of widespread pansinusitis. Persistent opacification of a sphenoid sinus alone is an unusual problem.

WHEN SHOULD YOU OBTAIN RADIOGRAPHS OF THE SINUSES?

A patient with a few-day history of symptoms suggestive of sinusitis is treated on the basis of the clinical examination. Cultures of the nose are of no value. Because most cases of acute sinusitis are due to *Pneumococcus*, *Streptococcus*, or *Hemophilus influenzae*, appropriate antibiotics are selected. When there is a complication or suspected complication developing, such as acute ethmoiditis, periorbital cellulitis, or a failure to show some evidence of response after 48 hours of treatment, a series of radiographs should be requested.

The most useful x-ray view is the upright Waters view, which, in acute sinusitis, will demonstrate a level of fluid (Fig 17–5). When the patient is lying down, the entire sinus should appear opacified, as the fluid will then layer out. The lateral view is also helpful, as it demonstrates the sphenoid and frontal sinuses. Mucosal thickening or levels of fluid will be seen in acute sinusitis.

The Caldwell view is taken with the forehead and nose touching the x-ray plate. It is the most useful view for evaluating the frontal sinus. Whenever there is any suspicion that a tumor could be present, the submentovertex view is extremely helpful. This view shows all of the sinuses as well as the posterior walls of the maxillary sinus and the foramina of the base of the skull. It is the most helpful view of the sinuses, but it is frequently omitted from a routine series because it is an uncomfortable position for the patient.

What Should You Look for on the Radiograph?

In acute sinus disease, there is generally diffuse mucosal thickening. Seldom is only one sinus involved. Mucosal thickening is present when there is more than 5 mm of thickness, measured along the lateral border of the maxillary sinus. When looking for malignancy, bony destruction is of key importance (Fig 17–6). Lack of definition of the bony rims of the sinuses suggests bony erosion. In the ethmoid region, the fine labyrinthine cells making up the ethmoid sinus should be identifiable. Bony destruction is not an absolute indication of malignancy; however, it is a red flag.

Until recently, tomographic views of the sinus (Figs

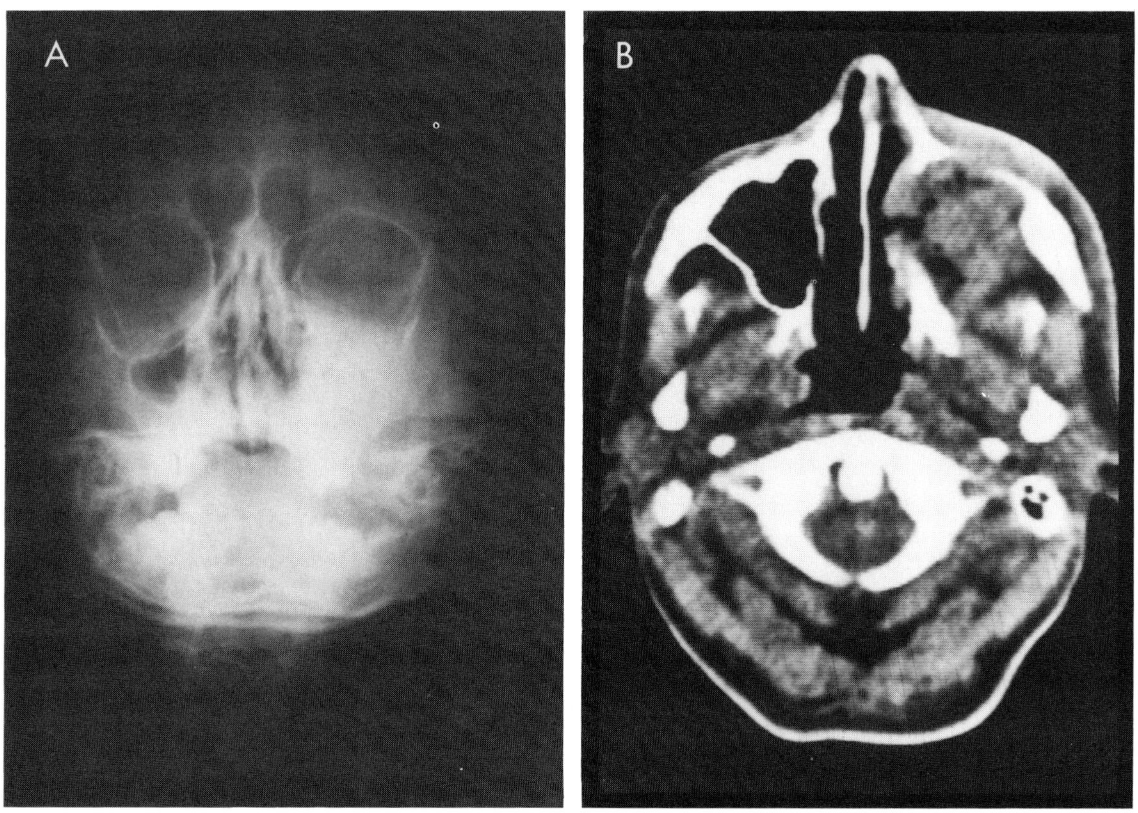

Fig 17–5.—A, upright Waters x-ray film demonstrates complete opacification of the left maxillary sinus. There is a suggestion of bony erosion of the medial and lateral sinus walls. Biopsy revealed squamous cell carcinoma. **B,** preoperative CT scan of large left maxillary sinus, confirming squamous cell carcinoma. The pterygoid plates are intact. There is no extension into the infratemporal fossa. The posterior wall of the maxilla is missing. The anterior wall of the maxilla is eroded.

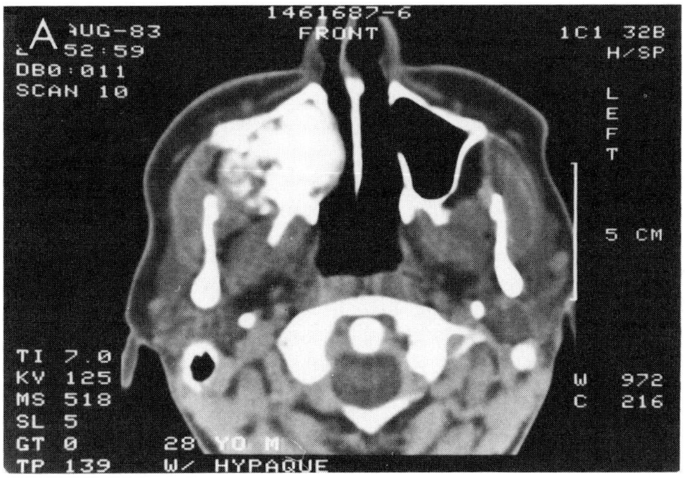

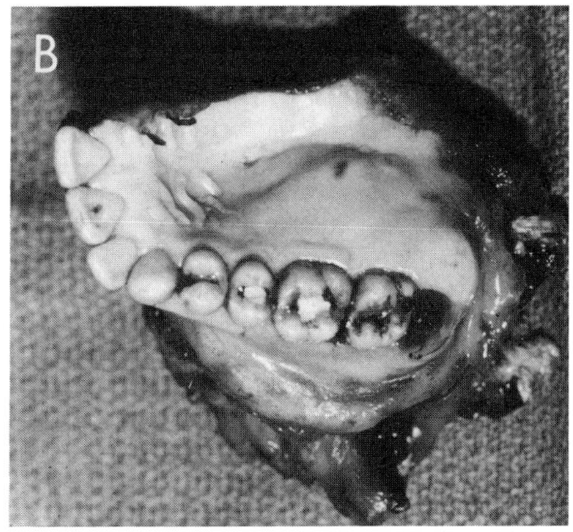

Fig 17–6.—A, CT scan of a 28-year-old man with an osteogenic sarcoma of the right maxilla. Note extension into nasal cavity and into soft tissues. **B,** resected specimen. More than 75% of the hard palate was resected.

17–7,A and B) were the most important form of radiologic evaluation. Bone erosion could be better detected on tomography. Direct tomography still plays an important role, even though the computerized tomographic (CT) scan has become the primary means of diagnosis of the extent of the disease (Figs 17–7,C and D) (see Chap. 3). Radiologic diagnosis of malignancy of the sinus still has a certain degree of inaccuracy. Even the best CT scans cannot distinguish between hyperplastic mucosa and tumor. The tumor may grow sufficiently to obstruct orifices of the sinus; then there is a secondary obstructive sinusitis. Radiologically, this looks like the extension of tumor.

Extensive bone erosion, however, should not occur with benign disease (see Fig 17–5,B). CT scans in the coronal view have been helpful in demonstrating whether the tumor has eroded the area of the cribriform plate and may be extending into the anterior cranial fossa. Coronal-view CT scans may demonstrate posterior extension through the region of the pterygomaxillary fossa toward the base of the skull. Even early orbital involvement can be appreciated on CT scans. Radiographs should always be obtained prior to any surgical intervention. Even nasal polypectomies and Caldwell-Luc procedures may cause enough edema and reaction to give misleading information when CT scans, tomograms, and routine radiographs are taken postoperatively.

MALIGNANT TUMORS OF THE MAXILLA

Management

The majority of cancers of the paranasal sinuses arise in the maxillary sinus, but may secondarily extend medially into the ethmoid area, posteriorly into the pterygomaxillary fossa, anteriorly into the cheek, superiorly into the orbit, or inferiorly into the palate. The important relationships at the base of the skull are shown in Figure 17–8. The routes of spread are illustrated in Figures 17–9 and 17–10. The TNM staging of maxillary sinus cancer is given in Table 17–2.

WHAT PHYSICAL SIGNS INDICATE EXTENSION OF DISEASE?

Physical examination may provide significant clues to the extent of the disease. A tumor extending inferiorly will widen the superior alveolar ridge and may cause loosening of the teeth (Fig 17–11). In fact, a malfitting denture or other indication may cause a dentist to be the first to recognize the disease (Fig 17–12). A tumor may extend out into the skin of the overlying cheek. Usually its appearance is like that of an inflammatory reaction of the overlying skin. In these circumstances, there is infraorbital nerve invasion (V_2), with the numbness of the cheek.

The most common direction of extension is superiorly, into the ethmoid region, involving the anterior ethmoid cells. Intranasal examination may show an exophytic lesion, medial displacement of the lateral nasal wall, or deformity of the middle turbinate. When that occurs, the ethmoid region is the preferable site for bi-

TABLE 17–2.—TNM CLASSIFICATION OF CARCINOMA OF THE MAXILLARY SINUS: PRIMARY TUMOR (T)

T_X	Minimum requirements to assess the primary tumor cannot be met
T_0	No evidence of primary tumor
T_1	Tumor confined to the antral mucosa of the infrastructure with no bone erosion or destruction
T_2	Tumor confined to the suprastructure mucosa without bone destruction, or to the infrastructure with destruction of medial or inferior bony walls only
T_3	More extensive tumor invading skin of cheek, orbit, anterior ethmoid sinuses, or pterygoid muscle
T_4	Massive tumor with invasion of cribriform plate, posterior ethmoids, sphenoid, nasopharynx, pterygoid plates, or base of skull

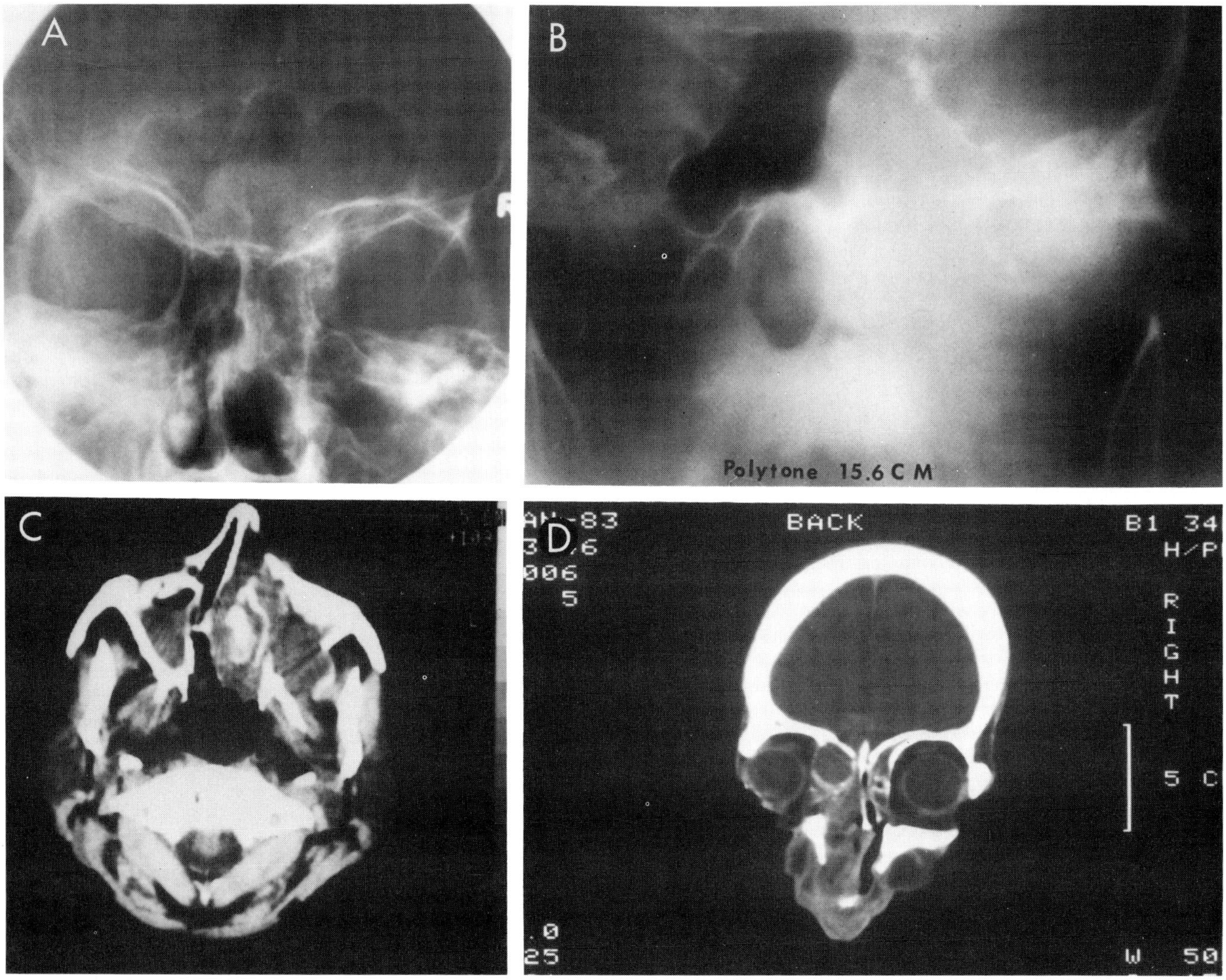

Fig 17–7.—A, upright Waters sinus x-ray film demonstrating opacification of the left maxillary sinus and a portion of the frontal sinus in a 68-year-old man complaining of nasal blockage and some bleeding. How much of the opacification is due to obstruction by the tumor? **B,** tomogram showing erosion of the medial maxillary wall, erosion into the septum, and extension into the ethmoid sinuses. Tomography is helpful for establishing bony erosion by tumor. **C,** CT scan demonstrating erosion of the posterior wall of the maxillary sinus. Biopsy demonstrated esthesioneuroblastoma. **D,** coronal-section CT scan demonstrating intercranial extension into the frontal lobe. Therefore, the patient was treated with irradiation only.

opsy, because it can be done in the office in order to avoid actually opening the sinus, as would be done in the Caldwell-Luc procedure. Tumorous extension into the pterygomaxillary fossa will cause trismus. However, there can be considerable extension and erosion of the pterygoid plates with no clinical symptoms. Invasion becomes evident only on CT scan or tomographic x-ray. Tumors may also extend into the infratemporal fossa, causing a bulge in the area just superior to the parotid gland. Extension to this area is a criterion of nonresectability. Tumors may extend posteriorly and then medially into the nasopharynx, pushing the lateral nasopharyngeal wall medially.

WHAT ARE THE CRITERIA FOR INOPERABILITY?

There are no absolute indications that a patient's tumor is inoperable. This is because some surgeons believe that there is a place for palliative maxillectomy. They recognize that large, fungating tumors soon become infected with extensive necrosis with a long delay before directly killing the patient. The majority of surgeons, however, believe that in such situations, therapeutic irradiation with a drainage procedure is sufficient treatment for palliation. A common indication for nonsurgical treatment is posterior extension of the tumor to

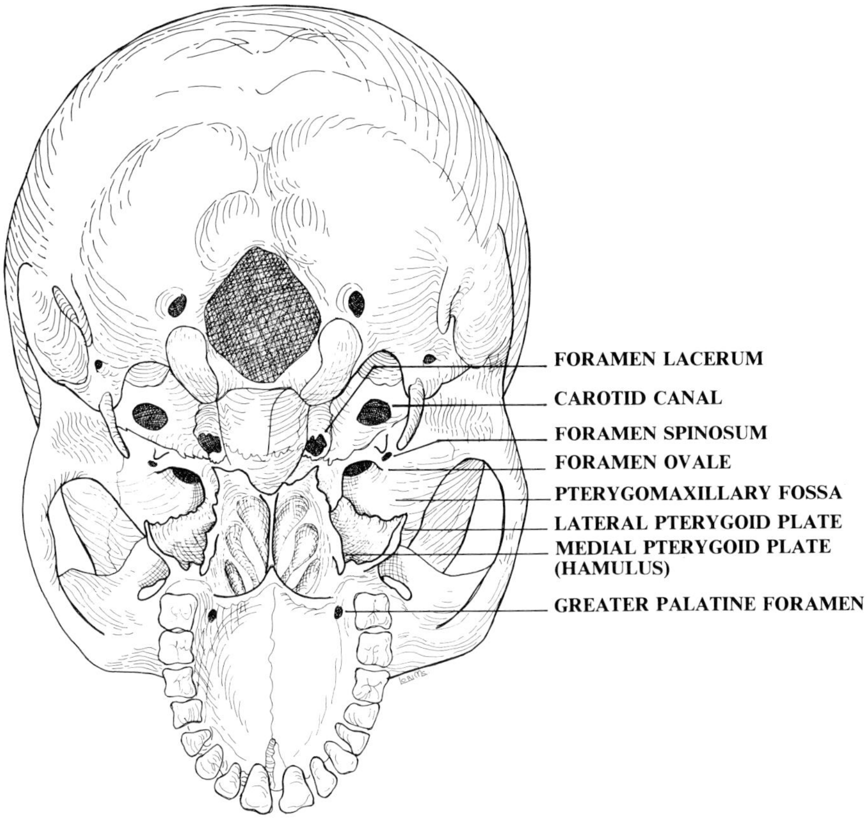

Fig 17–8.—Normal landmarks seen on x-ray or CT scan of the base of the skull. Determination of operability is based on defining the extent of disease in this area.

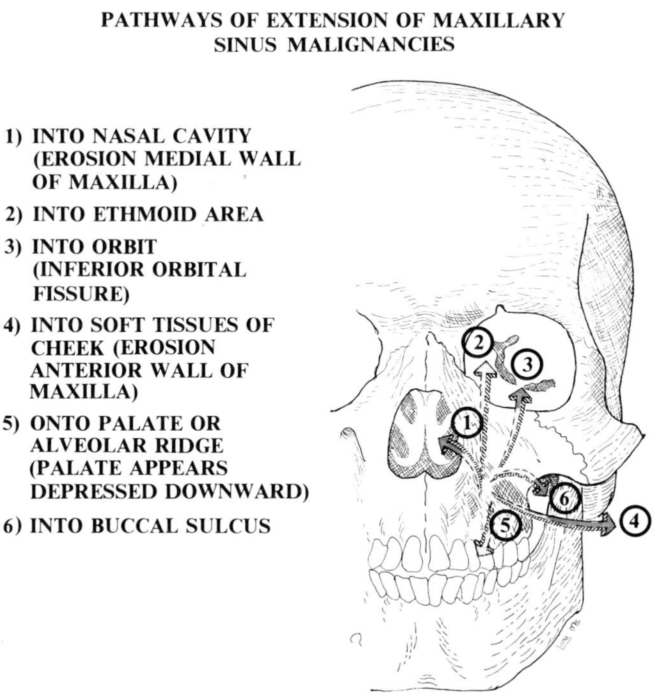

Fig 17–9.—Frontal view of the skull showing possible pathways of extension of a maxillary sinus cancer.

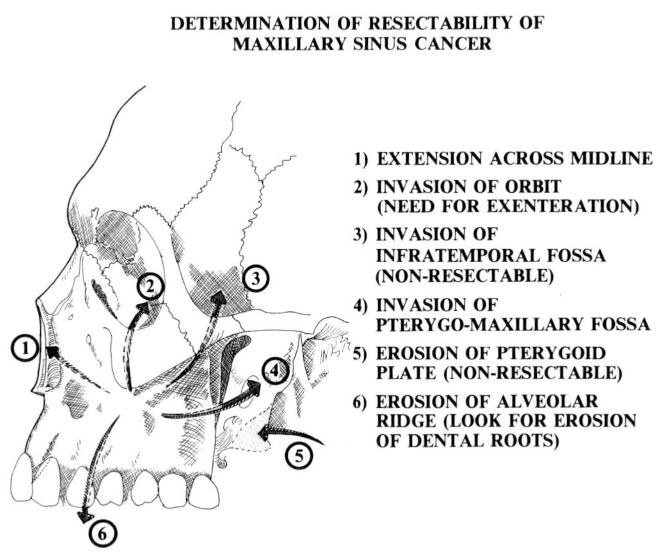

Fig 17–10.—Side view of areas of possible extension that should be considered in determining resectability.

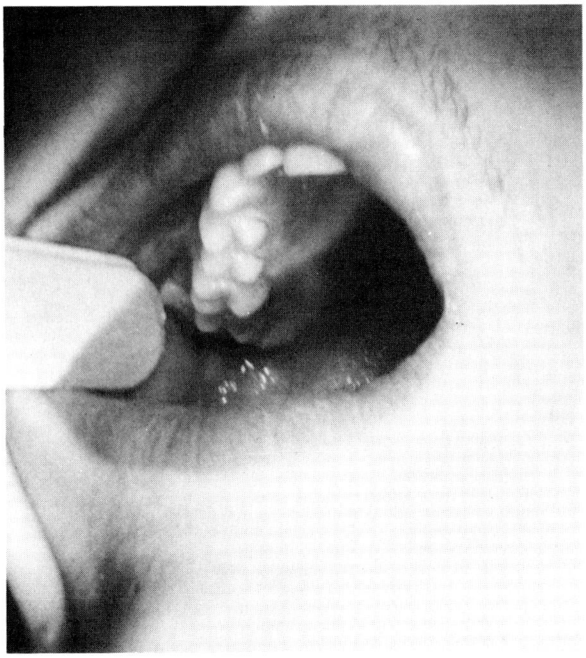

Fig 17–11.—Note deviation of the right third molar and enlargement of the maxillary alveolar ridge. These findings would be typical of a slow-growing benign or malignant tumor.

the base of the skull. This can be demonstrated by erosion of the pterygoid plates or erosion of the skull in the region of the foramen ovale (see Fig 17–8). While it is theoretically possible to resect this area of the base of the skull, the survival rate was not enhanced by resection. The surgical morbidity and mortality were not acceptable.

Radiologic evidence of erosion of the posterior wall of the maxillary sinus is not an indication of nonoperability but suggests that at the time of surgery, tumor will be found extending into the pterygomaxillary fossa. Plans must be made preoperatively to remove the pterygoid plates close to the base of the skull so as to "clean out" the pterygoid musculature. Tumors extending into the infratemporal fossa have invaded so much of the area at the base of the skull that they are generally not considered resectable. Tumorous extension across the midline, while not an indication of inoperability, makes it extremely difficult for the oral prosthodontist to create any type of usable prosthesis. If at least some of the teeth on the opposite side can be preserved, the prosthesis can be anchored to them. Tumor extending out into the cheek will require simultaneous resection of the skin of the cheek and closure with a direct cheek and cervical skin advancement flap.

The most difficult decision is whether to remove the orbital contents by orbital exenteration. When there is obvious tumor extending through the orbital floor and onto the periorbita, the eye must be removed. This determination cannot always be made preoperatively. While CT scans of the orbit are very useful when they demonstrate obvious destructive disease, early extension is not apparent. It may require frozen sections at the time of surgery to prove invasion of the orbital contents. In a very limited number of cases it is possible, using frozen sections as a control, to excise the periorbita and replace it with a split thickness skin graft (STSG) and preserve the eye. A preoperative CT scan that demonstrates erosion of the orbital floor, or anesthesia of the infraorbital nerve, or any form of diplopia or proptosis, suggests that the orbital contents will have to be removed. In any large cancer of the maxillary sinus, consent for orbital exenteration should be obtained preoperatively, because clinically inapparent tu-

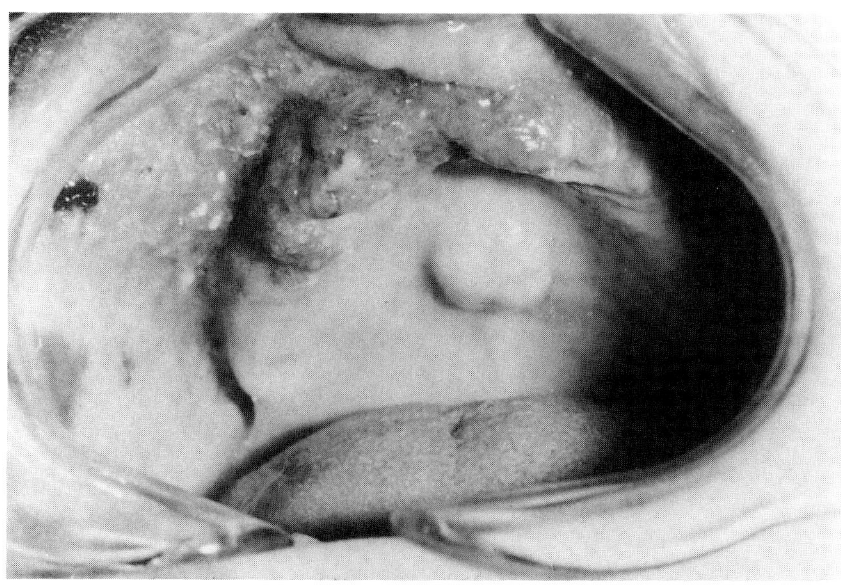

Fig 17–12.—Superficial squamous cell carcinoma of the right alveolar ridge. Eventually such tumors will erode into and involve the maxillary sinus. This tumor has extended across the midline. Note the typical location and appearance of a torus palatinus near the center of the palate.

mor may be found to be extending into the orbit at surgery.

Tumor extending into the anterior ethmoids will require a maxilloethmoidectomy. Tumor extending farther posteriorly, into the posterior ethmoid cells, generally cannot be removed. Unfortunately, when a CT scan shows clouding of the ethmoid cells and sphenoid sinus, even the experienced interpreter may not be able to distinguish whether this is due to invasion by tumor or to secondary obstructive sinusitis. Significant anterior ethmoid invasion or primary tumors of the ethmoid sinus are best treated by a combined craniofacial resection.

WHAT IS A CRANIOFACIAL RESECTION?

This en bloc operative procedure combines a frontal craniotomy with a "dropout" of the maxilla and ethmoid sinuses from below.[19] First, the neurosurgeon uses a coronal incision to approach from above the region of the olfactory groove and ethmoid labyrinth. The burr hole should be sufficiently superior as not to enter the frontal sinus. The dura and brain are gently elevated from the region of the cribriform plate. The dura may be adherent in this area, and a fascia graft to repair the dura may be required.[20] Now the ethmoid cells are outlined from above and the chisel cuts are made. The amount of tissue removed will depend on the site and size of the primary malignancy. Generally the resection crosses the midline to include the cribriform plate, the rostrum, and the fovea ethmoidalis. More limited tumors, such as the neuroesthesioblastoma, can be treated by resection of the base of the skull and cribriform sinus and ethmoid area, with dural repair achieved through a wide transfacial approach.

Preparation for a Maxillectomy

Preoperative
- Obtain a biopsy specimen, preferably transnasally. Await permanent pathologic confirmation.
- Obtain CT scan to document extent of disease and determine resectability.
- Obtain oral surgery and prosthodontic consultation with impression of palate.
- Obtain ophthalmologic consultation for involvement of eye and to establish condition of contralateral eye.
- Provide a thorough explanation to patient and family of extent of procedure, with special reference to orbital involvement.

Operative preparation
- Use a large-bore needle for administering fluid and blood.
- Prepare the entire face and neck.
- Use bilateral tarsorraphy sutures to protect the patient's eyes.
- The site and length of the incision are determined by extent of disease.
- Prepare the thigh for STSG.

Postoperative care
- A prosthesis can be placed immediately.
- The patient is allowed a liquid diet on the second postoperative day, with packs in place.
- The patient should be ambulatory on the first postoperative day.
- Systemic prophylactic antibiotics are maintained until packs are removed.
- Packing is usually removed in 1 week to 10 days.
- Modify the obturator at that time.
- Instruct the patient on care of the cavity. A Water Pik-like apparatus with a modified nasal spray tip will help maintain a clean cavity.
- Wait 4 weeks before starting postoperative irradiation.

Steps in a Maxillectomy

1. *Incision in skin:* Weber-Ferguson incision (Figs 17–13 and 17–14); may be modified to include orbital exenteration; may be modified to include removal of skin of cheek. Round the incision at the medial canthus.

2. *Buccal incision:* Incision lies below buccal alveolar groove, especially if a previous Caldwell-Luc procedure

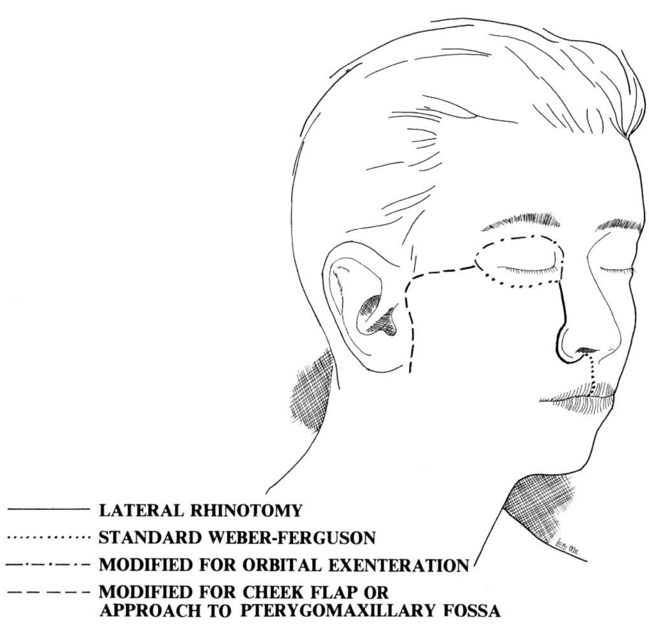

Fig 17–13.—Variations in incisions. A lateral rhinotomy is used in patients with cancer limited to the normal nasal cavity, or the ethmoid sinus. The Weber-Ferguson incision is used in patients with maxillary sinus cancer without orbital exenteration. The Weber-Ferguson incision may be modified if preoperative evaluation has established need for orbital exenteration. A cheek flap incision is used for tumor that has penetrated the anterior wall and facial skin. This incision also provides access for a posterolateral approach to the pterygomaxillary fossa.

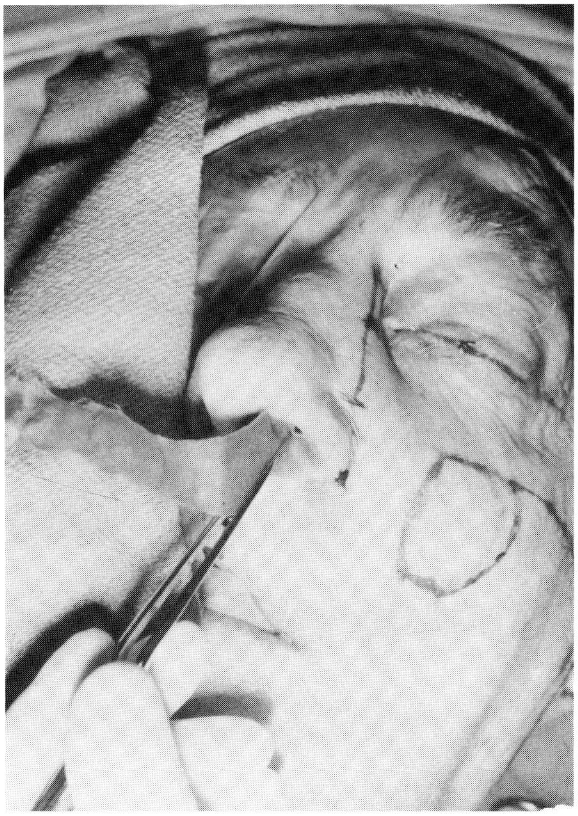

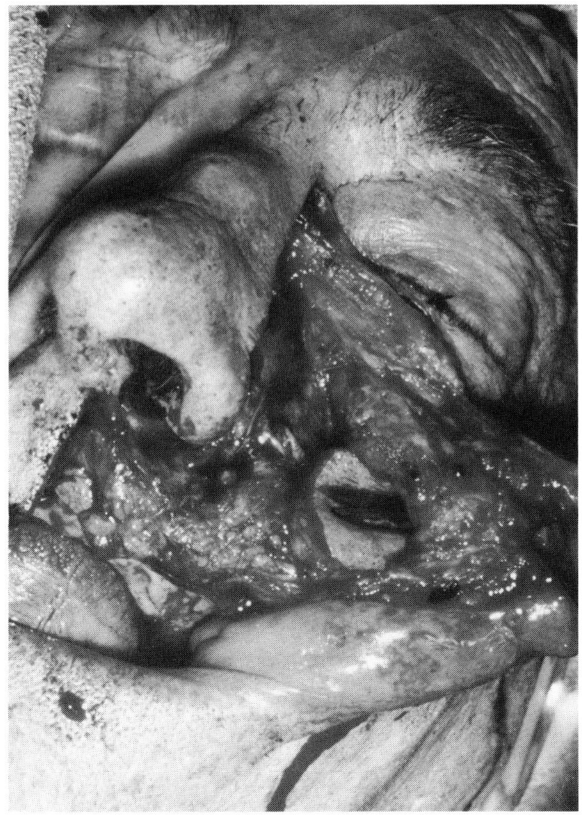

Fig 17–14 (left).—Patient whose x-ray film and CT scan are shown in Figure 17–5. The first step in maxillectomy is to plan the skin incisions. Because of erosion demonstrated on the CT scan, a segment of skin will be included in the specimen. The nose is packed with cocaine-impregnated gauze to reduce hemorrhage. A decision has not yet been made on preservation of the orbit.

Fig 17–15 (right).—Skin flap is elevated, leaving all muscular attachments to the maxilla as part of the specimen.

has been performed. Extend to posterior hard palate (maxillary tuberosity).

3. *Elevation of skin flap:* Deep muscle and soft tissue will remain attached to specimen (Fig 17–15).

4. *Identification of zygomatic arch and mandibular coronoid process:* The coronoid process is removed but left attached to the temporalis muscle for later reconstruction of the orbital floor.

5. *Lateral rhinotomy:* Nasal chisel is used to separate the maxilla and nasal bone. The middle and lower turbinates will be included in the specimen.

6. *Ethmoid:* Elevate the orbital periosteum. The incision is extended posteriorly along the suture line of the orbital process of frontal bone. The anterior and posterior ethmoid arteries are identified.

7. *Malar bone:* The inferior orbital fissure is identified by elevating the orbital periosteum. A right-angled clasp is placed through the fissure and used to pass the Gigli saw.

8. *Zygomatic arch:* In a similar manner, the Gigli saw is passed. In a variation of this technique, used in certain circumstances, the Gigli saw or right-angled oscillating saw is passed to permit preservation of the malar zygomatic eminence.

9. *Palate:* Elevate the nasal mucoperiosteum along the floor of the nose to the posterior aspect of the hard palate (Figs 17–16 and 17–17). A right-angled clamp is placed into the roof of the mouth at the posterior edge of the hard palate. A Gigli saw is passed. It may be possible to preserve the premaxilla and central and lateral incisors by changing the angle of the most anterior cut, as shown by the alternative dotted line in Figure 17–17.

10. *Pterygoid plate:* The external maxillary artery may be identified as it passes between the heads of the lateral pterygoid muscle. Removal of the coronoid process permits additional exposure. A finger is used to free the pterygoid muscle from attachments to the lateral pterygoid plate. The lateral and medial plates are exposed. The chisel cut is made under direct vision. If the posterior wall is involved, the chisel cut is placed high, toward the base of the skull (Figure 17–18).

11. *Complete the removal:* The entire specimen is "rocked" and the posterior orbital bony attachment will

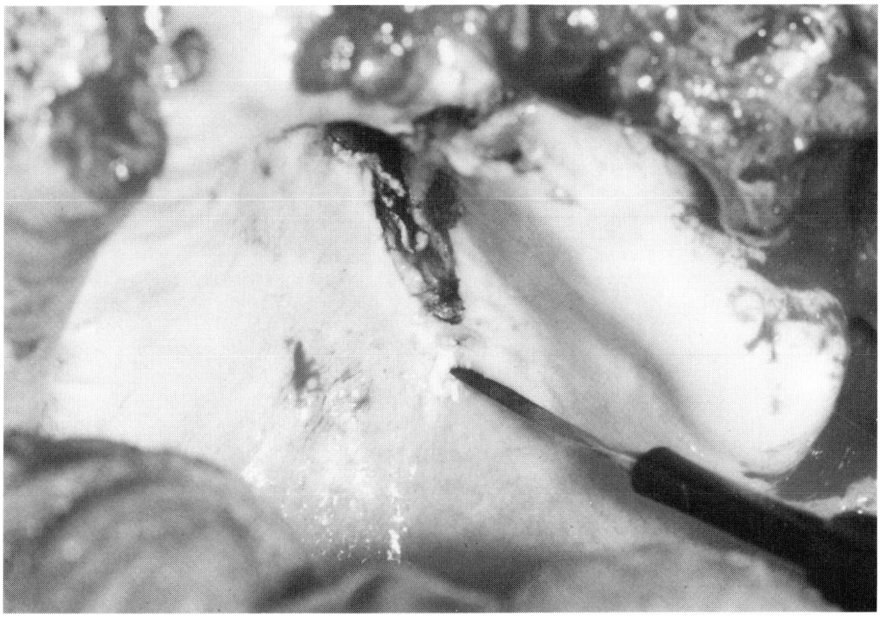

Fig 17–16.—The hard palate is incised with a cutting cautery.

fracture. Mayo scissor's are used to free the remaining soft tissue attachment.

12. *Examination of specimen:* The entire specimen is examined for completion of resection. The maxilla should remain as an enclosed "box." The posterior area of pterygomaxillary fossa is examined for tumor and ligation of vessels.

13. *Skin graft:* A split-thickness skin graft (15/1,000) is placed and sutured in position with absorbable suture.

14. *Packing:* The cavity is packed with 1-inch iodoform gauze with an antibiotic ointment. The skin flap is then replaced. The predesigned prosthesis can be placed. (Fig 17–19). If no prosthesis is possible, 0-0 silk sutures from the lateral wall to the remaining edge of the hard palate will hold the packing in place. When Silastic sheeting is placed above the sutures, the patient can eat on the first postoperative day.

Modifications

Under certain circumstances, the standard maxillectomy can be modified.

Palatal tumor: A malignant neoplasm on the palate may not extend upward into the area of the orbit. The orbital floor can be preserved. Unfortunately, whenever a partial maxillectomy is performed, the "box" tends to fracture like an eggshell and makes the thoroughness of the surgery less effective.

Ethmoid tumor: The palate may be preserved. A craniofacial approach may be considered.

Reconstruction

Overlying skin: If the skin over the maxilla has been invaded, it is outlined and removed as part of the specimen. The incision is extended laterally and slightly superiorly to the pretragal area, then downward to the neck. This will permit primary closure. There is a tendency in this situation for a fistula to develop in the medial canthal area. Make certain there is no tension on the thin skin in this region. Avoid sharp corners.

Orbital floor: The temporalis muscle with its fascia remains connected to the coronoid process. The incision is extended posterosuperiorly, splitting the tem-

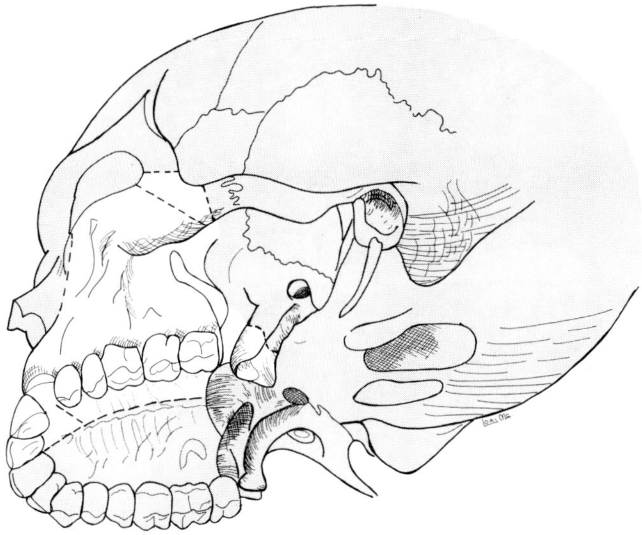

Fig 17–17.—Saw and chisel cuts along the skull base zygoma and maxilla. Note the following: an incision is made along the frontal process of the maxilla; malar bone can be resected by a single anterior cut or two separate incisions farther back; preservation of the premaxilla, when possible, will allow better obturator fit and stability; and the lateral and medial pterygoid plates are taken close to the skull base when the posterior maxillary wall is involved.

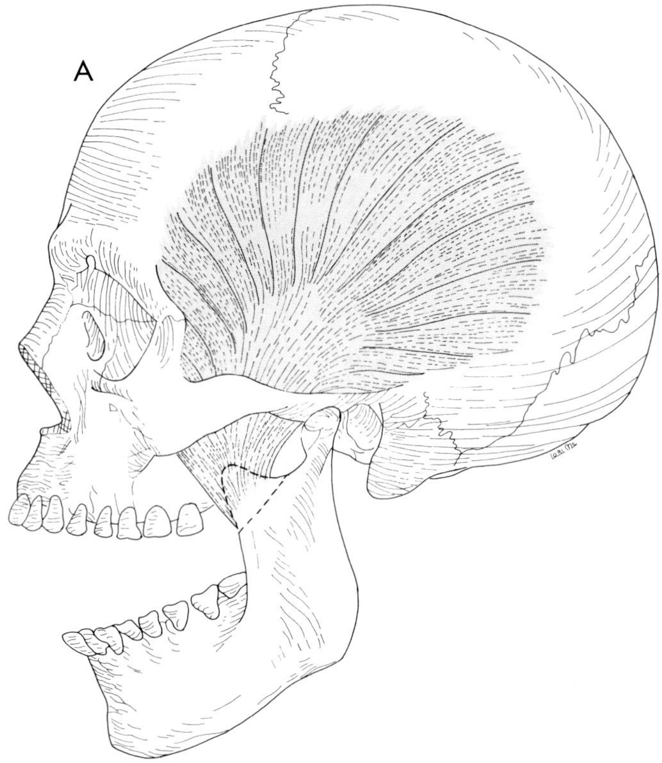

POSTERIO-LATERAL APPROACH TO THE MAXILLA
CHISEL INCISION SEPARATES THE CORONOID PROCESS WITH ATTACHED TEMPORALIS MUSCLE.

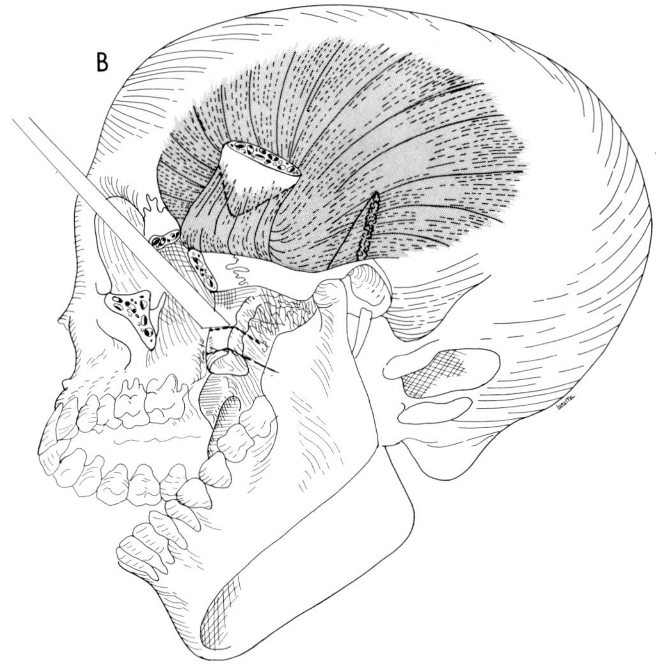

THE PTERYGOID PLATES ARE SEPARATED FROM THE BASE OF THE SKULL UNDER DIRECT VISION. HEIGHT OF THE CUT DEPENDS UPON EXTENT OF TUMOR.

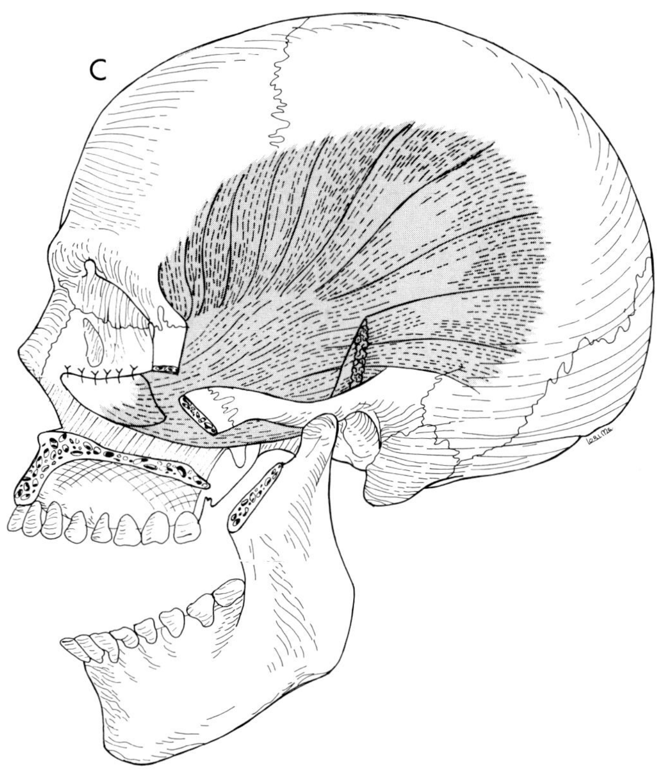

TEMPORALIS MUSCLE, FASCIA, AND CORONOID PROCESS FORM THE NEW ORBITAL FLOOR.

Fig 17–18.—Posterior lateral approach to the pterygomaxillary fossa with orbital floor reconstruction. **A,** coronoid process is divided, with the temporalis muscle attachment preserved. **B,** under direct visualization, a chisel cut is made in the pterygoid plate. The pterygoid plate is identified and soft tissue attachments to the plate are mobilized by finger dissection. Resection is performed closer to the base of the skull when the posterior sinus wall is involved; otherwise it is performed closer to the maxilla, as illustrated by the two alternative cuts. **C,** the coronoid process with attached temporalis fascia is brought forward to create a new orbital floor. Additional length is obtained by elevating more temporalis fascia and extending the incision along the temporalis muscle.

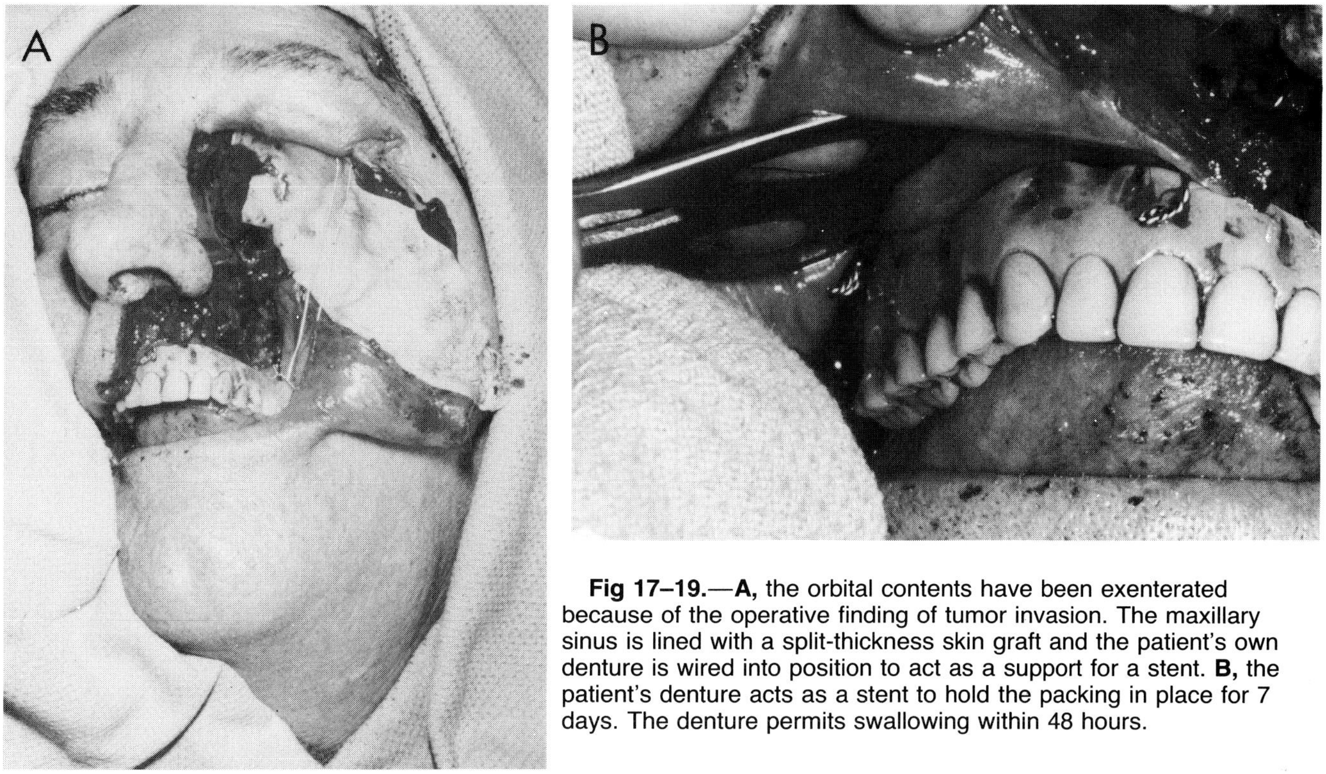

Fig 17–19.—A, the orbital contents have been exenterated because of the operative finding of tumor invasion. The maxillary sinus is lined with a split-thickness skin graft and the patient's own denture is wired into position to act as a support for a stent. **B,** the patient's denture acts as a stent to hold the packing in place for 7 days. The denture permits swallowing within 48 hours.

poralis muscle. The fasciae and muscle are sutured to the periosteum in the ethmoid area or to the lateral nasal wall. The segment of coronoid lies in the anteromedial area of the orbital floor (see Fig 17–18,C).

Orbital Exenteration

The decision to remove the orbital contents may have to be made at the time of surgery (see Fig 17–19,A). If there is evidence of orbital invasion on the CT scan, the decision is made preoperatively and incisions are planned accordingly. The orbital contents are removed en bloc by elevating the periosteum. Right-angled rhinoplasty scissors are used to incise the optic nerve and posterior attachments. Bleeding is controlled with packing. The entire bony orbit is skin grafted. The deep depression of the orbit is not covered. The remaining skin of the eyelid is sutured to the orbital margins. A patch or, later, prosthetic attachment will cover the defect (Figure 17–20).

What Are the Results of Treatment of Cancer of the Maxillary Sinus?

Table 17–3 summarizes some of the major series. Results are stratified by stage, presence or absence of node metastases, and treatment modality, when studied and reported by the authors. Where 5-year survival statistics were available, they are provided. It should be emphasized that malignant tumors involving the maxilla are rare in children. When they occur, they are of embryonal cell types (Fig 17–21).

TUMORS OF THE NOSE

Where Does Epidermoid Carcinoma of the Nasal Cavity Occur?

Malignant nasal tumors constitute only 3% of all malignancies of the head and neck. The most common site of nasal malignancy is the lateral nasal wall, and the second most common site is the nasal septum. These two sites alone account for more than 50% of primary nasal malignancies. The nasal vestibule and the posterior choana are uncommon sites of nasal malignancy. Tumors can become so large it is difficult to ascertain where they originated. Squamous cell carcinoma accounts for more than half of primary nasal malignancies, and adenocarcinoma is the second most common malignant tumor. All other nasal malignancies are rare.

NASAL SEPTUM

Primary squamous cell carcinoma of the septum is unusual.[21] When it does occur, the most common site is just posterior to the mucocutaneous junction, and all tumors are more common anteriorly than posteriorly. Malignancies of the nasal septum have been found at a higher frequency in persons with certain occupational exposure: nickel refiners and persons exposed to bis-

TABLE 17–3.—RESULTS OF TREATMENT OF CARCINOMA OF THE MAXILLARY SINUS

STUDY, YEAR, INSTITUTION	NO. OF PTS.	LENGTH OF FOLLOW-UP*	PROCEDURE AND RESULTS			
Sakai and Hamasaki,[21] 1967 (Japan)	226	5 yr	*Survival by cancer stage:*	I, II	III	IV
			Radiation + surgery	30%	32%	. . .
			Radiation alone	35%	9%	0
Frazell and Lewis,[32] 1963 (NY Memorial)	416	5 yr	*Overall 5-yr survival:*			24.7%
			Overall 5-yr cure:			35%
			Surgery (253 pts.):			
			Cervical recurrences			11
			Salvaged by radical neck			4
			Primary irradiation (98 pts.)			
			Cured			14%
			No. free of disease at primary site			17
Tabb,[33] 1957 (Charity Hosp., New Orleans)	60	. . .	Radiation (25 pts.)			Alive: 1
			Combined (20 pts.)			Alive: 2
			Palliation (7 pts.)			Alive: 0
			Surgery (8 pts.)			Alive: 4
Schall,[34] 1951 (Massachusetts Eye and Ear)	219	5 yr	*Overall 5-yr survival:*			27.8%
			Survival by cancer type:			
			Adenocarcinoma			7/22
			Undifferentiated			3/15
			Squamous cell (all grades)			29/108
			Survival by procedure:			
			Surgery alone			12/22
			Combined			14/41
			Radiation			8/59
			Overall survival, surgery and radiation combined:			35.1%
St. Pierre and Baker,[35] 1983 (Univ. of Michigan)	66	5 yr	*Overall 5-yr survival:*			
			With nodes			28.6%
			No nodes			32.6%
			Later nodes			15%
			Surgery			20%
			Radiation			15.7%
			Combined			58%
Lee and Ogura,[36] 1981 (Washington Univ., St. Louis)	96	5 yr	*Overall 5-yr survival, preop. radiation (5,000–6,000 rad):*			
			Combined:			
			T_1		3/5	18/47 (38%)
			T_2		5/11	
			T_3		5/18	
			T_4		5/13	
			Radiation			
			T_2		0/2	0/23
			T_3		0/6	
			T_4		0/15	

*For purposes of determining survival statistics.

chlormethyl ether, isopropyl oils, mustard gas, and hexamethyl phosphoramide. Presenting symptoms are bleeding, nasal obstruction, stuffiness, and headache. The more posterior the tumor, the more likely it is to present as obstruction.

Treatment is primarily by surgery or a combination of surgery plus irradiation. There are no data to ascertain whether preoperative or postoperative irradiation is favored. Our own preference is postoperative therapeutic irradiation, as it is very difficult to ascertain the full extent of these tumors after preoperative irradiation has been given. A lateral rhinotomy is utilized and an osteotomy of the nasal bones is performed if necessary for larger exposure. The amount of resection then depends on the extent of the tumor, but includes at least a septectomy. Postoperative radiation is administered to the cervical nodes as well as to the site of the primary and retropharyngeal nodes, which drain this area. Because irradiation is administered to both sides of the neck, prophylactic neck dissection is not performed.

In the Mayo Clinic's series, 25% of the patients de-

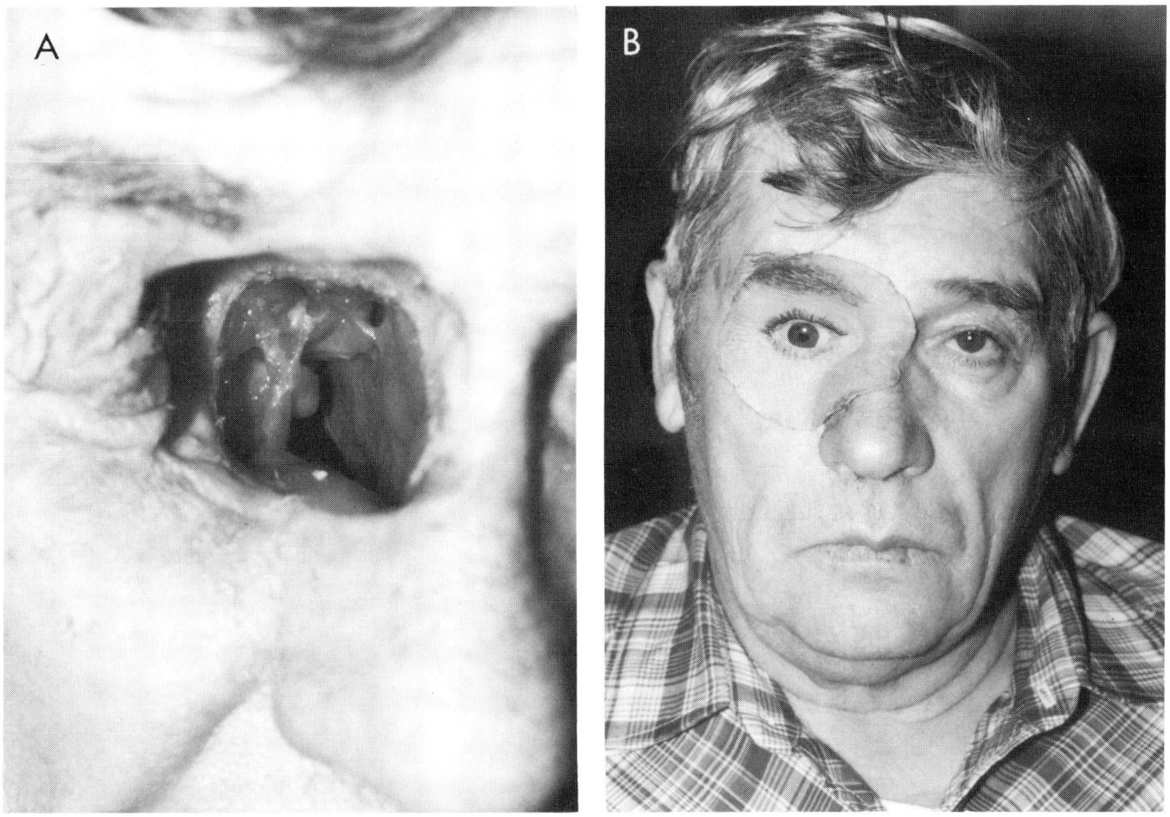

Fig 17–20.—**A,** a large medial canthal tumor extending into the ethmoid sinus is resected. Extension into the orbit required exenteration of the orbital contents. **B,** this defect is best repaired by a prosthesis rather than an extensive, reconstructive procedure. The prosthesis allows cleaning of the cavity and observation for possible recurrence.

veloped cervical metastases. The overall 5-year survival rate for patients with squamous cell carcinoma was 67%. Death usually results from uncontrolled local disease and extension superiorly to the orbit, extension to the paranasal sinuses, and extension upward toward the brain. Recurrent disease may require a second, very extensive operative procedure.

Chung et al. were able to obtain good local control with primary radiation therapy, especially for early lesions. Their report, however, does not specifically state where the tumors were located in the nose, only that they were limited to the nasal cavity without extension to the sinuses. Fourteen of 20 patients with squamous cell carcinoma were cured with irradiation alone. Chung et al. advocate a combination of radiation and surgery for larger lesions. They also recommend prophylactic radiation therapy to the neck, since 16% of their patients developed cervical metastases, but only one of 21 patients in whom the primary disease was controlled developed cervical metastases.

LATERAL NASAL WALL

The lateral nasal wall is the most common site for the development of nasal malignancy. Included in this area are malignancies that are thought to be directly related to occupational exposure, such as squamous cell carcinoma in nickel workers (40 times higher incidence than in the general population). Multiple other chemicals have also been incriminated as possible causes of such unusual malignancies. It is in this group of patients that prophylactic prevention of inhalation of such substances must be achieved.

While adenocarcinoma developing in the lateral nasal wall has been reported in furniture workers, in most series squamous cell carcinoma is by far the most common malignant tumor. The most common site is the anterior tip of the middle turbinate. Treatment requires a lateral rhinotomy extended to include a radical ethmoidectomy[22] and resection of a portion of the medial wall and frontal process of the maxilla. The operative procedure is enlarged as necessary, depending on the extent of the tumor. Postoperative radiation therapy is usually administered. The eye can often be preserved, although the lacrimal bone is resected as part of the ethmoid complex. It is difficult to find actual statistics on survival, because such tumors are generally grouped with other malignancies of the nose and paranasal sinuses or with the ethmoid malignancies because

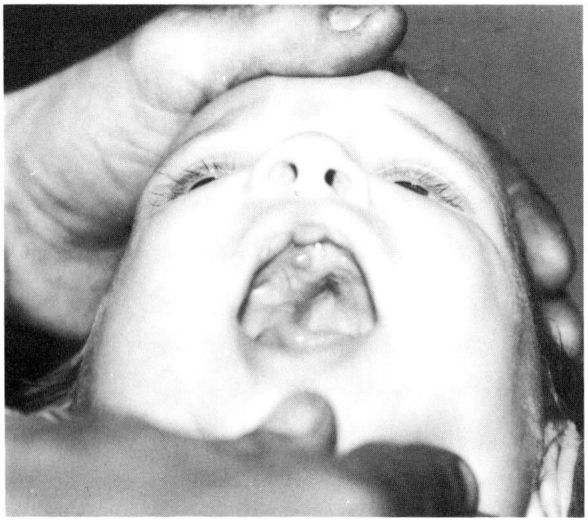

Fig 17–21.—Malignant tumors of the maxilla and nasal sinuses are uncommon in children. This 6-month-old infant has a pigmented neuroectodermal tumor of the right maxilla. A partial maxillectomy was performed. Three years later, there are no signs of recurrence. The area has closed with fibrosis.

of their early and immediate extension into this region. In general, the survival statistics are the same as those for maxilloethmoid carcinoma.[22]

CANCER OF THE NASAL VESTIBULE

The nasal vestibule is covered by skin and includes the area caudal to the septal cartilage, the membranous cartilage, the columella, and, laterally, the alae of the nose. It is the third most common site for the development of nasal malignancy. Squamous cell carcinoma is the most common malignancy to arise in this area. In early stages it is difficult to distinguish squamous-cell cancer from the more common papilloma or warty-like tumor that develops in this region. Squamous-cell cancer occurs most commonly in white men over the age of 60 who are very heavy smokers.

Small malignancies in the nasal vestibule are treated effectively by radiation or surgery. Regional surgical flaps and split-thickness skin grafts can effectively reestablish a normal nasal vestibule. Larger tumors are better treated by radiation therapy, with surgery reserved for salvage. Large cosmetic deformities are created; they may be so large that a prosthetic nose may be more effective than surgical flaps brought into a heavily irradiated area. A compounding difficulty in the management of these lesions is the propensity of the tumor to metastasize in the cervical area. Metastases may be unilateral or bilateral.

Two factors appear to be responsible for the poor prognosis: (1) invasion into the upper lip with its rich lymphatic supply, allowing for bilateral metastases, and (2) multiple areas of development of malignancy. The M. D. Anderson Hospital series of 26 patients revealed an absolute survival rate of 78%. Sixteen patients were treated by radiation therapy and ten by primary surgery. The M. D. Anderson Hospital group prefers radiation therapy for large tumors, reserving surgery for recurrent disease or cervical metastatic disease. The cure rate was directly affected by development of metastatic disease. Radical neck dissection with postoperative radiation therapy is recommended when neck disease develops. Of the 16 patients treated by irradiation, three experienced recurrence and underwent surgical salvage. Of the ten patients treated with surgery, one experienced recurrence and was cured by radiation. Cervical metastases developed in eight patients.

In Schafer's study, four of twelve patients with cancer of the nasal vestibule had multiple sites of involvement, and all four had a very poor prognosis, regardless of treatment method. Schafer advises wide surgical resection as a primary treatment, with postoperative radiation therapy to include the area of drainage of the lymphatics. These tumors tend to metastasize to the facial, submandibular, submental, and parotid lymph nodes, and later to the superficial and deep cervical nodes.

At the University of Minnesota, our preferred treatment is wide surgical resection utilizing regional and island flaps to reconstruct the defect. Postoperative therapeutic irradiation is given for large tumors if there was extension posteriorly, suggesting the possibility of lymphatic drainage to the retropharyngeal lymph nodes. Radiation is delivered to both sides of the neck even in the absence of clinical palpable cervical metastatic disease. Radiation portals are sufficiently high to include the parotid lymph nodes. Smaller lesions are handled effectively by either primary radiation therapy or primary surgical resection. Radical neck dissection is reserved for palpable cervical metastases and has not been done prophylactically.

Malignant Tumors Specific to the Nose

In addition to epidermoid carcinoma, which is by far the most common intranasal malignancy, there are three other important malignancies that are encountered only in the nasal cavity: (1) esthesioneuroblastoma, (2) the malignancy associated with malignant inverted papilloma, and (3) papillary adenocarcinoma. These three malignancies occur in the same location—high in the lateral nasal vault in the region of the middle and superior turbinate. The presenting symptoms are nasal stuffiness, loss of sense of smell, rhinorrhea, and epistaxis. All three tumors can grow to a large size with extension into the ethmoid sinus, and can even cause proptosis. Because of their high location, early extension to the region of the cribriform plate must be anticipated. Diagnosis is confirmed by both anterior and posterior rhinoscopy and by careful biopsy after appropriate radiographs have been obtained.

ESTHESIONEUROBLASTOMA

This rare nasal tumor was initially reported by Berger, Lu, and Richard in 1924. The tumor arises from the sustentacular or supporting cells of the olfactory epithelium located high in the nasal vault. The tumor rarely causes symptoms until it expands to produce obstruction or bleeding. It can extend directly through the cribriform plate into the anterior cranial fossa with involvement of the frontal lobe. The presenting symptom may be a personality change. It is slightly more common in males and can occur in childhood as well as in elderly persons.[23–26]

Elkon et al. reviewed 97 cases reported since 1966. They found the prognosis to be favorable in early cases.[24] Because tumor growth is slow, the 5-year survival may be excellent, reported as high as 50%, while the 5-year disease-free rate is less than 20%. Histologically, the tumors can be divided into three types: (1) olfactory neuroepithelioma,[25] (2) olfactory neurocytoma, and (3) neuroblastoma.[26] However, there is no apparent clinical correlation with the specific subclassification of tumor.

When Would You Suspect an Esthesioneuroblastoma?

The patient is usually a man between the ages of 20 and 40 years. He presents with signs of nasal obstruction, stuffiness, bleeding, headaches, and anosmia. The clinical examination reveals a fleshy mass high in the nasal vault. Radiographs are obtained first and may demonstrate bony erosion, although in early cases a radiologic examination will be normal. Polytomography may reveal bony destruction of ethmoid cells. This bony destruction would not occur in the presence of ethmoid sinusitis. If standard radiographs are not definitive, a CT-scan may provide additional information on the extent of the lesion.

How Do I Biopsy This Tumor?

If the radiologic evaluation shows extensive bony erosion or possible erosion of the base of the skull, biopsy should be performed in the operating room. This allows the examiner an opportunity to control the profuse bleeding that may occur.

What Is the Best Treatment for This Tumor?

No single institution has a large experience with this uncommon tumor. Recommendations are based on a composite of various reported series. While complete surgical resection would be the preferred treatment, the extent of disease at recognition may make the tumor inoperable. Early intracranial extension is the rule.

Fortunately, these tumors are radiosensitive, and a full course of therapeutic irradiation for inoperable tumors can be administered to the area. For early disease, the results of radiation or surgery appear to be equally effective. Large, operable tumors have, when feasible, been treated by a combined approach: anterior craniotomy with a radical ethmoidectomy followed by postoperative therapeutic irradiation. Some groups with large experience advise this as the preferred treatment. Metastases occur to the cervical nodes and may be bilateral. Radical neck dissection is effective for the short term in controlling the local disease. Chemotherapeutic agents are now being employed, but currently there is no evidence that any particular drug is effective.

What Is the Preferred Surgical Treatment?

When the tumor is limited to the nasal cavity and ethmoid region, without evidence of extension to the cribriform plate, a lateral rhinotomy is preferred. The exposure will include a complete ethmoidectomy with removal of the anterior wall to the sphenoid, up to and including the cribriform plate. Larger tumors require a combined neurosurgical approach. The fovea ethmoidalis is outlined, as well as the cribriform plate; then the entire tumorous mass is brought out from below. The dura is repaired and a fascia graft applied. Complications can include leakage of CSF, and meningitis.[20] There is a high rate of local recurrence, and postoperative irradiation is advised. There are currently no prospective data to indicate that this will improve the statistics for survival. In Bailey's series, however, the only patients with 5-year "cures" had been treated with this combined therapeutic approach.

INVERTED PAPILLOMA

The inverted papilloma is a benign tumor that occurs in the lateral nasal wall in the area of the middle turbinate or the ethmoid region. Only 10% of these tumors occur on the septum. It appears polypoid, but more fleshy than an ordinary allergic type of nasal polyp. In most other respects, its presentation is similar to that of the common nasal polyp. It causes nasal obstruction by gradually increasing in size. It received its name because of the inversion of the squamous or respiratory epithelium into the stroma. It occurs more commonly in men, usually in the fifth and sixth decades of life.[27, 28]

When Would I Suspect an Inverted Papilloma Rather Than the Common Nasal Polyp?

Inverted papillomas occur in patients with no preceding history of sinusitis, allergy, or other apparent cause. They are unilateral. Radiologic examination may show a destructive process in the region of the ethmoid sinus. Because of obstruction, sinusitis may coexist. The symptoms are similar to those of all nasal tumors: epistaxis, nasal obstruction, and resultant sinusitis. There is no absolute way of distinguishing a benign nasal polyp from an inverted papilloma other than by biopsy.

Why Are Benign Inverted Papillomas Included in a Discussion of Malignant Nasal Tumors?

Inverted papillomas have a high tendency to local, regional recurrence. The recurrence rate is reported to be as high as 40%. Simple polypectomy as performed for allergic polyps will result in a 100% recurrence rate. A complete ethmoidectomy and resection of the tumor with a margin of normal tissue are necessary for cure and control. Approximately 10% of these tumors have a coexisting malignancy—squamous cell carcinoma. A central question is whether these tumors are originally malignant or undergo malignant degeneration. Thus, the pathologist is obliged to examine multiple serial sections of every tumor specimen to make certain there are no areas within the tumor mass that have coexisting malignancy. Benign inverted papillomas may recur in a benign form or may undergo malignant change.

What Is the Recommended Treatment?

The pathologist is usually the first to recognize that the surgeon is dealing with an inverted papilloma rather than a common nasal polyp. Thus, polypectomy has already been performed either in the office or in the operating room. This will not be sufficient treatment. A lateral rhinotomy approach is required. The incision shown in Figure 17–13 can be extended or the procedure modified as necessary. This may require combining the procedure with a radical ethmoidectomy and even extending the resection to the region of the frontal sinus, if there is evidence that the tumor has extended up the frontal duct. Removal of the common wall between the maxillary sinus and nasal cavity, along with the middle and superior turbinates, is frequently necessary (Denker procedure). This creates a cavity that can easily be inspected for evidence of recurrence.

How Do You Manage a Recurrent Inverted Papilloma?

The treatment of recurrent tumor is similar to the initial operation. A much wider resection is always necessary. Benign inverted papilloma is always treated surgically. Surgical procedures for recurrent tumor may be similar to those for malignant tumors.

What Is the Treatment for an Inverted Papilloma That Has Evidence of Malignancy?

The tumor is treated as for a malignant tumor of the ethmoid or maxillary sinus. Wide surgical resection including radical ethmoidectomy, orbital exenteration if necessary, and maxillectomy is performed. The extent of resection of the tumor will have to be modified, depending on the extent and location of the tumor. Postoperative therapeutic irradiation is recommended in this situation.

PAPILLARY ADENOCARCINOMA OF THE NOSE

An unusual variant of adenocarcinoma arises high in the nasal vault or ethmoid sinus. It occurs more commonly in men. It can present as a small polypoid lesion that may bleed intermittently. It is clinically indistinguishable from the common benign allergic nasal polyp except for the following features: (1) it is higher than usual (in the superior meatus), (2) it is unilateral, and (3) it bleeds easily and copiously when biopsied. Biopsy will reveal a characteristic pattern of adenocarcinoma, papillary type.

Treatment requires wide surgical resection. This tumor is particularly slow-growing and locally and regionally invasive. It can extend directly through the cribriform plate into the frontal lobe. Ten-year survival after multiple procedures is not unusual. Metastases to cervical lymph nodes or to lungs are rare. The tumor kills by local invasion of the skull.

UNUSUAL MALIGNANCIES OF THE NOSE AND PARANASAL SINUS

Malignant Melanoma

Malignant melanoma occurring in mucous membranes accounts for only 10% of all melanomas of the head and neck, or approximately 0.5%–2.7% of all melanomas. It occurs most frequently in the area of the anterior nasal septum,[15, 16] on the palate,[17] or in the region of the middle or inferior turbinate. The signs and symptoms are identical to those of other malignant tumors. The majority of melanomas arise within the lateral nasal cavity and may then extend into the maxillary sinus.

Survival statistics correlate with the size of the initial lesion. Unfortunately, these tumors can reach a large size before any symptoms such as nasal obstruction or epistaxis appear. Survival statistics reported by Lund and Ihnen revealed that patients with tumors 0–2 cm in size had a 60% 5-year survival, but when the lesion reached 3–7 cm, the survival rate dropped to 11.8%[16]

A wide variety of treatments has been utilized for mucosal melanomas of the nose and paranasal sinuses. These have included such unusual practices as injection of rabies vaccine and cowpox vaccine around the site of the lesion. Electrocautery has also been reported to be effective. The role of therapeutic irradiation is still not definitely established. In our own experience and that of others, it is evident that such tumors do respond, initially dramatically, to radiation therapy. Cures are not obtained by this modality, but survival may be prolonged. Radiation therapy may be given as either an implant or by external beam. In addition, both preoperative and postoperative therapeutic irradiation have been combined with surgery for malignant melanoma.

There are no large series to establish the preferred means of combining radiation and surgery in the treatment of malignant melanoma. The standard treatment remains wide surgical resection en bloc. Unfortunately, satisfactory margins cannot always be obtained, and as with other malignant tumors of the nose and paranasal sinuses, the retropharyngeal lymph nodes are one of the first sites of metastases. The presence of palpable nodes in the neck carries an extremely poor prognosis. In this situation, these nodes are not the first line of defense, but the secondary nodes. Radical neck dissection has been advocated, since 50% of mucosal melanomas tend to metastasize to the cervical lymph nodes. Currently, most surgeons perform only radical procedures en bloc and do not perform a prophylactic neck dissection for malignant melanomas of the nose. Five-year survival rates have been reported, but this is not by any means the same as a cure rate. The overall 5-year survival is 16%. Death is generally due to local recurrence as well as invasion of adjacent structures and to distant, widespread metastases.

Malignancies of Minor Salivary Glands

Adenoidcystic carcinoma is the most common malignant tumor of minor salivary glands that occurs in the nose or sinuses. This tumor is known for its potential of extending along perineural lymphatic spaces and for vascular invasion. Its actual extent always exceeds its clinical appearance; that is, a biopsy specimen 3 cm or more away from the obvious tumor may show evidence of adenoidcystic carcinoma. Likewise, the direct invasion of surrounding bone may not be demonstrated on radiologic examination until extensive destruction occurs (Fig 17–22). It occurs with equal frequency in men and women and usually in a younger age group than the more common squamous cell carcinoma.

Adenoidcystic carcinoma has frequently been described as radiosensitive but not radiocurable. Wide surgical resection is the preferred method of treatment, but the necessity of combining radiation with surgery is not established. Some centers, including our own, prefer to treat such tumors by wide surgical resection followed by postoperative radiation therapy. If the tumor is initially found to be unresectable, a full course of external beam radiation therapy is administered.

Adenoidcystic carcinoma is also known to have a prolonged survival with a high rate of local recurrence. These prolonged survival statistics most likely have been influenced by the high incidence of this tumor in major salivary glands. Our experience with this tumor in the nose and sinus suggests that if it cannot be fully encompassed with a large en bloc procedure initially, the course rapidly causes death by widespread invasion and local extension.

Both cervical and pulmonary metastases can occur. It was once thought that cervical and pulmonary metastases did not occur prior to local recurrence; however, patients have presented with both regional and distant metastases. These tumors have been divided into high- and low-grade varieties, depending on the extent of the cribriform pattern on pathologic examination. Enroth demonstrated a difference in overall survival according to such a division. Our own experience has not supported a clear difference in survival when retrospective pathologic evaluation was performed.[12] It appeared that

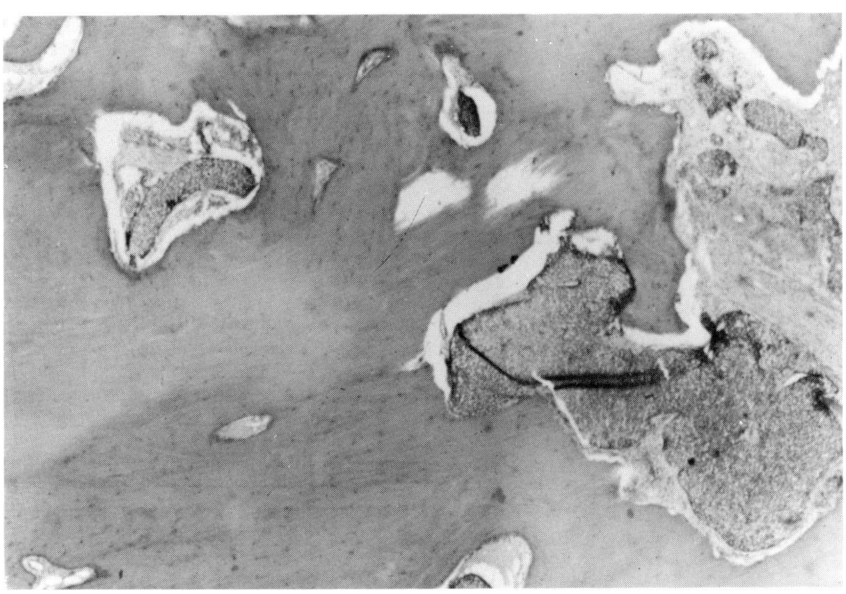

Fig 17–22.—Adenoidcystic carcinoma will directly invade bone interstices. Radiologic examination at this stage will fail to demonstrate bony erosion. Therefore, the margins required for resection of an adenoidcystic carcinoma must always be greater than those for squamous cell carcinoma. Frozen section of the outer soft tissue margins is essential.

the size, extent of the tumor on initial evaluation, location, and the feasibility of performing a wide, all-encompassing resection were the most important factors influencing the survival rate.

Conley reported on 19 cases of adenoidcystic carcinoma developing within the nasal cavity. He recommended surgical resection. Tumors were noted to extend submucosally and to invade the bone directly. Superior extension into the cranial cavity was not unusual. While his survival statistics are 64% for 5 years, this figure could be overly optimistic, because only one of 13 patients in the series was alive at 15 years. Radiation is generally employed to extend cancer control beyond surgical margins, which frequently are not sufficient. This is because of the extent and location of these tumors. Wide surgical margins are frequently not feasible in the area at the base of the skull. Radiation can provide some palliation for inoperable patients. Chemotherapy is currently being utilized, but its role in the management of this disease has not been established.

Malignant Fibrous Histiocytoma

The most common form of malignancy of soft tissue or connective tissue in both young and old is the malignant fibrous histiocytoma.[29] This rare tumor develops from the connective tissue histiocyte. Because of the cell's potential, several histologically similar tumors may be grouped under this classification. Included in the differential diagnosis of malignant fibrous histiocytoma are fibrosarcoma, liposarcoma, and spindle cell sarcomas. Another name, frequently used in the past, is fibroxanthosarcoma. This tumor may arise in areas of previous bone disorders such as Paget's disease, enchondroma, and fibrous dysplasia. It has been reported in patients who previously underwent irradiation to that area, and has been associated, in our own experience, with younger patients who received treatment for hereditary forms of retinoblastoma.

The tumor generally appears as an asymptomatic mass. An area of gradual expansion with such features as loosening of the teeth may be the presenting finding. Radiologic examination will show large areas of bony destruction. The tumor is nonencapsulated and invades bone and soft tissue. It extends posteriorly toward the base of the skull, which may make it nonresectable. It can appear in any of the structures of the head and neck, but has a particularly poor prognosis when it involves the mandible, maxilla, or larynx.

Wide surgical resection is the preferred and recommended treatment. Recent series have shown that preoperative chemotherapy can be utilized. The most popular drugs have been Adriamycin and high-dose methotrexate, with Citrovorum factor rescue and vincristine. While these drugs have improved the survival statistics, they have not been demonstrated to be curative. The tumors do show some sensitivity to radiation, but since it does not effect a cure, it is reserved only for inoperable patients.

Blitzer et al. were able to collect 87 case reports in which this disease involved deep structures of the head and neck.[30] Several factors were associated with poor prognosis: (1) development in an area of previous irradiation, (2) development in a patient with associated underlying diseases such as leukemia, (3) pain as an initial symptom, (4) multifocal origins of tumors, (5) a size greater than 3-cm on presentation, and (6) appearance in older men. The overall fatality rate of the entire collected series was 27%, with a 32% incidence of metastases. As with other sarcomas, both hematogenous and lymphatic spread are prominent. The most common distal metastatic site has been the lung.

Osteogenic Sarcoma

This form of sarcoma presents as an enlarging, firm mass involving either the nose or paranasal sinuses. Radiologic examination will show areas of bony destruction and formation of new bone. The mass is rock-hard on palpation. It appears to be well-defined by x-ray, but at the time of surgery there is always extension into the surrounding soft tissues. Surgical resection is made difficult because it is difficult to establish how much surrounding soft tissue to resect. Extension of tumor toward the base of the skull may be the limiting factor.

These tumors occur in both the maxillary ethmoid and the frontal sinuses. The poor prognosis is most likely related to direct extension of the tumor to the base of the skull. When this tumor develops in the mandible, the prognosis has been shown to be directly related to its location. The more anteriorly located sarcomas near the symphysis have a better prognosis. As with maxillary and palatal or sinus tumors, the more anteriorly the tumor is located, allowing resection of a large amount of normal tissue, the better the prognosis will be.

In almost all large institutions, osteogenic sarcoma is treated by wide surgical resection, followed by postoperative chemotherapy. Agents used include methotrexate in high dosages and Adriamycin. Like the previously discussed sarcomas, these tumors tend to have a high local recurrence rate as well as metastatic disease spread to the lung. Since they are relatively rare in the head and neck, the treatment protocols have been extrapolated from treatment experience of tumors originating in the extremities.

REFERENCES

1. Keen W.: The surgical operations on President Cleveland in 1893. *Saturday Evening Post*. Philadelphia, 1928.

Quoted by Morrells C.L., Jr.: New historic information on the Cleveland operations. *Surgery* 62:542–551, 1967.
2. Clark W.L.: Electrical desiccation as an adjunct to surgery. *Surg. Gynecol. Obstet.* 5:220, 1912.
3. New S.B.: The use of heat and radium in the treatment of cancer of the jaws and cheeks. *JAMA* 71:1369, 1918.
4. Quick D.: Treatment of malignant growths of the nasal accessory sinuses and nasopharynx. *Radiology* 14:191, 1930.
5. Frazell E.: The surgical treatment of cancer of the paranasal sinuses. *Laryngoscope* 65:557, 1955.
6. Frazell E., Lewis J.: Cancer of the nasal cavity and accessory sinuses. *Cancer* 16:1293, 1963.
7. Tabb H.G.: Maxillectomy in carcinoma of the antrum. *Laryngoscope* 69:119, 1959.
8. Smith R.R., Klopp C.T., Williams J.M.: Surgical treatment of cancer of the frontal sinus and adjacent areas. *Cancer* 7:991, 1954.
9. Adams G.L., Duvall A.J., Smith D., et al.: Malignant tumors of the paranasal sinuses. *Minn. Med.* 57:562–568, 1974.
10. Sisson G.A.: Symposium: Treatment of malignancies of the paranasal sinuses. *Laryngoscope* 80:945, 1970.
11. St. Pierre S., Baker S.R.: Squamous cell carcinoma of the maxillary sinus: Analysis of 66 cases. *Head Neck Surg.* 5:508–513, 1983.
12. Adams G.L., Duvall A.J.: Adenocarcinoma of the head and neck. *Arch. Otolaryngol.* 93:261, 1971.
13. Goepfert H., Luna M.R., Lindberg R.D., et al.: Malignant salivary gland tumors of the paranasal sinuses and nasal cavity. *Arch. Otolaryngol.* 109:662–668, 1983.
14. Brounson R.J., Ogura J.H.: Primary carcinoma of the frontal sinus. *Laryngoscope* 91:71, 1971.
15. Walker E.H., Snow J.B.: Management of melanoma of nose and paranasal sinuses. *Arch. Otolaryngol.* 89:652–670, 1969.
16. Lund R.A., Ihnen M.: Malignant melanoma. *Surgery* 38:652–662, 1955.
17. Bartkowski S.B., Panas M., Wilezanska H., et al.: Primary malignant melanoma of the oral cavity: A review of 20 cases. *Am. J. Surg.* 148:362–366, 1984.
18. Shaw H.J.: Combined therapy for cancer of the upper jaw and paranasal sinuses. *J. Laryng. Otol.* 80:105, 1966.
19. Ketcham A.S., Wilkins J.M., Van Buren J.M., et al.: A combined intracranial facial approach to the paranasal sinuses. *Am. J. Surg.* 106:698, 1963.
20. Ketcham A.S., Hoye R.C., Van Buren J.M., et al.: Complications of intracranial facial resection for tumors of the paranasal sinuses. *Am. J. Surg.* 112:591, 1966.
21. Lyons G.D.: Squamous cell carcinoma of the nasal septum. *Arch. Otolaryngol.* 89:47–49, 1969.
22. Ketcham A.S., Chretien P.B., Van Buren J.M., et al.: The ethmoid sinuses: A re-evaluation of surgical resection. *Am. J. Surg.* 126:469, 1973.
23. Hutter R.U.P., Lewis J.S., Foote F.W., et al.: Esthesioneuroblastoma. *Am. J. Surg.* 106:748–753, 1963.
24. Elkon D., Hightower S., Lim M., et al.: Esthesioneuroblastoma. *Cancer* 44:1087–1094, 1979.
25. Skolnik E.M., Massari F.S., Tenta L.T.: Olfactory neuroepithelioma. *Arch. Otolaryngol.* 81:644–653, 1966.
26. Bailey B.J., Barton S.: Olfactory neuroblastoma. *Arch. Otolaryngol.* 101:1–5, 1975.
27. Myers E.N., Schramm V.L., Barnes E.L.: Management of inverted papilloma of the nose and paranasal sinuses. *Laryngoscope* 91:2071–2084, 1981.
28. Hyams V.J.: Papillomas of the nasal cavity and paranasal sinuses: A clinicopathologic study of 315 cases. *Ann. Otol. Rhinol. Laryngol.* 80:192–206, 1971.
29. Urban C., Rosen G., Huvos A.G., et al.: Chemotherapy of malignant fibrous histiocytoma of bone. *Cancer* 51:795–802, 1983.
30. Blitzer A., Lawson W., Zak F.G., et al.: Clinical-pathological determinants in prognosis of fibrous histiocytosis of head and neck. *Laryngoscope* 91:2053–2070, 1981.
31. Sakai S., Hamasaki Y.: Proposal for the classification of carcinoma of the paranasal sinuses. *Acta Otolaryngol.* 63:42–48, 1967.
32. Frazell E.L., Lewis J.S.: Cancer of the nasal cavity and accessory sinuses. *Cancer* 16:1293–1301, 1963.
33. Tabb H.G.: Carcinoma of the antrum. *Laryngoscope* 67:269–341, 1957.
34. Schall L.A.: Malignant neoplasms of the nase, paranasal sinuses and nasopharynx: Evaluation of surgical treatment. *Trans. Am. Acad. Ophthalmol. Otolaryngol.* 55:209–213, 1951.
35. St. Pierre S., Baker S.R.: Squamous cell carcinoma of the maxillary sinus: An analysis of 66 cases. *Head Neck Surg.* 5:508–513, 1983.
36. Lee F., Ogura J.H.: Maxillar sinus carcinoma. *Laryngoscope* 91:133–139, 1981.

ADDITIONAL READINGS

1. McCarten A.B.: The combined transzygomatic approach in resection of maxilla. *Am. J. Surg.* 106:696–697, 1963.
2. Barbosa J.F.: Surgery of extensive cancer of paranasal sinuses. *Arch. Otolaryngol.* 73:129–138, 1961.
3. Rousch G.C.: Epidemiology of cancer of the nose and paranasal sinus: Current concepts. *Head Neck Surg.* 2:3–11, 1979.
4. Weber A.L., Stanton A.C.: Malignant tumors of the paranasal sinuses: Radiologic, clinical and histopathologic evaluation of 200 cases. *Head Neck Surg.* 6:761–776, 1984.
5. Schaefer S.D., Hill G.C.: Epidermoid carcinoma of the nasal vestibule. *Laryngoscope* 90:1631–1635, 1980.
6. Chung C.T., Rabuzzi D.D., Sagerman R.H., et al.: Radiotherapy for carcinoma of the nasal cavity. *Arch. Otol.* 106:763–766, 1980.
7. Goepfert H., Guillansondegui O.M., Jesse R.H., et al.: Squamous cell carcinoma of the nasal vestibule. *Arch. Otol.* 100:8–10, 1974.
8. Harrison D.: Surgical pathology of olfactory neuroblastoma. *Head and Neck Surg.* 7:60–64, 1984.
9. Appelblatt N.H., McClatchey K.D.: Olfactory neuroblastoma: A retrospective clinicopathologic study. *Head Neck Surg.* 5:108–123, 1982.
10. Batsakis J.G., Rapezi J.D., Solomon A.R., et al.: The pa-

thology of head and neck tumors: Mucosal melanoma. *Head Neck Surg.* 4:404–418, 1982.

11. Snow G.B., VanDerEsch E.P., Slotten E.A.: Mucosal melanomas of the head and neck. *Head Neck Surg.* 1:24–30, 1978.
12. Batsakis J.G.: The pathology of head and neck tumors: Nasal cavity and paranasal sinus. *Head Neck Surg.* 2:410–419, 1980.
13. Wilder W.H., Harner S.G., Banks P.M.: Lymphoma of the nose and paranasal sinus. *Arch. Otol.* 109:310–312, 1983.
14. Kelly J.H., Joseph M., Carroll E., et al.: Inverted papilloma of the nasal septum. *Arch. Otolaryngol.* 106:767–771, 1980.

18 / Odontogenic Tumors and Tumors of Bone

GRAEME A. BROWNE, B.SC., M.SC., B.D.S., F.R.C.D.

IN THE ENTIRE SPECTRUM of primary head and neck malignancies, cancers that arise in the odontogenic tissues and bone are relatively rare. Osteogenic sarcoma occurs in the head and neck area (most commonly the mandible and maxilla) in only 6% of all cases (see Chap. 24). Ewing's sarcoma rarely makes its first appearance in the head and neck region.[1] When a tumor is found in the jaws, the tissue of origin is still not commonly among the intrinsic dental tissues. In 54,534 dental specimens submitted to one oral pathology department over 41 years, Regezi et al. found 706 tumors of odontogenic origin, of which 78 (11%) were ameloblastomas.[2]

Invasive and aggressive tumors can arise de novo in bone, the dental apparatus, and the adjacent connective and mesenchymal tissues. The problems for the clinician are compounded because these tumors arise in a universe of cancers that may be metastatic to the head and neck or may be confused with an impressive array of cysts, infections, injuries, fibroses, and so forth that also produce skeletal radiographic abnormalities.

HOW SHOULD THE CLINICIAN APPROACH RADIOLUCENT AND RADIOPAQUE LESIONS OF THE JAW?

In a society where good dental care is common and dental x-ray equipment is ubiquitous, minimal dental symptoms or routine dental studies may disclose a radiographic abnormality.

The radiographic appearance of lesions of the jaws is a formidable clinical problem in diagnosis. The defects may represent local or metastatic neoplasms, inflammation or infection, developmental arrests, or even the secondary effects of metabolic diseases such as hyperparathyroidism. The infrequency of malignant disease does not justify an exhaustive discussion of each of the possibilities. Our objective is to give the reader a scaffold upon which to develop general clinical probabilities. Several texts in the references can provide details. If one considers anatomical location and radiographic characteristics, a reduced list remains for working diagnoses. Without some method of subclassification, however, the diversity is too great. We will sort the classifications later in a manner that parallels the clinical evaluation.

If a lesion is suspected or known to exist, a good x-ray study of the jaws or skeleton of the head is needed. For the jaws, an orthopantomogram (Panorex) is a useful preliminary radiograph. It is simple and easy to obtain for both the patient and the technician. The entire mandible, maxilla, and contiguous skeleton can be viewed on one film. An orthopantomogram is well suited to patients who would be unable to cooperate in the gymnastics and positioning that are required to get detailed views by other means. The symmetry of an orthopantomogram permits comparison of contralateral structures. Intraoral radiographs (e.g., occlusal and periapical dental views) can be taken to provide finer resolution of detail and to evaluate the minute characteristics of the bony trabeculation, the periodontal ligament, the lamina dura, the dentition, and the contour of the area under study.

Dental infections are very common. In general, *chronic* inflammation produces well-defined, sometimes sclerotic, bone margins. The cancellous bone trabeculae *will be* relatively dense. This is contrasted to the findings in *acute* inflammation, where there is frequently a loss of bone trabeculation and the peripheral margins of the lesion are not sclerotic, i.e., there is no reactive new bone formation. Chronic periodontal disease with acute exacerbations causes a unique extensive irregular resorption of alveolar crest bone.

When malignancy from contiguous structures infiltrates bone locally or when the cancer is metastatic, there is an irregular bone lysis that may be similar to that seen with acute or subacute infection. External malignant invasion typically destroys part of the structure of the tooth itself, an uncommon event with inflammatory disease. Hyperparathyroidism may cause radiopaque lesions in the gonial angle of the mandible (osteitis fibrosis cystica). Metastatic spread from prostatic cancer, breast cancer, or clear cell cancers (e.g., hypernephroma) may appear in the same gonial region.

Lesions that arise from the dentition and tooth primordia are the native suspects when a radiographic abnormality is found in the jaws. Since these are uncommon in the general surgeon's experience, we can discuss some of them without getting too embroiled in the controversies over histogenesis and classification.

WHAT ARE SOME OF THE TUMORS NOT DISCUSSED IN OTHER SECTIONS OF THE BOOK THAT ARISE IN THE ODONTOGENIC TISSUES OR THAT INVOLVE THE FACIAL SKELETON?

Remnants of progenitor cells from the dental lamina, the radicular epithelial projections of the tooth germ, or the ameloblastic layer of the tooth may all give rise to neoplasms and cysts.[3]

AMELOBLASTOMA.—Ameloblastoma may occur at all ages; the mean age at occurrence is 45 years. It is derived from the odontogenic epithelium, specifically the dental lamina.[4] It is thought that ameloblastoma in children arises in association with dentigerous cysts, which would explain its frequent association with impacted or unerupted teeth in the young. The vast majority of ameloblastomas (80%) occur in the mandible.[5] A painless swelling or the chance finding of a multilocular (soap bubble appearance) radiolucent area (Figs 18–1, 18–2) in bone is the presenting finding. If the examiner does not know the site of origin, the histologic pattern of ameloblastoma can be confused with craniopharyngioma. Treatment in adults is by en bloc excision with a normal border of bone. For larger aggressive lesions, hemimandibulectomy has been used. The childhood tumors are not considered to have malignant potential and rarely recur after conservative local excision, whereas adult tumors have a reported 50% to 90% recurrence after conservative treatment.[5, 6]

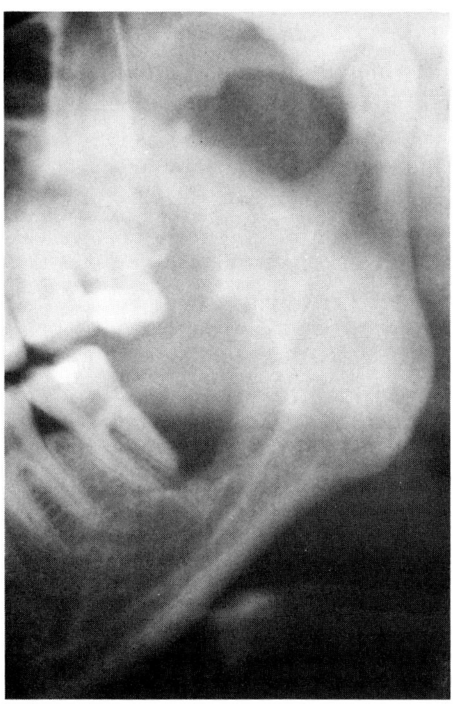

Fig 18–1.—Ameloblastoma. Lateral view shows characteristic cystic lucent lesion in the posterior mandible without dental erosion of the adjacent teeth.

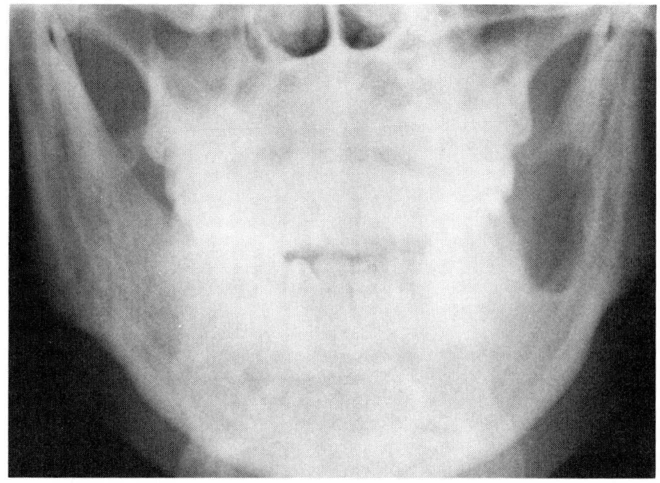

Fig 18–2.—Same patient as Figure 18–1. This view shows the characteristic medial cortical expansion and thinning of the mandible.

ADENOMATOID ODONTOGENIC TUMOR.—Adenomatoid odontogenic tumor is a rare tumor, accounting for less than 0.1% of tumors and cysts of the jaw.[2, 7] It occurs most commonly in children and young adults. Stafne originally proposed an origin in developmental cysts.[8] It is a slow-growing, cyst-like benign neoplasm that is generally painless. It is more common in females. It is usually noted around the maxillary incisor, cuspid, or premolar teeth (65/105) or at the angle of the mandible (40/105).[7] Since it is often associated with unerupted teeth, it is similar in radiographic appearance to a dentigerous cyst. It is easily enucleated without recurrence. However, it can be clinically confused with the more aggressive adamantinoma. Hence, all tissue removed should be submitted for careful histologic study.

CALCIFYING ODONTOGENIC CYST.—Calcifying odontogenic cyst (Gorlin's cyst) provokes discussion as to whether it is a neoplasm or a cyst. Gorlin from our institution described this lesion in 1962.[9] It generally occurs in young people and most commonly in the mandible, frequently anterior to the first molar. The "calcification" features may be prominent, patchy, or absent. Enucleation is curative and recurrence is rare. It is radiologically similar in appearance to the two previously discussed lesions.

AMELOBLASTIC FIBROMA.—Ameloblastic fibroma is also called soft mixed odontogenic tumor, or fibroadamantoblastoma. Again, this lesion predominates in the young. It creates a radiolucent bony defect. It is generally thought to be nonaggressive and easily treated by

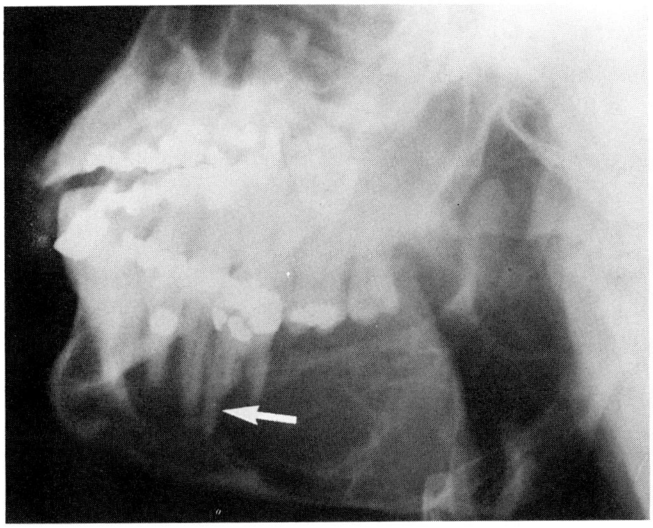

Fig 18–3.—Myxoma—in this case, an extensive multiloculated radiolucent lesion of the ramus and posterior body of the mandible. Note the dental root erosion *(arrow).*

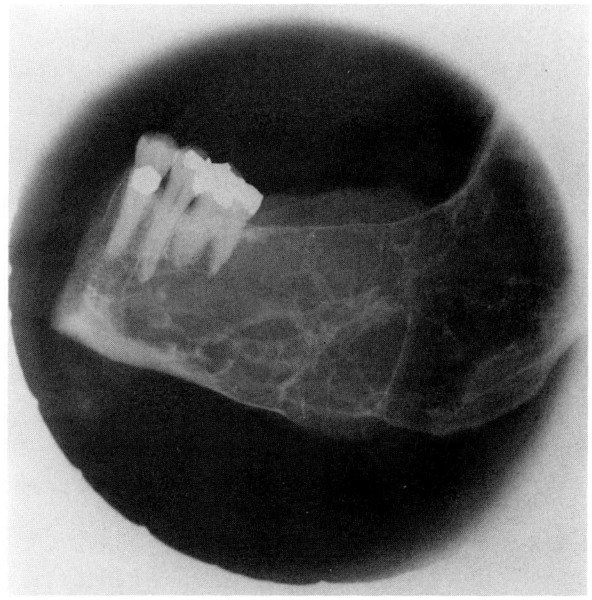

Fig 18–4.—Myxoma. Radiograph of the specimen removed from the patient in Figure 18–3 shows the extensive destruction of the mandible. The patient underwent reconstruction with multiple procedures.

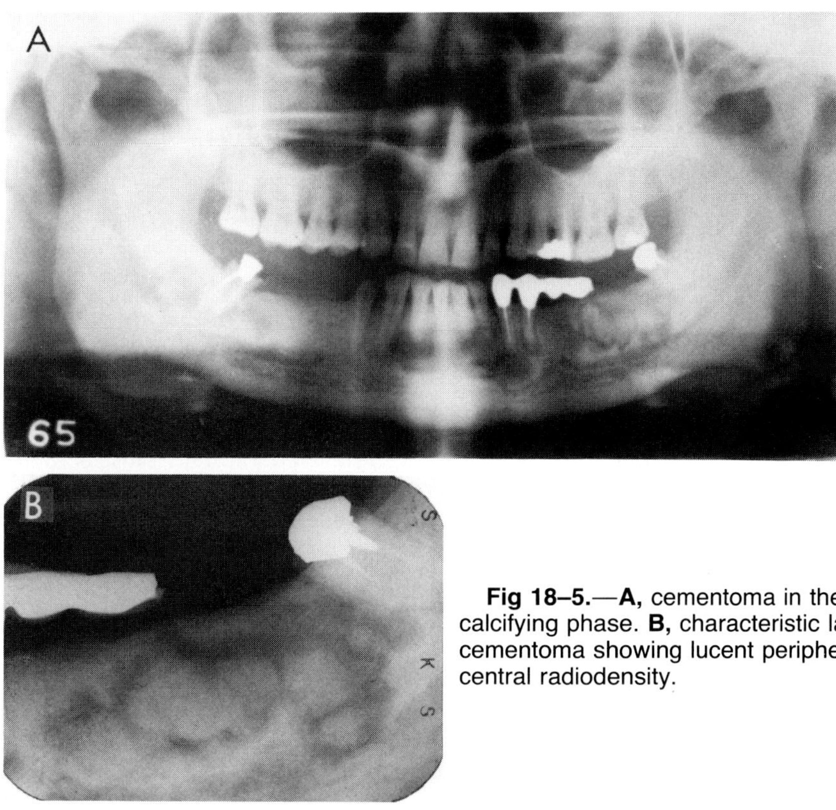

Fig 18–5.—**A,** cementoma in the lytic and calcifying phase. **B,** characteristic late stage of cementoma showing lucent periphery and central radiodensity.

enucleation. Recent reports have noted a recurrence rate of about 40%.[10, 11] This suggests that resection with a margin is desirable.

MYXOMA.—A myxoma is a lesion found in all age groups, with most cases occurring at 10–29 years. Myxoma is thought to be unique to the jaws and presumed to arise from primitive mesodermal tooth germ tissue.[12] It is slow-growing, multiloculated, nonpainful, and may resemble a dentigerous cyst on x-ray films. The trabeculae of bone may have a "sunburst" pattern at the periphery (Fig 18–3). There is no mortality related to the tumor, although in some cases the tumor may become extensively invasive (Fig 18–4).[3, 13] Patients who have wide local excision are reported by some to be free of recurrence. Other authors report recurrence rates of 25%–30%.[3, 14]

CEMENTOBLASTOMA (CEMENTOMA).—This tumor is usually fused to the root of the involved tooth. It can occur in any age group. It arises from the functioning mesenchymal cementoblasts. Pain occurs occasionally when the tumor encompasses the root apex. A conservative surgical approach is recommended. It does not recur.[15, 16] Initially it can be cystic (Fig 18–5); later it can develop the characteristic calcification fused to the root.

ODONTOMA.—When routine radiographic studies are done on young people, this is the most common primary odontogenic lesion found (about 20% of lesions).[2, 3] It is usually seen as a calcific radiopaque mass associated with an impacted tooth.

STAFNE'S DEFECT.—Stafne's defect represents an arrest in bone development that is occupied by salivary gland. It always lies below the neurovascular bundle in

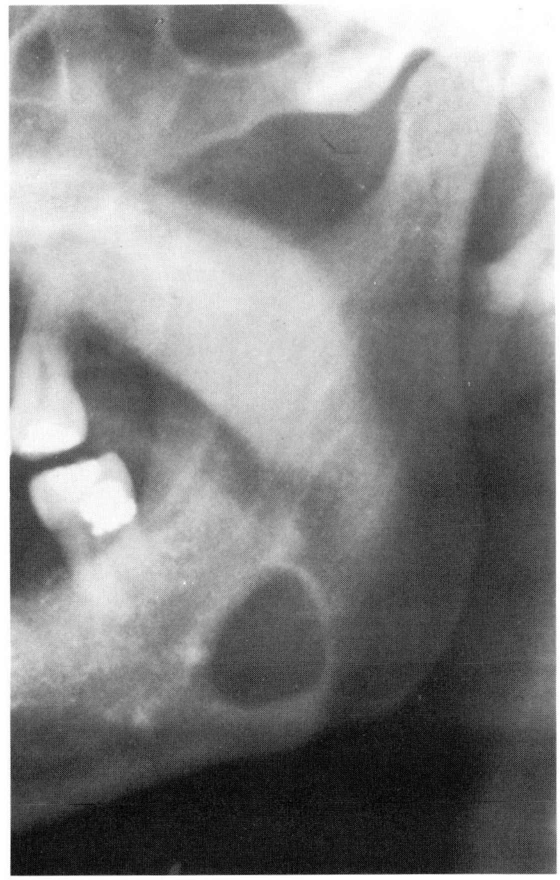

Fig 18–6.—Stafne's defect shows a circumscribed radiolucent area in the gonial angle. There is *not* a reactive periphery.

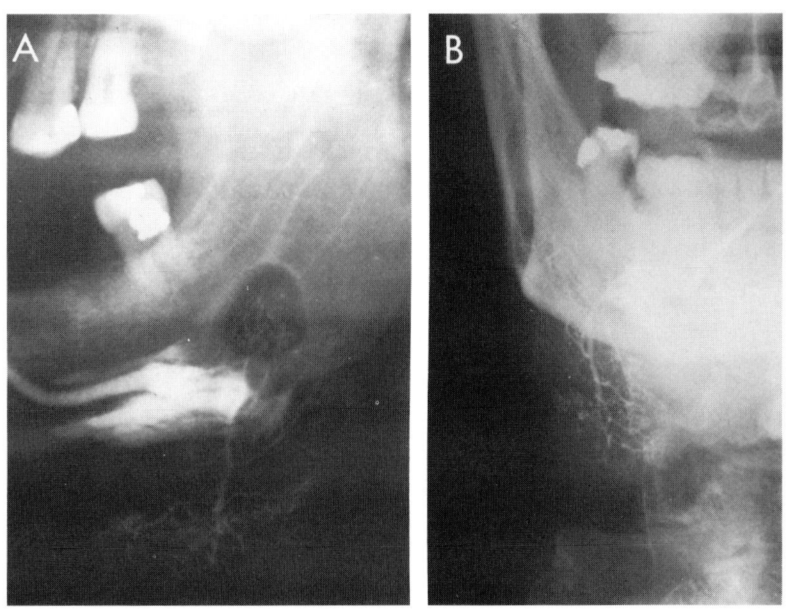

Fig 18–7.—Two views of stafne's defect. A sialogram shows the submandibular ductal structures entering the radiolucent defect, confirming that the tissue is salivary in origin.

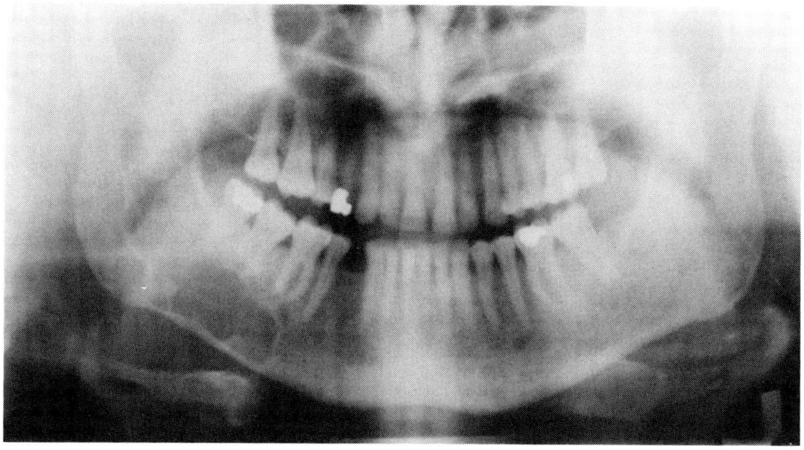

Fig 18–8.—Keratocyst. These lesions are multiloculated and have a reactive dense border. They may displace the teeth but not erode them.

the gonial angle. Biopsy shows the salivary gland. A sialogram is diagnostic (Figs 18–6, 18–7).

ODONTOGENIC CYSTS, KERATOCYSTS, DENTIGEROUS CYSTS, AND CALCIFYING EPITHELIAL ODONTOGENIC TUMOR (PINDBORG TUMOR).—These tumors are variable in size, are usually radiolucent, and present differential diagnostic problems.

The odontogenic primordial cyst and keratocyst (Fig 18–8) may recur if the lining is not completely removed by curettage. Recurrence is always a problem when epithelial remnants remain after surgery.

The dentigerous cyst (Fig 18–9) is one of the more common lesions. It is frequently unilocular and found predominantly in young people. Some 80%–90% are associated with impacted teeth. Rarely is there aggressive erosion of adjacent teeth.

NONODONTOGENIC TUMORS.—Nonodontogenic tumors may include the following:

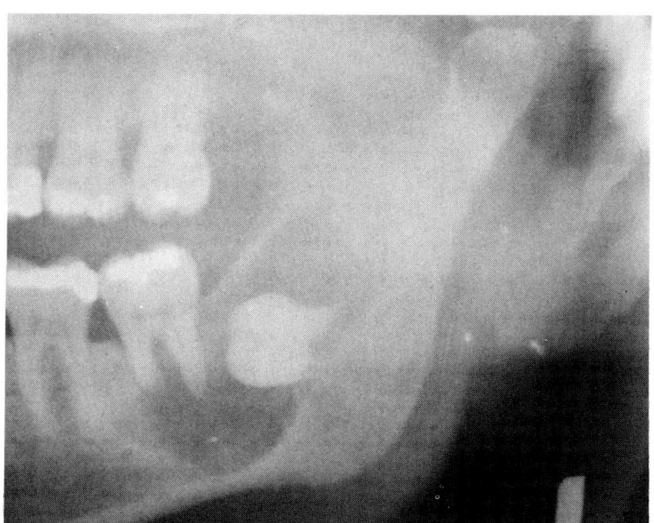

Fig 18–9.—Dentigerous cyst.

Osteomas. These may also be associated with Gardner's syndrome.

Osteoblastoma (osteoid osteoma).

Osteogenic sarcoma.

Chondrosarcoma. A chondrosarcoma is typically located at the mandibular symphysis or near the temporomandibular joint or coronoid process.

Fibrous dysplasia. Fibrous dysplasia (Fig 18–10) is occasionally familial, usually histologically benign and locally aggressive. Usually it stabilizes by the second or third decade. A few cases have undergone sarcomatous transformation.

Ossifying fibroma.

Ewing's sarcoma.

All of these are similar in behavior to their counterparts in other areas of the body. They are discussed in chapters 4 (Pathology) and 24. Dahlin's review is quite extensive.[17] Dehner reviewed the University of Minnesota experience in children with both benign and malignant lesions of the jaws.[18, 19] Vickers and Rosai have summarized the surgical pathology of the mandible.[20]

Table 18–1 summarizes the embryologic tissues of origin for the odontogenic tumors.

Table 18–2 lists the aggressive (recurring or invasive) benign odontogenic tumors.

Tables 18–3 through 18–5 list some other lesions of the jaws and skull that may produce radiographic abnormalities. There are numerous possible causes for a radiographic abnormality. Traumatic bone cyst (Fig 18–11) is a common lesion that is detected radiographically.

HOW DO YOU REACH A WORKING DIAGNOSIS FOR A SYMPTOMATIC OR RADIOLOGICALLY DETECTABLE LESION OF THE JAWS?

Assume that the radiographic studies show a definite lesion. Table 18–6 lists the potential lesions in an ap-

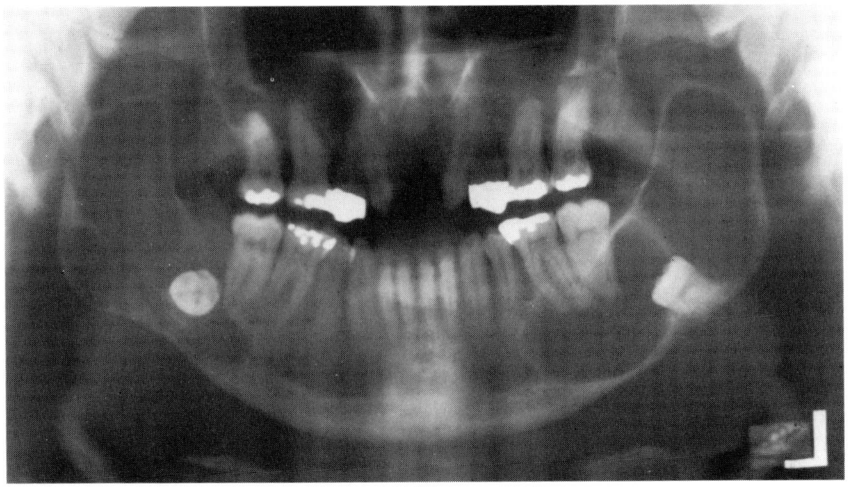

Fig 18–10.—Fibrous dysplasia in a teenager with cherubism and extensive fibrous dysplasia.

proximate order of frequency as they are found on radiographic studies. These can be further subdivided by appearance into three broad categories: radiolucent lesions, radiopaque lesions, and reactive bone margins. Further refinement will often permit subdivision of radiolucent lesions into unilocular or multilocular (the multilocular lesion is said to have the radiographic appearance of soap bubbles). Table 18–7 combines this subdivision into unilocular and multilocular lesions with several other conditions that may confuse the radiographic interpretation. Table 18–8 focuses on subdivision by the presence or absence of the characteristics of malignancy. These lists should be reviewed in connection with Figures 18–12 and 18–13. The location of the lesion, particularly within the mandible, gives additional clues that reflect some of the common locations for specific lesions. In dealing with these lesions, remember that common lesions are commonly found. The lists were arranged in our estimate of descending order of frequency.

TABLE 18–1.—Embryologic Origin of Odontogenic Tumors

ECTODERM
Periodontal cyst
Dentigerous cyst
Keratocyst
Primordial cyst
Ameloblastoma
Pindborg tumor
MESODERM
Cementoma
Myxoma
Fibroma
Dentinoma
Fibrosarcoma
MIXED
Odontoma
Teratoma
Ameloblastic fibroma

TABLE 18–2.—Locally Aggressive Benign Odontogenic Tumors

Myxoma*
Keratocyst†
Ossifying fibroma
Ameloblastoma* (less aggressive in children)
Pindborg tumor* (calcifying epithelial odontogenic tumor)

*High recurrence rate. Remove as a block of bone or tissue.
†Remove wall with bur or ablate with cryotherapy.

HOW DO YOU FINALLY ARRIVE AT A DEFINITIVE DIAGNOSIS AND PLAN FURTHER MANAGEMENT?

Biopsy can be both diagnostic and therapeutic. Very few lesions have characteristics that are pathognomonic to a point of more than 90% assurance. For some, there

TABLE 18–3.—Giant and Round Cell Lesions

GIANT CELL LESIONS
Peripheral
Central
Brown tumor
ROUND CELL LESIONS
Eosinophilic granuloma
Hand-Schüller-Christian disease
Letterer-Siwe disease
Myeloma

TABLE 18–4.—Syndromes Associated With Multiple Impacted Teeth and Dentigerous Cysts

Gardner's*
Bifib rib*
Multiple mucosal nevoid

*Associated with intestinal polyposis MEA II (Sipple's syndrome). Also may have bone involvement from hyperparathyroidism.

TABLE 18–5.—Nonodontogenic Cysts

MANDIBLE
Traumatic bone "cyst"
Aneurysmal bone cyst
Median mandibular cyst
MAXILLA
Nasopalatine duct cyst
Globulomaxillary
Median palatal
Nasoalveolar (Kledstadt's)

TABLE 18–6.—Mandibular Lesions, Listed in Estimated Declining Order of Radiologic Incidence

1. Osteosclerosis	17. Myeloma
2. Periodontal cyst	18. Neurofibroma
3. Impacted teeth	19. Pulmonary metastasis
4. Dentigerous cyst	20. Myxoma
5. Osteoma	21. Plasmacytoma
6. Keratocyst	22. Prostatic metastasis
7. Residual cyst	23. Primary squamous cell ca.
8. Primordial cyst	24. Ameloblastoma
9. Traumatic bone cyst	25. Renal metastasis
10. Cicatrix	26. Osteochondroma
11. Cementoma	27. Osteofibroma
12. Paget's disease of bone	28. Osteosarcoma
13. Aneurysmal bone cyst	29. Chondrosarcoma
14. Odontoma	30. Central hemangioma
15. Fibro-osseous lesions	31. Pindborg tumor
16. Giant cell lesions	32. Gorlin's cyst

is a tossup among the possible etiologies. A dentigerous cyst, a mural ameloblastoma, and an intraosseous squamous cell cancer may all look quite similar on x-ray films. Because of this, removal of the lesion and its lining should be planned. All tissue removed from the patient *must* be submitted for histologic examination. Where there is a high suspicion of malignancy and there is a soft tissue extension that can be sampled, an incisional biopsy specimen can be submitted for frozen section. This may occur where there are typical findings for a neoplasm such as a chondrosarcoma. For most lesions, bone and bony spicules are contained in the biopsy specimen or curettings. Consequently, the specimen must be decalcified before complete histologic section and study can be done several days later. The large majority of lesions are approached by a transoral route unless a lesion is far posterior in the mandible. Then it is appropriate to operate through an external posteroinferior inframandibular incision positioned in a skin crease.

Cystic lesions should first be aspirated through a small bur hole, particularly if there is any possibility of a high-pressure vascular lesion. The examiner should look for ipsilateral hypertrophy, visible pulsations, thrills, or unusual associated vasculature. If the lesion is vascular, one must have angiographic study and be prepared to control the vascular inflow at points outside the lesion margins. If the lesion is vascular, adequate blood replacement must be available before curettage is undertaken. For most cysts, the lesion is then unroofed with a dental drill and the contents evacuated and curetted. Small bleeding points away from the alveolar nerve can be controlled by electrocautery. Local packing and an adequate wait for clotting to occur will manage most bleeding. If soft tissue is obtained that is free of bone, some may be examined by frozen section.

Table 18–2 lists the locally aggressive benign tumors and indicates those with a high recurrence rate. These tumors include the keratocyst, which is found in approximately 35% of dentigerous cyst diagnoses. The

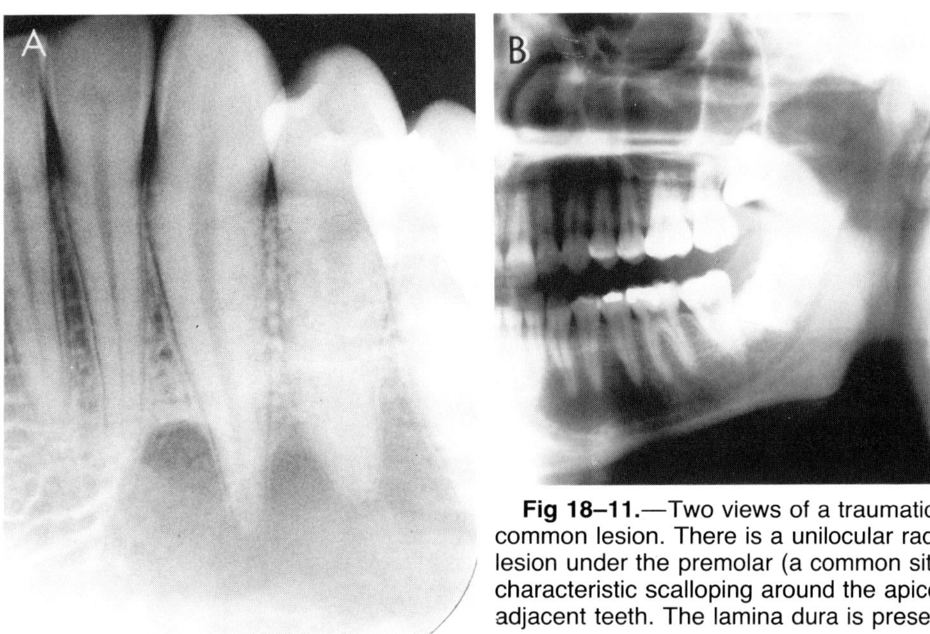

Fig 18–11.—Two views of a traumatic bone cyst, a common lesion. There is a unilocular radiolucent lesion under the premolar (a common site) with characteristic scalloping around the apices of the adjacent teeth. The lamina dura is preserved.

TABLE 18–7.—SUBDIVISION OF RADIOLOGIC LESIONS OF THE MANDIBLE

RADIOPAQUE MANDIBULAR LESIONS (Decreasing incidence)
Osteosclerosis
Impacted teeth
Osteoma
Cementoma (late)
Retained roots
Sialolith
Dystrophic calcification: nodes, tonsils, vascular
Odontoma
Fibro-osseous lesions (late)
Prostatic metastasis
Osteosarcoma
Renal metastasis
Pindborg tumor
RADIOLUCENT MANDIBULAR LESIONS (Decreasing incidence)
Unilocular
Tooth germ
Primordial cyst
Dental granuloma
Traumatic bone cyst
Cicatrix
Cementoma (early)
Fissural cysts
Giant cell lesions
Myeloma
Neurofibroma
Hemangioma
Brown tumor (osteitis fibrosis cystica)
Metastatic disease:
Pulmonary
Breast
Colon
Primary intra-osseous
Squamous cell carcinoma
Chondromas
Chondrosarcoma
Multilocular
Dentigerous cyst
Keratocyst
Fibrous dysplasia (early)
Myxoma
Ameloblastoma
Pindborg tumor
Fibroma
Hemangioma
Fibrosarcoma

multiple daughter cysts in bony loculi require complete excision and sclerosis of the nidus with a liquid nitrogen probe or bismuth paste. For the keratocysts, a follow-up is required at 6- to 9-month intervals looking for recurrence.

After evacuation, curettage, and any further treatment, the local osseous defect is slightly saucerized (the overhanging edges smoothed down) and closed primarily. A small Hemovac suction drain is placed. If the dead space exceeds 20–25 cc or if the mucoperiosteal flap lacks support, then the defect can be packed with vaseline gauze that is gradually withdrawn as the defect granulates from the bottom. Primary cancellous bone grafts provide another option for filling the defect. Some authors advocate marsupialization (removal of one wall) and decompression of extensive cystic lesions in order to avoid a pathologic fracture or nerve damage that may occur with extensive curettage. Ultimately, it is necessary to excise the cyst epithelium to prevent recurrence. It is also essential to assure that a mural ameloblastic lesion or a more ominous neoplasm is not present. This requires complete excision and thorough histologic examination. As most odontogenic tumors grow, the alveolar nerve is usually pushed aside and can be preserved.

Ameloblastoma, myxoma, and the very rare Pindborg tumor (calcifying epithelial odontogenic tumor) all require a clean local block excision of the investing bone and any contiguous soft tissue that may be involved. The other odontogenic tumors of ectodermal origin (see Table 18–1) are treated by curettage only. Some of the mesodermal tumors (e.g., cementoma) may require no treatment at all. Some require block resection (myxoma) or wide resection (fibrosarcoma).

For the odontogenic myxoma and the ameloblastoma, margins must be adequate. If the lesions perforate the cortical plate, the periosteum will be invaded. A margin of adjacent soft tissue must be removed. The absence of tumor at the margins should be confirmed by frozen section. Maneuvers that might lead to local seeding should be avoided.

Management of the traumatic unilocular bone cyst (a pseudocyst) is by simple aspiration or the creation of a surgical opening. An aneurysmal bone cyst is multilocular. It is usually treated by curettage or block excision, sparing the lower rim of the mandible, since it is usually free of involvement. The "brown tumor" (osteitis fibrosa cystica) of the jaws is an osseous manifestation of hyperparathyroidism (Fig 18–14). If this tumor is biopsied or if a diagnosis of central giant cell granuloma is made, one is obliged to look for and manage hyperparathyroidism.

Fibrous dysplasia may involve parts of the entire skeleton other than the jaws. Polyostotic fibrous dysplasia associated with café au lait spots and sexual precocity is known as Albright's syndrome. The variety without endocrine involvement is known as Jaffe's syndrome. Familial fibrodysplasia of the jaws is inherited as an autosomal dominant trait with variable expression that lacks endocrine involvement (see Fig 18–10). These esoterica are mentioned to stress the importance of carefully obtaining a family history *before* surgically attacking a radiographic finding. Fibro-osseous dysplasia is treated to correct esthetic defects or orthognathic dysfunction. Compressive effects destroy vision and function. For cranial or periorbital lesions, the involved bone has been successfully removed, resculptured, and

TABLE 18–8.—RADIOGRAPHICALLY DETECTABLE LESIONS OF THE JAWS

	SOLITARY				MULTIPLE			
	ODONTOGENIC		NONODONTOGENIC		ODONTOGENIC		NONODONTOGENIC	
	Benign	Malignant	Benign	Malignant	Benign	Malignant	Benign	Malignant
RADIOLUCENT LESIONS	Tooth germ Primordial cyst Keratocyst* Periodontal cyst Dental granuloma Cementoma (early) Myxoma* Ameloblastoma* Ameloblastic fibroma* Pindborg tumor* Fibroma Gorlin's tumor	Fibrosarcoma Primary intraosseous squamous cell cancer	Cicatrix Traumatic bone cyst Aneurysmal bone cyst Fissural cysts† Giant cell lesions Fibrous dysplasia (early) Neurofibroma Hemangioma *Anatomical* Stafne's defect† Foramina	Myeloma Histocytomas Chondrosarcoma Ewing's sarcoma	Cementomas (early) Gardner's‡ Bifid rib‡ MEA II‡	N/L	Neurofibroma Brown tumor *Anatomical* Nutrient canals	Histiocytosis X Plasmacytoma? Myeloma Pulmonary§ Breast§ Colon§
RADIOPAQUE LESIONS	Cementoma (late) Impacted tooth Supernumerary tooth Retained root Odontoma Ossifying fibroma Pindborg tumor†	N/L	Osteosclerosis Osteoma Sequestrum	Osteogenic sarcoma	Cementoma (late) Odontomas Impacted teeth	N/L	Dystrophic calcification: Tonsil Nodes Glands Vascular Epiglottis Osteomas Paget's d. Fibrous dysplasia (late) Foreign bodies Myelogram residua	Metastatic Prostate§ Hypernephroma§

*Locally aggressive growth, frequent recurrence
†Maxilla involved
‡Syndromes
§Metastatic

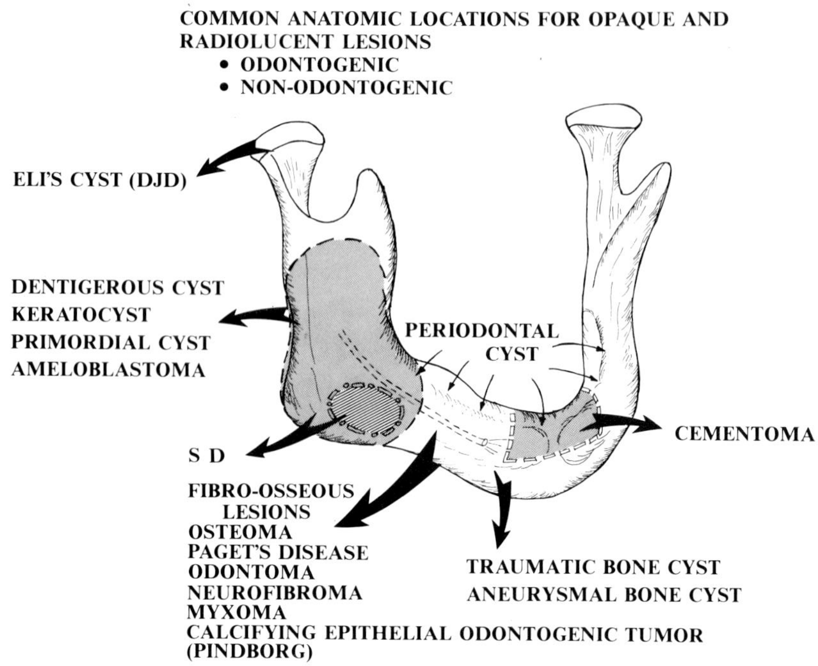

Fig 18–12.—The common locations for benign lesions of the mandible. Some of the lesions may be locally aggressive and recur. Eli's cyst may cause radiographic confusion with other radiolucent lesions. It is a pseudocyst composed of granulation tissue and represents degenerative joint disease of the temporomandibular joint.

replaced using cranio-facial reconstructive techniques.[21] The lesions can prove to be quite vascular during large remodeling surgical projects. In rare cases, sarcomatous degeneration has developed.

Plasmacytoma is managed by local excision with an uninvolved margin. This lesion presents two diagnostic problems. First, apical dental granulomas may be heavily populated with plasma cells, making histologic distinction difficult. Second, the plasmacytoma is histologically identical to multiple myeloma. Solitary plasmacytoma may have further progression over 5 years, and other lesions may appear at other sites. When the lesion is solitary, only a few (< 5%) are associated with splenomegaly, lymphadenopathy, or other cryptic bone lesions. Only a fraction (< 25%) will have M protein in the urine. The likelihood of positivity declines as the

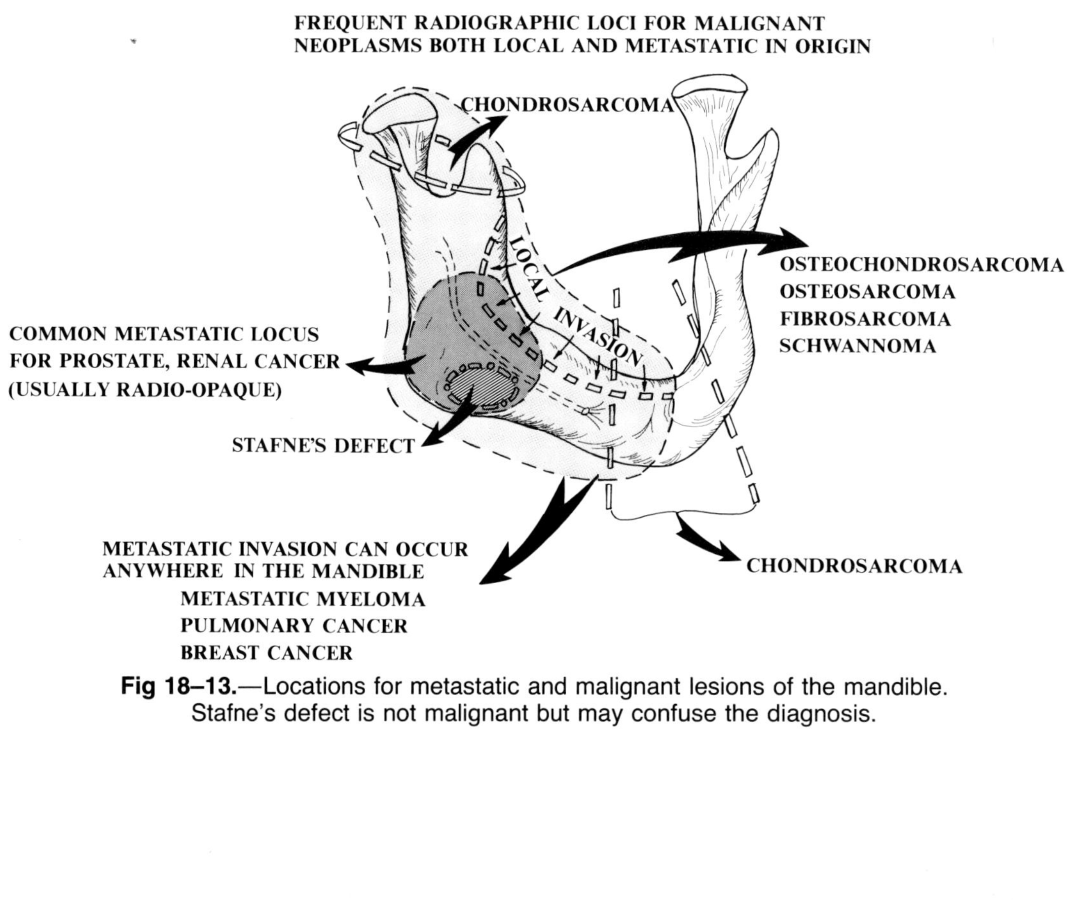

Fig 18–13.—Locations for metastatic and malignant lesions of the mandible. Stafne's defect is not malignant but may confuse the diagnosis.

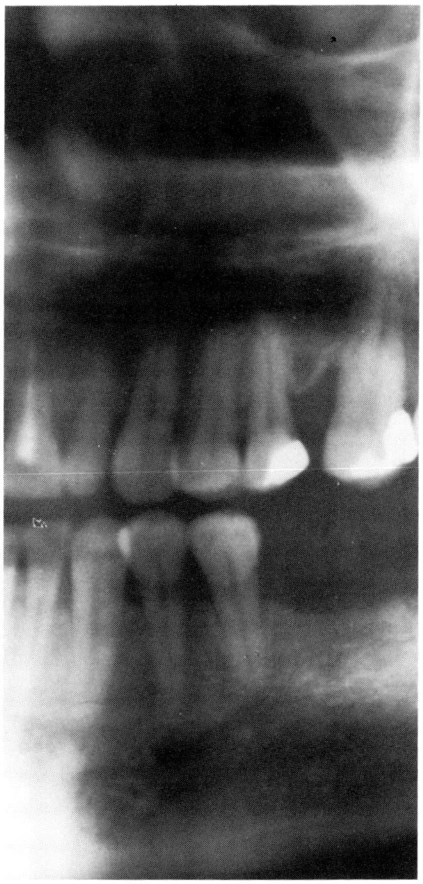

Fig 18–14.—Lytic lesion of osteitis fibrosa cystica, the "brown tumor." It is secondary to hyperparathyroidism.

lesions become smaller. Hence, M protein tests are rarely positive with the small lesions in the jaws.

WHAT TYPE OF BONE AND ODONTOGENIC NEOPLASMS NEED MORE EXTENSIVE SURGICAL PROCEDURES?

Looser and Kuehn[22] studied the cases in the Connecticut tumor registry from a period of about 35 years that were entered because of malignant or presumed malignant potential. They found 53 cases of primary tumors of the mandible. There were 21 *aggressive* ameloblastomas, 11 osteogenic sarcomas, 4 reticulum cell sarcomas (these would probably be classed as malignant fibrous histiocytomas today), 4 epidermoid cancers, 2 chondrosarcomas, 1 adenocarcinoma, 1 giant cell sarcoma, and 1 myxosarcoma. The ameloblastoma patients had an 87% survival rate. Cure was most often effected by excision with a margin. All of the patients who underwent enucleation and curettage experienced recurrence. The patients with osteogenic sarcoma had pain and/or numbness with nerve involvement, and only a 27% 5-year survival rate. Wide resection with upper neck node dissection had the highest degree of success. Two patients had positive regional nodes. Four of the eight patients who died had distant metastases. Shedev[5] found that simple curettage of ameloblastoma was followed by recurrence (90%). Block excision of ameloblastoma is required for cure. Radiation was ineffective.

Chondrosarcoma typically appears at the symphysis and rarely near the temporomandibular joint. Just as is seen with chondrosarcoma in a rib, mandibular involvement of any dimension will expand the bone cortex. The data from Looser and Kuehn parallels our own experience—i.e., wide local excision with clean borders of 2–3 cm is usually sufficient to prevent recurrence. This size of resection requires primary reconstruction of the mandible. Repair after resection of a limited midline lesion is a good place to employ the myo-osseous mandibular advancement illustrated in Chapter 6. Chondrosarcoma is rare in the maxilla. An appropriately designed maxillectomy is required.

Myxosarcoma probably deserves wide excision and reconstruction. Experience is so limited that one can only extrapolate from the fact that minimal excisions almost always end up in recurrence. Frequently, the lesion destroys the mandibular structure.

Looser and Kuehn found that treatment by radiation alone or in combination with resection was 50% successful in reticulum cell sarcoma. Of the four patients with fibrosarcoma, two failed with local excision, and one of two treated with wider resection and lymphadenectomy survived. All of the patients with primary intra-osseous epidermoid cancers died despite radiation or resection.

We tend to agree with Looser and Kuehn that for selected cancers—fibrosarcoma, epidermoid carcinoma, myxosarcoma, osteogenic sarcoma, and chondrosarcoma—an initial wide excision with primary reconstruction is desirable. Adjacent regional nodes should be included for osteogenic sarcoma. A complete lymphadenectomy is warranted for the rare intraosseous epidermoid carcinoma.

REFERENCES

1. Dahlin D.C., *Bone Tumors,* ed. 3. Springfield, Ill., Charles C Thomas, Publisher, 1978, pp. 274–287.
2. Regezi J.A., Kerr D.A., Courtney R.M.: Odontogenic tumors: Analysis of 706 cases. *J. Oral Surg.* 36:771–779, 1978.
3. Greer R.O. Jr., Mierau G.W., Favora B.E.: *Tumors of the Head and Neck in Children.* New York, Praeger Publishing Co., 1983.
4. Greer R.O., Richardson J.F.: Ameloblastoma of mucosal origin: A pathologic re-evaluation. *Arch. Otolaryngol.* 100:174–175, 1974.

5. Shedev M.K., Huvos A.G., Strong E.W., et al.: Ameloblastoma of the maxilla and mandible. *Cancer* 33:324–333, 1974.
6. Mehlish D.R., Dahlin D.C., Mason J.K.: Ameloblastoma: A clinicopathologic report. *J. Oral Surg.* 30:9–22, 1972.
7. Giansanti J.S., Someran A., Waldron C.A.: Odontogenic adenomatoid tumor. *Oral Surg.* 30:69–86, 1970.
8. Stafne E.C.: Epithelial tumors associated with developmental cysts of the maxilla: A report of three cases. *Oral Surg.* 1:887–894, 1948.
9. Gorlin R.J.: Calcifying odontogenic cyst, a possible analogue of cutaneous calcifying epithelioma of Malherbe (an analysis of 15 cases). *Oral Surg.* 15:1235–1243, 1962.
10. Trodahl J.N.: Ameloblastic fibroma, a survey of cases from the A.F.I.P. *Oral Surg.* 30:547–558, 1972.
11. Carr J.C.: Recurrent ameloblastic fibroma. *Oral Surg.* 29:85–90, 1970.
12. Gorlin R.J.: Odontogenic tumors, in Gorlin R.J., Goodman H.M. (eds.): *Thomas' Oral Pathology*, ed. 6. St. Louis, C.V. Mosby Co., 1970.
13. Farman A.G., et al.: Myxofibroma of the jaws. *Br. J. Oral Surg.* 15:3–18, 1977.
14. Fu Y.S., Perzin K.H.: Non-epithelial tumors of the nasal cavity, paranasal sinuses, and nasopharynx: VII. Myxomas. *Cancer* 39:195–203, 1977.
15. Corio R.L., Crawford B.E., Schaberg S.J.: Benign cementoblastoma. *Oral Surg.* 41:524–530, 1976.
16. Abrams A.M., Kirby J.W., Melrose R.J.: Cementoblastoma. *Oral Surg.* 38:394–407, 1974.
17. Dahlin D.C.: *Bone Tumors: General Aspects and Data on 6221 Cases*, ed. 3. Springfield, Ill., Charles C Thomas, Publisher, 1978.
18. Dehner L.P.: Tumors of the mandible and maxilla in children: A study in 14 primary and secondary malignant tumors. *Cancer* 32:112–120, 1973.
19. Dehner L.P.: Tumors of the mandible and maxilla in children: I. Clinicopathologic study of 46 histologically benign lesions. *Cancer* 31:364–384, 1973.
20. Vickers R.A., Rosai J.: Mandible and maxilla, in Rosai J. (ed.): *Ackerman's Surgical Pathology*, ed. 6. St. Louis, C.V. Mosby Co., 1981, chap. 6.
21. Edgerton M.T., Persing J.A., Jane J.A.: The surgical treatment of fibrous dysplasia (of the cranial or facial bones). *Ann. Surg.*, in press.
22. Looser K.G., Kuehn P.G.: Primary tumors of the mandible: A study of 49 cases. *Am. J. Surg.* 132:608–614, 1976.

GENERAL READING

1. Batsakis J.G.: *Tumors of the Head and Neck: Clinical and Pathological Considerations*, ed. 2. Baltimore, Williams & Wilkins Co., 1979.
2. Wirth H.N.: *Principles and Practice of Oral Radiological Interpretation*. Chicago, Year Book Medical Publishers, Inc., 1963.
3. Gorlin R.J., Chanhdry A.P., Pindborg J.J.: Odontogenic tumors: Classification, histopathology and clinical behavior in man and domesticated animals. *Cancer* 14:73–101, 1961.

19 / Thyroid and Parathyroid Cancer

DONALD G. McQUARRIE, M.D., PH.D. / CATHERINE C. LIMAS, M.D.

THE DIAGNOSIS and treatment of thyroid cancer defy the frequent attempts to capsulize management in one brief statement. The literature on thyroid cancer is extensive. Placing the topic on any program generates spirited discussion, especially if the participants include representatives of surgery, endocrinology, and nuclear medicine. The discussion in this chapter tries to identify major issues at decision junctions. The reader is urged to examine the literature to expand and adjust his decisions in light of present and future data. Newer diagnostic techniques such as tumor DNA content, nuclear magnetic resonance imaging, or high resolution computerized tomography (CT) scans may allow more precise decisions to be made.

HOW HAS THE TREATMENT OF THYROID CANCER EVOLVED?

The treatment of thyroid cancer has developed in a changing historical context. For centuries, a high frequency of large iodine-deficiency goiters cloaked the recognition of many thyroid cancers. The modern era has witnessed a miniepidemic of radiation-induced thyroid cancers superimposed on the base cancer rate. At the same time, colloid goiter has become less frequent because of the routine addition of iodine to table salt. This shift in historical patterns has colored attitudes toward the management of thyroid cancer.

Wharton gave a good anatomical description of the thyroid gland in 1656. The exact function of the thyroid prompted strange speculation. Wharton thought that the viscid fluid of the follicles somehow lubricated the trachea.[1] Others thought that the rich thyroid vascularity was a shunt in the cerebral circulation. Rush in 1820 made an observation that would have gotten him pilloried by modern women. He speculated that the larger gland in women was "necessary to guard the female system from the influence of the more numerous causes of irritation and vexation of the mind to which they are exposed than the male sex."

Goiter was endemic in higher mountainous or inland regions where leaching and water runoff removed most soil iodine. Unless seafood was a dietary staple, nontoxic goiter was common (> 25%). Adults require 100 μg/day of iodine. Seafish contain 200–1,000 μg/kg of iodine. On the other hand, 5 kg of vegetables contains only 100 μg of iodine. It was 1917 before Marine and Kimball showed, by administering exogenous iodine to thousands of schoolgirls in Akron, Ohio,[2] that endemic goiter could be virtually eliminated. Where endemic nontoxic goiters were common, thyroid cancers were usually recognized late and in an advanced stage. Surgery was difficult; complications were frequent.

During the 1800s the techniques of thyroid surgery developed slowly. Hemostasis was difficult to achieve and recurrent nerve damage was frequent. Total thyroidectomy produced "cachexia strumapriva" (myxedema) in 30 of Kocher's first 100 patients.[3] Kocher was the pioneer thyroid surgeon. His operative mortality for benign thyroid lesions fell from 6.9% in 1883 to 0.18% in 560 thyroidectomies reported in 1898. In all, he performed about 5,000 thyroidectomies in his career. Kocher's development of safe thyroidectomy and the demonstration of essential endocrine thyroid function were recognized with a Nobel Prize in Medicine in 1909. Kocher performed thyroidectomy in much the same manner as is done today except that he did not ligate the superior thyroid artery. After ligating the inferior thyroid artery he removed the major portion of the gland by cutting between crushing clamps. Kocher's work stimulated the interests of other surgeons; he counted among his friends Crile, Ochsner, Lahey, and the brothers Mayo.

Halstead and Kocher had many communications and visits. Halstead added ligation of the superior thyroid artery and fastidious ligation of small branches of the inferior thyroid artery in order to avoid the recurrent laryngeal nerve and preserve the parathyroids. Unfortunately, these technical refinements were slow to percolate through to the usual operating surgeons. Bloody, crush-and-clamp thyroidectomy persisted into the 1920s. Practitioners with questionable training and dubious skills persisted in attempting thyroidectomy until well into the 1930s. Surgery of the thyroid also got a bad reputation when thyroid storm from thyrotoxicosis was included in the reported mortalities of early surgical series. It was Plummer who made surgery easier. He produced a firmer, less friable gland with preoperative administration of iodine (as Lugol's solution) in 1923.[4] The early technical problems did leave a justified and lasting impression of frequent complications associated with thyroid surgery. Fortunately, competent training and technical developments in the last half-century have made thyroid surgery reliably simple and safe. Unfortunately, aversion to simple surgery still persists among diagnosticians.

HOW LARGE A PROBLEM IS THYROID CANCER?

The overall incidence of thyroid cancer in the United States is 3.6 per 100,000 population per year. Nevertheless, only an estimated 1,200 people die of thyroid cancer annually. Most deaths are from undifferentiated thyroid cancer. Papillary thyroid cancer is more common in women (0.42 male-female ratio). Thyroid cancer includes several distinct histologic varieties. They may vary from rapidly lethal (anaplastic spindle cell) to a slowly-growing papillary cancer that does not alter normal survival if treated at an early stage. The distribution of histologic types and corresponding survival rates in five larger series are given in Table 19–1. Examination of this table immediately underscores the necessity of being specific about cell type, sex incidence, and whether the tumor is intrathyroidal or extrathyroidal. Papillary cancer is the most frequent variety, followed by follicular cancer. Anaplastic thyroid cancer has an abysmal survival compared to other types. Medullary carcinoma is interesting because of its frequent association with the multiple endocrine neoplasia syndrome, type II (MEN II).

WHICH ARE THE MAJOR HISTOLOGIC TYPES OF THYROID CANCER, AND WHAT ARE THE PROBLEMS IN THEIR DIFFERENTIAL DIAGNOSIS?

Primary thyroid neoplasia may originate from any of the cellular components of the gland: follicular and parafollicular cells, vascular endothelium, stromal fibroblasts, and lymphocytes. The great majority of thyroid tumors arise from follicular cells; other histogenic types are rare. The only known neoplasm of parafollicular cell origin is the medullary carcinoma. Primary thyroid fibrosarcoma and angiosarcoma remain questionable entities, while malignant lymphomas are rare and usually arise in the setting of lymphocytic thyroiditis or Hashimoto's disease.

Follicular cell neoplasms can be classified into three major categories according to their resemblance to normal cells and the pattern of cell arrangement. These categories are *papillary* neoplasms, characterized by papillary formations and often psammoma bodies; *follicular* neoplasms, characterized by follicular formations similar to normal, immature or hyperplastic thyroid; and *anaplastic* neoplasms, which have no characteristic architecture and bear no resemblance to normal thyroid cells.

Subclassification of these major categories is possible on the basis of morphological details. For example, when the follicular cells contain abundant eosinophilic granular cytoplasm, the term oxyphil cell tumor (Hurthle tumor) may be used.

It is widely accepted that all papillary neoplasms have malignant potential. Consequently, the diagnosis of papillary carcinoma is established whenever clearcut papillary structures and/or psammoma bodies are found in any proportion. Papillary carcinoma has some peculiarities that should be taken into consideration for optimal therapy. It is very often multifocal (up to 80% of cases) and found in both lobes,[10] and it frequently metastasizes to regional nodes, which usually (60% of cases) do not appear clinically enlarged.[11]

Anaplastic neoplasms are aggressively malignant and have a high metastatic potential. They are subclassified into small cell, giant cell, and spindle cell types, depending on the predominant cell morphology. The differential diagnosis for the anaplastic carcinomas includes metastatic malignancies and lymphomas. It is uncommon to find metastatic neoplasms from other sites involving the thyroid. If they do occur, the most frequent sources of metastases are renal cell cancer or breast carcinoma.

Primary thyroid lymphomas are sometimes difficult to differentiate from the rare small cell type of anaplastic carcinomas. Electron microscopic studies are helpful in arriving at a correct diagnosis.

Real diagnostic problems are encountered frequently in the interpretation of *follicular* neoplasms. This is because the application of cytologic criteria for malignancy is not valid. The biologic potential of follicular neoplasia must be judged from the presence or absence of an invasive growth pattern. Regardless of cytologic features, a completely encapsulated follicular neoplasm is considered benign and is classified as an adenoma. In contrast, whenever any evidence of invasive growth is found, the follicular neoplasm is classified as carcinoma, although it may lack the cytologic characteristics of malignancy. An invasive pattern may be grossly obvious at surgery or on gross cross section. At the other extreme, invasion may be detected only after careful examination of an apparently encapsulated nodule and the vessels adjacent to the nodule. In the latter case, the term angioinvasive or low-grade follicular carcinoma with capsular invasion is often applied. These considerations lead to the following conclusions: (1) The differential diagnosis between benign and malignant follicular lesions is not possible on the basis of cytologic criteria. (2) The gross appearance is very important for the differential diagnosis of follicular neoplasia. (3) The diagnosis of follicular adenoma cannot be established without thorough evaluation of the capsule and surrounding vessels be-

TABLE 19–1.—DISTRIBUTION OF HISTOLOGIC TYPES OF THYROID CANCER WITH THE DETERMINANT 5- AND 10-YEAR SURVIVALS

	MAYO CLINIC[5] (1926–1960) (N = 1,181)				SEER TUMOR REPORTING REGISTRY[6] (N = 2,905)		MEMORIAL HOSPITAL, N.Y.[7] (N = 673)		M. D. ANDERSON[8] (N = 476)			FINLAND CANCER REGISTRY[9] (N = 227)		
	Distribution (N)		Survival (%)							Survival (%)			Survival (%)	
HISTOLOGIC TYPE			5 yr	10 yr	Distribution (N)	Survival (%) (5 yr)	Distribution (N)	Survival (%) (5 yr)	Distribution (N)	5 yr	10 yr	Distribution (N)	5 yr	10 yr
Papillary*														
Occult		35	98	95										
Intrathyroidal	62	50	97	94	44	95	65	80	19	80	78	43	83	81
Extrathyroidal		15	80	58										
Mixed† (where not categorized)	0				12	87			10	90	85			
Follicular														
Angioinvasive		50	95	92										
Invasive (1.5:1 F/M)	18	50	60	35	17	94	17	63	54	80	52	26	54	40
Medullary‡														
Neg. nodes	6		95	90 }			9	40	9	46	46	4	89	77
Pos. nodes			68	42 }										
Anaplastic	14		0	0			7	2	6	10	10	25	15	17
Unspecified	0				27		1		2	0	0	1		

*Male-female incidence 1/2.3.
†Most pathologists would classify these as papillary.
‡Male predominance, 4:1.

cause it is based on the exclusion of invasive growth pattern.

The diagnosis of medullary carcinoma is based on features highly specific for this neoplasm such as amyloid deposits in the stroma and positive immunoperoxidase reaction for calcitonin in the cell cytoplasm. In addition, medullary carcinoma is sometimes associated with other endocrine neoplasias in the context of MEN IIa or IIb.

WHAT IS THE BEST APPROACH FOR OBTAINING DIAGNOSTIC MATERIAL FROM THE THYROID?

Material for the histologic diagnosis of thyroid lesions may be obtained at surgery or prior to the operative procedure by either needle (cutting needle) core biopsy or needle (fine needle) aspiration. Each of these approaches has merits as well as limitations. Obviously, a thyroid lobectomy encompassing the lesion will yield quantitatively and qualitatively optimal material that can be evaluated grossly and microscopically. Surgery is the most invasive, least comfortable, and most expensive approach. Many patients might be spared the discomfort of surgery if a correct diagnosis could be attained using an alternative procedure.

Fine needle aspiration biopsy is the least traumatic, fastest, and most inexpensive procedure. These merits must be weighed against the limitations in diagnostic accuracy. Aspiration biopsy of the thyroid was introduced many years ago[12–14] but did not gain popularity in the United States until recently.[15] The fear of implantation of malignant cells has proved unjustified.[16] Fine needle aspiration biopsy is simple in principle and requires inexpensive equipment. It does require the key ingredient of expertise for both the procurement and the evaluation of the aspirated material. For the technique to be effective, the following are necessary:

1. A skilled person who can identify, immobilize, and reliably aspirate cellular material from the correct nodule.
2. A 22-gauge needle, a tight-fitting syringe, and a special syringe handle that allows the development of powerful negative pressure.
3. Three separately smeared cytologic specimens, obtained by expelling the needle contents on slides and pulling a smear with a cover glass to distribute the cells evenly (fixation is by immersion in 95% alcohol).
4. Careful staining of the specimens by the Papanicolaou method for the study of nuclear details.
5. Additional, air-dried slide preparations are used for other histochemical and, if needed, immunochemical procedures. The needle is then washed with normal saline and the washings are used for cell blocks or membrane filter preparations.
6. A trained cytologist who is experienced in fine needle aspiration biopsy specimens must stain and interpret the three slides. Some physicians prefer to augment the cytologic study with "minisliver" histologic study; the specimen is obtained by using a 15-gauge Tru-Cut needle or a radiologic 20-gauge "skinny needle."

The major limitations of aspiration biopsy cytology become evident if one considers the preceding discussion on the differential diagnosis of thyroid neoplasms. Since the biologic potential of follicular neoplasms cannot be determined on the basis of cytologic characteristics, it follows that a needle aspirate cannot differentiate between benign (hyperplasia and adenoma) and malignant (carcinoma) follicular growth. If the aspirate contains only follicular structures the diagnosis will be "consistent with follicular neoplasia" or "unremarkable thyroid," depending on the cellularity. If either papillary formation or psammoma bodies are found, a definitive diagnosis of papillary carcinoma is made. The demonstration of amyloid and/or intracellular calcitonin in the aspirated material establishes the diagnosis of medullary carcinoma. Whenever the majority of cells are highly pleomorphic with overt malignant cytologic features, primary anaplastic and metastatic malignancies are considered. Then the differential diagnosis of pleomorphic anaplastic aspirates requires clinical data and special histochemical procedures. Hurthle (oxyphil) cell tumors can be recognized in aspiration biopsy samples because of the characteristic cytoplasmic texture. However, this cytoplasmic characteristic is not diagnostic by itself because oxyphilic cytoplasm is often present in damaged follicular cells in Hashimoto's thyroiditis. The differential diagnosis between the two conditions is based on the absence or presence of inflammatory cells.

Overall, needle aspiration cytology is a potentially valuable procedure since a definitive diagnosis is attainable in a large number of cases. It does not completely substitute for the conventional open surgical approach.

WHAT CLINICAL FINDINGS AND SYMPTOMS SUGGEST THE PRESENCE OF A THYROID CARCINOMA?

Benign adenomatous goiter is the most common cause of thyroid enlargement. In low iodine areas, like the Central European Alps, nontoxic goiter was virtually universal in the early 1900s. Iodine therapy in the 1920s and 1930s reduced the incidence of goiter in Zurich schoolchildren from 92% to 28%.[17] In the Midwestern United States "goiter belt," a high frequency of iodine deficiency goiter is still to be expected in the older patient populations.

In the contemporary U.S. population, which receives adequate iodine in table salt, it is hazardous to dismiss all thyroid enlargement as benign adenomatous goiter. In one study, 21% of patients who were found to have thyroid cancer had a history of "goiter."[18] A stable multinodular goiter can usually be found and diagnosed by history and palpation. Beahrs and Pasternak estimated that 10%–20% of multinodular goiters are operated on because of size, compression, or enlargement.[5] In their patients, cancer was found in about 5% of "goiter" patients. There was a 14% incidence of cancer in goiters that had a suspicion of malignancy and a 4% incidence in goiters removed for other reasons.

A lump in the neck, either in the thyroid gland or the lymph nodes, is the major symptom in 41% of thyroid cancers. Other symptoms are hoarseness (13%), pressure on the airway or esophagus (8%), and pain (5%).[18] To this list we should add distant osseous or systemic metastases (3%–5% of cases) from follicular cancer. Rarely, a patient has hemoptysis when tumor invades the airway. Rapid growth of a mass and unilateral vocal cord paralysis are ominous signs. Nerve entrapment, rapid growth, and pain are seen in 72% of patients with anaplastic thyroid cancers.[19] Continued rapid enlargement is usually *not* hemorrhage into a colloid nodule. A suspected or truly solitary thyroid mass alone or in association with enlarged lymph nodes should trigger a complete evaluation.

How Important Is the Patient's Age in Determining the Possibility of Malignancy of a Thyroid Nodule?

Patient age is of critical importance. Figure 19–1 shows two curves. The heavy dotted line shows the increasing frequency of thyroid nodules with age, approximating a 20% incidence in the eighth decade. This is plotted with the data from six studies on the frequency of malignancy in thyroid nodules, which were clinically dominant or solitary.[20–25] The likelihood of malignancy is high in young patients, lessens in middle age, and increases again after age 50–60 years. Unfortunately, the incidence of *anaplastic* thyroid carcinoma increases after age 50–60 years. The higher value range probably represents better patient selection. The lower range reflects less diagnostic discrimination and/or a high rate of endemic goiter. The data from Hayles et al.[20] are divided into incidence in patients *before* frequent head and neck irradiation in children and the rate in children *after* irradiation was common. The patient population that received head and neck irradiation in childhood in the 1920–1940 period will be moving through the demographic distribution for decades to come.

The main lesson to be drawn from Figure 19–1 is that a thyroid nodule in a patient under 30 years old has a 15%–35% chance of malignancy. Of the 58 young patients described by Harness et al. two thirds had cervical node metastasis as the presenting finding.[26] Almost 88% were ultimately found to have cervical lymph node metastases. In an elderly male VA hospital population, the likelihood that a solid solitary mass is malignant is small, about 6%.

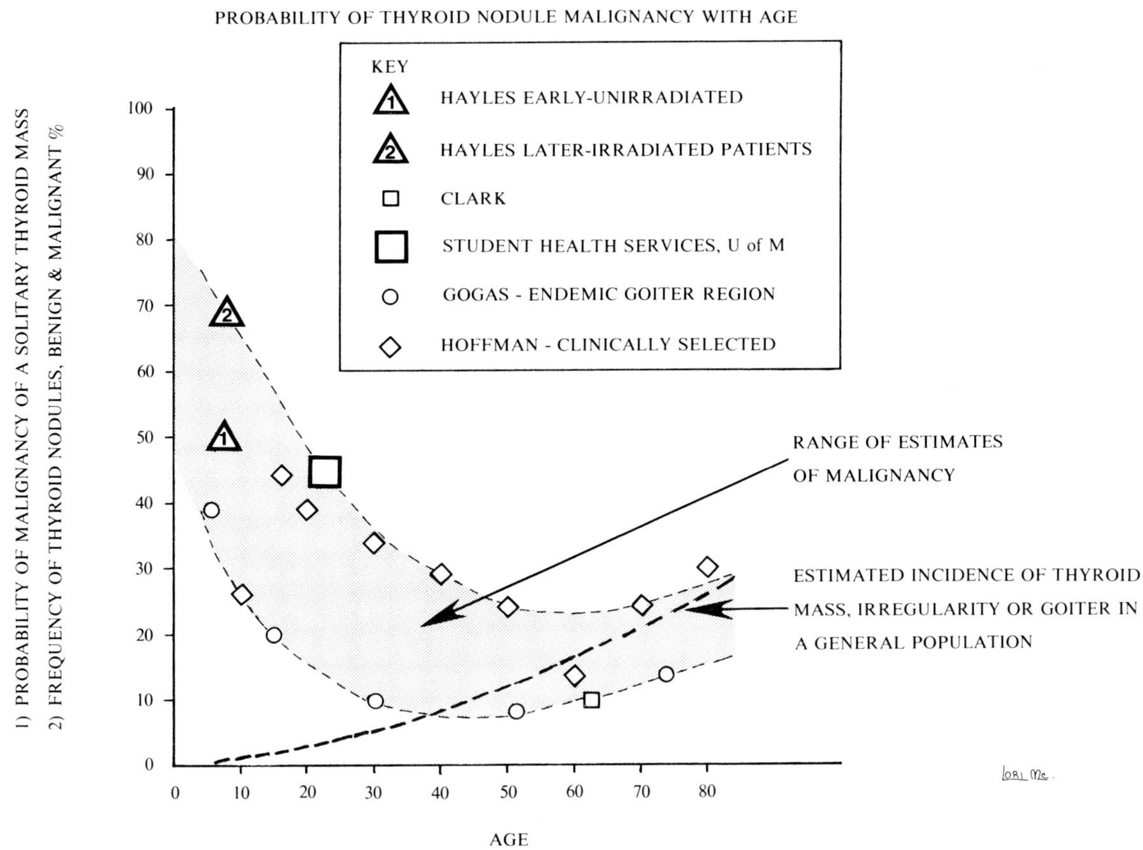

Fig 19–1.—The incidence of malignancy in clinically dominant or solitary thyroid nodules, plotted against age. The data are a composite of several series. Hayles' data are from groups treated before and after irradiation of the head and neck was frequent. A series from an area where goiter is endemic shows that the probability of cancer is "diluted" by the frequency of endemic colloid nodules.

What Are the Risks of Thyroid Cancer as a Result of Previous Irradiation of the Head and Neck Area?

In the past, young patients were treated by irradiation for any of the following reasons:

1. *To cause involution of the thymus.* The normally prominent childhood thymus was perceived as too large and thought to contribute to the frequent respiratory infections that were difficult to manage in the preantibiotic era.

2. *To cause involution of the tonsils and adenoids.* This was done using widely marketed radium capsules on a nasal carrier. The rod carrier was used to position the source in the nasopharynx. This was a poorly controlled wide-field gamma source.

3. *To treat adolescent acne.* Doses of 75–1,000 rad were given with primitive uncallibrated equipment in dermatologists' offices.

4. *To treat tuberculous cervical adenitis:* This disease used to be much more common in children. Radiation was reputed to be effective in controlling scrofulous nodes.

5. *To control unwanted facial hair.* About 600–1,200 rad was given for depilatory purposes.

6. *For valid therapy of other malignancies.* Ideally, this is the only persisting use.

It is important that the clinician actively seek a history of past head and neck irradiation treatment. Attempts to identify and recall irradiated patients have been minimally successful despite areawide publicity.

The association of irradiation with the subsequent development of thyroid cancer has been well documented over the past 30 years. The relationship was first detected by Duffy and Fitzgerald in 1950.[27] Others confirmed the association.[28–35] Winship and Rosvoll reviewed reports of childhood thyroid carcinoma from 1900 to 1960 and showed the rapid increase in number of cases in the 1950–1960 era.[36] The occurrence of this "epidemic"[30] in our age of roentgenophobia has made the public at large as aware of the problem as physicians. In general, only 3% of children have any suspicion of thyroid abnormality.[23, 37] Hempelmann et al. studied 2,872 young adults irradiated in infancy and 5,005 sibling controls.[38] They found 8.3 cases of thyroid cancer per 1,000 irradiated patients after a follow-up of 20 years. This exceeded the spontaneous rate by 100 times. The "high-dose" group had a rate 300 times that expected. Hempelmann et al. calculated that the cancer or thyroid nodularity due to irradiation would be 38 to 52 cases per 10^6 persons exposed per rad of thyroid dose per year.[38, 39] The latent period before cancers occur is 10–15 years, and the peak incidence is 20–30 years after exposure.[33, 34, 36] DeGroot and co-workers studied 416 patients irradiated in childhood. Of these, 113 had suspicious thyroid masses, and 41 (36%) of the masses were thyroid cancer. Of the 41, 59% were multifocal and 25% were node positive. DeGroot et al. made a prospective attempt to suppress development of abnormalities in the patients without thyroid masses by giving exogenous thyroid hormone. There was no effect. Abnormalities and cancer rate were comparable to those in the unsuppressed group.[40]

The actual rate of irradiation-induced cancers may be skewed by the diligence with which abnormalities are looked for. Wilson et al. studied 2,118 patients who had received head and neck irradiation and from whom varying amounts of thyroid and nodal tissue were removed at surgery for histologic sampling. They concluded that the varying incidence of cancer—from 21% to 59%— was due in part to the extent of the thyroidectomy, to whether or not cervical nodes were sampled, and to the amount of tissue processed and histologically examined.[41]

Is There a Thyroid Cancer Risk From Diagnostic Scans and Therapeutic Iodine 131?

Iodine 131 has an 8.9-day half-life. Over 99% of its energy is expended in 56 days. The ^{131}I emissions include β particles (low-energy particles that dissipate their ionizing effect in 1–2 mm of tissue). It is also a γ particle emittor. When used for scans, ^{131}I delivers significant irradiation to the thyroid. A therapeutic dose that gives a concentration of 80–150 Ci/gm of thyroid will deliver 7,000–10,000 rad to thyroid tissue. Even a fractional 1/100 scanning dose will deliver measurable radiation. To avoid this irradiation technetium 99 or iodine 123 are used for diagnostic scans because of the short half-life, measured in hours.

HOW DO YOU APPROACH A NECK MASS IN THE REGION OF THE THYROID?

Thyroid cancer patients are usually seen because of a cervical mass or some dysfunction of structures in the neck. A few patients present with findings that require expeditious workup, open biopsy, and appropriate surgery. Dysphagia, hoarseness (with vocal cord paralysis or palsy), proved osseous or systemic metastasis, and fixation of a mass to the trachea, paraspinous muscles, or other cervical structures all require direct surgical examination biopsy and treatment. In one half to two thirds of the younger patients the thyroid cancer is found on cervical lymph node biopsy. Anyone with a family history suggesting MEN II syndrome should be evaluated for thyrocalcitonin excess, hyperparathyroidism, and the presence of a cryptic pheochromocytoma. The associated pheochromocytoma may be synchronous or may appear in a symptomatic form as much as a decade before or after the medullary cancer. In older patients who smoke, oroairway squamous cell cancer is the leading diagnostic consideration when a neck mass is present. One is obliged to prove that squamous cell cancer is *not* present by careful examination, studies, and appropriate endoscopies. It is disappointing to see an obvious laryngeal, tonsillar, or retromolar trigone lesion missed while a "million-dollar" endocrine workup is done. It is always wise to consider a modest catalogue of esoterica: schwannoma of the vagus nerve, chemodectoma, hemangioma, cystic hygroma, rhabdomyosarcoma, parathyroid cancer, fibrous histiocytoma, and so on. The most useful diagnostic aid is still the physical examination to determine the boundaries of thyroid tissue and movement of the mass with the thyroid cartilage during swallowing. The texture of a mass is important. Cysts *feel* fluid-filled; colloid nodules have a gelatinous doughy deformability (as do follicular cancers). Papillary cancers and medullary cancers frequently feel like hard rubber nodules. A scintiscan is most useful in determining if the mass deforms the thyroid uptake pattern. In some instances a CT scan defines complex relationships in the neck. Ultrasound can demonstrate the location and presence of cystic characteristics.

When oroairway squamous cell carcinoma, metastatic lung cancer, common lymphomas, and lymphocytic leukemia have been excluded and physical examination confirms there is a thyroid mass that moves with swallowing, the physician is left with several diagnostic options: (1) adenomatous or colloid goiter, (2) benign adenoma, (3) thyroiditis, (4) thyroid cancer of some type, or (5) an esoteric entity that is an uncommon presentation of a common disease or a common presentation of an uncommon disease. Thyroiditis frequently has a characteristic history of pain and tenderness. One or more immunologic tests are positive. Usually both lobes are involved. Discrete nodules are uncommon. It must be kept in mind that thyroiditis and thyroid cancer can coexist.

Finally, we can identify thyroid masses that are suspicious for cancer by using the following guidelines:

1. Young person, less than 30–35 years old.
2. History of head and neck irradiation.
3. Enlarged cervical lymph nodes associated with thyroid abnormality.
4. Fixation to surrounding tissues.
5. Rubbery, hard thyroid mass.
6. Family history suggestive of MEN II.
7. A suspicious fine needle aspiration cytology or proved biopsy.

If these features are present, there is a high suspicion of malignancy. In the case of a young person or one that received cervical irradiation, the physician would still recommend exploration of the thyroid and a lobectomy for biopsy, despite other findings to the contrary, since operation carries minimal risk.

There remains a large group of patients (> 60%) who are not in the high-risk group but have a mass or dominant nodule in the thyroid. What other discriminating diagnostic tools are available?

How Good Is Thyroid Scanning in Diagnosis?

The scan basically defines an area of uptake of the scanning agent in the gland. For reasons of radiation dosage, ^{123}I or ^{99m}Tc is used. The information obtained falls into several categories:

1. Homogeneous uptake:
   Normal in speed and amount.
   Accelerated uptake.
2. One clearly defined solitary area of reduced uptake. Size can be estimated. Solitary "cold" nodule.
3. One or more areas of reduced uptake, less well defined.
4. Area of increased isotope uptake—"hot" nodule.
5. Absent or abnormally located gland tissue.

The definition of a thyroid mass by scan is dependent on the geometry of the mass and the gland. Smaller posterior nodules may be overlain by active thyroid tissue. Multiple small nodules may give a relatively homogeneous appearance. Hot nodules may be associated with general glandular hyperfunction. Autonomously functioning (hot) thyroid nodules are operated on to treat existing thyrotoxicosis or to prevent subsequent thyrotoxicosis in asymptomatic patients. They are not operated on for high suspicion of cancer. In one study, no cancers were reported in 101 hot nodules.[42] In a fat or thick muscular neck, the scan is of premier value in confirming equivocal palpatory findings. It will tell you whether a questionable cervical mass is associated closely with the thyroid or deforms the scan pattern.

There are real problems with scan accuracy of sizing and precision of location. Becker and Southwick compared preoperative scan reports and operative findings in 15 patients with papillary thyroid cancers. In 14 patients the scan did not locate accurately the location of the cancer in the thyroid parenchyma.[43] The majority of malignant lesions (95%) are hypofunctioning, i.e., cold nodules. The problem nodule shows normal or spotty uptake. Depending on prescan selection criteria, the incidence of malignancy in solitary cold nodules is 5%–30%.[21, 44–47] A scan tells absolutely nothing about histology. It can distinguish a multinodular lesion (3%–5% are malignant) from a uninodular lesion (10%–30% are malignant).[48, 49] We tend to agree with Nelson et al. that "unless the nodule is hyperfunctioning, clinical criteria rather than appearance of a scan should contribute most to the decision of whether to treat surgically."[49] Other scanning agents do not improve specificity.

Are There Other Examinations That May Help in Selected Instances?

SOFT TISSUE ROENTGENOGRAPHY OF THE NECK

Psammoma bodies are characteristic of papillary thyroid carcinoma. When these small bodies are calcified in more advanced papillary cancers, they may appear as finely stippled areas on soft tissue cervical films.[50] This type of calcification should be distinguished from the "cracked eggshell" calcification sometimes seen edging large degenerated colloid nodules, particularly in the upper mediastinum with retrosternal goiter.

ULTRASOUND

Ultrasonography can usually distinguish a purely cystic nodule. About 20% of smaller (1–3 cm) solitary nodules are cystic. Only rarely (2%–3% of cases) is a purely cystic nodule associated with a thyroid cancer. The interpretive problems are caused by large cystic degenerative areas in some tumors and variable liquefaction of colloid nodules. A cyst may be echogenically homogeneous, failing to disclose its cystic nature. Blum et al. ultrasonically scanned 800 patients with thyroid abnormalities; 122 with lesions were operated on. The scan correctly identified 13 cystic and 54 solid lesions in 67 solitary nodules.[51] Other studies have shown good accuracy in delecting cystic lesions in the 1- to 4-cm range.[52, 53] A recent study of 341 patients questions whether a "cystic lesion" can be regarded as benign when 16 of 71 cystic lesions harbored a cancer, and one third of 48 cancers had a significant cystic component.[54] Aspiration cytology, as we will see later, can reduce diagnostic error further.

COMPUTERIZED TOMOGRAPHY

This mode is of particular help in assessing the extent and relationships of larger thyroid lesions, particularly in the pudgy thick-necked patient.

Is a Trial of Suppression Desirable and Definitive in Detecting Malignancy in a Solid Solitary Thyroid Nodule?

The rationale behind an attempt at suppression is that an adenomatous goiter and/or nodule arises in response to an excess of thyroid-stimulating hormone (TSH) that is unchecked by negative feedback inhibition from thyroxine. Low serum levels of thyroxine result in elevated TSH levels that stimulate follicular proliferation and colloid accumulation in the thyroid. Administration of exogenous thyroxine (T_4) or 3,5,3-triiodothyronine (T_3) inhibits TSH production and probably has an additional inhibitory effect on hypothalamic secretion of thyrotropin-releasing hormone (TRH). When low levels of TSH are achieved by suppression, the proliferative drive on the thyroid is removed and a nodule of nonmalignant cells and colloid should involute and diminish in size. In contrast, a malignant nodule is presumed to be autonomous in its growth and will continue to enlarge. Advocates of a trial of suppression point to the slow progress of most thyroid cancers and believe that the treatment delay for the 2- or 3-month trial is justified. As stated by thoughtful advocates, the effort is made because "the problem in the management of the solitary thyroid nodule is not that the patients die or are incapacitated by thyroid cancer, but rather that too many benign nodules are excised and may be followed by unnecessary untoward surgical effects."[55] The statement is cited because it reflects broadly held views among some endocrinologists. Before proceeding, it is important to examine the statement for conceptual errors. As we will see later, patients do die of thyroid cancer. All the large series that show an excellent survival are *the result of judicious and effective surgery.* Finally, the "untoward surgical effects" do not occur in the course of thyroidectomy for the smaller benign solitary nodule. The problems of nerve loss and hypoparathyroidism occur where unyielding malignancy invades or totally embraces the recurrent nerve or parathyroid tissue.

The real question is whether suppression is diagnostically discriminating. Two proponents, Blum and Rothschild, ran a careful study.[55] The findings are diagramed in Figure 19–2. The authors gave doses of liothyronine which suppressed TSH to less than 2.5 IU/ml. Cystic lesions were excluded by echograms. Thirty percent of patients had clear indications for direct operation, with a 43% incidence of cancer. After a complete trial of suppression, 50 of 83 patients (60%) showed nodule regression. *But,* they are then asked to follow a program of lifelong suppression with 0.2–0.3 mg of levothyroxine per day. The cardiovascular risks of lifelong suppression are unknown. Blum and Rothschild have had patients insist on surgery because the side effects of tremor and irritability were not tolerated. The option of suppression is in lieu of a simple safe surgical procedure.[56]

Has suppression been effective in other series? Table 19–2 gives the results of some other suppressive trials. The majority of nodules do not suppress reliably. Both Beahrs[60] and Thompson et al.[61] have reported from surgical series that most of the observed reduction in size really represents a decrease in the surrounding extranodular thyroid parenchyma.

In conclusion, suppression has much variation. It in-

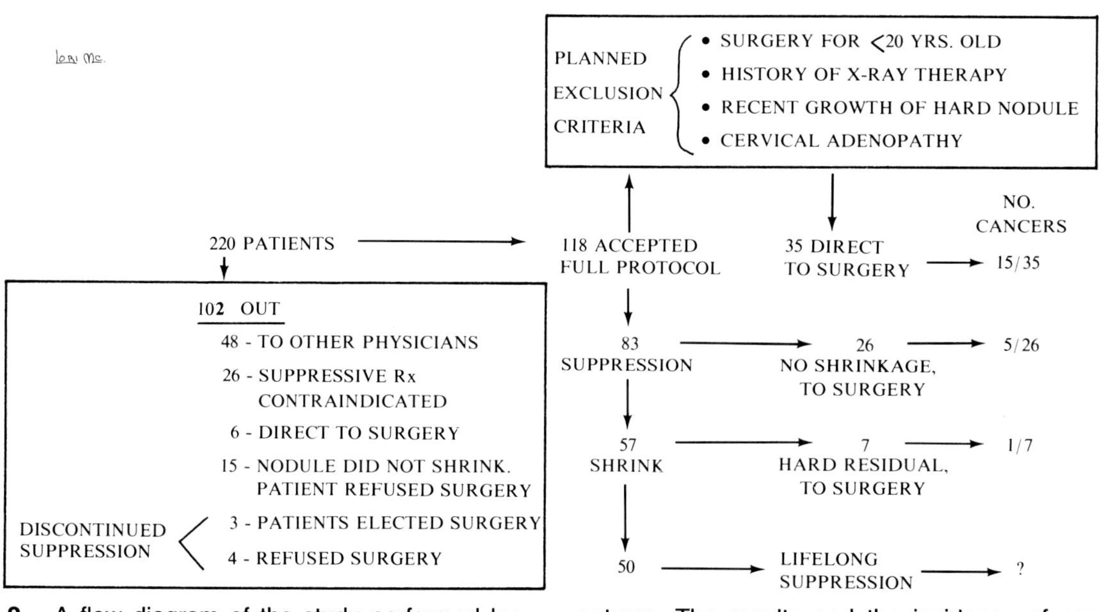

Fig 19–2.—A flow diagram of the study performed by Blum and Rothschild.[55] One group (30%) of their patients had findings that prompted immediate referral for thyroidectomy. The results and the incidence of cancer in the subgroups of patients undergoing a trial of suppression are shown on the far right.

TABLE 19–2.—RESULTS OF TRIALS OF SUPPRESSION TO REDUCE THE SIZE OF SOLITARY "COLD" THYROID NODULES

STUDY, YEAR	NO. OF PTS.	% SUPPRESSED
Mazzaferri et al.,[57] 1977	83	13
Miller et al.,[58] 1979	164	13
Astwood et al.,[59] 1960*	230	40
Blum and Rothschild,[55] (unselected) 1980	166†	30
Blum and Rothschild,[55] (selected) 1980	83	60

*Some were suppressed for long periods.
†Number includes those who started suppression and those in whom suppression was contraindicated (see Fig 19–2).

volves time loss, uncertainty, and the cumulative costs of medication and repeated examinations. It appears to have very little use in *routine* diagnosis, particularly when compared with the favorable experience now accumulating with fine needle aspiration cytology or fine needle biopsy.

How Effective is Fine Needle Aspiration Cytology and/or Needle Biopsy of the Suspicious, Solitary, Thyroid Nodule?

A fine needle aspirate produces a few clumps of cells for cytologic examination. The techniques and limitations were discussed earlier. Detailed atlases on techniques, histology, and cytology are available.[62]

Some of the published results are collected in Table 19–3. The results show a low incidence of false negative and false positive results, especially if the following three important points are observed.

1. An occasional cystic lesion will be associated with a cancer. The presence of any significant residual solid mass after aspiration should prompt repeat biopsy or aspiration. The cyst wall can be biopsied with a Tru-Cut needle.[68]

2. Hurthle cell lesions require effective surgery. Thompson et al. have shown that one cannot safely make a diagnosis of benign Hurthle cell adenoma. Their data, reported in 1974, on 25 patients supported the thesis that all such lesions are malignant in behavior, and patients should undergo a total thyroidectomy.[69] Extending their experience another decade and increasing the series to 62 patients continued to support aggressive surgical management.[70]

3. One must recognize the diagnostic limitations of the technique, particularly for follicular lesions, as was discussed earlier.

Some clinics go directly to fine needle aspiration biopsy when a thyroid nodule is detected. In 1982, Dr. P. O. Granberg from Stockholm, said that in his usual daily practice, the patient was sent directly to pathology for aspiration cytology after initial history and physical examination were concluded. The answer is obtained in an hour and the diagnoses were 90% correct.[71]

What Are the Specificity and Sensitivity of Various Diagnostic Tests For a Solitary Thyroid Nodule?

Ashcraft and Van Herle[72–74] and Solomon and Keeler[75] have reviewed and evaluated the data on diagnostic tests for thyroid cancer. Their reviews assigned both sensitivity and specificity to the tests in common use. A summary derived from their studies and illustrations is redrawn in Figure 19–3 to focus on major categories. Scans will never have specificity. Suppression also lacks specificity even when data from selected series are included. Of all the studies, the specificity of fine needle aspiration biopsy approximates that of lobectomy and tissue section most closely. The fine needle aspirate is a desirable discriminator in the truly solitary nodule with a low suspicion of malignancy. This assumes that morbidity is minimal and that the risk of dissemination

TABLE 19–3.—RESULTS OF FINE NEEDLE ASPIRATION (FNA) AND NEEDLE BIOPSY FOR THE CORRECT DIAGNOSIS OR EXCLUSION OF CANCER

	FNA			NEEDLE BIOPSY		
STUDY	False Neg. (%)	False Pos. (%)	Malig. Rate in Susp. (%)	False Neg. (%)	False Pos. (%)	Malig. Rate in Susp. (%)
Boey et al.[63] (N = 167)	2.2	0	33	7.8	0	36.4
Colacchio et al.[64] (N = 300)	1	1	. . .	NA	NA	NA
Crile and Hawk[65] (N = 135)	0*	4.0	NA	Needle used to confirm histology		
Wang et al.[66]	NA	NA	NA	5†	0	10
Gershengorm et al.[67] (N = 33)	3	9	NA	NA	NA	NA
Miller[58] (N = 455)‡	4	29	19	3	0	16

*Assumption of correct diagnosis because patients were observed for variable follow-up periods.
†Follicular lesions: known to be "suspicious" until capsule and entire nodule were examined.
‡Six patients with benign nodules had occult cancer (< 1 cm) elsewhere.

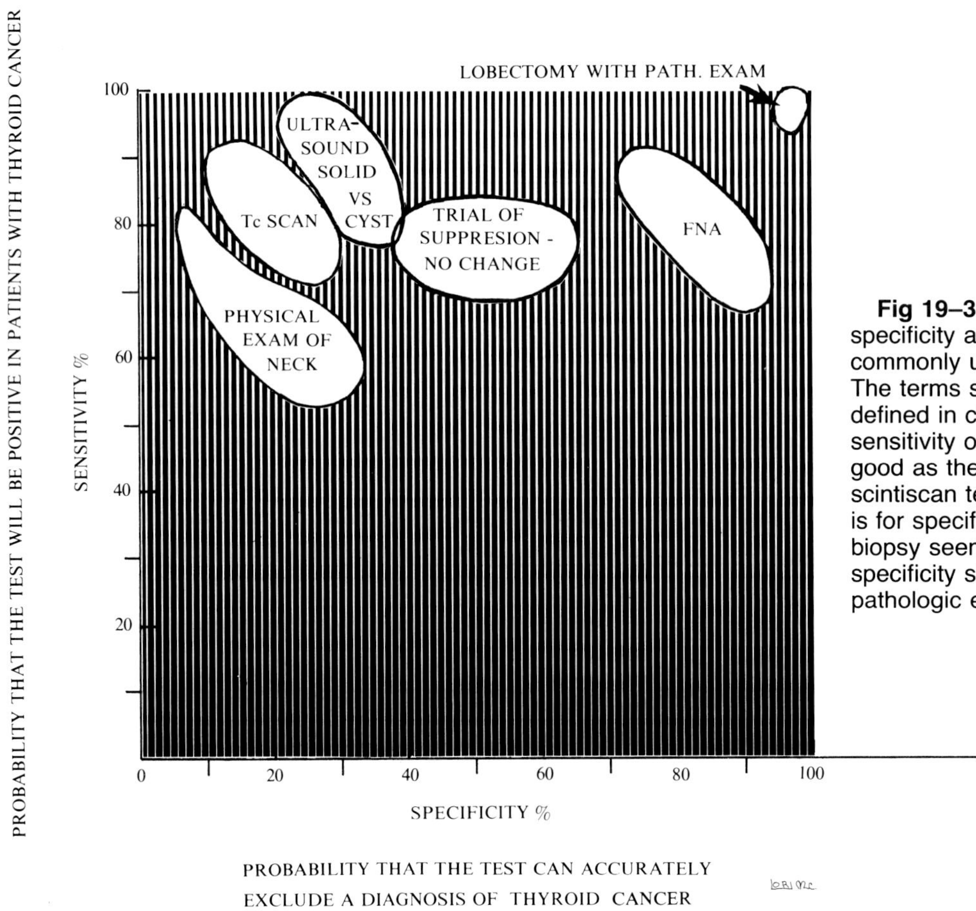

Fig 19–3.—The estimated zones of specificity and sensitivity of various studies commonly used to evaluate thyroid nodules. The terms sensitivity and specificity were defined in chapter 9 (see Fig 9–3). The sensitivity of palpation alone is about as good as the sensitivity of many of the scintiscan techniques. The real clinical need is for specificity. Fine needle aspiration biopsy seems to add the highest level of specificity short of a lobectomy and pathologic examination.

and implantation remains as small as has been reported to date.

When lobectomy carries a very small risk, long periods of suppression and multiple tests with poor specificity are not warranted. Kassirer and Pauker use the solitary thyroid nodule as an example in their editorial, "The toss-up."[76] Their analysis showed that minimal difference in patient risk was incurred by pursuing suppression or going directly to lobectomy, and that "the consequences of divergent choices are, on the average, virtually identical."

Based on the previous section on diagnosis, a very general summary evaluation outline is shown in Figure 19–4.

WHEN A DECISION IS MADE TO OPERATE ON A THYROID MASS, HOW DO YOU PROCEED?

We will discuss operative treatment beginning with the minimal solitary nodular lesion and progress in subsequent sections to larger and more complex cancers.

A lobectomy of the thyroid is the minimal biopsy technique for a thyroid nodule in a patient at high risk of malignancy or in a patient with a "positive" or "suspicious" fine needle aspiration cytology.

In 1964 I reviewed thyroid cancers on a university student health service covering a period dating back to 1940, when a number of nodule enucleations were performed by a nonfaculty surgeon. Fifteen of fifteen enucleated malignant lesions in young people persisted or recurred locally.[25] A lobectomy including the isthmus is safer, more definitive, tidier, and easier. Thompson and co-authors have illustrated the techniques of thyroidectomy with isthmusectomy.[77] Several principles guide this initial phase of the operation.

1. Use a long enough transverse incision. Don't fight skin stenosis.

2. Rough dissection tears veins on the thyroid. Be gentle, keep the field absolutely free of blood stain.

3. Both lobes should be mobilized and examined. Occasionally, the more significant lesion has not been recognized preoperatively.

4. When the appropriate lobe is selected for removal, the superior and inferior arterial supply is taken on the thyroid gland as advocated by Thompson et al.[77] Before any inferior thyroid artery branches are divided, it is necessary to identify the recurrent laryngeal nerve. On the right side, it is important to remember the variations in the recurrent laryngeal nerve, as shown in Figure 19–5.[78] Stewart reported six instances in 1,770

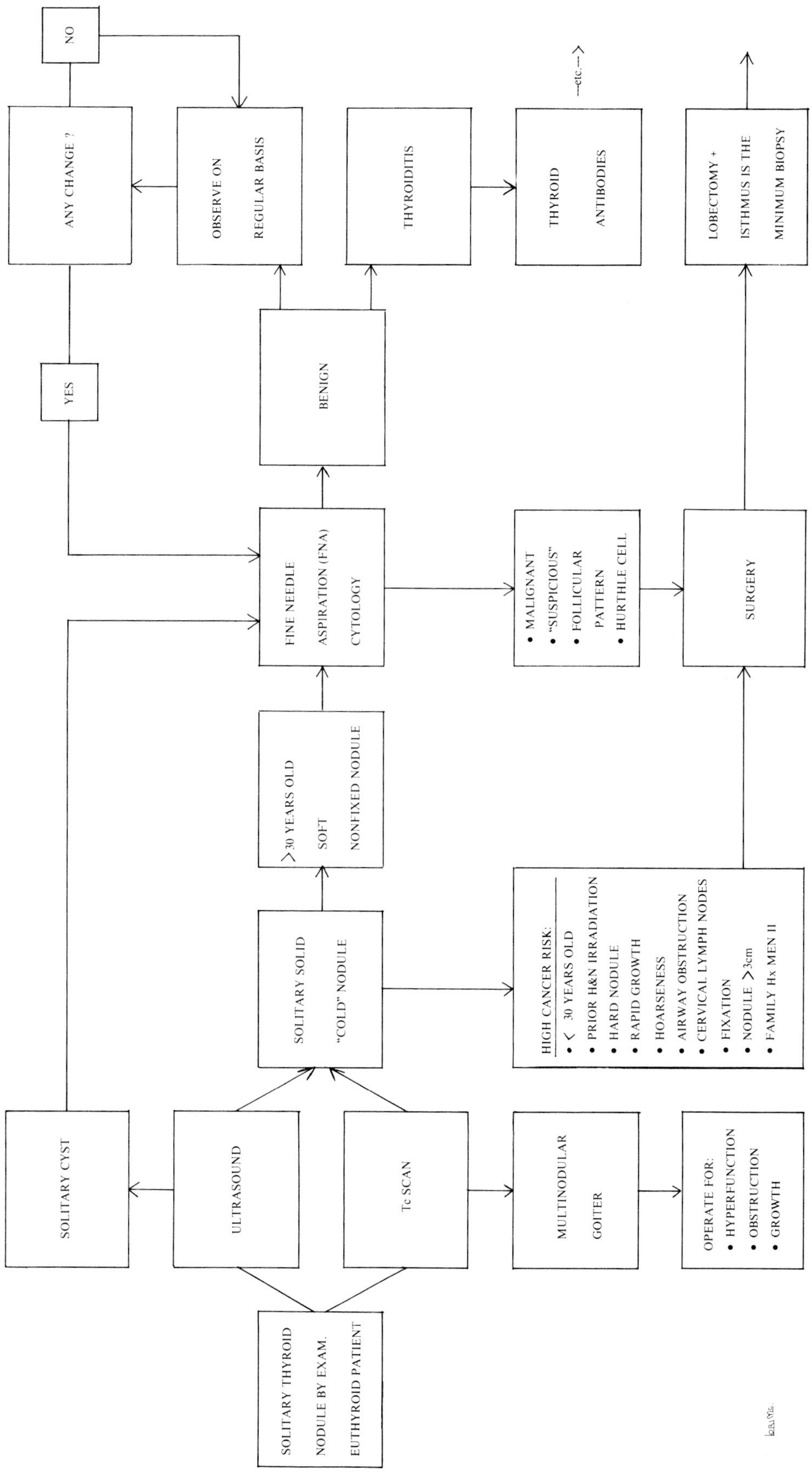

Fig 19–4.—A suggested decision scheme for evaluation of a solitary or dominant thyroid nodule.

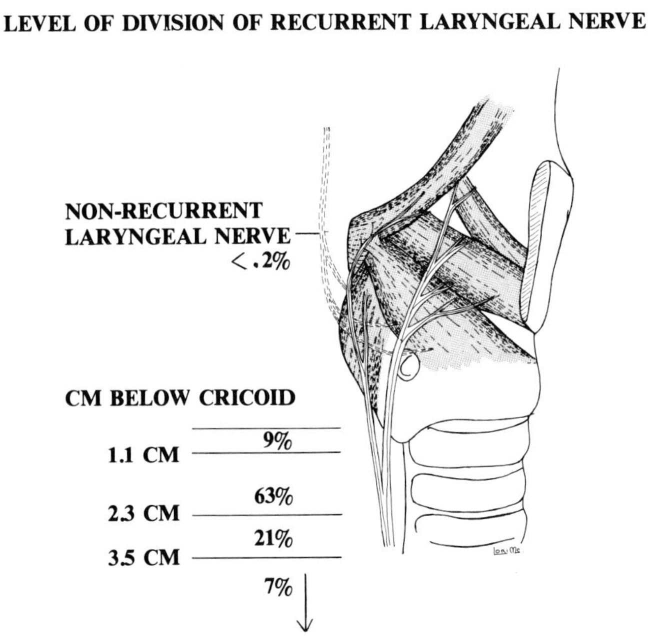

Fig 19–5.—Some of the variations in the location and extrathyroid division of the recurrent laryngeal nerve. The nerve is always recurrent on the left. On the right, it may not be recurrent, especially if there is other evidence of abnormalities in the great vessels. A nonrecurrent nerve is associated with a developmental anomaly of the fourth branchial arch and an abnormal origin of the right subclavian artery.

thyroidectomies on both sides where the recurrent nerve was *not* recurrent.[78] There may be extralaryngeal divisions as far as 3–4 cm below the inferior border of the cricoid.[79] In identification, the tissue is removed from the nerve. The recurrent nerve is not compressed with forceps or holding tools, and it should not be put on tension. Don't bruise it with surgical hardware.

5. If possible, identify and preserve the parathyroids with their blood supply intact. Some time—within an hour or years—their function may be important.

6. The entire lobe and isthmus are resected and submitted to pathology for frozen section diagnosis. The next set of decisions rest on the results of the pathologist's examination.

WHAT TYPES OF PRIMARY LESIONS OF THE THYROID CAN BE ENCOUNTERED?

Adenomatous goiter and colloid goiter with a dominant nodule are the most common findings, particularly in older patients. No further surgery is required. In women, usually over 40 years old, one of the forms of thyroiditis may be encountered, i.e., granulomatous thyroiditis (de Quervain's), subacute thyroiditis (Hashimoto's), or, in rare instances, invasive thyroiditis (Reidel's). The last type, Reidel's struma, may be quite adherent to nerves and parathyroids. If this firm woody variant is found throughout the gland, an incision biopsy rather than a lobectomy may be sufficient. Hashimoto's thyroiditis is an unlikely diagnosis in men. In an older series, 112 of 114 cases occurred in women.[80] A benign follicular adenoma is distinguished from a prominent nodule of follicular hyperplasia by being single, encapsulated, and having a different cellular and stromal pattern. Follicular lesions with benign-appearing cytology are treacherous. Any such solitary lesion over 3 cm is suspect and a careful microscopic search should be made for capsular or vascular invasion, both characteristic of cancer.

Papillary adenocarcinoma is the most frequent malignancy (60%). This includes any lesion with papillary components. Further treatment options are discussed below. Follicular cancer (15%–18%) is the next most common lesion. If the surgeon does not give the pathologist time to examine a number of pericapsular frozen sections, the malignant potential may not be appreciated until several days later, when capsular and/or vascular invasion are found on the permanent histologic sections. The correct diagnosis should be made at surgery. For follicular cancer, a total thyroidectomy is recommended since systemic metastases are more frequent. Effective treatment of metastases with ^{131}I requires that there be no functioning thyroid uptake to compete with uptake by metastases. Cervical node metastases from follicular cancer are rare, occurring in 3%–10% of cases.

Spindle cell and anaplastic giant cell cancers may be found associated with other cancer types. Nishiyama et al. confirmed that anaplastic thyroid cancers have a grim prognosis:[81] 49 of 53 patients (92%) were dead within a year of operation. Therapy of all types had little effect. Notable was the large number of patients in which the anaplastic cancer appeared to develop from a lower grade neoplasm (an estimated 30 of 53, or 57%).

Medullary thyroid carcinoma occurs in MEN syndrome, especially MEN IIa (47%) and MEN IIb (ganglioneuroma). Calcitonin levels (iCT) are elevated. The iCT levels for diagnosis may vary with the antiserum used and the sex of the patient. Medullary carcinoma (medullary carcinoma with amyloid stroma) is frequently bilateral (90% bilateral in MEN II syndrome and 20% in the sporadic group) so a total thyroidectomy is done. It is essential that parathyroid hyperplasia (from thyrocalcitonin excess) be suspected, sought, and properly treated (Fig 19–6 emphasizes the secondary origin of hyperparathyroidism). Cervical node metastases are more common in the MEN IIb and sporadic group (50%) and slightly less common in the MEN IIa group (25%). Nodes are examined and sampled. The minimal surgical procedure should be a total thyroidectomy with dissection of the bilateral central compart-

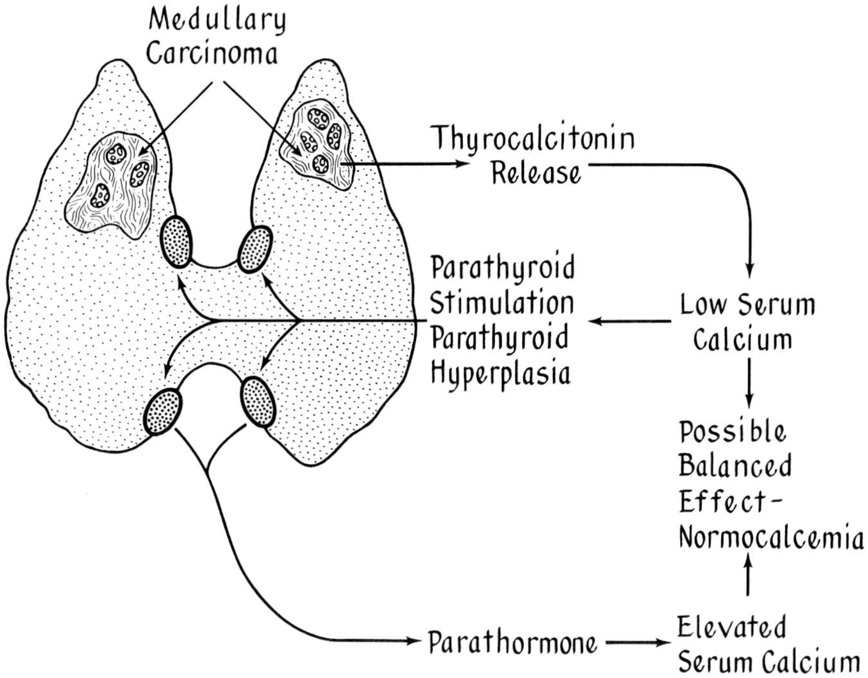

Fig 19–6.—Scheme of the probable evolution of enlarged parathyroids and hyperparathyroidism in the setting of a medullary carcinoma producing excess thyrocalcitonin. The competing effects of parathormone and thyrocalcitonin may give normal or near-normal values on an isolated calcium determination.

ment nodes. If nodes are positive, the dissection is extended to a formal cervical lymphadenectomy. A modified conservation dissection focusing on the lower central cervical compartment is preferred (see Chap. 9).

Although some people disagree, Hurthle cell cancers and neoplastic adenomas consisting *entirely* of Hurthle cells should be regarded as cancers and treated by total thyroidectomy.[69, 70]

Ultrastructural studies have shown that the lesion once called small cell undifferentiated cancer represents a lymphoma variant.[82] Restudy of 35 cases showed 34 to be lymphoma and one to be a misclassified medullary cancer. The 5-year survival with nonoperative treatment was 54%.

In treating all of these thyroidal cancers, with the possible exception of advanced cancers and larger medullary cancers, it is important to preserve parathyroid tissue on one side. Total parathyroidectomy and resultant tetany and Ca^{++} balance problems can be a much greater risk to life than some of the more indolent thyroid cancers.

WHAT ARE THE SURGICAL OPTIONS FOR PAPILLARY THYROID CANCER?

Three of every five thyroid malignancies are papillary cancer. When this diagnosis is made from frozen section study after lobectomy, a careful search is undertaken for grossly positive lymph nodes. Suspicious nodes and/or samples of the lower jugular and tracheoesophageal lymph nodes are submitted for frozen section examination. If papillary cancer is found in lymph nodes, a conservation neck dissection (sparing the spinal accessory nerve and/or sternocleidomastoid) is done in conjunction with a total or near-total thyroidectomy. There are two major reasons: First, the patient with *extrathyroidal* papillary cancer is more likely to have subsequent neck recurrence and consequent airway compromise (see causes of death, below). It is desirable to remove all papillary cancer from the juxta-airway location. Second, if ^{131}I therapy is to be employed postoperatively or at some time in the future, active thyroid tissue must be ablated to achieve ^{131}I uptake and identify metastases.

A third, less secure, reason for performing total or near-total thyroidectomy is that papillary thyroid cancer is frequently multifocal. Very small lesions in the contralateral lobe will be missed if a simple lobectomy is done. Tollefson and co-workers studied 261 patients with papillary cancer.[83] Two operations were done in the series; 45 patients had a total thyroidectomy and 216 had only a lobectomy. In the total thyroidectomy patients, the contralateral lobe contained "minute occult foci" of papillary cancer in 36% of specimens. Presumably, the patients who had only a lobectomy had a similar incidence of occult papillary cancer. However, after 5–35 years of follow-up, only 4.6% of the lobectomy only patients had clinically evident recurrence in the remaining lobe. A subgroup of 164 followed up for at least 14 years had a recurrence rate of only 4.2%. A number of other studies have had difficulty ascribing a high risk to the much discussed "minute occult foci" of papillary cancer.

Two other features can be used in deciding therapy: patients older than 40 have a higher cancer mortality,[9, 61] and males have a higher likelihood of recurrence and are more apt to need future treatment. Therefore, a more extensive thyroidectomy is usually recommended in males and in patients over 40 years old. It is obvious that I generally prefer a more extensive thyroidectomy. There are valid criteria for doing a lobectomy-isthmusectomy as the only procedure. These are: a female patient, less than 40 years old, with a circumscribed papillary thyroid cancer less than 2 cm in its largest dimension, nonadherent to any surrounding tissues, and completely contained within the thyroid. There must be no cervical nodes and the nodule should have no anaplastic or questionable histologic components. The reader may wish to adjust these criteria. The decision problem most often arises in treating patients who are referred after a lobectomy or in whom a histologic diagnosis is delayed. Beahrs and Pasternak followed 149 patients in whom *limited occult* cancer was found *after* thyroid lobectomy for other nonmalignant thyroid disease.[5] No subsequent nodal, cervical, or systemic cancer was found on long-term follow-up.

Where a definitive macrofocus of papillary cancer is found, Thompson et al. strongly recommend total thyroidectomy.[61] Their experience suggests that should carcinoma persist or recur in the remaining lobe, it is more likely to be invasive or anaplastic. The lobectomy versus total thyroidectomy decision hinges on the premise that complications are more frequent with total thyroidectomy. Katy and Bronson studied 630 operations and showed that this might be a false issue.[85] They found the incidence of tetany, recurrent nerve damage, and other complications was equivalent following either lobectomy or total thyroidectomy.

Beahrs and Pasternak[5] and others propose a "near-total" thyroidectomy for intrathyroidal papillary cancer. This small compromise is made in order to be more assured of preserving viable parathyroid tissue, to minimize thyroid replacement, and to help avoid recurrent nerve damage. The rationale is that removal of 90%–95% of the contralateral lobe will reduce proportionately the incidence of missed occult cancer foci. If ^{131}I treatment is required, the small amount of remaining thyroid can be ablated with radioiodine. Experience in a defined population in Malmo, Sweden confirmed the lack of survival difference when total and less than total thyroidectomy were compared.[84] A subtotal thyroidectomy is desirable if the patient is extremely elderly or unreliable to follow-up and will not be placed on suppression therapy. If there is any question, preservation of parathyroid tissue and recurrent nerve should take precedence over total thyroid ablation when there is no gross tumor in the contralateral lobe. A total thyroidectomy requires care in preserving parathyroid blood supply by ligating minute branches of the inferior thyroid artery on the gland, as illustrated by Attie and Khafif.[86]

DOES ANYONE DIE OF THYROID CANCER?

Anaplastic cancer is rapidly lethal. The best reported 5-year survivals are about 7%–8%.[87] In some series in which histologic review was not thorough and there were long-term survivors, there is a real question as to whether the series contains some misclassified medullary cancers or lymphomas. There is no adequate treatment. Extrathyroidal papillary cancer has a 58% 10-year survival.[5] Invasive follicular cancer has a 35% 10-year survival (see Table 19–1). Node-positive medullary cancer kills 33% of patients in 5 years and 60% of patients in 10 years. In the more favorable intrathyroidal, noninvasive, node-negative, well-differentiated thyroid cancers, the good survivals are achieved for the most part by judicious surgery. The results reflect low operative mortality, adequate operative treatment, and adequate follow-up treatment, not therapeutic nihilism. Sometimes this point is lost in interdisciplinary talmudic erudition.

Table 19–4 presents results in several series of lethal cases. Examination of failures can guide therapy. Local uncontrolled cervical recurrence is a common cause of death due to tissue compression and airway obstruction by the cancer. Anaplastic cancer predominates as the serious cell type, although papillary and follicular cancers cause significant numbers of fatal cases.

DOES ANAPLASTIC THYROID CANCER ARISE FROM MORE DIFFERENTIATED CELL TYPES?

Anaplastic cancer is a frequent autopsy finding in thyroid cancer patients. A fair number of such cancers are associated with areas of a more differentiated cancer pattern (usually papillary). The presumption is that the more differentiated cell type represents the tumor of origin and the anaplastic components represent further de-differentiation. Table 19–5 summarizes six autopsy series. Only one series[93] failed to demonstrate the phenomenon. It appears that between one third and one half of anaplastic cancers arise after years of preceding tumor or goiter which becomes anaplastic and grows rapidly.[81, 92] Ibanez et al. from M. D. Anderson Hospital approached the question in a different way. They identified 42 autopsied cases. Of these, 27 patients had had several previous operations. They traced these patients' records and found that half (13/27) the anaplastic cancers had developed in patients who had undergone

TABLE 19–4.—MAJOR ANATOMICAL AREA INVOLVED BY THYROID CANCER THAT CAUSED DEATH

STUDY, YEAR	NO. OF DEATHS	CELL TYPE	AREA OF INVOLVEMENT % Local Cervical	% Distant Systemic	Unrelated
Tollefson et al.,[88] 1964	70	Papillary and mixed	36	64	
Silverberg et al.,[89] 1970	54	Differentiated	5	18	18
		Undifferentiated	19	22	1
		Medullary	4	12	1
Fransilla,[90] 1975	42	All types	50	50	
Heitz et al.,[91] 1976	161	Papillary	4	4	
		Follicular	9	25	5
		Anaplastic	27	26	

*More than one area may be involved.

previous biopsies and resections for pure papillary or follicular cancer.[94] Over years, a significant proportion of recurrent or untreated thyroid cancer will be expected to develop anaplastic components, with rapid growth, invasion, and dissemination.

WHAT FACTORS FAVOR A LACK OF THYROID CANCER RECURRENCE?

Papillary Cancer

A widely quoted study by Mazzaferri et al. analyzed 576 patients in the Air Force tumor registry.[57] Stepwise multivariant analysis showed the items in Table 19–6 to be associated with significantly lower recurrence. In 20 years of follow-up there was a cumulative recurrence of nearly 30%. Presumably the recurrences were successfully managed, since actuarial survival approximated that of the population at large. Thompson et al. also stressed the features listed in Table 19–6.[61] The relationship of increased survival to routine postoperative use of thyroid hormone has recently been questioned[95] by Cady and others who had originally thought it was effective.[96] Their more recent study of 761 patients confirmed a good survival for patients with differentiated thyroid carcinoma. But the study failed to show any effect on survival from administration of thyroid hormone postoperatively.[95] At this time the issue is unresolved.

One cannot change the patient's age, the size of the lesion, or the local invasiveness of the lesion. One can do a more extensive thyroidectomy. Removing all the disease in the neck may reduce subsequent airway compression. In patients with larger and node positive tumors (about 20% of Mezzaferri's series), one may use ^{131}I when definite indications are present, as discussed below.

TABLE 19–5.—METAPLASIA IN THYROID CANCER

STUDY, YEAR	NO. OF AUTOPSIED CASES	CHANGE FROM DIFFERENTIATED TO ANAPLASTIC	% CHANGED
Tollefson et al.,[88] 1964	70	18/70	26
Silverberg et al.,[89] 1970	54	10/54	19
Harada et al.,[92] 1970	27	9/27	33
Nishiyama et al.,[81] 1972	53	42/53	79*
Heitz et al.,[91] 1976	161	By statement	25
Selzer et al.,[93] 1977	254	Unable to demonstrate; 17% anaplastic	0?

*Anaplastic areas associated with other well-differentiated thyroid cancers.

Follicular Cancer

This thyroid cancer rarely metastasizes to lymph nodes—13% in Cady's series[96] and 5% in Thompson's series.[61] It is generally conceded that women and younger patients have a longer survival than men and older patients.[97] The other factors in follicular cancer recurrence have not been as clearly related. The key decision determinant for adding ^{131}I therapy to surgery is the presence of angioinvasion. Tumor in blood vessels is associated with existing or subsequent metastases in over three fourths of patients.[96] After total thyroidectomy, replacement thyroid hormone is withheld for 6 weeks. A body scintiscan is done to search for metastases. If metastatic tissue uptake is discovered, ^{131}I is given in therapeutic amounts, i.e., about 175–200 mCi for an average adult. Beierwaltes repeats the scan annually and re-treats if metastatic uptake persists.[98, 99]

Medullary Cancer

The large Mayo Clinic series of 143 patients with medullary cancer defines the risk of recurrent medullary thyroid cancer.[100] They observed that the medullary cancer recurrence rate was low (4/67) in patients with tumor confined to the thyroid but was high (26/49) when nodes were invaded. Local soft tissue invasion was associated with 50% recurrence. Recurrence is least in lesions confined to the thyroid. Intrathyroidal medullary cancer is most often encountered when the diagnosis is made by doing screening tests in asymptomatic members of MEN II kinships. In this specific group, 86% of cancers were confined to the thyroid

TABLE 19–6.—FACTORS AFFECTING PAPILLARY THYROID CANCER RECURRENCE IN 576 PATIENTS*

VARIABLE	VALUE	RECURRENCE	P
Age	< 30 yr	44/266 (17%)	< 0.003
	> 30 yr	26/310 (8%)	
Primary lesion size	< 2.5 cm	5.8%	< 0.05
	> 2.5 cm	10.8%	
Surgical resection	Subtotal	48/261 (18%)	< 0.002
	Total	22/310 (7%)	
Local invasion beyond thyroid capsule	Present	28.6%	< 0.02
	Absent	11.1%	
Medical postop. therapy	None	40. %	< 0.001
	Thyroid hormone	10.9%	
	^{131}I	2.6%	

*When examined by stepwise analysis of variance, each variable was significant.

when the only finding was an elevated iCT level. All medullary cancers were intrathyroidal when the only finding was a pentagastrin-stimulated elevation of the iCT level. The best success comes from detecting early disease in other family members when the disease is first detected in the propositus. This is emphasized in two major series.[100, 101] The nonfamilial medullary cancers have a high recurrence rate (14/27). The presence of elevated iCT *and* CEA levels is predictive of recurrence.[102] When recurrence is detected, excision of a localized defined lesion is occasionally possible, but the opportunity to do so is rare.

Anaplastic Cancer

The spindle cell variety is usually impossible to resect when first treated. Treatment of recurrence is aimed at preservation of an airway.

WHAT SHOULD BE DONE FOR SMALL CELL CARCINOMA OF THE THYROID?

The histologic and ultrastructural studies of Burke, Butler, and Fuller showed this lesion to be a lymphoma in most instances (34/35).[82] The lymphomas should be staged and treated as with any other lymphoma. On the slight chance (1/35) that the tumor might be a cellular variant of medullary carcinoma, it is wise to have thyrocalcitonin determination and ultrastructural histology.

WHAT OPERATIVE PROCEDURES SHOULD BE DONE FOR INVASIVE AND EXTENSIVE THYROID CANCERS?

Long-term survival is frequently achieved with more differentiated thyroid cancers even though there is massive tumor and local tissue invasion. Therapy is usually surgical with adjuvant ^{131}I when uptake can be demonstrated in metastases. The treatment objectives with large invasive thyroid cancers are as follows:

1. To remove all gross tumor and metastasis from the neck.
2. To remove functioning thyroid tissue or, if necessary, to preserve essential structures, reduce thyroid tissue to a small minimum that can be ablated with ^{131}I.
3. To preserve parathyroid function.
4. To preserve the airway and voice function whenever possible.

Wanebo et al. have shown that the larger invasive thyroid cancers cause most of the deaths in most series.[103] Breaux and Guillamondigui reviewed 47 cases of thyroid cancer with extensive local tissue invasion.[104] The recurrent nerve was invaded or encased in 20%. Five percent required tracheal resection. Repeat operations were frequently required. Adjuvant ^{131}I was employed in 35 of the 47 patients. Survival was 62% at 10 years. The course of one of our patients is shown in Table 19–7. Long-term survival can be achieved in differentiated cancer by effective removal of recurrent cancer.

With extensive thyroid cancer, one must distinguish between attachment, encasement, and invasive destruction of adjacent tissues. Cervical musculature can almost always be sacrificed with no technical problems, as can the cervical veins. When a differentiated thyroid tumor is on the carotid, it can usually be separated in a subadventitial plane. If there is only close attachment to the perineurium of the recurrent laryngeal nerve, put on the Loupes and do a careful sharp preservative dissection. Thyroid and tracheal cartilage can be tangentially excised. In one report, 13 of 190 patients (6.8%) had airway invasion. Only 3 of the 13 have died of thyroid cancer, while 8 of the 13 have been free of

TABLE 19–7.—LONG-TERM SURVIVAL MAY REQUIRE SURGERY FOR RECURRENCE: REPRESENTATIVE CASE

S.D.K.—Hospitalized in mental institution for chronic schizophrenia.
1960—Total thyroidectomy performed for a papillary cancer, 3 × 3 × 3 cm, in the right lobe. Lymph node samples were negative. Parathyroids were preserved. Patient was maintained on replacement thyroid hormone.
1967—Massive recurrences after delayed recognition of disease while patient was hospitalized in mental institution. Bilateral modified neck dissection removed:
(1) 3 × 4 × 5 cm mass in right neck, attached to carotid and esophagus (peeled from periadventitial vascular plane). Tangential excision of esophageal wall with repair was performed.
(2) 3 × 4 × 4 cm retrosternal mass.
(3) 4 × 4 × 4 cm mass invading left jugular vein.
1967—External beam irradiation to the neck.
1970—A mass 3 × 4 × 5 cm (papillary cancer) was noted obstructing middle third of esophagus. Patient had esophagectomy and staged colon interposition.
1982—Patient alive without evidence of thyroid cancer (22 years).

recognizable disease for 5–20 years. Partial resection of laryngeotracheal involvement can be effective.[105] We have seen several patients with visible intralaryngeal or intratracheal thyroid cancer that required tracheal resection with laryngectomy or reconstruction. About 25%–30% of the tracheal circumference can be resected. Two or three tracheal rings can be resected and reapproximated without pulmonary mobilization. Partial laryngectomy can sometimes be used. Tovi and Gittot used a myoperiosteal flap in three cases to repair tracheal and laryngeal defects.[106] Djalilian et al. have reported good survivals after resection of intraluminal invasion.[107] It is worthwhile being aggressive in treating differentiated thyroid cancer. Preservation of the airway will prevent a significant number of deaths. Considerable effort should be made to preserve parathyroid tissue.

WHEN AND HOW IS ^{131}I THERAPY USED FOR THYROID CANCER?

Radioactive iodine is used to treat angioinvasive follicular cancer, invasive papillary cancer, lymph node–positive papillary cancer, and any recurrent or residual differentiated tumor that cannot be removed surgically. Beierwaltes has reviewed his experience with ^{131}I therapy.[108] He emphasizes that ^{131}I therapy is an adjunct to effective surgery. If one is to use ^{131}I, a total thyroidectomy should be done. Cady et al. studied recurrence rates in 631 differentiated cancers and identified high recurrence risks in men over 40 and women over 50 years old.[109] Fortunately, radioiodine cured 70% of recurrences in the low-risk group but only 10% of recurrences in the high-risk group. This older high-risk group had a 35% overall recurrence with a 27% mortality over a 15- to 45-year follow-up. Older age should prompt one to do a total thyroidectomy so that the 6-week postoperative scintiscan can detect metastases or residuals. If there is recurrence after a simple lobectomy, the remaining thyroid should be removed. A small residual remnant can be ablated with 100 mCi of ^{131}I. The patient is studied later. Any metastases are then treated with additional ^{131}I.

The ionizing radiation from ^{131}I is largely confined to the tissue with uptake. Radioiodine emits much of its energy as lower energy 609 keV β particles. The dose is about 10 rad/mCi/gm of tissue. The β irradiation dissipates its energy in a few millimeters of tissue. Even a small percentage uptake can produce high local radiation dose.

External beam therapy has been advocated only when there is known tumor with no demonstrable uptake after 6 weeks without thyroid hormone replacement in a thyroidectomized patient. External beam may control local disease but has not extended survival.[96–109]

The risks of ^{131}I therapy consist of (1) leukemia (1%–2%); the incidence is dose related and increases with repeated doses at less than 1-year intervals; (2) other malignancies (probably around 1%–3%[57, 109, 110]); there is a question as to how many second cancers are really fortuitous; and (3) pulmonary fibrosis, which has been observed with high single doses given for pulmonary metastases. It is rare when pulmonary uptake is less than 100 mCi.

The Atomic Energy Commission limits a single maximum dose to 200 mCi. When used appropriately, ^{131}I is effective.

HOW CAN WE CREATE A LOGICAL PATTERN OF CARE THAT ASSEMBLES THESE DIVERSE ELEMENTS?

One must consider histology, age, sex, history, time, cost, and so forth in the somewhat complex manner shown in Figure 19–7. A complex logical analysis of each patient's problem is required. Management cannot be based on generalities.

HOW CAN PARATHYROID CANCER BE RECOGNIZED AND TREATED?

Parathyroid cancer is rare, accounting for about 1%–2% of parathyroidectomy patients. Barnes and Cope described hyperfunctioning parathyroid cancer and reported 10 cases in 250 patients with hyperparathyroidism.[111] Immediate problems with the operation for parathyroid cancer are finding the parathyroids (one fourth may be in obscure sites) and then recognizing malignant characteristics in the glands. In a review of 70 cases, the presenting symptoms were usually those

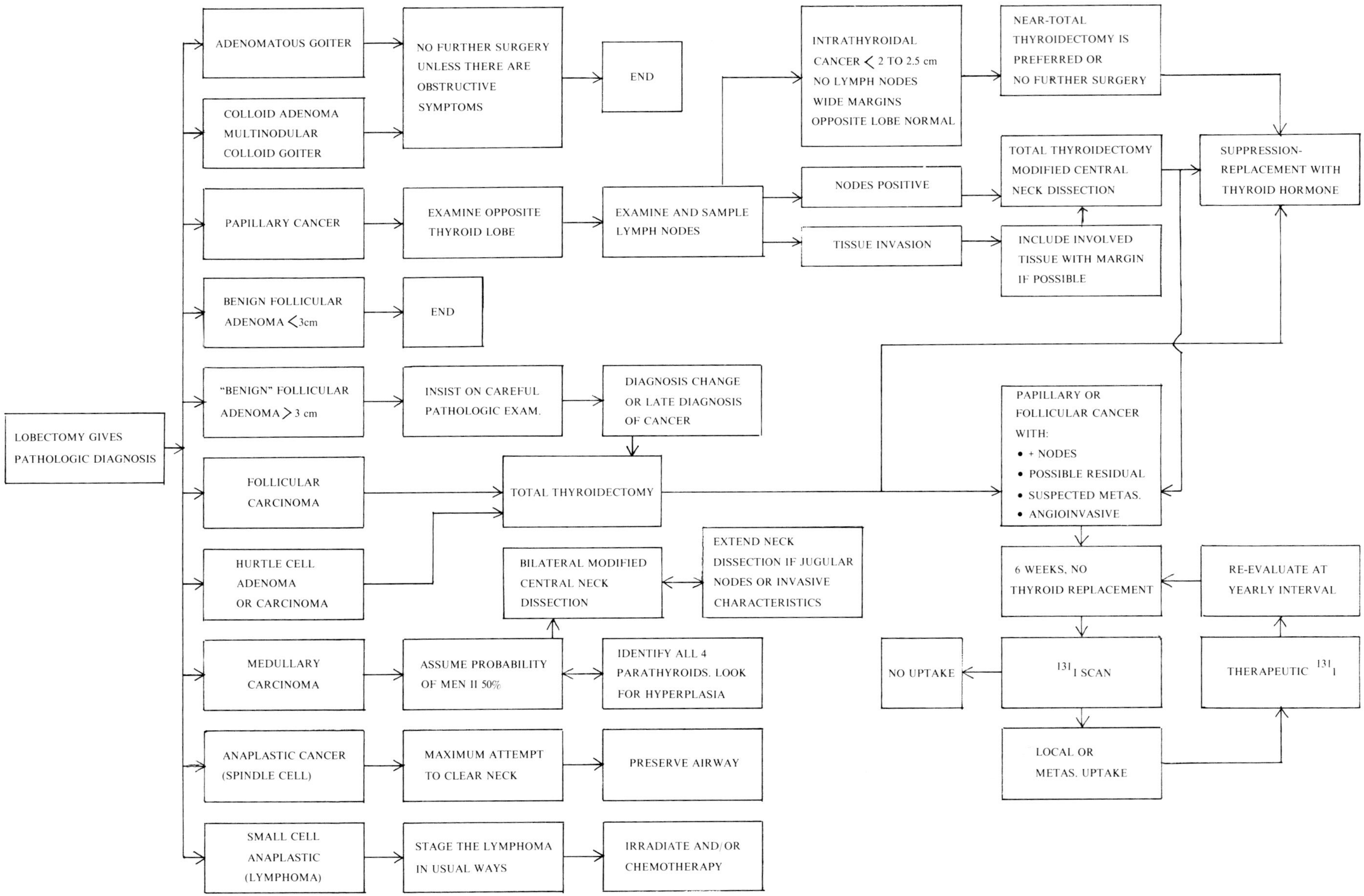

Fig 19–7.—A detailed consideration of treatment is required once the histologic diagnosis of thyroid cancer has been established. These options are not all-inclusive, and other factors may alter decisions.

of hyperparathyroidism. One third of the cancer patients had a palpable neck mass. The histologic criteria for malignancy were fibrous trabeculae (90%), mitotic figures (81%), capsular invasion (67%), and blood vessel invasion (12%).[112] Other clues to malignancy are local invasion or lymphatic metastases. Suspicion should be aroused when the serum calcium level is very high, above 14 mg/dl, or the parathormone level is high.[113] It is important to make the diagnosis at the time of surgery. Of 14 patients treated at the M.D. Anderson Hospital, 12 had hyperfunctioning parathyroid tissue. The nonfunctioning cancers were aggressive cancers. Only 3 of the 14 patients survived their malignancy free of disease at the time of report. Death resulted from hypercalcemia rather than from organ replacement by tumor. Some palliation can be obtained from resecting recurrent disease.[114] In general, re-exploration after delayed recognition resulted in fewer than 10% of patients surviving 2 years. Re-exploration was more effective in the Mayo Clinic series.[113] When a thorough dissection is done at initial operation, about 20%–30% of patients survive 5 years. At 10 years, recurrence has reduced the proportion of survivors to 15%.[112–115]

When parathyroid cancer is encountered on one side of the neck, the involved parathyroid tissue, the thyroid lobe, and a margin of uninvolved tissue should be removed. Since lymphatic metastases are common, a modified neck dissection is performed with particular attention to harvesting paratracheal, tracheoesophageal, and retrosternal lymphatic tissues. In 2 of 14 cases Van Heerden et al. reported more extensive resections with thoracic components.[113] Mediastinal metastases were resected in the M. D. Anderson Hospital series in 2 long-term survivors.[114]

REFERENCES

1. Harrington C.R.: Biochemical basis of thyroid function. *Lancet* 1:1199–1204, 1261–1266, 1935.
2. Marine D., Kimball O.P.: The prevention of simple goitre in man: A survey of the incidence and types of thyroid enlargements in the school girls of Akron, Ohio from the 5th to 12th grades inclusive. The plan of prevention proposed. *J. Lab Clin. Med.* 3:40–48, 1917.
3. Kocher T., cited in Thompson N.W., Olsen W.R., Hoffman G.L.: The continuing development of the technique of thyroidectomy. *Surgery* 73:913–922, 1973.
4. Plummer H.S.: Results of administering iodine to patients with exophthalmic goiter. *JAMA* 80:1955, 1923.
5. Beahrs O.H., Pasternak B.M.: Cancer of the thyroid gland. *Curr. Probl. Surg.* December 1969.
6. Axtell L.M., Asire A.J., Meyers M.H.: *Cancer Patient Survival.* Report No. 5, National Cancer Institute, DHEW publication No. (NIH) 77–992, 1976.
7. Frazell E.L., Schottenfeld D., Hutter R.V.P.: The prognosis and insurability of thyroid cancer patients. *CA* 20:270–275, 1970.
8. MacComb W.S., Fletcher G.H.: *Cancer of the Head and Neck.* Baltimore, Williams & Wilkins Co., 1967.
9. Fransilla K.O.: Prognosis in thyroid carcinoma. *Cancer* 36:1138–1146, 1975.
10. Russel W.O., Ibanez M.L., Clark R.L., et al.: Thyroid carcinoma: Classification, intraglandular dissemination and clinicopathologic study based upon whole organ sections of 80 glands. *Cancer* 16:1425–1460, 1963.
11. Frazell E.L., Foote F.W. Jr.: Papillary thyroid carcinoma: Pathological findings in cases with and without clinical evidence of cervical node involvement. *Cancer* 8:1165–1166, 1955.
12. Stewart F.W.: The diagnosis of tumors by aspiration. *Am. J. Pathol.* 9:801–812, 1933.
13. Soderstrom N.: Puncture of goiters for aspiration biopsy: A preliminary report. *Acta Med. Scand.* 144:237–244, 1952.
14. Soderstrom N.: Identification of normal tissues and tumors by cytologic aspiration biopsy. *Acta Soc. Med. (Uppsala)* 65:53–87, 1958.
15. Miller J.M.: Hamburger J.I., and Kini S.: Diagnosis of thyroid nodules: Use of fine-needle aspiration and needle biopsy. *JAMA* 241:481–484, 1979.
16. Lowhagen T., Granberg P.O., Lundell G., et al.: Aspiration biopsy cytology (ABC) in nodules of the thyroid gland suspected to be malignant. *Surg. Clin. North Am.* 59:3–18, 1979.
17. Foss H.L.: The evolution of our knowledge of the physiology and pathology of the thyroid gland. *West. J. Surg. Obstet. Gynecol.* 42:536–541, 1934.
18. Wanebo H.J., Andrews W., Kaiser D.L.: Thyroid cancer, some basic considerations. *CA* 33:87–97, 1983.
19. Beahrs O.H., Kubista T.B.: Diagnosis of thyroid cancer, in *Cancer Management: A Special Graduate Course on Cancer.* Philadelphia, J.B. Lippincott Co., 1968, pp. 573–579.
20. Hayles A.B., Johnson L.M., Beahrs O.H., et al.: Carcinoma of the thyroid gland in children. *Am. J. Surg.* 106:735–742, 1963.
21. Clark O.H., Demling D.: Management of thyroid nodules in the elderly. *Am. J. Surg.* 132:615–619, 1976.
22. Gogas J.G., Kalsikas D., Sechas M., et al.: Prediction of malignancy in solitary thyroid nodules in a country with endemic goiter. *Am. J. Surg.* 132:623–624, 1976.
23. Mantovinovic J., Hayner N.S., Epstein F.H., et al.: Goiter and other studies in Tecumseh, Michigan: Studies in a total community. *JAMA* 192:234, 1965.
24. Hoffman G.L., Thompson N.W., Heffron C.: The solitary nodule: A reassessment. *Arch. Surg.* 105:379–385, 1972.
25. McQuarrie D.G.: Incidence of thyroid malignancy in college students, 1965. Unpublished data.
26. Harness J.K., Thompson N.W., Nishiyama R.H.: Childhood thyroid carcinoma. *Arch. Surg.* 102:278–284, 1971.

27. Duffy B.J., Fitzgerald P.J.: Cancer of the thyroid in children: A report of 28 cases. *J. Clin. Endocrinol. Metab.* 10:1296–1308, 1950.
28. Wilson G.M.: Thyroid neoplasms following irradiation. *Br. Med. J.* 2:929–934, 1958.
29. Saenger E.L., et al.: Neoplasia following therapeutic irradiation for benign conditions in childhood. *Radiology* 74:889–904, 1960.
30. DeGroot L., Paloyan E.: Thyroid carcinoma and radiation: A Chicago epidemic. *JAMA* 225:487–491, 1973.
31. Block M.A., Miller M.J., Horn R.C. Jr.: Carcinoma of the thyroid after external radiation to the neck in adults. *Am. J. Surg.* 118:764–769, 1969.
32. Pifer J.W., Hempelmann L.H.: Radiation induced thyroid carcinoma. *Ann. NY Acad. Sci.* 114:838–848, 1964.
33. Raventos A., Winship T.: The latent interval for thyroid cancer following irradiation. *Radiology* 83:501–508, 1964.
34. Wagner D.H., Evans R.H.: A review of one hundred fifty thyroidectomies following prior irradiation to the head, neck, and upper part of the chest. *Surg. Gynecol. Obstet.* 147:903–908, 1978.
35. Nelson D.F., Reddy K.V., O'Mara R.E., et al.: Thyroid abnormalities following neck irradiation for Hodgkin's disease. *Cancer* 42:2553–2562, 1978.
36. Winship T., Rosvoll R.V.: Childhood thyroid carcinoma. 14:734–742, 1961.
37. Rallison M.L., Dobyn B.M., Keating F.R., et al.: Thyroid disease in children: A survey of subjects potentially exposed to fall out radiation. *Am. J. Med.* 56:457–463, 1974.
38. Hempelmann L.H., Hall W.J., Phillips M.: Neoplasms in persons treated with x-rays in infancy: Fourth survey in 20 years. *JNCI* 55:519–530, 1975.
39. Hempelmann L.H.: Risk of thyroid neoplasm after irradiation in childhood. *Science* 160:159–161, 1968.
40. DeGroot L.J., Reilly M., Pennameneni K., et al.: Retrospective and prospective study of radiation induced thyroid disease. *Am. J. Med.* 74:852–862, 1983.
41. Wilson S.D., Komorowski R., Cerletty J., et al.: Radiation-associated thyroid tumors: Extent of operation and pathology technique influence the apparent incidence of carcinoma. *Surgery* 94:663--669, 1983.
42. Eyre-Brook I.A., Talbot C.H.: Treatment of autonomous functioning thyroid nodules. *Br. J. Surg.* 69:577–579, 1982.
43. Becker F.D., Economou S.G., Southwick H.W.: Adult thyroid cancer after head and neck irradiation in infancy and childhood. *Ann. Intern. Med.* 83:347–351, 1975.
44. Burrow G.N., Mujtata W., LiVolsi V., et al.: The incidence of carcinoma in solitary cold nodules. *Yale J. Biol. Med.* 51:13–17, 1978.
45. Ashcraft M.W., VonHerle A.J.: Management of thyroid nodules: I. *Head Neck Surg.* 3:216–227, 1981.
46. ReMine W.H., McConahey W.M.: Management of thyroid nodules. *Surg. Clin. North Am.* 57:523–531, 1977.
47. Messaris G., Evangelow G.N., Toemtas C.: Incidence of carcinoma in cold nodules of the thyroid gland. *Surgery* 74:447–448, 1973.
48. Anderson P.O., Sumner H.W., Seigel B.A.: The single palpable thyroid nodule: Evaluation by ^{99m}Tc-pertechnetate imaging. *Cancer* 37:258–265,,1976.
49. Nelson R.L., Wahner H.W., Gorman C.A.: Rectilinear thyroid scanning as a predictor of malignancy. *Ann. Intern. Med.* 88:41–44, 1978.
50. Akisada M., Fujimoto Y.: *Soft Tissue Roentgenography in Diagnosis of Thyroid Cancer: Detection of Psammoma Bodies by Spot-Tangential Projection.* Tokyo, Igaku Shoin, 1973.
51. Blum M., Goldman A.B., Herskovic A., et al.: Clinical applications of thyroid echography. *N. Engl. J. Med.* 287:1164–1168, 1972.
52. Lees W.R., Vahl S.P., Watson L.R., et al.: The role of ultrasound scannings in the diagnosis of thyroid swellings. *Br. J. Surg.* 65:681–684, 1978.
53. Mishkin M., Rosen I.B., Walfish P.G.: B-mode ultrasonography in assessment of thyroid gland lesions. *Ann. Intern. Med.* 79:505–510, 1973.
54. Hammer M., Wortsman J., Folse R.: Cancer in cystic lesions of the thyroid. *Arch. Surg.* 117:1020–1023, 1982.
55. Blum M., Rothschild M.: Improved non-operative diagnosis of the solitary cold nodule. *JAMA* 243:242–245, 1980.
56. Colcock B., King M.L.: Mortality and morbidity of thyroid surgery. *Surg. Gynecol. Obstet.* 114:131–136, 1962.
57. Mazzaferri E.L., Young R.L., Oertel J.E., et. al.: Papillary thyroid carcinoma: The impact of therapy in 576 patients. *Medicine* 56:171–196, 1977.
58. Miller J.M., Hamburger J.I., Kini S.: Diagnosis of thyroid nodules: use of fine needle aspiration and needle biopsy. *JAMA* 241:481–484, 1979.
59. Astwood E.B., Cassidy C.E., Auerbach G.D.: Treatment of goiter and thyroid nodules with thyroid. *JAMA* 174:459–464, 1960.
60. Beahrs O.H.: Cancer of the thyroid: Its management. *Aust. NZ J. Surg.* 48:604–606, 1978.
61. Thompson N.W., Nishiyama R.H., Harness J.K.: *Thyroid Carcinoma: Current controversies.* Chicago, Year Book Medical Publishers, Inc., 1978.
62. Hamberger J.I., Miller J.M., Kini S.R.: *Clinical-Pathological Evaluation of Thyroid Nodules: Handbook and Atlas.* Southfield, Mich., Northland Thyroid Laboratory, 1982.
63. Boey J., Hsu C., Wong J., et al.: Fine-needle aspiration versus drill-needle biopsy of thyroid nodules: A controlled clinical trial. *Surgery* 91:611–615, 1982.
64. Colacchio T.A., LoGerfo P., Feind C.R.: Fine needle cytological diagnosis of thyroid nodules. *Am. J. Surg.* 140:568–571, 1980.
65. Crile G., Hawk W.A.: Aspiration biopsy of thyroid nodules. *Surg. Gynecol. Obstet.* 136:241–245, 1973.
66. Wang C., Vickery A.L., Maloof F.: Needle biopsy of the thyroid. *Surg. Gynecol. Obstet.* 143:365–368, 1976.
67. Gershengorn M.C., McClung M.R., Chu E.W., et al.: Fine needle aspiration cytology in the pre-operative diagnosis of thyroid nodules. *Ann. Intern. Med.* 87:265–269, 1977.

68. LoGerfo P., Ting W.: Method for biopsy of the wall of a thyroid cyst. *Am. J. Surg.* 146:383–384, 1983.
69. Thompson N.W., Dunn E.L., Batsakis J.G., et al.: Hurthle cell lesions of the thyroid gland. *Surg. Gynecol. Obstet.* 139:555–560, 1974.
70. Gundry S.R., Burney R.E., Thompson N.W., et al.: The importance of total thyroidectomy for Hurthle cell neoplasm of the thyroid. Presented at the 90th annual meeting of the Western Surgical Society, Nov. 16, 1982.
71. Granberg P.O.: Summaries of breakfast panels, in *State of the Art of Surgery:* Basel, International Association for Chirurgy, 1982, p. 69.
72. Ashcraft M.W., Van Herle A.J.: Management of thyroid nodules: I. History and physical examinations, blood tests, and ultrasonography. *Head Neck Surg.* 3:216–230, 1981.
73. Ashcraft M.W., Van Herle A.J.: Management of thyroid nodules: II. Scanning techniques. thyroid suppressive therapy, and fine needle aspiration. *Head Neck Surg.* 3:297–322, 1981.
74. Ashcraft M.W.: Analysis of techniques to evaluate thyroid nodules, in Van Herle A.J. (moderator): *The Thyroid Nodule: UCLA Conference. Ann. Intern. Med.* 96:221–232, 1982.
75. Solomon D.H., Keeler E.B.: Cost-effective analysis of the evaluation of thyroid nodule, in Van Herle A.J. (moderator): *The Thyroid Nodule: UCLA Conference. Ann. Intern. Med.* 96:221–232, 1982.
76. Kassirer J.P., Pauker S.G.: The toss-up, editorial: *N. Engl. J. Med.* 305:1467–1469, 1981.
77. Thompson N.W., Olsen W.R., Hoffman G.L.: The continuing development of the technique of thyroidectomy. *Surgery* 73:913–927, 1973.
78. Stewart G.R., Montain J.C., Colcock B.A.: Non-recurrent laryngeal nerve. *Br. J. Surg.* 59:379–381, 1972.
79. Nimeroff P.M., Katy A.D.: Extralaryngeal divisions of the recurrent laryngeal nerve: Surgical and clinical significance. *Am. J. Surg.* 144:466–469, 1982.
80. Marshall S.F., Meissner W.A.: Struma lymphomatosa (Hashimoto's disease). *Ann. Surg.* 141:737–746, 1955.
81. Nishiyama R.H., Dunn E.L., Thompson N.W.: Anaplastic spindle cell and giant cell tumors of the thyroid gland. *Cancer* 30:113–127, 1972.
82. Burke J.S., Butler J.J., Fuller L.M.: Malignant lymphomas of the thyroid: A clinical-pathological study of 35 patients including ultrastructural observations. *Cancer* 39:1587–1602, 1977.
83. Tollefson H.R., Shaw J.P., Huvos A.G.: Papillary carcinoma of the thyroid: Recurrence in the thyroid gland after initial surgical treatment. *Am. J. Surg.* 124:468–472, 1972.
84. Christensen S.B., Ljungberg O., Tibblin S.: Surgical treatment of thyroid carcinoma in a defined population: 1960–1977. *Am. J. Surg.* 146:349–354, 1983.
85. Katy A.D., Bronson D.: Total thyroidectomy: The indications and results in 630 patients. *Am. J. Surg.* 136:450–454, 1978.
86. Attie J.N., Khafif R.A.: Preservation of parathyroid glands during total thyroidectomy. *Am. J. Surg.* 130:399–404, 1975.
87. Aldinger K.A., Samaan N.A., Ifaney M., et al.: Anaplastic carcinoma of the thyroid: A review of 84 cases of spindle and giant cell carcinoma of the thyroid. *Cancer* 41:2267–2275, 1978.
88. Tollefson H.R., DeCosse J.J., Hutter R.V.P.: Papillary carcinomas of the thyroid. *Cancer* 17:1035–1044, 1964.
89. Silverberg S.G., Hutter R.V.P., Foote F.: Fatal carcinoma of the thyroid: Histology, metastases, and causes of death. *Cancer* 25:792–802, 1970.
90. Fransilla K.O.: Prognosis in thyroid carcinoma. *Cancer* 36:1138–1146, 1975.
91. Heitz P., Moser H., Staub J.J.: Thyroid cancer: A study of 573 thyroid tumors and 161 autopsy cases observed over a thirty-year period. *Cancer* 37:2329–2337, 1976.
92. Harada T., Ito K., Shimaoka K., et al.: Fatal thyroid carcinoma: Anaplastic transformation of adenocarcinoma. *Cancer* 39:2588–2596, 1977.
93. Selzer G., Kahn L.B., Albertyn L.: Primary malignant tumors of the thyroid gland: A clinicopathologic study of 254 cases. *Cancer* 40:1501–1510, 1977.
94. Ibanez M.L., Russell W.O., Albores-Saaverdra J., et al.: Thyroid carcinoma: Biological behavior and mortality. Postmortem findings in 42 cases, including 27 in which the disease was fatal. *Cancer* 19:1039–1052, 1966.
95. Cady B., Cohn K., Rossi R.L., et al.: The effect of thyroid hormone administration upon survival in patients with differentiated thyroid carcinoma. *Surgery* 94:978–983, 1983.
96. Cady B., Sedgewick C.E., Meissner W.A., et al.: Changing clinical pathologic, treatment and survival patterns in differentiated thyroid carcinoma. *Ann. Surg.* 184:541–553, 1976.
97. Crile G. Jr.: Diagnosis and management of thyroid cancer. *Hosp. Med.* 13:48–56, 1977.
98. Beierwaltes W.H.: The treatment of thyroid carcinoma with radioactive iodine. *Semin. Nucl. Med.* 8:79, 1978.
99. Varma V.M., Beierwaltes W.H., Nofal M.M., et al.: Treatment of thyroid cancer: Death rates after surgery and after surgery followed by sodium iodide ^{131}I. *JAMA* 214:1437, 1970.
100. Russell C.F., Van Heerden J.A., Sizemore G.W., et al.: The surgical management of medullary thyroid carcinoma. *Ann. Surg.* 197:42–48, 1983.
101. Jackson C.E., Talpos G.B., Kambouris A., et al.: The clinical course after definitive operation for medullary thyroid carcinoma. *Surgery* 94:995–1001, 1983.
102. Rougier P., Calmettes C., Laplanche A., et al.: The values of calcitonin and carcinoembryonic antigen in the treatment and management of nonfamilial medullary thyroid carcinoma. *Cancer* 51:855–862, 1983.
103. Wanebo H.J., Andrews W., Kaiser D.L.: Thyroid cancer: Some basic considerations. *Am. J. Surg.* 142:474–479, 1981.
104. Breaux E.P., Guillamondigui O.M.: Treatment of locally invasive carcinoma of the thyroid: How radical? *Am. J. Surg.* 140:514–517, 1980.

105. Shelton V.K., Skolick E.M., Berlinger F.G.: Laryngotracheal invasion by thyroid carcinoma. *Ann. Otol. Rhinol. Laryngol.* 91:363–369, 1982.
106. Tovi F., Gittot A.: Sternocleidomastoid myoperiosteal flap for the repair of laryngeal and tracheal wall defects. *Head Neck Surg.* 5:447–451, 1983.
107. Djalilian M., Devine K.D., DeSanto L.W., et al.: Intraluminal involvement of the larynx and trachea by thyroid cancer. *Am. J. Surg.* 128:500–504, 1974.
108. Beierwaltes W.H.: Radiation in the management of thyroid cancer, in Najarian J.S., Delaney J.P. (eds.): *Endocrine Surgery.* New York, Appleton-Century-Crofts, 1981, pp. 51–68.
109. Cady B., Sedgwick C.E., Meissner W.A., et al.: Risk factor analysis in differentiated thyroid cancer. *Cancer* 43:810–820, 1979.
110. Wyse E.D., Hill C.S., Ibanez M.L.: Other malignant neoplasms associated with carcinoma of the thyroid: Thyroid carcinoma, multiplex. *Cancer* 24:701–708, 1969.
111. Barnes B.A., Cope O.: Carcinoma of the parathyroid glands: Report of 10 cases with endocrine function. *JAMA* 178:556–559, 1961.
112. Schantz A., Castlemann B.: Parathyroid carcinoma: A study of 70 cases. *Cancer* 31:600–605, 1973.
113. Van Heerden J.A., Weiland L.H., ReMine W.H., et al.: Cancer of the parathyroid glands. *Arch. Surg.* 114:475–480, 1979.
114. Anderson B.J., Samaan N.A., Vassilopoulou-Sellin R., et al.: Parathyroid carcinoma: Features and difficulties in diagnosis and management. *Surgery* 94:906–915, 1983.
115. Holmes E.C., Morton D.L., Ketcham A.S.: Parathyroid carcinoma: A collective review. *Ann. Surg.* 169:631–640, 1969.

20 / Salivary Gland Neoplasms

THEODOR B. GRAGE, M.D., PH.D. / CHARLES E. MORROW, M.D.

THE parotid, submaxillary, and sublingual salivary glands constitute the major salivary glands. In addition, 400–700 very small minor or accessory salivary glands are present in the neck, oral cavity, lips, and parapa-rotid areas. This chapter emphasizes tumors of the major salivary glands.

HOW ARE MOST MAJOR SALIVARY GLAND TUMORS DETECTED?

The usual clinical history of a parotid or submaxillary gland tumor is that of a mass steadily increasing in size until the patient seeks medical attention. In many instances infectious lymphadenopathy is suspected on the first medical contact. A lengthy workup for lymphoma or a long course of antibiotics is common. Unfortunately, many patients with salivary tumors continue to be referred for surgical treatment following an inappropriate incisional biopsy.

WHAT ARE THE IMPORTANT HISTORICAL AND PHYSICAL FINDINGS IN A PATIENT WITH A SALIVARY GLAND TUMOR?

Specific attention should be directed to the patient's age and sex and the duration of symptoms. Historical information should include the rate of growth and the presence of pain. An inadequate history that neglects the subtle symptoms of keratoconjunctivitis, xerostomia, rhinolaryngitis, and rheumatoid arthritis (Sjögren's disease) may result in inappropriate surgical therapy. Other local and systemic diseases that may produce parotid enlargement will include tuberculosis, actinomycosis, lymphoma, mumps, suppurative parotitis, tonsillitis, Bell's palsy, and distant malignancies. For example, cervicofacial actinomycosis lesions may produce sinus tracts and florid desmoplasia that burrow into soft tissues and surrounding bone, mimicking the appearance of a malignant parotid tumor. A fluctuation in size of a parotid mass is unusual and may represent papillary cystadenoma lymphomatosum (Warthin's tumor).

Physical examination should look for evidence of fixation of the tumor to the skin or mandible, enlargement of cervical nodes, paralysis of the facial nerve, and distant metastases. Bimanual examination of the lateral wall of the oropharynx and retromandibular area is necessary in all patients with parotid lesions to detect deep lobe tumors. A common error is failure to detect other primary head and neck malignancies. If the patient is a smoker over 30, careful oral examination and indirect laryngoscopy are a minimum examination. With any voice changes, direct laryngoscopy should be done. Malignant tumors of the scalp, the upper lip, floor of the mouth, and nasopharynx frequently metastasize to lymph nodes that are in or surround the parotid and submaxillary glands.

AFTER NON-SALIVARY GLAND SOURCES ARE EXCLUDED, WHAT POSSIBLE TYPES OF TUMORS MAY BE FOUND?

The following facts aid the surgeon in the correct preoperative decisions and subsequent surgical treatment of salivary gland tumors. The most frequent neoplasm (60%) of the major salivary glands is the benign mixed tumor (pleomorphic adenoma). The most frequent *malignant* tumor of the parotid gland is mucoepidermoid carcinoma (6%–10% of all parotid tumors). Although capillary hemangioma is the most common salivary gland tumor in infants and children, mucoepidermoid carcinoma is the most frequent malignant salivary gland tumor in children.

Submaxillary gland tumors have a relatively higher ratio of malignant to benign lesions than tumors of the parotid gland. Adenoid cystic carcinoma is the most common malignant submaxillary gland tumor. Bilateral parotid tumors usually represent papillary cystadenoma lymphomatosum (Warthin's tumor) or benign lymphoepithelial lesions. Acinic cell carcinomas may also be bilateral and multicentric. Warthin's tumors occur predominantly in males (10:1 male-female ratio),[1] and all other major salivary gland tumors except pleomorphic adenoma (3:1 in females) occur with equal frequency in males and females.

The above facts often help in establishing the diagnosis of major salivary gland lesions preoperatively. However, the surgeon must also rely on the findings at the time of operation to establish the correct diagnosis (Fig 20–1). Table 20–1 lists the incidence of submaxillary and parotid tumors in several large reported series and our own recent review. In comparison, Table 20–2 lists the incidence of minor salivary gland tumors.[1a] Minor salivary gland tumors are often malignant (50%) and most frequently located in the palate, antrum, lips, tongue, or cheek.

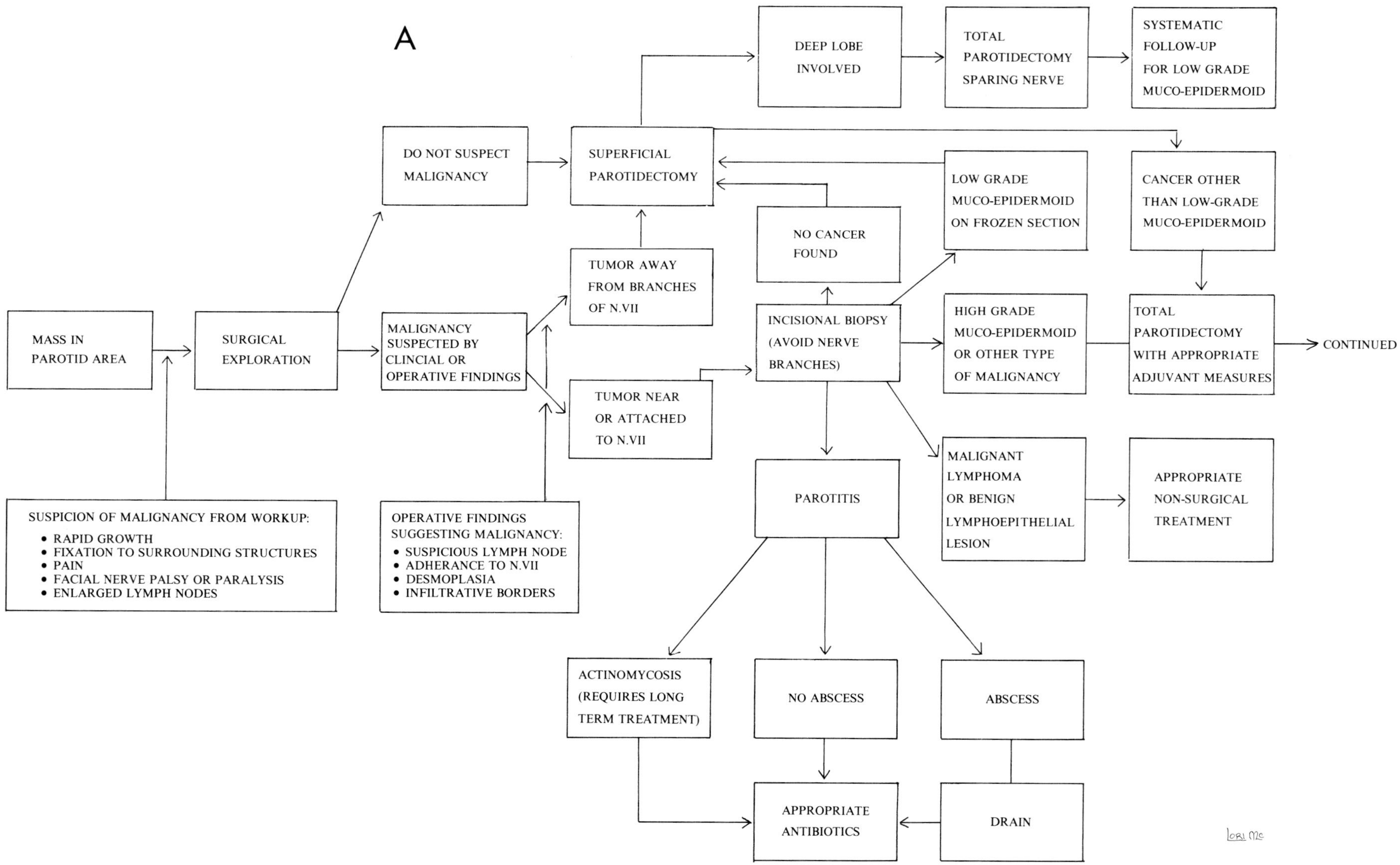

Fig 20–1.—A, a suggested decision plan for the diagnosis and management of a parotid mass when first seen and when the differentiation between benign and malignant neoplasms is uncertain.

B

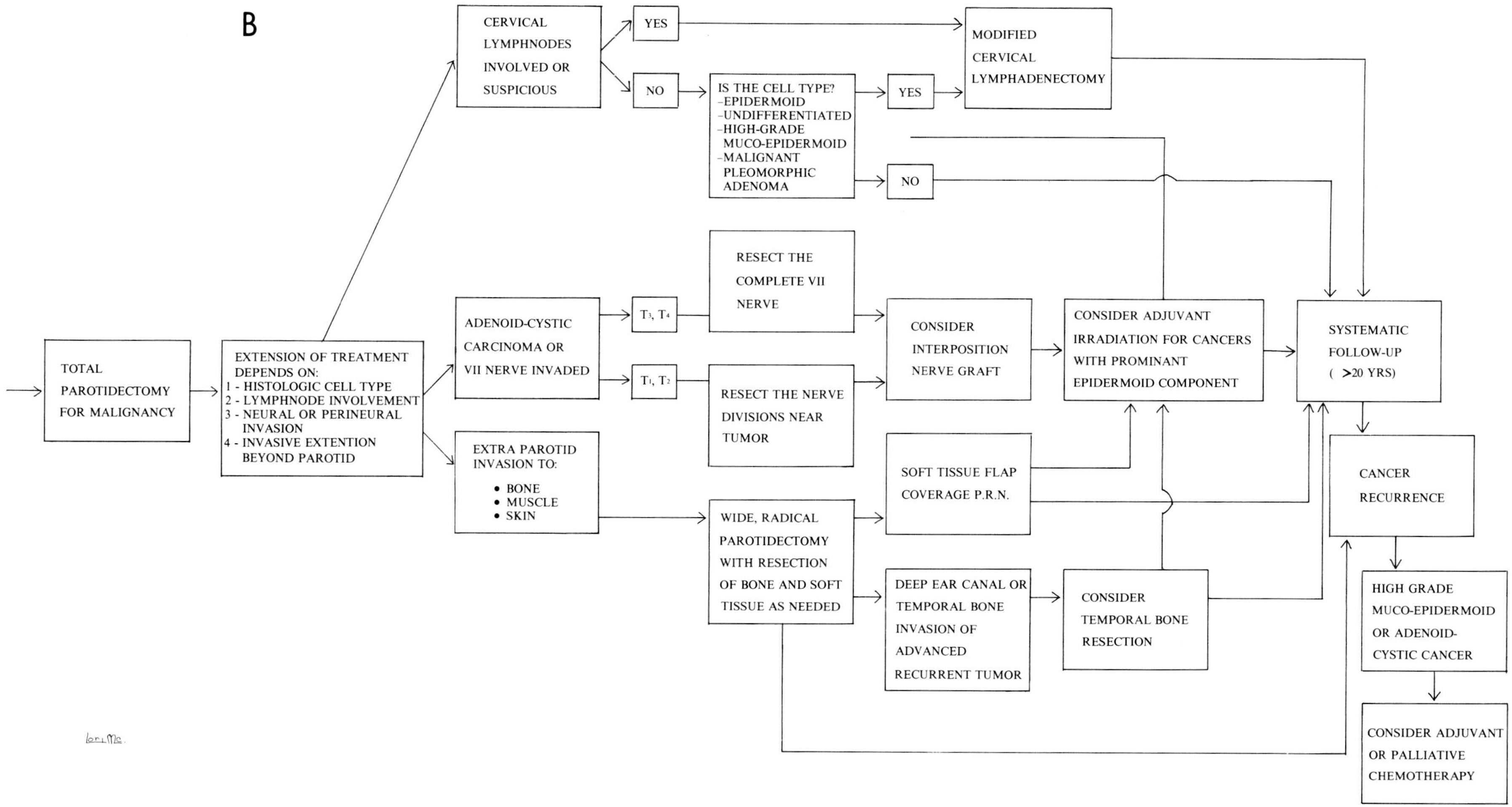

Fig 20–1. (cont.)—B, an extension of diagram **A** showing the key questions and options when a malignancy other than a low-grade mucoepidermoid cancer is found.

TABLE 20–1.—PERCENTAGE OF TUMORS OF THE PAROTID AND SUBMAXILLARY GLAND ACCORDING TO HISTOLOGIC TYPE

	SERIES					
	Parotid Gland			Submaxillary Gland		
HISTOLOGIC TYPE	Foote et al.[34] (N = 766)	Woods et al.[24] (N = 742)	Present Series (N = 366)	Eneroth et al.[35] (N = 170)	Attie et al.[22] (N = 62)	Present Series (N = 40)
BENIGN						
Benign mixed tumor	58	52	55	60	50	52.5
Papillary cystadenoma lymphomatosum (Warthin's)	6.4	27	6.3	. . .	. . .	. . .
MALIGNANT						
Mucoepidermoid	. . .	6	7.4	3.6	11.3	. . .
Low grade	5.8	. . .	5.5	. . .	. . .	. . .
High grade	5.8	. . .	1.9	. . .	. . .	. . .
Acinic cell	2.7	4.4	5.2	0.6	. . .	2.5
Adenoid cystic	2.1	2.6	4.1	15.0	16.1	7.5
Epidermoid	3.4	1.8	4.9	7.0	1.6	17.5
Adenocarcinoma	. . .	2.3	3.0	. . .	. . .	. . .
Malignant mixed tumor	5.9	1.6	1.1	1.8	3.2	. . .
Undifferentiated	. . .	0.7	1.4	9.0	1.6	. . .

WHY NOT JUST EXCISE SALIVARY GLAND MASSES DIRECTLY?

If it were not for associated and adjacent structures, treatment of salivary gland tumors would be a simple operation. The location of the functionally important facial nerve and its branches makes parotid biopsy more than a trivial matter. A brief description of the surgical anatomy is appropriate (Fig 20–2,A). Anatomically the parotid gland is a bilobed structure, and weighs 15–30 gm, and is divided into a superficial and deep lobe by the facial nerve (Fig 20–2,B). The parotid gland empties into contributory ductules that drain to Stensen's duct. Stensen's duct emerges from the anterior border of the superficial lobe, crosses the masseter muscle horizontally, penetrates the buccinator muscle, and empties into the oral cavity opposite the second maxillary molar.

The blood supply to the parotid gland arises from the external carotid artery and the transverse facial arteries. The external carotid artery lies deep to or within the deep lobe and bifurcates at the level of the mandible into the superficial temporal and the internal maxillary artery.

The facial nerve (cranial nerve VII) exits from the skull by the stylomastoid foramen and passes anterior to the posterior belly of the digastric muscle and lateral to the styloid process, external carotid artery, and posterior facial vein—all important landmarks. After coursing inferiorly and anterolaterally, the nerve enters the parotid gland and quickly divides into two main trunks: the temporofacial and cervicofacial portions. Each bifurcation further subdivides into five or six terminal branches—temporal, "ophthalmic," zygomatic, maxillary (buccal) mandibular, and cervical—which eventually emerge from beneath the superficial lobe and above the underlying masseter muscle (see Fig 20–2,A). The pattern of terminal branching and anastomotic connections is complex[2, 3] and frequently of surgical importance. The cervicofacial trunk has few cross-anastomoses and therefore, if the marginal mandibular nerve is cut, injury will produce motor paralysis of half of the lower lip. The temporofacial trunk has more plentiful cross-connections. Consequently, spontaneous return of function after injury in this division is more likely.[3] In its extraglandular position, the parotid duct

TABLE 20–2.—TUMORS OF THE MINOR SALIVARY GLANDS ACCORDING TO HISTOLOGIC TYPE

	INCIDENCE (%)	
HISTOLOGIC TYPE	Spiro et al. (N= 492)	Schell et al.* (N = 118)
BENIGN		
Benign mixed tumor	11.6	. . .
Oncocytoma	0.2	. . .
MALIGNANT		
Mucoepidermoid	15.5	23
Acinic cell	0.4	0.8
Adenoid cystic	35.4	57
Epidermoid	2.9	. . .
Adenocarcinoma	7.5	19
Malignant mixed tumor	2.6	0.8

*Adapted from Million R.R., Cassisi W.J., Wittes R.E.: Cancer in the head and neck, in DaVita V.T., Hellman S., Rosenberg S.A. (eds.): *Cancer: Principles and Practice of Oncology*. Philadelphia, J.B. Lippincott Co., 1982, Table 13–56.

A

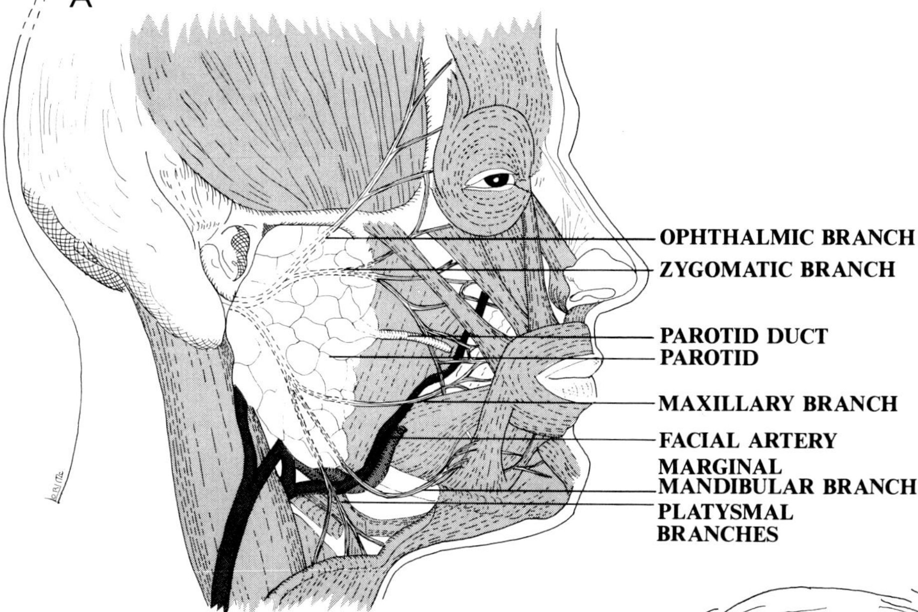

B

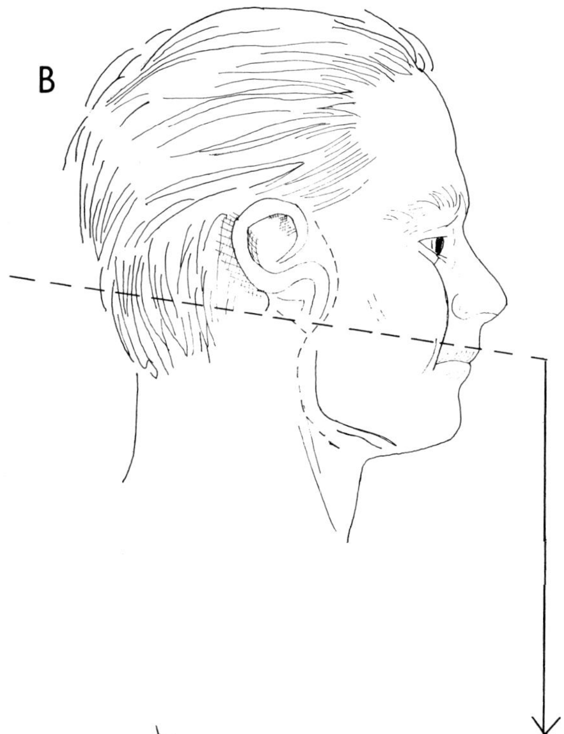

Fig 20–2.—**A,** side view of the parotid region showing the relationship of the key anatomical elements and the muscles of facial expression innervated by the facial nerve. An "ophthalmic" branch is usually not listed in the precise anatomical nomenclature. "Zygomatic" and "temporal" are official terms. The ability to close the eye is the important function. **B,** the usual parotidectomy incision. *Below,* a cross section in the line indicated showing the relationship of the facial nerve to the key structures. Note the increasing depth of the facial nerve as it courses posterior to the mandible.

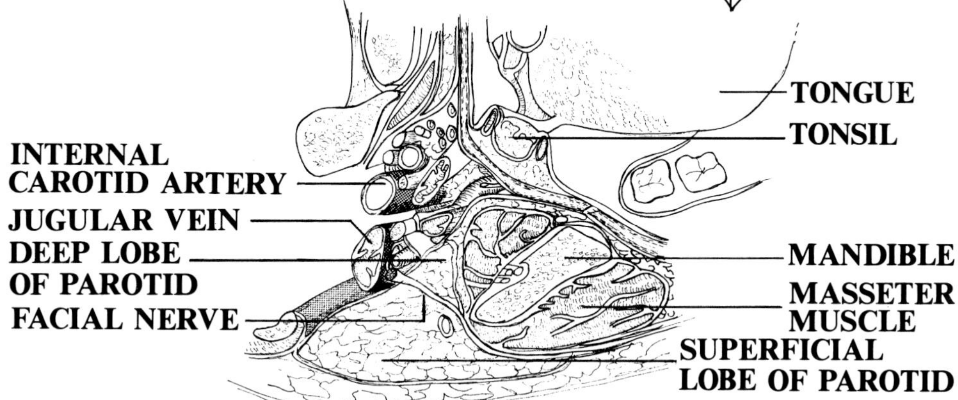

CROSS-SECTION ENLARGED AT PAROTID

is sometimes crossed by the closely applied maxillary (buccal) branch of cranial nerve VII, responsible for innervating the muscles of facial expression, including the perioral and circumoral muscles of the upper lip. Dissection near the parotid duct must therefore be done with precision to avoid injury to the maxillary (buccal) branch of the seventh nerve.

The submaxillary gland is located beneath the horizontal ramus of the mandible, bordered by the anterior and posterior parts of the digastric muscle. Wharton's duct drains saliva from the submaxillary gland into the floor of the mouth. The sublingual gland is located beneath the mucosa of the anterior mouth and empties saliva directly into the floor of the mouth. Submaxillary, intracapsular submaxillary, and submental lymph nodes drain the submaxillary and sublingual glands. The submaxillary gland is supplied by the external maxillary artery and its submental branch.

The submaxillary gland is juxtaposed to three important nerves. The marginal mandibular branch of cranial nerve VII crosses the upper portion of the gland, the lingual nerve lies deep to the upper inferior portion of the submaxillary gland, and the hypoglossal nerve lies beneath the submaxillary gland and the digastric tendon.

WHEN SHOULD A SALIVARY GLAND NEOPLASM BE BIOPSIED?

The only curative treatment for the majority of true salivary gland neoplasms is surgical removal. For the parotid a superficial parotidectomy is the safest and ideal biopsy when the tumor is in the superficial lobe, as it is in 80%–90% of cases. If the deep lobe is involved, it is excised after the superficial lobe is removed and the nerve and branches are identified. We generally limit incisional biopsy to intraoperative sampling during the course of a planned parotidectomy when signs of malignancy are present. The branches of the facial nerve can then be identified and avoided in taking the biopsy specimen. In such instances, histologic confirmation of the diagnosis will alter subsequent decisions regarding surgical therapy (see Fig 20–1). An incisional biopsy, avoiding branches of cranial nerve VII, provides adequate tissue for frozen section study. It is our procedure of choice in patients with suspected malignant lesions or possible benign lymphoepithelial lesions. Frozen section study of a superficial parotidectomy specimen should be routinely done at the time of surgery to rule out low-grade malignant lesions. One cannot safely rely on a gross specimen impression of benign or malignant. Needle biopsy or incisional biopsy should be performed in patients where surgical or anesthetic risks are large and where there is evidence of a malignant salivary tumor.

WHAT IS THE CORRECT SURGICAL PROCEDURE FOR PAROTID AND SUBMANDIBULAR GLAND TUMORS?

Enucleation of parotid tumors is not advisable, with the exception of benign lymphoepithelial lesions and Warthin's tumors located far down in the tail of the parotid. Benign mixed tumors have a pseudocapsule, and strands of cells often protrude into normal salivary tissue. The recurrence rate after simple enucleation varies from 10% to 50%, depending on the series. Recurrence can appear up to 20 years after an incomplete removal.

Malignant parotid tumors often invade surrounding salivary tissue. Adequate margins of normal salivary tissue must be resected to reduce the chances of local recurrence. In summary, a controlled superficial parotidectomy is the minimum biopsy required for lesions of the lateral lobe of the parotid gland. Total resection of the submandibular gland is the sampling technique of choice for all submandibular neoplasms.

What Are the Operative Techniques of Parotidectomy?

The initial surgical objectives for treating parotid neoplasms include complete removal of the tumor and preservation of the uninvolved facial nerve. An S-shaped skin incision is made extending from the middle of the ear to the posterior tip of the greater cornu of the hyoid bone in a skin crease one to two fingerbreadths below the mandible (see Fig 20–2,B). A skin flap is raised to expose the gland capsule up to the anterior border of the parotid gland. A short postauricular skin flap helps to expose the ear canal, the mastoid process, and the sternocleidomastoid muscle. The greater auricular nerve is identified, retracted, and preserved. At this point, dissection of the seventh nerve can take place in an antegrade manner from the main nerve trunk or by a retrograde technique beginning at the peripheral branches.

When the antegrade technique is used, the deep fascia is opened in the angle formed by the mastoid and the ear cartilage. The main trunk of cranial nerve VII is identified and dissected free of surrounding parotid tissue by blunt dissection in the area 1.0 cm deep and 1.5 cm above the tip of the mastoid process (Fig 20–3). Following identification of the main trunk of cranial nerve VII, blunt dissection is continued in the plane superficial to the nerve, with care taken to prevent pressure or undue tension on the nerve (Fig 20–4). Bleeding vessels are controlled with fine suture ligatures to avoid injury to the nerve. Blind electrocoagulation in the wound depth can cause extensive nerve damage. It should be avoided. Gentle dissection without traction is necessary at all times in the course of

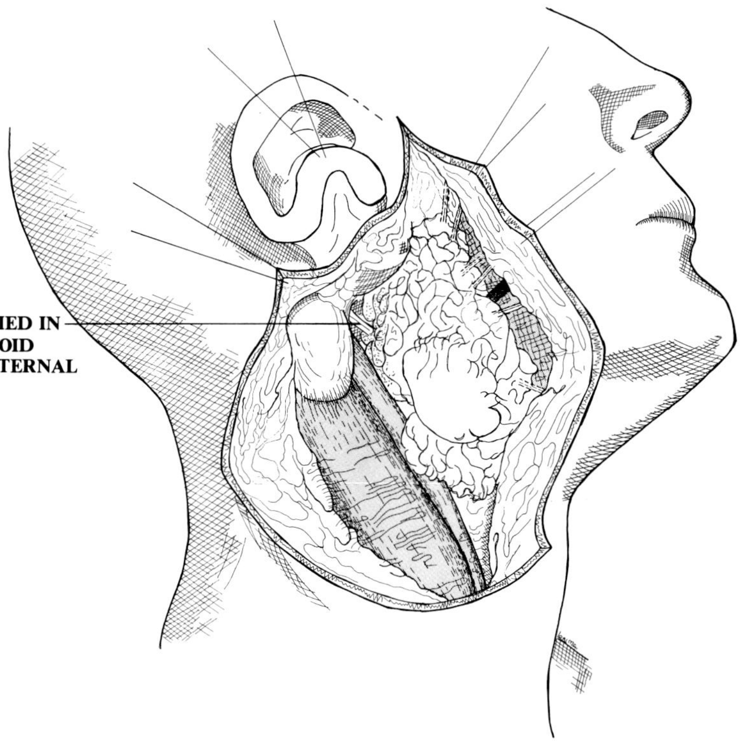

Fig 20–3.—In an antegrade dissection of a superficial lobe parotid tumor from the facial nerve, it is necessary to identify cranial nerve VII in the groove formed by the cartilage of the ear canal and the mastoid process. The areolar plane next to the ear cartilage is easily dissected. The facial nerve is quite deep at this point—1 to 2.5 cm, depending on the mass of parotid parenchyma and the location of the tumor.

superficial parotidectomy to eliminate postoperative nerve paresis. The posterior facial vein is divided and blunt dissection is continued peripherally beyond the cervicofacial and temporofacial trunks (Fig 20–5). Stensen's duct is dissected free of surrounding nerve branches and the lateral tributary is ligated. The skin incision is closed without drainage using absorbable superficial fascial sutures and fine interrupted skin sutures. The method of superficial parotidectomy described above is directed at safely and functionally preserving the branches of the facial nerve.

The superficial parotid gland may also be dissected free from the underlying facial nerve in a retrograde fashion by first individually identifying the temporal, ophthalmic, zygomatic, buccal, mandibular, and cervical peripheral branches (Fig 20–6). The peripheral branches can then be bluntly dissected from surrounding parotid tissue back toward the proximal divisions and main trunk. The technique requires careful horizontal division of the gland tissue between identified nerves. The technique does avoid undue tension on the nerve and allows earlier identification of a locus of adherent tumor. The gentle retrograde technique was originally described by Dr. D. State. Occasionally the size and location of parotid tumors mandate a retrograde dissection. Examples of such tumors include very large or partially fixed tumors near the mastoid, the ear canal, and the main nerve trunk. It is a useful technique for recurrent malignant tumors. Surgeons involved in the care of patients with parotid lesions should be familiar with both techniques. In certain instances a combination of both techniques may be required.

The operative procedure for *malignant* parotid lesions may require total parotidectomy, resection of involved portions of the facial nerve, adjacent muscles, ligaments, and bone, as well as modified or radical neck dissections (outlined below and in Fig 20–1,B) according to the characteristics of the particular parotid cancer.

Although superficial parotidectomy is indicated for all benign parotid tumors, occasional isolated small tumors in the tail of the parotid gland well away from the nerve or in the thin area of the gland overlying the masseter muscle require only complete removal of the tumor and a margin of normal salivary tissue.

What Is the Operative Technique of Submaxillary Gland Resection?

A submandibular skin incision is made and skin flaps are raised superiorly to the level of the mandible and

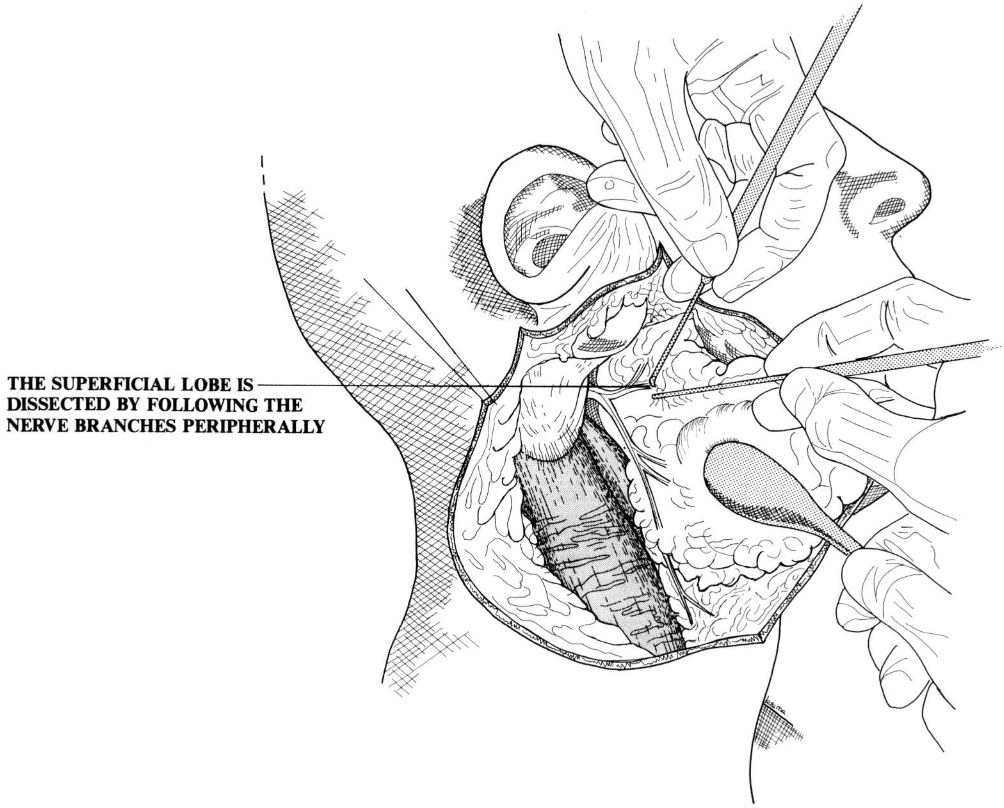

Fig 20–4.—The branches of the facial nerve are followed peripherally. The tissue is bluntly divided between *identified* nerve branches. Care is taken to not abrade, bruise, crush, or stretch the nerve. A large Headblom periosteal elevator makes a good retractor.

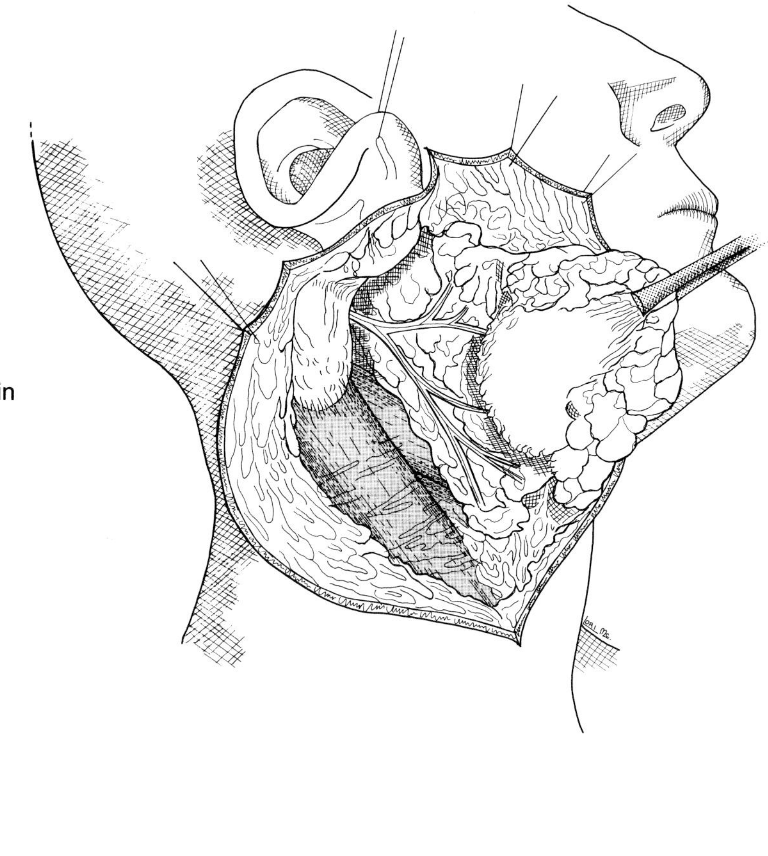

Fig 20–5.—The antegrade parotidectomy nearly completed. Care must be taken at this point not to apply undue tension or to sever small nerve branches that may be tented up in the retracted specimen.

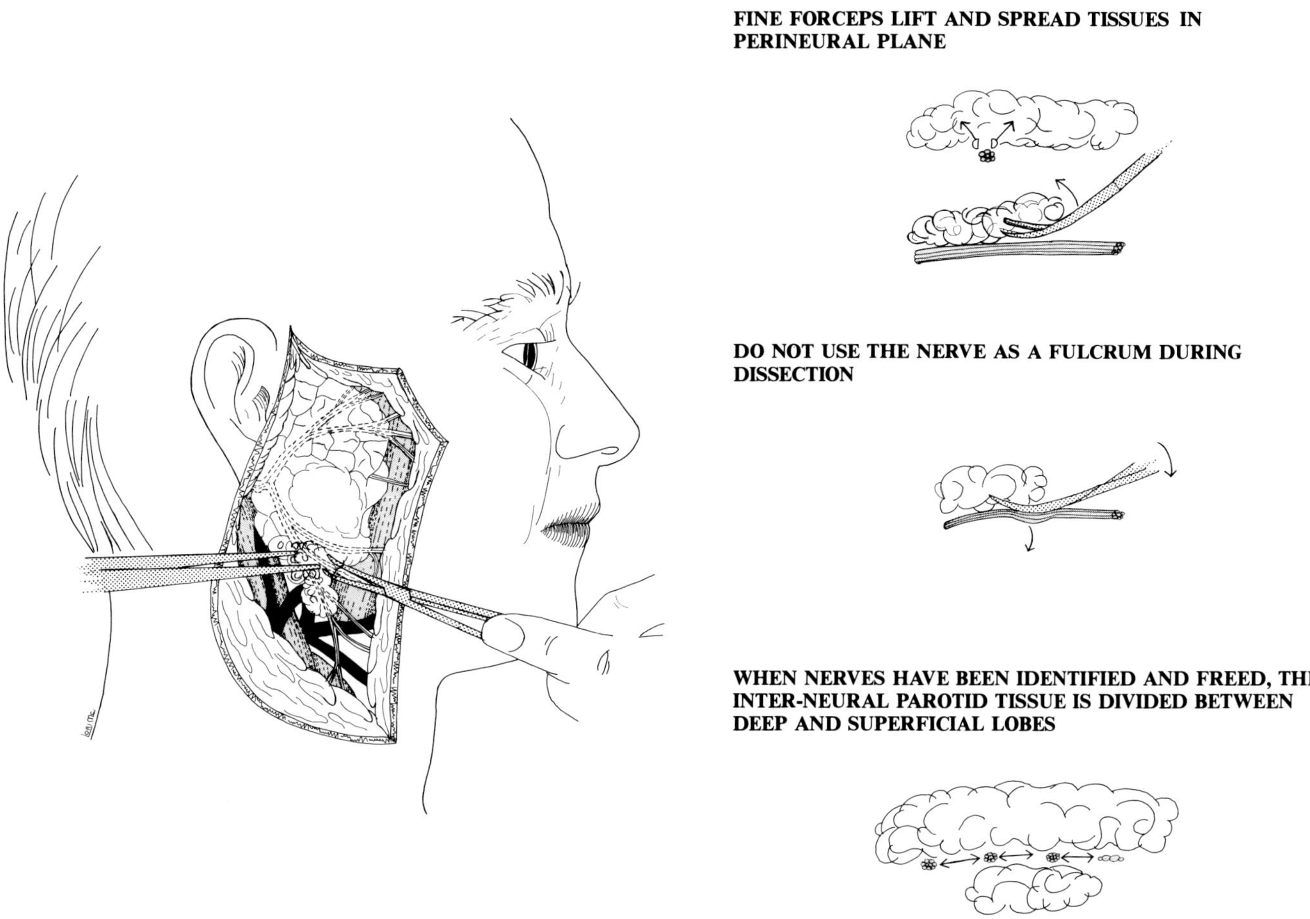

Fig 20–6.—A, retrograde resection of the parotid begins with identification of the peripheral branches of the facial nerve as they lie on the investing fascia of the masseter muscle. The parotid tissue is lifted from the nerve in a perineural plane. Care is taken not to lean heavily on the fine branches of the nerve. Cottonoids dipped in 1:1,000,000 epinephrine solution are used to protect the nerve branches if suction is used. After the branches are identified, a horizontal dissection plane is developed. This plane divides the deep and superficial lobes. When the main trunk is identified from the front, the posterior parotid tissues can be safely divided.

inferiorly to the hyoid bone. The marginal mandibular branch of cranial nerve VII is identified and carefully preserved. Next, the facial artery and vein are separately divided. The lower border of the submaxillary gland is dissected free. The anterior belly of the digastric, mylohyoid, and hyoglossus muscles are retracted to expose and identify the course of the hypoglossal nerve. The nerve is preserved. The lingual nerve is identified as the superior border of the submaxillary gland is dissected. With downward tension on the gland, the chorda tympani branch of cranial nerve VII which travels with the lingual nerve will tether the gland to the lingual nerve because secretory fibers pass to the gland. The lingual nerve will be pulled down in a V. Care must be exercised to preserve the lingual nerve and not cut off the apex of the V. Wharton's duct is visualized and ligated, with care taken to avoid injury to the adjacent hypoglossal nerve. After the anterior facial vein and facial artery are divided, thereby freeing the posterior superior aspect of the gland, the submaxillary gland and associated lymph nodes are removed and the wound is closed.

WHAT ARE THE IMPORTANT BENIGN NEOPLASMS OF THE MAJOR SALIVARY GLANDS?

In order to present a rational clinical decision-making scheme for treatment of salivary gland neoplasms, it is necessary to realize that usually the surgeon will be operating on a mass that is benign but may be malignant in about one fourth of cases. The following discussion examines the spectrum of decisions for management of benign and malignant tumors in the context of the surgical experience at the University of Minnesota spanning a period of 50 years, a period that encompassed the development of pioneer techniques in nerve dissection. Such a dip into the past gives us a view of less successful therapeutic options.

Benign mixed tumors (pleomorphic adenoma) are the most frequent salivary gland neoplasms. They accounted for 55% of all tumors and 80% of all benign tumors in patients surgically treated for salivary gland neoplasms at the University of Minnesota between 1932 and 1979 (Table 20–3). Characteristically, 60% of the patients were female, and the average age was 44 years. Nonetheless, benign mixed tumors can also be found in children[4] and elderly patients.

What Is the Clinical Presentation of Patients With Benign Mixed Tumors?

In our series, patients with benign mixed tumors had a long duration of symptoms (average, 4.5 yrs). The most common complaint was a slowly growing, nontender, palpable mass located either in front of or behind the ear. On physical examination the tumor was usually found to be a firm, smooth, distinct mass, freely movable and located in the superficial lobe of the parotid gland. Fourteen patients (7%) presented with involvement of the deep lobe.

Surgical treatment of benign mixed tumors of the parotid has evolved with time. Procedures have included excision or enucleation (54 patients), superficial lobectomy (102 patients), and total parotidectomy with preservation of the facial nerve (49 patients). The improvement in surgical techniques over time has given some insight into what maneuvers are *not* effective. Fifty-four early patients were treated in the 1930s by simple excision, enucleation, or piecemeal removal. Involved margins or spillage of tumor into the operative field was described in 16 (30%) patients. Following simple enucleation, five patients (10%) had recurrent tumor. More recently, the majority of patients with benign mixed tumors were treated by superficial parotidectomy (102 patients) or total parotidectomy (49 patients) with preservation of the facial nerve and its branches. Only two patients (1.3%) experienced recurrence, at 1 and 4 years after a superficial parotidectomy. In both cases the margins of the tumor had been violated at the time of primary resection.

Twenty-one patients with submaxillary benign mixed tumors were treated by complete excision of the submaxillary gland. Two patients also underwent en bloc removal of the contents of the submaxillary triangle. Only one patient (5%) with a supposed benign mixed tumor of the submaxillary gland experienced a recurrence. This case illustrates the difficulty in distinguishing between benign and malignant mixed tumors by histology only. The lesion subsequently recurred, invaded the mandible, and resulted in death 14 months later from extensive local spread.

What Determines Recurrence Rates of Benign Mixed Tumors?

The long-term recurrence rate following treatment for benign mixed tumor has been shown to be directly dependent on the initial surgical procedure. Recurrence rates are highest following simple enucleation or inadvertent operative spillage.[5] Unfortunately, the subsequent recurrences are often multiple and densely adherent to the nerve.[6] The proper surgical therapy for benign mixed tumors of the parotid entails complete removal of all neoplastic tissue, namely, the superficial lobe, or a total parotidectomy (in the case of deep lobe tumors) with careful preservation of the facial nerve.[7] If the pleomorphic adenoma is not inappropriately biop-

TABLE 20–3.—HISTOLOGIC CLASSIFICATION OF 279 BENIGN TUMORS OF THE MAJOR SALIVARY GLANDS SURGICALLY TREATED AT THE UNIVERSITY OF MINNESOTA HOSPITALS (1932–1979)

TUMOR TYPE	LOCATION			TOTAL	
	Parotid	Submaxillary	Sublingual	No.	(%)
Benign mixed tumors (pleomorphic adenoma)	201	21	0	222	(80)
Papillary cystadenoma lymphomatosum (Warthin's)	23	0	0	23	(8)
Oncocytoma (oxyphilic adenoma)	1	1	0	2	(1)
Benign lymphoepithelial lesion (Mikulicz's disease)	14	1	0	15	(5)
Hemangioma	10			10	(4)
Lipoma	3			3	(1)
Neurofibroma	2			2	(1)
Granular cell myoblastoma	0	1		1	(. . .)
Lymphangioma	1			1	
Total				279	100

sied or fragmented during the course of these procedures, the recurrence rate should be between 0 and 5%.

What Are the Expected Complications After Surgery for Benign Mixed Tumors?

The major complication following surgical therapy of all parotid lesions is facial nerve paralysis. In this series of 201 patients with benign mixed tumors of the parotid, 21 (10%) had partial facial weakness that resolved within 2 months. In the majority of patients the weakness was mild and involved the buccal, mandibular, or cervical branches of the facial nerve. In the 1930–1940 period, facial nerve paresis followed enucleation (3 patients), superficial lobectomy (1 patient), and total parotidectomy (2 patients). Facial nerve injuries were treated by primary nerve repair or interposition grafts using the greater auricular nerve.

Additional complications in this series included one instance of a salivary fistula and five instances of auriculotemporal (Frey's) syndrome. This syndrome, also called painful gustatory sweating, consists of flushing and sweating over the skin supplied by the auriculotemporal nerve after the ingestion of food. All five patients with the auriculotemporal syndrome had mild symptoms that did not require further surgical treatment.

What Is the Fate of Patients After Surgical Treatment for Benign Mixed Tumors?

The long-term prognosis of patients with benign mixed tumors is excellent. In this series only one of 222 (0.5%) patients died of local tumor. Since documented tumor-free intervals before recurrences have been as long as 27 years,[9] patients with benign mixed tumors must be followed up for life. Very rarely,[10] pleomorphic adenomas metastasize to the lung. Like the primary tumor, the metastasis may appear histologically benign. Of note, 2%–9% of all mixed tumors of the parotid gland may undergo malignant transformation.[6]

What Are the Clinical Characteristics of a Patient With Warthin's Tumor?

Papillary cystadenoma lymphomatosum and oxyphilic adenomas, or oncytomas, constitute the benign monomorphic adenomas of the major salivary glands. Both kinds of tumor are believed to originate from cells of the striated or excretory ducts.[11–13]

The so-called Warthin's tumor was well described by Albrecht and Artz 20 years before Warthin's description.[1] Warthin's tumor is the second most frequent benign tumor of the major salivary glands (see Table 20–3). It has several important distinctions from other salivary gland tumors. It occurs primarily in males (17 of 23 patients in this series). There is a 10:1 male-female ratio in many series. It is often bilateral (10% in this series), and frequently multicentric.[1] Up to 70% of all *bilateral* salivary gland neoplasms are Warthin's tumors.[12] For unknown reasons, Warthin's tumors are found only in the parotid gland. The usual complaint of 23 patients with Warthin's tumors was of a slowly growing, nontender, movable mass.

Surgical treatment of the 23 patients with Warthin's tumor treated at the University of Minnesota included simple excision in 11 patients, superficial parotidectomy in 9 patients, and total parotidectomy in 3 patients. Although simple excision of this lesion is considered curative, 2 patients (9.7%) in this series developed recurrences or new neoplasms following limited excision.

Two patients with oxyphilic adenomas, or oncocytomas, were treated by total parotidectomy and wide local excision and have remained free of disease after 5 years.

What Is the Presentation and Treatment of Patients With Benign Lymphoepithelial Lesions of the Major Salivary Glands?

This tumor, or parotid enlargement, should be well known to the head and neck surgeon. Historically this entity has been misclassified as a malignant disease. Unfortunately some patients have undergone needlessly aggressive surgical therapy. Benign lymphoepithelial lesions of the major salivary glands are part of a greater symptom complex known as Sjögren's syndrome.[14] This syndrome includes xerostomia, keratoconjunctivitis sicca, rheumatoid arthritis, and hypergammaglobulinemia. Mikulicz's disease is characterized by bilateral and asymptomatic swelling of the major salivary and lacrimal glands.[15] Our series included 15 patients with benign lymphoepithelial lesions. Nine (60%) of the patients had associated abnormalities of Sjögren's syndrome. Thirteen (87%) of the patients were women, with an average age of 45 years. The site of involvement was the parotid gland in 14 patients (bilateral in 6) and the submaxillary gland in one patient. The usual presenting history was a gradually enlarging, nontender parotid mass.

Surgical therapy for benign lymphoepithelial lesions included biopsy only (2 patients), wide excision (4 patients), superficial lobectomy (5 patients), or total parotidectomy (3 patients). The one patient with a submaxillary lesion was treated by wide excision. In the early years, surgical procedures were usually performed, owing to the difficulty of differentiating benign lymphoepithelial lesions from other benign or malignant neoplasms. To date the clinical course of all 15 patients has been unremarkable. The patients in whom the gland was simply biopsied have demonstrated persistent enlargement but little discomfort. Of the 13 patients that underwent surgical removal of the lesion, only one patient reports intermittent swelling of the remnant of the parotid gland at 6 years following wide excision. We believe that a reasonable surgical approach is to perform a superficial lobectomy with preservation of the facial nerve in patients with an isolated nodule and to obtain an immediate frozen section for diagnosis. In patients with the likely diagnosis of benign lymphoepithelial lesions due to multiple gland involvement, or clear-cut Sjögren's syndrome, a biopsy may be all that is necessary.

What Other Benign Lesions of the Salivary Glands Can Be Expected?

Benign capillary hemangiomas (hemangioendotheliomas) usually occur in the parotid glands of infants and children and may spontaneously regress.[4] In our series eight of ten hemangiomas of the parotid gland occurred in children ranging in age from 7 weeks to 12 years. Of clinical importance, in eight of the patients the chief complaint was a firm, palpable mass with no visible characteristics of a hemangioma. The lesion involved the deep lobe of the parotid in two patients.

Surgical therapy included simple excision (6 patients), superficial parotidectomy (1 patient), or total parotidectomy (3 patients) with preservation of the facial nerve. Four patients experienced a transient facial weakness and one patient developed a salivary fistula in the immediate postoperative period that spontaneously closed. There have been no recurrences following surgical removal after a follow-up of 8 years.

Other uncommon benign lesions of the parotid gland in our series included lipoma (3 patients), lymphangioma (1 patient), and neurofibroma (2 patients).

Summary of Surgical Treatment of Benign Major Salivary Gland Tumors

Between 1932 and 1979, 279 patients were surgically treated for benign major salivary gland tumors at the University of Minnesota Hospitals. Surgical treatment included biopsy only (2 patients), wide excision or enucleation (99 patients), superficial lobectomy (119 patients), or total parotidectomy (62 patients). The incidence of complications following these procedures was low (Table 20–4) and included temporary seventh nerve paresis (7.8%), complete seventh nerve injury (1.8%), Frey's syndrome (2.5%), and salivary fistula (0.4%). These surgical results, together with the very low recurrence rates for benign mixed tumors, papillary cystadenoma lymphomatosum, and hemangiomas, suggest that superficial lobectomy, or total parotidectomy for deep lobe tumors, is the treatment of choice for benign parotid lesions. If recognized, iatrogenic injury to the seventh nerve occurring during the surgical treatment for benign parotid tumor should be immediately repaired by primary reanastomosis or nerve interposition using the greater auricular or sural nerve.

WHAT CLINICAL AND OPERATIVE FINDINGS SUGGEST MALIGNANCY?

As outlined in Figure 20–1, the surgical decision-making process for treatment of salivary gland neoplasms begins with determining if the lesion is benign or malignant. Clinical signs of malignancy include a large size, rapid growth, skin fixation, pain, facial nerve paralysis, and firm palpable cervical lymph nodes. The most important operative finding that suggests malignancy is adherence to adjacent structures, especially the facial nerve. When the tumor adheres to the facial nerve branches or other structures, the alert surgeon should be suspicious of malignancy and obtain a frozen section pathologic diagnosis in order to determine subsequent definitive therapy.

Not shown in most reviews of parotid tumors is the frequency of lymphoma. In some patients, an enlarged node in the lower parotid is the presenting lesion of lymphoma. One should always be suspicious and examine the subdigastric and midjugular lymph nodes during early dissection of the lower portion of the parotid. If multiple enlarged nodes are obvious, a node

TABLE 20–4.—INCIDENCE OF COMPLICATIONS OF SURGICAL TREATMENT OF 279 PATIENTS WITH BENIGN MAJOR SALIVARY GLAND TUMORS

	TRANSIENT* NERVE VII PARESIS	COMPLETE NERVE VII INJURY	FREY'S SYNDROME	SALIVARY FISTULA
	No. (%)	No. (%)	No. (%)	No. (%)
Superficial parotidectomy	14 (5)	2 (1)	4 (1.5)	1 (0.4)
Total parotidectomy	8 (3)	3 (1)	3 (1)	0
Total	22 (8)	5 (2)†	7 (2.5)	1 (0.4)

*lasting < 30 days
†Does not include two cases in which the facial nerve was knowingly sacrificed during the course of operation for a presumed malignant tumor.

may be sent for biopsy before one proceeds with a facial nerve dissection.

What Are the Important Malignant Neoplasms of the Major Salivary Glands?

Although malignant tumors constitute less than 25% of all major salivary gland tumors, they pose special problems for the surgeon. These problems often relate to three questions: (1) Should the facial nerve be sacrificed? (2) What should be the extent of wide-field resection? (3) Should a cervical lymphadenectomy be performed? In the postoperative period, the benefits of regional irradiation and adjuvant chemotherapy must be evaluated in view of the potential for distant metastasis and local recurrence, depending on the particular malignant tumor type.

Mucoepidermoid carcinoma is the most frequent malignant tumor of the parotid gland[16] and the most common malignant salivary gland tumor in children.[4] These tumors must be subdivided into low-grade and high-grade types, as each type has a strikingly different biologic behavior. Twenty-seven patients (17 women and 10 men) with mucoepidermoid carcinoma of the parotid gland (Table 20–5) have been treated at the University of Minnesota. Twenty patients (74%) had a low-grade malignancy with mucin cells predominating and 7 patients (26%) had a high-grade malignancy with an atypical squamous cell histology. Patients with low-grade mucoepidermoid tumors ranged in age from 21 to 73 years. Clinically, they could not be distinguished from patients with benign mixed tumors. Patients with low-grade mucoepidermoid carcinomas had a slow-growing, nontender, cystic preauricular mass. In marked contrast, the seven patients with high-grade mucoepidermoid tumors presented with hard and large (>3 cm) masses with fixation to surrounding soft tissue (3 patients) or obvious involvement of the facial nerve (1 patient).

Seven of eight patients with low-grade parotid mucoepidermoid tumors treated by simple excision with a margin of normal salivary tissue remain tumor free after a follow-up of 12 years. The remaining patient treated by simple excision had two local recurrences 2 and 4 years later treated by re-excision. He has remained disease free for 23 years. Ten patients underwent more extensive parotid resections, including superficial parotidectomy (5 patients) or total parotidectomy (5 patients). In addition, three patients underwent radical neck dissection, but no evidence of metastatic tumor deposits was found in the resected regional lymph nodes. All ten patients treated with more aggressive resection are alive and well without tumor recurrence after 4–11 years.

TABLE 20–5.—HISTOLOGIC CLASSIFICATION OF 128 MALIGNANT TUMORS OF THE MAJOR SALIVARY GLANDS SURGICALLY TREATED AT THE UNIVERSITY OF MINNESOTA HOSPITALS (1932–1979)

TUMOR TYPE	LOCATION			TOTAL
	Parotid	Submaxillary	Sublingual	No. (%)
Mucoepidermoid carcinoma	27	0	0	27 (21)
Acinic cell carcinoma	19	1	0	20 (16)
Adenoid cystic carcinoma (cylindroma)	15	3	1	19 (15)
Epidermoid carcinoma	18	7	0	25 (20)
Malignant lymphoma	6	2	0	8 (6)
Adenocarcinoma	11	0	0	11 (9)
Malignant mixed tumor	4	0	0	4 (3)
Undifferentiated	5	0	0	5 (4)
Metastatic tumor	6	3	0	9 (7)
Total				128 (100)

In contrast to the patients with low-grade mucoepidermoid cancers, the seven patients with high-grade mucoepidermoid carcinomas died within 2 years despite aggressive surgical therapy. Four patients were treated by radical total parotidectomy with sacrifice of the facial nerve and en bloc radical neck dissection. Metastatic deposits in the resected lymph nodes were present in two (50%) patients. In addition, three of these patients received irradiation to the parotid and neck regions. In the remaining three patients the lesions had invaded the base of the skull and were not completely resected. Extensive pulmonary metastases developed in four patients with high-grade mucoepidermoid tumors.

What is the Expected Survival Rate for Patients With Mucoepidermoid Carcinoma?

Actuarial 2- and 5-year survival rates for patients with low-grade mucoepidermoid cancer of the parotid are excellent (Table 20–6, Fig 20–7) and range from 89% to 97% in collected series.[17] Patients with high-grade mucoepidermoid cancers have a 5-year survival rate of 22%–56%.

What Is the Treatment of Choice for Patients With Mucoepidermoid Cancers of the Parotid Gland?

Because of their excellent survival patterns and the infrequent involvement of the facial nerve or metastases to subparotid or digastric lymph nodes, patients with low-grade mucoepidermoid cancers of the parotid gland

TABLE 20–6.—ACTUARIAL PATIENT SURVIVAL ACCORDING TO MALIGNANT PAROTID TUMOR TYPE*

TUMOR (N)	2-YEAR SURVIVAL (%)	5-YEAR SURVIVAL (%)
Mucoepidermoid carcinoma, low grade (20)	88 ± 6	80 ± 7
Acinic cell carcinoma (20)	100	68 ± 10
Adenoid cystic carcinoma (19)	47 ± 11	36 ± 11
Epidermoid carcinoma (25)	66 ± 9	47 ± 10

*Cumulative patient survival ± SE.

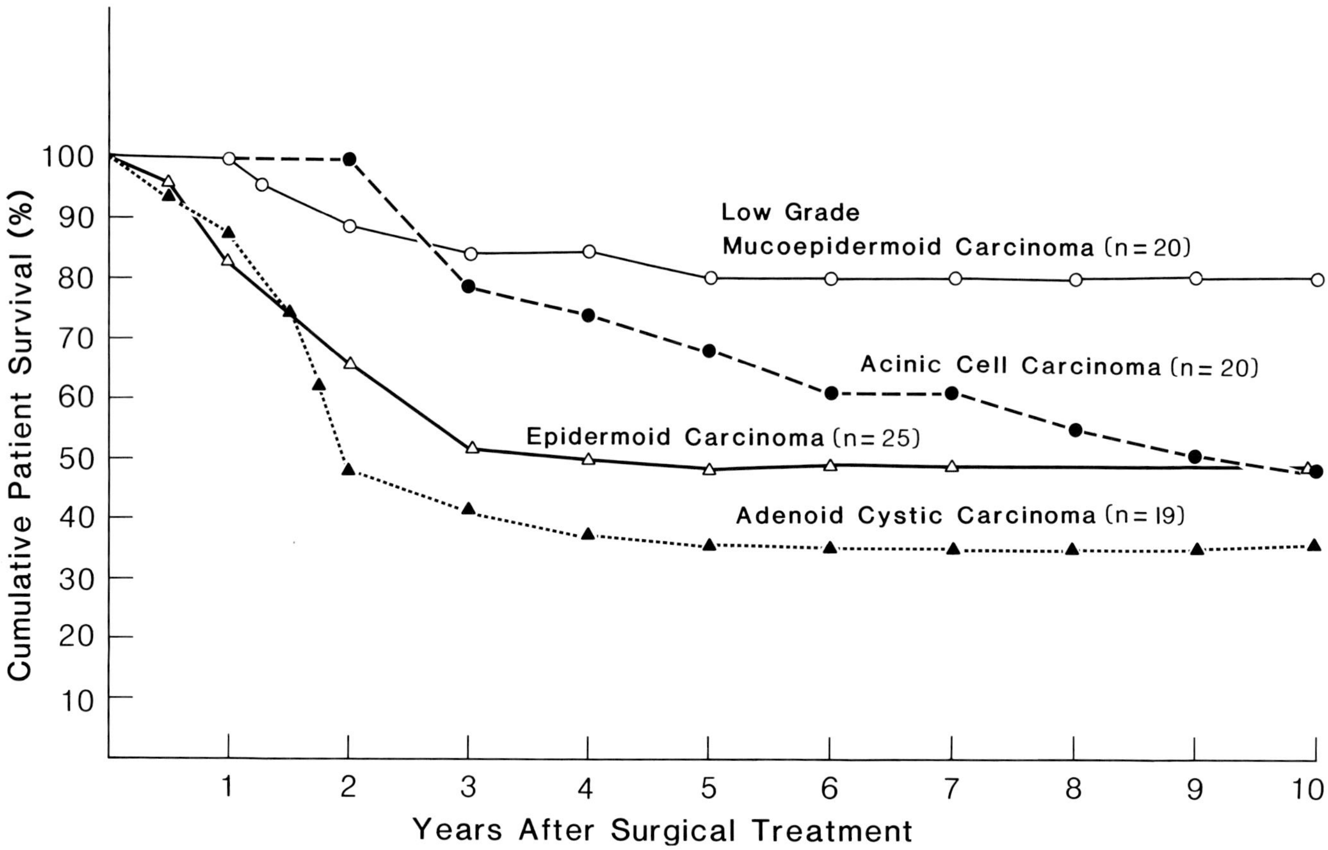

Fig 20–7.—Actuarial patient survival curve after surgical therapy for major salivary gland malignant tumors. The series spans a large number of years.

are adequately treated by removal of the tumor with a cuff of normal salivary tissue (usually superficial parotidectomy), with preservation of the facial nerve when the tumor and nerve are easily separated (see Fig 20–1). The subdigastric lymph nodes should be inspected at the time of surgery.[18]

In contrast, high-grade mucoepidermoid cancers have a higher incidence of facial nerve involvement (10%)[17] and lymph node metastases (44%).[18] Adequate treatment for these patients includes total parotidectomy and regional dissection (see Chaps. 22 and 23). The facial nerve is sacrificed if it is grossly involved by tumor. Full-dose postoperative radiation therapy is added. Local recurrences are best controlled with local surgical therapy. Chemotherapy including methotrexate and cisplatin has been reported to have some benefit.[19]

What Are the Characteristics of Patients With Acinic Cell Carcinoma?

Acinic cell carcinomas usually occur in the parotid gland and are slow-growing.[20] Although acinic cell tumors are usually considered low grade, they frequently recur locally, in the regional lymph nodes, or in distant sites.[21] In this series acinic cell tumors were present in 20 patients (14 women and 6 men). The site of involvement was the parotid gland in 19 and the submaxillary gland in one patient. Symptoms were long standing (average duration, 7.5 years) and included a nontender palpable mass in 19 patients. Grossly the tumors ranged in size from 1 to 15 cm. They appeared to have a friable capsule at the surgery. In some patients the neoplastic tissue had infiltrated beyond the capsule. Metastases were present in regional lymph nodes in six patients (30%).

Unfortunately, the inadequacy of simple excision of acinic cell tumors became obvious very early in our series. Four of five patients (80%) treated by simple excision experienced prompt recurrences. In contrast, seven patients had wide local excisions (superficial lobectomy) with preservation of the seventh nerve. Only one patient had a local recurrence at 2 years. Eight patients with more advanced tumors underwent total parotidectomy with sacrifice of all or a portion of the facial nerve. Six patients had an en bloc standard radical neck dissection at the time of total parotidectomy. The tumor recurred locally in five of eight patients treated by total parotidectomy. One patient with an acinic cell carcinoma of the submaxillary gland was treated by radical resection and radical neck dissection, but the tumor recurred locally at 12 months.

What Is the Surgical Treatment of Choice for Patients With Acinic Cell Carcinoma of the Major Salivary Glands?

Although patients with acinic cell carcinoma had a 100% 2-year survival, local recurrences and metastatic disease resulted in only a 68% 5-year survival (see Table 20–6). Radiation therapy was unsuccessful in controlling recurrent local disease in five patients. Radical surgical treatment including total parotidectomy and sacrifice of any part of involved facial nerve is justified[20] in patients with acinic cell carcinoma (see Fig 20–1). Patients with clinically palpable or questionably involved lymph nodes should undergo modified neck dissections;[21] however, the incidence of lymph node metastases is low.

What Is the Clinical Presentation of Patients With Adenoid Cystic Carcinoma of the Major Salivary Glands?

Adenoid cystic carcinomas are slow-growing yet highly malignant tumors. In addition, they frequently demonstrate perineural invasion. In our series, 19 patients (11 men and 8 women) with adenoid cystic carcinoma have been treated. The tumor originated in the parotid gland in 15 patients, the submaxillary gland in three patients, and the sublingual gland in one patient. While eight patients presented with symptoms of a slowly growing (average duration, 10 years) mass, five patients presented with a painful lesion, and six patients demonstrated facial nerve paresis. Unfortunately, 11 patients with adenoid cystic carcinomas had advanced lesions following inadequate treatment elsewhere. The previous treatments were biopsy alone (4 patients) radiation therapy (4 patients), or incomplete wide excision (3 patients). Ten of these 11 patients died of local or distant recurrence within 3 years. Removal of all obvious tumor was possible in eight patients. Two patients were treated by superficial lobectomy and preservation of the seventh nerve; one remains tumor free after 5 years and the other suffered a local recurrence at 15 years. Four patients were treated by total parotidectomy and sacrifice of the seventh nerve. After this radical therapy two remain tumor free at 4 and 12 years; however, two developed distant metastases at 1 and 6 years. Three patients with submaxillary lesions were treated with wide local excision and en bloc radical neck dissections but experienced recurrences at 2, 4, and 8 years. The 5-year determinant patient survival for all 19 patients with adenoid cystic carcinoma was only 36% (see Fig 20–7).

What Is the Treatment of Choice for Patients With Adenoid Cystic Carcinoma of the Major Salivary Glands?

Other authors have documented the poor prognosis of patients with adenoid cystic carcinoma,[22] especially of the solid histologic type.[23] Facial nerve paralysis (17%), local recurrence (60%),[24] and pulmonary metastases are frequent. Surgical therapy should include total parotidectomy, sacrifice of involved seventh nerve, and immediate nerve grafting.[33] Modified neck dissection should be performed in patients with palpable nodes. The benefit of radiation therapy postoperatively is controversial, with reports of temporary remission,[25] improvement,[26] and no effect[22] on patient survival after its use. Of recent interest, cisplatin, Adriamycin, and 5-FU appear to have efficacy, especially in relieving pain, in patients with adenoid cystic carcinomas.[19] Partial and complete responses have been shown in patients with both local and regional disease using cisplatin[34] as well as 5-FU.[27]

How Do You Treat Patients With Epidermoid Carcinoma of the Major Salivary Glands?

Although the majority of epidermoid carcinomas of the parotid or submaxillary gland are metastatic from another source, 25 patients in our series (17 men and 8 women) had salivary gland epidermoid carcinomas. Their ages ranged from 47 to 82 years, and 13 patients (52%) were more than 60 years old. The site of involvement was the parotid (18 patients) or submaxillary gland (7 patients). Three of the tumors originated in Stensen's duct, and the squamous portion of a mucoepidermoid carcinoma may have been the origin of others.[11]

Surgical treatment in our patients included radical total parotidectomy with sacrifice of the seventh nerve and postoperative irradiation in seven patients. Radical neck dissections were included in seven of the above 11 patients. A wide en bloc excision of the tumor in seven patients with submaxillary gland epidermoid carcinoma was combined with a radical neck dissection in five patients and postoperative irradiation in four patients. Results of surgical treatment were surprisingly good in patients who underwent curative resections, with eight patients remaining disease-free after 7 years' follow-up (see Table 20–6). Seven patients with unresectable epidermoid carcinomas due to extension to the pharynx or base of the skull died within 1 year despite irradiation or incomplete surgical resection.

What Is the Treatment of Choice in Patients With Epidermoid Carcinoma of the Major Salivary Glands?

Patients with epidermoid cancers of the parotid and submaxillary gland have a high incidence of occult cervical lymph node metastases (40%).[18] There is a benefit from the addition of modified cervical lymphadenectomy to a total parotidectomy. Resection of the seventh nerve is also indicated if it is adjacent to or involved by tumor. Epidermoid cancers are also relatively radiosensitive. Adjunctive postoperative irradiation can be added.

What Is the Surgical Treatment for Patients With Adenocarcinoma and Malignant Mixed Tumors of the Salivary Glands?

Adenocarcinoma of the major salivary glands is a heterogeneous pathologic entity that includes malignant pleomorphic adenomas, papillary adenocarcinoma, and some gland-forming tumors that cannot be classified into other categories. Malignant transformation of a mixed tumor is uncommon (2%–9%).[28–31] Undifferentiated carcinoma, epidermoid, and mucoepidermoid carcinomas can also develop from a mixed tumor. In this series 11 patients (6 men and 5 women) were surgically treated for adenocarcinoma (10 solid and 1 papillary tumor) of the parotid gland. Also, four patients had malignant pleomorphic adenomas of the parotid gland with distinct pathologic evidence of both benign mixed tumor and foci of poorly differentiated adenocarcinoma. Clinically, a suddenly increased rate of growth in a longstanding tumor mass was noted in three patients.

Surgical treatment of the 11 patients with adenocarcinoma of the parotid gland included superficial lobectomy in five patients and total parotidectomy in six patients. Four patients had radical neck dissection, in three the facial nerve was sacrificed, and ten were treated with postoperative irradiation. Excellent results have followed this aggressive treatment protocol, with eight patients tumor-free after an average follow-up of 9 years. The four patients with malignant mixed tumors were treated by superficial lobectomy (4 patients), irradiation (3 patients), and chemotherapy, including 5-FU, methotrexate, vincristine, and Cytoxan (2 patients). Nevertheless, three died with local recurrence within 7 years.

How Are Patients With Malignant Lymphoma and Metastatic Carcinoma of the Major Salivary Glands Treated?

Malignant lymphoma, a rare neoplasm of the major salivary glands, may involve the parotid gland as part of a disseminated process or in the clinical setting of Sjögren's syndrome.[29] In our series eight patients (5 women and 3 men) were treated for malignant lymphoma of the salivary gland located in the parotid gland (6 patients) and the submaxillary gland (2 patients). Treatment included wide local excision (3 patients), superficial parotidectomy (2 patients), or total parotidectomy (3 patients) and included irradiation in all patients. Despite the presence of generalized lymphoma, three patients have survived 7–14 years since the date of last treatment.

The major salivary glands contain a large number of lymph nodes and can be the infrequent site of metastatic disease. In this series nine patients were treated for apparent parotid tumors that subsequently proved to be metastatic spread from other head and neck primaries: from squamous cell cancer (6 patients), malignant melanoma (2 patients), and adenocarcinoma (of a meibomian gland, 1 patient).

What Is the Fate of Patients With Undifferentiated Tumors of the Salivary Glands?

Five patients in this series presented with undifferentiated tumors of the parotid glands. All of the tumors were unresectable and treated with local irradiation and chemotherapy, including 5-FU, Cytoxan, and Adriamycin. All five patients died of persistent or recurrent tumor within 2 years. Undifferentiated tumors may mimic adenoid cystic carcinoma pathologically, but must be treated very aggressively owing to their high local recurrence rate (64%)[24] and the frequent involvement of the facial nerve (24%).[17]

Summary of Surgical Treatment of Malignant Major Salivary Gland Tumors

Between 1932 and 1979, 128 patients with malignant major salivary gland tumors were surgically treated at the University of Minnesota Hospitals (see Table 20–5). The sites of involvement were the parotid gland (111 patients), submaxillary gland (16 patients), and sublingual gland (1 patient). Malignant tumors of the parotid gland were treated by wide excision (35 patients), superficial lobectomy (26 patients), or total parotidectomy (37 patients); the remaining 11 patients with malignant parotid tumors had nonresectable lesions. In addition, 26 patients (23%) had all or part of the seventh nerve sacrificed and 31 (28%) had radical neck dissections. Sixteen patients with submaxillary malignant tumors were treated by wide local excision, including a radical neck dissection in eight patients.

Patients with malignant parotid gland tumors can be broadly considered as two separate biologic populations. The first group consists of patients with low-grade mucoepidermoid tumors who are adequately treated by excision of the neoplasm with a margin of surrounding normal salivary tissue. The second population consists of patients with high-grade mucoepidermoid, acinic cell, adenoid cystic, epidermoid, malignant pleomorphic adenoma, adenocarcinoma, and undifferentiated carcinomas. These tumors demonstrate extreme local invasiveness, frequent perineural involvement (especially the adenoid cystic carcinoma), and may metastasize to regional lymph nodes. Based on the majority of the reported long-term survival figures (see Fig 20–7), these patients are candidates for aggressive surgery, including total parotidectomy, sacrifice of the seventh nerve, and elective radical neck dissection on a *selective* basis, depending on the anatomical findings and type of carcinoma (see Fig 20–1).

WHAT ARE THE INDICATIONS FOR DELIBERATE RESECTION OF PART OR ALL OF THE FACIAL NERVE?

Patients with small, localized, high-grade mucoepidermoid, acinic cell, adenoid cystic, epidermoid malignant pleomorphic adenoma, adenocarcinoma, and undifferentiated tumors of the parotid gland should only undergo resection of immediately involved nerve branches, and receive immediate nerve interposition grafts.[36] If the above tumors have advanced to the T_3 stage (> 4 cm, multiple neck nodes, deep fixation, skin ulceration, or dysfunction of the facial nerve) radical parotidectomy and total sacrifice of the facial nerve are indicated. Frozen sections should verify free nerve margins. If there is evidence of facial nerve involvement into the mastoid bone, the skull should be resected until free nerve margins are obtained (see Chap. 21). Any patient with seventh nerve paralysis or recurrent malignancy should be treated by total sacrifice of the seventh nerve.

WHEN IS A WIDE-FIELD (MUSCLE, SKIN, MANDIBLE, MASTOID TIP, TEMPORAL BONE, ETC.) RESECTION OF THE PAROTID REGION INDICATED?

Any large parotid malignancy with extraparotid spread (T_4 lesion) but confined to the locally resectable area should be treated by aggressive surgery to achieve adequate margins. Surgery in this group of patients may include resection of soft tissues including skin, masseter muscle, and buccal fat pad, as well as mandible, zygoma, mastoid, or temporal bone. Current myocutaneous flap procedures allow an uncompromised resection of broad areas of soft tissue and bone (see Chap. 21)

WHICH PATIENTS WITH PAROTID TUMORS DERIVE CURATIVE BENEFIT FROM CERVICAL LYMPHADENECTOMY?

Any patient with palpable cervical lymph nodes should be treated with concomitant modified cervical lymphadenectomy. Lymph nodes, both occult or palpable, occur in 18%–25% of all patients with tumors of the major salivary gland at the time of treatment. Lymph nodes most likely to harbor metastatic disease include the subparotid, infraparotid, and subdigastric groups. To date, evidence does not exist to demonstrate clear curative benefit from routine elective cervical lymphadenectomy of a N_0 neck. Our series and several others have included patients with occult cervical lymph node metastases (found on pathologic tissue examination). A number of these patients are among the long-term survivors. The role of routine prophylactic neck dissection in patients with salivary gland cancers is controversial.[32] One must individualize on the basis of tumor histology, tumor stage, and clinical findings. In the absence of controlled trials, we recommend modified cervical lymphadenectomy for all patients with palpable cervical nodes. Patients with facial nerve paralysis or large tumors with deep fixation (T_3 lesions) have a higher incidence of lymph node metastasis; similarly, patients with aggressive biologic tumors of the epidermoid, malignant mixed tumors, and high-grade mucoepidermoid type may benefit from prophylactic lymph node dissections. All patients with submaxillary tumors should undergo modified cervical lymphadenectomy.

WHICH PATIENTS AND WHICH SPECIFIC TUMOR TYPES BENEFIT FROM POSTOPERATIVE RADIATION THERAPY?

It has recently been reported[26] that radiation therapy is beneficial in the treatment of patients with recurrent salivary gland malignancies. There are no clear data to support or refute the benefit of radiation therapy for patients suspected of harbouring residual microscopic foci. Evidence of perineural involvement, large tumors (T_3 or T_4 lesions), high-grade cancers (undifferentiated, malignant mixed tumors, adenocarcinoma, adenoid cystic, high-grade mucoepidermoid, and epidermoid), positive regional lymph nodes, or deep lobe location has been cited as reason for adding postoperative irradiation.[17, 30]

Response rates of observable parotid cancers to photon beam therapy have been under 33% despite pushing doses to the maximum tissue tolerance.[37] A single report of excellent local tumor control with neutron beam therapy (80%–90% response, all histologic cell types) is encouraging.[38] The future may hold more promise if this report is confirmed by others.

REFERENCES

1. McQuarrie D.G., Winter L.: Papillary cystadenoma lymphomatosum: An unusual incidence. *Arch. Surg.* 93:511–516, 1966.

1a. Spiro R.H., Koss L.G., Majdu S.I., et al.: Tumors of minor salivary origin: A clinicopathologic study of 492 cases. *Cancer* 31:117–129, 1973.
2. McCormack L.J., Cauldwell E.W., Anson B.J.: The surgical anatomy of the facial nerve: With special reference to the parotid gland. *Surg. Gynecol. Obstet.* 80:620–630, 1945.
3. Davis R.A., Anson B.J., Budinger J.M., et al.: Surgical anatomy of the facial nerve and parotid gland based upon a study of 350 cervicofacial halves. *Surg. Gynecol. Obstet.* 102:385–412, 1956.
4. Krolls S.O., Trodahl J.N., Boyers R.C.: Salivary gland lesions in children. A survey of 430 cases. *Cancer* 36:145–155, 1972.
5. Malett K.J., Harrison M.S.: The recurrence of salivary gland tumors. *J. Laryngol. Otol.* 85:439–448, 1971.
6. Frazell R.L.: Observations in the management of salivary gland tumors. *Cancer* 18:235–241, 1968.
7. Baker D.C., Conley J.: Treatment of massive deep lobe parotid tumors. *Am. J. Surg.* 138:572–575, 1979.
8. Grage T.B., Lober P.H., Shahon D.B.: Benign tumors of the major salivary glands. *Surgery* 50:625–633, 1961.
9. State D, Grage T.B.: Surgical treatment of parotid tumors. *Curr. Probl. Surg.* January 1966, pp. 3–67.
10. Chen K.T.K.: Metastasizing pleomorphic adenoma of the salivary gland. *Cancer* 42:2407–2411, 1978.
11. Rosai J.: Major and minor salivary glands, in *Ackerman's Surgical Pathology*. St. Louis, C.V. Mosby Co., 1981.
12. Turnbull A.D., Frazell E.L.: Multiple tumors of the major salivary gland. *Am. J. Surg.* 118:787–789. 1969.
13. Gray S.R., Cornog J.L. Jr., Seo I.S.: Oncocytic neoplasms of salivary glands. A report of fifteen cases including two malignant oncocytomas. *Cancer* 38:1306–1317, 1976.
14. Kassan S.S., Gardy M.: Sjögrens syndrome: An update and overview. *Am. J. Med.* 64:1037–1046, 1978.
15. Grage T.B., Lober P.H.: Benign lymphoepithelial lesions of the salivary glands. *Am. J. Surg.* 108:495–499, 1964.
16. Grage T.B., Lober P.H.: Malignant tumors of the major salivary glands. *Surgery* 52:284–294, 1962.
17. Johns M.E.: Parotid cancer: A rational basis for treatment. *Head Neck Surg.* 3:132–144, 1980.
18. Spiro R.H., Huvos A.G., Berk R., et al.: Mucoepidermoid carcinoma of salivary gland origin. *Am. J. Surg.* 136:461–468, 1978.
19. Sven J.Y., Johns M.E.: Chemotherapy for salivary gland cancer. *Laryngoscope* 92:235–239, 1982.
20. Grage T.B., Lober P.H., Arhelger S.W.: Acinic cell carcinoma of the parotid gland. *Am. J. Surg.* 102:765–768, 1961.
21. Eneroth C.M., Jakobsson P.A.: Acinic cell carcinoma of the parotid gland. *Cancer* 19:1761–1772, 1966.
22. Attie J.N., Sciubba J.J.: Tumors of major and minor salivary glands: Clinical and pathologic features. *Curr. Probl. Surg.* February 1981, pp. 67–155.
23. Perzin K.H., Gullane P., Clairmont A.C.: Adenoid cystic carcinomas arising in salivary glands: A correlation of histologic features and clinical course. *Cancer* 42:265–289, 1978.
24. Woods J.E., Chang G.C., Beahrs O.H.: Experience with 1360 primary parotid tumors. *Am. J. Surg.* 130:460–462, 1975.
25. Cummings C.W.: Adenoid cystic carcinoma (cylindroma) of the parotid. *Ann. Otol.* 86:280–292, 1977.
26. Guillamondegui O.M., Byers R.M., Luna M.A., et al.: Aggressive surgery in the treatment for parotid cancer: The risk of adjunctive radiotherapy. *AJR* 123:49–54, 1975.
27. Tannock I.F., Sutherland D.J.: Chemotherapy for adenoid cystic carcinoma. *Cancer* 46:452–454, 1980.
28. Eneroth C.M., Zetterberg A.: Malignancy in pleomorphic adenoma. *Acta Otolaryngol.* 77:426–432, 1974.
29. Anderson L.G., Talal N.: The spectrum of benign to malignant lymphoproliferation in Sjögren's syndrome. *Clin. Exp. Immunol.* 9:199–221, 1971.
30. Krause C.J.: The management of parotid neoplasms. *Head Neck Surg.* 3:340–343, 1980.
31. Spiro R.H. Huvos A.G., Strong E.W.: Malignant mixed tumor of salivary origin: A clinicopathologic study of 146 cases. *Cancer* 39:388–396, 1977.
32. Perzik S.L., Fisher B.: The place of neck dissection in the management of parotid tumors. *Am. J. Surg.* 120:355–358, 1970.
33. Ronkow R.M.: Surgical decisions in the treatment of major salivary gland tumors. *Plast. Reconstr. Surg.* 51:514–523, 1973.
34. Foote F.W., Frazell E.L.: Tumors of the major salivary glands. *Cancer* 6:1065–1133, 1953.
35. Eneroth C.M.: Salivary gland tumors in the parotid gland, submandibular gland, and the palate region. *Cancer* 27:1415–1418, 1971.
36. Woods J.E.: The facial nerve in parotid malignancy. *Am. J. Surg.* 146:493–496, 1983.
37. Kagan A.R., Nussbaum H., Handler S., et al.: Recurrences from malignant parotid salivary gland tumors. *Cancer* 37:2600–2604, 1976.
38. Kaul R., Hendrickson F., Cohen L., et al.: Fast neutrons in the treatment of salivary gland tumors. *Int. J. Radiat. Oncol. Biol. Phys.* 7:1667–1671, 1981.

21 / Cancers Involving the Middle Ear and Temporal Bone

George L. Adams, M.D.

Malignant tumors involve the temporal bone in one of four ways: (1) primary malignancy of the external canal, (2) primary malignancy of the middle ear and mastoid, (3) metastasis from a distant site, or (4) direct extension from a parotid malignancy.

Primary malignant tumors of the temporal bone are rare. The rarity of this tumor can be seen from the following data:

1. At the Royal Victoria Hospital in Montreal, there were nine cases in 8 years.
2. Newhart found 34 cases described prior to 1917.
3. Furstenberg found an additional 14 cases described by 1924 and reported on two cases of adenocarcinoma seen at the University of Michigan.[1]
4. In 1964, Tabb reported on nine cases at New Orleans Charity Hospital in a 15-year period.
5. Goodwin and Jesse reported on 85 cases of squamous cell carcinoma of the external canal and middle ear treated at M. D. Anderson Hospital between 1967 and 1974.[2] Twelve additional patients had involvement of the temporal bone from primary tumors of the salivary gland.
6. Lodge et al. reported six malignant cases in a population of 1 million over a 3-year period.[3]
7. In a 15-year period, there were 16 patients with primary malignant tumors of the external ear canal or mastoid treated at the University of Minnesota.[4, 5] During the same period, there were ten patients with disease metastatic to the temporal bone and four patients with direct extension from tumors of the salivary glands.

WHAT IS THE MOST COMMON TYPE OF MALIGNANCY?

As in other areas of the head and neck, squamous cell carcinoma is the most common form of carcinoma (> 50% of cases). Malignant tumors arising in the external canal also include basal cell carcinoma (second most common) and melanoma, and the middle ear can be the site of primary squamous cell carcinoma or adenocarcinoma.

IN WHAT AGE GROUP DO THESE TUMORS OCCUR?

Both squamous cell and basal cell cancers are most common over age 60, with basal cell cancer more common in the even older group. There is a slight male preponderance, 60:40.

WHERE DO THESE TUMORS ARISE?

At least 90% and perhaps all squamous cell carcinomas of the canal and middle ear arise in the external canal and extend into the middle ear. Tumors arising in the conchal area may extend down the canal and invade the surrounding bone. Fissures through the cartilaginous canal allow anteriorly located tumors of the canal to extend into the parotid area. Unusual tumors such as adenocystic carcinoma and carcinoma of the ceruminous glands arise in the glandular structures of the external canal. For practical purposes, they are managed in much the same way as is squamous cell carcinoma. Tumors that arise on the auricle and then invade the temporal bone, causing facial paralysis, have a very poor prognosis.

WHAT ARE THE MOST COMMON SYMPTOMS?

A chronically draining ear is by far the most common symptom. There is often a longstanding history of chronic drainage of more than 20 years' duration. The drainage is foul-smelling, frequently painless, and very similar to that seen in chronic otomastoiditis. Signs and symptoms include (1) an aural polyp or chronic infection, (2) pain, (3) cranial nerve VII paralysis, (4) other cranial nerve pareses, (5) hemorrhage, (6) hearing loss, (7) vertigo, (8) tinnitus, (9) hemotympanum, and (10) acute otitis media or mastoiditis.

HOW CAN I DISTINGUISH A PRIMARY TUMOR FROM A METASTATIC TUMOR?

The clinical presentation may be the same.[6–8] Past history of a malignancy is the most important key. Biopsy in the office will be sufficient in the case of a thyroid, kidney, or breast cancer. If the tumor is an adenocarcinoma or squamous cell carcinoma, a metastatic survey is indicated. This should include a chest x-ray, bone scan, and liver and spleen scan. These examinations serve a twofold purpose. If there is a primary cancer, it is important to make certain metastases do not exist; if it is metastatic, it is essential to determine the primary site. Figures 21–1 through 21–3 show three different presentations of primary squamous cell and basal cell cancers of the ear canal.

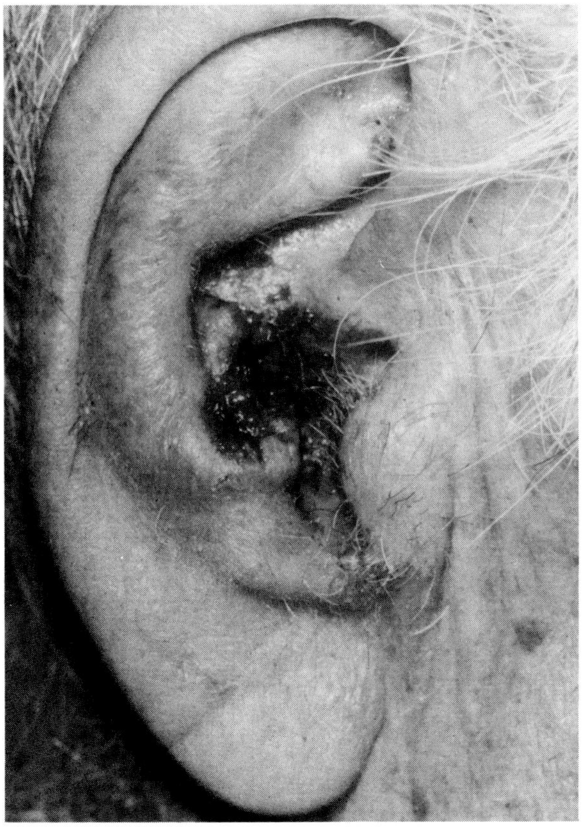

Fig 21–1.—Basal cell carcinoma of the conchal area with invasion into underlying bone. A sleeve resection of the canal, mastoidectomy, and resection of a large segment of the pinna were required.

WHAT ARE THE MALIGNANCIES THAT MOST COMMONLY METASTASIZE TO THE TEMPORAL BONE?

The lung and breast are the most common sites of primaries that metastasize to the temporal bone, followed by the kidney, stomach, and thyroid. In addition, the temporal bone and mastoid can be involved by lymphoma and leukemia. Proctor and Lindsay pointed out that the marrow of the petrous bone serves as a filter.[9] Thus, many secondary malignancies will arise in the petrous area, extend to the mastoid, and cause the symptoms in the middle ear.

HOW DO PAROTID MALIGNANCIES SPREAD TO THE TEMPORAL BONE?

In advanced cases, it is sometimes difficult to distinguish whether the tumor arose deep in the canal and then invaded the parotid, or vice versa. Embryologic pathways exist from the parotid region to the external canal (Huschke's canal). A history of a long standing parotid mass or a previous parotidectomy for a malignant tumor is usually obtainable. Tumors of the inferior alveolar ridge, tonsillar area, and nasopharynx can extend to the temporal bone.

HOW ARE THESE TUMORS CLASSIFIED?

Primary malignancies of the temporal bone are classified by location—outer ear canal, deep canal, and middle ear. The outer canal also includes the conchal area, and it should be noted whether the malignancy is

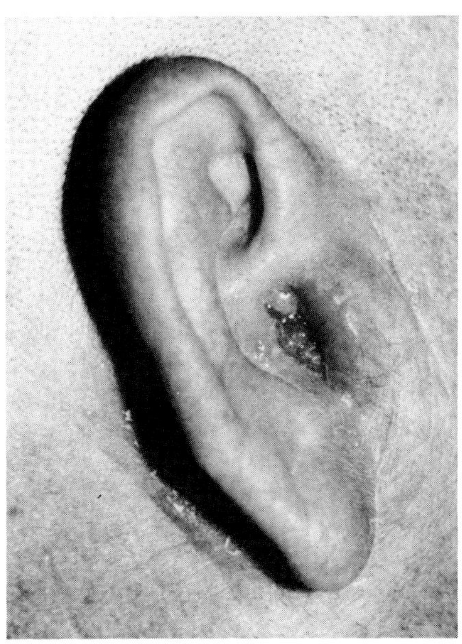

Fig 21–2.—Squamous cell carcinoma of the external canal. A lateral temporal bone resection was required.

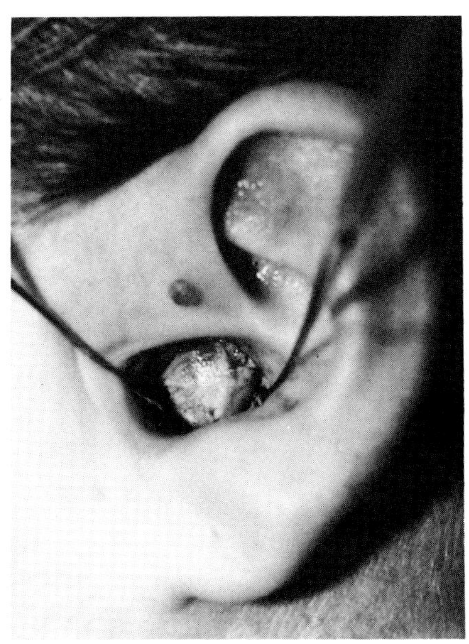

Fig 21–3.—Squamous cell carcinoma. Every aural polyp requires a biopsy.

anterior or posterior. Both the treatment and the prognosis are dependent on the site of involvement.[10–12] Tumors of the outer third of the canal and conchal area are associated with the best prognosis—a 50% 5-year survival. Patients with tumors of the middle ear have approximately a 27% 5-year survival. When the temporal bone is involved extensively by a malignancy of the parotid gland, the survival rate is very poor despite extensive surgery. Such surgery may prolong life but is generally more palliative than curative.

WHAT IS THE PREFERRED TREATMENT?

Currently, surgery is the preferred treatment, in combination with preoperative or postoperative irradiation. Occasional patients present with disease that cannot be resected with negative margins, and surgery may be performed for palliation and relief of pain and otorrhea. Radiation is delivered postoperatively to enhance the survival rate when the margins are clear. When radiation is delivered in the presence of positive margins, the survival rate is not increased. Radiation is not used as the primary modality when cartilage or bone is involved because there is a significant risk of osteonecrosis and brain damage. Even basal cell carcinoma of the ear canal can invade bone and become resistant to radiation. (In the ear canal, the skin lies directly upon bone; there is no subcutaneous tissue.)

HOW IS IT DETERMINED THAT THE PATIENT HAS RESECTABLE DISEASE?

This is the most important and most difficult portion of evaluation of a patient with malignancy of the temporal bone. Most important, a patient with chronic external otitis, chronic drainage, and aural polyps or granulation tissue needs a biopsy in the office to determine the possibility of the existence of a malignancy (see Figs 21–1 through 21–3). Early diagnosis is crucial. These tumors tend to invade the temporal lobe or cerebellum. They do extend down the eustachian tube and to the carotid artery. They may extend along tissue planes along the base of the skull without any clinical or radiologic findings.

Although routine mastoid x-ray studies are helpful for eliciting evidence of bone destruction, until recently polytomography was the single best diagnostic tool. The computerized tomographic (CT) scan has become the preferred diagnostic tool for establishing whether there is intracranial extension.[13] Erosion of the petrous bone alone suggests that one is dealing with a metastatic tumor or inoperable primary tumor. The base of the skull where the carotid and jugular enter must be evaluated by CT scan. This triangular area of bone must be intact if surgery is to be considered.

Clinical examination of cranial nerves IX, X, XI, and XII is important. Loss of function occurs if there is extension or metastases to the transverse process of C1–2 (node of Ranvier). X-ray films of the base of the skull are obtained to look for destruction of the spine of the sphenoid. Any destruction medial to this is a sign of inoperability.

WHAT IS THE INCIDENCE OF CERVICAL METASTASES?

All series are small, but for squamous cell carcinoma, the incidence of cervical metastases is 12%–18%. Tumors of the deep canal have the highest incidence of metastasis.

WHAT SURGERY IS PERFORMED?

The extent of the surgical procedure must be specifically tailored to the size, type, and location of the tumor of the temporal bone.[14–19]

1. Malignant tumors of the outer third of the canal and conchal area are treated by an expanded sleeve resection of the area. In all anterior tumors, the parotid is included as part of the resection. The canal is then resected en bloc, just lateral to the tympanic membrane. If the facial nerve is paralyzed, the resection includes the nerve. If there is no evidence of facial involvement, the facial canal can be identified from behind and lifted from the canal, the resection completed, and the nerve laid into a new area.

2. Tumors lying deep in the canal require a more aggressive approach. If there is evidence of invasion of the middle ear or mastoid, a formal resection of the temporal bone is required. Tumors of lesser size can be resected by a lateral temporal bone resection. This includes a mastoidectomy and resection of the entire bony and cartilaginous canal, the tympanic membrane and ossicles, the parotid gland, and frequently the condyle or portion of the ascending ramus of the mandible[15, 19] The facial nerve can seldom be preserved. A facial-hypoglossal anastomosis may be performed.

3. Tumors of the middle ear or mastoid and large tumors of the external canal require resection of the total temporal bone. This procedure was initially reported by Ward et al.[19] and Campbell[14] in 1951. Campbell's operation required a piecemeal resection of the temporal bone. Parsons and Lewis removed the temporal bone en bloc in 11 cases reported in 1954.[15] There were two postoperative deaths.

Conley reported on 36 cases in 1965.[10] He had no operative deaths, but ten patients (31%) had significant operative complications including leakage of CSF, herniation of the brain, wound infection, and meningitis.

The incidence of cervical metastasis was 16% and elective dissection of the neck was not advised.

Hilding and Selker made a major contribution to surgery on the temporal bone when they described their techniques in 1969.[17] These techniques added the needed safety to the resection by providing a means of defining and protecting the carotid artery as the first portion of the procedure. This is the technique currently employed as they described it:

1. An extended parotidectomy incision is made. If the tumor involves the canal, a core of skin from the canal is retained as part of the specimen. Extensive involvement of the conchal area requires total resection of the auricle with a scalp-rotation flap or split thickness skin graft (STSG) for closure (Fig 21–4).
2. The facial nerve is identified and divided after it enters the parotid gland.
3. A parotidectomy is performed and includes cervical nodes in the upper neck area.
4. The zygomatic process is identified and a portion of the arch removed.
5. The ascending ramus of the mandible is divided and removed. This permits the necessary access to the condylar fossa (Fig 21–6 and 21–7).
6. The carotid artery and jugular vein are identified in the neck by retracting soft tissue in the area of the mastoid.

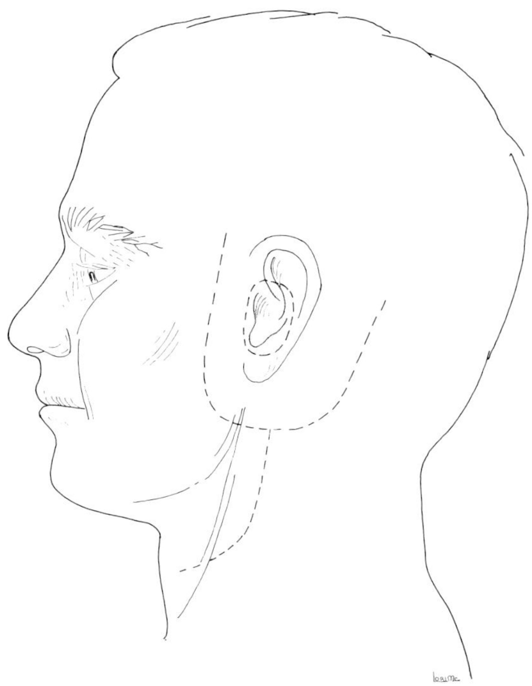

Fig 21–4.—Incision for partial or total temporal bone resection. A conchal incision for a smaller tumor of the external canal permits preservation of pinna; an anterior limb permits parotidectomy; an inferior extension permits upper neck dissection and allows identification of the carotid artery and jugular vein.

7. The microscope and mastoid drill are now utilized. The condylar fossa is carefully drilled away, exposing the carotid artery. The chorda tympani, tensor tympani, and eustachian tube are exposed. The entire length of the carotid artery can now be traced.
8. An approach through the middle cranial fossa is used to expose the tegmen tympani from above. Keeping the head of the table elevated will reduce pressure from CSF and permit safer retraction of the temporal lobe. Figure 21–5 shows a top view and cross section of the area.
9. The lateral sinus and the jugular bulb are exposed by removing bone in the posterior mastoid. Heavy bleeding can occur from the petrosal sinus. This is controlled by packing with Gelfoam. Persistent bleeding is controlled with pledgets of free muscle sutured to the sinus or dura, in much the same manner by which hemorrhage of the liver or spleen is controlled.
10. A chisel is placed medial to the arcuate eminence and a controlled fracture is made. This is very similar to a transverse fracture of the temporal bone (Fig 21–7).
11. The specimen is removed and, if feasible, an anastomosis of the facial-hypoglossal nerve is performed. Figure 21–8 shows the completed resection.

Invasive tumors extending from the oral cavity, parotid gland, or adjacent tissues are handled in a similar manner. It is imperative that a thorough evaluation be done to determine resectability. Because of the low cure rate and high morbidity, performing such extensive surgery requires a great deal of forethought. More commonly, portions of a temporal bone resection are performed with radical parotidectomy: that is, resection of the tympanic segment, identification of the facial nerve with resection of the tip of the mastoid, and resection of a segment of the mastoid for a high ligation of the jugular vein.

WHAT IS THE ROLE OF THERAPEUTIC IRRADIATION?

C.C. Wang delivered postoperative therapeutic irradiation to 20 patients.[20] All four patients with lateral tumors of the canal were alive at 5 years, and seven of ten patients with deeper tumors were also alive. In that series, five patients had osteonecrosis. Surgery for recurrent disease after full-course radiation therapy has a particularly high rate of complications. In Conley's series, these complications included meningitis, hernia of the brain, and delayed healing.[21]

SUMMARY

Resection of the temporal bone with postoperative therapeutic irradiation is the preferred treatment for

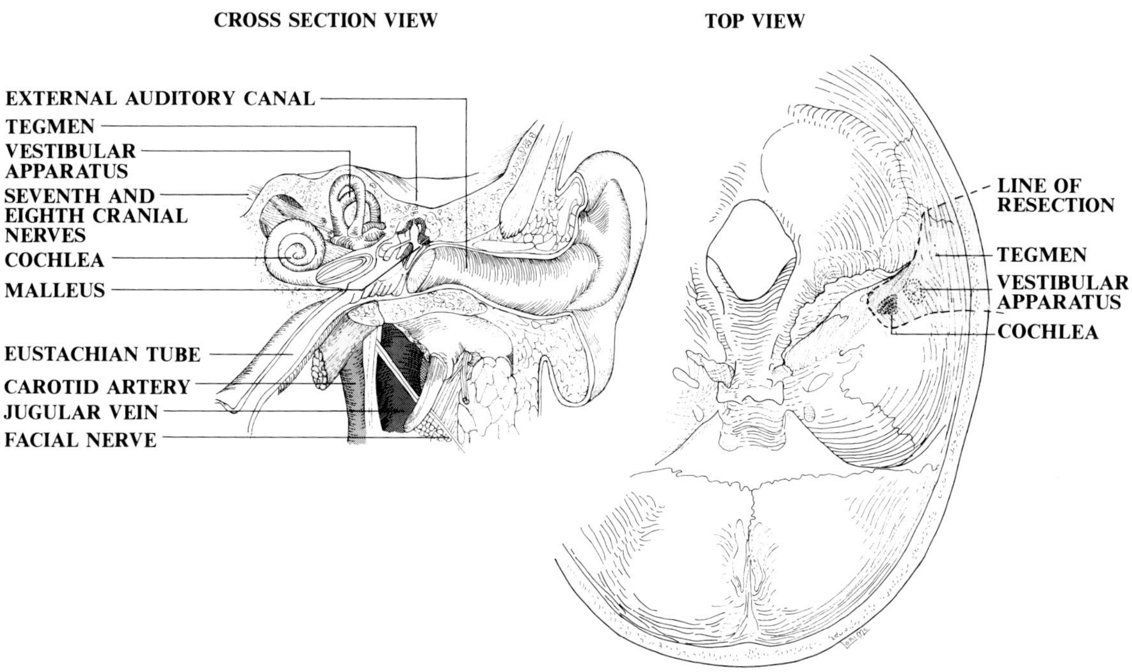

Fig 21–5.—Temporal bone resection. A partial temporal bone resection includes en bloc removal of the external auditory canal and middle ear contents. For a total temporal bone resection, a chisel cut is made medial to the superior semicircular canal (arcuate eminence).

malignant tumors of the deep canal with involvement of the middle ear. Tumors located more laterally can be resected by a lateral temporal bone resection, generally with a total parotidectomy and condylectomy. Prior to any resection, polytomography and CT scanning are required to define the extent of disease. It is not unusual to encounter more tumor than was appreciated preoperatively. Resection of the temporal bone, even as made safer by the method of Hilding and Selker, is associated with significant loss of blood, prolonged oper-

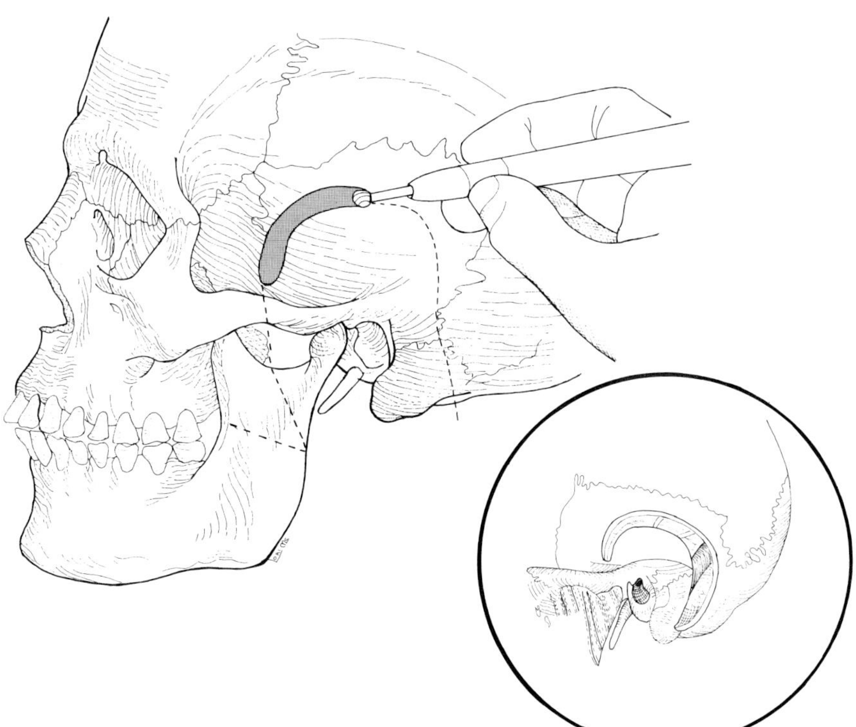

Fig 21–6.—Temporal bone resection: Delineation of en bloc resection of the temporal bone. Resection of the mandibular condyle provides an anterior margin and access to the internal carotid artery. The middle fossa and posterior fossa durae are exposed. The sigmoid sinus can be pushed posteriorly. Bleeding from the sinus is controlled by suturing muscle pledgets to any vessel wall lacerations.

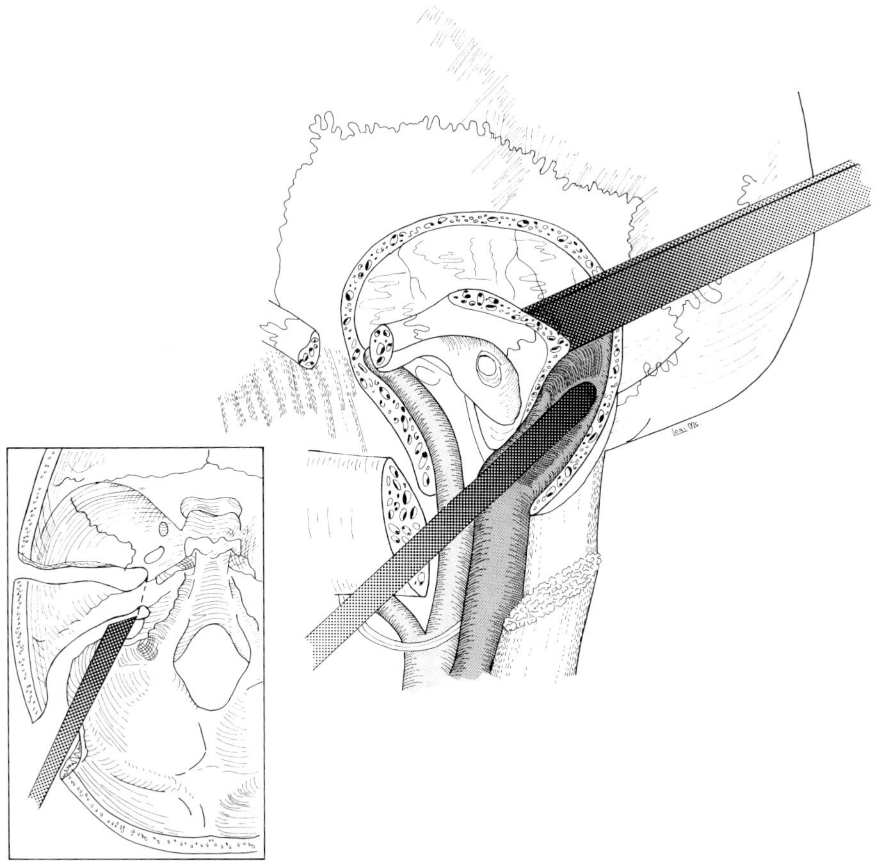

Fig 21–7.—Temporal bone resection. The carotid artery has been defined and protected. The transverse incision is made from above. A carefully executed posterior chisel cut completes the en block resection.

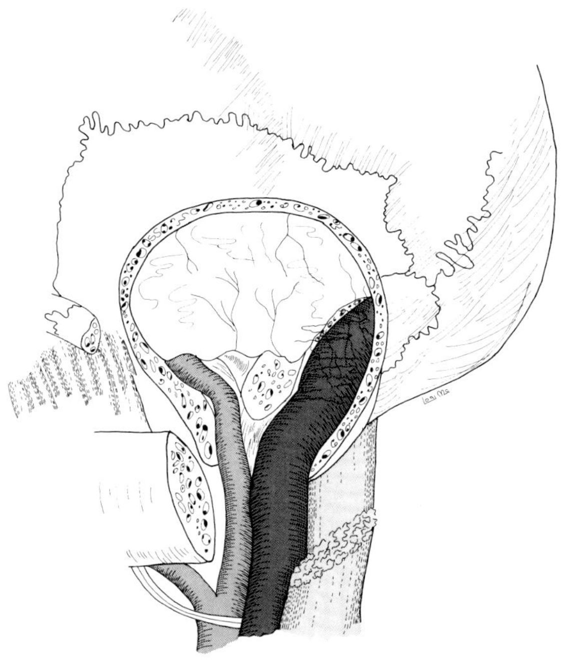

Fig 21–8.—Completion of a total temporal bone resection. Included in the specimen are the lateral portion of the petrous bone; the mastoid, middle ear, and external canal; the condyle of mandible; and all of the parotid gland. The facial nerve has been sacrificed. Repair can be performed with regional rotation flaps or a pectoralis major myocutaneous flap.

ative procedure (10–15 hours), a high operative morbidity, and significant mortality. Patients with positive margins die of disease, despite postoperative irradiation. The possibility that the tumor is metastatic to the temporal bone should be considered. Tumors of the lung, heart, and kidney tend to metastasize to the petrous portion of the temporal bone.

REFERENCES

1. Furstenberg A.C.: Primary adenocarcinoma of the middle ear and mastoid. *Ann. Otol.* 33:677, 1924.
2. Goodwin J.G., Jesse R.H.: Malignant neoplasms of the auditory canal and temporal bone. *Arch. Otol.* 106:675–679, 1980.
3. Lodge W.O., Jones H.M., Smith M.E.: Malignant tumors of the temporal bone. *Arch. Otolaryngol.* 61:535, 1955.
4. Berlinger N.T., Koutroupas S., Adams G., et al.: Patterns of involvement of the temporal bone in metastatic and systemic malignancy. *Laryngoscope* 90:619–627, 1980.
5. Adams G.L., Paparella M.M., Elfiky F.M.: Primary and metastatic tumors of the temporal bone. *Laryngoscope* 82:1273–1285, 1971.
6. Mawson S.R.: *Diseases of the Ear*, ed. 2. London, Edward Arnold, Ltd., 1967.
7. Schuknecht H.F., Allam A.F., Yoshihiko M.: Pathology

of secondary malignant tumors of the temporal bone. *Ann. Otol.* 77:5, 1968.

8. Maddox H.E.: Metastatic tumors of the temporal bone. *Ann. Otol.* 76:149, 1967.
9. Proctor B., Lindsay J.R.: Tumors involving the petrous pyramid of the temporal bone. *Arch. Otolaryngol.* 46:180, 1947.
10. Conley J.J.: Cancer of the middle ear. *Ann. Otol.* 74:555, 1965.
11. Lederman M.: Malignant tumors of the ear. *J. Laryngol.* 79:85, 1965.
12. Frew I., Finney R.: Neoplasms of the middle ear. *J. Laryngol.* 77:415, 1963.
13. Olsen K.D., DeSanto L.W., Forbes G.S.: Radiographic assessment of squamous cell carcinoma of the temporal bone. *Laryngoscope* 93:1162–1167, 1983.
14. Campbell E.: Total resection of the temporal bone for malignancy of the middle ear. *Ann. Surg.* 134:397, 1951.
15. Parsons H., Lewis J.S.: Subtotal resection of the temporal bone for cancer of the ear. *Cancer* 7:995, 1954.
16. Lewis J.S., Page R.: Radical surgery for malignant tumors of the ear. *Arch. Otolaryngol.* 83:114, 1966.
17. Hilding D.A., Selker R.: Total resection of the temporal bone for carcinoma. *Arch. Otolaryngol.* 89:636, 1969.
18. Hilding D.A., Selker R.: Total resection of the temporal bone for carcinoma. *Arch. Otolaryngol.* 89:636–645, 1969.

19 Ward G.E., Loch W.E., Lawrence W.: Radical operation for carcinoma of the external auditory canal and middle ear. *Am. J. Surg.* 82:169–178, 1951.

20. Wang C.C.: Radiation therapy in the management of carcinoma of the external auditory canal, middle ear and mastoid. *Radiology* 116:713–715, 1975.
21. Conley J., Schuller D.: Malignancies of the ear. *Laryngoscope* 86:1147–1163, 1976.

22 / Melanoma of the Head and Neck

MICHAEL L. SCHWARTZ, M.D., PH.D.

IS MELANOMA A RARITY? WILL I EVER SEE ONE?

APPROXIMATELY 17,400 new cases of melanoma were diagnosed in 1983.[1] This figure represents 2% of all cancers diagnosed in the United States. About 20% of all melanomas occur in the head and neck area. The frequency with which melanoma is diagnosed is rapidly increasing in almost all parts of the world (Table 22–1). The reasons for the increased number of cases are not clear but may be related to increased recreational activity in the sun, changes in clothing, migration to the "sun belts," and an increase in ultraviolet light exposure from a decrease in the atmospheric ozone layer. The rate of increase in melanoma is unparalleled by that of any cancer except lung cancer. It is probably not due to an increase in the reporting of cases.

WHAT LESIONS ARE CLINICALLY SUSPECT FOR MELANOMA?

Melanomas occur primarily in whites. Whites have an average of 15–20 pigmented moles over their entire body surface. Since there are six new melanomas diagnosed per 100,000 population per year, approximately 1 in 250,000 moles will be a melanoma. Obviously some guidelines are necessary in attempting to decide which lesions to biopsy.

The key to recognizing a melanoma is irregularity. The color is often irregular. Shades of gray, brown, red, pink, blue, white, and black may be present in the lesion, or there may be no pigmentation at all. The outline of the lesion is also irregular—notching is a particular characteristic. There may also be an indistinct margin or even satellite lesions. The surface of the lesion is often irregular in height and texture. Ulceration may be present. Changes in size and color are the earliest changes noted in melanomas (Table 22–2). Ulceration, bleeding, and itching occur in thicker lesions.

TABLE 22–1.—INCIDENCE OF MELANOMA

	EARLIER PERIOD (per 100,000 Population)	LATER PERIOD* (per 100,000 Population)	TIME INTERVAL (yr)
United States			
New York[2, 3]	1.2	4.3	27
Texas[4]	2.6	7.0	18
Norway[5]	1.9	5.0	18
Sweden[5]	1.6	4.5	18

*Later reporting period was 1966–1972 for all series.

TABLE 22–2.—SIGNS AND SYMPTOMS OF MELANOMA ACCORDING TO TUMOR THICKNESS: % OF PATIENTS*

	THICKNESS (MM)			
SIGN/SYMPTOM	<.85	0.85–1.69	1.70–3.64	>3.65
Increase in size	55	49	51	72
Color change	49	47	45	58
Increase in height	36	51	59	82
Bleeding	13	25	48	63
Ulcer	5	15	33	50
Itching	20	30	29	46

*Percent of patients (total, 598) having a particular sign or symptom.
From Sober et al.[6] Reproduced by permission.

Changes in any mole such as ulceration, bleeding, color change, itching, size, contour change, or infection are highly suspicious of a melanoma. Several beautifully illustrated, highly descriptive monographs have been published on the clinical recognition of melanoma.[7, 8]

A number of articles have addressed the clinical accuracy of diagnosing a melanoma. Epstein et al.[9] made the clinical diagnosis of melanoma 31 times in the course of examining 559 black lesions. Biopsy proved the diagnosis in only 12 instances (38%). Kopf et al.[10] studied the diagnostic accuracy in 99 melanomas. Twenty-three were not diagnosed as melanoma, and 19 benign lesions were thought to be melanoma, for a diagnostic accuracy of 64.4%. One should remember that even the experts are often incorrect in diagnosing melanoma clinically. Biopsy should be used liberally with any suspicious lesion to avoid the grave error of allowing a melanoma the opportunity to grow and metastasize.

IS IT HARMFUL TO PERFORM EXCISIONAL OR INCISIONAL BIOPSIES ON A MELANOMA?

There is no evidence that biopsy of a melanoma adversely affects the ultimate prognosis of the lesion. On the contrary, the first step in treating melanoma is to make the diagnosis.

Records of the California tumor registry were analyzed retrospectively to determine the role of biopsy in the prognosis of melanoma.[9] The 10-year crude survival rate was 55.8% in patients who underwent radical excision without biopsy, compared to 65.4% in patients who underwent biopsy before definitive treatment. Ames et al.[11] analyzed the cases of 166 patients with clinical stage I melanoma of the head and neck and found no difference in survival if patients underwent biopsy prior to referral to M. D. Anderson Hospital for treatment. Knutson et al.[12] analyzed the cases of 230 patients with melanoma of all sites and found no difference in long-term survival. Jones et al.[13] noted a 33% 5-year survival in patients who underwent incisional biopsy versus a 36% 5-year survival for all patients in his series. Finally, Cascinelli et al.[14] compared survival curves in 553 patients with (63) and without (490) previous biopsy and found no difference at 10 years. The information gained from biopsy far outweighs the theoretical disadvantages of biopsy.

When an excisional biopsy may be mutilating, an incisional biopsy should be performed. This is especially true for lesions about the face. When an excisional biopsy is possible, such as on the neck or scalp, a conservative biopsy, not one through the platysma muscle, is recommended. An excisional biopsy is not appropriate therapy. The depth of the lesion is of utmost importance in planning further therapy. A shave or curettage biopsy will not yield this information and should not be used to diagnose a melanoma.

ARE THERE DIFFERENT CLINICAL TYPES OF MELANOMA?

Three different types of melanoma occur in the head and neck region: lentigo maligna melanoma, superficial spreading melanoma, and nodular melanoma. Lentigo maligna melanoma (Fig 22–1), the least common form of melanoma (10% of cases), usually occurs on the cheek or temple of an elderly woman. It develops in a benign Hutchinson's freckle (lentigo maligna) (Fig 22–2). This lesion is usually an extensive, irregularly pigmented but smooth lesion. Thickening within the freckle signals the development of malignancy. Superficial spreading melanoma is the most common type of melanoma (70%). It has the typical irregular coloration, margins, and ulceration. It often grows superficially for some time (horizontal growth stage, Fig 22–3,A) before becoming deeply invasive (vertical growth phase, Fig 22–3,B). Nodular melanoma (15% of melanomas) is the most aggressive type of melanoma. Generally dark brown or black in color, it is deeply invasive at the onset and has usually metastasized by lymphatic or hematogenous routes by the time of diagnosis (Fig 22–4).

WHAT ARE THE USEFUL METHODS OF CLASSIFYING MELANOMA?

The American Joint Committee on Cancer has published guidelines for staging head and neck melanoma (Table 22–3).[15] Necessary for staging is a careful physical examination that includes inspection of the primary tumor for size, ulceration, and nodularity. Satellite nodules and in-transit metastases should be sought in surrounding skin. Regional nodes should be carefully palpated. Chest films and hemograms are required. Liver function studies are encouraged. Scanning the liver, brain, or bone is not useful in asymptomatic patients.[16] As can be seen from Table 22–3, microstaging by both Breslow's[17] and Clark's[18, 19] systems is included in the TNM classification scheme.

Before microstaging criteria were developed, clinical stage I melanoma had a highly variable outcome. Both the Breslow and the Clark systems allow the clinician to accurately identify the patients at greater risk of lymph node and systemic metastasis.

Clark et al.[18, 19] described five different levels of invasion by melanoma (Fig 22–5), as follows:

Level I: Tumor cells are confined to the epidermis without invasion of the basement membrane. This is not an invasive cancer.

Level II: Invasion of melanoma cells through the basal lamina into the papillary dermis.

Level III: Invasion of melanoma cells fills the papillary dermis and impinges on but does not invade the reticular dermis.

Level IV: Invasion of melanoma cells into the reticular dermis.

Level V: Invasion of melanoma cells into the subcutaneous tissue.

Breslow measured the depth of invasion of melanoma with an ocular micrometer. Specimens were fixed and sectioned at right angles to the skin surface. The depth of invasion was measured from the skin surface to the deepest point of invasion. Although both methods of microstaging are used in the TNM classification, the Breslow method seems to be in more widespread use. It is simpler to use and results are probably more reproducible than with the Clark method. Balch et al.[20, 21] noted that Clark levels III and IV include markedly different depths of invasion (>.76 mm to 4.00 mm) with markedly different survival rates (Table 22–4). Using a multifactorial method of analysis, Balch et al. also noted that when Clark levels were controlled for depth of invasion (Breslow's method), the level of invasion was not significant.

AFTER DIAGNOSIS AND MICROSTAGING, WHAT OPERATION IS APPROPRIATE TO CONTROL THE PRIMARY LESION?

The standard answer to this question is a wide excision that includes the deep fascia. Wide excision means 5-cm gross margins for lesions on the trunk and extrem-

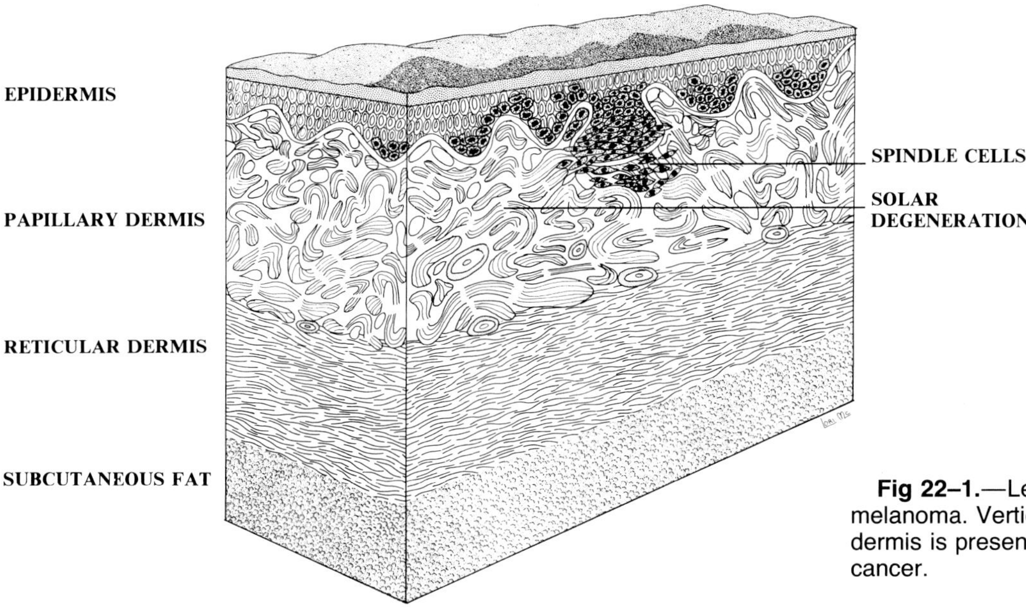

LENTIGO MALIGNA MELANOMA

Fig 22–1.—Lentigo maligna melanoma. Vertical growth into papillary dermis is present. This is an invasive cancer.

ities. Surgical margins of 5 cm are possible for lesions on the scalp and neck but are disfiguring for lesions on the face.

Breslow and Macht[22] excised 62 thin melanomas (< .76 mm depth of invasion) with less than 5-cm margins. The margin was 1.0 cm or less in 32%. None of these patients developed local recurrences or distinct metastases. Balch et al.[23] noted no recurrences when thin melanomas (< 0.76 mm) were excised with margins as narrow as 0.5 cm. They recommend 2-cm margins for thin melanoma. Das Gupta[24] noted eight local recurrences in ten patients with Clark level IV or V lesions but no local recurrences in 33 patients with lesions that extended into the papillary dermis (Clark level II). The WHO study[25] analyzed 281 patients with thin melanomas (< 2 mm). Local recurrence was noted in 4.4% when the primary lesion was excised with a 2-cm margin or less. The local recurrence rate was 1.3% when a margin greater than 2 cm was used. The difference was not statistically significant. With thick lesions, more

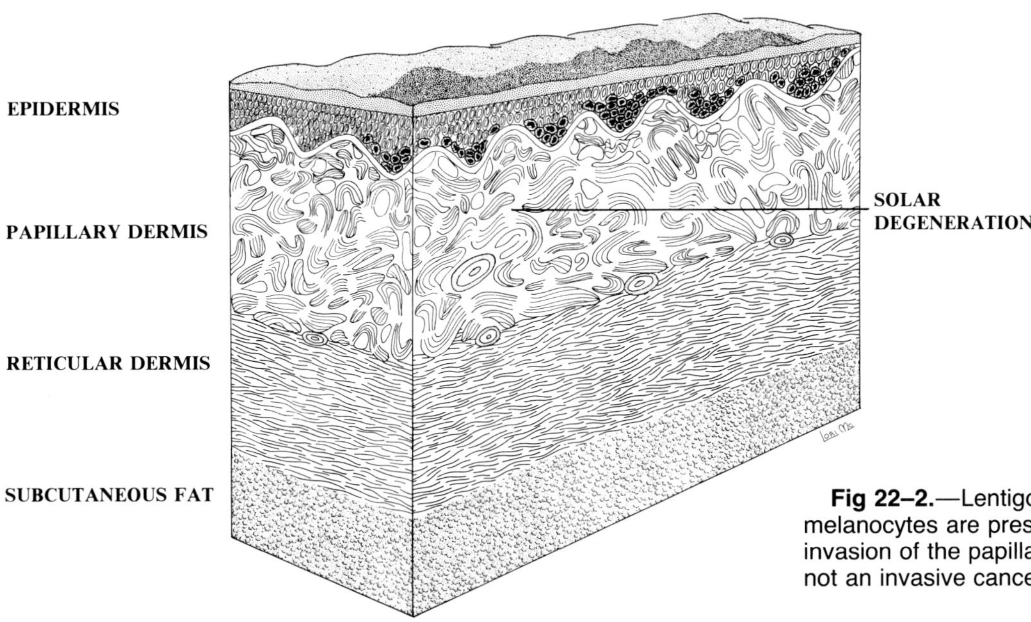

LENTIGO MALIGNA

Fig 22–2.—Lentigo maligna. Abnormal melanocytes are present, but there is no invasion of the papillary dermis. This is not an invasive cancer.

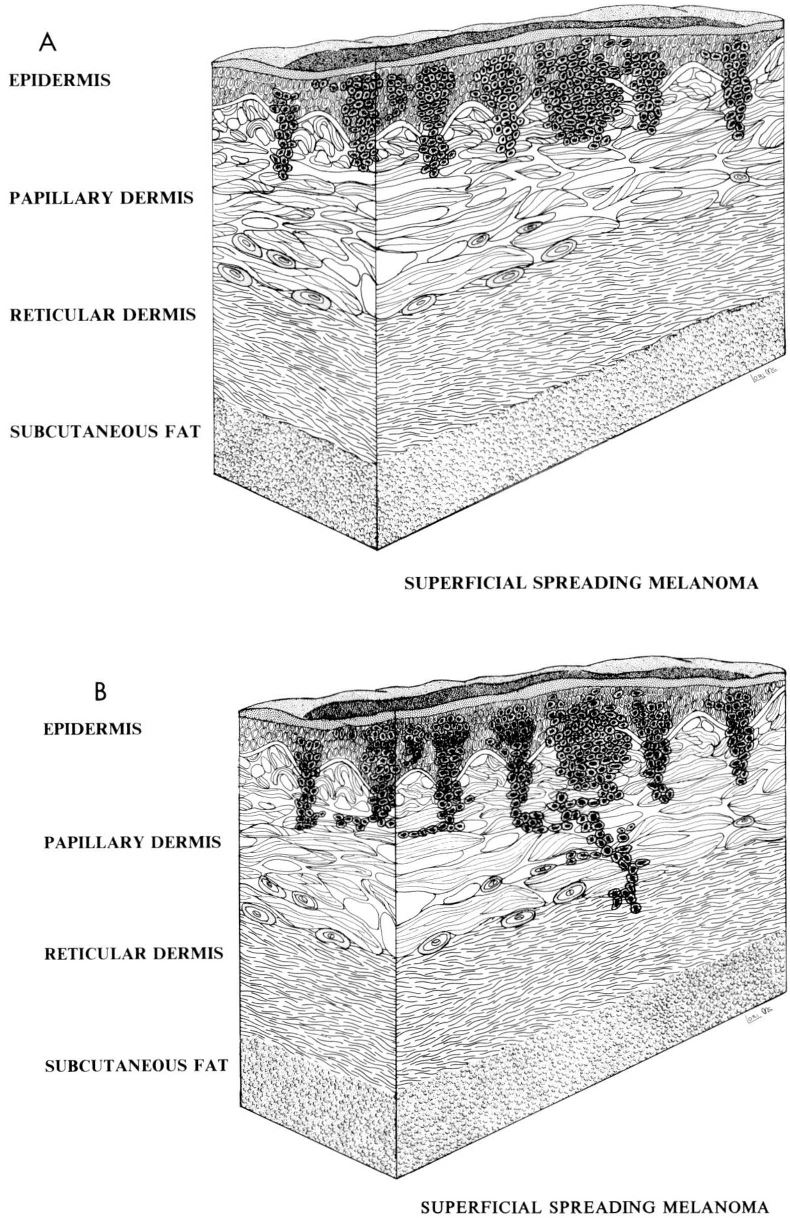

Fig 22–3.—Superficial spreading melanoma. Horizontal **(A)** and vertical **(B)** growth phases are illustrated.

than 2 mm in thickness, there was a significant difference in local recurrences: 12.1% with the smaller, 2-cm resection margin, versus 4.2% with wider margins.

It is apparent that the doctrine of 5-cm margins has fallen. The extent of resection is determined by the level of invasion as well as by the natural barriers on the face. Thicker lesions require a wider margin of resection, while thin melanomas may be completely excised with narrower margins. The narrowest margin of resection with thin lesions should probably be 2 cm. Larger resection margins, up to the classic 5-cm margin, are still warranted for thicker lesions on the neck and scalp where a large resection would not be mutilating.

The method of closure does not affect the cure rate if the lesion is completely excised.[11, 25] Therefore, where appropriate for the size of the defect after wide excision, split-thickness skin grafts, full-thickness skin grafts, flaps, or primary closure may be used to obtain the most cosmetic skin closure.

WHAT ABOUT DEEP MARGINS? IS IT NECESSARY TO REMOVE DEEP FASCIA?

Virtually every expert in the field of melanoma surgery recommends removal of the deep fascia along with the primary lesion. A single study by Olsen[26] gave a contrary view. He found a greater number of subse-

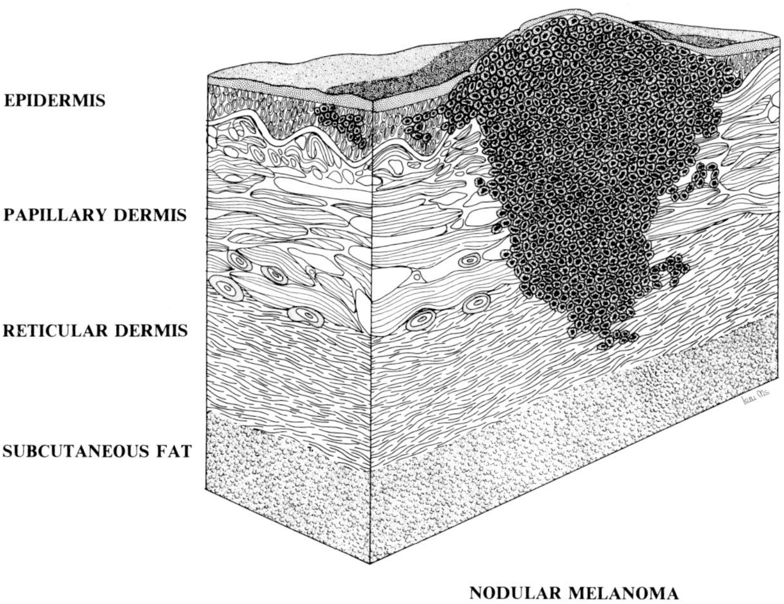

Fig 22–4.—Nodular melanoma. This melanoma is deeply invasive from inception.

quent node metastases when the deep fascia was removed. Olsen's study was retrospective and not controlled for depth of invasion. No other data exist on this still controversial issue.

WHEN SHOULD A RADICAL NECK DISSECTION BE PERFORMED ON A PATIENT WITH CLINICALLY POSITIVE NODES?

If a careful search for distant metastases is negative, clinically positive nodes should be resected by an appropriate neck dissection (Fig 22–6).

WHEN SHOULD A RADICAL NECK DISSECTION BE PERFORMED FOR CLINICALLY NEGATIVE NODES?

The answer to this problem is not perfectly clear, despite a wealth of literature on the subject. As Knutson et al. put it, "It would be of little comfort to a patient to realize the magnitude of the lack of concensus among surgeons regarding the best management of the regional lymph nodes of a patient with melanoma."[27] However, some answers can be synthesized by analyzing retrospective studies on head and neck lesions and prospective randomized studies on extremity lesions.

Four recent articles (Tables 22–5 and 22–6) examine the survival rates of head and neck melanoma patients. Comparing crude survival rates, Conley and Hamaker[28] and Ballantyne[29] found 16%–17% higher 5-year survival rates when elective radical neck dissection was performed along with wide local excision. Simons[30] and Ames et al.[11] noted strikingly similar rates of neck metastases in head and neck melanoma (see Table 22–6) but only a slightly greater survival rate when neck dissection was performed for microscopic disease rather than for the delayed development of clinically positive nodes. Figure 22–7 outlines some of the major decisions to be made.

The two randomized studies conducted thus far (Table 22–7) both fail to show an increase in survival following elective radical lymph node dissection. Unfortunately, both studies included only extremity lesions. There are no randomized studies of head and neck lesions. The Mayo clinic study[30] included a large proportion of thin melanomas (two thirds of cases), and there were very few patients—only seven—with microscopic node metastases. These two factors weight the study groups with patients who would most likely not benefit from regional node dissection. In addition, the follow-up period is short. Other authors have shown that the differences between groups may not be apparent until 5–8 years after treatment.[23]

The WHO prospective randomized study,[31] conducted by Veronesi et al., did not show a significant difference in survival between groups. The study has been widely quoted and widely criticized for (1) excluding lesions on the proximal limb, where lymph node dissection could be of great benefit, (2) including more women (450) than men (103), (3) including more lower extremity (458) than upper extremity (95) lesions, and (4) staging only 60% of the lesions according to Clark's and Breslow's methods. The only valid criticism is the last one, but the study began in 1967 before microstaging was proved to be useful. The patients that were staged did show a greater 5-year survival (70.1% vs. 58.3%) for Clark level IV lesions treated by node dis-

TABLE 22–3.—TNM CLASSIFICATION OF MELANOMA

Primary tumor	
Tx	No evidence of primary tumor (unknown primary or primary tumor removed and not histologically examined)
T_0	Atypical melanocytic hyperplasia (level I). Not a malignant lesion
T_1	Invasion of papillary dermis (level II) and/or 0.75-mm thickness or less
T_2	Invasion of the papillary-reticular-dermal interface (level III) and/or 0.76-to 1.5-mm thickness
T_3	Invasion of the reticular dermis (level IV) and/or 1.51- to 4.0-mm thickness
T_4	Invasion of subcutaneous tissue (level V) and/or more than 4.0 mm in thickness *or* satellite(s) within 2 cm of any primary melanoma
Nodal involvement (N)	
N_X	Nodes cannot be assessed
N_0	No regional lymph node involvement
N_1	Involvement of only one regional lymph node station; nodes(s) movable and not over 5 cm in diameter *or* negative regional lymph nodes and the presence of less than five in-transit metastases
N_2	Any one of the following: Involvement of more than one regional lymph node station Regional node(s) over 5 cm in diameter or fixed Five or more in-transit metastases or any in-transit metastases with regional lymph node involvement
Distant metastases (M)	
M_X	Not assessed
M_0	No known distant metastases
M_1	Involvement of skin or subcutaneous tissue beyond the site of primary lymph node drainage Specify ________
M_2	Visceral metastases (spread to any distant site, other skin or subcutaneous tissues) Specify ________
Specify sites according to the following notations: Pulmonary (PUL) Osseous (OSS) Hepatic (HEP) Brain (BRA) Lymph nodes (LYM) Bone marrow (MAR) Pleura (PLE) Skin (SKI) Eye (EYE) Gastrointestinal (GI) Subcutaneous (SUBC) Other (OTH)	
Recurrent tumor (r) Recurrent tumor is not to be considered the same as residual tumor left after biopsy or incomplete resection. Residual tumor calls for no special recognition because it is such a common clinical circumstance. The development of local recurrence at the site of previous surgery calls for specific recognition when staged by using the prefix "r" (rTNM).	
Stage grouping	
Stage 1	T_1 or T_2, N_0, M_0
Stage IIA	T_3, N_0, M_0
IIB	T_4, N_0, M_0
Stage III	Any T, N_1, M_0
Stage IV	Any T, N_2, M_0
	Any T, any N, M_1, or M_2[15]

section than with wide local excision alone. There was also a greater survival for 1.6-mm to 4.5-mm lesions (78.5% vs. 69.7%) treated by node dissection versus wide local excision. Neither difference was statistically significant. However, these differences may become significant after a longer follow-up period.

The data on head and neck melanoma seem to indicate that a neck dissection may be helpful in stage I disease, but the randomized studies for extremity melanoma do not identify patient groups helped by node dissection. If one assumes there are groups of patients in whom the benefits of node dissection (survival) outweigh the risks of the procedure, examination of the frequency of nodal involvement and survival by Clark's and Breslow's microstage methods may identify these groups. As can be ascertained from Table 22–8, Clark

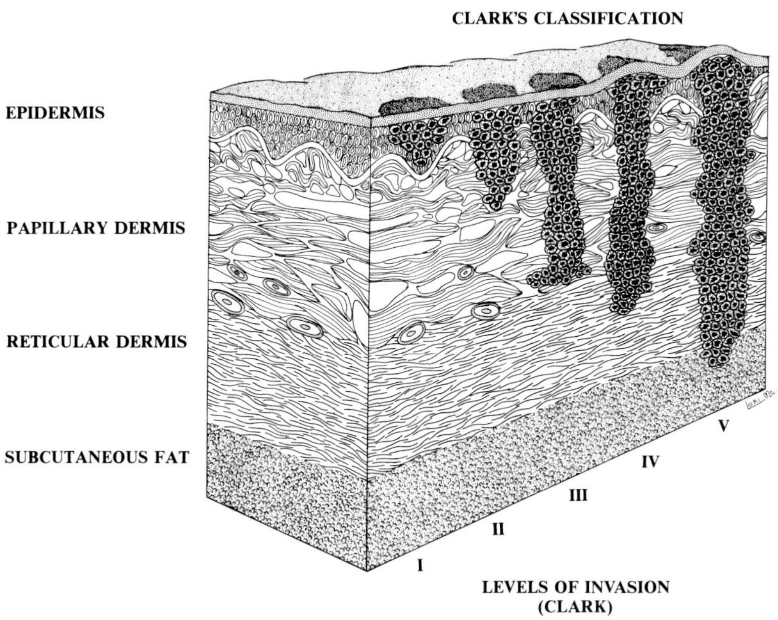

Fig 22–5.—Clark levels of invasion. See text for explanation.

level III, IV, and V lesions are associated with an appreciable number of metastases in clinically negative nodes. Table 22–9 gives similar data about microstaging by Breslow's method. It is obvious from these tables that theoretically there is a point where the potential gains from doing a neck dissection far outweigh the potential morbidity and mortality from the procedure. According to Beahrs,[39] the mortality from a neck dissection is about 1% and the morbidity is about 5%. If we accept these levels of morbidity and mortality, a neck dissection would be indicated for Clark level III, IV, and V lesions or for a tumor more than 1.5 mm thick.

Balch et al.[20] recently published a retrospective study of 1,786 patients who had microstaging and long-term follow-up. In both Australia and Alabama, significant differences were observed when a node dissection was carried out in conjunction with wide local excision (Table 22–10). Improvement in survival was greater in the 1.50-mm to 3.99-mm group and also occurred in the 0.76-mm to 1.49-mm group. This is the most persuasive evidence that node dissection is potentially helpful. Approximately 330 of the patients had head and neck lesions, although they are not described separately. A prospective study should confirm these results. Veronesi has planned a study to include "other sites" (extremities) not included in his first study.

WHICH LYMPH NODES SHOULD BE REMOVED WHEN A REGIONAL NODE DISSECTION IS CONSIDERED NECESSARY?

It is far easier to decide which nodes should be removed than to decide when to remove them. Posterior scalp lesions require a modification of the standard neck

TABLE 22–4.—MELANOMA PROGNOSIS IN ALABAMA AND AUSTRALIA: TEN-YEAR SURVIVAL RATES FOR CLINICAL STAGE I PATIENTS SUBGROUPED BY MELANOMA MICROSTAGE*

LEVEL OF INVASION	TUMOR THICKNESS (MM) 0.76	0.76–1.49	1.50–2.49	2.50–3.99	4.00
II	92% ± 3% (N = 230)	90% ± 6% (N = 48)	. . .	. . .	. . .
III	33% ± 7% (N = 81)	76% ± 6% (N = 145)	51% ± 7% (N = 108)	53% ± 9% (N = 50)	40% ± 17% (N = 17)
IV	83% ± 9% (N = 46)	70% ± 7% (N = 192)	62% ± 5% (N = 181)	43% ± 6% (N = 145)	24% ± 8% (N = 92)
V	. . .	. . .	. . .	47% ± 15% (N = 20)	22% ± 6% (N = 72)
Total pts.	357	388	295	218	184

*From Balch et al.[20] Reproduced by permission. Ellipses in table indicate sample was too small for statistical calculations.

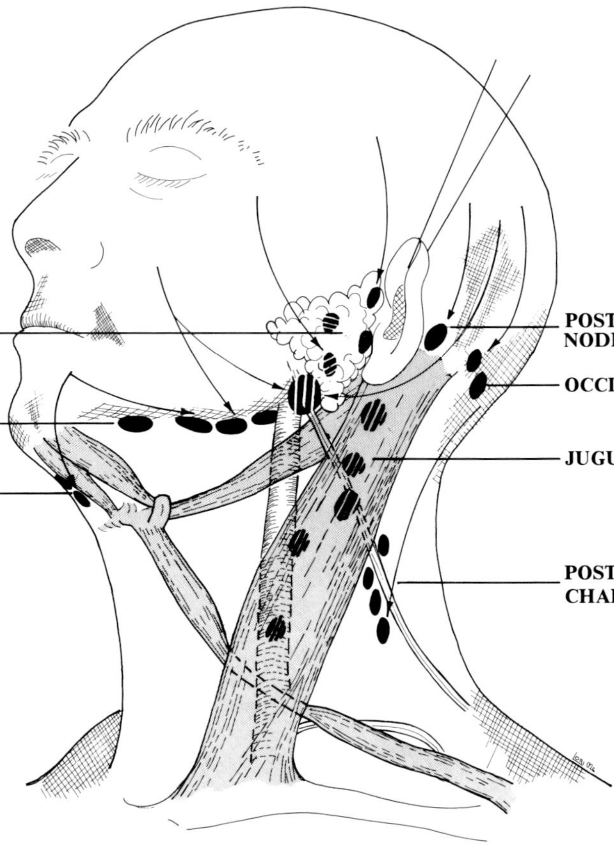

Fig 22–6.—Lymph node drainage. General areas of lymph node drainage emphasize the importance of posterior neck dissection and parotidectomy when appropriate.

TABLE 22–5.—SURVIVAL AFTER EXCISION OF MELANOMA*

STUDY	WIDE LOCAL EXCISION PLUS ELECTIVE RADICAL NECK DISSECTION No.	(%)	WIDE LOCAL EXCISION, NO DISSECTION No.	(%)
Conley and Hamaker[28]	62	(55)	113	(38.5)
Ballantyne[29]	73	(76.9)	115	(60.8)

*Numbers and percentages in Table refer to 5–year survival.

dissection (Beahrs) to include removal of the postauricular and occipital nodes (see Fig 22–6). Anterior scalp lesions and cheek lesions drain into the parotid nodes before the jugular nodes and require a superficial parotidectomy in addition to the standard neck dissection. Midline lesions can spread in either or both directions. There are no natural barriers in the midline to lymphatic spread (see chapter 9).

WHAT IS THE PROGNOSIS FOLLOWING EXCISION OF A MELANOMA?

The prognosis following excision of clinical stage III melanoma is not good. The average survival is less than 1 year, and 5-year survival is rare.[40] The prognosis following excision of clinical stage II melanoma also is not good. The 5-year survival is 24%, but the 10-year survival is 0%. Patients with clinical stage I, pathologic stage II (micrometastases) disease have a 5-year survival rate of 48%. In clinical stage I, pathologic stage I disease, the prognosis varies greatly with the thickness of the tumor and site of the primary tumor (Table 22–11).[40] The lesions are separated into BANS (upper back, posterolateral arm, posterior and lateral neck, and posterior scalp) and non-BANS groups because of the differences in prognosis. The thickness measurements are different from the usual Breslow measurements because the authors have directed a step-function in survival at these points.[41] The survival rates are averages. Slightly higher or slightly lower rates may occur when

TABLE 22–6.—SURVIVAL AFTER EXCISION OF POSITIVE LYMPH NODES

STUDY	PTS. WITH MICROSCOPIC POSITIVE NODES: Elective Dissection (%)	Survival No.	(%)	PATIENTS THAT DEVELOPED CLINICALLY POSITIVE NODES AFTER WIDE LOCAL EXCISION: Excision (%)	Survival No.	(%)
Simons[30]	15	5	(20)	20	30	(16)
Ames et al.[11]	19	15	(33)	21	21	(24)

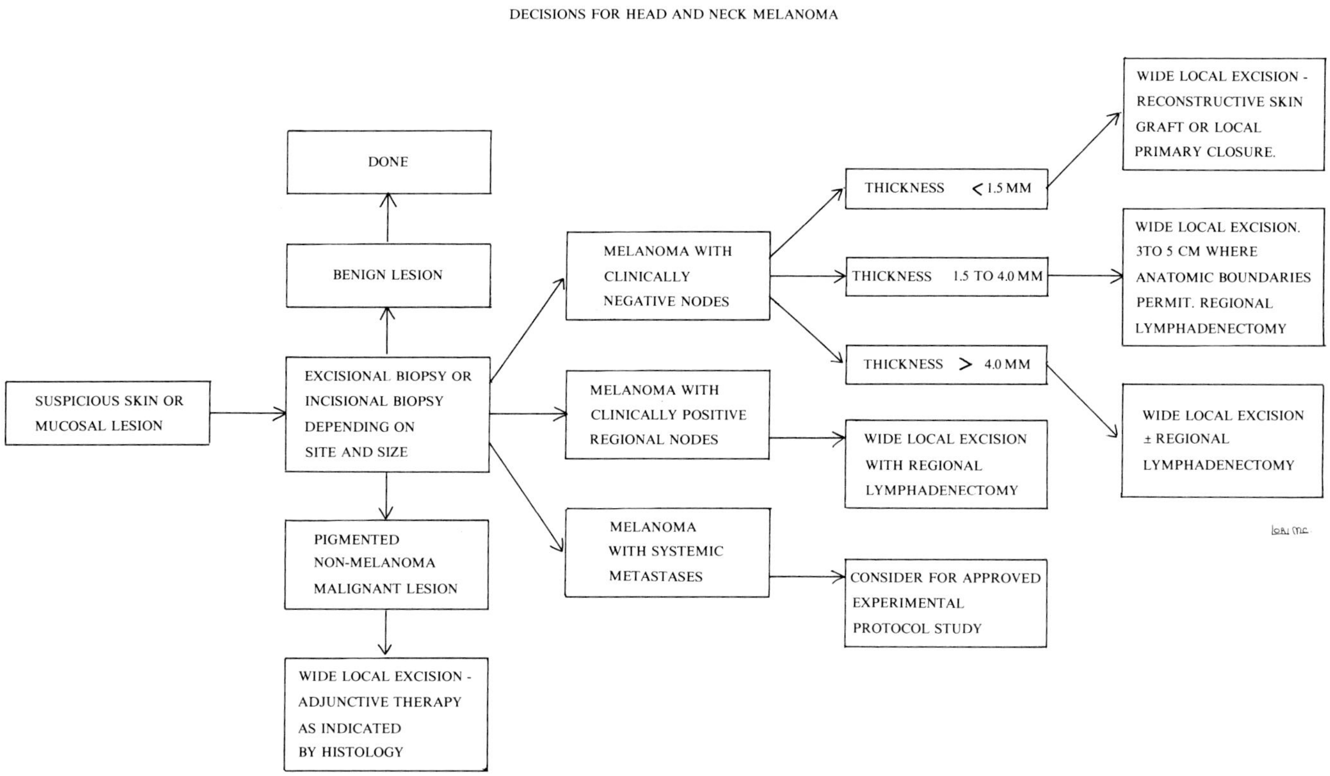

Fig 22–7.—Decisions for managing head and neck melanoma.

TABLE 22–7.—PROSPECTIVE RANDOMIZED STUDIES OF NON-HEAD AND NECK MELANOMA

		SURVIVAL (%)	
STUDY	NO. OF PTS.	Wide Local Excision	Wide Local Excision Plus Regional Node Dissection
Veronesi et al.[31]	553	70	71
Sim et al.[32]	117	86	86*

*Approximate 3-year survival.

regional node dissection is added or omitted with the thicker lesions (≥ 1.69 mm). Table 22–12 gives 5-year survival figures by site without regard to microstaging. There is great variability in survival rates because of the lack of microstaging.

DOES MELANOMA OCCUR ELSEWHERE IN THE HEAD AND NECK REGION?

Melanoma also occurs in the eye and on mucous membranes. The eye is a common site of melanoma. Diagnosis and treatment of melanoma of the eye are usually performed by ophthalmologists and will not be considered further here. Mucosal melanomas are a special problem. They account for 10%–15% of head and neck melanomas.[42] They most frequently occur in the oral cavity (50%), on the palate or alveolar ridge. The nasal cavity (35%) and sinuses are the next most frequent sites. Unfortunately, mucosal melanomas frequently do not cause symptoms until they are quite large. Treatment is by wide local excision. Local recurrence rates are very high (25%–40%), and 5-year cure rates are low (10%–15%).

Attempts are now being made to stage mucosal melanomas. Clark's method is not useful because the reticular and papillary layers do not exist in the mucous membranes. Shah and Goldsmith[42] attempted to measure depth of invasion, and there appears to be a relationship with survival. Node dissection is indicated for

TABLE 22–8.—PERCENTAGE OF PATIENTS WITH POSITIVE LYMPH NODES, CLINICAL STAGE I, BY CLARK LEVEL

	CLARK LEVEL				
STUDY	II	III	IV	V	NO. OF PTS.
Wanebo et al.[34]	4	7	25	70	169
Fortner et al.[35]	0	14	31	33	162
Cohen et al.[36]	15	14	35	33	140
Holmes et al.[37]		29	42	58	250
Donnellan et al.[38]*	6	29	32	63	104
Median	6	14	32	58	825

*Head and neck lesions only.

TABLE 22–9.—PERCENTAGE OF PATIENTS WITH POSITIVE LYMPH NODES, CLINICAL STAGE I, BY BRESLOW'S METHOD

STUDY	THICKNESS (MM) <.75	0.75–1.5	1.5–4	>4.0	NO. OF PTS.
Wanebo et al.[34]*	6	7	22	39	151
Holmes et al.[37]		10	{20}		120
Balch et al.[23]	0	25	51	62	287

*Thickness categories do not fit exactly.

clinically positive nodes. While the incidence of metastasis is similar to that for cutaneous melanoma, too little data are available to make recommendations about node dissection, although dissection would seem to be indicated with larger lesions.

ARE OTHER FORMS OF TREATMENT (IRRADIATION, CHEMOTHERAPY, IMMUNOTHERAPY) HELPFUL IN TREATING MELANOMA?

Irradiation has not proved helpful as adjuvant treatment of melanoma,[33] but it may be helpful in treating recurrent skin or nodal disease.[43] Chemotherapy using dimethyl triazeno imidizole carboxanide (DTIC, dacarbazine) or nitrosoureas is associated with partial remission in 15%–20% of patients. Trials with adjuvant chemotherapy have been quite disappointing.[44–46] Immunotherapy using BCG is helpful when injected into a skin or subcutaneous melanoma lesion, causing regression in 90% of such lesions and in 17% of distant lesions.[47] Immunotherapy alone or in combination with chemotherapy has not been useful as adjuvant therapy in prolonging survival[44, 48] (see chapter 31).

Although patients with thick melanomas and/or node metastases are at great risk (50%–85%) of tumor recurrence, there is presently no effective means of decreasing that risk.

CAN ANYTHING BE DONE TO PREVENT MELANOMA?

Because melanoma is related to sun exposure, limiting exposure to the sun by use of protective clothing and effective sun screens (PABA) should decrease the incidence of melanoma. And because two thirds of melanomas develop from benign preexisting lesions, removal of these lesions could reduce the risk of melanoma.

TABLE 22–10.—PERCENTAGE OF PATIENTS SURVIVING 10 YEARS, BY THICKNESS OF LESION

THICKNESS (MM)	Alabama WLE*	Alabama WLE + RND*	New South Wales WLE	New South Wales WLE + RND
<0.76	90	90	90	90
0.76–1.49	45	85	60	90
1.50–3.99	15	65	40	70
>4.00	25	35	25	25

NOTE: Percentages are approximate readings from four graphs, Figure 1 in Balch et al.[20]
*WLE, wide local excision, RND, regional node dissection.

TABLE 22–11.—PROBABILITY OF DEATH (%) FROM MELANOMA IN 7½ YEARS WITH CLINICAL STAGE I DISEASE*

LESION THICKNESS (MM)	NON-BANS HEAD/NECK	BANS
<.85	0	2
0.85–1.69	0	22
1.79–3.64	36	42
>3.65	35	67

*BANS = upper back, posterolateral arm, posterior and lateral neck, and posterior scalp.[35]

TABLE 22–12.—FIVE-YEAR SURVIVAL (%) BY SITE OF MELANOMA

SITE	STUDY Catlin[49]	Ballantyne[29]	Ariel[50]
Cheek	43		
Neck	39	69.5	28
Scalp	39	53.2	31.8
Ear	56		32.6
Forehead	23		
Nose	50		60
Face		65.8	32.6

REFERENCES

1. Silverberg E.: Cancer statistics 1983. *CA* 33:9, 1983.
2. Elwood J.M., Lee J.A.H.: Recent data on the epidemiology of malignant melanoma. *Semin. Oncol.* 2:149, 1975.
3. Cosman B., Heddle S.B., Crikelair G.F.: The increasing incidence of melanoma. *Plast. Reconstr. Surg.* 57:50, 1976.
4. MacDonald E.J.: *Neoplasms of the Skin and Malignant Melanoma.* Chicago, Year Book Medical Publishers, Inc., 1976.
5. Magnus K.: Incidence of malignant melanoma of the skin in the five Nordic countries: Significance of solar radiation. *Int. J. Cancer* 20:477, 1977.
6. Sober A.J., Day C.L., Kopf A.W., et al.: Detection of "thin" primary melanomas. *CA* 33:160, 1980.
7. Kopf A.W., Bart R.S., Rodriguez-Sains R.S., et al.: *Malignant Melanoma.* New York, Masson Publishing USA, Inc., 1979.
8. Clark W.H., Goldman L.I., Mastrangelo M.J.: *Human Malignant Melanoma.* New York, Grune & Stratton, 1979.
9. Epstein E., Bragg K., Linden G.: Biopsy and prognosis of malignant melanoma. *JAMA* 208:1369, 1969.
10. Kopf A.W., Mintzis M., Bart R.S.: Diagnostic accuracy in malignant melanoma. *Arch. Dermatol.* 111:1291, 1975.

11. Ames F.C., Sugarbaker E.V., Ballantyne A.J.: Analysis of survival and disease control in stage I melanoma of the head and neck. *Am. J. Surg.* 132:484, 1976.
12. Knutson C.O., Hori J.M., Spratt J.S. Jr.: Melanoma. *Curr. Probl. Surg.* December 1971, pp. 3–55.
13. Jones W.M., Williams W.J., Roberts M.M., et al.: Malignant melanoma of the skin: Prognostic value of clinical features and the role of treatment in 111 cases. *Br. J. Cancer* 22:437, 1968.
14. Cascinelli N., van der Esch E.P., Breslow A., et al.: Stage I melanoma of the skin: The problem of resection margins. *Eur. J. Cancer* 16:1079–1085, 1980.
15. American Joint Committee on Cancer: *Staging of Cancer of Head and Neck Sites and of Melanoma.* 1980, pp. 34–37.
16. Thomas J.H., Panoussopoulous D., Liesmann G.E., et al.: Scintiscans in the evaluation of patients with malignant melanoma. *Surg. Gynecol. Obstet.* 149:574, 1979.
17. Breslow A.: Thickness, cross-sectioned area and depth of invasion in the prognosis of cutaneous melanoma. *Ann. Surg.* 172:902, 1970.
18. Clark W.H. Jr., From L., Bernadino E.A., et al.: The histogenesis and biologic behavior of primary human malignant melanomas of the skin. *Cancer Res.* 29:705, 1969.
19. Clark W.H., Ainsworth A.M., Bernadino E.A., et al.: The developmental biology of primary human malignant melanomas. *Semin. Oncol.* 2:83, 1975.
20. Balch C.M., Soong S., Milton G.W., et al.: A comparison of prognostic factors and surgical results in 1,786 patients with localized (stage I) melanoma treated in Alabama, USA and New South Wales, Australia. *Ann. Surg.* 196:677, 1982.
21. Balch C.M., Murad T.M., Soong S., et al.: A multifactorial analysis of melanoma: Prognostic histopathological features comparing Clark's and Breslow's staging methods. *Ann. Surg.* 188:732, 1978.
22. Breslow A., Macht S.D.: Optimal size of resection margins for thin cutaneous melanoma. *Surg. Gynecol. Obstet.* 145:691, 1977.
23. Balch C.M., Murad T.M., Soong S., et al.: Tumor thickness as a guide to surgical management of clinical stage I melanoma patients. *Cancer* 43:883–888, 1979.
24. Das Gupta T.A.: The results of treatment of 269 patients with primary cutaneous melanoma: A five year prospective study. *Ann. Surg.* 186:201, 1977.
25. WHO Collaborating Centres for Evaluation of Methods of Diagnosis and Treatment of Melanoma: Stage I melanoma of the skin: The problem of resection margins. *Eur. J. Cancer* 16:1079, 1980.
26. Olsen G.: Removal of fascia: Cause of more frequent metastases of malignant melanomas of the skin to regional lymph nodes. *CA* 17:1159, 1964.
27. Knutson C.O., Hori J.M., Watson F.R.: Melanoma of the head and neck. *Am. J. Surg.* 124:543, 1972.
28. Conley J., Hamaker R.C.: Melanoma of the head and neck. *Laryncoscope* 87:760, 1977.
29. Ballantyne A.J.: Malignant melanoma of the skin of the head and neck. *Am. J. Surg.* 120:425, 1970.
30. Simons J.N.: Malignant melanoma of the head and neck. *Am. J. Surg.* 124:485, 1972.
31. Veronesi V., Adamus J., Bandiera D.C., et al.: Inefficacy of immediate node dissection in stage I melanoma of the limbs. *N. Engl. J. Med.* 297:627, 1977.
32. Sim F.H., Taylor W.F., Ivins J.C., et al.:A prospective randomized study of the efficacy of routine elective lymphadenectomy in management of malignant melanoma. *Cancer* 41:948, 1978.
33. Creagan E.T., Cupps R.E., Ivins J.C., et al.: Adjuvant radiation therapy for regional nodal metastasis from malignant melanoma: A randomized prospective study. *Cancer* 42:2206, 1978.
34. Wanebo H.J., Woodruff J., Fortner J.G.: Malignant melanoma of the extremities: A clinicopathologic study using levels of invasion (microstage). *Cancer* 35:666, 1978.
35. Fortner J.G., Woodruff J., Schottenfeld D., et al.: Biostatistical basis for elective node dissection for malignant melanoma. *Ann. Surg.* 186:101, 1977.
36. Cohen M.H., Ketcham A.S., Felix E.L., et al.: Prognostic factors in patients undergoing lymphadenectomy for malignant melanoma. *Ann. Surg.* 186:635, 1977.
37. Holmes E.C., Moseley H.S., Morton D.L., et al.: A rational approach to the surgical management of melanoma. *Ann. Surg.* 186:481, 1977.
38. Donnellan M., Seemayer T., Huvos A., et al.: Clinicopathologic study of cutaneous melanoma of the head and neck. *Am. J. Surg.* 124:450, 1972.
39. Beahrs O.H.: Surgical anatomy and technique of radical neck dissection. *Surg. Clin. North Am.* 57:663, 1971.
40. Day C.L., Mihm M.C., Lew R.A., et al.: Cutaneous malignant melanoma: Prognostic guidelines for physicians and patients. *CA* 32:113, 1982.
41. Balch C.M., Soong S., Murad T.M., et al.: A multifactorial analysis of melanoma: III. prognostic factors in melanoma patients with lymph node metastasis (stage II). *Ann. Surg.* 193:377, 1981.
42. Shah J.P., Goldsmith H.S.: Prognosis of malignant melanoma in relation to clinical presentation. *Am. J. Surg.*
43. Habermaltz H.J., Fisher J.J.: Radiation therapy of malignant melanoma. *Cancer* 38:2258, 1976.
44. Veronesi V., Adamus J., Aubert C., et al.: A randomized trial of adjuvant chemotherapy and immunotherapy in cutaneous melanoma. *N. Engl. J. Med.* 307:913, 1982.
45. Fisher R.I., Terry W.D., Hodes R.J., et al.: Adjuvant immunotherapy as chemotherapy for malignant melanoma. *Surg. Clin. North Am.* 61:1267, 1981.
46. Pinsky C.M., Oettgen H.F.: Surgical adjuvant therapy for malignant melanoma. *Surg. Clin. North Am.* 611:1259, 1981.
47. Morton D.L., Eilber F.R., Malmgren R.A., et al.: Immunologic factors which influence response to immunotherapy in malignant melanoma. *Surgery* 68:158, 1970.
48. Kaiser L.R., Burk M.W., Morton D.L.: Adjuvant therapy for malignant melanoma. *Surg. Clin. North Am.* 61:1249, 1981.
49. Catlin P.: Cutaneous melanoma of the head and neck. *Am. J. Surg.* 112:512, 1966.
50. Ariel I.M.: *Malignant Melanoma.* New York, Appleton-Century-Crofts, 1981.

23 / Large Nonmelanoma Skin Cancers of the Head and Neck

ALAN R. SHONS, M.D., PH.D.

HOW IMPORTANT AND HOW COMMON ARE SKIN CANCERS OF THE HEAD AND NECK?

THE MOST COMMON FORM of malignancy is cancer of the skin. The majority of these lesions are seen in the sun-exposed head and neck area. Their easy accessibility and early recognition usually result in definitive cure with little morbidity or cosmetic deformity. Skin cancers develop most frequently in blond persons of fair complexion and rarely in Orientals or blacks. About 60% of all cancers of the skin are basal cell cancers and 30% are squamous cell cancers. The remaining 10% are less common histologic types. The median age of patients at the time of first diagnosis of skin cancer is greater than 65 years.

These relatively innocuous cancers can become therapeutic and reconstructive challenges if initial treatment is delayed or if initial treatment is inadequate, resulting in a more invasive recurrent lesion. With recurrence or neglect, an easily handled surface cancer can become a deeply invasive tumor that encroaches on important functional or cosmetic structures. Before discussing the treatment of advanced skin tumors of the head and neck, a brief review of the general features is useful.

WHAT ARE THE CHARACTERISTICS OF BASAL CELL CARCINOMA, AND HOW IS IT USUALLY TREATED?

Basal cell cancers are locally invasive and can be elusive. They occur most frequently in exposed areas of the face, neck and ears. The seborrheic midportion of the face is a common site. They tend to occur at a younger age than squamous cell cancers. The most common appearance is a round, firm, slightly raised cutaneous lesion. There may be a shallow ulceration in the center of the grayish or pink lesion. The morphea type tends to be macular with indistinct margins and is whitish in color. Because of its benign appearance it may be ignored by the patient or physician for long periods of time. A particularly aggressive variant is the "rodent ulcer." This is a painless ulcerative lesion characterized by early extensive subepidermal local invasion and tissue destruction. The basal cell nevus syndrome is an autosomal dominant genetic disorder in which multiple basal cell carcinomas begin to appear in childhood and adolescence and continue to appear throughout life. Associated signs of the syndrome include palmar pits, dentigenous cysts, a broad nasal root, and an increased interpupillary distance.[1, 2]

Local recurrence is rare following excision of basal cell carcinoma. Cure rates exceeding 90% are achieved with x-ray therapy, curettage, and electrodesiccation, surgical excision, or chemosurgical excision[7] (Table 23–1). Even when the gross margins of excision are clear but the microscopic margins show tumor involvement, the local recurrence rate is only 35%. Very rarely, metastases may occur.[8]

WHAT ARE THE CLINICAL CHARACTERISTICS OF SQUAMOUS CELL CARCINOMA?

Seventy-five percent of all squamous cell carcinomas occur in the sun-exposed head and neck area. The lesions frequently develop in areas of previous skin change such as the proliferative keratoses. A precise time of cancer formation is not easily recognized. Squamous cell cancers frequently develop at the junction of skin and mucous membranes such as on the lower lip, the nostrils, and the eyelids. A comparison with basal cell carcinoma shows the growth rate of squamous cell carcinoma to be faster, with more widespread local invasiveness. Unlike basal cell carcinomas, squamous cell carcinomas can be expected to metastasize in late stages. Metastases occur by lymphatics. Hematogenous spread is rare. The typical lesion has an indistinct solid infiltrating margin and a friable ulcerative center. Differentiation between squamous cell carcinoma and basal cell carcinoma may be difficult clinically. Biopsy of suspicious lesions is imperative. The pathologic characteristics of squamous cell carcinoma are detailed in chapter 4.

WHAT IS MOHS CHEMOSURGERY TECHNIQUE? WHEN AND HOW SHOULD IT BE USED?

Mohs chemosurgery is a technique of microscopically controlled excision developed by Mohs.[9, 10] The original technique involves application of a zinc chloride paste to produce a chemical fixation of the tissue surface. Several hours after zinc chloride application, seg-

TABLE 23–1.—RATE OF CURE OF BASAL CELL SKIN CANCERS WITH FOUR MODES OF TREATMENT

STUDY, YEAR	NO. OF LESIONS	5-YR CURE RATE (%)	TREATMENT
Bart et al.,[3] 1970	50	92.7	X-ray therapy
Tromovitch,[4] 1965	75	96	Curettage
Lauritzen et al.,[5] 1965	2,900	96.6	Excision
Mohs,[6] 1978	4,000	99.1	Chemosurgical excision

ments of tissue 1–3 mm thick are removed and examined by frozen section techniques. The excision is within the area of tissue fixation. The specimens are carefully oriented for microscopic examination, and precise localization of tumor is possible. Sections are taken repeatedly until all of the cancer is removed. The technique most commonly employed today is a fresh tissue modification of the classic technique. Local anesthesia is used; zinc chloride fixation is omitted and sequential layer excision with microscopic control of the margins is performed. The fresh tissue technique is a more rapid procedure.

Chemosurgical extirpation is the technique of choice for recurrent lesions in the inner canthal and nasolabial fold area. The technique allows precise removal of tumor with preservation of uninvolved important surrounding structures.

TREATMENT OF ADVANCED LESIONS:

What Is an Adequate Excision for Basal Cell Carcinoma?

At present, the number of patients who delay treatment because of ignorance or fear of surgical mutilation is decreasing. Most of the advanced basal cell carcinomas are now seen after repeated failure of initial therapy. Inadequate initial therapy occurs most frequently in compromised excision of lesions that develop in the inner canthal and alar base areas. There is an understandable but treacherous reluctance to remove cosmetically important eyelid and nasal structures, to the detriment of adequate cancer treatment. If there is a consequent deep-seated tumor recurrence, then the basic structures of the nose and orbit will be more seriously jeopardized.

For the large primary lesion (> 2 cm), a 1 to 1½-cm lateral margin is advised, especially for the ulcerative-invasive type of basal cell carcinoma. Deep excision of the first mesodermal barrier and of the underlying structure is recommended in this type of tumor (e.g., fascia and underlying muscle for a lesion of the temple). Surgical and chemosurgical excision procedures are the treatments of choice for large primary and recurrent lesions. Large cancers that invade cartilage or bone will require full-thickness cartilage excision when there is gross involvement. If there is no actual invasion of bone, removal of the periosteum may be adequate.

As in any cancer operation, cosmetic factors should *not* compromise the adequacy of tumor resection. Frozen sections should be used liberally to ensure that there are tumor-free margins before a major reconstructive procedure is started. If possible, reconstruction should be delayed until all of the permanent histologic sections are processed and adequate margins have been confirmed, to preclude the possibility of burying persisting cancer under a reconstructive project. If there is a question of adequacy of resection, the area can be temporarily covered with a split-thickness skin graft and closely observed for 4–6 months before reconstruction.

What Is the Role of Irradiation in the Treatment of Advanced Basal Cell Cancer?

Basal cell cancer is responsive to radiotherapy. Large noninvasive lesions of the face and neck can be treated by irradiation. Radiation therapy has been advocated as the treatment of choice for lesions involving the tip of the nose, the ala, the vermillion margins of the lips, and the eyelid margins. With well-designed fields and shielding it is possible to preserve functional structural components of the eyelids and nose using radiation therapy. If the lesions are removed from these areas by excision, a reconstructive procedure is required. The disadvantage of irradiation is that the adequacy of tumor eradication is uncertain. Postirradiation fibrosis may result in considerable distortion of the area. Radiation therapy should not be used for lesions that deeply invade cartilage and bone because of the difficulty of eradicating the tumor completely from cartilage or bone. Chondritis and osteoradionecrosis may also result from radiation therapy. Radiation therapy should not be used for lesions that are recurrent failures of primary radiation therapy.

How Does Management of Cutaneous Squamous Cell Carcinoma Differ From Management of Basal Cell Carcinoma?

The management of large squamous cell carcinomas involves many of the principles of accurate biopsy, adequate margins, and effective ablative treatment outlined above. Failure to identify precisely the extent of the tumor is a more common error in the treatment of cutaneous squamous carcinoma than in the treatment of basal cell carcinoma. This error in judgment can have disastrous consequences. Glass et al. identified and reported 34 cases of squamous cell carcinoma that were found to be inadequately excised although initially thought to be completely excised by the operating surgeon. There was a 50% recurrence rate after reexcision. Ultimately a 25% mortality resulted.[11] The depth of invasion of squamous cell cancer is difficult to define by gross observation. Extension to underlying bone and cartilage may be missed in the early stages. Clinically palpable fixation occurs long after microscopic invasion of cartilage or bone by tumor cells.

Histologic grading is important in the prognosis of squamous cell carcinoma. Less-differentiated tumors tend to be more invasive and have a higher incidence of metastases.[12] It is true that larger tumors are more frequently less differentiated, so that size and the degree of dedifferentiation may not be independent variables.

Excision of large or recurrent squamous cell carcinomas requires wide lateral margins (1–2 cm in all planes). Frozen section and permanent section evaluation of margins is mandatory. Underlying bone or cartilage must be removed if the tumor is fixed to the deep structures. Fixation of a scalp tumor to the underlying calvarium without radiographic or computerized tomographic (CT) evidence of bone invasion necessitates at least removal of the outer table of the skull. If bony invasion is grossly apparent at operation or shown to be present by radiography or CT scan, a full thickness of the skull should be removed. Dural involvement necessitates dural excision as well. Reconstructive procedures should be performed only when there is absolute confirmation of the adequacy of the tumor excision. The reader is referred to chapter 6 for reconstructive techniques.

What Is the Role of Radiation Therapy in the Treatment of Advanced Squamous Cell Carcinoma?

The role of irradiation in the treatment of *advanced* cutaneous squamous cell cancer is not as clear as it is with the usual small lesion. Control of advanced squamous cell carcinoma may be achieved with radiotherapy if bone or cartilage invasion is not present. The role of radiation therapy in the treatment of squamous cell cancer may be more limited than in the treatment of basal cell cancer because squamous cell cancers are frequently deeply invasive. Radiation therapy can be considered for patients who have had previous surgical excision or recurrent disease with uncertain margins and perineural invasion.

HOW DO YOU PLAN TO TREAT POTENTIAL LYMPH NODE METASTASES THAT MAY OCCUR WITH ADVANCED SQUAMOUS CELL CANCER?

Metastases to regional nodes may occur at any time with cutaneous squamous cell carcinoma. Lymph node metastases tend to occur relatively late in the evolution of squamous carcinoma of the skin of the head and neck when compared to squamous carcinoma of the tongue or oral mucosa. Metastases generally occur when the cancer burrows deeply through the dense reticular dermis to invade the subcutaneous lymphatic system. The pattern of metastases is determined by the location of the primary lesion. In general, the progression of lymph flow in the head and neck is from superficial to deeper nodes and from above downward. Thus, early metastases from carcinoma of the skin of the lower lip or chin are most frequently found in the superficial submental or submaxillary nodes. Subsequently, midjugular and deeper nodes become involved (Fig 23–1).

Although the overall incidence of metastasis from head and neck skin cancer is low, the incidence is increased in longstanding tumors, large tumors (> 2 cm), invasive tumors, and relatively undifferentiated tumors. In a study by Binder et al., nine of 114 patients with carcinoma of the nose developed cervical metastases. All patients with metastases had symptoms for more than 1 year, and all but one had lesions larger than 3 cm. All lesions were invasive to bone or cartilage.[13] Conley reported that four of 24 patients with squamous cell carcinoma of the scalp subsequently developed cervical node metastases. Metastatic lesions all came from large invasive tumors.[14]

Because the incidence of metastatic disease from squamous cell carcinoma is low in all reported series, elective node dissection is not indicated at the time of primary tumor resection in the majority of patients. Elective node dissection should be considered in patients with deeply invasive tumors over 2 cm in diameter. Elective node dissection is recommended in large (> 4 cm) invasive or recurrent tumors.

Total or subtotal parotidectomy may be necessary to control metastatic disease from tumors in areas that drain through the parotid lymphatics. Until recently the results of later dissection and parotidectomy for proved metastases were uniformly poor, with a 5-year survival of 12.5%–25% in patients who underwent surgery alone for skin cancer metastatic to the parotid gland. In a recent series reported by Jackson and Ballantyne,[15] 196 patients underwent parotidectomy-lymphadenectomy during the course of primary treatment for skin cancer (see Fig 22–6). Aggressive operative therapy with sacrifice of necessary structures (preserving the facial nerve when feasible) was found to

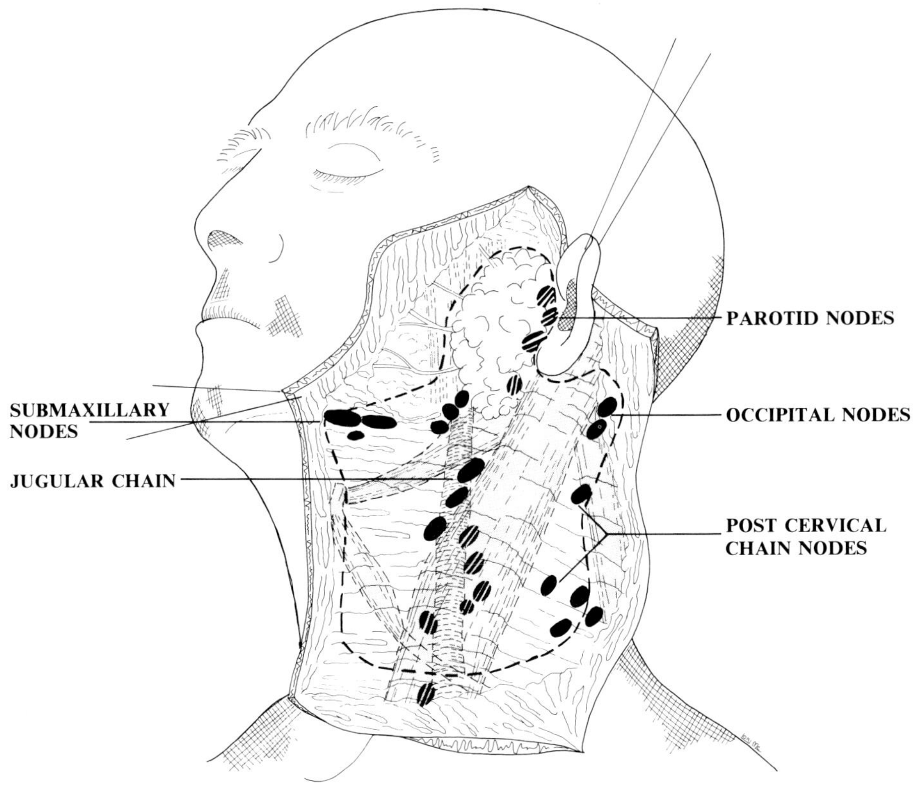

Fig 23–1.—Some important lymphatic drainage of the skin of the head. Note the nodes in the paraparotid area and the tail of the parotid gland. The posterior auricular and occipital nodes may also be involved by metastases from skin cancers. Therefore, the design of an adequate lymphadenectomy must be individualized.

result in satisfactory control, with an overall local or regional control rate of 70.9%. Jackson and Ballantyne recommend the addition of some form of neck dissection to the therapeutic parotidectomy because of a 24% incidence of occult metastases in clinically negative necks. In their series the most frequent site of recurrence was the parotid gland or skin in the primary regions.

WHAT IS THE TREATMENT OF SKIN APPENDAGE CARCINOMAS?

Carcinoma of the sebaceous gland is the most frequent of the skin appendage carcinomas that occur in the head and neck. This lesion occurs most frequently on the eyelid. The clinical appearance is widely variable, but an ulcerated nodule or growth is the most common presentation. The growth of this cancer on the eyelid is often associated with widespread aggressive metastatic disease. The same histologic type of lesion when it appears elsewhere on the head and neck is less aggressive in behavior.

Carcinomas of the exocrine and apocrine sweat glands can appear on the head and neck. Both lesions are locally invasive and rarely metastasize. Treatment principles for these lesions are the same as for the basal and squamous cell carcinomas. In most instances wide surgical excision is adequate for cure.

REFERENCES

1. Howell J.B., Caro M.R.: The basal cell nevus: Its relationship to multiple cutaneous cancers and associated anomalies of development. *Arch. Dermatol.* 79:67, 1959.
2. Gorlin R.J., Goltz R.W.: Multiple nevoid basal cell epithelioma, jaw cysts and bifid rib: A syndrome. *N. Engl. J. Med.* 262:908, 1960.
3. Bart R.S., Kopf A.W., Petratos M.A.: X-ray therapy of skin cancer: Evaluation of standardized method for treating basal cell epithelioma, in *Sixth National Cancer Conference Proceedings.* Philadelphia, J.B. Lippincott Co., 1970, p. 559.
4. Tromovitch T.A.: Skin cancer: Treatment by curettage and dessication. *Calif. Med.* 103:107, 1965.
5. Lauritzen R.E., Johnson R.E., Spratt J.S.: Pattern of recurrence in basal cell carcinoma. *Surgery* 57:813, 1965.
6. Mohs F.E.: Chemosurgery: Microscopically controlled surgery for skin cancer—past, present, and future. *J. Dermatol. Surg. Oncol.* 4:41, 1978.
7. Paletta F.X.: Tumors of the skin: A plastic surgeon's viewpoint, in Converse J.M. (ed.): *Reconstructive Plastic Surgery*, ed. 2. Philadelphia, W.B. Saunders Co., 1977.
8. Wernmuth B.M., Fajardo L.F.: Metastatic basal cell carcinoma. *Arch. Pathol.* 90:458, 1970.
9. Mohs F.E.: Chemosurgery: Microscopically controlled method of cancer excision. *Arch. Surg.* 42:279, 1941.
10. Mohs F.E.: The chemosurgical method for the microscopically controlled excision of cancer of the skin. *NY State J. Med.* 56:3481, 1956.

11. Glass R.L., Spratt J.S., Perez-Mesa C.: The fate of inadequately excised epidermoid carcinoma of the skin. *Surg. Gynecol. Obstet.* 122:245, 1966.
12. Warren S., Hoerr S.O.: A study of pathologically verified epidermoid carcinomas of the skin. *Surg. Gynecol. Obstet.* 69:726, 1939.
13. Binder S.C., Cady B., Catlin D.: Epidermoid carcinoma of the skin of the nose. *Am. J. Surg.* 116:506, 1968.
14. Conley J.J.: Malignant tumors of the scalp. *Plast. Reconstr. Surg.* 33:1, 1964.
15. Jackson G.L., Ballantyne A.J.: Role of parotidectomy for skin cancer of the head and neck. *Am. J. Surg.* 142:464, 1981.

24 / Connective Tissue Malignancies of the Head and Neck

MELODY J. O'CONNOR, M.D. / DALE C. SNOVER, M.D. / A.D.J. PEARSON, M.D. / M.E. NESBIT, M.D.

I. Soft Tissue Sarcomas of the Head and Neck in Adults

MELODY J. O'CONNOR, M.D. / DALE C. SNOVER, M.D.

THIS CHAPTER expands upon the pathologic types of connective tissue tumors presented in chapter 3. Soft tissue sarcomas in children are different enough from soft tissue sarcomas in adults that they are discussed separately in Part II of this chapter.

WHAT ARE THE GENERAL CHARACTERISTICS OF SOFT TISSUE SARCOMAS?

Soft tissue sarcomas are malignant tumors that arise from nonskeletal connective and supportive tissues. These tissues, derived embryologically from the mesoderm, include skeletal muscle, adipose tissue, and fibrous tissue surrounding the blood vessels serving these tissues. The vessels themselves, along with endothelial cells, pericytes, and smooth muscle cells, are also included. Tumors of the peripheral nervous system, which are derived embryologically from neuroectoderm, are also considered to be among the soft tissue sarcomas.[1]

Soft tissue sarcomas are relatively rare tumors with an expected yearly incidence of 4,500 new cases in the United States (NCI survey). These tumors represent 0.7% of cancers for all age groups and 6.5% of cancers in patients younger than 25 years of age.[1]

WHAT IS THE DISTRIBUTION OF SOFT TISSUE SARCOMA TYPES?

The histologic classification of individual soft tissue sarcomas is based on the adult tissue type toward which they are differentiating. Table 24–1 lists the relative incidence of individual soft tissue sarcomas in all locations, based on data compiled by the American Joint Committee for Cancer Staging and End Results. The data were reported from 13 hospitals over a period of 15 years (1954–1968).[2] Fibrosarcoma, rhabdomyosarcoma, and liposarcoma were the three most commonly diagnosed soft tissue sarcomas, each accounting for about 20% of the whole. While the most common locations for soft tissue sarcomas were in the upper and lower extremities (40%), 15% occurred in the head and neck. The most common head and neck soft tissue sarcoma was rhabdomyosarcoma (7%), occurring predominantly in children (see Part II). It should be remembered, however, that in any one series, the relative incidence of each of these tumors will vary considerably from the above figures owing to the small number of patients within a series, the age range of the patient population, and the relative incidence of tumors at various locations.

WHAT PROBLEMS ARISE IN PLANNING THERAPY FOR SOFT TISSUE SARCOMAS?

In view of the rarity of these tumors, it is not surprising that a single institution is unable to accumulate enough experience to suggest a comprehensive management plan and method of predicting the prognosis, based on a single series of patients. Recommendations regarding therapy are frequently based on a minimal personal experience influenced by a literature review. Similarly, data from experience with soft tissue sarcomas in other sites are often extrapolated to tumors in the head and neck. Nevertheless, there *are* valid general behavioral characteristics that apply to soft tissue sarcomas as a group, regardless of location: many soft tissue sarcomas are slow-growing, rather indolent tumors that tend to invade locally, spreading along fascial planes far past perceived borders of gross tumor involvement; soft tissue sarcomas frequently have a deceptive "pseudocapsule" with multiple projections of tumor beyond the obvious confines of the mass; the tumors have a remarkable tendency to recur locally; they rarely metastasize to regional lymph nodes, with a few notable exceptions (synovial sarcoma, rhabdomyosarcoma); and they have a definite tendency toward blood-borne spread to lung, liver, and bone. An overall recurrence (local and distant metastases) rate of 30%–

TABLE 24–1.—SOFT TISSUE SARCOMAS, ALL LOCATIONS

MALIGNANT TUMOR TYPE	TISSUE OF ORIGIN	BENIGN COUNTERPART	MOST COMMON LOCATION	% OCCURRING IN HEAD/NECK	AGE
Fibrosarcoma	Fibrous	Fibromatoses	Extremities	16	0–2 yr Mid-adult
Dermatofibrosarcoma protruberans	Fibrous	Dermatofibroma	Trunk	14	Young adult
Malignant fibrous histiocytoma	?	Fibrohistiocytoma (xanthoma)	Trunk Extremities	7	Mid-adult
Liposarcoma	Adipose	Lipoma	Extremities	5	Mid-adult
Rhabdomyosarcoma	Skeletal muscle	Rhabdomyoma	Extremities	34	Childhood
Leiomyosarcoma	Smooth muscle	Leiomyoma	Extremities	3	Mid-adult
Malignant schwannoma	Schwann cell	Neurofibroma	Extremities	25	Mid-adult
Synovial cell sarcoma	?	?	Extremities	1	Early adult
Angiosarcoma	Blood vessel	Hemangioendothelioma	Head and Neck	15	Late adult

50% can be expected following definitive wide local excision. As an aggregate group, patients with soft tissue sarcomas have a general overall 5-year survival rate of about 40%.

The potential for malignant behavior in soft tissue sarcomas, and hence the necessity for aggressive therapy, is determined by a number of factors identifiable at the time of first diagnosis: histogenetic type of tumor, size, and location, evidence of direct extension into adjacent tissues (bone, nerves, blood vessels), involvement of lymph nodes, presence of distant metastatic lesions, and, most important, histologic grade of tumor.

The following discussions draw on data applicable to a particular class of tumor, and the examples confined to the head and neck area are not segregated from the other anatomical sites. Where available, data for the head and neck area are segregated.

HOW IS THE DIAGNOSIS OF SOFT TISSUE SARCOMA ESTABLISHED?

The diagnosis of the "unknown primary" is discussed in chapter 25. Most of the precautions discussed there must be observed. Many times, clinical features will raise suspicion of a soft tissue sarcoma.

Principles of diagnosis of tumors of the soft parts have been outlined in detail by Fortner in a review of therapy of all soft tissue tumors[6] and by Das Gupta in a review of adipose tumors.[7] Fortner recommends generous incisional biopsy under general anesthesia, with meticulous attention to hemostasis, gentle handling of tumor tissue, and closure of the biopsy incision by layers. The biopsy technique for soft tissue sarcomas of the head and neck is determined by the specific location of the tumor. Biopsy skin incisions are planned so that they will lie within the boundaries of wide excision of the tumor and not interfere with incision and flap design for subsequent resective and reconstructive surgery. The proximity of tumor to vital structures (arteries, bone, nerves) will limit both the biopsy and the extent of ultimate tumor resection. Paraganglionomas, for example, are intrinsically highly vascularized. They may surround and intimately involve the carotid artery. Injudicious biopsy of paraganglioma leads to massive bleeding and can be disastrous if the carotid artery is sectioned or obstructed in desperate attempts to control bleeding. The diagnosis is based on gross appearance or angiographic findings. With the exception of this one caveat, the size of the biopsy specimen of a soft tissue sarcoma should be as generous as possible to allow accurate diagnosis without compromising the eventual adequacy of resection. Areas of hemorrhagic and necrotic tumor should be avoided since such tissue is frequently nondiagnostic. Generally, the solid areas of the tumor will represent the actively growing, most easily diagnosable tissue.

Regional variations in histologic patterns may lead to minor discrepancies in the subtyping of the tumor when the biopsy interpretation and final diagnosis based on the resection specimen are compared. Because of this regional variation, it is generally recommended that a minimum of one section per centimeter of tumor diameter be examined from the resection specimen.

Needless to say, the entirety of any biopsy specimen should be examined. Frozen section may be used to determine if adequate tissue for diagnosis has been obtained, but the final diagnosis must rest on the permanent section. If frozen section is used, the entire biopsy specimen should not be frozen. Enough well-fixed representative tissue must be retained for accurate interpretation. In addition, tissue fixed in gluteraldehyde for ultrastructural examination may be useful for confirming the subtype of tumor, although it is not absolutely necessary. Wider availability of the immunoperoxidase techniques will provide an additional tool for diagnosis. Ethanol fixation of a portion of the tissue may provide better retention of some markers, although immunoperoxidase studies can be performed on routine Formalin-fixed, paraffin-embedded tissue.[8]

The ultimate purpose of careful histologic study is to provide some idea of the expected behavior and treatment of the tumor. When older literature is examined, it is good to know that the terminology of soft tissue sarcomas has changed with time, with the identification of new subtypes of sarcoma and the alteration and refinement of criteria for diagnosis. Diagnoses that at one time were quite common (e.g., pleomorphic rhabdomyosarcoma) have been replaced by new terms (e.g., malignant fibrous histiocytoma), although the tumors themselves have not changed. Soft tissue sarcomas are usually categorized by the type of normal tissue which they most closely simulate histologically, i.e., the normal tissue which the more differentiated elements of the tumor seem to resemble. Hence, a leiomyosarcoma is a tumor that differentiates toward smooth muscle. It is easy to understand how confusion and disagreement may persist regarding tumors that are very poorly differentiated. While most soft tissue sarcomas will fall into one of the well-defined categories, some tumors will show divergent differentiation; these tumors are best treated as their most aggressive component would be treated.[9]

The histologic grade of the tumor is a useful predictor of the overall behavior, which can guide the necessary treatment planning. Low-grade tumors (e.g., well-differentiated liposarcomas) tend to recur locally without metastasis, whereas high-grade neoplasms (e.g., pleomorphic liposarcomas) are known to metastasize frequently and therefore require more aggressive therapy. While numerous grading schemes have been reported, using such criteria as degree of pleomorphism, mitotic activity, etc.,[2] each specific histologic subtype has its own particular major determinants of "grade." With many subtypes (e.g., pleomorphic liposarcoma), no other grading is necessary, although with a few tumors (e.g., synovial sarcoma), individual tumor variation based on mitotic activity and other features can be useful.[10] It behooves the clinician, therefore, to be familiar with the aggressive potential of each type of sarcoma and to communicate freely with the pathologist if there is any question as to the grade of a given neoplasm.

WHAT ARE SOME PRINCIPLES OF THERAPY FOR SOFT TISSUE SARCOMAS OF THE HEAD AND NECK?

Most authors agree that the primary determinant of successful operative therapy (as measured by survival and local recurrence) of soft tissue sarcomas in *adults* is the adequacy of local excision of tumor.[5, 6, 11–13] This observation applies both to accessible tumors (head and neck, extremities, trunk) and to relatively inaccessible tumors (retroperitoneum). Unfortunately, the success of multimodal therapy that has revolutionized the treatment of rhabdomyosarcoma in children has not yet been effectively applied in the adult counterparts.

Overall local recurrence rates in several series of all types of soft tissue sarcomas range from 13%[3] to 18%.[14] Simon and Enneking, citing an overall recurrence rate of 16% in soft tissue tumors of the extremities,[11] noted a 2% recurrence rate following "adequate" local excision and a 100% recurrence rate following "inadequate" excision. Most other series cite similar trends of high recurrence rates with inadequate local excision of tumor.[3, 14] The classic definition of "adequate" local excision of soft tissue sarcomas was originally described for tumors of the extremities by Bowden and Booker[13] in 1958 and includes the following steps: wide excision of surrounding grossly normal tissue, the removal of entire muscle bundles involved by tumor, including points of origin and insertion, the use of sharp rather than blunt dissection, and the ligation of major venous tributaries early in the procedure. Bowden and Booker[13] and others[5, 6, 14] go on to state that when these maneuvers are not feasible, i.e., when major vessels, bones, or joints compromise wide resection, amputation should be performed. Obviously, this final therapeutic coup de grace is not feasible for head and neck soft tissue sarcoma.

While radiation therapy alone has proved inadequate for cure for almost all soft tissue sarcomas,[15] there are reports of success when wide local resection, adjunctive radiation, and/or chemotherapy are used. These protocols have allowed limb salvage in some soft tissue sarcomas of the extremities.[16–18] Data from comparable combined protocols for head and neck soft tissue sarcomas are anecdotal at this time.

Regardless of plans for future adjunctive therapy, careful pathologic examination of the margins of the resection specimen should be performed to ensure the adequacy of resection. Any histologic involvement of the margin of resection line, whether it is located in a tissue plane, vascular bundle, or nerve, will compromise a cure. Thorough extirpation is particularly important for certain tumors, such as neurofibrosarcomas, which will extend for some distance along the nerve of origin. Pathologically negative margins do not necessarily insure a good prognosis. It should always be kept in mind that it is impossible to sample the entire margin of a tumor, which leaves some room for doubt in all cases of "margins negative for tumor."

Wide excision of soft tissue sarcoma in the head and neck region is frequently hindered by proximity to bone, nerve, or major blood vessels. These circumstances lead to the adjuvant or primary use of irradiation or chemotherapy, depending on the expected response rate for the particular tumor type. Prophylactic lymph node dissection is rarely indicated except for rhabdomyosarcoma or synovial sarcoma, in which spread to regional lymphatics is more common. A lymphadenectomy type of operation is useful in carrying out wide-field dissection in an appropriate fascial compartment. Clinically involved lymph nodes, regardless of primary tumor type, should be removed at the time of wide-field tumor excision.

WHAT SPECIFIC SOFT TISSUE SARCOMAS OCCUR IN THE HEAD AND NECK AREA?

Tumors of Fibrous Tissue

FIBROSARCOMA

Fibrosarcomas are malignant tumors of fibrous tissue. They account for 15%–20% of all soft tissue sarcomas.[2, 19] Histologically, these tumors are composed of spindle-shaped cells arranged in fasicles, sometimes showing a "herring bone" pattern. Most of these tumors are histologically low grade, with minimal nuclear pleomorphism. Many tumors that would have been designated as high-grade fibrosarcomas by earlier classification systems are now designated as malignant fibrous histiocytoma (see below).

Peak incidence occurs in middle age (40–60 years), with an earlier, smaller peak in infants (age 0–2 years). The usual presentation of head and neck fibrosarcomas is that of a painless superficial mass. The poorly differentiated tumors will invade deeply into subjacent tissues and may cause pain and symptoms related to cranial nerve involvement. Fibrosarcomas of the head and neck occur most commonly in the soft tissues of the face and neck, followed by occurrence in bony structures (mandible, maxilla, sinuses) and oropharyngeal cavities.[20–23] An association between prior radiation therapy and the development of aggressive fibromatoses and fibrosarcomas has been reported.[24]

The natural history of fibrosarcomas includes a tendency to be locally invasive (nearly 100% of cases), to recur locally after surgical excision (50%–75%), and to metastasize to lungs, bone, and liver (50% in the adult age group).[20] These tumors rarely metastasize to regional lymph nodes (5%) (Table 24–2).[22] The overall 5-year survival is 45%.[19]

DERMATOFIBROSARCOMA PROTUBERANS

Dermatofibrosarcoma protuberans tumors are tumors of young adults (aged 20–40 years) that generally present as a painless, slow-growing purple or dark blue mass located on the trunk; less commonly they are found on the head and neck.[25, 26] Histologically they are characterized by a uniform proliferation of spindle cells arranged in a cartwheel or "storiform" pattern, hence the alternative designation, storiform fibrous histiocytoma. Mitotic activity may be present but tumor giant cells or anaplasia are not found. The proliferation is confined to the dermis (hence, *dermatofibrosarcoma*) which may be expanded to produce a plaque-like elevation of the skin (hence, *protuberans*). In a review of the literature and a report of a single patient, Sauter et al. cited the occurrence of dermatofibrosarcoma protuberans in the head and neck in seven (2%) of 344 reported cases.[27] These tumors demonstrate a marked tendency to recur (33%) and therefore should be widely resected.[25] Lymph node metastases have been reported but are decidedly rare (5%). Burkhardt et al. reported the use of adjuvant radiation therapy for recurrent tumor but found it to be of little benefit.[25] Patients with dermatofibrosarcoma protuberans have a good survival—95% at 5 years.[25]

MALIGNANT FIBROUS HISTIOCYTOMA

In the past, malignant fibrous histiocytomas were relatively rare tumors, constituting 10% of all soft tissue sarcomas.[2] The apparent incidence should increase in contemporary series since many of these tumors were previously classified under different histologic categories (see Chap. 17 for additional discussion on maxillary sinus involvement).

TABLE 24–2.—SOFT TISSUE SARCOMAS OF THE HEAD AND NECK

	METASTATIC POTENTIAL			RESPONSE TO:	
	Distant (%)	Regional Lymph Node (%)	RECURRENCE RATE (%)	Radiation	Chemotherapy
Fibrosarcoma	50	5	50–75	±	±
Dermatofibrosarcoma protruberans	5	< 1	33	–	–
Malignant fibrous histiocytoma	42	50–75	73	±	±
Liposarcoma (varies with cell type)	20–80	< 10	50–80	+	–
Rhabdomyosarcoma	50	15–74	50	+	+ +
Leiomyosarcoma	10–50	25	< 50	±	±
Malignant schwannoma	60–70	< 10	63–78	±	±
Synovial cell sarcoma	80	23	28–77	±	±
Angiosarcoma	28	57	?	±	±

The histologic features of malignant fibrous histiocytoma vary, but the most typical examples are characterized by proliferation of spindle cells that are arranged focally in a storiform pattern with interspersed anaplastic giant cells. Mitotic activity is usually brisk. Several important variants exist, including one with a predominance of myxoid areas resembling myxoid liposarcoma.[28] This myxoid variant is characterized by a better prognosis than the more solid variant. A second variant, the inflammatory fibrous histiocytoma, has a prominent component of polymorphonuclear cells scattered throughout the tumor; this variant may carry a worse prognosis,[29] although this has been denied by others.[30]

When a tumor with histologic features of malignant fibrous histiocytoma is identified in the anterior neck, the differential diagnosis includes anaplastic carcinoma of the thyroid, a diagnosis that can be confirmed by identifying preexisting papillary or follicular carcinoma within the tumor or by identifying tumor within the thyroid.

Malignant fibrous histiocytomas present as a painless mass in the extremities (68%) and retroperitoneum (17%).[30, 31] There are several reported cases of maxillary and paramandibular presentation.[32, 33] There is a 73% incidence of recurrence after excision,[31] and a high incidence of nodal metastasis (50%–70%).[30, 31] While not specifically recommended by most authors, routine removal of regional nodes seems to be both valid and justified. In a study by Soule and Enriquez, the 5-year survival after wide local excision was 50%, with no 10-year survivors.[31] A single case report of malignant fibrous histiocytoma in the maxilla claimed some tumor shrinkage from radiation therapy prior to wide local excision.[32] Sasaki et al. demonstrated tumor shrinkage and a change from a pleomorphic tumor to a xanthoma-like tumor is response to irradiation.[34] There are no long-term follow-up data for either case report.

Sarcomas of Muscle Tissue

RHABDOMYOSARCOMA

Rhabdomyosarcomas, derived from skeletal muscle, are the most common soft tissue malignancy in patients 15 years of age or younger.[35] These are discussed in more detail in Part II of this chapter, on sarcomas of childhood. Unfortunately, the prognosis for adults has not improved as much as for the pediatric age group.

The clinical presentation, malignant behavior, and treatment responses of rhabdomyosarcoma depend in part on the histologic subtype of tumor: embryonal, alveolar, botryoid, or pleomorphic. The embryonal, botryoid, and alveolar types are histologically composed of small uniform cells with scant cytoplasm. Mitotic activity is variable. Occasional cells with more abundant eosinophilic cytoplasm (presumably representing attempts at rhabdoid differentiation) may be found and allow distinction from the other "small blue cell" tumors of childhood. The identification of definite cross-striations is not necessary for the diagnosis of these three types of rhabdomyosarcoma, but such cross-striations are necessary for the diagnosis of pleomorphic rhabdomyosarcoma. The latter is characterized by a spindle cell population with abundant eosinophilic cytoplasm, numerous bizarre tumor giant cells, abundant mitotic activity, and cells with cross-striations. Tumors without cross-striations are now categorized as malignant fibrous histiocytoma, which accounts for the decreasing incidence of pleomorphic rhabdomyosarcoma in recent series. The embryonal or the botryoid form is the most common variety of rhabdomyosarcoma of the head and neck, occurring predominantly in young children. The clinical presentation most commonly is that of a painless retroorbital mass (31%), a retropharyngeal mass (29%), or a soft tissue mass of the face and neck (24%).[36] Pleomorphic rhabdomyosarcomas *occur in older age groups* (55–70 years old) and are most often located in the extremities (76%), less frequently in the head and neck (7.4%).[37] Rhabdomyosarcoma occurring in parameningeal areas (nasopharynx, paranasal sinuses, middle ear) carry the worst prognosis, and extension of tumors into the CNS has been considered a "death warrant."[35]

Rhabdomyosarcomas are locally aggressive tumors with a propensity for distant or nodal metastasis (50% at the time of the original diagnosis).[36] Rhabdomyosarcoma of the orbit, however, has a much lower rate of metastasis, both nodal and distant.[38] Initial workup for nonorbital rhabdomyosarcoma of the head and neck should include a search for metastatic disease. For accessible tumors in adults, the primary lesion should be widely excised, in conjunction with regional lymph node dissection. In patients in whom excision is not feasible, biopsy should be performed to firmly establish the diagnosis and cell type, and should be followed by a combination of irradiation and chemotherapy.[36] Further treatment may include debulking of tumor, depending on tumor response to irradiation or chemotherapy. Response to therapy depends on stage of disease at the time of initial treatment and on histologic subtype.[35] A combination of surgery, irradiation, and multiple-drug chemotherapy (vincristine, actinomycin D, cyclophosphamide, adriamycin, dacarbazine) for embryonal rhabdomyosarcoma has yielded 50%–70% disease-free 2-year survivals, compared to prior results with surgery and/or radiation therapy of only 5%–9%.[36]

LEIOMYOSARCOMA

Extragastrointestinal sarcomas of smooth muscle are extremely rare. They are characterized by a proliferation of spindle cells with elongated cytoplasmic extensions arranged in bundles. The nuclei tend to be rounded at the ends ("cigar-shaped" nuclei), a feature allowing some distinction from fibroblasts. Nuclear pleomorphism and mitotic activity may vary. Distinction from tumors showing neural or fibroblastic differentiation may be difficult; consequently, ultrastructural examination for neurosecretory granules may be necessary to arrive at a definitive diagnosis. In a series of 256 patients with nonepithelial tumors of the nasal cavity, six were leiomyosarcomas.[39] Stout and Hill reported results in a series of 36 leiomyosarcomas of the superficial soft tissues, of which 9 were in the head and neck.[40] A tendency toward recurrence and metastasis, particularly in large tumors, has been reported.[39–41] The mainstay of therapy is wide local excision. Response to radiation therapy has been variable, but irradiation has been advocated as therapy for recurrent disease.[39]

Sarcomas of Adipose Tissue

Liposarcomas occur in middle-aged adults with a slight male predominance and constitute about 15% of all soft tissue sarcomas.[42] The tumors are noticed as a painless mass, most commonly located in the lower (59%) or upper (16%) extremity. Two percent of all liposarcomas occur in the head and neck.[7, 43] The natural history of liposarcomas corresponds to the subtype (myxoid, round cell, well differentiated, or pleomorphic).[44] The most common subtype occurring in the head and neck is myxoid liposarcoma, followed by the well-differentiated variety.[42, 45]

Particularly judicious selection of treatment is needed for tumors of the well-differentiated "lipoma-like" categories in the neck. Recent studies show that most tumors previously placed in the category of *well-differentiated* liposarcoma do not grow or spread rapidly. Recurrence is rare and metastases are nonexistent. Most such tumors are now classified as pleomorphic lipomas[46] or spindle cell lipomas,[47] both characteristically found in the neck or shoulders of older males.

As is typical for liposarcomas in other locations, those that occur in the head and neck also have a tendency to recur (50%–80%), particularly if they are incompletely excised.[40, 48] Metastasis occurs predominantly to lungs, liver, CNS, and bone,[44] at rates depending on tumor subtype. The treatment of choice is wide local excision. Because lymph node metastases are infrequent, routine lymph node dissection is not used unless palpable suspicious nodes are clinically evident. Typically, authors will say that radiation therapy may be used for recurrence or for radiosensitive tumors that are locally unresectable.[42] The only way to determine radiosensitivity for this or any other soft tissue sarcoma is to deliver the irradiation and see if there is a response.

In general, liposarcomas are considered resistant to chemotherapy. Overall survival for liposarcomas in all locations ranges from 20% to 85%, being worst for pleomorphic and round cell varieties.[49, 50]

Synovial Sarcoma

Synovial sarcomas occur in young adults (20–30 years) most commonly in the extremities (93%).[51] The typical histologic pattern is that of a biphasic tumor with a spindle cell component and a glandular epithelioid component. Both spindle and epithelioid monophasic variants have also been described, although distinction from fibrosarcoma and metastatic carcinoma, respectively, can be a difficult if not impossible task. The grade of tumor varies and is related to the mitotic activity. Recently a peculiar calcified variant of low grade has been described.[52] Synovial sarcomas are rare in the head and neck, but may arise in the cervical prevertebral connective tissue space or in the superficial soft tissues of the neck.[53] Symptoms relate to mass effect in the retropharyngeal area—dysphagia, dyspnea, or hoarseness. These tumors demonstrate a marked tendency to recur after local excision. Unlike most soft tissue sarcomas, synovial sarcomas have a high frequency of lymph node metastasis (23%).[53] The majority of tumors (81%) ultimately metastasize to lung.[53] For this reason, recommended therapy includes wide local excision and prophylactic resection of regional lymph nodes.[53] Variable responses to radiation and chemotherapy have been observed.[10, 51, 53] The 5-year survival ranges from 25% to 62%, and the 10-year survival from 11% to 30%. Deaths are usually due to late distant metastasis.[10]

Soft Tissue Sarcoma of Neural Origin

MALIGNANT SCHWANNOMA

Malignant schwannomas represent 10% of all soft tissue sarcomas. They occur in middle-aged adults, with a slight predominance in men.[54, 55] A clear histologic distinction between fibrosarcoma, leiomyosarcoma, and malignant fibrous histiocytoma may present critical diagnostic problems because all of these tumors are characterized by spindle cell proliferation. Clear-cut evidence of neural differentiation in the form of nuclear palisading, a "wavy" configuration to the nuclei, or alternating myxoid and solid areas may be useful. Frequently the diagnosis rests on the clinical situation (i.e., a high-grade spindle cell sarcoma in a patient with von Recklinghausen's disease) or on the finding of preexisting benign neurofibroma or nerve from which the sarcoma is arising. These tumors present most often as painless, slow-growing masses in the upper or lower extremities (68%). Less than 10% arise in the head and neck region. Malignant schwannomas have a high rate of local recurrence (63%–78%) after simple excision. They should be widely excised. These sarcomas rarely metastasize to lymph nodes, but do spread to distant sites in 60%–70% of patients. Unpredictable responses to radiation or chemotherapy have been noted.[56] Overall, the 5-year survival in these patients is about 35%.[55, 56]

A moderate proportion of malignant Schwannomas occur in patients with von Recklinghausen's disease (less than half). In patients with familial neurofibromatosis, the malignant schwannomas tend to arise at an earlier age than in patients in whom the tumors arise de novo.[57] Mortality is significantly greater (75% 5-year) in patients with von Recklinghausen's disease who develop malignant schwannoma than in patients with solitary tumors.[58]

MALIGNANT CHEMODECTOMAS

Paraganglionomas or chemodectomas are tumors that arise from chemoreceptors (carotid body, glomus jugulare complex).[59, 60] Histologically they are similar to the more common pheochromocytoma of adrenal origin, with polygonal cells with abundant cytoplasm arranged in nests or "zellballen." The nests are separated by a vascular stroma. The vast majority of chemodectomas are benign. Only 6% are considered to be malignant tumors, although malignancy cannot be distinguished by histology. They present as neck masses that cause symptoms related to pressure on adjacent structures. Carotid body tumors present with hoarseness, cough, or dysphagia. Glomus jugulare tumors may cause hearing loss, tinnitus, ear discharge or infections, and facial nerve paralysis.[61] These tumors behave in a locally aggressive fashion and rarely metastasize (4% of all paraganglionomas).[60] They are highly vascular tumors. The vascularity makes them slightly compressible. Incision biopsy will produce brisk bleeding that is difficult to control. Chemodectomas are intimately associated with major vessels. For this reason preoperative angiography is recommended in order to display the characteristic vascular blush, confirm the diagnosis, and help the surgeon plan the subintimal resection of chemodectomas with complete vascular control or with installation of an intravascular shunt when the tumor is in the characteristic location at the carotid bifurcation.

The treatment of choice is surgical removal when technically feasible. We have had one patient with multiple cervical and upper mediastinal metastases treated by excision of all grossly malignant tissue. Surgery was followed by mediastinal irradiation. Survival (N.E.D.) exceeded 5 years. Surgery may require a temporary vascular Sundt shunt, depending on the extent of carotid artery involvement. Radiation therapy is recommended as a "poor alternative" therapy in the rare case where carotid artery dissection is technically impossible.[61]

RARE SOFT TISSUE SARCOMAS OF NEURAL ORIGIN

MALIGNANT EPITHELIOID SCHWANNOMAS.—Malignant epithelioid schwannomas are rare soft tissue sarcomas that have features of melanoma and malignant schwannoma. They occur in exposed areas of the head and neck in adult patients. Their behavior is like that of most soft tissue sarcomas, with a tendency to recur locally after excision; however, they have a predilection for lymphatic metastasis as well as hematogenous dissemination.[57]

MALIGNANT TRITON TUMOR.—Malignant triton tumor (malignant schwannoma with rhabdomyoblastic differentiation) is a rare, locally aggressive neural soft tissue sarcoma that occurs in young patients with von Recklinghausen's disease. It occurs in the neck, back, and extremities and presents as a progressively enlarging soft tissue mass with an associated neurologic deficit.[57]

NEUROBLASTOMAS.—Neuroblastomas rarely occur in the head and neck. Peak age incidence is at less than 3 years of age, but a second smaller peak exists in young adults. These tumors fall into the general category of "small blue cell tumors." Ultrastructural examination may be necessary to distinguish them from rhabdomyosarcoma, lymphoma, or Ewing's sarcoma. Tumors occurring in the older age group are thought to behave in a less aggressive fashion than those in children. Neuroblastomas demonstrate a fairly good response to multiple-drug chemotherapy (cyclophosphamide, vincristine, Adriamycin, and dacarbazine).[62, 63]

ESTHESIONEUROBLASTOMAS.—Esthesioneuroblastomas (olfactory neuroblastomas) are "low-grade" malignant neurogenic tumors that present with symptoms of nasal obstruction, epistaxis, or localized pain. More advanced tumors may present with headache or visual symptoms. These tumors are locally invasive, have a metastatic potential of 14%, and have a fairly good 5-year survival (50%).[64, 65] Treatment of choice is a combination of surgical excision and radiation therapy. Single-drug adjunctive chemotherapy with thiotepa is of possible value, but reports substantiating this are few (see Chap. 17).[66]

Soft Tissue Sarcomas of Blood Vessel Origin

ANGIOSARCOMA

Angiosarcomas are rare tumors of the skin and soft tissue that most commonly present as soft or ulcerated painless masses of the scalp or face.[67, 68] Reported series are small. Angiosarcomas of the head and neck are most frequently tumors of the skin with extension into the subcutaneous soft tissue. True noncutaneous soft tissue angiosarcomas are very rare. The distinguishing histologic feature of these tumors is the presence of anastomosing vascular spaces lined with atypical endothelial cells. These atypical cells may extend into vessels outside the gross margins of the neoplasm. Perivascular extension is the chief factor responsible for the frequent recurrence of this tumor. Angiosarcomas have also been reported to occur in the mandible, maxillary sinus, oral mucosa, skull, and thyroid.[69, 70]

Cutaneous angiosarcomas occur in middle age with a slight male predominance. They often display locally invasive growth. Bardwill et al. reported on a series of seven patients, of whom four had lymph node metastasis and two had distant metastases.[71] For this reason they recommended complete local excision plus lymph node removal when lymph nodes are clinically suspicious and when the primary tumor can be completely resected. Three of Bardwill's patients died of their disease. These three showed no response to chemotherapy and an equivocal response to radiation therapy.[71] Cochran and Fee reported a favorable response in one of four patients treated with a multiple-drug chemotherapy regimen (Cytoxan, vincristine, Adriamycin, and dacarbazine). Cochran and Fee also stated that 5-year disease-free survival in patients with angiosarcoma is rare.[68]

HEMANGIOPERICYTOMA

Hemangiopericytomas are tumors showing pericytic differentiation and having a pronounced vascular component. Histologically they bear a resemblance to the glomus tumor, although the cells are more oval to spindle-shaped than the glomus tumor. Many hemangiopericytomas are histologically benign; malignant characteristics can usually be predicted by increased mitotic activity and nuclear pleomorphism. These tumors most commonly occur in the trunk, with up to 30% arising in the head and neck.[72] Rhodes et al. reported on a group of five patients with hemangiopericytomas of the nasal cavity who presented with nasal obstruction and expistaxis. In these five cases, the tumors behaved in a benign fashion.[73] Nasal hemangiopericytomas must be distinguished from the majority of hemangiopericytomas, which present as painless mass, usually late in life.[72, 74] The usual tumors are slow-growing, are locally invasive, rarely metastasize to lymph nodes, and tend to spread in a hematogenous fashion. Treatment of choice is wide local excision, with high-dose radiation therapy reserved for recurrent or unresectable tumor.[74] Five-year survival varies from 50% to 70%.[72, 74]

Rare Soft Tissue Sarcomas of the Head and Neck

EPITHELIOID SARCOMA

These tumors arise primarily from subcutaneous tissue of the fingers, hands and forearms; less than 4% arise in the head and neck.[75] They are composed of epithelioid-appearing malignant cells frequently arranged in a nesting or "granulomatous" pattern that may cause diagnostic problems. Many of the epithelioid sarcomas are originally misdiagnosed as granuloma annulare or metastatic carcinoma. They are most frequent in young adults (aged 15–35 years) with a slight male predominance. Clinically they present as a slow-growing painless mass. As with other soft tissue sarcomas, epithelioid sarcoma tends to recur (76%) and metastasize to lungs, lymph nodes, skin, and CNS (47%).[75] Recommended therapy is wide excision with regional lymph node dissection, followed by radiation or chemotherapy for recurrent disease.

ALVEOLAR SOFT PART SARCOMA

Of 143 cases of alveolar soft part seen at the Armed Forces Institute of Pathology, 39 were in the head and neck (27%).[75] Histologically they are composed of plump eosinophilic cells arranged in a nested or "alveolar" pattern. The cells characteristically have a prominent central nucleolus, which distinguishes them from the granular cell tumor, to which they are *not* related. These tumors occur as slow-growing painless masses in adults (predominant location, lower extremity) or children (orbit, tongue). These tumors are highly vascular, subject to hemorrhage on resection. They rarely metastasize to lymph nodes. They frequently recur after excision. Local recurrence or hematogenous metastatic disease may be treated with chemotherapy (thiotepa), although experience is small due to the rarity of the tumor.[76]

MALIGNANT GRANULAR CELL MYOBLASTOMA

Despite the ominous name of myoblastoma, most of these tumors with characteristic pink granular cytoplasm are benign. Benign and malignant types of granular cell myoblastoma are both thought to be derived from primitive neurogenic elements. The rare malignant tumors are important to this chapter. Hunter and Dewar reported a literature review of 12 patients where the majority of tumors occurred in the head and neck and extremities. Prognosis was poor, and lymph node and hematogenous metastases were frequent.[77]

EXTRASKELETAL MESENCHYMAL CHONDROSARCOMAS

These rare tumors, derived from primitive cartilaginous mesenchyma, are primarily tumors of the head and neck, including the orbit, neck, and nasopharynx.[78, 79] They occur in young adults and present as slow-growing painless masses. Recurrence is common, as is distant metastasis. Wide local excision is recommended and occasional responses to radiation and chemotherapy are reported.[78]

NONOSSEUS OSTEOGENIC SARCOMA

Of 60 reported cases of nonosseus osteogenic sarcoma, one was located within the soft tissues of the neck.[80] These tumors also have been reported to occur as a polypoidal lesion of the larynx. They occur in older patients, more often in males, and behave in a highly malignant manner. Wide local excision followed by chemotherapy has been recommended.[81]

WHERE DOES TREATMENT OF HEAD AND NECK SOFT TISSUE SARCOMAS FAIL?

The preceding review of reported series indicates that local recurrence is the predominant problem that is amenable to improvement. The message is clear. Attempt to achieve wide margins around soft tissue sarcomas at the initial excision. Irregular invasive extension beyond gross tumor is common for most cell types. Pseudocapsules of compressed adjacent tissues are easy to dissect, but only deceivingly reassuring. One should dissect well outside of such pseudocapsules when they exist. Controlled compartmental resections give the best chance of encompassing localized soft tissue sarcoma.

REFERENCES

1. Enzinger F.M., Weiss S.W. (eds.): *Soft Tissue Tumors.* St. Louis, C.V. Mosby Co., 1983, pp. 1–13, 103–124, 519–549, 625–656, 780–813.
2. Russell W.O., et al.: A clinical and pathological staging system for soft tissue sarcomas. *Cancer* 40:1562–1570, 1977.
3. Suit H.D., Russell W.O., Martin R.G.: Sarcoma of soft tissue: Clinical and histopathological parameters and response to treatment. *Cancer* 35:1478–1483, 1975.
4. Sears H.F., Hopson R., Inouye W., et al.: Analysis of staging and management of patients with sarcoma. *Ann. Surg.* 191:488–493, 1980.
5. Gerner R.E., et al.: Soft tissue sarcomas. *Ann. Surg.* 181:803–808, 1975.
6. Fortner J.G.: Operative management of soft tissue sarcomas, in Najarian J.S., Delaney J.P. (eds.): *Advances In Cancer Surgery.* New York, Grune & Stratton, 1976, pp. 393–399.
7. Das Gupta T.K.: Tumors and tumor-like conditions of the adipose tissue. *Curr. Probl. Surg.* March 1970, pp. 1–60.
8. Osborn M., Weber K.: Biology of disease: Tumor diagnosis by intermediate filament typing: A novel tool for surgical pathology. *Lab. Invest.* 48:372–394, 1983.
9. Snover D.C., Sumner H.W., Dehner L.P.: Variability of histologic pattern in recurrent soft tissue sarcomas originally diagnosed as liposarcoma. *Cancer* 49:1005–1015, 1982.
10. In Enzinger F.M., Weiss S.W. (eds.): *Soft Tissue Tumors.* St. Louis, C.V. Mosby Co., 1983, pp. 227–295.
11. Simon M.A., Enneking W.F.: The management of soft tissue sarcomas of the extremities. *J. Bone Joint Surg.* 58A:317–327, 1976.
12. Campbell D.A., Eckhauser F.E., Oechler J.R., et al.: Liposarcoma of the lower extremity. *Surgery* 88:453–460, 1980.
13. Bowden L., Booker R.J.: The principles of technique of resection of soft parts sarcoma. *Surgery* 44:963–977, 1958.
14. Shiu M.H., Castro E.B., Hadju S.I., et al.: Surgical treatment of 297 soft tissue sarcomas of the lower extremity. *Ann. Surg.* 182:597–602, 1975.
15. Suit H.D.: Soft tissue sarcomas: The role of radiation therapy. *Hosp. Pract.* July 1982, pp. 114–120.
16. Fine G., Hajdu S.I., Morton D.L., et al.: Soft tissue sarcomas: Classification and treatment (a symposium). *Pathol. Annu.* 17:155, 1982.
17. Lindberg R.D., et al.: Surgery and postoperative radiotherapy in the treatment of soft tissue sarcomas in adults. *Am. J. Roentgenol. Radium Ther. Nucl. Med.* 123:123–129, 1975.
18. Rosenberg S.A., et al.: The treatment of soft tissue sarcomas of the extremities. *Ann. Surg.* 196:305–315, 1982.
19. In Enzinger F.M., Weiss S.W. (eds.): *Soft Tissue Tumors.* St. Louis, C.V. Mosby Co., 1983, pp. 103–124.
20. Batsakis J.G., Rice D.H., Howard D.R.: The pathology of head and neck tumors: Spindle cell lesions (sarcomatoid carcinomas, nodular fasciitis, and fibrosarcoma) of the aerodigestive tracts. Part 14. *Head Neck Surg.* 4:499–513, 1982.
21. Conley J., Stout A.P., Healy W.V.: Clinicopathologic analysis of eighty-four patients with an original diagnosis of fibrosarcoma of the head and neck. *Am. J. Surg.* 114:561–569, 1967.
22. Swain R.E., Sessions D.G., Ogura J.H.: Fibrosarcoma of the head and neck: A clinical analysis of forty cases. *Ann. Otol.* 83:439–444, 1974.
23. Van Blarcom C.W., et al.: Fibrosarcoma of the mandible. *Oral Surg.* 32(3):428–439, 1971.
24. Pettit V.D., et al.: Fibromatosis and fibrosarcoma following irradiation therapy. *Cancer* 7(1):149–158, 1954.
25. Burkhardt B.R., et al.: Dermatofibrosarcoma protuberans. *Am. J. Surg.* 3:638–644, 1966.
26. McPeak C.J., et al.: Dermatofibrosarcoma protuberans: An analysis of 86 cases—five with metastasis. *Ann. Surg.* 166(5):803–816, 1967.
27. Sauter L.S., DeFeo C.P.: Dermatofibrosarcoma protuberans of the face. *Arch. Dermatol.* 104:671–673, 1971.
28. Weiss S.W., Enzinger F.M.: Myxoid variant of malignant fibrous histiocytoma. *Cancer* 39:1672–1685, 1977.
29. Kyriakos M., Kempson R.L.: Inflammatory fibrous histiocytoma. *Cancer* 37(3):1584–1606, 1976.
30. Weiss J.W., Enzinger F.M.: Malignant fibrous histiocytoma: An analysis of 200 cases. *Cancer* 41:2250–2266, 1978.

31. Soule E.H., Ehriquez P.: Atypical fibrous histiocytoma, malignant fibrous histiocytoma, malignant histiocytoma and epithelioid sarcoma. *Cancer* 30:128, 1972.
32. Spector G.J., Ogura J.H.: Malignant fibrous histiocytoma of the maxilla. *Arch. Otolaryngol.* 99:385–387, 1974.
33. Solomon M.P., Sutton A.L.: Malignant fibrous histiocytoma of the soft tissues of the mandible. *Oral Surg.* 35(5):653–660, 1973.
34. Sasaki R., et al.: Malignant fibrous histiocytoma in the maxillary sinus: Xanthoma-like changes of the tumor after radiotherapy. *Laryngoscope* 93:202–204, 1983.
35. Batsakis J.G., et al.: The pathology of head and neck tumors: Fibroadipose tissue and skeletal muscle. Part 8. *Head Neck Surg.* 3:145–168, 1980.
36. Healy G.B., et al.: Rhabdomyosarcoma of the head and neck: Diagnosis and management. *Head Neck Surg.* 1:334–339, 1979.
37. Keyhani A., Booher R.J.: Pleomorphic rhabdomyosarcoma. *Cancer* 22(5):956–967, 1968.
38. Dito W.R., et al.: Rhabdomyosarcoma of the head and neck. *Arch. Surg.* 84:112–118, 1962.
39. Fu Y.S., Perzin K.H.: Nonepithelial tumors of the nasal cavity, paranasal sinuses, and nasopharynx: A clinicopathologic study. *Cancer* 35(5):1300–1308, 1975.
40. Stout A.P., Hill W.T.: Leiomyosarcoma of the superficial soft tissues. *Cancer* 11(4):844–854, 1958.
41. Rosen L., et al.: Leiomyosarcoma of the superficial soft tissues. *Mount Sinai J. Med.* 46(2):181–184, 1979.
42. Saunders J.R., Maj M.C., et al.: Liposarcomas of the head and neck. *Cancer* 43(1):162–168, 1979.
43. Enterline A., et al.: Liposarcoma: A clinical and pathological study of 53 cases. *Cancer* 13:932–950, 1960.
44. O'Connor M., Snover D.C.: Liposarcoma: A review of factors influencing prognosis. *Am. Surg.* 49(7):379–384, 1983.
45. Batsakis J.G., et al.: The pathology of head and neck tumors: Fibroadipose tissue and skeletal muscle. Part 8. *Head Neck Surg.* 3:145–168, 1980.
46. Shmookler B.M., Enzinger F.M.: Pleomorphic lipoma: A benign tumor simulating liposarcoma. A clinicopathologic analysis of 48 cases. *Cancer* 47:126–132, 1981.
47. Enzinger F.M., Harvey D.A.: Spindle cell lipoma. *Cancer* 36:1852–1859, 1975.
48. Kindblom L.G., et al.: Liposarcoma of the neck: A clinicopathologic study of 4 cases. *Cancer* 42:774–780, 1978.
49. Enzinger F.M., Winslow D.J.: Liposarcoma: A study of 103 cases. *Virchows Arch. [Pathol. Anat.]* 335:367–388, 1962.
50. Kindblom L.G., et al.: Liposarcoma: A clinicopathologic, radiographical and prognostic study. *Acta Pathol. Microbiol. Scand. Suppl.* 253:1–71, 1975.
51. Shmookler B.M., et al.: Orofacial synovial sarcoma. *Cancer* 50:269–276, 1982.
52. Varela-Duran J., Enzinger F.M.: Calcifying synovial sarcoma. *Cancer* 50:345–352, 1982.
53. Roth J.A., et al.: Synovial sarcoma of the neck: A follow-up study of 24 cases. *Cancer* 35:1243–1253, 1975.
54. Das Gupta T.K., Brasfield R.D.: Solitary malignant schwannoma. *Ann. Surg.* 171:419–425, 1970.
55. Ghosh B.C., Ghosh L., Huvos A.G., et al.: Malignant schwannoma: A clinicopathologic study. *Cancer* 31:184–198, 1973.
56. D'Agostino A.N., et al.: Primary malignant neoplasms of nerves (malignant neurilemmomas) in patients without manifestations of multiple neurofibromatosis (von Recklinghausen's disease). *Cancer* 16:1003–1014, 1963.
57. in Enzinger F.M., Weiss S.W. (eds.): *Soft Tissue Tumors.* St. Louis, C.V. Mosby Co., 1983, pp. 625–656.
58. D'Agostino A.N., et al.: Sarcomas of the peripheral nerves and somatic soft tissues associated with multiple neurofibromatosis (von Recklinghausen's disease). *Cancer* 16:1015–1026, 1963.
59. Howell A., et al.: Chemodectomas of the head and neck. *Surg. Clin. North Am.* 53(1):175–177, 1973.
60. Borsanyi S.J.: Glomus jugulare tumors. *Laryngoscope* 71:1336–1345, 1961.
61. Irons G.B., et al.: Paragangliomas of the neck: Clinical and pathologic analysis of 116 cases. *Surg. Clin. North Am.* 57(3):575–583, 1977.
62. Fortner J., et al.: Neuroblastoma: Natural history and results of treating 133 cases. *Ann. Surg.* 156(1):132–142, 1968.
63. Lopez R., et al.: Treatment of adult neuroblastoma. *Cancer* 45:840–844, 1980.
64. Hutter R.V.P., et al.: Esthesioneuroblastoma. *Am. J. Surg.* 106:748–753, 1963.
65. Kadish S., et al.: Olfactory neuroblastoma: A clinical analysis of 17 cases. *Cancer* 37:1571–1576, 1976.
66. Grahne G.: Olfactory neuroblastoma. *Acta Otolaryngol.* 60:37–48, 1954.
67. Jones E.W.: *Malignant Angioendothelioma of the skin.* London, Institute of Dermatology, 1960, pp. 21–39.
68. Cochran J.H., Jr., Fee W.E. Jr.: Angiosarcoma of the head and neck. *Otolaryngol. Head Neck Surg.* 87:409–416, 1979.
69. Farr H.W., et al.: Malignant vascular tumors of the head and neck. *Am. J. Surg.* 120:501–504, 1970.
70. Bankaci M., et al.: Angiosarcoma of the maxillary sinus: Literature review and case report. *Head Neck Surg.* 2:274–280, 1979.
71. Bardwill J.M., et al.: Angiosarcomas of the head and neck region. *Am. J. Surg.* 116:548–553, 1968.
72. O'Brien P., Brasfield R.D.: Hemangiopericytoma. *Cancer* 18:249–252, 1965.
73. Rhodes R.E. Jr., et al.: Hemangiopericytoma of nasal cavity. *Arch. Otolaryngol.* 79:505–511, 1964.
74. Gerner R.E., et al.: Hemangiopericytoma. *Ann. Surg.* 179:132, 1974.
75. in Enzinger F.M., Weiss S.W. (eds.): *Soft Tissue Tumors.* St. Louis, C.V. Mosby Co., 1983, pp. 780–813.
76. Spector R.A., et al.: Alveolar soft part sarcoma of the head and neck. *Laryngoscope* 89:1301–1306, 1979.
77. Hunter D.T., Dewar J.P.: Malignant granular-cell myoblastoma: Report of a case and review of literature. 26:554–559, 1960.
78. Guccion J.G., et al.: Extraskeletal mesenchymal chondrosarcoma. *Arch. Pathol.* 95:336–340, 1973.

79. Salvador A.H., et al.: Mesenchymal chondrosarcoma: Observations on 30 new cases. *Cancer* 28:605–615, 1971.
80. Jussawalla D.J., Desai J.G.: Primary osteogenic sarcoma arising in extra-skeletal soft tissues of the neck. *Br. J. Surg.* 51(7):504–505, 1964.
81. Dahm L.J., et al.: Osteosarcoma of the soft tissue of the larynx. *Cancer* 42:2343–2351, 1978.

II. Connective Tissue Malignancies of the Head and Neck Region in Children

A.D.J. PEARSON, M.D. / M.E. NESBIT, M.D.

THE DIFFERENT PATTERNS of head and neck cancer in children and the differences in therapeutic approach warrant a separate discussion from adult connective tissue malignancies.

The recent improvement in the treatment results for connective tissue tumors in children is a major success story. It exemplifies the benefit of multidisciplinary care. It shows how well-designed, multi-institution clinical trials can be used to evaluate and improve treatment. The quality of management and decision-making has progressed rapidly in a system of randomized trials which are conscientiously performed and quantitatively analyzed.

WHAT ARE THE MALIGNANT NEOPLASMS THAT AFFECT THE HEAD AND NECK REGIONS IN CHILDREN?

Excluding intracranial neoplasms, between 5% and 10% of all malignant solid tumors in children occur in the head and neck region. Malignant lymphomas and soft tissue sarcomas are the most frequent neoplasms in children. In contrast to adults, children have relatively few carcinomas, although 68% of all carcinomas in children arise in the head and neck region.[1–4] The types of soft tissue sarcomas in children are also different. Rhabdomyosarcoma and its variants predominate, with the head and neck region and genitourinary tract being the most frequent sites. In adults, liposarcoma, fibrosarcoma, and malignant fibrous histiocytoma are more frequent, occurring most commonly in the retroperitoneum and extremities.[5] The relative incidence of the different primary malignant neoplasms in the head and neck in children are given in Table 24–3.

In the pediatric age group, malignant lymphomas represent 40% of the malignancies in the head and neck region.[7] Hodgkin's disease and non-Hodgkin's lymphoma are equally frequent. Hodgkin's disease usually affects older children with a mean age of 11 years. They are more often male. Between 60% and 90% of Hodgkin's disease patients present with nontender cervical lymphadenopathy. Enlargement of the lower cervical nodes is often associated with mediastinal involvement.

TABLE 24–3.—PRIMARY MALIGNANT HEAD AND NECK TUMORS IN CHILDREN, EXCLUDING RETINOBLASTOMA AND PRIMARY INTRACRANIAL NEOPLASMS*

TUMOR	NO	(%)
Malignant lymphoma	169	(41)
Hodgkin's disease	86	
Non-Hodgkin's	83	
Rhabdomyosarcoma	74	(17.8)
Fibrosarcoma / Malignant schwannoma	41	(9.8)
Thyroid malignancies	31	(7.5)
Neuroblastoma	18	(4.3)
Squamous cell carcinoma	17	(4.1)
Malignant melanoma	10	(2.4)
Ewing's sarcoma	7	(1.7)

OTHER TUMORS
- Malignant fibrous histiocytoma
- Osteogenic sarcoma
- Chondrosarcoma
- Malignant hemangiopericytoma
- Malignant hemangioendothelioma
- Malignant teratoma
- Neuroepithelioma (atypical neuroblastoma, primitive neuroectodermal tumor)
- Synovial cell sarcoma
- Melanotic neuroectodermal tumor of infancy
- Histiocytosis X
- Liposarcoma
- Leukemic deposits, including granulocytic sarcoma

*Compiled from three series totaling 416 malignant head and neck tumors.[3, 4, 6]

In 6% there is preauricular lymphadenopathy that may simulate parotid swelling. Extranodal involvement is relatively uncommon compared to non-Hodgkin's lymphoma.[3, 4, 8, 9] There are four histologic types, in decreasing order of frequency: nodular sclerosis, mixed cellularity, lymphocyte predominance, and lymphocyte depletion.[8, 9]

Non-Hodgkin's lymphoma tends to occur at a younger age of 6–10 years. Again, there is a male predominance.[10] Only one third of patients have localized disease at presentation. Widespread involvement of the mediastinum and abdomen is quite common. About 20% of patients also have bone marrow or CNS involvement.[11] Extranodal sites such as the tonsil or nasopharynx contain lymphoma four times more commonly at diagnosis than with Hodgkin's disease. In children with non-Hodgkin's lymphoma, nodular histology is unusual. There are four main subtypes: lymphoblastic, undifferentiated Burkitt's lymphoma, undifferentiated pleomorphic non-Burkitt's lymphoma, and large cell type (histocytic).[12]

Rhabdomyosarcoma, the commonest soft tissue sarcoma in childhood,[13] is the second most common malignant neoplasm of the head and neck region (17%). This tumor is derived from the primitive mesenchyme with varying degrees of myogenous differentiation. Its occurrence is not limited to sites of skeletal muscle. Rhabdomyosarcoma has a tendency to disseminate widely to the lung, bone marrow, and lymph nodes.[14]

The next two common soft tissue sarcomas, fibrosarcoma and malignant schwannoma, are locally aggressive but have a lower metastatic potential.[13]

Fibromatoses, which are localized proliferation of fibroblasts, often have a histologic picture which is difficult to distinguish from that of a fibrosarcoma. They may be locally aggressive.[15]

Thyroid carcinomas represent less than 3% of all childhood cancers and occur in increasing frequency in the second decade.[16] The three most common histologic variants are the differentiated medullary, papillary, and follicular types, with anaplastic variants being uncommon.[17] As discussed in chapter 19, previous radiation exposure is an important etiologic factor. Thyroid cancer can arise as a second primary malignancy following the treatment of another pediatric tumor or leukemia, or following irradiation to the thymus.[18, 19]

Neuroblastomas are derived from the embryonic neural crest. They can show evidence of differentiation into ganglioneuromas. Some 70% of cases that present in the head and neck region represent metastases from a distant primary.[3] Primary cervical neuroblastomas occur, especially in younger children. They are usually associated with a good prognosis and often do not require adjuvant therapy.[20]

Nasopharyngeal carcinomas represent only 20%–35% of primary nasopharyngeal neoplasms and are most common in children of Oriental or African nationality.[21] The Ebstein-Barr virus has been implicated as an etiological agent. Ebstein-Barr virus DNA has been found incorporated into all tumors examined.[22] These tumors are locally invasive and can spread to the meninges, producing cranial nerve palsies in 50% of patients. Lymph node metastases from nasopharyngeal cancer are very common. They occur in virtually all afflicted children. Distant metastases to the lungs and bone are less frequent.[23] Nasopharyngeal carcinomas together with malignant lymphoma and rhabdomyosarcoma are the main causes of malignant cervical lymphadenopathy in a child.

Although malignant melanoma is a rare pediatric malignancy, 43% of all cases arise in the head and neck region.[4]

WHAT ARE THE BENIGN AND MALIGNANT NEOPLASMS OCCURRING IN DIFFERENT SITES OF THE HEAD AND NECK REGION IN CHILDREN?

The types of neoplasms are best presented in tabular form. They are shown in Table 24–4.

WHAT ARE THE PATHOLOGIC SUBTYPES OF RHABDOMYOSARCOMA?

Rhabdomyosarcoma is an embryonal mesenchymal tumor in which myoblastic differentiation may occur. The variable degree of muscle differentiation can be detected by the presence of cross-striations or by electron microscopic ultrastructural studies that show the thick intracytoplasmic filaments. The presence of myoglobin can be shown by immunoperoxidase studies.[34–36] There are three major histologic variants of rhabdomyosarcoma: embryonal, alveolar, and pleomorphic. Tumors with mixed histology can occur. The data from the cooperative Intergroup Rhabdomyosarcoma Study (IRS) has contributed to the understanding of the clinical behavior of the different subtypes.[37] The embryonal pattern constitutes 75% of all head and neck rhabdomyosarcomas[38] and tends to occur in younger children between the ages of 3 and 5 years.[39] The tumor is composed of small dark round or spindle cells with little scanty acidiophilic cytoplasm; cross-striations or longtitudinal striations can be detected in 40%–60% of cases.[40, 41] A more differentiated variant of embryonal rhabdomyosarcoma has larger cells and more prominent cross-striations. This variant has a predilection for the orbit and middle ear but does have a better prognosis.[5]

The botryoid rhabdomyosarcoma is essentially a further subdivision of the embryonal variant. It differs be-

TABLE 24–4.—Benign and Malignant Neoplasms in Children, by Site of Origin

SITE	BENIGN	MALIGNANT
Nasal cavity, nasopharynx[24–26]	Nasal polyps Teratoma Papillomas Angiofibroma polyp Juvenile nasopharyngeal angiofibroma Meningoma Angioma Neurofibroma	Rhabdomyosarcoma Malignant lymphoma Nasopharyngeal carcinoma Esthesioneuroblastoma Histiocytosis X Granulocytic sarcoma Metastatic Neuroblastoma Wilms' tumor Retinoblastoma
Paranasal sinuses[26, 27]	Osteoma Ossifying fibroma Giant cell granuloma	Rhabdomyosarcoma Lymphoma Malignant fibrous histiocytoma Fibrosarcoma Osteogenic sarcoma
Jaw: mandible, maxilla[28, 29]	Odontogenic cysts Hemorrhagic bone cyst Hemangioma Aneurysmal bone cyst Ondontogenic tumors Giant cell granuloma Fibro-osseous tumors, including fibromatosis	Metastatic lesions (most frequent) Neuroblastoma Malignant lymphoma Rhabdomyosarcoma Osteogenic sarcoma Ewing's sarcoma Mesenchymal chondrosarcoma (rare) Fibrosarcoma
Middle ear and temporal bone[24]	Meningoma Glomus jugulare	Rhabdomyosarcoma Histiocytosis X Granulocytic sarcoma
Soft tissue[24]	Branchial cleft cyst Cystic hygroma Hemangiomas Aggressive juvenile fibromatosis Neurofibroma	Malignant lymphoma Rhabdomyosarcoma
Larynx[24]	Juvenile laryngeal papillomatosis Hemangioma Granular cell myoblastoma Neurofibroma	Rhabdomyosarcoma Fibrosarcoma Epidermoid carcinoma
Oral cavity[24]	Pyogenic granuloma Peripheral giant cell tumor Peripheral ossifying fibroma Granular cell tumor Pigmented neuroectodermal tumor of infancy Focal epithelial hyperplasia Squamous papilloma Hemangioma Lymphangioma Neurofibroma Neurilemmoma Leiomyomas	Rhabdomyosarcoma Fibrosarcoma Histiocytosis X Epidermoid carcinoma Leukemic infiltrates
Orbit[30–33]	Dermoid cyst Hemangioma Optic nerve glioma Neurofibroma Lymphangioma Inflammatory pseudotumor Lipoma	Rhabdomyosarcoma Neuroblastoma Retinoblastoma (involving orbit) Leukemia Granulocytic sarcoma Lymphoma Histiocytosis X Ewing's

cause it occurs in mucosal sites with normal mucous membrane covering it. The tumor usually presents as a polypoid "grape-like" mass. Microscopically there is an abundant gelatinous myxoid matrix. All types of embryonal rhabdomyosarcoma have a tendency to metastasize to the lung and other sites, to recur locally, and to infiltrate along tissue planes.[40] Lymph nodes metastases are uncommon. They occur in 5% of all head and neck rhabdomyosarcomas.[42]

The alveolar rhabdomyosarcoma tends to occur in older children at a mean age of 10 years. It has a predilection for the extremities, with only 15% of cases originating in the head and neck.[38] The characteristic histologic feature is the presence of "alveoli" which are separated by fibrous connective tissue trabeculae. These alveoli, which may be empty, are lined by layers of tumor cells in which cross-striations may be detected.[43] The prognosis for the alveolar variant is worse than that for the embryonal type even when treated with multimodal therapy. Alveolar rhabdomyosarcoma disseminates widely, especially to bones and marrow. It can produce a clinical picture of a leukoerythroblastic anemia with multiple osteolytic lesions from a small inapparent primary.[44] In contrast, relatively few metastasize to the lung, liver, or brain. A recent study showed that tumors of alveolar histology respond to initial chemotherapy as often as do tumors of other histologies. However, there were increased numbers of local, regional, and distant relapses. The difference was most marked in children who had had complete gross resection of the primary tumor and adjuvant chemotherapy. The 4-year mortality was 44% in children who had alveolar histology, compared to 13.5% in children with the embryonal type.[45]

Pleomorphic rhabdomyosarcoma is rare in children. It occurs most frequently in the extremities. These tumors are composed of a mixture of strap-like, racket-shaped, large or multinucleated cell types that contain granular or acidophilic cytoplasm.[41]

The IRS study has identified three additional histologic types of soft tissue sarcomas that were initially classified as rhabdomyosarcomas. Two of these are thought to be extraskeletal Ewing's sarcoma (soft tissue Ewing's sarcoma) because of a histology similar to that of Ewing's sarcoma of bone. Type I (classic Ewing's sarcoma) of bone is composed of uniform-sized round or oval anaplastic cells with scant glycogen-positive cytoplasm. Type II (large cell Ewing's sarcoma) is composed of larger, more irregular cells with less dense chromatin characteristics.[46] Early treatment results in patients on rhabdomyosarcoma protocols suggest that the therapeutic prognosis is similar to that for classic rhabdomyosarcoma. The final histologic type has been classified as small cell undifferentiated mesenchymal sarcoma, type indeterminate. These tumors consist of small primitive, round or spindle-shaped cells that exhibit no differentiation.[46]

A recent development is a pathologic classification system defined by cytologic features. Tumors with unfavorable histology, either anaplastic with enlarged bizzare mitotic figures and nuclear pleomorphism or monomorphous round cell types, are associated with a worse survival rate than those with a mixed histology.[47]

DO RHABDOMYOSARCOMAS AT DIFFERENT SITES IN THE HEAD AND NECK REGION HAVE A DIFFERENT CLINICAL BEHAVIOR?

Recently it has been demonstrated that rhabdomyosarcomas in different sites have different clinical behaviors and prognoses. There are four groups, according to anatomical area. These are discussed below.

Orbit

Rhabdomyosarcoma is the commonest malignant neoplasm of the orbit in children.[31] Some 10% of all rhabdomyosarcomas and 26% of those arising in the head and neck region occur in the orbit or eye.[38, 48, 49] These neoplasms usually present with exopthalmos (100%), ptosis (33%), or a mass (25%). Other symptoms that occur less often include pain (10%), and epistaxis (10%).[50] At diagnosis only 35% of lesions can be completely resected. Biopsy or limited resection is possible in the remainder.[51] Orbital tumors have always been associated with a better prognosis than tumors in other regions.[52, 53] With surgery alone, approximately 50% of patients survived,[50] compared to 6% of patients with tumors at all other sites. When clean-margin radical surgery (orbital exenteration) was possible, 70% survived.[50] Using radiotherapy, 5,000–6,000 rad following biopsy alone, local control was produced in 90%; however, the 5-year survival rate was 68%, with 30% experiencing recurrence at distant sites.[54, 55] The addition of chemotherapy to radiation has now produced relapse-free survival rates of 77%–96%.[51, 56]

The better prognosis of orbital rhabdomyosarcoma is related to the lower incidence (30%) of hematogenous metastatic spread as compared to other sites (51%).[14, 57] At presentation only 6% of patients have metastatic disease, compared to 20% of patients with rhabdomyosarcomas at all other sites.[48, 51] With modern therapy, biopsy, irradiation, and chemotherapy in the IRS-I study, the incidence of metastases has been reduced to 6%.[51] Lymph node spread is very unusual, occurring in 0%–6% of patients.[42, 51, 56] Meningeal extension and therefore dissemination to the CNS are also rare (3%–15%).[14, 51, 58] Meningeal extension probably occurs only if the disease advances to where there is radiologic or computerized tomographic (CT) demonstration of erosion of the bony orbit.[51, 58, 59] The reduced incidence of hematogenous metastases and meningeal extension has been related to the limiting barrier of the bony orbit that produces early symptoms and prevents meningeal extension.[60] The poor lymphatic drainage of the orbit may explain the rarity of lymphatic spread.

About 79% of orbital rhabdomyosarcomas have the more favorable embryonal histology, compared to 59% of rhabdomyosarcomas in all sites.[38, 40] Conversely, tumors with the less favorable alveolar histology constitute only 6% of orbital rhabdomyosarcomas, compared to 21% at all sites. This leaves 15% that have an undifferentiated histology and 2% that represent an extraosseous Ewing's sarcoma.[38, 40]

Neck

Rhabdomyosarcomas that arise in the cervical soft tissues between the mastoid process and the clavicle have recently been identified as having a worse prognosis than rhabdomyosarcomas that arise in other nonorbital, nonparameningeal sites when treated by the combined modality treatment that is recommended by the IRS.[61] Fewer of the midcervical tumors have an embryonal histology (46%) compared by other nonorbital, nonparameningeal sites (74%). When the patients first seek medical attention, they tend to have a greater tumor diameter. More patients (29%) have proved involvement of regional lymph nodes. The 5-year relapse-free survival is only 54%, with local and distant relapse contributing equally to failure.[61] It has been suggested that improved pretreatment definition of the extent of these tumors by CT scan will improve the treatment planning for surgery and radiotherapy for tumors of the neck.

Parameningeal Sites

Rhabdomyosarcomas that arise in the middle ear, paranasal sinuses, pterygoid region, mastoid, infratemporal fossa, and nasopharynx have a tendency to be locally invasive along fascial planes. They may erode the bone at the base of the skull and then spread directly to the meninges and, hence, disseminate through the CNS.[62–65] Because these anatomical areas have the ominous implication of involvement of the CNS, they have been termed "parameningeal sites."[62] Rhabdomyosarcomas that arise in parameningeal areas constitute 46% of all head and neck cases.[38] The incidence of meningeal extension of these tumors has been reported as 7%, 35%, and 60% in different series.[58, 62, 63] Certain features seen at presentation have been of value in predicting later meningeal extension of these tumors.[62, 64, 66, 67] These are:

1. Evidence on CT scan or plain radiographs of bony erosion of the base of the skull. Bone erosion has been shown to be a major discriminant feature. Often, changes are detected only on CT scan (see Chap. 3).
2. Evidence of intracranial extension of the tumor.
3. Any cranial nerve palsy.

Cranial nerve palsies are especially common with middle ear lesions that may produce deafness and a facial palsy.[65] Nasopharyngeal tumors can produce multiple lower cranial nerve palsies (see illustration of regional cross section in Chap. 15).

Overt disseminated meningeal disease has been shown to have a very poor prognosis, with only 10% of children with known disease alive in one series.[62] Once meningeal disease is established, aggressive treatment with intrathecal chemotherapy and craniospinal irradiation is not effective, which suggests that prophylaxis is required to prevent dissemination.[58, 62, 68] Disseminated CNS rhabdomyosarcoma may present with (1) symptoms and signs of increased intracranial pressure,[64] (2) spinal cord compression,[69, 70] and (3) posterior fossa signs, including ataxia and cranial nerve palsies.[64] In these cases malignant cells may be present in the cerebrospinal fluid (CSF),[64] although determination of their malignant nature may be difficult.[68, 69] Meningeal disease with or without intradural tumors can occur without local relapse at the primary site,[40, 64, 70] as well as when there is persistent or recurrent local disease.[58, 71]

The overall 3-year relapse-free survival for children with parameningeal rhabdomyosarcoma has been reported to be 45% in the IRS-I study.[38] Similar poor survival rates have been reported by other groups.[58, 71]

In addition to the problems of meningeal extension, large parameningeal rhabdomyosarcomas also have a high local relapse rate.[38, 71] It has been suggested that the frequency of treatment failure is due to (1) poor penetration of chemotherapeutic agents across the blood-brain barrier to reach the intracranial disease,[62] (2) lack of appreciation of the extent of the disease without a CT scan, and (3) inadequate radiation.[62, 71] In their first study, the IRS group found that in 58% of patients with meningeal extension, inadequate volumes of tissue had been incorporated into the irradiated field. Retrospectively, 68% received an inadequate dose, which suggests that there is a tendency to undertreat because of the tumor's position adjacent to the CNS.[62]

Rhabdomyosarcomas of the middle ear have been associated with a particularly poor prognosis, with no survivors among those diagnosed before 1969.[72] In a recent analysis, the prognostic importance of signs indicating meningeal extension was again confirmed. When there was absence of meningeal extension, 66% survived, compared to 33% who had evidence of intracranial tumor or bone erosion.[73]

Other Sites

Rhabdomyosarcomas that arise in the oral cavity, oropharynx, larynx, and parotid gland, cheek, or scalp have been reported to have a 90% retained complete, durable, remission rate when treated with multimodal therapy.[61] Laryngeal rhabdomyosarcomas are rare, comprising 0.3% of all laryngeal tumors. Patients with laryngeal rhabdomyosarcomas appear to have a very good survival without laryngectomy.[74, 75]

WHAT ARE THE OTHER MALIGNANT SOFT TISSUE SARCOMAS IN THE HEAD AND NECK REGION IN CHILDREN?

The histologic characteristics of the connective tissue tumors were discussed in Part I of this chapter (adult sarcomas).

Fibrosarcomas together with malignant schwannomas are the next most frequent malignant soft tissue sarcomas in the head and neck region in children. About 13%–20% of all fibrosarcomas arise in this region.[76, 77] There are two age peaks for fibrosarcomas of all sites: 62% occur in the first 5 years of life, with half of these developing in the first 5 months; another 26% occur at ages 10–15 years.[76, 77] The commonest sites for fibrosarcomas are over the chin and mandible, nasopharynx, paranasal sinuses, and sinuses. They also occur in the facial bones, especially the mandible. Fibrosarcoma is rare in the oral cavity, the tonsil, and hypopharynx.[76, 77] These tumors usually are seen as a rapidly growing mass or as a diffuse destructive radiolucency if the bone is the site of the primary.[77, 78] It is not possible to predict the clinical behavior of fibrosarcoma from the histologic pattern. In children less than 4 years old, tumors with an anaplastic histologic picture do not behave in an aggressive manner.[76, 79] The morphological differentiation of fibrosarcomas from aggressive fibromatoses (localized proliferation of fibroblasts) can be very difficult.[15,79] The best prognostic histologic indices in childhood fibrosarcoma appear to be nuclear pleomorphism, mitotic activity, and vascular invasion. Metastases occur in only 8% of childhood fibrosarcomas,[76] a lower rate than in the adult counterparts. Although 43% of patients may experience local recurrence,[76] the 5-year survival rates range from 86% to 92%.[76, 77, 80]

Malignant schwannomas or neurogenic sarcomas are malignant neoplasms of the nerve sheath that arise from Schwann cells. Between 36% and 61% arise in neurofibromas in children who have von Recklinghausen's disease.[81–83] It has been suggested but not confirmed that these tumors have a greater degree of anaplasia and a worse prognosis.[81, 82] A malignant schwannoma usually presents as a rapidly expanding mass arising in a previously stationary neurofibroma in the neck. Between 2% and 29% of patients with neurofibromatosis will develop a malignant schwannoma.[84] These tumors tend to recur after inadequate primary excision, just as do fibrosarcomas. The required margin is traditionally underestimated or technically impossible to achieve. There is conflicting evidence as to the metastatic potential of malignant schwannoma. Frequencies vary from 21% to 71% in different series.[81–83, 85]

Malignant fibrous histocytomas are common soft tissue malignancies in the adult but account for only 2%–5% of all soft tissue sarcomas in children.[13] Most of those that occur in the first two decades of life do so in the *second* decade.[86] There is a male predominance. These neoplasms are frequently associated with prior irradiation. Malignant fibrous histiocytoma has been reported to occur following the treatment of a retinoblastoma.[5] The distinction between benign and malignant fibrous histiocytomas may be difficult to make. The position, invasiveness, and size of the tumor are better predictors of malignant behavior than are nuclear pleomorphism or mitotic activity. Small lesions found in the superficial soft tissues behave in a more benign manner than do deeper lesions, especially those in the sinonasal regions.[5, 86–88]

Angiosarcomas, either malignant hemangiopericytomas or hemangioendotheliomas, are rare in children. The most common site in the head and neck region is the face and scalp.[89] Synovial cell sarcomas constitute 5%–10% of all soft tissue sarcomas.[13] When found in a young person, they occur most commonly in adolescents and young adults. The three commonest sites in the head and neck regions are the cervical soft tissues, the occipital region, and the nasopharynx. The usual presentation is that of a soft tissue mass, which in 25%–30% of instances shows calcification on x-ray studies.[90]

Osteogenic sarcoma constitutes 20% of all primary bone neoplasms,[91] but only 10% occur in the head and neck region.[91] The peak age for neoplasms of the jaw is 25–35 years, which makes these malignancies uncommon in children. The mandible is the most common site, followed in frequency by the maxilla, then other skull bones.[92] Radiation therapy is one etiologic factor that has been established.[93] In children, tumors are osteoblastic or chondroblastic; a few are fibroblastic. Hematogenous metastases to the lungs occur less commonly from jaw primaries than from the long bones. Survival rates on the order of 35% have been reported.[92]

In a series of 251 patients with Ewing's sarcoma, only 2.4% of cases occurred in the head and neck.[94] The peak age incidence is between 10 and 20 years, and males are more often affected.[91] This is probably a neoplasm of a primitive uncommitted mesenchymal cell. It can present diagnostic problems because it is composed of a uniform population of cells with round nuclei with occasional vacuolated cytoplasm due to the presence of glycogen.[5] Ultrastructure reveals the presence of cell junctions in about 50% of cases.[5] Metastases to the lung and bone occur frequently, and indeed the bones of the skull may often be metastatic sites.[95]

Only 8% of all chondrosarcomas occur in the first two decades, predominantly in the second. A similar distribution of sites is assumed as in adults, where 9% occur in the skull and facial bones.[91] The most common sites are the anterior maxilla and posterior mandible.[96] The prognosis of head and neck chondrosarcomas is poor, with late local relapse occurring in up to 85% at 10 years.[97] Two thirds of cases of the mesenchymal variant of chondrosarcoma occur in children and adolescents. The facial bones are one site of predilection, and 43% are extraosseous.[5, 91]

WHAT NEUROECTODERMAL TUMORS OCCUR IN THE HEAD AND NECK REGION IN CHILDREN?

Neuroblastoma

This malignant embryonic tumor of the nervous system with neuroblastic differentiation is the fourth most common malignancy of children.[4, 16] The majority (70%) of neuroblastomas that are discovered in the head and neck region are metastatic lesions to the cervical lymph nodes, cranial bones, or retroorbital area.[3] Despite the frequency of metastatic origin, *primary* neuroblastomas are the sixth most common childhood head and neck malignancy.[3] There is a major difference in the clinical behavior of primary versus metastatic head and neck neuroblastomas.

Primary neuroblastomas in the neck account for only 6% of all neuroblastomas and usually arise in the cervical sympathetic ganglia.[20] They occur predominantly in the first 3 years of life, with a preponderance in the first 6 months.[20, 98] The usual presentation is that of an enlarging neck mass, which may be associated with respiratory distress or difficulty in feeding. Because the tumor originates in the sympathetic ganglia, early neurologic deficit may include a Horner's syndrome.[98, 99] Some 75% of these tumors show histologic evidence of differentiation toward a ganglioneuroma (ganglioneuroblastoma).[3] They are usually stage I (tumors confined to the organ or structure of origin) or stage II (tumors extending in continuity beyond the organ or structure of origin), according to the Evan staging system.[98–100] As a group, these tumors have an excellent prognosis: 80%–90% become relapse-free survivors.[20, 98, 99] The adverse prognosis of stage II patients with lymph node metastases has been recently reported.[101]

Widely disseminated neuroblastoma (stage IV) has a poor prognosis when there are metastases to the bone, bone marrow, and lymph nodes.[20] Lung metastases are rare. Some infants may have a metastatic distribution that involves liver and skin predominantly—this has been classified as stage IVS. It has been proposed that these cases represent multiple primary tumors rather than metastatic spread.[102] The 3-year survival rate of 70% for stage IVS tumors with minimal treatment contrasts sharply with the 10% survival for stage IV.[20]

Esthesioneuroblastoma (Olfactory Neuroblastoma)

This is an uncommon tumor that is composed of epithelium and nerves of the olfactory mucosa and arises high in the nasal vault on the lateral wall adjacent to the ethmoid labyrinth. It is composed of epithelium and nerves of the olfactory mucosa. The peak age of occurrence in the young is between 11 and 20 years, with 5%–25% of patients being less than 15 years old, and males predominating.[103, 104] These lesions usually present with unilateral nasal obstruction, epistaxis, or excessive lacrimation. Macroscopically, a reddish gray polypoid mass that easily bleeds is seen. The adult presentation of esthesioneuroblastoma is discussed in chapter 17.

Over 50% of tumors are locally advanced at the time of discovery, with extension to the paranasal sinuses. The natural history of the tumor is one of repeated local recurrence with intracranial extension and a slow growth pattern. Distant metastases to the cervical nodes and lungs occur only in 22%, and mostly in patients with advanced disease. Only 18% are 5-year relapse-free survivors, although an additional 32% are alive with disease at 5-year follow-up.[103–105]

Melanotic Neuroectodermal Tumor of Infancy

This tumor has many synonyms, including melanotic prognoma and retinal anlage tumor. About 71% arise in the anterior portion of the maxilla in children in the first year of life, and especially in the first 6 months. It can occur at other sites, including the mandible, skull, and non-head and neck region. It presents as a soft tissue mass with an intact overlying mucosa. Growth rate is variable.[5, 106] Blue and black pigmentation is usually present. Histologically, rosettes are not present. There are two cell types—a larger melanocytic cell with pale cytoplasm with melanin pigment, and a small neuroblastic cell with a dark-staining nucleus and little pale cytoplasm. It is believed that the tumor arises from migrating neural crest tissue from which neuroblastic and melanocytic differentiation occurs.[5, 106] This concept is supported by the finding of increased urinary VMA levels in some cases. The tumor is usually benign, although 15% can be locally invasive with recurrence after excision. Metastases have been very rarely observed and are confined to tumors that appear to behave as neuroblastomas.[5]

Primitive Neuroectodermal Tumors

Primitive neuroectodermal tumors of the CNS are composed of poorly differentiated small, dark cells that probably arise from primitive neuroepithelium. They appear to have potential for neuronal and astroglial differentiation. These highly malignant tumors usually arise in supratentorial locations and have a fatal outcome in more than 80% of cases.[107] These primary CNS tumors may involve the head and neck regions by local contiguous invasion or, rarely, by metastatic spread. Primary non-CNS primitive neuroectodermal tumors may also occur.[108]

ARE THERE ANY FAMILIAL SYNDROMES THAT INCLUDE SOFT TISSUE SARCOMAS IN CHILDREN?

In 1969 Li and Fraumeni identified a family cancer syndrome in which siblings or cousins have rhabdomyosarcomas and the mother develops breast carcinoma at a young age.[39, 109] This constellation of tumors was subsequently extended to include brain tumors and adrenal-cortical carcinomas. Later, leukemia in children and other adult tumors were added. The characteristics of this syndrome appear to be an aggregation of childhood tumors with an increased incidence of malignancy in young family members. Both the childhood and adult malignancies present at a younger age than in the general population, and there is a tendency for multiple neoplasms. A second tumor in the same patient tends to be of the same type as that which occurs in the sibling.[109, 110] In some kinships, despite the appearance of the full constellation of tumors in several siblings in a short period of time, there is not a true excess of other family members with a malignancy.[110]

Children with the inherited condition of neurofibromatosis have an increased incidence of various malignant tumors outside the CNS: malignant schwannomas, rhabdomyosarcomas, and Wilms' tumor.[84] Also, survivors of bilateral and hereditary retinoblastoma have been found to have an increased incidence of second tumors, with 60% being within the previous radiation fields.[111] Osteogenic sarcomas and malignant fibrous histiocytomas have been the most frequently reported types of second malignancy.[5, 111]

WHAT IS THE RATIONALE FOR MULTIMODAL TREATMENT OF HEAD AND NECK RHABDOMYOSARCOMA?

In 1961 the reported 5-year relapse-free survival rate of 170 cases of rhabdomyosarcoma of the head and neck in children was 8.2%.[57] Up to that time, treatment was largely surgical. Radiation therapy and chemotherapy were rarely used in a coherent program. Approximately half of the relapses were local, and the remainder of the deaths were from distant metastases.[49, 57] Since the 1960s, improvement in local control for some sites has principally been achieved by carefully planned radiation therapy.[112, 113] For example, a 90% *local* control rate has been obtained for rhabdomyosarcoma of the orbit with radiation alone after biopsy.[55] However, in all areas, including the orbit, survival rates have been substantially lower owing to the presence of distant disease in patients who presented with what appeared to be local disease. It has been estimated that 50% of all patients in whom all the gross cancer is removed will have distant micrometastases at the time of diagnosis, as compared to 75% in those patients in whom the cancer is incompletely removed.[80] In 1961 Pinkel and Pickren suggested the use of adjuvant chemotherapy for patients with apparently localized rhabdomyosarcoma in order to eradicate distant and regional micrometastases.[114] Their proposal followed the demonstration that gross metastatic disease would respond to vincristine, actinomycin D, and cyclophosphamide, used either singly or in combination.

Since then, various groups have shown improved survival rates using surgery, radiation, and adjuvant chemotherapy. Relapse-free survival rates range from 66% to 76%.[48, 56, 60, 112, 113, 115] Further refinements of therapy include modification of the treatment schedules according to the stage and site of the tumor, as well as determination of the optimum duration and combination of chemotherapy. For example, a randomized study of children who have had complete removal of microscopic and macroscopic tumor and received postoperative irradiation found that addition of adjuvant chemotherapy with vincristine and actinomycin D increased the 2-year survival from 53% to 82%.[116] A subsequent study by the IRS showed that the addition of postoperative radiation therapy did not increase the 92% survival rate when these children were treated with a combination of vincristine, actinomycin D, and cyclophosphamide.[37, 48] The second IRS study attempted to reduce chemotherapy in this group and reported that the addition of cyclophosphamide to vincristine and actinomycin D did not produce an increase in the 2-year survival rate.[117, 118] Thus, these three studies have tried to define the minimally effective adjuvant chemotherapy required for cure while reducing toxicities caused by radiation and cyclophosphamide.

The large IRS-I study of 633 patients also showed no advantage from the addition of cyclophosphamide to the combination of postoperative irradiation with intensive vincristine and actinomycin D in the subgroup of children with residual *microscopic* disease.[37, 48] Recently, a more intensive combination of these three drugs again failed to be superior to the two-drug regimen.[117, 118] However, in patients with residual *macroscopic* disease, increasing the intensity of chemotherapy by using a pulsed rather than a cyclical schedule of vincristine, Adriamycin, actinomycin D, and cyclophosphamide has increased the frequency of complete remissions and improved survival curves, indicating that different scheduling of the same drugs may increase efficacy.[119] Children with metastatic rhabdomyosarcoma at first presentation do poorly, with only 45% achieving a complete remission and 14% achieving a 4-year relapse-free survival in IRS-I.[37, 48] Those children with bone marrow metastases at presentation are usually older and have a worse prognosis than those with metastases to other sites.[120] Three possible alternative future treatments for poor-prognosis groups would be: use very intensive initial chemotherapy in the preoperative or preirradiation period; use a high-dose alkylating agent, for example high-dose melphalan, and autologous marrow rescue after a period of conventional chemotherapy[56]; and use additional chemotherapeutic agents, cisplatin or VP-16.[121]

Some European groups, including the Société Internationale d'Oncologie Pediatrique (SIOP), have employed a different approach to rhabdomyosarcomas, including those of the head and neck region. They have attempted to avoid the disadvantages of extensive surgery and radiation therapy. They have used chemotherapy primarily. Surgery and radiation are used only if there is an incomplete response.[122–125] The overall survival rate has been 53%, but parameningeal sites have fared poorly, supporting the need for radiation therapy in these tumors.[122] The current SIOP III study is a randomized trial comparing primary chemotherapy with conventional multimodal therapy. It excludes parameningeal sites. At present, there are no conclusive results.[123] Also, a new primary chemotherapy regimen substituting ifosphamide for cyclophosphamide in combination with vincristine and actinomycin D has recently showed some promising early results.[125] However, two other series evaluating the effect of chemotherapy alone found that only 29%–62% of tumors completely responded.[126, 127]

In summary, with multimodal therapy, the most recent 2-year relapse-free survival rates are 85%–94% for orbital tumors,[38, 56] 68% for all parameningeal sites (86% for those without risk of meningeal involvement and 55% for those at risk),[128] 56% for neck sites, and 78% for other sites.[61]

WHAT IS THE TREATMENT PLAN FOR NONPARAMENINGEAL RHABDOMYOSARCOMA OF THE HEAD AND NECK IN CHILDREN?

The IRS suggests using a multimodal approach for all rhabdomyosarcomas. A combination of surgery, radiation therapy and chemotherapy is employed in view of the potential for metastatic spread. There are five usual phases of treatment and assessment: surgery, staging, initial chemotherapy, radiation, followed by further chemotherapy for 1–2 years.[117, 131]

The surgical objective is to remove the primary tumor with a wide margin of normal tissue.[129] This is rarely possible because of the location, the proximity to vital structures, and for cosmetic reasons. In practice, the maximum amount of tumor is removed without excessive destruction of adjacent tissues. This may require two operations if microscopic evidence of tumor is found at the margins and the area can be re-excised without risk.[129] Biopsy of adjacent tissue may define the extension of the tumor if there are narrow margins around the primary tumor.[129] Radical lymph node dissection has not been routinely recommended because head and neck rhabdomyosarcoma has a low incidence (5%) of lymph node metastasis.[42] If there are enlarged nodes, these should be removed.[129] Orbital lesions have been considered as a special management problem. In view of their good prognosis, an incisional biopsy is often recommended as the initial step, with orbital exenteration reserved for local relapse.[56, 129]

Two staging systems are shown in Table 24–5. In both schemes there is discrimination in prognosis between the different stages.[48, 56] In the more widely used IRS system, determination of whether the disease is stage I, II, or III depends on the surgeon's observations at operation, the microscopic evidence of involvement of the margins of the excision, and the postoperative examination of the region by CT scan. The CT scan can also determine if there is any unsuspected bony erosion of the cranial base indicating invasive parameningeal disease.[66] Chest x-ray films and CT scans are required to detect pulmonary metastases. Both bone marrow aspiration and trephine biopsy are done for marrow metastases. A skeletal survey and isotope bone scan complete the search for bone metastases.

Following staging, the appropriate chemotherapeutic regimen is followed, depending on stage, as is shown in

TABLE 24–5.—STAGING SYSTEMS FOR RHABDOMYOSARCOMA

STAGE		DESCRIPTION
		IRS System
I		Localized disease, complete macroscopic and microscopic removal, regional nodes not involved
	1.	Confined to muscle or organ of origin
	2.	Contiguous involvement with infiltration outside the muscle or organ of origin, as through fascial planes
II	1.	Grossly removed tumor with microscopic residual disease; no evidence of regional node involvement
	2.	Regional disease, completely removed (regional nodes involved and/or extension of tumor into an adjacent organ; no microscopic residual disease)
	3.	Regional disease with involved nodes, grossly removed, but with evidence of microscopic residual disease
III		Incomplete removal or biopsy with gross residual disease
IV		Distant metastatic disease present at onset
		Barts/Marsden System
I		Localized disease confined to tissue of origin
	A	Completely resected
	B	Not resected
II		Regional disease
	A	Extending outside tissue of origin to involve contiguous bone or nerve
	B	With nodal metastases
III		Generalized disease
	A	Without marrow involvement
	B	With marrow involvement

Figure 24–1, which is based on the IRS-II recommendations. Various combinations of vincristine and actinomycin D (with or without the addition of cyclophosphamide and Adriamycin) are given for 6 weeks prior to radiation therapy.[117] Preirradiation chemotherapy is employed to treat micrometastases or overt metastases in stage IV disease. If intensive chemotherapy and radiation therapy were to be administered concomitantly, severe mucositis and myelosuppression would result. This would prolong radiation therapy and reduce the chance of delivering an adequate program of systemic chemotherapy. It is generally agreed that radiation therapy should be in the dose range of 4,000–6,000 rad delivered over 6 weeks to the area of the primary tumor. Because rhabdomyosarcoma may extend beyond the detectable margins, a wider radiation field is recommended so that the field includes a 5-cm margin of normal tissue. All measurements are determined by the prechemotherapy tumor sizes. The first IRS study shows that radiation therapy delivered to the tumor bed after a microscopically confirmed total excision did not statistically increase the chance of relapse-free survival.[48] Analysis of data from this study suggests that local control can be obtained in stage II patients if the radiation dose is in the range 4,000–4,500 rad.[130] For patients with stage III cancer, larger tumors (>5 cm in diameter), and for older children, higher radiation doses are suggested, as follows: For patients less than 6 years old and with tumor diameters of 5 cm or less, radiation doses of 4,000–4,500 rad are used; these are increased to 4,500–5,000 rad for tumor diameters of more than 5 cm. For patients older than 6 years and with tumor diameters of 5 cm or less, radiation doses of 4,500–5,000 rad are used; these doses are increased to 5,000–5,500 rad for tumor diameters of more than 5 cm.

Following the radiation treatment cyclical or pulsed chemotherapy is started, using a combination of two or more agents: vincristine, actinomycin D, cyclophosphamide, and Adriamycin. Chemotherapy is continued for 1–2 years to eradicate micrometastatic disease or treat overt metastases.[117]

WHAT IS THE TREATMENT PLAN FOR PARAMENINGEAL RHABDOMYOSARCOMA?

The previously mentioned studies have demonstrated that there is a poor survival of children with parameningeal rhabdomyosarcomas due to a combination of meningeal extension and local relapse.[58, 62, 71] Present therapy concentrates on improved control of these two problems. Surgery in the parameningeal sites is limited to removal of as much tumor as is possible without damage to essential structures. In many cases surgery is limited to biopsy only.[51] Staging is of paramount importance both for determining the extent of local disease and for deciding on the likelihood of meningeal extension. A search is made for distant metastases by the same means as are recommended for nonparameningeal tumors. The degree of CNS invasion as it relates to clinical features is shown in Table 24–6. Evidence of actual or potential meningeal extension is obtained by: (1) CT scan to detect intracranial extension of the tumor as well as local bony erosion, (2) plain radiographs of the base of the skull, (3) testing of cranial nerve function, and (4) examination of the CSF for cell count and cell types.[131] The CT scan has produced improvement in radiotherapy planning by defining tumor margins accurately.[66] Previously, the lack of good visualization may have produced judgmental errors leading to some local relapses. If there is evidence of meningeal extension, therapy is altered, as discussed below. The general systemic chemotherapy is determined by the staging of the tumor irrespective of meningeal extension.

If there is no *evidence* of a high likelihood of meningeal extension, radiation therapy is started 6 weeks after the commencement of chemotherapy. The initial tumor volume—the volume prior to chemotherapy—is irradiated, together with an adjacent margin of tissue

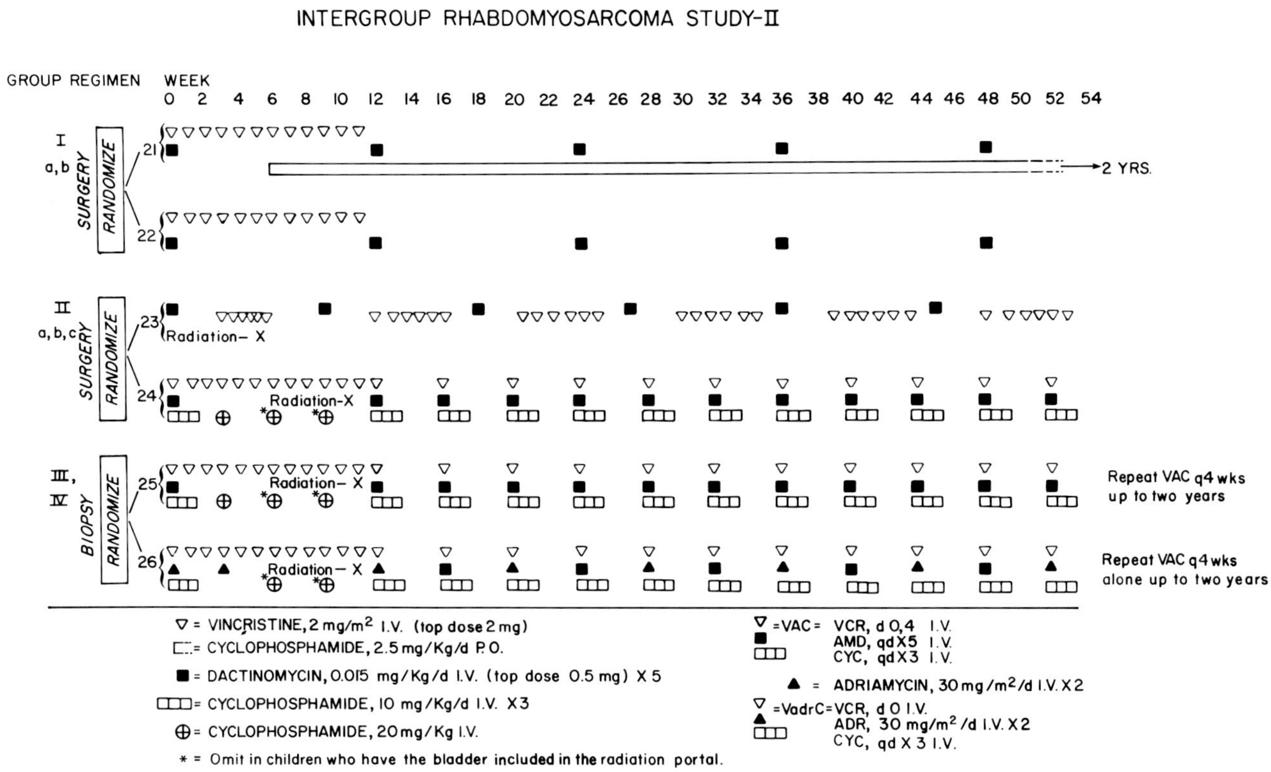

Fig 24–1.—Details of the treatment protocols for the Intergroup Rhabdomyosarcoma Study II. This is particularly good for the details of chemotherapy administration.

and a 2-cm margin of adjacent meninges.[131] When an emphasis is placed on avoiding a reduction in the irradiation dose and the field volume, then an 86% complete response rate with relapse-free survival has been achieved in patients *without* evidence of meningeal involvement.[128]

Patients who have *evidence of intracranial extension* or are at high risk of meningeal extension (with either erosion of bone of the cranial base or cranial nerve palsies) are treated with immediate radiation therapy because it is believed that systemic chemotherapy does not cross the blood-brain barrier in sufficient concentration to reach intracranial disease with an effective dose.[62, 131] When chemotherapy and *local* irradiation are used, the meningeal relapse has occurred as an isolated event, without any local or systemic relapse being observed.[63, 70] This suggests that CNS micrometastases are present and are not effectively treated by systemic chemotherapy. Because of the need to control intracranial diseases, radiation to the whole brain is advised. Despite these aggressive measures, relapse in the CSF or spinal cord has been reported.[68] Therefore, periodic installation of intrathecal chemotherapy by lumbar puncture has been advised using methotrexate, hydrocortisone, and cytosine arabinoside, or methotrexate alone.[117, 131] This technique for treating the CNS with intrathecal agents is similar to that used for acute lymphoblastic leukemia. Intrathecal therapy is modified because of the less radiosensitive nature of rhabdomyosarcomas.

TABLE 24–6.—DEGREE OF CNS INVASION WITH PROGNOSTIC IMPORTANCE RELATED TO CLINICAL FEATURES*

CLINICAL FEATURE	DEGREE OF CNS INVASION				
	I	II	III	IV	V
CSF positive cells	–	–	–	–	+
Spinal cord involved	–	–	–	–	+
Intracranial extension	–	–	–	+	±
Erosion of bone base of skull	–	–	+	±	±
Cranial nerve palsy	–	+	±	±	±

*Data from Tefft et al.[62] and Raney et al.[128]

With this combined approach to all parameningeal disease, the meningeal relapse rates in the IRS study patients was reduced to 7% from a previous 35%. Relapse-free survival improved from 33% to 68%.[128] This increase in survival was confirmed by another study, using similar therapy, with an improvement from 8% to 66% in survival and a reduction in meningeal relapse (isolated or associated with local relapse) from 66% to 9%.[71] From these studies, however, it is difficult to determine if all the components of therapy—early irradia-

DESCISION DIAGRAM FOR TREATMENT OF HEAD AND NECK RHABDOMYOSARCOMAS. BASED ON IRS II RECOMMENDATIONS (117, 118, 131).

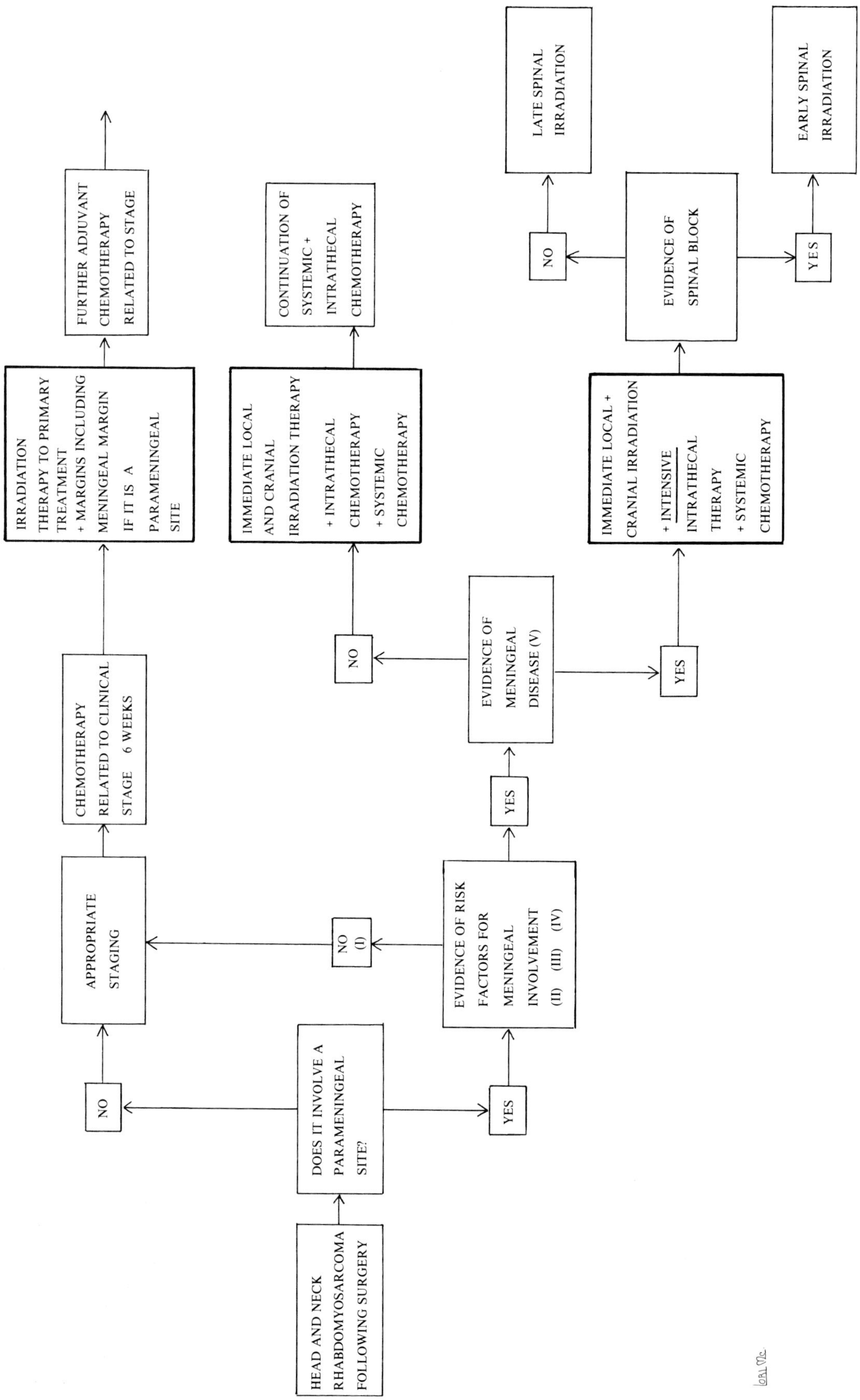

Fig 24–2.—Summary decision points for head and neck rhabdomyosarcoma management.

tion, strict adherence to dose and volume of irradiated tissue, cranial irradiation, and intrathecal chemotherapy—are vital to the achievement of improved survival and reduced incidence of meningeal extension in this group of children.[58, 63, 71]

Disseminated meningeal involvement has a very poor prognosis in all series. Various suggestions for management include weekly intrathecal chemotherapy until malignant cells are no longer present in the CSF, followed by combined craniospinal radiation. However, if a tumor is causing a spinal cord block, then spinal radiation, with or without laminectomy, is given first.[131]

The therapeutic recommendations from the IRS group are summarized in Table 24–7 and Fig 24–2.

WHAT IS THE APPROACH TO OTHER SOFT TISSUE SARCOMAS OF THE HEAD AND NECK IN CHILDREN?

With the exception of rhabdomyosarcoma, other soft tissue sarcomas are relatively rare in children. Because of their infrequent occurrence, our knowledge of the natural history, the metastatic tendency, and the sensitivity to chemotherapy is imprecise. For this reason, some oncology groups recommend that all other soft tissue sarcomas should be treated by the same regimen as rhabdomyosarcoma.[67, 132] Their overall survival rates have been reported to be similar to that for rhabdomyosarcomas.[132] However, this group of sarcomas is quite heterogeneous. Consequently, the results may be weighted by inclusion of cancers such as fibrosarcomas that have a low metastatic potential.

The main therapeutic challenge for fibrosarcomas is local control. In view of their low metastatic potential and poor chemosensitivity, surgical removal with, if possible, a wide margin followed by radiation therapy to any remaining tumor has been the recommended approach.[80] Reported results show an 82% survival rate with a median follow-up of 11 years. A similar approach with initial radiotherapy followed by subsequent surgery appears to have equivalent results.[133] Full evaluation of these patients requires a long follow-up period since metastases appear late.[76]

Neurogenic sarcoma survival rates with surgery alone or with radiation therapy have been 17% and 16%, respectively. Relapses have initially been local, followed by the later development of distant metastases.[81–83] Because of this, some groups have advocated the use of multimodal therapy that includes surgery, radiation therapy, and chemotherapy.[83] Recommended therapy has emphasized radiation with doses in excess of 4,000 rad when there is microscopic or gross evidence of residual tumor after surgery. The added chemotherapy includes multidrug treatment with vincristine, actinomycin D, Adriamycin, and cyclophosphamide. The multimode regimen has resulted in preliminary relapse-free survival rates in excess of 60%, but only a small number of patients have been studied, and the follow-up periods have been short.[83]

The behavior and chemosensitivity of malignant fibrous histiocytoma seems to depend on whether it originates in bone or soft tissue.[134, 135] Good response to chemotherapy has been reported recently for fibrous histiocytomas originating in bone. The treatment regimens use high-dose methotrexate with vincristine and Adriamycin[135] or cisplatin.[136] By contrast, fibrous histiocytomas arising in the soft tissue have a poor response to vincristine, actinomycin D, cyclophosphamide, and Adriamycin.[134]

Thus, the best general recommendations at this time would support treating all soft tissue sarcomas in children with a multimodal approach using chemotherapy and adequate radiation doses, with the exceptions of fibrosarcoma and those sarcomas that are totally and widely resected. With such a regimen, an overall 75% 5-year relapse-free survival rate has been reported for

TABLE 24–7.—IRS SUGGESTIONS FOR TREATMENT OF RHABDOMYOSARCOMA IN A PARAMENINGEAL SITE

SITE	RADIATION	SYSTEMIC CHEMOTHERAPY	INTRATHECAL CHEMOTHERAPY
Parameningeal site (no meningeal extension risk factors present)	Primary tumor at 6 weeks, including 2-cm margins of meninges; strict adherence to dose and volume	Vincristine + actinomycin ± cyclophosphamide ± Adriamycin, depending on stage	None
Parameningeal site (with meningeal extension risk factors present)	Primary tumor radiation on day 0 Cranial radiation on day 0 3,000 rad if >5 yr 2,400 rad if <5 yr	As above	Periodic intrathecal methotrexate, cytosine, hydrocortisone
Meningeal involvement (malignant cells in CSF)	As above; spinal radiation, when CSF clear of tumor cells	As above	Weekly intrathecal chemotherapy until CSF clear
Meningeal involvement; spinal block	As above + immediate local spinal radiation	As above	Intrathecal chemotherapy

head and neck soft tissue sarcoma, with no difference between rhabdomyosarcoma and other soft tissue sarcomas.[67]

Recently, the use of chemotherapy with Adriamycin and dacarbazine has been described for initially unresectable fibromatosis in the head and neck region. This has produced enough tumor shrinkage to allow delayed resection in some patients.[137]

WHAT ARE THE LONG-TERM SEQUELAE OF TREATMENT?

With the improved survival of children with head and neck soft tissue sarcomas, attention has focused on the long-term effects of the therapy on the survivors. Most data are available on children treated for orbital rhabdomyosarcoma.[56, 138, 139] There is high incidence of cataract formation (83%) and facial bone asymmetry (57%).[138] It must be remembered that therapeutic irradiation impairs bone growth in the treatment field. Other complications have included corneal changes, ptosis, and enophthalmos. The rate of late enucleation of the eye is about 10%.[56, 138] Most of these sequelae have resulted from tissue changes induced by radiation therapy. However, on the positive side, the majority of survivors are functioning as average students at school.[138] For children receiving radiation therapy, endocrine sequelae have been described, including growth hormone deficiency, and hypothalamic-pituitary dysfunction affecting thyroid, gonadal, and adrenal hormones.[140]

Finally, second malignant neoplasms have been reported in these survivors. The latency period may be quite long and may extend well into the adult years.[93, 138]

REFERENCES

1. Jones P.G., Campbell P.E. (eds.): *Tumors of Infancy and Childhood.* Oxford, England, Blackwell Scientific Publications, 1976, p. 14.
2. Jaffe B.F., Jaffe N.: Head and neck tumors in children. *Pediatrics.* 51:731–740, 1973.
3. Jaffe B.F.: Pediatric head and neck tumors: A study of 178 cases. *Laryngoscope* 83:1644–1651, 1973.
4. Marsden H.B.: The pathology and natural history of childhood tumors, in Duncan W. (ed.): *Paediatric Oncology: Recent Results in Cancer Research.* New York, Springer-Verlag, 88:11–25, 1983.
5. Dehner L.P.: Soft tissue sarcoma of childhood: The differential diagnostic dilemma of the small blue cell. *Natl. Cancer Inst. Monogr.* 56:43–59, 1981.
6. Conley J.J.: Tumors of the head and neck in children, in *Concepts in Head and Neck Surgery.* New York, Grune & Stratton, 1970, pp. 181–192.
7. MacComb W.S., Fletcher G.H.: Pediatric tumors, in *Cancer of the Head and Neck.* Baltimore, Williams & Wilkins, Co. 1967, pp. 428–446.
8. Tan C., D'Angio G.J., Exelby P.R., et al.: The changing management of childhood Hodgkin's disease. *Cancer* 35:808–816, 1975.
9. Norris D.G., Burgert E.O., Cooper H.A., et al.: Hodgkin's disease in childhood. *Cancer* 36:2109–2120, 1975.
10. Murphy S.B.: Classification, staging, and end results of treatment of childhood non-Hodgkin's lymphomas: Dissimilarities from lymphomas in adults. *Semin. Oncol.* 7:332–339, 1980.
11. Anderson J.R., Wilson J.F., Jenkin R.D.T., et al.: Childhood non-Hodgkin's lymphoma: The results of a randomized trial comparing a four drug regimen (COMP) with a ten drug regimen (LSA2L2). *N. Engl. J. Med.* 308:559–565, 1983.
12. Wilson J.F., Jenkin R.D.T., Anderson J.R., et al.: Studies on the pathology of non-Hodgkin's lymphoma in childhood: I. The role of routine histopathology as a prognostic factor. A report from the Children's Cancer Study Group. *Cancer* 53:1695–1704, 1984.
13. Soule E.H., Mahour G.H., Mills S.D., et al.: Soft tissue sarcomas of infants and children: A clinicopathological study of 135 cases. *Mayo Clin. Proc.* 43:313–326, 1968.
14. Okamura J., Sutow W.W., Moon T.E.: Prognosis in children with metastatic rhabdomyosarcoma. *Med. Pediatr. Oncol.* 3:243–251, 1977.
15. Greer R.O., Mierau G.W., Favara B.E.: *Tumors of the Head and Neck in Children: Clinicopathological Perspectives.* New York, Praeger Publications, 1983, pp. 200–217.
16. Young J.L., Miller R.W.: Incidence of malignant tumors in US children. *J. Pediatr.* 86:254–258, 1975.
17. Winship T., Rosvoli R.V.: Childhood thyroid carcinoma. *Cancer* 14:734–743, 1961.
18. Schneider A.B., Favus M.J., Stachura M.E., et al.: Incidence, prevalence and characteristics of radiation-induced tumors. *Am. J. Med.* 64:243–251, 1978.
19. Roggli V.L., Estrada V., Fechner R.E.: Thyroid neoplasia following irradiation for medulloblastoma. *Cancer* 43:2232–2238, 1979.
20. Coleman A.J., Fryer C.J.H., Elwood J.M., et al.: Neuroblastoma: Influence of age at diagnosis, stage, tumor site, and sex on prognosis. *Cancer* 46:1896–1901, 1980.
21. Greene M.H., Fraumeni J.F., Hoover R.: Nasopharyngeal cancer among young people in the United States: Racial variations by cell type. *JNCI* 58:1267–1270, 1977.
22. Glaser R., Monoyama M., Szymanowski R.T., et al.: Human nasopharyngeal carcinomas positive for Epstein-Barr virus DNA in North America. *JNCI* 64:1317–1319, 1980.
23. Pick T., Maurer H.M., McWilliams N.B.: Lymphoepithelioma of childhood. *J. Pediatr.* 84:96–100, 1974.
24. Dehner L.P.: *Pediatric Surgical Pathology.* St. Louis, C.V. Mosby Co., 1975, pp. 106–158.
25. Straka J.A., Bluestone C.D.: Nasopharyngeal malignancies in children. *Laryngoscope* 82:807–816, 1972.
26. Heffner D.K.: Problems in pediatric otorhinolaryngic pathology: I. Sinonasal and nasopharyngeal tumors and

masses with myxoid features. *Int. J. Pediatr. Otorhinolaryngol.* 5:77–91, 1983.
27. Wright J.L., Phelps P.D., MacIver A.G.: Sarcoma of the ethmoid in children. *J. Laryngol. Otol.* 85:57–67, 1971.
28. Dehner L.P.: Tumors of the mandible and maxilla in children: I. Clinicopathological study of 46 histologically benign lesions. *Cancer* 31:364–384, 1973.
29. Dehner L.P.: Tumors of the mandible and maxilla in children: II. A study of 14 primary and secondary malignant tumors. *Cancer* 32:112–120, 1973.
30. Henderson J.W.: *Orbital Tumors.* New York, Brian C. Decker, 1980, p. 73.
31. Iliff W.J., Green W.R.: Orbital tumors in children, in *Ocular and Adenexal Tumors.* Birmingham, Aesculapius, 1978, p. 669.
32. Youssefi B.: Orbital tumors in children: A clinical study of 62 cases. *J. Pediatr. Ophthalmol.* 6:177–181, 1969.
33. Eldrup-Jorgensen P., Fledelius H.: Orbital tumors in infancy: An analysis of Danish cases from 1943–1962. *Acta Ophthalmol.* 53:887, 1975.
34. Khan H.J., Yeger H., Kassim O., et al.: Immunohistochemical and electron microscopic assessment of childhood rhabdomyosarcoma. *Cancer* 51:1897–1903, 1983.
35. Bale P.M., Parsons R.E., Stevens M.M.: Dignosis and behavior of juvenile rhabdomyosarcoma. *Hum. Pathol.* 14:596–611, 1983.
36. Mierau G.W., Favara B.E.: Rhabdomyosarcoma in children: Ultrastructural study of 31 cases. *Cancer* 46:2035–2040, 1980.
37. Maurer H.M., Moon T., Donaldson M., et al.: The Intergroup Rhabdomyosarcoma Study: A preliminary report. *Cancer* 40:2015–2026, 1977.
38. Sutow W.W., Linberg R.D., Gehan E.A., et al.: Three-year relapse-free survival rates in childhood rhabdomyosarcoma of the head and neck. *Cancer* 49:2217–2221, 1982.
39. Li F.P., Fraumeni J.F.: Rhabdomyosarcoma in children: Epidemiologic study and identification of a familial cancer syndrome. *JNCI* 43:1365–1373, 1969.
40. Gaiger A.M., Soule E.H., Newton W.A.: Pathology of rhabdomyosarcoma: Experience of the Intergroup Rhabdomyosarcoma Study 1972–78. *Natl. Cancer Inst. Monogr.* 56:19–27, 1981.
41. Gonzalez-Crussi F., Black-Schaffer S.: Rhabdomyosarcoma of infancy and childhood: Problems of morphologic classification. *Am. J. Surg. Pathol.* 3:157–171, 1979.
42. Lawrence W., Hays D.M., Moon T.E.: Lymphatic metastasis with childhood rhabdomyosarcoma. *Cancer* 39:556–559, 1977.
43. Enzinger F.M., Shiraki M.: Alveolar rhabdomyosarcoma: An analysis of 110 cases. *Cancer* 24:18–31, 1969.
44. Henderson D.W., Raven J.L., Pollard J.A., et al.: Bone marrow metastases in disseminated alveolar rhabdomyosarcoma: Case report with ultrastructural study and review. *Pathology* 8:329–341, 1976.
45. Hays D.M., Newton W., Soule E.H., et al.: Mortality among children with rhabdomyosarcoma of the alveolar histologic subtype. *J. Pediatr. Surg.* 18:412–417, 1983.
46. Soule E.H., Newton W., Moon T.E., et al.: Extraskeletal Ewing's sarcoma. *Cancer* 42:259–264, 1978.
47. Palmer N.F., Foulkes M.: Histopathology and prognosis in the second intergroup rhabdomyosarcoma study IRS-II. *Proc. Am. Soc. Clin. Oncol.* C897:2:229, 1983.
48. Mauer H.M.: The intergroup rhabdomyosarcoma study: Update, November 1978. *Natl. Cancer Inst. Monogr.* 56:61–68, 1981.
49. Masson J.K., Soule E.H.: Embryonal rhabdomyosarcoma of the head and neck. *Am. J. Surg.* 110:585–591, 1965.
50. Jones I.S., Reese A.B., Kraut J.: Orbital rhabdomyosarcoma: An analysis of 62 cases. *Am. J. Ophthalmol.* 61:721–736, 1966.
51. Raney R.B., Donaldson M.H., Sutow W.W., et al.: Special considerations related to primary site in rhabdomyosarcoma: Experience of the Intergroup Study 1972–1976. *Natl. Cancer Inst. Monogr.* 56:69–76, 1981.
52. Sutow W.W., Sullivan M.P., Reid H.L., et al.: Prognosis in childhood rhabdomyosarcoma. *Cancer* 25:1386–1390, 1970.
53. Pratt C.B., Smith J.W., Woerner S., et al.: Factors leading to delay in the diagnosis and affecting the survival of children with head and neck rhabdomyosarcoma. *Pediatrics* 61:30–34, 1978.
54. Sagerman R.H., Tretter P., Ellsworth R.M.: Orbital rhabdomyosarcoma in children. *Trans. Am. Acad. Ophthalmol. Otol.* 78:602–605, 1976.
55. Sagerman R.H., Tretter P., Ellsworth R.M.: The treatment of orbital rhabdomyosarcoma of children with primary radiation therapy. *Am. J. Roentgenol. Radium Ther. Nucl. Med.* 114:31–36, 1972.
56. Kingston J.E., McElwain T.J., Malpas J.S.: Childhood rhabdomyosarcoma: Experience of the Children's Solid Tumor Group. *Br. J. Cancer* 48:195–207, 1983.
57. Dito W.R., Batsakis J.G.: Rhabdomyosarcoma of the head and neck. *Arch. Surg.* 84:112–118, 1962.
58. Berry M.P., Jenkin R.D.T.: Parameningeal rhabdomyosarcoma in the young. *Cancer* 48:281–288, 1981.
59. Fusner J., Pizzo P.A., Poplack D.G., et al.: Meningeal relapse of orbital rhabdomyosarcoma. *Med. Pediatr. Oncol.* 4:247–251, 1978.
60. Donaldson S.S., Castro J.R., Wilbur J.R., et al.: Rhabdomyosarcoma of the head and neck in children. *Cancer* 31:26–35, 1973.
61. Wharam M.D., Foulkes A.A., Lawrence W., et al.: Soft tissue sarcoma of the head and neck in childhood: Nonorbital and non-parameningeal sites. *Cancer* 53:1016–1019, 1984.
62. Tefft M., Kernandez C., Donaldson M., et al.: Incidence of meningeal involvement by rhabdomyosarcoma of the head and neck in children: A report of the IRS. *Cancer* 42:253–258, 1976.
63. Chan R.C., Sutow W.W., Lindberg R.D.: Parameningeal rhabdomyosarcoma. *Radiology* 131:211–214, 1979.
64. Gerson J.M., Jaffe N., Donaldson M.H., et al.: Meningeal seeding from rhabdomyosarcoma of the head and neck with base of the skull invasion: Recognition of the clinical evolution and suggestions for management. *Med. Pediatr. Oncol.* 5:137–144, 1978.

65. Leviton A., Davidson R., Gilles F.: Neurologic manifestations of embryonal rhabdomyosarcoma of the middle ear cleft. *J. Pediatr.* 80:596–602, 1972.
66. Raney R.B., Zimmerman R.A., Bilaniuk L.T., et al.: Management of craniofacial sarcoma in childhood assisted by computed tomography. *Int. J. Radiat. Oncol. Biol. Phys.* 5:529–534, 1979.
67. Littman P., Raney B., Zimmerman R., et al.: Soft tissue sarcomas of the head and neck in children. *Int. J. Radiat. Oncol. Biol. Phys.* 9:1367–1371, 1983.
68. Hutchinson R.J., Raney R.B.: Meningeal extension of head and neck rhabdomyosarcoma. *J. Pediatr.* 91:516–517, 1977.
69. Raney R.B.: Spinal cord "drop metastases" from head and neck rhabdomyosarcoma: Proceedings of the Tumor Board of the Children's Hospital of Philadelphia. *Med. Pediatr. Oncol.* 4:3–9, 1978.
70. Humphreys R.P., McGreal D., Fitz C.R., et al.: Rhabdomyosarcoma of the head and neck in children. *Can. J. Neurol. Sci.* 10:119–125, 1983.
71. Gasparini M., Lombard F., Gianni C., et al.: Childhood rhabdomyosarcoma with meningeal extension: Results of combined therapy including central nervous system prophylaxis. *Am. J. Clin. Oncol.* 6:393–398, 1983.
72. Jaffe B.F., Fox J.E., Batsakis J.C.: Rhabdomyosarcoma of the middle ear and mastoid. *Cancer* 27:29–37, 1971.
73. Raney R.B., Lawrence W., Maurer H.M., et al.: Rhabdomyosarcoma of the ear in childhood: A report from the Intergroup Rhabdomyosarcoma Study-I. *Cancer* 51:2356–2361, 1983.
74. Abramowsky C.R., Witt W.J.: Sarcoma of the larynx in a newborn. *Cancer* 51:1726–1730, 1983.
75. Kedar A., Kuten A., Joachims H.Z., et al.: Rhabdomyosarcoma of the larynx treated by laser surgery, combined with radiotherapy and chemotherapy. *Med. Pediatr. Oncol.* 11:279–280, 1983.
76. Soule E.H., Pritchard D.J.: Fibrosarcoma in infants and children: A review of 110 cases. *Cancer* 40:1711–1721, 1977.
77. Chung E.B., Enzinger R.M.: Infantile fibrosarcoma. *Cancer* 38:729–739, 1976.
78. Van Blarcom C.W., Masson J.M.K., Dahlin D.C.: Fibrosarcoma of the mandible. *Oral Surg.* 32:428–439, 1971.
79. Dehner L.P., Askin F.B.: Tumors of fibrous tissue origin in childhood: A clinicopathologic study of cutaneous soft tissue neoplasms in 66 children. *Cancer* 38:888–899, 1976.
80. Jenkin D., Sonley M.: Soft tissue sarcoma in the young. *Cancer* 46:621–629, 1980.
81. Sordillo P.D., Helson L., Hajdu S.I., et al.: Malignant schwannoma: Clinical characteristics, survival and response to therapy. *Cancer* 47:2503–2509, 1981.
82. Ghosh B.C., Ghosh L., Hvvos A.G., et al.: Malignant schwannoma: A clinicopathological study. *Cancer* 31:184–190, 1973.
83. Raney R.B., Littman P., Jarrett P., et al.: Results of multimodal therapy of children with neurogenic sarcoma. *Med. Pediatr. Oncol.* 7:229–236, 1970.
84. Hope D.G., Mulvihill J.J.: Malignancy in neurofibromatosis, in Riccardi V.M., Mulvihill J.J. (eds.): *Neurofibromatosis (von Recklinghausen Disease).* New York, Raven Press, 1981, pp. 33–55.
85. Markhede G., Angervall L., Steiner B.: A multivariate analysis of the prognosis after surgical treatment of malignant soft tissue sarcomas. *Cancer* 49:1721–1733, 1982.
86. Weiss S.W., Enzinger F.M.: Malignant fibrous histiocytoma: An analysis of 200 cases. *Cancer* 41:2250–2266, 1978.
87. Blitzer A., Lawson W., Biller H.F.: Malignant fibrous histiocytoma of the head and neck. *Laryngoscope* 87:1479–1499, 1977.
88. Blitzer A., Lawson W., Zak F.G., et al.: Clinicopathological determinates in prognosis of fibrous histiocytomas of the head and neck. *Laryngoscope* 91:2053–2069, 1981.
89. Girard C., Waine C.J., Graham J.H.: Cutaneous angiosarcoma. *Cancer* 23:868–883, 1970.
90. Roth J.A., Enzinger F.M., Tannerbaum M.: Synovial sarcoma of the neck: A follow-up study of 24 cases. *Cancer* 35:1243–1253, 1975.
91. Spjut H.J., Ayala A.G.: Skeletal tumors in children and adolescents. *Hum. Pathol.* 14:628–642, 1983.
92. Greer R.O., Miereau G.W., Favara B.E.: *Tumors of the Head and Neck in Children: Clinicopathological Perspectives.* New York, Praeger, 1983, pp. 125–133.
93. Meadows A.T., Strong L.C., Li F.P., et al.: Bone sarcomas as a second malignant neoplasm in children: Influence of radiation and genetic predisposition. *Cancer* 46:2603–2606, 1980.
94. Perez C.A., Tefft M., Nesbit M.E., et al.: Radiation therapy in the multimodal management of Ewing's sarcoma of bone: Report of the Intergroup Ewing's Sarcoma Study. *Natl. Cancer Inst. Monogr.* 56:263–271, 1981.
95. Nesbit M.E., Perez C.A., Tefft M., et al.: Multimodal therapy for the management of primary non-metastatic Ewing's sarcoma of bone: An Intergroup Study. *Natl. Cancer Inst. Monogr.* 56:255–262, 1981.
96. Greer R.O., Mierau G.W., Favara B.E.: *Tumors of the Head and Neck in Children. Clinicopathologic Perspectives.* New York, Praeger, 1983, pp. 134–142.
97. Vener J., Rice D.H., Newman A.N.: Osteosarcoma and chondrosarcoma of the head and neck. *Laryngoscope* 94:240–242, 1984.
98. Orr J.D.: Cervical neuroblastoma in childhood: A better prognosis? *Clin. Oncol.* 4:353–358, 1978.
99. Cushing B.A., Slovis T.L., Philipart A.I., et al.: A rational approach to cervical neuroblastoma. *Cancer* 50:785–787, 1982.
100. Evans A.E., D'Angio G.J., Randolph J.: A proposed staging for children with neuroblastoma. *Cancer* 27:374–378, 1971.
101. Ninane J., Pritchard J., Morris-Jones P.H., et al.: Stage II neuroblastoma: Adverse prognostic significance of lymph node involvement. *Arch. Dis. Child.* 57:438–442, 1982.

102. Evans A.E., Chatten J., D'Angio G.J., et al.: A review of 17 IVS patients at the Children's Hospital of Philadelphia. *Cancer* 45:833–839, 1980.
103. Ferlito A., Michaeu C.: Infantile olfactory neuroblastoma. *ORL J. Otorhinolaryngol. Relat. Spec.* 41:40–50, 1979.
104. Elkon D., Hightower S.I., Lion M.L., et al.: Esthesioneuroblastoma. *Cancer* 44:1087–1094.
105. Wade P.M., Smith R.E., Johns M.E.: Response of esthesioneuroblastoma to chemotherapy: Report of five cases and a review of the literature. *Cancer* 53:1036–1041, 1984.
106. Karma P., Rasanen O., Karja J.: Melanotic neuroectodermal tumor of infancy. *J. Laryngol. Otol.* 91:973–979, 1977.
107. Dehner L.P.: Primitive neuroectodermal tumors of the central nervous system in childhood: Retrospective and overview, in Humphrey G.B. (ed.): *Pediatric Oncology*. Boston, Martinus Nijhoff, Publishers, 1981, pp. 277–288.
108. Hashimoto H., Enjoji M., Nakajima T., et al.: Malignant neuroepithelioma (peripheral neuroblastoma): A clinicopathological analysis of 15 cases. *Am. J. Surg. Pathol.* 7:309–318, 1983.
109. Li F.P., Fraumeni J.F. Jr.: Soft tissue sarcoma, breast cancer and other neoplasms: A familial syndrome. *Ann. Intern. Med.* 71:747–752, 1969.
110. Pearson A.D.J., Craft A.W., Ratcliffe J.M., et al.: Two families with the Li-Fraumeni cancer family syndrome. *J. Med. Genet.* 19:362–365, 1982.
111. Kitchin F.D., Ellsworth R.M.: Pleiotrophic effects of the gene for retinoblastoma. *J. Med. Genet.* 11:244–246, 1974.
112. Schuller D.E., Lawrence T.L., Newton W.A.: Childhood rhabdomyosarcoma of the head and neck. *Arch. Otolaryngol.* 105:689–694, 1979.
113. Liebner E.J.: Embryonal rhabdomyosarcoma of head and neck and children. *Cancer* 37:2777–2786, 1976.
114. Pinkel D., Pickren J.: Rhabdomyosarcoma in children. *JAMA* 1975:293–298, 1961.
115. Malpas J.S., Freeman J.E., Paxton A., et al.: Radiotherapy and adjuvant combination chemotherapy for childhood rhabdomyosarcoma. *Br. Med. J.* 1:247–249, 1976.
116. Heyn R.M., Holland R., Newton W.A., et al.: The role of combined chemotherapy in the treatment of rhabdomyosarcoma in children. *Cancer* 34:2128–2142, 1974.
117. Maurer H.M.: The Intergroup Rhabdomyosarcoma Study II: Objectives and study design. *J. Pediatr. Surg.* 15:371–372, 1980.
118. Maurer H.M., Foulkes M., Gehan E.: Intergroup Rhabdomyosarcoma Study (IRS)-II: Preliminary report, in *Proceedings of the XV International Study of Pediatric Oncology* 1983. York, England, September 20–26.
119. Raney R.B., Gehan E.A., Maurer H.M., et al.: Evaluation of inherited chemotherapy in children with advanced rhabdomyosarcoma (clinical groups III and IV). *Cancer Clin. Trials* 2:19–28, 1979.
120. Ruymann F.B., Newton W.A., Ragab A.B., et al.: Bone marrow metastases at diagnosis in children and adolescents with rhabdomyosarcoma: A report from the Intergroup Rhabdomyosarcoma Study. *Cancer* 53:368–373, 1984.
121. Baum E.S., Gaynon P., Greenberg L., et al.: Phase II trial of cisplatinum in refractory childhood cancer: Children's Cancer Study Group report. *Cancer Treat. Rep.* 65:815–822, 1981.
122. Voute P.A., Vos A., deKraker J., et al.: Rhabdomyosarcomas: Chemotherapy and limited supplementary treatment program to avoid multilation. *Natl. Cancer Inst. Monogr.* 56:121–125, 1981.
123. Flamant F., Rodary C.H.: Rhabdomyosarcoma Trial SIOP III, in *Proceedings of XV International Society of Pediatric Oncology*. York, England, September 20–24, 1983.
124. Carli M., DeBernadi B., Ceci A., et al.: Primary chemotherapy in childhood rhabdomyosarcoma (RMS): Preliminary data of the Italian Co-operative Group for RMS, in *Proceedings of XV International Society of Pediatric Oncology* York, England, September 20–24, 1983.
125. Voute P.A., Vos A., deKraker J.: Chemotherapy as initial treatment in rhabdomyosarcoma, abstract C 341. *Proc. Am. Soc. Clin. Oncol.* 3:87, 1984.
126. Tefft M., Fernandez C.H., Moon T.E.: Rhabdomyosarcoma: Response with chemotherapy prior to radiation in patients with gross residual disease. *Cancer* 39:665–670, 1977.
127. Pratt C.B., George S.: Response of childhood rhabdomyosarcoma (RMS) to combination chemotherapy, abstract 723. *Proc. Am. Assoc. Cancer Res.* 21:181, 1980.
128. Raney R.B., Tefft M., Maurer H., et al.: Results of intensive treatment of children with cranial parameningeal sarcoma: A report from the Intergroup Rhabdomyosarcoma Study (IRS), abstract 47. *Proc. Am. Assoc. Cancer Res.* 31:120, 1982.
129. Lawrence W. Jr., Hays D.M.: Surgical lesions from the Intergroup Rhabdomyosarcoma Study. *Natl. Cancer Inst. Monogr.* 56:159–163, 1981.
130. Tefft M., Lindberg R.D., Gehan E.A.: Radiation therapy combined with systemic chemotherapy of rhabdomyosarcoma in children: Local control in patients enrolled in the Intergroup Rhabdomyosarcoma Study. *Natl. Cancer Inst. Monogr.* 56:75–81, 1981.
131. Raney R.B., Handlee S.D.: Management of neoplasms of the head and neck in children: II. Malignant tumors. *Head Neck Surg.* 3:500–507, 1981.
132. Flamant F., Rodary C.H., Voute T., et al.: Malignant mesenchymal tumors: Registration and follow-up, in *Proceedings of XV International Society of Pediatric Oncology*. York, England, September 20–24, 1983.
133. Suit H.D.: Soft tissue sarcomas (excluding rhabdomyosarcoma): Radiotherapy applications. *Natl. Cancer Inst. Monogr.* 56:245–249, 1981.
134. Leite C., Goodwin J.W., Sinkovics J.G., et al.: Chemotherapy of malignant fibrous histiocytoma. A Southwest Oncology Group Report. *Cancer* 40:2010–2014, 1977.

135. Weiner M., Sedlis M., Johnson A.D., et al.: Adjuvant chemotherapy of malignant fibrous histiocytoma of bone. *Cancer* 51:25–29, 1983.
136. Benjamin R.S., Chawla S.P., Plager C., et al.: Primary malignant fibrous histiocytoma of bone—a chemotherapy-responsive tumor, abstract 569. *Proc. Am. Assoc. Cancer Res.* 24:144, 1983.
137. Cangir A., Jaffe N., Goepfert H.: Chemotherapy for aggressive "benign" tumors of the head and neck in children, abstract C322. *Proc. Am. Assoc. Clin. Oncol.* 4:83, 1984.
138. Heyn R., Ragab A., Raney B., et al.: Late effects of therapy in orbital rhabdomyosarcoma (RMS): A report from the Intergroup Rhabdomyosarcoma Study I (IRS I), abstract C257. *Proc. Am. Assoc. Clin. Oncol.* 1983, vol. 66.
139. Nadola R.P., Evans R.G., Gilchrist G.S., et al.: Morbidity and mortality of pediatric orbital rhabdomyosarcoma, abstract C297. *Proc. Am. Assoc. Clin. Oncol.* 1983, vol. 76.
140. Bajorunas D.R., Ghavimi F., Jereb B., et al.: Endocrine sequelae of antineoplastic therapy in childhood head and neck malignancies. *J. Clin. Endocrinol. Metab.* 50:329–335, 1980.

25 / Decisions and Management of Metastatic Cancer With an Unknown Primary Site

George L. Adams, M.D.

This chapter provides a practical approach to the evaluation and management of a patient with a neck mass when the cause of the mass is not immediately apparent on careful physical examination. Figure 25–1 briefly outlines the logical approach to a cervical mass.

In most cases, an explanation for a mass in the neck is clinically evident. Examples of specific neck masses include a mass adjacent to the thyroid gland, a midline cystic mass attached to the hyoid bone, a mass in the tail of the parotid gland, and a swollen lymph node in the setting of a large intraoral malignancy. A node may also be palpable in patients with an established history of lymphoma or chronic leukemia. The workup and evaluation of these specific neck masses are well established.

Let us concentrate on the mass for which no immediate cause is found and which lies in the upper two thirds of the neck. It is firm and 2 cm in diameter. It can be further delineated as to location in the anterior, posterior, or submandibular triangle (see Chap. 2). If it feels like a lymph node (firm, mobile, along the jugular vein), its specific size and location should be charted.

The evaluation begins with a careful history that accentuates the most likely explanations for a cervical mass. The patient is asked about:

1. Age.
2. Duration of the mass.
3. Pain in the mass.
4. Fluctuation in size of the mass.
5. Infections of pharynx or of dental origin.
6. Past medical problems.
7. Smoking and drinking habits.
8. Exposure to infectious disease.
9. Weight loss.
10. Dysphagia.
11. Hoarseness or change in voice.
12. Otalgia or middle ear symptoms.

A complete physical examination is performed, with special attention to the head and neck region. A thorough examination may be more difficult in a child than in an adult, but the principle remains the same.

Specific hints to aid in the examination are listed.

Oral cavity

1. Note status of dentition.
2. Tongue elevated to bimanually palpate floor of mouth and submandibular triangle.
3. Check tongue function (cranial nerve XII).

Oropharynx

1. Note appearance of tonsils (palpate for any difference in size).
2. Palpate base of tongue (the most important and frequently overlooked area).

Nasopharynx

1. Especially important if mass is in upper posterior triangle
2. A normal-appearing nasopharynx does not exclude the possibility of malignancy.
3. Fifty percent of patients with nasopharyngeal carcinoma will present with a neck mass.[1]

Nasal cavity

1. Check for ulceration of septum.
2. Check for polypoid lesions, especially if they bleed easily when palpated with a suction tip.
3. Shrinkage of the nasal mucosa with a topical decongestant spray permits a much better examination.

Larynx

1. Note vocal cord mobility.
2. Make certain the anterior commissure is visualized.
3. Do not look right past the epiglottis.
4. Try to observe the subglottic region.

Hypopharynx

1. Note ulceration.
2. Note pooling of secretions.

GENERAL HEAD AND NECK EXAMINATION

Because the mass may represent a malignant melanoma or a metastatic scalp lesion, the fundi, scalp, ear canal, and facial skin must be examined.

When a complete pharyngeal examination is not possible because of a hyperactive gag reflex, do not hesitate to apply a topical anesthetic. The flexible fiberoptic laryngoscope can be passed transnasally. It is especially useful for examining the nasopharynx and larynx. Even in a cooperative patient it can be used to supplement the mirror examination. Remember, there are still areas in the piriform sinuses and base of the tongue that are not well seen without laryngoscopic manipulation.

Concentrate last on the examination of the neck. This way you will be certain you did not overlook any area.

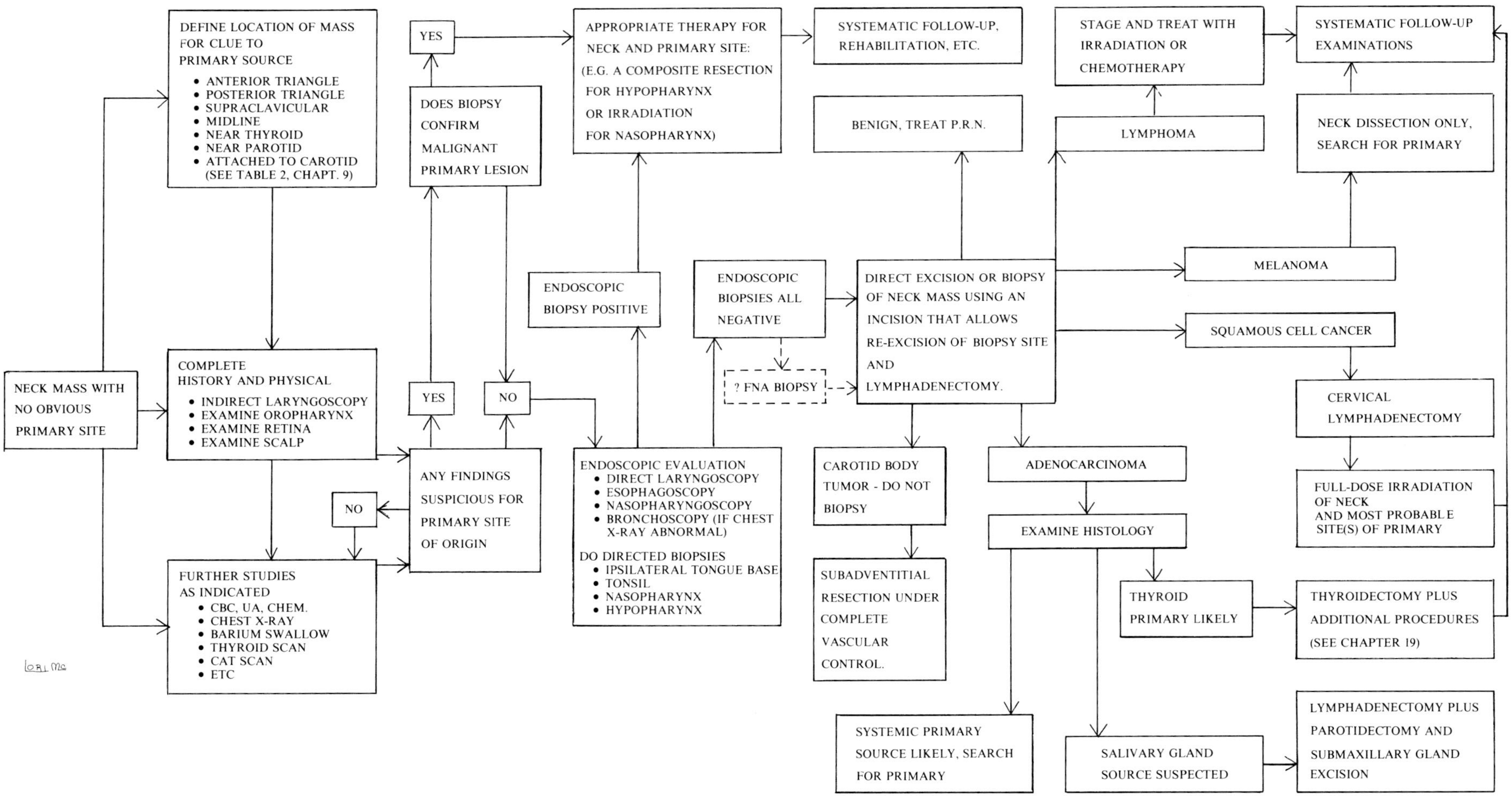

Fig 25–1.—Management of the "unknown primary" for a non-tender mass in the upper two-thirds of the neck in an adult over 40 years old.

Record the following information:

1. Location in triangle of the neck.
2. Palpation of thyroid gland.
3. Relationship to the carotid artery on auscultation.
4. Fixation or mobility. Does it move with swallowing?
5. Soft or cystic versus firm.
6. Is there more than one mass?
7. Tenderness.
8. Dimensions of mass in centimeters.

A thorough history and physical examination will lead to a correct tentative diagnosis in the vast majority of cases. It is estimated that 80% of head and neck malignancies can be detected on physical examination.

A number of laboratory and radiologic studies are available to assist in diagnosis. Consequently, specific studies from the large repertoire are selected so they provide the most productive information. The history and physical examination provide the base information that guides in the selection of appropriate studies. For example, a neck mass that moves on swallowing or is associated with a unilaterally enlarged thyroid gland indicates that a radioactive iodine thyroid scan should be obtained. A possible mass in the subglottic area or larynx can be demonstrated by a laryngeal CT scan. Tomograms are used less frequently but have helped in demonstrating masses in the upper trachea and subglottic area. A history of dysphagia suggests the need for a barium swallow. Paranasal sinus radiographs have not been of value.

In other words, radiology studies other than chest x-ray films are used selectively.

The remainder of the evaluation is based on statistics and facts accumulated at large centers on the incidence of diagnosis based on age, history, and location of the neck mass.

Concern will be limited to the upper two thirds of the neck, since low-lying supraclavicular masses are more often associated with primary diseases of the lungs or gastrointestinal (GI) tract.

HOW CAN YOU DIFFERENTIATE A BENIGN FROM A MALIGNANT MASS?

The likelihood of malignancy increases with age. Malignancy should be suspected when the mass occurs in a heavy smoker or in an individual over 40. The suspicion of malignancy continues to increase with age, so that a neck mass in a 60-year-old person has almost a 90% likelihood of being malignant.[2] The suspicion of malignancy is multiplied in tobacco users.

Children and young adults are more likely to have benign than malignant masses, but persistence of a mass, regardless of age, mandates a histologic diagnosis.

The most common benign masses include the following:

1. Inflammatory lymph node. This is often associated with existing or recent infection.
2. Thyroglossal duct cyst. This is a midline mass associated with the hyoid bone. It rises on swallowing.
3. Pharyngeal cleft cyst. A pharyngeal cleft cyst is found along the anterior border of sternocleidomastoid muscle. Because it fluctuates in size a tract may develop that may become acutely infected.
4. Deep neck abscess. This is most often seen in a patient with a history of recent pharyngeal or oral infection and in the setting of fever and an elevated WBC count. The area is tender on palpation.
5. Granulomatous disease, enlarging lymph nodes. This may be atypical tuberculosis. You should consider tuberculosis (scrofula) in those ethnic or socioeconomic populations with a high incidence of pulmonary tuberculosis.

THE EXPLANATION FOR THE NECK MASS IS STILL NOT APPARENT. WHAT'S THE NEXT STEP?

The next step depends on the age of the patient and the history. In an adult over age 40, it is more judicious to consider the mass as a potential metastatic malignancy than as a benign lymph node. If thyroid masses are excluded, 80% of neck masses in adults are malignant.

A persistent mass in a child requires excisional biopsy. If the mass is not of congenital origin, it is most likely an enlarged lymph node. Pathologists prefer to receive the entire node undisturbed by surgical manipulation. They can then proceed with appropriate evaluation.

In an adult, excisional biopsy is not performed without prior endoscopic evaluation. In the case of a malignant mass in the neck of an adult, the primary will be found in the head and neck area in 50%–60% of cases. Therefore, a thorough upper aerodigestive tract endoscopic evaluation is justified prior to excision.

What Endoscopic Procedures Are Advised?

Again, the history and physical examination will allow selectivity. When the chest x-ray film has been normal and when there is an absence of pulmonary symptoms, then bronchoscopy has not yielded positive results with sufficient frequency to justify routine use.

Dysphagia, weight loss, or questionable findings on barium swallow indicate the need for esophagoscopy—all the way to the gastroesophageal junction. The suggestion of a mass in the nasopharynx or a high or posterior neck mass requires nasopharyngoscopy.

These procedures are combined with direct laryngoscopy, which is the single most useful evaluation. The laryngoscope blade permits evaluation of the piriform sinus and allows the examiner to lift the larynx anteriorly to examine the postcricoid region. With the patient anesthetized, complete palpation of the tongue base and pharynx is repeated.

During endoscopy, the site of the primary malignancy is often found and a generous biopsy specimen is obtained using cup forceps. Biopsy specimens of any other suspicious areas are also obtained in case of a synchronous lesion, and when needed to establish the extent of resection necessary or the size of the field for radiation therapy.

What If No Abnormality Is Found?

This is a controversial question. Some surgeons believe that biopsies are not justified when tissues appear normal. They hold that biopsy only adds to morbidity. We perform "directed biopsies," as distinguished from "blind biopsies," or more random sampling of sites.

Directed biopsies are performed on the same side of the pharynx or hypopharynx as the location of the neck mass. Selection of the biopsy sites must consider the compartmentalization of the neck and recognize that there is some predictability in the lymphatic drainage pattern. The location of the neck mass determines the biopsy sites. For example, posterior and high neck masses require a biopsy of the vault of the nasopharynx and fossa of Rosenmüller. When the mass is in the jugulodigastric region, a biopsy of the tongue base and hypopharynx is performed. In our experience most of the initially unapparent primaries have been found by endoscopy to be located in the base of the tongue or piriform sinus area. Occasionally an area of leukoplakia, superficial ulceration, or easy bleeding (when brushed by the laryngoscope) is encountered. Such areas are biopsied.

Is Tonsillectomy of Value?

In the case of a visible suspicious tonsillar lesion, the strong preference is to perform a biopsy with a large cup forceps (4–5 mm). Tonsillectomy requires at least 2 weeks to heal and will impede the evaluation. In certain circumstances, however, tonsillectomy may be necessary. Tonsillectomy is employed when there is a unilaterally enlarged tonsil or when palpation indicates that the tonsil on the side of the node is definitely more firm. Tonsillectomy may provide the diagnosis of lymphoma or Hodgkin's disease. However, it is not part of a routine evaluation.

SUPPOSE THERE IS STILL NO DETECTABLE PRIMARY MALIGNANCY OR EXPLANATION FOR THE NECK MASS?

Even after a thorough examination and directed biopsies, no explanation for the neck mass will be found in 3%–8% of patients. At this point, open excisional biopsy is performed. The incision is transverse so that it can be incorporated into an H or horizontal limb of a neck dissection. A benign mass is removed in its entirety. A cervical lymph node is removed as undisturbed as possible and sent for immediate pathologic evaluation. Preliminary communication with the pathologist is essential. He may wish to perform "touch" preparations, culture, or electron microscopy. If the report is a benign lymph node and there are several other large nodes in the immediate area, it is worth while removing additional nodes for evaluation.

The one exception to excisional biopsy is the inadvertent finding of a carotid body tumor. Location, vascular appearance, compressibility, and fixation to the carotid bifurcation are sufficient criteria on which to base a diagnosis of carotid body tumor. Unless one had planned to deal with a chemodectoma, it is preferable not to proceed but to close the incision and obtain a confirming carotid arteriogram. The patient should understand the risks and benefits of excision. Resection of a small chemodectoma may not be indicated at all in an individual over 50 years of age. The arteriogram may demonstrate the true extent of the tumor to be larger than anticipated. At surgery, sufficient blood units should be available in the operating room to replace any blood lost. Surgeons experienced with safe vascular control, intra-arterial shunting, and carotid artery replacement should be available to come to the operating room before proceeding with tumor removal.

Why Not Perform an Open Incisional Biopsy Before Starting an Extensive Diagnostic Workup?

When excisional biopsy yields a malignant tumor, the surgeon should be prepared to proceed with an appropriate resection.[3] The patient should accept the plan of management and should give informed preoperative consent. Premature biopsy or incisional biopsy of a neck mass without definite resection increases the incidence of wound necrosis from 11% to 20%, the incidence of regional recurrence in the neck from 24% to 32%, and the incidence of distant metastasis from 24% to 40%.[4]

IF THE MASS IS METASTATIC EPIDERMOID CARCINOMA, HOW DO YOU PROCEED?

This is why it is important to be certain that the primary site is "unknown." Radiation therapy or a composite resection would have been performed if the primary site had been located. Now it may be reasonable to perform a radical neck dissection without knowing the primary site. Different centers have accumulated data to provide some statistics on how to proceed.

There are five options:

1. Close the wound and continue searching for the primary. This is not advised.
2. Close the wound and administer radiation therapy to the neck and suspected site of the primary lesion.
3. Convert the incision into an appropriate incision for a neck dissection. Proceed with a standard radical neck dissection.
4. Same as 3. Administer postoperative full-dose irradiation to the pharynx and regions most likely to metastasize to this site.
5. Excise the lymph node, close the incision, administer a full course of irradiation, and then perform a radical neck dissection.

Our own preference is No. 4. The philosophy behind the approach described is based on the fact that the majority of malignancies that metastasize to the lymph nodes of the upper two thirds of the neck arise in the upper aerodigestive tract. It is assumed that the primary is so small that it remains elusive but will be encompassed in the radiation field. Option 5 is preferred at some centers, but in some reports, 50% of patients so treated had had the biopsy performed before referral.

We prefer combined therapy for all nodal disease N_1–N_3. The idea is that the primary will be included in the radiation field. Most likely the primary site is in the nasopharynx, base of the tongue, or piriform sinus. Some centers prefer surgery alone for N_1 disease, reserving combined therapy for N_2 and N_3 disease.[5, 6]

Both Leipzig et al.[5] and Fried et al.[7] prefer full-course radiation therapy followed by radical neck dissection as their method of combined therapy.

In the M. D. Anderson Hospital series,[8] radiation therapy was the most frequent treatment, with combined therapy used less often. Surgery was preferred for a single node in the subdigastric triangle so as to protect the larynx from radiation. In that series 52% of the patients had had a biopsy of the neck mass performed prior to referral. Excluding patients with supraclavicular nodes, the 3-year survival was 53%.

In our series, when neck dissection alone was performed and the primary was found later (usually in the base of the tongue), no patient had a longer survival whether treated by surgery or radiation therapy, see Table 25–2. Jesse et al.[9] reported a 3-year survival of 58% when the primary was never found, compared to a 31% 3-year survival when it later became evident. Acquarelli et al.[10] and Coker et al.[6] likewise reported decreased survival when the primary grew in the posttreatment period until it was recognized and an attempt was made at definitive treatment.

In the New York Memorial Hospital Series reported by Barrie et al.,[11] the primary was later found in 38 of 103 patients. Treatment then included surgery or surgery and irradiation. The primary was eventually found in a subset of five patients with adenocarcinomas. Only one of the patients with adenocarcinoma survived 5 years. In this same series, the location of the primary in patients with metastatic squamous cell carcinoma did not affect survival. Regardless of whether or not the primary was found, the 5-year survival rate was approximately 30%. Fried et al.[7] reported no survivors when the lymph node was larger than 4 cm.

Coker et al.[6] provide statistics to justify postoperative radiation therapy for N_2 and N_3 nodal disease. They too prefer surgery alone for N_1 disease. They compared the 5-year survival rate by stage for squamous cell carcinoma (54%) and anaplastic carcinoma (32%). For N_1 disease, the 5-year survival rate with surgery alone was 68%. The survival of patients with N_1 disease treated with radiation only was 40%. Coker's combined 5-year survival statistics are given in Table 25–1.

Can the Neck Dissection Be Modified?

Specific criteria for modifying a neck dissection in this situation do not exist. How extensive a resection to perform is a matter of judgment. The existence of a large (> 4 cm) node or multiple-level nodes requires a standard neck dissection. A single small, mobile node in the anterior neck may permit preservation of cranial nerve XI or a modified Bocca neck dissection. This modification is acceptable if postoperative irradiation will be administered.[12]

WHAT IF THE BIOPSY REVEALS ADENOCARCINOMA?

In certain instances, the pathologist may be able to identify the adenocarcinoma as possibly arising from salivary gland tissue. Certainly a mass adjacent to the submandibular gland would be treated as if the primary

TABLE 25–1.—5-YEAR SURVIVAL OF PATIENTS WITH METASTATIC CANCER IN CERVICAL LYMPH NODES TREATED WITH LYMPHADENECTOMY AND POSTOPERATIVE IRRADIATION*

STAGE	SQUAMOUS CELL CARCINOMA (%)	ANAPLASTIC CARCINOMA (%)
N_1	81	100
N_2	60	42
N_3	12	15

*Data from Coker et al.[6]

were in that gland. Parotidectomy combined with upper neck dissection is performed for a mass adjacent to the parotid gland area.

One special situation is metastatic adenocarcinoma of the thyroid gland. In this situation, modified neck dissection accompanied by total thyroidectomy is advised. The detailed management of metastatic carcinoma of the thyroid gland under various circumstances is outlined in chapter 19. Most patients have a good chance for survival.

In another circumstance, radical neck dissection has not been found to be beneficial to the patient.[13] Adenocarcinoma in the lower half of the neck is treated by excisional biopsy only. The area is irradiated postoperatively, and after a search for the primary has been completed. Most metastatic adenocarcinomas in the lower third of the neck arise from primaries in the breast, lung, or GI tract. The search for a primary should include the breast, ovary, prostate, and stomach. No radical procedure is advised because the cervical metastasis implies systemic dissemination of the adenocarcinoma.

WHAT IF THE BIOPSY REVEALS MALIGNANT MELANOMA?

A careful search for a primary lesion should have already been completed. Specifically, the scalp, conjunctivae, internal nose, and fundi should have been thoroughly examined. If no primary can be found, radical neck dissection is appropriate. Careful follow-up will eventually establish the primary site, but in some patients, this may be a matter of several years.

SUPPOSE THE MASS IS A LYMPHOMA?

Pathologists prefer the node to be removed without disturbing the capsule. If a good specimen is obtained, special procedures can be performed and the classification of Hodgkin's disease or lymphoma can be established. Approximately two thirds of lymphomas arising in the head and neck region are of the histiocytic type. The pathologist will want the entire node with an intact capsule so he can perform imprint studies. Electron microscopy is often required to distinguish between a poorly differentiated carcinoma and lymphoma. A carcinoma is determined by the presence of desmosomes and intracellular bridges.

WHAT IF THE MASS IS A POORLY DIFFERENTIATED OR UNDIFFERENTIATED CARCINOMA OR AN ANAPLASTIC CARCINOMA?

Our policy has been to resect the lesion and administer radiation therapy. Numbers are too small to allow evaluation of this group of patients, but in some cases survival has been better than with the more differentiated lesions.[6] Many of these patients present with such a large, fixed mass that no surgery is feasible.

WHY NOT PERFORM A NEEDLE BIOPSY OF THE NECK MASS AND DETERMINE IMMEDIATELY IF THE MASS IS MALIGNANT?

Thin needle aspiration biopsy is a useful procedure that is gaining acceptance. If it is performed with a No. 22 needle and a satisfactory sample is obtained, the accuracy of diagnosis is 80%–90%.[14] Thin needle aspiration biopsy has not led to seeding of the tumor, and may be cost-effective. There is one probable advantage of a needle biopsy: when it is done by someone not trained as a head and neck specialist, the diagnosis of malignancy will usually result in prompt referral of the patient, without an extended trial of antibiotics or an endless sequence of systemic studies. An inappropriate open biopsy can be avoided. The patient is placed on a correct path of management.

Thin needle biopsy does have certain limitations. (1) It is not effective in a rock-hard solid mass. (2) The study may have to be repeated if an inadequate sample is obtained. (3) If there are technical errors, the aspirate may contain only normal tissue or tissue from an adjacent node, leading to false conclusions. When the examining physician is knowledgeable about head and neck problems and is able to conduct all of the appropriate examinations, the usefulness of *routine* needle biopsy can be seriously questioned.

The reasons we do not uniformly recommend the procedure are as follows:

1. It should not replace a thorough head and neck evaluation.
2. It will often give information on whether the mass is benign or malignant, but will not be sufficiently specific so that the treatment plans will be changed.
3. Often thin needle biopsy does not eliminate the need for open biopsy or additional procedures.

An explanation of this last statement is necessary. If, as discussed earlier, 90% of firm neck masses in persons over the age of 60 are malignant, then using aspiration biopsy-cytologic study to establish that a lesion is malignant only confirms what is already assumed. If the aspirate shows squamous cell carcinoma, a search for the primary continues. If the aspirate shows adenocarcinoma, a search for the primary continues. If the aspirate shows a lymphoma, the pathologist will request that a complete, intact node be excised. If the aspirate from a mass in an older patient who smokes is benign, there is sufficient residual uncertainty that one would still recommend excision biopsy.

When is a Needle Aspiraton Biopsy Considered?

Nevertheless, there are certain circumstances when an aspiration biopsy is useful. These include the following:

1. A supraclavicular mass where the primary is most likely below the clavicle, a diagnosis is needed, but there are no plans for surgery.
2. To establish that the neck mass is metastatic tumor in a patient already known to have had a cancer, e.g., a patient with a past history of treatment for breast or colon cancer.
3. To establish a diagnosis in a patient who would not be a candidate for a complete evaluation or surgery, e.g., an elderly patient, a patient with recent cardiac problems.
4. A patient with a history of head and neck cancer who now has a suspected recurrence and biopsy is required before initiating a radiation therapy or chemotherapy regimen.
5. To document recurrence of lymphoma.
6. To evaluate a suspected node in the posterior neck or contralateral neck that may determine that the patient's tumor is not resectable.
7. It is especially helpful in the differential diagnosis of thyroid neoplasms, e.g., cyst versus carcinoma (see Chap. 19).
8. To evaluate a fixed mass that would not be considered resectable.

WHAT IS THE AVERAGE 5-YEAR SURVIVAL IN PATIENTS TREATED FOR A METASTATIC NECK NODE WHEN THE PRIMARY SITE OF ORIGIN IS UNKNOWN AT THE TIME OF TREATMENT?

Results are often reported in terms of 3-, 4-, and 5-year survival and include lesions of all sizes. They also include more than one modality of treatment. These survival rates for squamous cell carcinoma range from 15%* to 40%†, with the majority of authors reporting a 30% 5-year survival. Treatment is effective. The patient should not be denied treatment when metastatic squamous cell cancer is found. The results of treatment in 44 of our patients in whom the primary site was truly unknown at time of treatment are shown in Table 25–2. The results are stratified by treatment. The site of primary, when found, is shown in Table 25–3. The causes of failure in patients treated for cure are reported in Table 25–4.

*Winegar's Michigan University study included supraclavicular masses.

†Jesse's high rate includes patients with a single node in the upper neck.

TABLE 25–2.—RESULTS OF TREATMENT OF SQUAMOUS CELL CANCER IN CERVICAL LYMPH NODES WHERE THE PRIMARY LOCUS OF THE CANCER WAS NOT DETECTABLE AT THE TIME OF TREATMENT*

TREATMENT	N	ALIVE	DD	LIVED ≥3 YR‡	DOC
RND + postop. XRT	20†	12	6	7	2 NED
Preop. XRT + RND	5	3	2	3	
RND only	4	1	3	3	
XRT for cure	5	2	2	4	1 NED
XRT for palliation	7	0	7	0	
Total	41	18	20	17	3

*Total group included 44 patients; 34 were treated for cure. DD, dead of disease; DOC, dead of other causes; NED, no evidence of disease.

†Three patients are less than 1 year postoperative.

‡To date, at least four patients have lived longer than 8 years without evidence of disease.

SUMMARY

A neck mass in an individual over age 40 is suspected of representing metastatic disease. A neck mass in an individual over age 60 is assumed to be malignant until proved otherwise. Heavy smokers warrant a higher suspicion of malignancy. A full physical examination with specific diagnostic and radiologic tests is required prior to biopsy. The tests that are ordered are selected on the basis of greatest yield. They are selected according to the location of the neck mass and any suggested sources provided by the patient's history. Needle aspiration biopsies are cost-effective and productive in certain circumstances, especially in documenting recent diseases and in supraclavicular neck masses. In approximately 5% of patients a malignant neck mass represents metastasis from an unknown primary. After eliminating lower third or supraclavicular masses, previously biopsied or partially excised masses and patients with large fixed masses, there are no large series to prove that one particular regimen of treatment (i.e., biopsy + irradiation or lymphadenectomy + irradiation) is preferable.

At this time our preferred treatment for metastatic squamous cell carcinoma when no primary is found is excisional biopsy, followed immediately by radical neck dissection. Lymphadenectomy is followed by postoperative irradiation of the neck and probable primary sites.

TABLE 25–3.—PRIMARY FOUND LATER (5/34 PATIENTS)

LOCATION	N	NO. ALIVE	INTERVAL
Base of tongue	2	0	1 yr; 5 yr
Nasopharynx	1	0	3 mo.
Floor of mouth	1	0	7 yr
Mandibular alveolus	1	1	2 yr

TABLE 25–4.—CAUSES OF DEATH IN PATIENTS TREATED FOR CURE (15/34)

CAUSE OF DEATH	N
Uncontrolled primary	4
Local disease (neck)	6
Distant metastases	2
Intercurrent disease	3
Total	15

This is done because it is thought that excising cervical metastatic masses larger than 3 cm has a better chance of tumor control. Studies reveal that in 50%–60% of patients, the primary carcinoma will never become evident.

Certain conclusions are evident, however, from these series. A relatively *good* prognosis can be expected when:

1. The mass is solitary.
2. The mass is less than 2 cm in size.
3. The mass is in the upper third of the neck, especially the submandibular triangle.
4. The metastasis is squamous cell carcinoma.
5. The primary is never found.
6. The mass has not been previously biopsied or excised.
7. The mass represents metastatic adenocarcinoma of the thyroid.

Conversely, the prognosis is *poor* when:

1. The mass is more than 4 cm in size.
2. There are multiple-level nodes.
3. The mass is in the lower half of the neck.
4. The mass is an adenocarcinoma of other than thyroid origin.
5. Bilateral nodes are present initially.

Preferred treatment is surgical excision of the mass. Incisional biopsy is to be avoided. Radical neck dissection in combination with radiation therapy appears to provide the longest survival.

REFERENCES

1. Fitzpatrick P.J., Kotalik J.: Cervical metastases from an unknown primary tumor. *Radiology* 110:659–663, 1974.
2. Winegar L.K., Griffin W.: The occult primary tumor. *Arch. Otol.* 98:159–163, 1983.
3. Martin H.: Untimely lymph node biopsy. *Am. J. Surg.* 102:17–18, 1961.
4. McGuirt W.F., McCabe B.F.: Significance of node biopsy before definitive treatment of cervical metastatic carcinoma. *Laryngoscope* 88:594–603, 1978.
5. Leipzig B., Winter M., Hokanson J.A.: Cervical nodal metastases of unknown origin. *Laryngoscope* 91:593–597, 1981.
6. Coker D.D., Casterline P.F., Chambers R.G., et al.: Metastases to lymph nodes of the head and neck from an unknown primary site. *Am. J. Surg.* 134:517–522, 1977.
7. Fried M.P., Diehl W.H., Brownson R.J., et al.: Cervical metastasis from an unknown primary. *Ann. Otol.* 84:152–157, 1975.
8. MacComb W.S.: Metastatic cervical nodes of unknown primary origin. *CA* 24:229–232, 1974.
9. Jesse R.H., Perez C.A., Fletcher G.H.: Cervical lymph node metastases: Unknown primary cancer. *Cancer* 31:854–859, 1973.
10. Acquarelli M.J., Matsunaga R.J., Cruze K.: Metastatic carcinoma of the neck of unknown primary origin. *Laryngoscope* 71:962–974, 1961.
11. Barrie J.R., Knapper W.H., Strong E.W.: Cervical nodal metastases of unknown origin. *Am. J. Surg.* 120:466–470, 1970.
12. Krause J.C., Schuller D.E.: Treatment with radical neck dissection, in Snow J.B. (ed.): *Controversy in Otolaryngology.* Philadelphia, W.B. Saunders Co., 198, pp. 197–201.
13. Templer J., Perry M.C., Davis W.E.: Metastatic cervical adenocarcinoma from unknown primary tumor. *Arch. Otolaryngol.* 107:45–47, 1981.
14. Weymuller E.A., Kiviat N.B., Duckert L.G.: Aspiration cytology: An efficient and cost-effective modality. *Laryngoscope* 93:561–564, 1983.

26 / Multiple Primary Epidermoid Carcinomas of the Upper Aerodigestive Tract

DONALD G. MCQUARRIE, M.D., PH.D.

IN the United States, tobacco and its combustion products, alone or combined with alcohol, are the major causes of epidermoid cancer of the aerodigestive tract. It is not surprising to find similar cancers arising in widely separated areas of similar epithelium that have had identical carcinogen exposure. Because the parts of the aerodigestive tract that are at risk are above and below the clavicle, the head and neck cancer surgeon must expand his scope of diagnostic interest to search for other cancers in the lung and esophagus.

HOW COMMON ARE SYNCHRONOUS OR METACHRONOUS CANCERS OF THE UPPER AERODIGESTIVE TRACT?

The phenomenon of multiple primary carcinomas was recognized in the early 1930s. In 1932, Warren and Gates[1] reported a 3.7% incidence of two or more malignancies in a series of 1,078 autopsies performed on cancer patients. One year later Lund[2] reported a 6% incidence of second primaries in the head and neck area in 1,548 patients with carcinoma of the buccal mucosa. In 1946 Slaughter[3] reported an 18% incidence of multiple epidermoid carcinomas in the head and neck. He postulated that intraoral carcinoma was frequently of multicentric origin. In the past two decades Bross and Coomb,[4] Rothman and Keller,[5] and Wynder and co-workers[6] have reported on series of patients with two or more primary carcinomas in the upper aerodigestive tract.

A variation ranging from 6% to 24% in the incidence of multiple primary epidermoid carcinomas of the aerodigestive tract has been reported in recent series by Derrick and co-workers,[7] Farr and associates,[8] and Vrabec.[9] The wide range of incidence may be due to multiple factors, including accuracy of follow-up, duration of follow-up, and difficulty in differentiating between subsequent primaries and metastases. It is obvious that if second primaries continue to develop, the series with a longer follow-up will show a higher aggregate incidence. Marchetta and associates[10] have distinguished between a subsequent primary and a metastasis on the basis of location (separated by normal tissues), histologic characteristics of the tumor (arising in an area of mucosal dysplasia), the natural history of the tumor, and the expected course of malignancy at each respective site.

The principles of management discussed in chapter 10 stressed the importance of recognizing the "condemned mucosa" which may have widespread dysplastic changes. The multifocal squamous metaplasia in the bronchial epithelium of heavy smokers is well known. The decree of condemnation of the susceptable mucosa is determined by prolonged carcinogen exposure.

To arrive at the frequency and timing of multiple upper aerodigestive cancers, we reviewed and interchecked the records of 405 patients with epidermoid head and neck cancer, 250 patients with esophageal cancer, and 2,350 patients with lung cancer for the 1965–1980 period. Of the 405 patients who had a head and neck cancer as their first primary, 52 (13%) had a synchronous or subsequent cancer.

IS THE SITE OF THE FIRST PRIMARY CANCER RELATED TO THE FREQUENCY OF A SYNCHRONOUS OR METACHRONOUS SECOND CANCER?

Table 26–1 shows the location of the first tumor. With the exception of a lower incidence of laryngeal cancers, it matches the usual head and neck cancer distribution. Different anatomical sites for the first primary have a varying incidence of subsequent primaries. Kogelnik and colleagues[11] found an incidence of a second primary ranging from 5% for vocal cord squamous cell carcinoma to 33% for carcinoma of the soft palate. Derrick and co-workers[7, 12] concluded that patients with supraglottic carcinoma are at higher risk for the development of a secondary primary than patients with glottic carcinoma. Patients with lung and esophageal cancer have a much lower cure rate. There will be a much smaller proportion of patients who survive to remain at risk for the development of a second cancer in a head and neck site.

Despite this variation in incidence, it is important that the clinician be aware that a patient with one head and neck epidermoid carcinoma is at high risk for the development of a second primary in the area. New symptoms should not be always attributed to the original tumor.

TABLE 26–1.—LOCATION OF THE FIRST PRIMARY TUMOR

SITE	PATIENTS No.	(%)
Tongue	11	(21)
Floor of the mouth	15	(28)
Larynx	9	(17)
Pharynx	5	(10)
Tonsil	5	(10)
Retromolar trigone	3	(6)
Lower lip	3	(6)
Soft palate	1	(2)
Total	52	(100)

WHEN DO PATIENTS DEVELOP A SECOND PRIMARY?

Table 26–2 gives the interval between diagnosis of the first and second cancers. The second cancers that come to the examiner's attention within the first 6 months most likely would have had some recognizable minimal lesion at the time the first cancer was treated if a more diligent examination had been done. Almost half of second cancers are seen within 2 years after the first. Our results are in agreement with the reports of Gluckman and associates[13] and Marchetta and associates[10] indicating that approximately half of the second primaries develop within 2 years of the first primary. However, in our series, patients continued to develop second primaries as late as 10 years after the first. Jesse and Sugarbaker[14] have reported a 37% incidence of second primaries in patients who survived more than 5 years after diagnosis of the original tumor. The risk appears to be directly proportional to the dose and duration of exposure to carcinogens.[15] It has been shown that successfully treated patients who continue smoking after the development of a primary in the head and neck area have a 40% lifetime chance of developing another oroairway cancer. A subsequent malignancy develops within 5 years in only 6% of patients who quit smoking. Unfortunately, most of the reported data are not in a form that allows one to calculate an accurate risk per year with and without continued smoking.

TABLE 26–2.—INTERVAL BETWEEN DIAGNOSIS OF THE FIRST AND SECOND PRIMARY TUMOR

INTERVAL	PATIENTS No.	(%)
0	5	(10)
< 6 mo.	8	(15)
6 mo. to 2 yr	12	(23)
2–5 yr	15	(29)
5–10 yr	9	(17)
>10 yr	3	(6)
Total	52	(100)

WHERE ARE SUBSEQUENT AERODIGESTIVE PRIMARIES LIKELY TO BE FOUND?

Table 26–3 lists the location of subsequent cancers. We found a nearly even distribution of subsequent primaries in the head and neck, esophagus, and lungs. The subsequent primary will most likely be the cause of death. Only 7 of our 52 patients survived a second cancer to develop a third. In 3 patients a fourth primary developed.

HOW CAN SECOND SYNCHRONOUS PRIMARIES BE FOUND?

The data from Table 26–3 make it clear that confining an examination to the head and neck area alone is inadequate to detect related synchronous or subsequent cancers in the lung and esophagus. In the days of rigid tube endoscopy, the risk of esophageal and bronchial examination was significant. Fiberoptic endoscopy is both simpler and safer. Gluckman and associates[13] have demonstrated the efficacy of panendoscopy in the initial evaluation of head and neck cancer patients. We have come to believe that all patients with epidermoid carcinoma of the upper aerodigestive tract should have a complete examination, including endoscopy. The 3%–15% likelihood of a silent synchronous primary justifies the cost of adding panendoscopy to the initial evaluation. The exception is that bronchoscopy has not been rewarding in the patient with both a normal chest X-ray and a complete absence of chest symptoms. See the precautions for patients with laryngeal lesions discussed in chapter 16.

McGuirt and co-workers, from the heart of the mid-South tobacco country, did a prospective panendoscopic study of 81 consecutive new patients with head and neck cancer.[16] Fourteen patients (17%) had multiple synchronous primary lesions. The higher rate probably reflects the diligence of their search. Their data are summarized in Table 26–4. There is little question in the study that triple endoscopy was effective in identifying lesions and was essential in confirming the malignancy by biopsy. Esophagoscopy was particularly effective. McGuirt et al. concluded that the risk of triple endoscopy was small (no complications in 81 patients) and that "every effort should be made to find all primary [cancer] sites before treatment of the index tumor is begun." Those conclusions were maintained when the series was extended to 100 patients.[17] From Table 26–4 it is clear that laryngoscopy should be performed in anyone with any laryngeal or hypopharyngeal symp-

TABLE 26–3.—LOCATION OF SUBSEQUENT PRIMARY TUMORS

SUBSEQUENT PRIMARY	HEAD & NECK		LUNG		ESOPHAGUS		TOTAL	
	No.	(%)	No.	(%)	No.	(%)	No.	(%)
Second primary	18	(29)	20	(32)	14	(22)	52	(83)
Third primary	3	(5)	2	(3)	2	(3)	7	(11)
Fourth primary	1	(2)	1	(2)	1	(2)	3	(6)
Total	22	(36)	23	(37)	17	(27)	62	(100)

toms, as well as in anyone with abnormal chest x-ray films. If one were to select a group in whom screening esophagoscopy should be applied, these are the patients to consider.

WHAT SHOULD BE DONE IN FOLLOW-UP TO SEARCH FOR SUBSEQUENT PRIMARIES?

Patients who continue to smoke remain at high risk. The highest recurrence rate is seen in the first 2 years. The primary objection to uniform panendoscopy for follow-up is the cost of the procedures. If we could ignore cost, then endoscopy could be more liberally applied for follow-up.

For the follow-up of a heavy smoker, re-examination of the oropharynx, bronchi, and esophagus should be repeated at 6 months to a year. On subsequent examinations one should search for pulmonary and esophageal symptoms. Any time the chest x-ray film is abnormal or the symptoms and signs *suggest* any new tumor symptoms, a thorough endoscopic examination is required. Early diagnosis offers the only hope of improvement in survival following the development of a subsequent primary.

WHEN TWO OROAIRWAY CANCERS COEXIST, WHICH ONE DO YOU TREAT FIRST?

When particular circumstances allow the election of treatment plans for two coexisting cancers, it is logical to treat first the lesion with the higher treatment failure rate or the more rapid mortality.

Patients with uncontrolled lung and esophageal cancer have a survival measured in months. Treatment cannot be delayed. If the head and neck primary were treated first, there would be very little time to treat, reconstruct, and rehabilitate a head and neck cancer patient before thoracotomy. If, after treatment of a coexisting lung or esophageal cancer, long-term survival seems likely, the head and neck cancer is indepen-

TABLE 26–4.—ENDOSCOPIC AND DIAGNOSTIC RESULTS IDENTIFYING SYNCHRONOUS PRIMARY CANCERS OF THE AERODIGESTIVE TRACT IN 81 PATIENTS*

STUDY THAT IDENTIFIED THE CANCER	NO. OF PTS. Subgroup	Group
Esophagoscopy		6
Esophagogram abnormal	3	
Esophagography not done	3	
Laryngoscopy		5
Synchronous tumor may have been found in evaluating symptoms	4	
Synchronous tumor would not have been found except for planned laryngoscopy	1	
Bronchoscopy		3
Chest radiograph "abnormal"	2	
Chest radiograph "normal"	1	
Total synchronous cancers		14/81 (17%)
No. of unsuspected cancers found only on prospective planned endoscopy		5/81 (6%)

*Adapted from McGuirt et al.[16]

TABLE 26–5.—PATIENT SURVIVAL AFTER FIRST AND SECOND PRIMARY TUMORS*

PERIOD	NO. OF PTS. (%) OF TOTAL GROUP OF 52 AT RISK WHO SURVIVED FOR: <2 yr	2–5 yr	5–10 yr	>10 yr
After first primary	11 (21)	16 (31)	18 (35)	7 (13)
After second primary	38 (73)	8 (15)	4 (8)	2 (4)
			14 (27)	
				6 (12)

*Only two patients were still alive at the time of the study.

TABLE 26–6.—LOCATION OF, AND SURVIVAL FROM SECOND PRIMARY TUMOR

SITE OF SECOND PRIMARY	NO. OF PTS. (%) OF TOTAL GROUP OF 52 AT RISK WHO SURVIVED <2 yr	2–5 yr	5–10 yr	> 10 yr
Head/neck	9/18 (50)	6/18 (33)	2/18 (11)	1/18 (6)
Esophagus	13/14 (93)	. . .	1/14 (7)	. . .
Lung	16/20 (80)	2/20 (10)	1/20 (5)	1/20 (5)
Total	38/52 (73)	8/52 (15)	4/52 (15)	5/52 (4)

TABLE 27–7.—CAUSE OF DEATH IN 50/52 PATIENTS

CAUSE OF DEATH	FIRST PRIMARY		SECOND PRIMARY		THIRD PRIMARY		FOURTH PRIMARY		UNRELATED CAUSE		TOTAL	
	No.	(%)	No.	(%)	No.	(%)	No.	(%)	No.	(%)	No.	(%)
Lung Ca.			16	(32)	2	(4)	1	(2)			19	(38)
Esophagus Ca.			12	(24)	2	(4)	1	(2)			15	(30)
Head/neck Ca.	3	(6)	6	(12)							9	(18)
Unrelated cause									7	(14)	7	(14)
Total	3	(6)	34	(68)	4	(8)	2	(4)	7	(14)	50	(100)

dently treated as promptly as possible with no compromise in the curative attempt. In some instances a massive head and neck cancer that threatens the airway may force a reversal of policy.

IS THERE A DECENT SURVIVAL IN THE FACE OF A SYNCHRONOUS OR A SUBSEQUENT CANCER?

Table 26–5 summarizes our experience with crude survival of the 52 patients after first and second aerodigestive cancers. The second primary was treated by resective surgery (41%), irradiation (29%), or a combination of modalities (9%). Eleven (21%) patients were beyond treatment or refused further treatment when the second cancer was found. The second primary was the cause of death in 34 of the 50 patients who died.

The survival is related to the site of the subsequent cancer in Table 26–6. Causes of death are given in Table 26–7. These data show the much shorter patient survival from a second primary when it occurs in the esophagus or lung. In only three patients was the first primary in the head and neck the cause of death.

Crude survival rates after the second primary of 27% at 2 years and 12% at 5 years (see Table 26–5) are similar to those reported by Marchetta and associates.[10] The lowest survival occurs when the second primary develops in the lungs or esophagus. In the subgroup where the second primary develops in the head and neck area, there is a somewhat higher proportion of survivors at 5 years (17%), although it is far below the aggregate crude 5-year survival after the first primary (48%).

Jesse and Sugarbaker[14] have reported that the subsequent primary was the cause of death in 66% of their patients who had subsequent cancers. This figure is somewhat lower than our figure of 80%.

IS IT WORTHWHILE TREATING SECOND OROAIRWAY CANCERS?

In terms of reasonable quality of survival, it is worthwhile to treat subsequent head and neck primaries. We have not achieved cures in second cancers in the esophagus, but our experience was drawn from a past era when a diligent search was not made. McGuirts' most recent report found esophagoscopy to be the high-yield study. Although not specifically identified for the esophagus, early lesions (T_1) were common.[17] We must wait to see if early diagnosis can be converted to long-term cure. Panendoscopy appears to be an important tool, as was demonstrated in a parallel study of other populations in our area.[18]

The simple chest radiograph is an important follow-up tool. A *solitary* pulmonary nodule that shows up on follow-up chest radiography is a new primary more often than a metastasis. The difficulty lies in ascertaining that the nodule is truly solitary. Pulmonary tomography or a CT scan is helpful. We do not wait more than 4 weeks before performing thoracotomy if the patient is otherwise healthy.

The importance of a functioning cancer registry with effective follow-up is crucial if second primaries are to be found at an early and treatable stage. Most of our patients who had significant survival were among the patients who were carefully followed up and in whom the second lesion was found in an asymptomatic stage.

REFERENCES

1. Warren S., Gates D.C.: Multiple primary malignant tumors: A survey of the literature and statistical study. *Am. J. Cancer* 16:1358, 1932.
2. Lund C.C.: Second primary cancer in cases of cancer of the buccal mucosa. *N. Engl. J. Med.* 209:1144, 1933.
3. Slaughter D.O.: Multicentric origin of intraoral carcinoma. *Surgery* 20:133, 1946.
4. Bross J.D., Coomb S.J.: Heavy drinking, smoking linked with oral cancer. *JAMA* 236(5):435, 1976.
5. Rothman K., Keller A.: The effect of joint exposure to alcohol and tobacco on risk of cancer of the mouth and pharynx. *J. Chron. Dis.* 25:711, 1972.
6. Wynder E.L., Dodo H., Block D.A., et al.: Epidemiologic investigation of multiple primary cancer of the upper alimentary and respiratory tracts. *Cancer* 24(4):730, 1969.
7. Derrick J.H., Wagenfeld M.B., Harwood A.R., et al.:

Second primary respiratory tract malignant neoplasms in supraglottic carcinoma. *Arch. Otolaryngol.* 107:135, 1981.

8. Farr H.W., Goldfarb P.M., Farr D.M.: Epidermoid carcinoma of the mouth and pharynx at Memorial Sloan-Kettering Cancer Center, 1965–1969. *Am. J. Surg.* 140:563, 1980.
9. Vrabec D.P.: Multiple primary malignancies of the upper aerodigestive system. *Ann. Otolaryngol.* 88:846, 1979.
10. Marchetta F.C., Sako K., Camp F.: Multiple malignancies in patients with head and neck cancer. *Am. J. Surg.* 110:537, 1965.
11. Kogelnik D.H., Fletcher G.H., Jesse R.H.: Clinical course of patients with squamous cell carcinoma of the upper respiratory and digestive tracts with no evidence of disease 5 years after initial treatment. *Radiology* 115:423, 1975.
12. Derrick J., Wagenfeld M.B., Harwood A.R., et al.: Second primary respiratory tract malignancies in glottic carcinoma. *Cancer* 46(8):1833, 1980.
13. Gluckman J.L., Crissman J.D., Donegan O.J.: Multicentric squamors cell carcinoma of the upper aerodigestive tract. *Head Neck Surg.* 3:90, 1980.
14. Jesse R.H., Sugarbaker E.V.: Squamous cell carcinoma of the oropharynx: Why we fail. *Am. J. Surg.* 132:435, 1976.
15. The Surgeon General Report: *The Health Consequences of Smoking, Cancer*, 1982. U.S. Department of Health and Human Services. Rockville, Md., 1982. DHHS (PHS)82–50179.
16. McGuirt W.F., Matthews B., Koufman J.A.: Multiple simultaneous tumors in patients with head and neck cancer: A prospective, sequential panendoscopic study. *Cancer* 50:1195–1199, 1982.
17. McGuirt W.F.: Panendoscopy as a screening examination for simultaneous primary tumors in head and neck cancers: A prospective sequential study and review of the literature. *Laryngoscope* 92:569–576, 1983.
18. Maisel R.H., Vermeersch H.: Panendoscopy for second primaries in head and neck cancer, (abstract). Presented at the American Laryngological Society Meeting, Vancouver, May 10, 1981.

27 / Early Recognition and Planned Management of Complications of Head and Neck Cancer Treatment

DONALD G. MCQUARRIE, M.D., Ph.D. / ALAN R. SHONS, M.D., PH.D.

The best-laid schemes o' mice an' men gang aft agley.

Robert Burns (1759–1796)
"To a Mouse"

IN OLD Scottish dialect, the term "agley" meant "askew" or "crosseyed." Both the recognition and the management of complications are seen distortedly, which skews the best clinical planning. This chapter discusses some complications that are either peculiar to head and neck cancer care or seen with some frequency.

WHO HAS COMPLICATIONS?

Everyone treating head and neck cancer will encounter complications with any effective therapy. On the other hand, there are careful, thoughtful surgeons[1] and therapists whose anticipation and skills allow them to sidestep many disasters where others would blunder into predictable problems. One must actively seek the early symptoms of complications and institute prompt treatment. The surgeon must be familiar with what can go wrong in a variety of scenarios and have contingency plans for correcting untoward developments in the perioperative period.

A number of factors are associated with a predictable likelihood of complications. The small-vessel disease of diabetes and the changes produced by irradiation predispose to wound infection and flap vascular problems. Tumor remaining at the line of resection is a positive predictor of increased infection, fistula, and wound breakdown.[5] In a heavily irradiated field, carotid exposure and rupture are more frequent and much more difficult to manage. Large tumors requiring extensive resection or precarious reconstruction are likely to be associated with complications.[4, 5] Pulmonary, cardiovascular, and metabolic complications increase with age. The actual incidences of common complications in several series are given in Table 27–1. One would expect studies that span recent years to show a moderate reduction in incidence.

Since the physician cannot remain constantly at the bedside, other members of the care team must be actively involved in the recognition and management of complications. The hours a physician spends teaching his associates how to recognize early signs of complications—or better, how to prevent complications—pays off when an untoward event threatens.

ARE THERE PARTICULAR ANESTHETIC PROBLEMS IN HEAD AND NECK CANCER SURGERY?

Head and neck cancer surgery presents a special challenge to anesthesia skills. Long-acting anesthetics are required in high-risk older patients. Airway access may be difficult to establish and maintain. Blood loss can be rapid. Air can enter the venous system. The surgeon's position in the operative field puts anesthesia at an uncomfortable distance.

Monitoring should be carried out on the basis of complicating disease, and in the anticipation of the worst possible complications. Monitoring can be done by means of an arterial pressure line, a central venous pressure (CVP) catheter, or a Swan-Ganz catheter. The patient should be adequately hydrated. A common error is to attempt a procedure on a poorly nourished, poorly hydrated patient. Hypotension from loss of vasomotor tone occurs on induction of anesthesia. Anoxia and low flow in a diseased vascular tree exacts a toll in myocardial infarction and stroke. It is always difficult to distinguish a simple hypotensive event from an anesthetic- or operation-related myocardial infarct in an elderly population. If severe hypotension does occur, cardiodepressant anesthetic agents are discontinued. If the CVP or left atrial wedge pressure (LAWP) is low, rapid fluid repletion is started. If the hypotension persists more than 10–15 minutes or if cardiac output responds sluggishly to resuscitative efforts, surgery is cancelled. The patient is continuously monitored and returned to an intensive or critical care unit until serial electrocardiograms on 3 successive days and enzyme levels (CPK-MB) confirm or refute a myocardial infarct. Our experience suggests that 25%–30% of such hypotensive episodes in older patients (> 60–65 years) represent unsuspected heart disease or a myocardial infarction.

Manipulation of the oropharynx and upper airway during endoscopy or the induction of anesthesia is fraught with peril in the head and neck cancer patient. Tumor and irradiation stiffen the tissues. Tumor bulk obstructs the airway. Trismus precludes an adequate laryngoscopic view. The difficulty in establishing a safe,

TABLE 27–1.—FREQUENCY (%) OF COMPLICATIONS OF HEAD AND NECK CANCER SURGERY*

COMPLICATION	McGuirt et al.[2] Univ. of Iowa 1979 (1964–1975)	Robbins et al.[3] Vancouver Gen. 1975 (20 yr)	Joyce and McQuarrie[4] Minnesota 1976 (1964–1975)	Gall et al.[5] Washington U., St. Louis 1977 (1955–1972)			
	Tumor All Sites	Oral Tumors (All Irradiated)	Oral Tumors (<25% Irradiated)	Total Laryngectomy Without Irrad.	Total Laryngectomy With Irrad.	Subtotal Supraglottic, Without Irrad.	Subtotal Supraglottic, With Irrad.
% of patients without complications	50	N.A.	82	65	71	77	66
Fistula	13.5	6	3	6	2	2	6
Carotid exposure or rupture	1.3	1	0	3	3	4	2
Wound infection	22		4	1.5	3	0.3	.5
Wound necrosis	17	28	2	3	4	2	7
Chylous fistula	2	3	0				
Hematoma or flap elevation	6	13	1.7	0.5	2	1	1.5
Pulmonary	11	21	7				
Cardiovascular	4.3	4	3	16.5	12	12	17
Misc.: Nerve injury delirium tremens, unspec.	18	12	8				
Deaths	3	7	2	3.5	4	2	3.5
No. of pts. reported	788	100	178	198	106	315	195

*In some series more than one complication per patient is reported.

controlled airway usually requires more than usual manipulation of the oropharynx, larynx, and cervical structures. This stimulation occasionally provokes profound neurovagal reflexes, with bradycardia and hypotension.[6] The afferent fibers are in the superior laryngeal nerve and the carotid sinus nerve. The effector limb is in the cardioinhibitory portions of the vagus.[7] The resulting bradycardia and hypotension are functionally the same as other vagally mediated cardiac effects, such as the Bezold-Jarisch reflex[8] and the Aschner phenomenon (marked slowing of the pulse following pressure on the eyeball). The pharyngeal reflex effect was described first by François Granck in 1876 and confirmed by Brodie and Russel in 1900.[9] The bradycardia and hypotension are potentiated by continued surgical manipulation, hypoxia, and hypercarbia.[6] In a series of 540 patients undergoing laryngeal microsurgery, Strong et al. found reflex-induced cardiac problems in 7 (1%) and some acute cardiac complications in 19 (3.5%). In our experience, two such episodes of unremitting hypotension and bradycardia have required external cardiac massage to maintain perfusion. Higher doses of preoperative atropine tend to block the effect, but topical anesthetics applied to the laryngopharynx do not inhibit the afferent stimulus arc. Beta-adrenergic stimulating agents are minimally effective or not effective.

Prevention is the key to avoiding reflex cardiovascular events. Give adequate doses of preanesthetic atropine. Use minimal stimulation during intubation. Use a fiberoptic intubation technique if necessary. Maintain good respiratory exchange. A pulse of less than 40 beats per minute and a systolic pressure of less than 60–80 mm Hg require immediate correction or external cardiac massage.

WHAT PROBLEMS ARISE IN MAINTAINING RESPIRATORY EXCHANGE DURING HEAD AND NECK CANCER PROCEDURES?

Endotracheal anesthesia was a major advance in head and neck cancer treatment. Securing and maintaining a controlled, protected airway avoids most of the complications of inadequate exchange or aspiration of blood, saliva, and gastric contents. It bears repeating that placement of the endotracheal tube is made difficult by trismus, nasal deformity, or massive tumor. Some tumors may swell acutely during intubation attempts. Both the surgeon and anesthesiologist should anticipate the problems and work in concert. The surgeon should be in the room during induction of anesthesia. A sterile but unopened tracheostomy set should be available in the room, not in some central supply department in the bowels of the hospital. The installation of a nasotracheal tube over a fiberoptic scope has eliminated a number of tense scenes. In selected circumstances a planned tracheotomy must be done first. A routine preliminary tracheostomy may not be required or wise. Baluyot and Shumrick suggest that a preliminary tracheostomy in laryngeal cancer is associated with an increased incidence of stomal recurrences.[10] They do not hesitate to recommend prompt laryngectomy should it be needed.

After the endoctracheal tube or tracheostomy tube is installed, the surgeon must assist in securing an uncompromised airway since the head may have to be repositioned many times. Whenever the surgeon or anesthesiologist questions good airway function, the procedure is halted until the problem, usually a leaky coupling, is resolved. Some causes of inadequate ventilatory exchange during and after surgery arc listed in Table 27–2. Rapid correction of inadequate ventilation is required. Check all connectors. Observe the movement of both hemithoraces. Disconnect the airway from the respirator and manually ventilate the patient with 100% oxygen. Pass a long suction catheter down and well through the airway tube to check for resistance. Listen to both sides of the chest over each major lobe for breath sounds, looking for pneumothorax, atelectasis, wheezing, obstructed bronchus. Deflate and reinflate the cuff. Listen for heart sounds—the gallop of heart failure, the "heart-beat-in-Rice-Krispies" sound of air embolism. If air embolism is highly suspected, immediately turn the patient right side up and aspirate the right atrium through a sterile transvenous catheter. Percuss the abdomen and chest to detect an air-filled stomach or pneumothorax. Check blood gases for an adequately elevated Pa_{O_2} (> 300 mm Hg) on an FI_{O_2} of 100%. If no cause of the poor ventilatory exchange is immediately evident, obtain a chest x-ray film to look for pneumothorax, pulmonary edema, poor tube position, atelectasis, large gastric bubble, etc. If postoperative respirations are poor, exchange volume should be measured by flow spirometry. Excessive relaxants can be reversed by edrophonium. Excessive narcotics can be reversed by antagonists (nalorphine) or respiratory support. The surgeon must be assured of adequate exchange volumes and confirm his impressions with blood gas dcterminations. A central arterial line makes arterial sampling easy and safe.[11] On more than 40% FI_{O_2} in a closed circuit, the PA_{O_2} should be above 200 mm Hg. If any question remains, change the tube.

TABLE 27–2.—COMMON CAUSES OF INADEQUATE VENTILATORY EXCHANGE DURING AND AFTER SURGERY FOR HEAD AND NECK CANCER

1. Mechanical problems, loose coupling, leaking cuff on tube.
2. Tube not in trachea.
3. Tube kinked.
4. Balloon cuff overexpanded or displaced over tip of tube.
5. Inspissated secretions plugging tube.
6. Endotracheal tube too far down bronchus, usually down right bronchus and obstructing left main-stem bronchus.
7. Atelectasis, usually due to bronchial obstruction with secretions, blood, etc.
8. Aspirated foreign body, teeth, tumor, small piece of anesthesia apparatus.
9. Pneumothorax from ruptured bleb, overinflation, dissection at root of neck.
10. Bronchospasm due to irritation, sensitivity, or adrenergic blockers.
11. Air embolism: bronchospasm is an early symptom.
12. Pulmonary edema due to:
    - Excessive fluid loading.
    - Acute myocardial infarct.
    - Chronic heart failure, cardiomyopathy.
13. Pulmonary embolism.
14. Severe chronic obstructive pulmonary disease plus any minimal complication.
15. Respirator failure or malfunction.
16. Acute gastric dilation that compromises respiration and produces reflex "shock-like" hypotension.
17. Excessive or persisting muscle relaxants.
18. Excessive sedation or narcotics.

If a patient is not anesthetized, mental confusion with combative anxious behavior is the first symptom of anoxia. Until the surgeon can prove that such a patient is well oxygenated, it is a grevious error to give sedatives or narcotics, which may impair oxygenation further. In a hard-drinking population, one must rely on blood gas values to make an early distinction between delirium tremens (high respiratory volume, good Pa_{O_2}) or anoxia (decreased Pa_{O_2}). Obstruction of a tube or bronchus is common. Atelectasis produces a decrease in Pa_{O_2} because of pulmonary venous admixture. This prevents elevation of the aterial oxygen pressure on increased FI_{O_2}. If atelectasis does not respond to simple suctioning, one should be ready and able to bronchoscope the patient. A tracheostomy makes bronchoscopy simple.

WHICH PATIENTS REQUIRE A TRACHEOSTOMY TO HELP PREVENT AIRWAY COMPLICATIONS?

Tracheostomy is done to ensure an unquestionably patent upper airway. It avoids upper airway obstruction from tissue edema and helps prevent aspiration. Suction can be easily used to remove lower airway secretions. A cuffed tube allows ventilator support. A tracheostomy reduces airway dead space, which may benefit patients with limited pulmonary reserve.

Most commonly, tracheostomy is performed in a controlled elective manner over a previously placed endotracheal tube. This is the safest method of tracheostomy. Why not do a preliminary tracheostomy on everyone? An operation may not proceed because of anesthetic complications, early discovery of signs of unresectability, or change to a lesser procedure. More than 90% of the tracheostomies we perform are done at the conclusion of the operation (or in the course of a laryngectomy). In an occasional patient, tracheostomy is done electively and preoperatively when tumor bulk or upper airway problems suggest that attempts at intubation during the procedure will pose a critical hazard. The desperate "crash" tracheostomy on the ward under poor conditions probably represents an acute accident or decision error. In head and neck cancer patients, tracheostomy has a low morbidity and minimum (< 1%) mortality (none of 264 consecutive patients in our experience). Tracheostomy's bad reputation arose in cardiovascular and plmonary surgery patients in whom it was done for various forms of pulmonary insufficiency or adult respiratory distress syndrome requiring positive pressure respiratory support.[12, 13] When we assume thoracic surgery responsibilities, we use endotracheal intubation for several days in preference to tracheostomy. The bacterial pneumonia superinfection rate is lowered if tracheostomy can be avoided in the setting of respiratory insufficiency.

For head and neck cancer patients, the need for tracheostomy can be assigned to one of three levels of priority.

First: Some patients unquestionably need a tracheostomy. Total laryngectomy is obvious (end-on stoma). Other indications include simultaneous bilateral neck dissection; any large resection of the mandibular arch that impairs functional support of the tongue, allowing the tongue to fall backward; large glossectomies that preclude effective handling of oral secretions; pharyngeal resection; any patient in whom the laryngeal protective reflexes are impaired; patients with a poor cough (i.e., $FEV_1 < 1.4$ L); patients undergoing bulky intraoral or pharyngeal flap reconstructions.

Second: Some patients may be strongly considered for tracheostomy, depending on clinical circumstances. Patients with smaller resections may be managed by endotracheal protection for 24 hours and the need for tracheostomy reevaluated on the basis of the amount of pharyngeal edema and oral function. Such a patient must be cared for in an intensive care unit where a surgeon or anesthesiologist is immediately available on 24-hour call. If at the end of 24 hours of endotracheal protection there is no obstructive oropharyngeal edema, the patient can be extubated and monitored another 24 hours, with blood gas confirmation of adequate oxygenation. The physician and intensive care unit staff should be able to reintubate the patient and/or perform a tracheostomy swiftly and safely. When this level of support is not available, a tracheostomy is advisable for patients who are to undergo major resctions, a hemiglossectomy, or a larger floor of the mouth resection, and for patients who have received therapeutic doses of irradiation before oropharyngeal resection.

Third: Some patients rarely need a tracheostomy. Included in this group are patients undergoing parotidectomy and submaxillary gland removal, with or without neck dissection; unilateral simple neck dissection (first side); superficial limited oral resection; and so forth. A rare episode of acute orofacial edema or hematoma may occur with minimal manipulation in this group of patients. Vigilance is required. In general, if there is any doubt, it is safer to err on the side of performing a tracheostomy under controlled conditions.

WHAT ARE THE COMPLICATIONS OF TRACHEOSTOMY?

The great bugaboo of tracheostomy is tracheal ulceration with consequent erosion into esophagus or a major vessel. Most commonly this is traced to poor tracheostomy placement (too low), poor tube fit, an overinflated high-pressure balloon cuff, or an improperly shaped "standard" tube. At the time of tracheostomy the lower edge of the wound is felt for a high-lying innominate artery. In stocky patients, it may arch quite high. The position of the tracheal opening and the curvature of the tube should avoid any pressure on the major vessels. If the tracheostomy tube transmits a prominent pulse heave with every heartbeat, the implication of potential erosion is obvious. Another tube position, tube configuration, or wire-reinforced soft tube must be used. The correct tube position is checked with x-ray studies. If it is not corrected beyond doubt, a wire-wound endotracheal tube must be substituted. Conversion to cricothyroidotomy has been used by some as a less desirable alternative.

If vascular erosion by a tube does occur, there may be a small sentinel bleed before a severe exsanguinating and asphyxiating hemorrhage occurs. Survival is rare if torrential bleeding occurs. The tracheostomy tube is left in place to protect the airway. The skin incision is enlarged as necessary, and one or two fingers are inserted anterior to the trachea to compress the innominate artery against the anterior chest wall. In the operating room a midline sternotomy is made with or without a fourth interspace extension to gain additional exposure. Vascular clamps are used for control. The artery must be ligated and oversewn in good tissue. A viable muscular flap must be interposed between the vessel and the tracheal erosion. An extrathoracic subclavian-subclavian shunt can be constructed to restore flow.

Simple tracheal erosion is usually due to cuff configuration and pressure on the tracheal wall, aggravated by the abrasive force of a positive-pressure respirator.[13] Fortunately, the need for respiratory support is short in most head and neck cancer patients. The cuff is used to minimize aspiration. Cuff pressures of 10–20 mm Hg are usually satisfactory with the newer low-pressure cuffs. The cuff should be deflated every 2 hours or so.

A simple ward-care oversight frequently negates the protective effect of a cuffed tube. One must avoid aspiration of the "goober bomb." When the cuff is inflated, blood and secretions accumulate above the cuff. When the cuff is deflated, this bacteria-laden "bomb" falls and may be aspirated. For prevention, one should aspirate at the tip of the tracheostomy tube during deflation to catch the pooled secretions.

Bleeding may force early tracheostomy tube replacement. Bleeding around the stoma should be controlled in the operating room with a good light, a tracheostomy set, suture, ligature, and electrocautery.

Some difficulties attend the elective change of a tracheostomy tube or the replacement of a dislodged tube. Most of the problems occur in replacing tracheostomy tubes in the obese patient and in the patient with a recent tracheostomy. Disaster comes in several ways. The airway is essential. If the tube is dislodged, the soft tissue surrounding the tracheostomy wound obstructs the air flow. If the tube is erroneously placed in the pretracheal space, an inflated cuff blocks the airway. The mediastinum can be insufflated with air from a respirator. Such errors compromise venous return while failing to maintain adequate oxygen exchange. Continuing, forceful attempts to replace the tube will compress the trachea and block any air exchange. In obese patients, an erroneously selected short tracheostomy tube may be placed into the trachea. Subsequently the short tube dislodges into the pretracheal space when the patient's head is repositioned.

If difficulty is encountered in replacing or changing a tube, several simple means can be used without the delay required to locate lights or instrument set. There are three methods that have proved useful in the safe routine management of tracheostomies.[14] These methods are illustrated in descending order in Figure 27–1.

The blade of a standard anesthesia infant laryngoscope is used as a lighted retractor to explore a new tracheostomy, as shown in diagram *1a*. The tracheostomy site can be easily located even in a fat neck. The blade of the infant laryngoscope is small enough to be

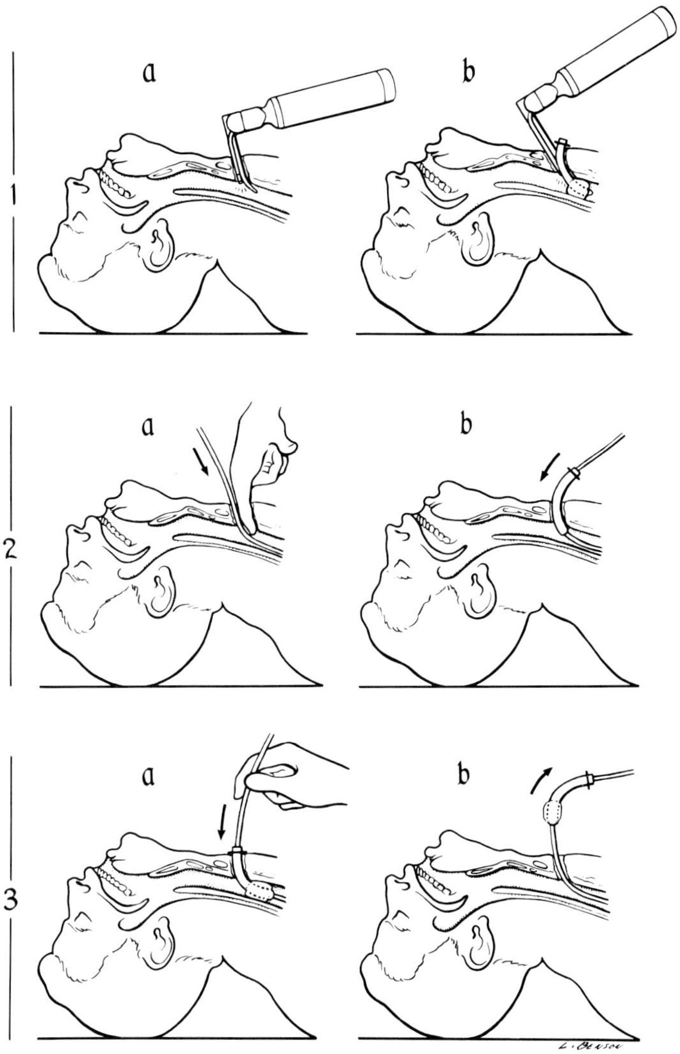

Fig 27–1.—1a, an infant laryngoscope makes an excellent lighted tool to explore a recent tracheostomy site in order to rapidly identify the tracheostoma and establish effective exchange. **1b,** with the blade used as a guide, a new tube is inserted under direct vision. **Diagram 2a,** a palpating finger guides the catheter into a recently made tracheostoma. **2b,** a tube is guided into the orifice over the suction catheter. **Diagrams 3a** and **b,** a catheter is used as a guide to remove and reinsert a tracheostomy tube. (From McQuarrie.[14] Reproduced by permission of *Surgery, Gynecology, & Obstetrics.*)

placed into the tracheostomy. The lower part of the trachea is lifted upward. If the patient is breathing spontaneously, this maneuver allows adequate air exchange. It is then relatively simple to insert the tracheostomy tube into the trachea under direct vision, using the open side of the laryngoscope as a smooth guide (diagram *1b*).

In the absence of a laryngoscope, digital exploration of the tracheostomy wound will allow palpation of the tracheostoma (diagram *2a*). A suction catheter can be guided by finger palpation into the trachea. A tracheostomy tube can then be slid over the catheter and inserted into the trachea, as shown in diagram *2b*.

When the tube in a new tracheostomy is changed, a suction catheter can be inserted through the tube to be removed (diagram *3a*). The tube is then removed over the catheter, leaving a good length of the catheter in the trachea. The new tracheostomy tube may then be slid into proper position over the catheter (diagram *3b*).

In all of these maneuvers, it is helpful to have the neck of the patient slightly hyperextended so that the tracheal orifice returns to the same position relative to the overlying soft tissue as when the tracheostomy was performed. After the tracheostomy tube is placed, it is essential to demonstrate that a suction catheter will enter the trachea easily and without resistance.

Of the techniques described, use of the infant laryngoscope blade is most reliable. The light at the tip of the blade is of major advantage. The smaller 2-inch blade has been used as an excellent retractor for performing an emergency tracheostomy if lighting on the unit is poor.

Personnel managing the patient must realize that simply holding back the soft tissue from the tracheostoma with a hemostat will allow some air exchange. Persistent use of brute force and awkwardness will compromise any residual airway.

Tracheostomy may contribute to complications with postoperative deglutition. The inflated balloon compresses the esophageal lumen through the compliant posterior wall of the trachea. Inexperienced staff will try to get the patient to swallow with a tracheotomy cuff tube snuggly inflated. A second problem occurs when the tracheostomy has diverted the air flow and the patient is unable to speak. On inspection the vocal cords are seen to rest in partial abduction and are poorly responsive to local sensory stimuli. The patient tends to aspirate easily until the vocal cords have had several days of "workout" to establish rapid response and firm closure. Finally, the tracheostomy and the inserted tube may keep the hyolaryngeal structures from elevating on swallowing. This makes swallowing more difficult and aspiration more likely. It is usually best to have the patient delay swallowing food until edema has subsided, a smaller metal (bypass) tracheostomy tube has been substituted for the cuffed tube, and the patient has been talking for several days.

HOW DO YOU CONTROL UNANTICIPATED INTRAOPERATIVE AND POSTOPERATIVE BLEEDING?

Most head and neck cancer surgery is conducted through a panorama of critical vascular scenery. As Professor Harold Hill said in "The Music Man," "you gotta know the territory." Utilization of common vascular surgical skills prevents most problems. One should be familiar with vascular instruments, their use, and the dissection repair and anastomosis of large and small vessels.

Preventive Technical Advice

The periadventitial level is the safest dissection plane for the carotid, jugular, and other large vessels. The vascular surgery admonition is to get in the periadventitial plane and stay in it, then you always have the vessels and branches in sight. Do not force a clamp blindly behind larger vessels. They may have a branch coming off posteriorly. Thin-walled veins tend to fold over the tip of a clamp. Moderate force is all that is needed to tear a gaping hold. Veins are most often torn or entered in the lower neck near the thin-walled valves, at the middle thyroid vein, in the parapharyngeal plexus near the hypoglossal nerve, and on the very thin upper internal jugular.

A standard hemostatic clamp will slide off the end of a big divided thin-walled vein very easily. Large vessels are best ligated in continuity. All bigger vessels must have an additional suture ligature placed. If not suture ligated, one pleat in a puckered ligated vein may slide through the ligature, more vein wall slips loose, and minimal pressure forces the tie loose. A second distal suture ligature will transfix the vein and prevent tissue sliding under the first tie.

Prevention of Air Embolism and Venous Injury

A hole in the veins of the lower neck poses more danger from aspiration and air embolism than from bleeding. Mild pressure or compression will temporarily control bleeding. If the head is elevated, it must be immediately lowered so the venous system is under continuous pressure. A Debakey vascular needle grasping forceps can be used to compress the defect while it is exposed, cleaned, and sutured with a running whip stitch of 5-0 or 6-0 vascular suture. Veins are a low-pressure system and minimal compression will staunch the flow. Grabbing with a standard hemostat will tear the veins. Use instruments with noncrushing serrated teeth designed to handle blood vessels.

High at the base of the skull, the internal jugular vein may be damaged getting around high-lying nodes or tumor. Circumdissection and closure are inhibited by the mastoid and surrounding tissues. If inadequate vein wall remains for suture closure after the specimen has been removed, a roll of levator scapulae muscle can be packed into the defect between deeply placed mattress sutures. If an intracranial sinus is entered in a craniofacial resection, a piece of muscle is used to obturate the defect since there is no elasticity in the walls. Cardiovascular sutures with small Ivalon felt pledgets also hold well.

Control of Arterial Injuries

Major arterial lacerations should be controlled with a vascular clamp. A Derra clamp or vascular bulldog clamp can be applied to allow one to inspect the defect and make a decision on ligation or repair. Unintentional injury to the carotid system should be rare. The problem areas are transsinus injury or vessel laceration near the base of the skull. Sobel et al. review the management and results of such injuries.[15]

Postoperative Hematoma

If bleeding collects under the closure in the postoperative period, it is futile to try to aspirate the clotted accumulation by using needles or catheters. Leaving potentially contaminated clot in a combined orocervical resection almost guarantees either infection or wound complications. Return the patient to the operating room. Open the flaps under sterile conditions. Clean out all clot. Locate, ligate, and control all bleeding points. A particular search should be made for intermittent venous bleeding by lowering the patient's head and raising the intrathoracic pressure. Many times a specific bleeding point will not be found. Irrigate the wound until it is clean. Replace the suction drainage catheters and close the wound carefully.

Coagulopathy

Diffuse intravascular coagulopathy is a consequence of severe anoxic episodes, transfusion reaction, sepsis, and acidosis. Thrombolysis is rare in head and neck surgery patients. Surgeons who encounter many "bleeding disorders" are usually short of ligatures, hemostasis, and patience. Some cirrhotics may have reduced but adequate vitamin K–dependent clotting factors to yield normal preoperative prothrombin time and partial thromboplastin time values at the beginning of a procedure. Subsequent transfusion with large amounts of banked blood can dilute vitamin K–dependent factors the point that clotting is prolonged. Fresh frozen plasma should be reserved for these patients and for patients with identifiable factor deficiency.

Late Postoperative Hemorrhage

Late bleeding is associated with deep wound infection or an oropharyngeal-cutaneous fistula. Vulnerable vessels and previous sites of ligature lie in an infected area. Some events that appear to be carotid blowouts originate in the ligated facial artery or a ligated external carotid artery. In these events, emergency control is achieved by applying direct pressure or a vascular clamp until light, suction, good venous lines, tools, blood for transfusion, monitoring devices, and assistance are available, preferably in the operating room. One maneuver is to place a larger vascular Fogarty balloon embolectomy catheter into the the lumen and inflate it. Upstream and downstream catheters may be needed. One can then restore blood pressure and assess the defect. In the setting of infection or previous irradiation, the vessel cannot be safely repaired in the local area. The vessel must be ligated and oversewn in a clean area with good arterial wall. A simple suture ligature placed through infected or irradiated tissue is doomed to failure in most instances. If the internal carotid artery is ligated and oversewn, the risks of stroke and cerebral defect are parallel to the risks on primary ligation (see Chap. 9). If stump pressure is low, there are isolated instances of success with a sweeping saphenous vein bypass outside the infected area, from good proximal artery to a good area on the internal carotid.

Massive carotid blowout is associated with tissue loss and wound problems following irradiation in over 80% of instances.[2] In McGuirt's series, three of ten patients in whom the internal carotid was ligated at the time of rupture ultimately survived.[2] Four of four additional patients underwent ligation at the first "warning bleed" and survived. Three of 16 patients treated by Ketcham and Haye died.[16] Those that survived returned to preligation status except for five with Horner's syndrome. The authors emphasized the need to heed a small sentinal bleed. Moore et al. reported 44 strokes (50%) and 33 deaths (38%) in 87 patients with nonelective ligation, in contrast to 15 strokes (23%) and 11 deaths (17%) in 64 patients with elective ligation.[17] The implication is that the hypotension that occurs with a massive blowout makes a major contribution to the morbidity and mortality. Fortunately, newer surgical techniques and a reduction in the number of patients operated on late after irradiation have reduced the frequency of late carotid artery blowout.

WHAT DO YOU DO FOR A CHYLOUS FISTULA?

If a lymphadenectomy is done, lymphatic channels are cut. Some lymph will enter every lymphadenectomy field. In the left side of the neck, the lower nodes and channels are contiguous with those around the thoracic duct. The thoracic duct usually enters the posterior lateral wall at the junction of the internal jugular and subclavian veins. A large valve of the internal jugular is situated just above this point. The thoracic duct may loop upward for a variable distance into the lower neck. It can usually be clearly identified. It does not tolerate much dissection without tearing. If the thoracic duct is identifiably injured in the dissection, it can be carefully oversewn with running 6-0 cardiovascular suture. Care is taken to avoid incorporating the phrenic nerve or the sympathetic chain in the multiple fine sutures. There is a smaller, more variable duct on the right. It may require the same management. About 15%–20% of late chyle collections are on the right. If excessive lymph accumulates in the lower neck during the operation, the surgeon must identify the point of leak and carefully oversew it.

It is difficult to distinguish serous and chylous drainage in the immediate postoperative period. If identifiable excessive lymph loss (> 200–300 cc/day) occurs immediately postoperatively, re-exploration of the lower neck under sterile conditions could be considered. Usually lymph is not distinguished from serous drainage until feeding is started. If there is doubt as to the nature of the drainage, the lymph triglyceride level is determined. Values above 110 mg/dl are diagnostic of lymph while values below 50 mg/dl are usually indicative of transudate fluid.[18] Intermediate values are indeterminate.

A late lymphatic accumulation under the flaps after removal of suction drainage catheters is managed by inserting a short length of a small Hemovac catheter into the collection and placing it on constant suction for 3–4 days until the fluid loss is less than 25 cc/day. The objective is to keep the flaps closely opposed. If lymph loss exceeds 500 cc/day after 5–10 days, exploration and suture closure are necessary. Most fistulas close with continuous suction drainage.

HOW DO YOU PREVENT OR MANAGE OROCUTANEOUS FISTULAS OR PHARYNGOCUTANEOUS FISTULAS?

Orocutaneous or pharyngocutaneous fistulas are common complications after extended composite surgical resections. Table 27–3 augments the data of Table 27–1 and shows the incidence in irradiated and unirradiated patients in several series. The frequency increases in parallel with four variables: increasing dose of irradiation, more elapsed time since irradiation, increasing size of the resection, and increasingly dependent and deep location of the cancer within the oropharynx. Large oropharyngeal and laryngeal cancers have a higher frequency of fistula.[21]

The oropharyngeal cutaneous fistula is a good example of the need to prevent complications in the preoperative planning and in the operative phase of care. Early recognition of potential complications and prompt management prevent some of the multiple catastrophes of a delayed salvage effort. Figure 27–2 is a composite plot of the presumed etiologic factors and the consequent complicating problems. Pedestrian preoperative and intraoperative preventive steps have a much greater payoff than brilliantly executed salvage efforts (see Chaps. 5 and 11).

Avoidance of complications starts by reducing the oral bacterial flora through good dental care and hygiene (see Chaps. 5 and 11). A combined orocervical operation is, at best, grossly contaminated. Dental plaque is virtually solid live and nonviable bacteria. The live bacteria counts in dental plaque reach 10^{10}/gm of mixed aerobic and anaerobic organisms. Bacterial counts of saliva are only slightly diluted, containing 10^7 to 10^8 bacteria per milliliter.[24, 25] The perioperative steps discussed in chapter 11 regarding preoperative antibiotics and nutrition are important.

When there are infectious complications, it is fortunate that *Bacteroides fragilis* is not a normal cohabitant of the upper airway.[25] As discussed in chapter 11, preoperative and intraoperative antibiotics have a proved clear benefit in several well-conducted trials.[26] Agents of choice should achieve prolonged high tissue levels.[24] The subject has been reviewed by Herzon. He emphasized the common contamination of *Staphylococcus aureus*, which is seeded from the skin.[27] Prophylactic preoperative, intraoperative, and postoperative antibiotics are essential, but their administration must be coupled with every effort to reduce the bacterial count in the operative field. Careful handling of tissues and prevention of wound drying will avoid unnecessary cell injury. Hemostasis should be impeccable. Finally, the wound is copiously irrigated with a cephalosporin solution before closure to try to reduce bacteria counts to below 10^4/ml. Diabetic patients present the double problem of small-vessel disease in flaps and increased susceptibility to infection.

If the resection is sizable and safe primary closure is nearly impossible, a controlled planned pharyngostoma is more desirable and effective than allowing a massive necrotizing infection to become established. As early as 1890, Butlin advocated a controlled fistula after orocervical resection.[28] Planned controlled fistulas are more common with extended pharyngeal resections (see Chap. 16).

If primary closure is accomplished, it is important that airtight closure be maintained by subflap suction until all parts of the closure are adherent. Leaks from the oral closure, around the tracheostomy site, or at the corners of the external tissue closure will prevent tight tissue-tissue apposition. The nonadherent areas will be seeded by bacteria and become infected. All noncontinent areas of the closure must be promptly repaired or corrected.

Figure 27–2 shows an "early action phase." Operating room time spent controlling bleeding is a good investment. The data from our institution show that iron-containing hemoglobin is a powerful inducement to

TABLE 27–3.—OROPHARYNGOCUTANEOUS FISTULAS

STUDY, YEAR	SITE/TREATMENT	NO. OF PTS.	% IRRADIATED > 3,000 RAD	% WITH FISTULAS	% OF FISTULAS REQUIRING CLOSURE
Joyce and McQuarrie,[4] 1976	Oral	178	11	3	50
Ching et al.,[13] 1974	Oral	100	100	6	NA
Daly and Strong,[19] 1974	Larynx/No prior treatment	465	NA	6	24
	Larynx/Prior treatment	57	NA	16	
Harwick[20] 1975	Pyriform sinus/Primary closure	43	NA	42	NA
	Pyriform sinus/Pharyngostomy	45	NA	Planned secondary closure	
Marchetta et al.,[21] 1967	Mixed sites/irradiated	83	100	16	NA
	Mixed sites/Unirradiated	81	0	2	NA
Schechter,[22] 1983	Mixed sites/Reconstructive flaps	100	100	7	
Dedo et al.,[23] 1975	Jaw and neck:	120	30	10	40
	Partial laryngopharyngectomy	72		17	71*
	Subtotal supraglottic laryngectomy	60		8	40
	Total laryngectomy	117		9	89*
	Total laryngectomy with reconstruction	7		100% planned	NA

*Some patients never had fistula closed.
NA, data not available.

bacterial growth.[29] If flaps are not viable because of irradiation or other conditions, fallback procedures for full-thickness coverage must be used for tension-free closure. Chapter 6 illustrates a few of the many options. If honest *pessimistic* evaluation says a flap has failed, the patient is returned promptly to the operating room and a second-choice procedure is used to provide the coverage. If all else fails, some full-thickness coverage of the carotid artery is achieved by viable flap or muscle.

Even when best efforts have been made, an occasional patient may enter the "obligatory action" phase (see Fig 27–2). The early clues to infection, fistula, or tissue necrosis should be sought: (1) redness or cellulitis, (2) flap necrosis internally or externally, (3) high fever and leukocytosis with findings absent outside of the wound area, (4) a sudden increase in wound pain or edema that was not present in the immediate postoperative period, (5) saliva or a continuous air leak in a suction drain, and (6) a fetid smell to the breath, which is a product of anaerobic bacterial growth.[25] A small leak will allow contaminated saliva into a bacteriologically hospitable space. All previous dissection planes may be contaminated. Bacterial exotoxins facilitate access. Indeed, pathogenic staphylococci are characterized by their production of coagulase. *Borrelia vincentii* and *Fusobacterium necrophorus* are among the common oral organisms that produce a synergistic infection characterized by interstitial invasion and tissue necrosis. Other oropharyngeal organisms can create a florid necrotizing infection. The richness of oral bacterial varieties has been documented by Bartlett and Gorbach[25] and by Becker et al.[24] Almost all of the significant infections involve multiple organisms.

Mladick et al. discussed the management of the massively infected oropharyngeal fistula.[30] Effective management requires inspection of oral closure on suspicion of leak, debridement of any necrotic tissue, diversion of drainage to the outside (i.e., creating a pharyngostoma), and washing out and draining all blind pockets. In a late stage, the carotid area may be so grossly infected that direct coverage would fail. Frequent (hourly) changes of saline-soaked gauze sponges (some add antibiotics to the saline) along with removal of gross debris will clean the area in 2–3 days. Unirradiated tissues can then be skin grafted or covered by local tissue. If the tissues have been heavily irradiated (more than 6 months previously), tissue with a normal blood supply may have to be brought to the area. A myocutaneous flap is ideal. It is fixed to the underlying structures immediately adjacent to the exposed carotid after maximal cleansing. The flap must be arranged so that no saliva can dissect under it. Further apposition of the tissues is not sought. Mladick et al. discourage attempts at flap coverage,[30] but for heavily irradiated exposed carotid it may be effective. The only other course is elective ligation of the carotid system.

Bone exposure condemns the infected osseous components. Early debridement and resection of infected bone may let the soft tissues collapse slightly and hasten the cleaning and debridement phase.

When there is a pharyngocutaneous fistula with a small opening, a narrow linear tract, good surrounding flap adhesion, and no necrosis, some authors have used

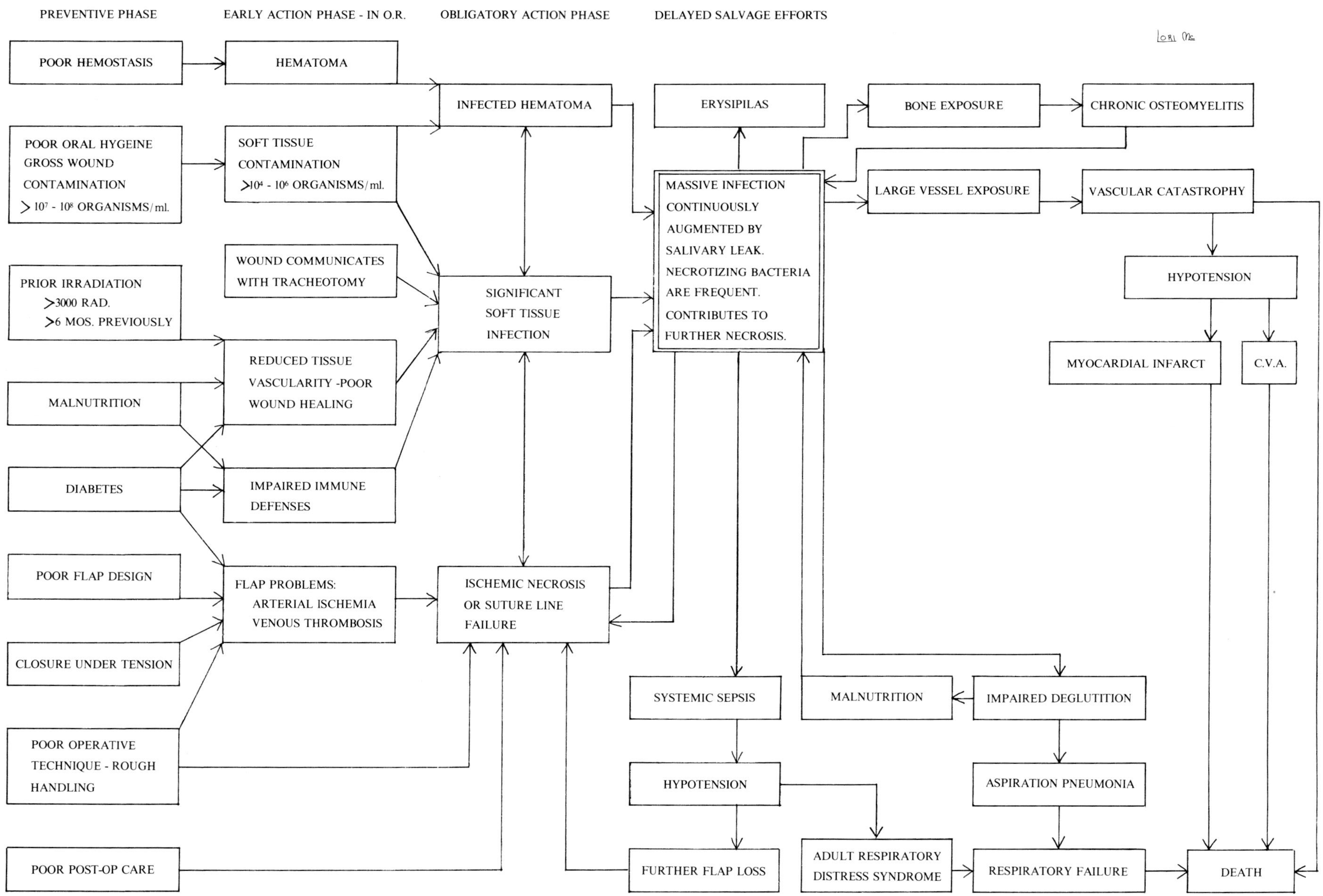

Fig 27–2.—Early recognition and prompt management of potential operative complications are the best way to prevent them. Problems that arise in the operating room and are not attended to may lead to catastrophe.

a through-and-through catheter drainage after opening the lowest area of the skin incision.[31] For fistulas after laryngectomy one group reported the use of a special flanged nasopharyngeal-esophageal tube to divert the saliva.[32] We have not found that these techniques give reliable control to the serious subflap infection.

When the fistula is clean and healing well, the physician must decide if it needs closure, and how closure is to be accomplished. If there were abundant internal and external tissues, small 1 to 2-cm defects will frequently close or may be easily closed with a local "turnover" flap, as illustrated by McGuirt et al.[2] Larger defects remaining after tissue necrosis will require bringing vascularized distant tissues to the area. If radiation injury is severe, the imported tissue must bring and maintain its own vascular supply (e.g., a myocutaneous flap). Occasionally two flaps are required, one for mucosal lining and one for external coverage.[33]

WHAT ARE THE COMMON COMPLICATIONS FOLLOWING THE USE OF GRAFTS AND FLAPS IN RECONSTRUCTION?

Each general category of reconstructive technique has unique pitfalls. Complications can be minimized by an awareness of potential problems and by taking necessary steps to prevent them.

Skin Grafts

The two most common causes of skin graft loss are subgraft hematoma and inadequate immobilization of the graft. For aesthetic reasons, sheet grafts are preferred for the head and neck area. Absolute hemostasis must be achieved in the recipient area prior to application of the unperforated skin graft. Any blood or serum collection beneath the graft will result in partial or total loss of the graft. If absolute hemostasis cannot be achieved at the time of the extirpative procedure, secondary split-thickness skin grafting 3–5 days later may be indicated.

Skin grafts in the head and neck area are best immobilized by a stent dressing. A layer of adaptic gauze is placed over the skin graft and saline-soaked absorbent cotton is then tied over the graft in a bulky fashion. When meticulously applied, a stent dressing can provide the absolute immobilization required for the graft.

Problems of skin graft healing may also be related to the thickness of the graft. A full-thickness skin graft does not reliably achieve vascularization of the graft, which may result in a partial or complete loss of the graft. Split-thickness skin grafts placed on the head and neck area are best taken at thicknesses of 12–15 thousandths of an inch. Thicker grafts may be poorly vascularized and have a tendency to develop irregular surface contours. Thinner grafts are difficult to handle and may heal in an irregular fashion. Very thin skin graft areas will tend to have islands of irregular hypertrophy over the 1-year healing period. Split-thickness skin graft infection is rare in the absence of hematoma formation or oral contamination.

Skin Flap

Skin flap complications can result from poor planning or operative and postoperative events.

PLANNING.—The vascular input to the base area of the flap is critically important for survival of a local rotation flap or a direct distant deltopectoral flap. Previous regional surgery or irradiation will alter the normal vascular anatomy of the base of the planned flap. If a skin flap design exceeds the normal base to length ratio guidelines for a particular area, preliminary delay of the flap should be considered. For example, the deltopectoral flap can be raised in a single stage to the lateral aspect of the shoulder (2.25:1 length to base ratio). If additional tissue is required from the posterior aspect of the shoulder or the proximal arm, this random portion of the flap should be outlined, raised, and replaced in the donor bed for 7–10 days prior to transfer of the flap.

Significant transposition of rotational advancement flaps will require some backcut, which will impinge on the base of the flap. The vascularized base must be wide enough *after* the required backcut.

OPERATIVE.—Compression of the flap tissue must be avoided in raising a full-thickness skin flap. The flap should be handled carefully with skin hooks. Holding the flap with the fingers places enough compression on the flap that echymotic injury may develop and cause occlusion of segments of the subdermal plexus and produce subsequent flap necrosis. In the early postoperative period capillary perfusion pressure may be half of normal (normal = 40 mmHg). One must be aware of the location of the axial vessels when elevating an axial-pattern flap. For example, in the deltopectoral flap the axial vessels lie just superficial to the fascia pectoralis. If the fascia pectoralis is raised with the flap, injury to the axial vessels will be avoided.

The flap must be set into a dry recipient area. A hematoma beneath the flap may produce direct pressure-related necrosis. Secondary compression from an inflammatory response to the sequestered blood will also be compressive. To avoid blood accumulation, a suction drain can be placed beneath the area of flap inset and removed at 24–48 hours. Care must be taken when a direct distant flap, such as the deltopectoral flap, is formed into a tube. Edema of the flap is inevitable in the first 12–24 hours following surgery. A flap that is sutured under moderate tension in the operating room may subsequently fail to survive due to edema and resulting vascular impairment in the first postoperative hours. The lower capillary perfusion pressure of a flap is easily exceeded. A hematoma within the tube will also create pressure that causes vascular impairment. We advise placement of a through-and-through Penrose drain in a tubed flap.

The perfusion of a skin flap can be assessed in the operating room by the use of intravenous fluorescein solution. Twenty minutes is allowed for vascular spasm to subside. Following this, a Woods light is used to examine the flap. Areas that do not fluoresce are inadequately perfused and will subsequently necrose. Nonfluorescing areas should be trimmed and the flap revised. Many pharmacologic techniques have been proposed to salvage a failing flap. There is no technique that is of proved benefit. Skin flaps fail primarily because of design and judgment errors. The problem must be solved by operative means.

POSTOPERATIVE.—The two principal concerns in the postoperative period are (1) prevention of a hypotensive episode that would stop adequate perfusion of the flap, and (2) avoidance of any pressure applied to the base of a flap. Constrictive dressings, straps, and ties are not permitted. Patient positioning can be of critical importance. A "fold crease" across a flap constricts subdermal blood flow.

Infection is uncommon unless there is oral contamination of the area. Infection of a flap will usually result in cellulitis, edema, and ultimately necrosis of an otherwise well-vascularized flap.

MYOCUTANEOUS FLAPS

PLANNING.—The principal blood supply of the musculocutaneous unit must remain intact. One must know when previous surgery or irradiation may have destroyed critical vessels. Under good circumstances, musculocutaneous flaps provide a reliable, well-vascularized skin-muscle unit. They are not the first choice for every purpose. Myocutaneous flaps are frequently bulky. In the obese patient the extreme bulk of the flap may make operation technically difficult or impossible.

OPERATIVE.—The skin island on a musculocutaneous flap is very loosely attached to the underlying muscle. Minimal manipulation during flap elevation can avulse the tenuous areolar vascular attachments. A skin island should be sutured to the underlying muscle fascia prior to elevation of the muscle unit (see illustrations in Chap. 14).

The vascular supply of the muscle must be carefully preserved during elevation. A precise knowledge of the anatomy of the vascular pedicle will prevent injury during flap elevation. When the flap is transferred, kinking of the vascular pedicle must be avoided. Intravenous fluorescein can be employed to assess the vascularity of the skin island. The test is unreliable for assessing muscle perfusion.

POSTOPERATIVE.—Compressive dressings are avoided. Careful patient positioning is critical to prevent pressure.

The vascularity of the musculocutaneous unit that makes it a reliable reconstructive flap also makes it more vulnerable to hematoma beneath the flap in the postoperative period. Tight closure of confined spaces should be avoided. We use soft Jackson-Pratt drains beneath such flaps for the first 24–48 hours. Without gross oral contamination, the well-vascularized musculocutaneous flap is subject to few infectious complications.

Microvascular Free Flap

Free flap transfers represent the most complex reconstructive procedure. The principal complication is loss of vascular perfusion of the flap.

PLANNING.—Certain free graft donor sites have reliable vascular pedicles. The latissimus dorsi and rectus muscles, the jejunum, and the omentum are examples of sites with dependable vascular anatomy. Previous regional surgery can eliminate these flaps as reconstructive options. For example, a prior mastectomy may have sacrificed a thorocodorsal vessel to the latissimus dorsi muscle, midline or paramedian abdominal incisions may have impaired the rectus muscle vascular supply, and intra-abdominal procedures may have divided the omentum or altered the bowel anatomy.

OPERATIVE.—Adequate donor and recipient vessels must be identified and prepared prior to transfer of the free flap. The recipient vessels must allow expeditious vascular anastomoses. The need for vein grafts must be anticipated and the veins harvested prior to division of the donor pedicle. Muscle flaps are extremely sensitive to warm ischemia, and any technical problem that adds as much as an hour to the flap transfer time may result in failure of the flap. Following revascularization, the reactive hyperemia of a muscle flap may lead to considerable surface bleeding. Hematoma beneath the flap is a real possibility in the first 24 hours and must be avoided. Use loose suturing of the flap and placement of appropriate drains.

POSTOPERATIVE.—Compression dressings must be avoided. The flap must be observed carefully for the first several days postoperatively. The flap may be lost due to venous congestion or arterial inflow failure.

Some vascular problems can be corrected if they are *immediately* recognized and the patient is returned with haste to the operating room for exploration and correction of the vascular pedicle problem. Temporizing delays almost always result in flap loss. Pharmacologic manipulation has not proved of benefit in the salvage of a failing flap.

If there is excellent vascularity, infectious complications are rare.

WHAT NERVES CAN BE DAMAGED DURING HEAD AND NECK CANCER SURGERY?

Any nerve in or around an operative field can be damaged. Many times the nerve is deliberately taken in the course of an effective cancer resection. When the nerve passes through the planned block of resected tissue, it should not be dissected free of immediately adjacent cancer. Table 27–4 lists the nerves, the operations in which they might be resected or damaged, the functional loss, and some comments on management. In many instances, the nerve is resected with the end organ, i.e., the lingual branch of nerve V and the hypoglossal nerve (XII) with a large hemiglossectomy. Nerve grafting has had equivocal success with nerves VII, XI, and XII. The best results are with nerve VII. If a critical repairable nerve is sectioned, immediate repair or grafting is best. Late repair lowers the success rate.

Nerve injury can occur in many ways. Direct surgical cutting is the most obvious. When nerve section is not planned, the injury is due to failure to know normal or abnormal anatomy. Fibrosis and scar around a nerve may obscure tissue planes and impede dissection. In-

TABLE 27–4.—NERVES THAT MAY BE SACRIFICED OR INJURED IN SURGICAL TREATMENT OF HEAD AND NECK CANCER

NERVE	OPERATION	FUNCTIONAL LOSS	TREATMENT, REHABILITATION, MANAGEMENT
Olfactory (I)*	Nasal sinuses	Anosmia if removed bilaterally	None
Optic (II)*	Orbital exenteration (about 30–40% of nasal cancers)	Loss of vision Usually unilateral cosmetic loss	Deformity can be partially corrected with ocular prosthetics
Oculomotor (III)* Trochlear (IV)* Abducens (VI)*	Orbital exenteration, removes muscles and distal nerve; sinusectomy	Abnormal eye movements	None in cancer patients
Trigeminal (V)*	Almost any oropharyngeal or cephalic resection removes branches; submandibular gland, lingual, mandibular operations	Muscles of mastication and facial sensation Usually unilateral loss of taste to anterior 2/3 of tongue	None
Facial (VII)*	Parotidectomy; resective procedures in area of mastoid, upper jugular, temporal bone	Paralysis of muscles of facial expression; unable to close eye	Can be partially restored by free autogenous graft, crossover graft from hypoglossal nerve, muscle transplantation; tarsorrhaphy is used to protect cornea
Acoustic (XIII)*	Temporal bone operations	Hearing and balance	Compensation and adjustment of vestibular functions in 4–6 weeks
Glossopharyngeal (IX)	Radical operations in tonsil, palate, pharynx, and posterior tongue.	Temporary dysphagia	Adaptation 2–4 weeks
Vagus (X) Recurrent laryngeal	Any cervical resective procedure; thyroid operations	Vocal cord paralysis, loss of supraglottic sensation	Nerve grafting rarely effective; Teflon injection of cord to give opposition; right recurrent may not be recurrent
Spinal accessory (XI)	Biopsy of posterior cervical node; radical neck dissection	Paralysis of trapezius	Free autogenous graft has been tried; physiotherapy to strengthen alternate muscles and prevent frozen shoulder is important
Hypoglossal (XII)	Oral procedures and resection of oropharyngeal lesions; submandibular gland	Paralysis of half of tongue	Severely impaired speech and swallowing if lost bilaterally; moderate loss if unilateral
Phrenic nerve	Any cervical procedure	Paralysis of diaphragm; atelectasis, pneumonia	Nerve graft not effective
Sensory cervical nerves	Any cervical or cranial carcinoma	Loss of certain sensations post head, ear, shoulder	Requires protection to avoid frostbite in cold climate
Cervical sympathetic chain	Operations deep in the neck	Horner's syndrome	None

*Nerves that may be damaged by high-dose tumor irradiation, i.e., for nasopharyngeal cancers.

direct injury is more subtle and more common. Overzealous electrocautery, excessive tension on nerves, prying on the nerves during dissection, and prolonged retractor pressure all produce permanent interruption of fascicles. Even applying neural tip suction to an unprotected nerve is too traumatic. If suction is needed, the nerve is protected by a cottonoid.

Not all nerve injuries are permanent, but even a transient phrenic nerve injury can impair oxygenation in patients with restricted pulmonary volumes. Recent case reports document the seriousness.[34]

Effective rehabilitation is crucial when nerve function has been lost. Removal of the spinal accessory nerve poses a functional problem. Without active planned rehabilitation, a frozen shoulder results. Painful joint rigidity is added to abductor muscle loss in 1–2 weeks of shoulder inactivity. Good rehabilitative programs maintain shoulder function and motility.[35]

WHAT ARE SOME OF THE INFECTIOUS COMPLICATIONS OF FACIAL, SINUS, AND CRANIAL RESECTIONS?

Some of the infrequent but most devastating complications are associated with facial, nasal, sinus, and cranial bone infections. If untreated and unrecognized, they can be deadly.

Cavernous Sinus Thrombosis

Cavernous sinus thrombosis is now a rare entity. It is associated with nasal and midfacial infections. One must be cognizant that midfacial infectious lymphangitis represents a true emergency (erysipelas). The septic thrombophlebitis in this area extends to the cavernous sinus. There is facial and orbital edema, proptosis, and impaired supraduction of the eyes. Nerves III, IV, and VI are involved early because they are embedded in the lateral cavernous sinus wall[36] (see Chap. 15). Intensive antibiotics are required. The need for anticoagulation is controversial. Steroids have little use except to mask fever and leukocytosis and to make the doctor feel better. For such infectious complications one must suspect the organisms involved and select high-dose intravenous antibiotics accordingly.[37] Beta-lactamase-producing *Staphlococcus* must be covered. Culture material is hard to obtain and culture results will be obtained too late to be useful.

Infection of the Brain and Meninges

When the brain and meninges are exposed during a procedure, brain abscess, subdural abscess or empyema, extradural abscess, pachymeningitis externa, and meningitis may occur.[38] A continuous cerebrospinal fluid (CSF) leak is a certain invitation to infection. With the exception of cancer operations on the nasal sinuses, a short trial (1–3 days) of antibiotic coverage and hopeful waiting is all that should be allowed before enlisting the operative aid of neurosurgical associates. CSF leak after treatment of nasal sinus cancer is discussed in chapter 17.

WHY SHOULD WE BE CONCERNED ABOUT ACUTE GASTRIC DILATION AND ILEUS IN HEAD AND NECK PROCEDURES?

These two complications occur and may be unrecognized in head and neck surgery patients. Almost any painful injury or procedure may induce gastric atony and/or reflex ileus of the bowel. It is more common in children. If reflex atony occurs, swallowed or insufflated air accumulates along with gastrointestinal fluids. Acute massive distention of the stomach produces hypotension and vagal-vagal reflex cardiac inhibition. Vomitus may be aspirated in patients with impaired swallowing mechanisms. Cuffed tubes are only partially protective.

Percussion of the upper abdomen for a tympanitic stomach is a simple diagnostic procedure. A nasogastric tube prevents and/or treats the distention. Improvement in cardiovascular and respiratory status occurs in minutes unless large amounts of gastrointestinal fluids are lost.

Since many head and neck patients are fed by tube postoperatively, we advocate the liberal use of a nasogastric tube. After major resections, the tube is kept on suction (and patency is checked) until good bowel sounds or bowel function is assured.

WHAT ARE SOME OF THE FLUID AND ELECTROLYTE PROBLEMS SEEN IN HEAD AND NECK CANCER PATIENTS?

This topic has been discussed in detail elsewhere.[39] The most frequent postoperative "fluid" complication is failure to empty the urinary bladder. Many male patients with head and neck cancer are elderly and have some obstructive component to prostatic enlargement. Occasionally a Foley retention catheter may be misplaced or obstructed. Percussion of the area of bladder dullness in the lower abdomen is easy to do.

Fortunately, most head and neck cancer patients do not have problems of fluid and electrolyte balance. This is a mixed blessing. The rarity of a severe fluid problem simplifies the working day, but it tends to produce a complacency that will lead to an unquestioning, stereotyped fluid management.

The goal is not to employ dazzling therapeutics in the salvage of a disaster, but to understand the underlying fluid and electrolyte physiology, to recognize which patients require more alert management, to balance the patients' fluids and electrolytes from the beginning of care, and finally to learn to deal with established fluid and electrolyte problems that may be encountered. One useful way of individualizing management is to use a fluid balance sheet that can be constructed on any sheet of lined paper. Coupled with a few simple estimates of the electrolyte composition of the body fluids that may be lost, intelligent estimates can be made of net change. Fluid orders are individualized! Besides the usual assortment of problems seen on any surgical service, head and neck cancer patients have some unique problems. These are described below.

The Nutritionally Deprived

It is often necessary to operate on a thin, wasted patient with a recent 20- to 30-lb weight loss. The weight loss is a predictable consequence of impaired deglutition. When such a patient is first studied, a chronically low serum sodium level is the prominent measurable abnormality. Unlike acute dilutional hyponatremia, serum sodium levels in the chronic low sodium state are relatively well tolerated even when the serum sodium hovers around 125 mEq/L. The low sodium level reflects a loss of lean body mass. The dangers of management come from a narrow-minded focus on the serum sodium concentration alone. The inexperienced person will follow a simplistic cycle of "low sodium, give concentrated saline or salt." This produces edema, which further complicates the debilitated state. The problem is more complex. The real question is, why is the extracellular sodium low? In chronic starvation the energy sources must come from fat and the lean body mass. The total body cell mass, particularly muscle, is depleted. The protein content of the remaining muscle cells is reduced. Since intracellular protein contributes a significant portion of the intracellular osmotic activity, the total osmotic activity of the extracellular *and* intracellular environment is decreased.

Hyponatremia by itself will impair the kidney's ability to secrete a water load. Any exogenously administered Na^+ will be distributed primarily in the extracellular water. Since the body osmolality is determined in this instance by the osmolality of the cell, there will be an osmotic balance reestablished by water leaving the cell. This will expand the extracellular fluid volume. If the amount of added Na^+ is sizable, edema will result, and the serum sodium level will still be low. The best treatment of a chronic low sodium state is to restore a positive nitrogen balance by establishing oral alimentation, by using parenteral supplementation, or by controlling septic processes. If acute edema has been produced in a starved patient with a low serum sodium level, the only recourse is to restrict water and use mild diuretics to remove enough sodium to achieve an appropriate-sized extracellular water space.

Acute Water Intoxication

Acute water intoxication is most commonly seen in the postoperative period, either alone or in conjunction with some nutritional impairment. This problem requires the intervention of medical personnel for its production. In the postoperative period, vasopressin (ADH) levels in the blood go from resting values to 2–5 pg/ml to as high as 50–150 pg/ml following a major operative procedure. ADH causes increased permeability of the distal tubule with the resultant transfer of water into the medullary interstitium. A level of 7–10 pg/ml produces a near-maximum ADH effect. ADH levels usually stay elevated for 24–72 hours postoperatively following a major procedure such as a gastrectomy. There are no direct data concerning the ADH blood levels following more routine oral and cervical surgical procedures. We have observed that hyperosmolality of the urine usually fades by 48 hours after major ablative oropharyngeal and cervical surgery.

Dilutional fluid retention occurs when a large hypo-osmolar fluid load is given to the debilitated patient while there is a significant ADH effect and the kidneys are actively retaining the water. In this circumstance body solutes are acutely diluted and osmolality is reduced. Acute water intoxication is most commonly seen 12–48 hours after surgery. When the serum sodium level is acutely lowered to 125–115 mEq/L, rapidly changing stupor, mental confusion, irrationality, and even generalized seizures may occur. One sure way of lowering the epileptic seizure threshold is to administer vasopressin and give water.

Management is by one of two modes. The first thought is to give hypertonic sodium. This can be tolerated by a young, vigorous patient. In an elderly patient with marginal cardiopulmonary reserve, however, an acute massive expansion of vascular fluid volume will result. The cardiovascular and pulmonary consequences can be deadly. The second and more desirable method is water restriction. Water intoxication begins with excessive water load in the operating room and is perpetuated by overzealous postoperative water administration.

There is a special circumstance that we have observed in head and neck surgery in which severe water retention is more than a transient problem. When cerebrovenous pressure is increased after ligation or obstruction of both internal jugular veins (as seen with a simultaneous bilateral neck dissection or with tumor occlusion in a superior vena caval obstruction), there is a marked ADH effect. Data from one such patient undergoing simultaneous bilateral neck dissection are shown in Figure 27–3. This patient experienced confusion and seizure when too much water was administered during a time of ADH excess. The patients whose

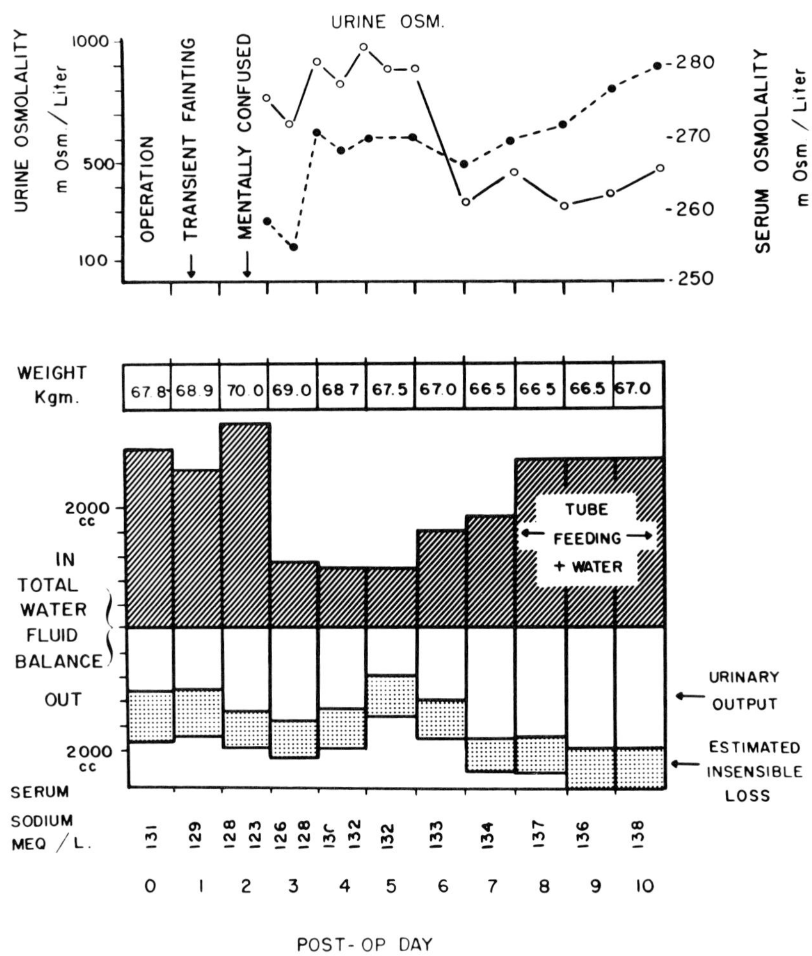

Fig 27–3.—Graphed data clearly show the effect of excess ADH in a patient who underwent a simultaneous bilateral neck dissection. An excessive volume of water (a volume usually considered "routine") was administered. Water intoxication resulted. Compare this Figure with Figure 9–20. The physiologic changes and possible consequences are schematized in Figure 9–21. (From McQuarrie et al.[40] Reproduced by permission of *Arch. Surg.*)

data are shown in Figure 9–20 were correctly managed. With the elevation of cerebral venous pressure, there is a marked antidiuretic effect (elevated urine osmolality with normal or reduced plasma osmolality). This antidiuresis persists until adequate venous collaterals have developed. (See discussion of bilateral neck dissection in chapter 9 and references 40 and 41.)

Early Recognition of Renal Failure

Therapeutic misadventures with excess water loads, excessive Na^+ administration, and acute pulmonary edema are frequently the result of faulty attempts to diagnose suspected renal failure. The usual postoperative oliguric head and neck surgery patient may lack good preoperative data on renal function (such as creatinine clearance data). The pattern of disaster is typical. The patient is brought into the hospital before surgery for workup and diagnostic tests over a period of several days and nights and given nothing by mouth. The night of surgery he is given nothing by mouth and no supplementary hydration. He may receive variable amounts of fluid and blood transfusion during surgery. There may have been a hypotensive episode during surgery. Postoperatively, oliguria is noted. A misguided enthusiast gives 3–4 L of fluids on the day of the patient's surgery with no results. This can be followed by a 500-ml water "flush," topped off by an assortment of diuretics.

All these trial-and-error steps are taken in an attempt to distinguish between acute tubular damage, ADH effect, simple dehydration, inadequate circulating blood volume, and chronic marginal renal function. By the time a clear answer is obtained, the patient has a fluid overload of 4–6 L. What is a better approach? First, use the clinical history. Try to pick out patients with previous diseases suggesting renal involvement, i.e., pyelonephritis, diabetes, obstructive uropathy. Recognize those patients in whom there is a higher risk of renal damage as a result of blood loss, bacteremia, hypotensive episodes, and so forth. When oliguria is noted, the distinction between dehydration or ADH effect and acute tubular necrosis is relatively simple. With simple dehydration there is maximal water conservation by functioning renal tubules. The serum osmolality will be normal or slightly elevated (290–297 mOsm/L). The serum sodium level will be normal to elevated. *The urine osmolality will be high*—usually 600–900 mOsm/L. One notes the clear difference between the concentrated urine and the serum values. With acute tubular necrosis from any cause, the tubules do no osmotic work on the small amount of urine that is formed. Therefore, it has the same osmolar values as an ultrafiltrate of plasma, about 300 mOsm/L. In the example of the water-loaded patient with oliguria, the low serum sodium concentration provides a clue. In a nondebilitated patient, dilution of the extracellular water resulting from failure of free water excretion is reflected in a lowered serum sodium level as well as a lowered osmolality. Urine specific gravity determination is next to worthless for assessing renal tubular function.

What steps can be taken to prevent acute tubular necrosis? First, avoid dehydration. Many studies have shown that the hydrated secreting tubule is less suceptible to the damage of transient hypoexemia and reduced renal blood flow. The patient scheduled for a major procedure should arrive in the operating room with an established water diuresis. Second, recognize and treat bacteremic episodes promptly. Third, treat hypotension promptly. Finally, when oliguria occurs, arrive at a definitive diagnosis early and begin active management before a patient has been pushed to pulmonary edema. Often a patient can be managed without dialysis through a period of tubular recovery if he has not had a fluid overload.

Tube Feeding Problems

When a patient is unable to swallow and requires all feeding by gastrostomy or by nasogastric tube, an unusual situation is established: the patient's internal environment is controlled by the attending physician. The patient cannot respond to thirst by drinking water. It should be unnecessary for every physician to discover iatrogenic hyperosmolar, hypernatremic dehydration for himself.

The normal adult on a 2,000 calorie/day diet excretes about 60 gm of solid per day, which corresponds roughly to 1,200 mOsm of solute. The metabolism of food (tube feeding) breaks it down into smaller, osmotically active metabolites. Because of metabolic fractionation the osmolar load of the urinary efflux is much higher than the osmolality of the feeding which was given. The newer iso-osmolar tube feedings remain iso-osmolar only until they are used by the metabolic processes. The osmotic load can be sharply increased if the diet is high in sodium. Thirty grams of urea will contribute about 500 mOsm/L; by contrast, 30 gm of NaCl will contribute about 1,200 mOsm/L. A rough calculation of solid load that a patient is receiving can be made from the following:

$$\frac{\left(\begin{array}{l}\text{Last 2 values of specific}\\ \text{gravity at 25° C}\end{array}\right) \times (2.6) \times \left(\begin{array}{l}\text{24-hour}\\ \text{urine vol.}\end{array}\right)}{1{,}000} = \text{Total solids (gm/day)}$$

When specific gravity is 1.020 and the urine volume is 1,000 ml, the solids amount to:

$$(\text{gm}/24\text{ hr}) = 20 \times 2.6 \times \frac{1{,}000}{1{,}000}$$
$$= 52 \text{ gm (If all urea, this would be about 900 mOsm)}$$

The physiology textbooks suggest there is a maximum ability to concentrate urine to 1,400 mOsm/L with water deprivation. These data were obtained by Dr. Pitts on healthy young males deprived of water while doing heavy labor on a hot day in a desert environment. In children the maximum urinary concentration may approach only 800 mOsm/L. Similarly, older hospitalized patients rarely show an ability to concentrate urine above 800 mOsm/L.

When high-calorie liquid feedings are given to an adult in the concentration of 1 calorie/ml, a 2,000 calorie diet is contained in much less than 1,800 ml of water, even when the 300 ml of water of combustion is considered. Insensible water loss then accounts for 500–600 ml of water. This leaves 1,200 ml of water to excrete the obligatory urinary osmotic load. The usual 2,000-calorie, high protein tube feeding produces about 1,200 mOsm or solute that must be excreted. Heavier calorie loads will push the osmotic load higher. Assuming a maximum ADH effect and no further aggravation of free water loss by hypotonic sweating, 1,200 mOsm in 1,200 ml would allow urine excretion at a rate of about 1,000 mOsm/L. This degree of concentration can be achieved only with excellent kidney function. The problem can be aggravated further if the tube feedings have a higher solute load because of the use of partially hydrolyzed products, soluble carbohydrates, and more electrolytes.

It can be seen that if the osmotic load is high and the ability to concentrate urine is limited, there will be a deficit of water, which must be made up from the total body water, both intracellular and extracellular. Clinically the patient usually loses weight and becomes somnolent. Muscle weakness supervenes. Ataxia and tremulousness occur. These effects are both peripheral and central in origin.[42] Oral and respiratory mucous membranes are desiccated. Cough and respiration are impaired. Coma, seizures, and death occur at levels above 400 mOsm. Even if the condition is recognized early, the patient is already severly jeopardized. The most usual complication is pneumonia. Prevention of the hyperosmolality is the key to therapy. When the patient is unable to augment his water needs by oral intake, adequate water volume must be provided with the feedings. Two approaches are satisfactory: First, never give tube feedings greater than ½ calorie/1 ml; or second, give enough plain water by gastrostomy or tube (or IV as 5% dextrose in water) to produce a net water excess. Usually this is a volume approximately equal to the concentrated 1 calorie/ml feeding. When there is a question, keep urine diluted to under 500 mO/L. An understanding of this simple problem can prevent the frequent lethal complications that follow pushing a serum sodium concentration to 165 mEq/L.

A second problem follows the use of concentrated tube feedings, and this is a simple osmotic diarrhea. When more than 50% of tube feeding calories are present as small carbohydrate molecules, they represent a large hyperosmolar load and act just as a saline cathartic. Again, management consists of making these feedings nearer the osmolarity of body fluids. New commercial tube feeding preparations have a lower osmolality and are quite satisfactory.

Adult Respiratory Distress Syndrome

This syndrome is not a fluid and electrolyte problem per se. Nevertheless, knowledge of the circumstances under which it may occur, its early recognition, and precise, judicious fluid management are essential for patient survival.

The syndrome is characterized by a delay in onset. It typically occurs 12–24 hours following injury, shock, and/or a successful resuscitative effort. This is a period when the clinician is confident of having surmounted the acute problems and when he may be most complacent and least suspicious. Injudicious fluid loading at this time ensures progressive pulmonary disaster. The clinician must anticipate that the syndrome may occur following any of the causative mechanisms listed in Table 27–5.

TABLE 27–5.—POSSIBLE CAUSES OF ADULT RESPIRATORY DISTRESS SYNDROME

1. Septic shock:
   - Direct bacterial toxin endothelial damage.
   - Secondary effects of infection that release vasoactive substances or cause platelet microaggregation.
2. Extrathoracic trauma. Etiological theories include:
   - Pulmonary vasospasm—increased pulmonary venous pressure—pulmonary vascular capillary disruption
   - Circulating substance (vasoactive) released elsewhere in the body directly or indirectly increases pulmonary capillary permeability.
   - Multiple microemboli (platelet aggregation).
3. Neurogenic pulmonary edema (frequent in head injury: CNS hemorrhage, CNS neoplasm, CNS infection):
   - Neurogenically controlled pulmonary arteriovenous (AV) shunting.
   - Eliminated by spinal cord section.
   - Eliminated by pharmacologic systemic ganglionic blockade.
4. Massive blood transfusion.
5. Pulmonary contusion.
6. Circulating activated enzymes (lipase), as from pancreatitis.
7. Inhalation of hot gases or bronchial burn.
8. Oxygen toxicity.
9. Fat embolism.

The early phase is characterized by bilateral patchy pulmonary infiltrates that may resemble mild pulmonary edema on chest x-ray films. If one could observe the lung at this stage, there would be pulmonary capillary and venous engorgement, microhemorrhages, and an increase in interstitial tissue fluid. Blood gas analysis typically shows a Pa_{O_2} less than 60 Torr. The Pa_{CO_2} remains low, in the range of 35–45 Torr. In the early phases, the syndrome is best characterized by a low arterial oxygen pressure out of proportion to the patient's clinical symptoms. By any means of measurement, there is an increasing pulmonary venous admixture, i.e., shunt fraction. This is a measure of the perfused lung with decreased areas of ventilation and impaired alveolar to arterial diffusion.

If the syndrome progresses, one will note an increasing pulmonary infiltrate, increasing pulmonary density, and decreased arterial Pa_{O_2} levels, even with supplemental oxygen, and respiratory support. Lactate levels increase. Pulmonary compliance measurements show increasing "stiffness" of the lungs. If volume-cycled respiratory assistance is employed, higher and higher pressures are required to maintain adequate tidal volume. Pneumothorax and its attendant complications may occur.

The management remedies are few and are aimed at (1) maintaining adequate oxygenation and respiratory support until there is resolution and restoration of pulmonary capillary integrity, (2) minimizing interstitial extravasation of fluid and blood elements, and (3) possible reduction of further pulmonary vascular injury.

The key to therapy is suspicion that pulmonary capillary damage may have occurred. Document the reduced oxygen level. Monitor the blood gases, and recognize that a falling Pa_{O_2} may be the earliest reliable clue. *Carefully avoid fluid overloading.* Typically, the syndrome can and does occur in the setting of a normal or low central venous pressure. If the syndrome is suspected, fluids should be curtailed to equal insensible loss plus output. If the patient is overloaded, total fluid restriction can be employed. If Pa_{O_2} is falling rapidly, infiltrates are increasing, or the Pa_{O_2} is less than 50 Torr, additional oxygen and volume-cycled respiratory assistance are used to keep Pa_{O_2} levels at 55–65 Torr or higher. Levels of inspired oxygen above 40% should be used only as needed. One should attempt to keep levels of inspired oxygen above 80% for no more than 12–24 hours, or only as absolutely required.

The aids to patient survival remain: (1) early suspicion and recognition, (2) avoidance of fluid overload in the vulnerable patient, (3) precise control of respiratory support for the duration of the pulmonary capillary injury, and (4) administration of antibiotics to minimize bacterial superinfection in the atelectatic areas.

Patients Who Retain Salt and Water

The body responds to surgery by the adrenal excretion of increased amounts of aldosterone. The excretion is magnified in several conditions; two examples are cirrhosis of the liver and congestive heart failure. The more sensitive cardiac patients are those with rheumatic valvular disease of the left ventricle.

There are many empirical data and a confusion of opinion regarding cirrhotic patients, particularly those with ascites. The term "hepatorenal syndrome" has been used to place the patient in a particular category without explaining mechanisms. The ascitic cirrhotic patient's predilection to retain salt and water usually results from (1) weeping of protein-rich fluid from the diseased liver surface, (2) lowered plasma volume, or (3) lowered renal glomerular filtration rate (GFR). Acutely raising plasma volume with the installation of a LaVeen shunt and increasing the GFR produces a brisk diuresis. The kidneys are perfectly functional. Small contributions to sodium retention can come from increased ADH activity, altered permeability of membranes, and altered tubular sodium resorption associated with increased aldosterone secretion. The fact is, sodium is easily retained in the usual cirrhotic patient.

The second large group of patients who require vigilance in management consists of those who have congestive heart failure, who have had marginal myocardial function in the past, or who have valvular disease with marginal cardiac reserve such that congestive failure can be easily induced by minimal blood volume expansion.

In reviewing fluid and electrolyte misadventures in a teaching hospital, we find that the most common cause is the unthinking application of a "formula" to the "routine" fluid orders hastily written on morning rounds. A "routine" order for a postoperative patient with moderate mitral stenosis may be something like "2,500 cc D5W with 75 mEq NaCl/L and 20 ml KCl/L." This is topped off with a dash of some vitamin preparation containing ascorbic acid, and the fluid for the day is started without the physician's cerebral cortex having once been stirred by the process. Yet if you told the same physician that you were ordering a diet containing 12 gm of salt for this same patient with mitral heart disease, he would have fits of consternation over this equivalent sodium load.

In the patient with congestive heart failure there is a total body excess of sodium. This sodium may be within cells as well as in the extracellular fluid. Decreased Na^+ excretion is partially due to decreased renal blood flow and to elevated aldosterone levels. Nevertheless, the practical message is clear: more sodium is retained in a patient with congestive failure, and an excess sodium load is not excreted as well.

Hypercalcemia

Elevated calcium levels can be produced by epidermoid carcinoma of the head and neck by two mechanisms. First, some tumors secrete parathormone-like substances which elevate the serum calcium. Goodwin and Chandler found 2 of 307 patients in their series who had elevated calcium levels which returned to normal after an epidermoid cancer was resected.[43] They were shown to have no bony metastases and normal parathyroids when they died some time later with no further elevation of the calcium level. One other similar patient is still alive after resection. Second, 139 of their patients had recurrences and metastases. Of these, 10 ultimately developed hypercalcemia. About half (5/139) had bony metastases that were thought to raise the serum calcium level by rapid release from resorbed bone. The other half were thought to have parathormone-like hormones produced by metastases. The lesson is clear: calcium elevation is not always associated with extensive systemic or bony metastases, although the likelihood is 50%–80%. A treatable patient with no proved metastases should not be denied therapy because of hypercalcemia. The hypercalcemia does need some correction before treatment. Patients with a calcium level above 12 mg/dl will be symptomatic. Nausea, vomiting, and severe muscle weakness supervene, with increasing mental changes progressing to coma at levels above 15 mg/dl. Renal failure may occur. The myocardial atony and contractile failure with high calcium levels are well known and are probably the ultimate cause of death. Very high levels—above 15 mg/dl—constitute a true medical emergency unless the patient is terminally ill.

Patients with hypercalcemia will be more active, feel better, and have better muscular strength if calcium can be reduced to near-normal levels. Temporary treatment of tumor-related hypercalcemia consists of hydration and diuretics. This is a short-term emergency measure that may buy some time. Definitive treatment requires eradication of the tumor. Mithramycin has been successfully used in patients with advanced neoplasms. This cytotoxic drug is used only as a last resort. It must be used with *extreme caution* and with *careful monitoring of blood elements*. By the time the patient has his first nosebleed, the marrow is destroyed. The complications and mortality of this drug are related to the cumulative dose. The slightest decline in platelet count or elevation of prothrombin time or partial thromboplastin time requires that the drug be stopped. The patient must have good renal function.

Steroids will sometimes lower the calcium level in patients with advanced metastatic bone disease.

WHAT CAUSES FACIAL EDEMA, AND HOW CAN IT BE MANAGED?

Edema of the lower face is a consequence of interrupted lymphatics after a lymphadenectomy. It is much more likely to occur after both cervical lymphatic systems have been extirpated. Following a single-sided lymphadenectomy, significant edema is rare or short-lived because of collateral crossover. The most effective step is to maintain the patient in an upright position as soon as possible for most of the day. Edema will develop rapidly if the head is level or dependent. Once edema is established it is slow to clear. Other helpful measures are adequate feeding to keep serum proteins up. Avoid salt loading. Ultimately, adequate collateral channels develop. Following bilateral neck dissection, this varies between 14 and 35 days. A rare patient with a massive resection may be edematous longer.

OSTEOMYELITIS OF THE SKULL

This complication used to be much more frequent as a result of older techniques of irradiation. It is still seen when large areas of skull are stripped of soft tissue and periosteum and the bone remains uncovered. If the areas have received irradiation, any denuded bone will die. Bare bone becomes secondarily infected and osteomyelitis is established. The treatment of such osteonecrosis is debridement of all nonviable bone after intensive antibiotics. Delay will allow meningeal and CNS infection. The debrided area requires coverage with a vascularized full-thickness flap. If complications produce exposure of *unirradiated* skull, a granulating bed can be established in limited areas by drilling multiple holes through the exposed outer table into cancellous marrow.

HOW DO YOU MANAGE OSTEORADIONECROSIS?

In most institutions the surgeon, otolaryngologist, or oral surgeon must manage osteoradionecrosis. Osteoradionecrosis is a pathologic process that sometimes follows irradiation of osseous tissue.[44] It is an occasional but recognized sequel to appropriate curative radiation. Dosage is crucial, as it is with mucositis, epidermitis, and depilation.

The term osteonecrosis encompasses two conditions—an aseptic process, which is asymptomatic, and a septic process, which presents with marked pain and distress secondary to infection. This septic form may be highly debilitating, with severe pain (trismus), fistula formation, abnormal fractures, and loss of soft and osseous tissues.[45, 46] The incidence following irradiation is variable, as shown in Table 27–6. Numerous factors have been implicated as causative agents in irradiated tissues. The following list is representative:

Quality of radiation
Quantity of radiation
Fractionation of total dose
Portals utilized
Site of the lesion
Quality of the dental, periodontal, and osseous tissue
Degree of trauma inflicted on irradiated tissues
Introduction of sepsis

A recent review of 100 patients treated between 1971 and 1977 for cancer involving the oral cavity, oropharynx, and nasopharynx had an overall incidence of osteoradionecrosis of 22%.[47] These patients received megavoltage external beam therapy and/or interstitial radium or iridium implants. Dentulous patients had a higher incidence of osteonecrosis (24.4%) than edentulous patients (13.6%). In the same study the incidence of osteoradionecrosis seemed to be a direct result of the radiation dose to the bone. Osteoradionecrosis did not occur at doses less than 6,500 rad. Those patients receiving 6,500–7,500 rad developed osteonecrosis at a frequency of 20%. At doses over 7,500 rad the rate was 76%. The size of the tumor at diagnosis did not appear to significantly influence the subsequent development of osteonecrosis.[47] Time at which dental extractions are done will directly influence the incidence of osteonecrosis. Extraction of teeth provides a portal of entry to the devitalized bone in the postirradiation period. The risk of osteoradionecrosis soars to 61% when the teeth were pulled at a significant time (20 months, average) after high-dose radiation treatment.

Bedwinek and co-workers at M. D. Anderson Hospital showed that the rate of osteoradionecrosis was 9.4% when the tumor was near bone, but only 2.1%

TABLE 27–6.—REPORTED INCIDENCE OF OSTEONECROSIS IN PATIENTS IRRADIATED FOR HEAD AND NECK CANCER*

STUDY, YEAR	NO. OF PTS.	YEARS OF STUDY	DOSAGE (rad)	OSTEONECROSIS No.	(%)
Bedwinek et al.,[44] 1976	381	1966–1971	6,000–7,500	54	(14)
Dodson, 1962[48]	108	1948–1960	5,000–9,500	10	(9)
Beumer, 1972[49]	278	1961–1969	5,000–7,000	10	(4)
Carl, 1973[50]	47	1968–1972	3,600–12,900	2	(4)
Morrish et al.,[47] 1981	100	1971–1977	4,950–9,755	22	(22)

*From Morrish et al.[47], with his series added.
Cancers of the oral cavity, nasopharynx, and oropharynx.

when the tumor was not adjacent to bone.[44] Conservative treatment should avoid mechanisms that injure mucosa. This includes abstinence from drinking hot and cold fluids, smoking, consuming alcohol, or wearing dentures. Acute infection is treated with broad-spectrum antibiotics (e.g., tetracycline, doxycycline, clindamycin). Mouth rinse and pain medication should be initiated. Irrigation, packing, minor surgical procedures (sequestrectomy or saucerization), and hyperbaric oxygen have been successfully utilized. We are quite conservative in treating the complication. Surgical management other than minor procedures should be reserved for patients with intractable pain, trismus, and severe infection. The goal is to eliminate the remaining devitalized irradiated bone. An intraoral approach is preferred. Extraoral manipulation of irradiated tissues will usually break through into the mouth, leading to the development of orocutaneous fistulas.[4]

If mucosal breakdown is avoided and there is no introduction of microorganisms, postirradiation necrosis is usually of little concern. The devitalized bone functions to provide support. The patient is asymptomatic. The key is to prevent bone exposure or infection. Once infection does occur the process can be chronic and debilitating.

Everyone treating head and neck cancer should be thoroughly familiar with the morphological and pathological changes induced in normal and malignant tissues by ionizing irradiation.[51]

REFERENCES

1. Beahrs O.H.: Hayes Martin Lecture: Factors minimizing mortality and morbidity rates in head and neck surgery. *Am. J. Surg.* 126:443–451, 1973.
2. McGuirt W.F., McCabe B.F., Drause C.J.: Complications of radical neck dissection: A survey of 788 patients. *Head Neck Surg.* 1:481–487, 1979.
3. Robins R.E., Budden M.K., MacDougal J.A.: Analysis of mortality and morbidity in 100 composite resections for oral cancer. *Am. J. Surg.* 130:178–181, 1975.
4. Joyce L.D., McQuarrie D.G.: Applications of contemporary reconstructive techniques in head and neck surgery for anterior oral-facial cancers. *Surgery* 80:373–378, 1976.
5. Gall A.M., Sessions D.G., Ogura J.H.: Complications following surgery for cancer of the larynx and hypopharynx. *Cancer* 39:624–631, 1977.
6. Strong M.S., Vaughan C.W., Mahler D.L. et al.: Cardiac complications of microsurgery of the larynx: Etiology, incidence, and prevention. *Laryngoscope* 84:908–918, 1974.
7. Suzuki M., Kirschner J.A.: Laryngeal reflex pathways related to rate and rhythm of the heart. *Ann. Otol. Rhinol. Laryngol.* 76:774–780, 1967.
8. Schaefer H.: Central control of cardiac function, in Eichna L.W., McQuarrie D.G. (eds.): *NAS-NRC Symposium on the Central Nervous System Control of the Circulation. Physiol. Rev.* 40; suppl. 4, April 1960.
9. Brodie T.G., Russel A.E.: On reflex cardiac inhibition. *J. Physiol.* 26:92–106, 1900.
10. Baluyot S.T., Shumrick D.A., Everts E.C.: Emergency laryngectomy. *Arch. Otolaryngol.* 94:414–417, 1971.
11. McQuarrie D.G., Johnson C., Monsees L., et al.: Modular development of patient-care oriented data processing system: A three year experience, in *Proceedings of the San Diego Biomedical Symposium*, vol. 13. Univ. Cal., San Diego, February 1974.
12. Aass A.S.: Complications to tracheostomy and long-term intubation: A follow-up study. *Acta Anaesthesiol. Scand.* 19:127, 1975.
13. Ching N.P.H., Ayres S.M., Spina R.C., et al.: Endotracheal damage during continuous ventilatory support. *Ann. Surg.* 179:123–130, 1974.
14. McQuarrie D.G.: Safe replacement of tracheostomy tubes. *Surg. Gynecol Obstet.* 140:769–770, 1975.
15. Sobel S.M., Freeman R., Thawley S., et al.: Management of inadvertent injury to the carotid artery during head and neck surgery. *Head Neck Surg.* 4:475–482, 1982.
16. Ketcham A.S., Haye R.C.: Spontaneous carotid artery hemorrhage after head and neck surgery. *Am. J. Surg.* 110:649–655, 1965.
17. Moore O.S., Karlan M., Sigler L.: Factors influencing the safety of carotid ligation. *Am. J. Surg.* 118:666–668, 1969.

18. Staats B.A., Ellefson R.D., Beedahn L.L., et al.: The lipoprotein profile of chylous and non-chylous pleural effusions. *Mayo Clin. Proc.* 55:700–704, 1980.
19. Daly C.J., Strong E.W.: Carcinoma of the glottic larynx, *Am. J. Surg.* 130:489–495, 1975.
20. Harwick R.D.: Carcinoma of the pyriform sinus. *Am. J. Surg.* 130:493–495, 1975.
21. Marchetta F.C., Sako K., Maxwell W.: Complications after radical head and neck surgery performed through previously irradiated tissues. *Am. J. Surg.* 114:835–838, 1967.
22. Schechter G.L.: Complications of flaps and grafts in the oral cavity and pharynx. *Laryngoscope* 93:306–309, 1983.
23. Dedo D.D., Alonso W.A., Ogura J.H.: Incidence, predisposing factors and outcome of pharyngocutaneous fistulas complicating head and neck cancer surgery. *Ann. Otol. Rhinol. Larynngol.* 84:833–840, 1975.
24. Becker G.D., Parell J., Busch D.F., et al.: Anaerobic and aerobic bacteriology in head and neck cancer surgery. *Arch. Otolaryngol.* 104:591–594, 1978.
25. Bartlett J.G., Gorbach S.L.: Anaerobic infections of the head and neck. *Otol. Clin. North Am.* 9:655–678, 1976.
26. Dor P., Klatersky J.: Prophylactic antibiotics in oral, pharyngeal, and laryngeal surgery for cancer: A double blind study. *Laryngoscope* 83:1992–1998, 1973.
27. Herzon F.S.: The prophylactic use of antibiotics in head and neck surgery. *Otol. Clin. North Am.* 9:781–787, 1976.
28. Butlin H.T.: *Diseases of the Tongue*. London, Cassel & Co. 1885.
29. Eaton J.W., Brandt P., Mahoney J.R., et al.: Haptoglobin: A natural bacteriostat. *Science* 215:691–693, 1982.
30. Mladick R.A., Horton C.E., Adamson J.E., et al.: Management of catastrophic postoperative breakdown after massive oropharyngeal cancer surgery. *Plast. Reconstr. Surg.* 49:316–322, 1971.
31. Monihan R.M., Lipshutz H.: Method for closure of a pharyngocutaneous fistula. *Plast. Reconstr. Surg.* 47:394–395, 1971.
32. Hicks J.N., Peters G.E.: A saliva-shunting technique for low anterior neck pharyngeal fistulas after laryngectomy: An emergency procedure. *Laryngoscope* 92:594–595, 1982.
33. Maizel R.H., Liston S.L.: Combined pectoralis major myocutaneous flap with medially based deltopectoral flap for closure of large pharyngocutaneous fistulas. *Ann. Otol. Rhinol. Laryngol.* 91:98–100, 1982.
34. Moorthy S.S., Gibbs P.S., Losasso A.M., et al.: *Laryngoscope.* 93:642–644, 1983.
35. Saunders W.H., Johnson E.W.: Rehabilitation of the shoulder after radical neck dissection. *Ann. Otol Rhinol. Laryngol.* 84:812–816, 1975.
36. Sofferman R.A.: Cavernous sinus thrombophlebitis secondary to sphenoid sinusitis. *Laryngoscope* 93:797–800, 1983.
37. Kisch A.L.: Principles of the antimicrobial therapy of head and neck infections. *Otol. Clin. North Am.* 9:751–769, 1976.
38. Kaplan R.J.: Neurological complications of infections of the head and neck. *Otol. Clin. North Am.* 9:729–749, 1976.
39. McQuarrie D.G.: Fluids and electrolytes, in Paparella M.M., Shumrick D.A. (eds.): *Otolaryngology*, ed. 2. Philadelphia, W.B. Saunders Co., 1980, Chap. 27.
40. McQuarrie D.G., Mayberg M., Ferguson M., et al.: Reduction of free water clearance with cephalic venous hypertension. *Arch. Surg.* 113:573–580, 1978.
41. McQuarrie D.G., Mayberg M., Ferguson M., et al.: A physiologic appraoch to the problems of simultaneous bilateral neck disssection. *Am. J. Surg.* 134:455–460, 1977.
42. Arieff A.I., Guisado R., Lazarowitz. Pathophysiology of hyperosmolar states, in Andreoli T.E., Grantham J.J., Rector F.C. (eds.): *Disturbances in Body Fluid Osmolality*. Bethesda, Md., American Physiological Society, 1977, Chapt. 11.
43. Goodwin W.J., Chandler J.R.: Hypercalcemia in epidermoid carcinoma of the head and neck. *Am. J. Surg.* 132:444–448, 1976.
44. Bedwinek J.M., et al.: Osteonecrosis in patients treated with definitive radiotherapy for squamous cell carcinoma of the oral cavity and naso oropharynx. *Radiology* 119:665–667, 1976.
45. Guttenberg S.A.: Osteoradionecrosis of the jaw. *Am. J. Surg.* 127:326–332, 1974.
46. Maindus E.G., Hart G.B.: Osteoradionecrosis of the mandible: Treatment with hyperbaric oxygen. *Otolaryngology*, vol. 101, 1975.
47. Morrish R.B., et al.: Osteonecrosis in patients irradiated for head and neck carcinoma. *Cancer* 47:1980–1983, 1981.
48. Dodson W.S.: Irradiation osteomyelitis of the jaws. *J. Oral Surg.* 20:467–474, 1962.
49. Beumer J., Silverman S.Jr., Benak S.: Hard and soft tissue necrosis following radiation therapy for oral cancer. *J. Prosth. Dent.* 27:640–644, 1972.
50. Carl W., Schoff N.G., Sako K.: Oral surgery and the patient who has radiation therapy for head and neck cancer. *Oral Surg.* 36:651–659, 1973.
51. Fajardo L.F.: *Pathology of Radiation Injury*. New York, Masson Publishing, 1980.

28 / Management of Recurrent or Uncontrolled Head and Neck Cancer

DONALD G. MCQUARRIE, M.D., PH.D.

WHEN CANCER recurs in the head and neck region, many physicians assume that further treatment would not be beneficial. It is even more tragic if the unfortunate patient is relegated to a homeopathic trial of chemotherapy and then abandoned by his doctors to suffer his last days in miserable seclusion.

Our most comfortable role as medical professionals is directed appropriately toward achieving a high level of therapeutic cure. When cure is not achieved, we still have an obligation to the patient to accept and manage the recurrent disease. We are plagued with the possibility that our faulty judgment and skills rather than the perversities of malignant disease underlie the recurrence. But lack of initial success in a patient under our care should not impair good logical planning—the patient should have as many remaining days of high quality life as possible. The treatment of recurrent cancer is associated with considerable uncertainty. The experience that others report is scanty and gives us few guides. The medical care team must, of necessity, establish a closer personal relationship with the patient while keeping a balanced objectivity. It is a challenging medical problem.

WHAT IS THE MAJOR DECISION WHEN RECURRENT HEAD AND NECK CANCER IS ENCOUNTERED?

Recurrent head and neck cancer requires a diagnostic effort and analysis to determine which of the five following circumstances may obtain:

1. Despite recurrence, the cancer is still localized, amenable to some mode of curative treatment (surgery or irradiation), and there is a reasonable probability of long-term control.
2. The likelihood of achieving long-term survival is minimal, but a therapeutic attempt would also be of significant palliative benefit. For example, an unsightly malodorous exposed cancer can be removed; a partially obstructed airway can be freed.
3. Long-term survival cannot be expected. Further therapy may prolong life or add to patient comfort and activity.
4. No further therapy will be beneficial. Significant active living is expected with good supportive care.
5. The patient has entered the period of rapid deterioration and death.

When a minimal recurrence is detected early, it is wise to err on the side of assuming some possibility of cure. At the other end of the spectrum, if a patient has massive widespread recurrence, it is meddlesome and bad practice to continue extensive diagnostic studies and debilitating treatment into the few short weeks before death. The unpredictability of malignant disease makes it nearly impossible to give a single patient an accurate prognosis. The wide variation in survival time does give the patient an element of hope and forces the physician to plan the care regimen on an ad hoc basis.

HOW COMMON IS RECURRENCE?

Quite simply, the majority of patients who are not cured do die of cancer. Recurrences are more common after treatment of larger cancers with nodal metastases and relatively infrequent after treatment of early T_1N_0 patients. Retreatment for cure is more effective in the small recurrence after a small cancer. In aggregate, one third to one half of head and neck cancer patients will present with recurrence. Our cured patients have a brief convalescence and are then seen periodically in follow-up. These happy cases command only a few hours of time in our working week to supervise follow-up and rehabilitation. On the other hand, patients with recurrence return again and again. They require frequent attention and consume a disproportionate amount of the medical team's effort. The prolonged efforts on the patients' behalf should be approached with the same intensity and good spirits as they received in their initial clinical encounter.

We must not dismiss a curative opportunity. Recurrence requires as much decision effort as the initial treatment, or more. Figure 28–1 shows a general plan of approach to patients with recurrent cancer.

HOW EFFECTIVE IS RE-TREATMENT OF SQUAMOUS CELL CANCERS?

Chapter 26 documented modest success in treating second and subsequent *new* oroairway primary cancers when they appear in the head and neck region. Unfortunately, re-treating *recurrent* cancers does not meet

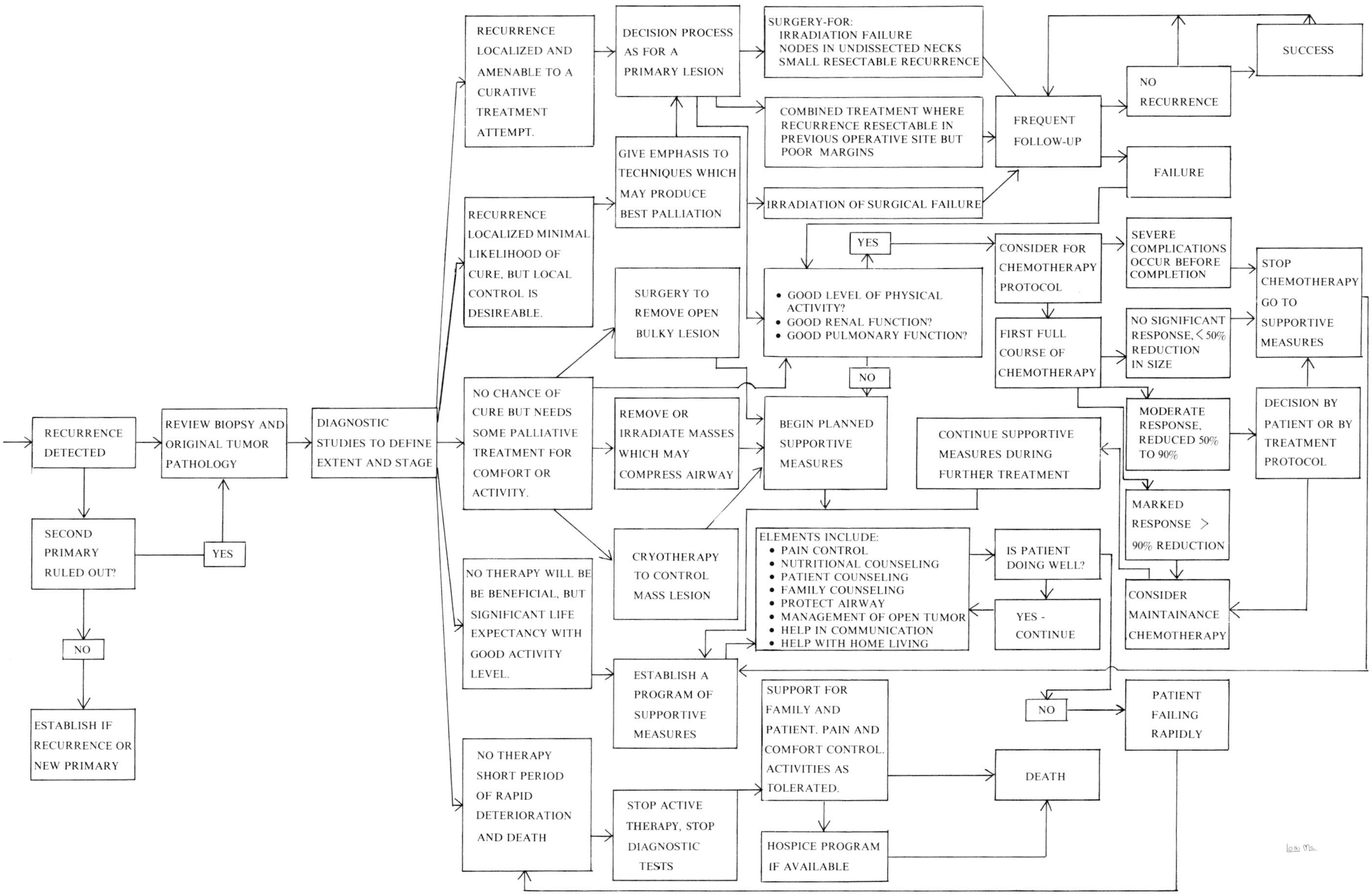

Fig 28–1.—The decisions that must be made when a patient has a recurrence are more complex than those for treatment of the primary cancer. A major effort is needed to ascertain when additional curative attempts are no longer beneficial. If the cancer is beyond local control, a planned program for palliation and supportive care is established.

with the same modest success. Two specific kinds of recurrent disease can be treated with a modicum of success: (1) recurrence or persistence after irradiation—treatment is by surgical salvage; and (2) contralateral cervical metastases that appear after initial treatment—treatment is by neck dissection.

To achieve any salvage of recurrent cancer one must detect it early. Try to cultivate the internal demon of pessimistic paranoia that will accompany you when you examine the "cured" patient in follow-up. The original site of the primary lesion and any remaining nodal drainage areas must be scrutinized carefully. Suspicious mucosal areas are biopsied early. Any enlarged node that appears in the neck should be assumed to contain metastases. The decision to re-treat is made as early as possible. For treatment planning, the physician must again diagnose the stage and extent of disease. In some instances the re-treatment attempt is nothing more than full-dose irradiation or the extensive wide-margin surgical procedure that should have been performed as the initial treatment. After larger extensive cancers, the recurrence may occur deeply and be widely infiltrated before detection.

Kokal et al. reviewed a typical experience with 67 patients who had recurrent oropharyngeal cancers.[1] Of 34 patients in whom surgery was the principal treatment, only 24 were amenable to a second curative attempt. Four of the 24 treated patients (17%) were tumor-free for more than 2 years. The four were treated by irradiation. Thirty patients experienced tumor recurrence after irradiation treatment. Thirteen of the 30 were operated on for cure. Five of these survived more than 2 years without detectable cancer. We have had a somewhat better result in cancers confined to the oral cavity in patients initially treated by irradiation.[2] Spiro and Strong reported a 5% long-term success rate in re-treatment of cancer of the tongue.[3] Cady and Catlin reported a 19% cure rate for recurrent alveolar ridge cancers.[4]

The literature varies in defining where the program of continuing management ends, and how much of a gap there must be between initial treatment and tumor reappearance before the lesion is called recurrent. If cancer persists at the same site or appears in appropriate lymph nodes, it is all persistent disease. As noted earlier, recurrence in the untreated ipsilateral neck or contralateral neck has a high reported success rate, in the 30%–50% range when other sites are free of cancer.[5–7] Chapter 16 reviewed the high level of effectiveness of treating laryngeal recurrence after irradiation or partial laryngectomy. Less promising results are seen after extensive surgery for stomal recurrences after laryngectomy. If one were to select a group of cancers that have a poor prognosis on re-treatment, it would include initially large and bulky cancers, cancers with multiple positive nodes, hypopharyngeal cancers, and the oropharyngeal cancers that extend behind the circumvallate papillae. Saxena reported extended tumor-free survival in only 6 of 128 patients (5%) with recurrent tongue cancers that had been initially stages as T_3 or larger.[8] Only 8% of patients with recurrent advanced oropharyngeal cancers who were re-treated by Kokal survived 2 years without evidence of disease.[1]

The following can be concluded:

1. Early detection and lymphadenectomy for N_1 or N_2 recurrent or persistent metastatic cancer in either undissected ipsilateral or contralateral neck nodes has a reasonably good salvage rate (30%–50%).
2. Surgical or irradation *re-treatment* of lower stage oropharyngeal cancers that recur in the primary site has a definite curative yield (10%–20%), depending on site.
3. Re-treatment of primary site recurrence after a larger cancer or of diffuse recurrence in a dissected neck has a much lower success rate (< 5%).
4. Laryngeal recurrence after partial laryngectomy or irradiation of glottic tumors can be treated with success.
5. Selected stomal recurrences after laryngectomy can be treated with some success.

HOW EFFECTIVE IS RE-TREATMENT OF NON-SQUAMOUS CELL CANCERS?

In general, it is worthwhile re-treating many thyroid cancers that recur in the neck. Recurrent low-grade parotid cancers can be cured with a significant frequency. Low-grade connective tissue malignancies can be palliated with re-treatment, although they are difficult to obliterate completely when they recur next to vital cervical structures.

WHAT ARE THE PROBLEMS OF THE UNCURED PATIENT?

When patients are deemed beyond cure, the role of the therapist changes. There are new problems. The Roswell Park group tabulated some of their experience with a representative group of terminal head and neck cancer patients.[9] Table 28–1 lists some of the preterminal conditions they reported. This list can serve as a guide to management priorities. It tells you what to expect and what to plan for. Pain is the most frequent problem. It typically occurs in the facial and neck area. It is severe enough to require opiates in about half of patients in the period just before death.

About 60% of Shedd's group ultimately needed feeding tubes or a tracheostomy to manage oral and airway problems. Bleeding and serous drainage from a bulky tumor can be most distressing to patients because of its

TABLE 28–1.—PRETERMINAL PROBLEMS IN 60 PATIENTS WITH HEAD AND NECK CANCER*

PROBLEM	% OF PTS.
Pain	85
Feeding problems	62
Pneumonitis	27
Draining tumor	20
Bleeding tumor	18
Respiratory distress	17
Change in mental status	13
Hypercalcemia	8
Other	3
None	5

*Adapted from Shedd et al. Reproduced by permission.

visibility, odor, and bleeding, and because it hinders oral function.

Table 28–2 lists the mechanisms that cause death in patients with cancer. These are the physical problems. The emotional sequelae are harder to quantify. Depression is common,[9, 10] occurring in about one third of patients. It can be ameliorated but not completely eliminated by treatment or understanding care. It is obvious that most patients have more than a single significant problem that requires supportive care. Emotional and physical problems are interrelated. The physician's ability to fix a physical problem is a powerful tool for creating positive patient attitudes toward active living.

WHAT ARE THE OPTIONS FOR MANAGING HEAD AND NECK CANCER THAT IS BEYOND CURE?

First, it is necessary to be aware of and to emphasize the wide variations in disease progression. The survival from histologically similar cancers with the same observable cell mass may vary from weeks to years. An occasional patient may seem to live in symbiosis with the cancer for years and then suddenly succumb in a few short weeks. Most pursue a relentless downhill course, with survival times clustered around the published mean survival times. The clinician can best help his patient by having an active and effective plan for managing the symptoms during the decline. It involves the same multidisciplinary support. The armamentarium consists of:

1. Good available personal contact from the team, with one person serving as the primary physician.
2. Judicious use of palliative treatment by surgery, irradiation, chemotherapy, and cryotherapy.
3. Effective management of pain by analgesics, nerve block, neurosurgical sensory interruptions, and irradiation.
4. Management of esthetics: control of tumor odor and bleeding as well as bandage concealment of lesions.
5. Preservation of airway with tracheostomy or, rarely, laryngectomy.
6. Maintenance of nutrition with varied food preparation, nutritional supplements, tube feeding, gastrostomy, or feeding jejunostomy.
7. Reinforcement of positive patient attitudes, which fosters a higher level of socialization and activity.
8. Support for patient home living by educating the family and the patient on how to manage simple care in a domestic setting. Home nursing visits are helpful and can be used to monitor the patients needs.
9. Emotional support of patient and family. They need praise and recognition for their positive efforts at meeting a challenge.

TABLE 28–2.—MECHANISMS OF DEATH IN PATIENTS WITH RECURRENT HEAD AND NECK CANCER*

MECHANISM OF DEATH	% OF PTS.
Respiratory failure	60
Hemorrhage	12
Cardiac failure	10
Tumor	7
Sepsis	5
Hepatic failure	3
Unknown	3

*Adapted from Shedd et al. Reproduced by permission.

IS FURTHER PALLIATIVE TREATMENT OF THE RECURRENT CANCER WORTHWHILE?

There is no strong evidence that survival is prolonged by giving noncurative palliative treatment to incurable head and neck cancer patients. Shedd's study of 60 terminally ill patients found no survival difference between those who accepted palliative treatment and those who did not.[9] To be useful, surgery, irradiation, and cryotherapy are specifically targeted to reduce compressive tumor bulk, protect the airway, reduce pain, provide a feeding conduit, or treat specific problems caused by distant metastases.

Chemotherapy and immunotherapy still are tantalizing and variable modalities. All of us have had occasional patients with a good temporary response and a rare patient in whom a response seemed to be the direct reason for prolonged survival. Each mode of chemotherapy has some of these anecdotes of success which tend to disappear if tested with a long analysis in a sizable randomized control series. For some years methotrexate was used by us and by others.[11] Combinations with bacille Calmette Guérin (BCG) and isoniazid (INH) produced no significant improvement in head and neck cancer patient survival.[12] Most recently single-course high-dose cisplatin, bleomycin, and high-dose methotrexate have been popular.[13] In a typical pilot study, 65% of 51 head and neck cancer patients had some measurable tumor response. Ten percent of these (three patients) had a *striking* regression of the visible tumor. The average duration of a response was 8–12 weeks. Three of five of the complete responders and four of the partial responders survived 2 years. Most of these patients also received further surgery and irradiation treatment. On the down side, two patients died as a result of chemotherapy treatment, 22 of the 51 patients had renal impairment from cisplatin; and nausea and vomiting were universal during treatment. No pulmonary damage from bleomycin was noted. Bone marrow suppression was documented.[13] If one is to consider chemotherapy for uncontrolled head and neck cancer, the patient must be reasonably well nourished, free of systemic infection, and must possess good renal and pulmonary function. The antineoplastic drug treatment is given to select the one or two patients in 20 who will have a marked response. These patients may benefit from subsequent maintenance therapy. If there is no marked cancer involution, or if there are complications, or if there is strong patient objection to the side effects and malaise, then it is not worth continuing the trial. Chemotherapy for palliation trades some mortality risk and considerable morbidity and discomfort for a marginal likelihood of extended survival. The best result to be desired occurs in a marked involution in a large, messy, hopeless cancer mass.

All *new* combinations of chemotherapy should be tested within the framework of a sanctioned randomized clinical trial so that the marginal differences in therapy can be evaluated as a guide to improved future treatments for others.

HOW CAN YOU MANAGE PAIN DUE TO RECURRENT CANCER?

More than half of preterminal head and neck cancer patients experience pain that demands medical management.[9] About one fourth of patients require more than mild analgesics during the period when they are active. The greatest help a physician can give a patient and the family is the continuing reassurance that cancer pain is manageable and that the patient should not anticipate any long period of excruciating physical pain. The various therapeutic tools available are the following.

1. Encouragement and support for very minimal discomfort.
2. Aspirin, acetaminophen, Darvon, and nonsteroidal anti-inflammatory agents for skeletomuscular pain.
3. Carbemazepine (Tegretol) for neuritic "stabbing" pains.
4. Nerve block.
5. Permanent nerve block with alcohol or neural section by steriotactic techniques.
6. Methadone plus enhancement with low dose chlorpromazine for moderate pain. Codeine and oxycodone (Percodan) are of limited usefulness.[14]
7. Medullary tractotomy by steriotactic methods with rigorous control (evoked potentials) in highly selected patients.
8. Morphine, meperidine, Percodan, Dilaudid and Brompton mixture for more severe pain.
9. Subcortical stimulation with an implanted electrode.
10. Pharmacologic "lobotomy" with high-dose chlorpromazine and analgesics.

Each of these measures is directed toward control of increasing levels of pain. Unfortunately, infiltrative head and neck cancer has very easy access to branches of the cranial nerves, extracranial ganglia, sympathetic fibers, and branches of the cervical plexus, If one is to be effective, the involved nerves or neural pathways should be accurately identified. A widespread infiltrative tumor may involve both somatic sensory and autonomic components. When simple analgesia has failed and anticipated survival is long, a neural block for focal pain may be the better choice to avoid the obtundation of narcotics.If narcotic analgesia is required, a low dose of chlorpromazine with methadone is a good first choice. It can be taken orally, and it allows the patient to remain alert and active. The chlorpromazine adds its own effects and potentiates the analgesia of the methadone. It must be remembered that all of the natural and synthetic opiates rapidly promote tachyphylaxis. If they are used indiscriminately, there may be no dosage reserve for the terminal period. Using oral preparations will prevent dependence on inpatient hospital care by the patient and family.

Irradiation is useful in specific control of pain due to a localized bony metastasis. The exact mechanism of effect is unknown.

On the final approach to death, titrated doses of analgesics may be used as necessary to prevent pain. The physician should not wait until the pain becomes agonizing; *no patient should ever wish for death because of his physician's reluctance to use adequate amounts of effective narcotics.* "Such patients, while they may be physically dependent, are not considered as 'addicts' even though they may need large doses on a regular basis."[15] The Brompton Hospital mixture is used by some centers to control pain and produce mild euphoria. It consists of 15 cc of a syrup containing 15 mg of morphine, 10 mg of cocaine, and a small amount of alcohol and chloroform for solubility and flavor.[16]

HOW DO YOU HELP PRESERVE THE AIRWAY?

Careful follow-up should search for recurrent lesions that threaten the airway. The specific role of palliative laryngectomy in removing a principal focus of recurrent tumor and establishing a tumor-free tracheostomy at some distance is discussed in chapter 16. When a paratracheal mass can be surgically removed with minimal risk, it is desirable to do so. If there has been no prior irradiation, focal irradiation of paratracheal masses can be effective. If it is obvious that upper oroairway tumor is going to be an obstructing mechanism, it is better to do a tracheotomy early rather than wait for stridor discomfort and a dramatic emergency fiasco. Recently, endoscopic carbon dioxide laser surgery has been used in some centers for maintaining airway in highly selected patients.

HOW DO YOU MAINTAIN NUTRITION IN PATIENTS WITH RECURRENT CANCER?

Chapter 11 discussed the general programs of nutritional maintenance in the perioperative period. Many of those concepts can be applied to the patient with recurrent cancer. Starvation is rarely a direct cause of death. Respiratory problems and sepsis account for roughly two thirds of deaths. Nutritional insufficiency and tumor burden do make a patient more susceptible to pneumonitis and systemic infections. Impaired deglutition and attempts to eat may produce aspiration. Protein and blood loss from open tumor surfaces create a continuous metabolic loss. A patient in a chronic catabolic state wastes muscle mass, becomes anemic, feels weak, and experiences a general malaise. Adequate nutrition helps to produce a sense of normalcy and well-being. Ultimately, 25%–50% of patients will require supplemental nutrition. There are graded options for nutritional maintainance, as described below:

1. Change the composition, bulk, and texture of food to those that taste best, are easiest to swallow, and please the patient. Commercial supplements can be used.
2. Use tube feeding for short periods, usually less than 3–4 weeks. Chronic tube feeding has a definite mortality and morbidity from aspiration if proper precautions are not taken.
3. Pharyngostomy for a long-term transesophageal feeding tube.
4. Gastrostomy.
5. Feeding jejunostomy if previous abdominal surgery limits ability to expose the stomach.

Weights should be recorded and noted at each visit during follow-up. If the patient is failing to maintain weight, especially in the absence of a correctable cause or widespread disease, then one of the options listed above should be employed to add calories.

HOW DO YOU MAINTAIN HIGH LEVELS OF SOCIALIZATION AND ACTIVITY?

The chapter on rehabilitation emphasizes the need for the care team to actively encourage social interchange on the ward and then extend it to hospitalwide and community contacts. Easy social interaction requires a modest desensitization on the part of the patient in order to deflect the reactions and questions of others about facial and oropharyngeal functional changes. The uncured patient has the same set of problems to a greater degree. The problems progress and are not stable. The problems of most concern to patients are listed in Table 28–3, along with suggested steps to help. It has been helpful to provide speech therapy and nonmasking prosthetics to patients who are expected to survive only 6 months to a year. Remember the wide variation in survival between individuals.

WHAT EMOTIONAL SUPPORT IS REQUIRED?

It is useless to try to conceal the facts of recurrent cancer from the patient. Herzon and Boshier have discussed the "crumbling belief systems" of patients.[17] To the patient, the recurrence represents "a failure of the health care team to accomplish its goal: to restore health." Both the physicians and the patients must accept the new circumstances and find a new basis for effective collaboration. If no further attempt at cure is to be undertaken, the facts of the situation must be presented to the patient along with a parallel coherent plan

TABLE 28–3.—SOURCES OF PROBLEMS INHIBITING SOCIAL CONTACTS FOR PATIENTS WITH RECURRENT HEAD AND NECK CANCER

1. Change in physical appearance of the face.
   Suggestions: Masking prostheses, clean bandages, masking cosmetics, long hair, high collars.
2. Difficulty speaking.
   Suggestions: Speech therapy, written messages.
3. Inability to manage saliva.
   Suggestions: Banthine, atropine, parotid duct transplant, absorptive paper tissue in mouth (changed frequently).
4. Visible tumor.
   Suggestions: Appropriate bulky bandage changed three to four times daily.
5. Malodorous tumor.
   Suggestions: Cleanse often with gentle hand spray or bulb syringe with dilute 1% hydrogen peroxide; suppress anaerobic growth with antibiotics, povidone iodine on external surfaces; use chlorpactin-soaked dressing on external surfaces.
6. Difficulty eating (see discussion)
7. Depression. Consider using amitriptyline HCl (Elavil) or fluphenazine HCl (Prolixin).

for managing the disease problems. It is necessary to anticipate the fears and anxieties of the patient since only a few strong patients can even bring them forward into consciousness to ask questions and discuss them.

The patient and the doctors become slowly aware that cure is not a possibility and that death from the cancer is inevitable. The course of cancer is highly variable. This uncertainty about expected survival makes problems, but it also adds some hope.

The patient will usually pick the person in the care team he wishes to relate to most closely. The care team, working through that person, should aim to make the uncertain time that remains as easy and pleasant as possible. In beginning to cope with all the problems, there is no advantage to an all-out assault on the patient's psyche. Do not try to cover every potential problem in 1 day's discussion. Do schedule three to four discussions with the patient over 7–10 days. Share some information each time. The first several discussions should be directed by the patient's questions. Patients will ask the questions for which they are prepared to receive answers. If you rush the timing or heap up problems in 1 day, the patient is forced to handle his anxieties by total rejection of help, by transferring his hostilities about the disease to his care-givers, by focusing a neurotic hysteria on minimal symptoms, and by conducting a full retreat from reality. Effort and timing can help avoid precipitating a crisis.

Do not be surprised if the patient tests your answers and plans by asking questions many times in different ways. Assure facilitated consultation if the patient wishes other opinions. The patient should be aware that you have planned for his further care. The patient is reassured that you are thinking ahead and accepting the responsibility for future care. Dr. J. E. Dunphy wrote about caring for the patient dying of cancer from the perspective of a patient and a knowledgeable surgeon.[18] It is important to "emphasize to the patient and family how variable the course of disseminated cancer may be. . . . The patient is vulnerable. He expects the worst. Frightened and uneasy, he needs more than anything to be recognized as a human being, not as a disease. He wants the compassion and understanding only his doctor can provide. A casual remark, a hurried examination or a brusque manner may affect the patient throughout his entire illness."

"The patient is not afraid of death, but he is terribly afraid of being abandoned by his physician in the face of death. . . . One should ask the patient about his pain (or problem). . . . Do a gentle examination and then make recommendations for changes in management. Attention to the little details such as food, drink, bowels (medications, bandages, etc.) brings big emotional dividends. Above all, touch the patient, shake hands, take the pulse, and gently palpate any areas of pain."

It is also important to maintain the self-esteem of the patient and the patient's family by commending them for their efforts, fortitude, and accomplishments in coping with trying problems. Patients and family like to have outside reinforcement that they are doing the right thing.

At least once, the physician has a responsibility to discuss the "cold facts of life" with the patient. Encourage the patient to get a lawyer, make a will, review his assets and liabilities, his insurance, and get his personal affairs in order. This frequently eases many practical burdens. After all of the questions and discussions are done, it is not necessary for the patient to work through his full range of fears and emotions at each visit. Most cancer patients develop a bicameral thinking. They deal with the unpleasant realities and then drop them into the background as soon as they can. They employ some appropriate element of denial to screen the unpleasantness of disease from routine consciousness.

You should assist the patient to approach the sequence of problems with a resolve to continue living and to enjoy life. Frequently, this resolve is rewarded by a long period, characterized by the patient as his most useful time. One patient (Fig 28–2) felt his long active survival with metastases was because "I think positive and go on down the road."

HOW DO YOU MANAGE THE FINAL DYING EPISODE?

A physician must decide when specific or customary therapies cannot add to comfort or achieve more days of functional pleasant life. There is a rapidly rising tumor burden. The accelerated phase of the dying process has begun. "The physician's role is to treat symptoms, avoid further diagnostic procedures when complications arise, explain the reasons for the symptoms and offer alternatives to deal with them. Reinforce the patient and family on the soundness of their decisions, support the nursing staff in their evaluations and opinions in helping the patient and family through the process of dying."[19] About 75% of the dying patient's terminal time can be spent outside the hospital setting with minimal daily assistance from a skilled nurse or health care team. Some cities have both outpatient and inpatient hospice programs. The former teach home care to the patients and their families. The latter are for those without families or homes. A good program avoids euphemisms and deals directly with the issues of dying. Avoidable symptoms are managed, particularly the treatment of pain. Extensive efforts at diagnosis and treatment are avoided during the dying period. They

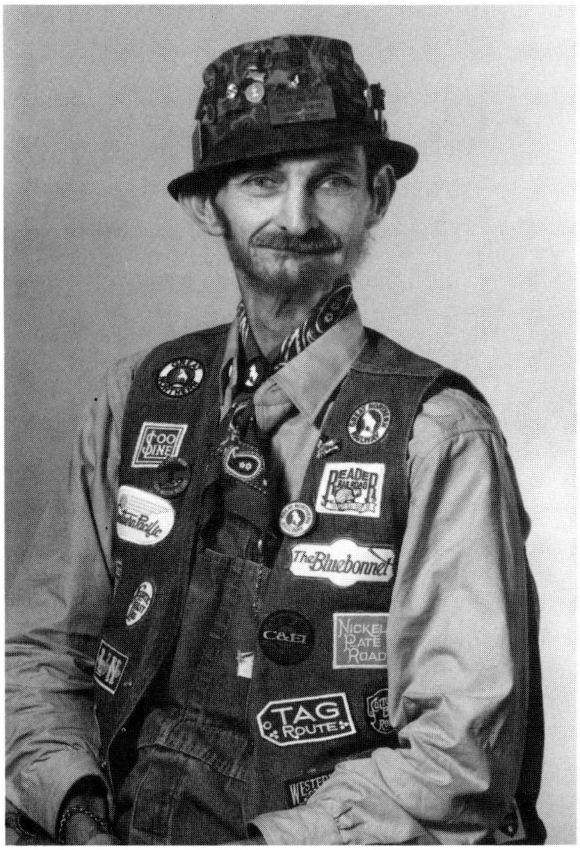

Fig 28–2.—Mountain Dew, King of the Hobos. He wanted his picture in this book to show other cancer patients that you can enjoy a lot of useful life despite persisting cancer. Although he lived 5 years free of head and neck disease after combined treatment of a T_2N_2 floor of mouth cancer, he had multiple bilateral biopsy-proved pulmonary metastases for 3 years before his death. The metastases responded to chemotherapy. The patient ascribed his long active survival to "thinking positive and going on down the road." He spent most of his survival time helping friends and giving cheerful supportive counsel to other cancer patients.

kindle false hopes that rapidly produce a feeling of failure in both patient and physician when the course is unchanged. When complications arise, laboratory testing, x-ray studies, and periods in intensive care units will only interfere with the patient's ability to deal with the emotional distress. "Death holds no fearful threat. Living without life is hell. Death is natural; it may be just; it is often easy and merciful; it ought always be dignified."[18]

REFERENCES

1. Kokal W.A., Neifeld J.P., Eisert D.R., et al.: Management of locoregional recurrent oropharyngeal carcinoma. *Am. J. Surg.* 146:436–440, 1983.
2. Mulholland M.W., Magallanes F., Press B.H.J., et al.: Aggressive surgical therapy after irradiation failure in treatment of cancer of the oral tongue. *Arch. Surg.* 119:394–399, 1984.
3. Spiro R.H., Strong E.W.: Epidermoid carcinoma of the mobile tongue. *Am. J. Surg.* 122:707–710, 1971.
4. Cady B., Catlin D.: Epidermoid carcinoma of the gum, a 20 year survey. *Cancer* 23:551–569, 1969.
5. Jesse R.H., Barkley H.T., Lindberg R.D., et al.: Cancer of the oral cavity: Is elective neck dissection beneficial? *Am. J. Surg.* 120:505–508, 1970.
6. Mendelson B.C., Wood J.E., Beahrs O.H.: Neck dissection in the treatment of carcinoma of the anterior two-thirds of the tongue. *Surg. Gynecol. Obstet.* 143:75–80, 1976.
7. Shah J.P., Tollefson H.R.: Epidermoid carcinoma of the supraglottic larynx: Role of neck dissection in initial surgical treatment. *Am. J. Surg.* 128:494–499, 1974.
8. Saxena V.S.: Cancer of the tongue: Local control of the primary. *Cancer* 26:788–794, 1970.
9. Shedd D.P., Allen C., Shedd C.: Problems of terminal head and neck cancer patients. *Head Neck Surg.* 2:476–482, 1980.
10. Nahum A.N., Golden J.S.: Psychosocial problems of laryngectomy. *JAMA* 186:1136–1142, 1963.
11. Neel H.B. III, Wood J.E.: Adjunctive therapy in treatment for head and neck cancer. *Surg. Clin. North Am.* 57:763–768, 1977.
12. Woods J.E., DeSanto L.W., Ritts R.E. Jr.: A controlled study of combined methotrexate, BCG and INA therapy for squamous cell carcinoma of the head and neck. *Surg. Clin. North Am.* 57:769–778, 1977.
13. Coker D.D., Elias E.G.S., Chretien P.B., et al.: Combination chemotherapy for advanced squamous cell carcinoma of the head and neck. *Head Neck Surg.* 4:111–117, 1981.
14. Mullen S.: Surgical management of pain in cancer of the head and neck. *Surg. Clin. North Am.* 53:203–210, 1973.
15. Goodman L.S., Gilman A.: *The Pharmacologic Basis of Therapeutics*, ed. 5. New York Macmillan Publishing Co., 1975, pp. 261–262.
16. The Brompton cocktail. *Lancet* 1:1220–1221, 1979.
17. Herzon F.S., Bashier M.: Head and neck cancer: Emotional management. *Head Neck Surg.* 2:112–118, 1979.
18. Dunphy J.E.: Annual Discourse: On caring for the patient with cancer. *N. Engl. J. Med.* 295:313–319, 1976.
19. Fortuny I.E., Hansen N., Dwyer P., et al.: Hospice care program. *Minn. Med.* 66:577–580, 1983.

29 / Ward Care of the Head and Neck Cancer Patient

DONALD G. MCQUARRIE, M.D., PH.D.

THE HOSPITAL EXPERIENCE of a head and neck cancer patient takes place on the ward, with only short episodes in the operating room or in the radiation therapy department. Physician contact periods are usually brief. In the total hours of the day, it is the ward nursing team that provides the care contact with the patient.

The ward experience of a head and neck cancer patient is a prolonged period of anxiety, insecurity, fear, pain, and emotional realignment. The patient must simultaneously cope with the therapeutic episode and a total change in perspective on his life and future. The possibility of death from cancer hangs over him like the sword of Damocles. Cure is uncertain. There will be functional losses from treatment. There are usually some changes in appearance, the face, and the self-image the patient holds. Emotional demons must be met and dispatched. The members of the ward team are needed allies.

On the practical side, the technology of care falls to the ward team. They translate, interpret, or augment the written order and convert it to action.

Finally, the ward nursing team carries the major responsibility for teaching and helping the patient with simple requirements of daily living, i.e., diet, stoma care, medical supplies, contacting local support groups, teaching other family members, etc. These crucial elements of care are frequently and appropriately delegated to nursing staff with only general guidance from physicians. Good ward nurses usually assume the leadership role in the areas covered by this chapter.

WHAT ATTITUDES SHOULD BE FOSTERED BY HEAD AND NECK CANCER WARD PERSONNEL?

The ward staff must have a positive attitude toward cancer cure. For all but the most advanced cancers, total control of the cancer presages an ability to achieve some degree of functional and cosmetic rehabilitation.

Even if a head and neck malignancy cannot be cured, patients usually have long periods of good quality living. One of the best discussions was Dr. J. Englebert Dunphy's "Annual Discourse—On caring for the patient with cancer,"[1] portions of which were quoted in chapter 28. This was written by a "caring surgeon" who knew at the time that he was dying of cancer.

With the average ward staff turnover, it is impossible for all ward personnel to have enough longitudinal experience to know the different consequences of aggressive treatment versus benevolent therapeutic nihilism. A young, inexperienced person may be shocked or horrified at the first unreconstructed surgical deformity he sees. If the staff member is personally upset by the slightest facial blemish on himself, he may quite audibly and forcefully declare the he "would rather die than have any treatment like that!" When such an expression is uttered within the earshot of patients or tacitly conveyed by attitude, the patients assume that adjustment will be intolerable outside of a health care setting. This same health care staff member is soon mellowed by seeing the *real* disaster of uncured head and neck cancer and experiencing the dying patients' daily agonies with them. It is important for the more seasoned members of the team to accept and guide the younger staff members by sharing with them some past experiences and reasons for decisions. The patient is the person *within* an epithelial envelope, not just the superficial features.

A positive attitude toward cure is reinforced when the tumor-free rehabilitated patient returns to visit the ward. As a policy, it is good to have some well-rehabilitated patients make follow-up visits in the ward environs where the ward staff can be involved. A distant clinic robs them of the "psychic" pay of success.

Conversely, if a patient needs terminal hospital care, he should not be hidden in some hospital backwater. The staff should participate in the patient's care. The patient is then able to associate episodes of care with a continuing positive effort and without experiencing the despair of abandonment.

Contemporary nursing standards stress coherent detailed care plans. Continuity of care is maintained by a primary care nurse. Reassurance and guidance of patients require familiarity and trust. Many repetitive contacts and some emotional bonding are required for the patient to feel secure and confident. Long-term complex care cannot be encapsulized in a terse note at the end of a shift. Familiarity with the patient's responses fosters early recognition of complications and care problems. A good nursing care plan actively anticipates and prevents many potential problems. The *initial* care plan extends to the early planning for ultimate rehabilitation and discharge.

WHAT ARE WARD CARE RESPONSIBILITIES IN THE PRETREATMENT PERIOD?

The objectives are to prepare the patient so that complications are minimized and optimal treatment can be employed.

Help the Patient Stop or Reduce Smoking

The most common postoperative complications are in the respiratory tract. Radiation irritation of oropharyngeal mucosa is severely aggravated by smoking. If smoking is heavy, then pulmonary secretions are continuously stimulated. The likelihood of postoperative atelectasis and pneumonia are increased tremendously (by a multiple of 4 or 5) if we extrapolate from thoracic surgery data. In many patients the benefit of even 7–10 days of "nearly stopping" can be easily documented by a simple spirometry test. The patient is never as easy to motivate to stop smoking as in the pretreatment period. A strong effort should be made. One tragedy is to have significant numbers of the ward staff health professionals who smoke. Admonitions and advice from staff are useless if patients see the same nurses and doctors smoking in ward offices and conference rooms. The patients follow the visual message and professional example.

Oral Hygiene

Along with the dental service, the ward personnel must reinforce good, three-times-a-day oral hygiene after professional cleaning. This is important if teeth are to be saved. Large necrotic tumors may require more frequent oral cleansing. Protocols with fluoride-retaining molds require coordination with dentists when teeth are retained in patients undergoing irradiation.

Acute Alcohol Withdrawal

Many patients need support and some medication in the first days of hospitalization because of acute alcohol withdrawal symptoms. Support must be coordinated with an active chemical dependency staff. Early preoperative referral is frequently rewarded by long-term posttreatment abstinence.

Personal Hygiene

Some head and neck cancer patients are not spontaneously fastidious about personal hygiene. Many have severe seborrhea of the scalp and face. They accumulate dandruff. Massively contaminated skin flakes will contaminate wounds. Infection is predictable. The operating room surgical scrub is not satisfactory by itself. A nonprescription antidandruff shampoo (Tegrin, Selsun) is used for daily shampoo and showers for 2–3 days before surgery. A germicidal soap shower is required on the night before surgery.

Nutritional Repletion

Some patients with larger cancers may need an adequate caloric and supplemental feeding (see Chap. 11). Ward and dietetic coordination is essential in getting proper taste, texture, and timing of feedings that will deliver the needed food. Routine vitamin supplementation may displease some purists, but in a heavily alcoholic population it is justified. Ascorbic acid deficiency is the one deficiency that impairs healing. Adequate supplementation of 1,000–2,000 mg/day is easy, nontoxic, and cheap. Large weeping ulcerating wounds or tumors can increase ascorbic acid requirements to levels above 1,000 mg/day.

Patients' appetites frequently fail because they are depressed. It is an appropriate situational depression. Gentle encouragement to eat does help. It is necessary to document that adequate calories are being taken. Positive nutrition is reflected in weight gain. Tube feeding and hyperalimentation are used as last efforts in the preoperative period (see Chap. 11).

Pretreatment Education

The amount of education varies with the disease. A parotidectomy patient needs a much lighter instruction sequence than a patient facing extensive ablation and reconstruction. Each service should assemble groups of appropriate teaching aids. We find that locally produced, simple, inexpensive multilithograph brochures are most appropriate. They can reproduce the ward practices exactly. Locally produced materials can be easily changed and updated. The educational aids that are presented must be consonant with local care practices. If commercially prepared educational materials are used, they should be carefully reviewed and edited. If there is any disparity between what the educational materials show and what the patient has been told or will experience, the patient becomes confused and scared by the conflict. The horrible example is to have a slick production slide show or video tape about laryngectomy shown to a patient who will not have such a procedure in his treatment.

In our institutions, the ward nursing staff prepare and update appropriate brochures with the consulting staff's approval of content. The working nurses have the best perception of patients' questions and problems. They keep the material simple and direct. It is couched in nontechnical terms. For example, a 16-page (6 x 8-inch) folder for laryngectomy patients covers the changes that result from surgery and defines terms such as "larynx," "laryngectomy," and "stoma." It presents simple diagrams and illustrations. It outlines stoma care, how to maintain a clear airway, how to provide humidity, how to cough, when to notify a doctor or nurse, and what options exist for communication in the early and late rehabilitative phases. Practical warnings such as don't swim, protect the stoma when your hair is cut, and the like are included, along with hints on clothing, protective stomal covering, expected changes in the sense of smell and taste, and managing the inevitable drippy nose. A list of needed supplies is added.

PRETREATMENT INTRODUCTION TO TREATMENT AND CARE AREAS

Booklets, slide shows, video tapes, and the like are generally informative, but the patient is much more reassured when he can meet the people in anesthesia, the operating room, and the intensive care area who will be caring for him. Waking up for the first time in a contemporary intensive care unit would frighten and confuse all but the most medically experienced person. A quick visit, a warm greeting by a person, and a look around can make this a period of reassurance rather than terror.

Informed Consent

The primary care nurse, ward physician, and senior consultant should all participate in informed consent discussions with patients (see Chap. 10).

Early Recognition of Failed Communication

Alert ward staff members make a large contribution when they identify a patient as confused or troubled or as misinterpreting information. Occasionally the patient's family has received a "mangled message." The primary care nurse is usually the most perceptive listener on the team. The physician should heed the nurses when they feel that the patient has communication problems or is upset. Many cancer patients can only assimilate a small amount of threatening information at one time. The physician must be willing to deliver information in small portions, repeat explanations, and deal tolerantly with misconceptions. Patients on a ward communicate extensively with each other. Occasional misconceptions arise when one patient interweaves his own particular fears, problems, and disabilities with those of another patient whose lesion or experience is totally different.

WHAT ARE THE IMPORTANT WARD FUNCTIONS IN THE POSTOPERATIVE AND POST-INTENSIVE CARE PERIOD?

The common complications are discussed in chapter 27. A large measure of responsibility for prevention, detection, and management rests with the ward staff. Major attention is directed toward maintaining excellent airway and pulmonary function, monitoring vital signs, recognizing complications in the early stages, and preventing infections.

Airway and Pulmonary Function

All ward personnel should receive formal instruction in tracheostomy and airway care. Suctioning is done with sterile catheters and gloved hands to prevent cross-contamination. Bronchial secretions are aspirated every 2 hours, or more frequently if necessary, until the patient can clear his own secretions. All modern tracheostomy tubes have inner cannula fittings that allow a volumetric rotary spirometer to be attached. An adult patient requires a resting exchange of 300–500 cc x 15/minute to meet oxygen demand. Maximum single-breath volumes should exceed 1,200 cc for all but the most severe pulmonary disease. An adult patient needs a forced maximal 1-second expiratory volume of more than 800 cc to clear secretions. If these volumes cannot be developed, regular suctioning will be required. Blood gas values are used to confirm adequate oxygenation if there is any question whatsoever.

Tracheostomy bleeding must be promptly corrected by the surgeon. Tracheostomy ties will constrict blood flow in cervical flaps if the patient lies improperly and creates tension on the ties for 10–30 minutes. Because of this possibility, we use sutures to secure the tube and eliminate ties around the neck until the late postoperative period.

Monitoring Vital Signs

Temperature, blood pressure, pulse rate, daily weight, fluid intake and output, and blood indices are monitored regularly and charted on a graph or flowsheet. The format is not critical as long as it provides an easy means to recognize trends. Fluid excess in the first 24–48 hours is common. If the patient has diabetes, heart disease, or liver disease, additional indices must be monitored and *responded to.*

Wound Observation, Wound care, and Suction Drains

In general, no wound dressings are required, with the exception of a split-thickness graft stent. It is best to leave the entire area open for easy observation. Because of the wide variety of incisions, flaps, grafts and so forth used on the ward, each person's experience is usually limited. Our nurses have created a very useful looseleaf "Wound Care Resource Manual." The manual is kept at the nurses' desk. Resource material includes a short discussion of procedures, methods of care, precautions, methods of prevention, and recognition of potential wound complications. It includes 8 × 10-inch color photographs that illustrate the normal healing appearance in serial sequence, as well as many examples of complications. It covers a variety of routine incisions, split-thickness skin grafts and donor sites, rotation flaps, myocutaneous flaps, and tube pedicle flaps. Armed with this information, an inexperienced person can make much better judgments about the significance of different appearances in a wound.

Suction catheter drains are most appropriately used in head and neck surgery to maintain tissue apposition and to remove serous exudates. They do not provide as easy a conduit for bacteria and air as does a Penrose drain. We prefer continuous suction through a chest-type continuous vacuum water-seal suction. The small accordion or bulb suction units are used when the patient is up and about. To avoid introducing contamination, the suction drains are never irrigated. A 2- to 3-foot length of sterile rubber tubing is interposed into the commercially supplied kit to alow the tubes to be stripped like chest tubes. *Any* air regularly passing through the suction drains should signal an incisional leak or failure of the oral closure. Fistula formation will occur if such a leak is not closed in 1–2 hours.

Duskiness or cyanosis of skin flaps or transfer flaps requires prompt action. Flap ischemia can result from minimal compression of the base of the flap, from unrecognized hypotension, from subflap infection, or from localized cooling.

Patient Communications

After laryngectomy, or if an endotracheal tube or cuffed tracheostomy tube is in place, the patient is forced to communicate in writing or by gesture. Writing materials (paper, pen, pencils, firm writing surface) should be at hand. If the patient cannot write, a pictograph board can be used. There are commercially made units, or appropriate action pictures can be laminated on artist's layout board. Preoperative discussion and practice of signals can make postoperative communication easier.

Positioning

Keeping the head and upper torso slightly elevated at all times will help reduce facial edema. When extensive reconstruction has been done and positioning is critical to flap success, a "vacuum plastic bean bag" called a Vac-Pac (Olympus Corp.) or sand bags are useful in keeping the head in position (sand bags made with two thirds sand and one third rice by volume are easier to mold and use). During the day, a lounge chair is a nice amenity.

Patient Attitudes

Patients must contend with the discouragement of a puffy edematous face, difficulty in controlling saliva, and inability to speak. Pain is annoying but usually quite minimal. Tubes and suction drains get in the way. It is not unexpected to see some depression and withdrawal. Preoperative discussion of this "discouraging phase" can do much to keep a positive attitude. A television set can be a welcome distraction. However, it is the unhurried nurse and physician visits that provide reassurance and support. Let the patient know if the convalescence is progressing as expected. A noncommittal "everything is right on schedule" can be reassuring. Emotional care varies with the outcome of the treatment. Herzon and Coshier discuss the attitude change when tumor recurrence is detected.[3]

WHAT WARD PROBLEMS OCCUR IN THE LATER POSTOPERATIVE PERIOD?

When immediate postoperative wound and respiratory problems have been managed, the early phases of rehabilitation begin immediately.

Shoulder Care

If the spinal accessory nerve has been resected in treatment, it is necessary to begin early an active program to maintain shoulder joint motility and strengthen residual muscle function. In adults, 10 days to 2 weeks of shoulder immobilization usually results in a frozen shoulder. Six weeks of immobility will virtually ensure a frozen shoulder. To avoid loss of shoulder function, exercises are started before 1 week postoperatively. They consist of "walking" the fingers up the wall ten times with the patient facing the wall and ten times with the patient standing at right angles to the wall, three times a day. Each time the arm is raised until the upper arm is fully extended along side the head. At about 3 weeks, a physical therapist prescribes some simple weight training exercises to strengthen the levator scapulae and other residual muscles. The rest of the time, the patient is encouraged to support the shoulder in a pocket in a robe or jacket to minimize drooping shoulder. The patient should avoid lifting more than 20 pounds with that arm (that is the weight of 2½ gallons of water).

Tracheostomy Care After the Acute Period

After 10 days or so, most temporary tracheostomies have served their functional purposes. An uncuffed tube or a bypass tube can be substituted so that the patient can speak by placing a finger over the tube. As soon as the patient is ambulatory, the younger alert patients are taught to care for their own tracheostomy tube. Before removing a tracheostomy tube we have preferred to have a wound tract with an established perimeter of mature fibroblastic activity. This healing is present at about 3 weeks postoperatively.

Unless a small tracheotomy tube (No. 5) has been substituted, as is done for partial laryngectomy patients, we actively discourage a plug in the end of a larger nonbypass tracheostomy tube because (1) improvised plugs can be and have been aspirated when made too small, (2) the total cross-sectional area of the trachea is reduced by the interposed defunctionalized tube, and (3) secretions adhere and dry on the tube end without being sensed. Patients are less diligent about cleaning the inner cannula. When they do, the plug of inspissated secretions may be loosened and aspirated.

If facial edema persists or if further reconstructive surgery is contemplated, the tracheostomy tube is best left in place. Reinstallation and multiple tracheostomies will ultimately narrow the tracheal lumen. For the temporary tracheostomy, an instruction period, written instructions, and a kit of prepared supplies are fairly simple. More detailed teaching and support are required for a laryngectomy patient with an end-on tracheostomy. The patient and/or family must learn all the methods of care and prevention of problems with maintenance of humidity, hydration, cleaning, and protecting the stoma.

HOW DO YOU REESTABLISH DEGLUTITION POSTOPERATIVELY OR MAINTAIN ORAL FUNCTION DURING RADIATION THERAPY?

The effectiveness of any nutritional program must be monitored by daily weight and an occasional check of serum protein levels, electrolyte levels, and appropriate serum chemistries.

There are definite treatment and posttreatment consequences of surgery and radiotherapy of head and neck cancer. Surgery produces abrupt changes in ability to take in food. The effect of radiation therapy on deglutition tends to occur in a more subtle way and may be missed. Chenchardic and Mossman studied 74 patients irradiated for head and neck cancer.[4] Some 80% of the patients had swallowing and nutritional problems. Most had lost some weight in the pretreatment period. During treatment, three of every four patients lost weight. The patients reported that abnormal tastes were most frequently present with high protein foods. They experienced difficulties while chewing and eating meats, fried foods, salads, and vegetables. Good dietetic consultation will assist in trial-and-error adjustments of food, texture, and tastes. It is a necessary ward task to find pleasing-to-eat foods to maintain nutrition. Synthetic saliva used between meals minimizes the discomfort of dry mouth.

Surgical ablation of most head and neck cancers abruptly alters the finely timed complex swallowing mechanism. Miller's monumental review of the physiology of deglutition provides the normal background for understanding the changes caused by cancer treatment.[5] The complex sequence is simplified in Table 29–1. As can be ascertained from this table, therapy that removes tissue, alters position, prevents pharyngeal movement, eliminates chewing and salivation, and changes glottic position and closure will have an effect on swallowing.[6, 7] Which changes cause bad problems? The particular problems with partial laryngectomy were discussed in chapter 16. Doberneck and Antoine studied 15 oral cancer patients by postoperative cineradiography.[8] They found that tissue loss rather than impaired mobility most closely correlated with clinical dysphagia. Loss of tongue mass was most critical in the four patients with dysphagia. Some comparable patients were able to swallow to their own satisfaction. Doberneck and Antoine agreed with Conley[9–11] that patient motivation is the major determinant of success. Conley has analyzed the effect of loss of particular oropharyngeal tissues.[9] In general, if only half of a midline structure is removed, swallowing is usually satisfactory. With to-

TABLE 29–1.—NORMAL STEPS IN DEGLUTITION

I. Preparation of the food.
   a. Chewing.
   b. Mixing with saliva.
   c. Division into smaller parts.
II. Passage from mouth through the pharynx (1⅓ seconds).
   a. *Collection phase:* Dorsum of tongue forms a depression in the midline, collecting the bolus. Soft palate forms a partition to the base of the tongue.
   b. *Anterior alveolar phase:* The tongue is raised to the hard palate anteriorly.
   c. *Midpalatal phase:* The bolus is moved progressively posteriorly on the tongue. The soft palate elevates and allows the bolus to pass through the faucial isthmus and prevents regurgitation into the epipharynx.
   d. *Posterior compression phase:* The hyoid complex is elevated. Respiration is temporarily arrested. The glottis closes. The bolus enters the pharynx, propelled by the tongue. Elevation of the bolus and tongue tips the epiglottis backward.
   e. *Pharyngeal phase:* True and false cords close to form the major protection of the laryngeal vestibule. The bolus is channeled around both sides of the epiglottis. The pharyngeal constrictors propel the bolus through the pharynx with a descending peristaltic wave. The hypopharyngeal sphincter (cricopharyngeus muscle) relaxes, allowing the bolus to enter the esophagus.
   f. *Clearing of the pharynx:* The palate relaxes, the larynx descends, the glottis opens, and respirations resume with an ascending column of air. This helps clear the cords.
III. Esophageal transport, by spontaneous organized peristalsis.

tal glossectomy and a functional pharynx, a number of patients are able to tip their head up and gulp like a collegian chug-a-lugging beer. The problems were discussed in chapter 14. Time should be spent in analyzing what the surgical defect or alteration has done to normal swallowing. Then, the partial solution can frequently be found by introducing changes in head position, in techniques of breathing and swallowing, and in diet, and by motivating the patient.

WHEN AND HOW DO YOU START FOOD AND LIQUIDS BY MOUTH?

It is important for the patients' attitudes that there be some element of success on early attempts. If premature attempts produce a drooling mess and a lot of uncomfortable choking, the patient looses confidence and is unwilling to try again. The following guidelines have proved useful: (1) Oral and pharyngeal edema should be nearly gone. (2) The tracheostomy tube has been changed to a noncuffed type and the patient has practiced speaking for several days (unless a laryngectomy has been done). (3) All incisional closures, particularly in the mouth, are well healed. Remember that the tongue can place strong tension on fresh suture lines. (4) The patient should be able to swallow most of his own saliva. (5) The patient is at least 10 days postoperative.

First attempts are made with a small amount of saline and/or a soft milk-based pudding. The patient is told to inhale and put the food in the middle of the mouth. The chin is elevated to lift the hyoid complex. The patient should be told to swallow twice with each bolus before exhaling and breathing and before taking additional sips.

Double-swallowing helps clear the cords so that food is not aspirated when the patient resumes breathing. The patient must learn these new motor skills. Those with minimal functional loss may be successful on first try. Older patients and patients with extensive functional changes will need 5–7 days of practice. Some of the more impaired patients may need to wait until all edema is gone and pharyngeal pliancy returns, (2 months or so) before they can swallow adequately enough to maintain nutrition. Occasionally 3 inches of rubber tubing on an aseptic bulb syringe can be used to place liquid feedings in the back of the mouth for easier control. Some patients will benefit by a cricopharyngeal myotomy if there is spasm of the superior constrictor mechanism.

A few patients (4%–6%) will ultimately require a gastrostomy for nutritional support. If there is a question, we wait. About one third of the tumor-free gastrostomy patients are taking all of their nutrition by mouth at 1 year and the gastrostomy is discontinued. If the patient requires gastrostomy, he or his family is instructed in feeding administration, diet preparation, keeping batches of food sanitary, use of a blender, and the use of various commercial preparations and supplements. The simplest and least expensive feedings are made in a family setting. Regular portions of the family meal (minus high-fiber items) can be deboned and liquified in a commercial heavy-duty blender with enough water or milk to adjust the consistency. The patient is instructed to take adequate additional water. When traveling, a gastrostomy patient can use a nutritionally balanced canned liquid diet food for short-term convenience. These canned preparations are generally available in urban and remote locations.

WHAT ARE SOME OF THE WARD PROBLEMS ENCOUNTERED WITH PATIENTS RECEIVING CHEMOTHERAPY?

Chemotherapy is usually given as a component of an approved planned experimental protocol (see Chap. 8). For most patients, intensive chemotherapy produces unpleasant symptoms and side effects. Herenz et al.[12] found that side effects were frequent. The emotional distress was associated with the number of symptoms rather than their duration. Diffuse weakness and pain (found in one third to one half of patients) caused more emotional disturbance than did the more specific problems of hair loss, odd food taste, diarrhea, or stomatitis. They showed that nausea on subsequent treatment cycles was largely a conditioned response (chapter 8 details several protocols to minimize nausea). They found that the emotional distress was best controlled by keeping the patient objectively informed about the progress and results of the chemotherapy so that patients did not erroneously attribute side effects to the recurrence or progress of disease. They recommended showing to the patients their x-rays, scans, and so forth so that the location and extent of disease are known, which removes "much of the mystery and potential for [fearful] fantasy."

HOW DO YOU SOCIALLY REINTEGRATE PATIENTS WITH SIGNIFICANT POSTSURGICAL DEFORMITIES?

About 20% of our surgical patients were treated at a late stage of disease. Severe deformity is a predictable consequence of treatment of advanced disease. Plastic surgical repair and prosthetic replacement can do much to help rehabilitate the patient. Coping with the remainder of the deformity requires adjustment by the patient. The help and positive attitudes of ward personnel are crucial. The early hospital experience is the first place to start. The patient's first ventures make a test presentation of the altered self-image to people in other parts of the hospital when patients go to other areas for care, counseling, and rehabilitation. The patients measure the response of strangers. The patient should be encouraged to move about in the supportive hospital environment. In the early periods a simple clean bandage can cover the recent deformity. The bandage carries the message, "valid medical problem under treatment—not a freak." Society usually accepts this message in a positive way. Usually the patient will spontaneously abandon props and seek more extensive social encounters. Many times there must be directed support to help the patient understand the difference between deformity and a change in appearance. For example, when the anterior mandibular arch has been marginally resected or prosthetically replaced, the patient is not repugnant, but the lip-to-chin height has been reduced, giving the patient a cherubic appearance. The face is definitely different. With severe ablative tissue loss, reconstruction or a prosthesis is required. Palatal, nasal, otic, and ocular prosthetics alone or in various combinations can be fabricated and are functionally excellent.[13] Newer materials have improved on older techniques.[14] The principles remain the same. Prostheses basically "fill" defects. Intraoral losses are replaced first. External facial prostheses required adhesion to dry, nonmucosal epithelium. The prosthetist must make appropriate specialized decisions about materials, flexibility, and technical approach. Consultation, measurements, and photographs should be secured before treatment to facilitate planning.

Ward personnel are crucial in teaching the successful use of adherent prosthetic devices. Basic skills with simple makeup can obscure junctions and periprosthetic scars. For the very particular patient, a short session with a skilled makeup person and a variety of makeup blends for several seasons can cover many textural flaws, with and without prostheses.

Support groups are available for speech loss. There are also support groups for cancer patients with other disabilities and for those with incurable disease. These can be contacted through the local chapters of the American Cancer Society.

The care of the uncured patient is discussed in chapter 28. Voice and speech rehabilitation for laryngectomy are discussed in chapter 16.

REFERENCES

1. Dunphy J.E.: Annual discourse: On caring for the patient with cancer. *N. Engl. J. Med.* 295:313–319, 1976.
2. Hickey A.J., Drane J.B.: Prosthetic treatment and rehabilitation: Use in patients with cancer of head and neck. *Curr. Probl. Cancer* 11(10):6–12, 1978.
3. Herzon F.S., Coshier M.: Head and neck cancer: Its emotional management. *Head Neck Surg.* 2:112–118, 1979.
4. Chenchardic J.D., Mossman K.L.: Nutritional consequences of radiotherapy of head and neck surgery. *Cancer* 51:811–815, 1983.
5. Miller A.J.: Deglutition. *Physiol. Rev.* 62:129–184, 1982.
6. Shedd D.P., Scatliff J.H., Kirchner J.A.: A cineradiographic study of postresectional alterations in oropharyngeal physiology. *Surg. Gynecol. Obstet.* 110:69–78, 1960.
7. Lirchner J.A.: Pharyngeal and esophageal dysfunction. *Minn. Med.* 50:921–925, 1967.
8. Doberneck R.C., Antoine J.E.: Deglutition after resection of oral, laryngeal and pharyngeal cancers. *Surgery* 75:87–90, 1974.
9. Conley J.J.: Swallowing dysfunctions associated with radical surgery on the head and neck. *Arch. Surg.* 80:602–612, 1960.
10. Conley J.J.: The crippled oral cavity. *Plast. Reconstr. Surg.* 30:469–478, 1962.
11. Conley J.J., Seaman W.: Function in the crippled laryngopharynx. *Ann. Otol. Rhinol. Laryngol.* 72:441–451, 1963.
12. Herenz D.R., Leventhal H., Love R.R.: Factors contributing to emotional distress during cancer chemotherapy. *Cancer* 50:1020–1027, 1982.
13. Desjardins R.P., Laney W.R.: Prosthetic rehabilitation after cancer resection in the head and neck. *Surg. Clin. North Am.* 57:809–822, 1977.
14. Robinson J.E., Niiranen V.J.: Maxillofacial prosthetics, in *Proceedings of an Interprofessional Conference.* Washington, D.C., United States Public Health Service publication No. 1950, 1966.

30 / Rehabilitation

DONALD G. MCQUARRIE, M.D. PH.D.

SINCE the 1950s most centers have stressed incorporating structural rehabilitative maneuvers into the initial plan of treatment and surgery.[1] Therefore, if we have done our work well in previous chapters, this should be a short chapter. This chapter reiterates the multidisciplinary requirements of good patient care outlined in chapter 10. The discussion addresses alternative and follow-up management which may improve oral function, speech rehabilitation, cosmetic reconstruction, prosthetic replacement, social adjustment, and vocational rehabilitation. Since it is best to integrate rehabilitation into each treatment plan, the discussion will focus on aspects of rehabilitation that are common to most head and neck cancer patients.

Rehabilitation aimed at cosmesis and structural function usually requires multiple surgical steps or revisions. Consequently, patient motivation must be regularly reinforced because a large dose of "tincture of time" is frequently required for surgically healed tissues to return to a more pliant state.

Tumor variations, primary reconstructive imperfections, therapeutic complications, or planned reconstructive staging demand considerable ingenuity in the subsequent rehabilitative course. Methods can be discussed only in general terms which need specific modification for each patient.

HOW CAN OROPHARYNGEAL FUNCTION BE IMPROVED?

The oropharyngeal complex is the starting point of deglutition and the final point of speech formation. Functional impairment is directly related to the size of the tumor and how close the tumor is to the more mobile functional elements. After resection of larger tumors, total correction is rarely possible; improvement is almost always possible. Rehabilitation stops at a compromise when marginal improvement requires extensive and risky efforts.

Initial reconstruction should give priority to the correction of specific defects of deglutition or speech. The requisite mechanisms of deglutition can be analyzed. Good data and an excellent review are available (see Chap. 13).[2] High-speed intelligible speech is much richer in complexity and physiologic subtlety than swallowing. Glottic vibrations are changed in overtones, shape, added sounds, augmented resonance, and gated flow by the anatomical complex spanning the distance from the terminal bronchi up through the mobile oropharynx, the resonating oropharynx, and the nasopharynx.[3] Deglutition and speech both require an oral cavity that can be completely closed, i.e., there must be no fistula. Lips must have sensation and be capable of closure. The tongue must be of adequate size and mobility to reach all portions of the teeth and mouth and sweep the buccal surface. There must be a competent functional division between oral and nasal cavities. The anterior tongue must be supported by the mandible. The hyoid complex must be mobile and capable of elevation. Oropharyngeal tissues should be pliant. There should be an adequately sized pharyngeal channel. Restoration of dentition is very desirable. These considerations set the agenda for rehabilitation. There is always a large degree of compromise due to tissue loss and failure of neuromuscular oropharyngeal function. Structural rehabilitation of oropharyngeal function is directed to specific correctable problems. Several practical hints found in Table 30–1 can avoid wasted time and patient discomfort. The full range of reconstructive techniques described in chapter 6 can be used.

THINGS TO LOOK FOR IN REHABILITATIVE PROCEDURES

Closure of Any Orocutaneous Fistula

Closure is delayed until infection is controlled and spontaneous healing is well progressed. Corso set the admonition to rhyme:[4] "With fistulae large and wide / Let time and patience ebb the tide, / For what was once a staggering gap / Is often closed with a minimal flap." With good drainage, it takes approximately 30 days to achieve a clean wound and establish initial healing fibroplasia. Wound contracture progresses at an accelerated rate from day 30 to day 60. Closure should be considered at 6–10 weeks. The defect may ultimately contract to a small cicatrical opening. Preparing the defect for closure will release some of the contracture at the edge. One should anticipate that the defect may enlarge to twice its initial size after the edges are prepared for closure. Whatever technique is used—local or distant rotational flap, pedicle flap, or myocutaneous flap—the maneuver must provide adequate interior lining and exterior full-thickness skin and subcutaneous tissue coverage. Closure under any tension is a wasted

TABLE 30–1.—PRACTICAL OBSERVATIONS IN REHABILITATIVE CANCER RECONSTRUCTIVE SURGERY

1. After 3–6 months, irradiated tissues (3,500 rad) have a reduced blood supply. An important deficiency is the scarcity of fibroblastic stem cells that lie along the small blood vessels. They are crucial to healing. Consequently, any tissue that is placed in an irradiated field must come from an unirradiated site and must bring and retain its own blood supply, with adequate perfusion and sufficient functional stem cells to achieve tissue healing and maintain viability.
2. Split-thickness skin grafts placed in the oral cavity may undergo as much as 50% contraction with healing.
3. One cannot mobilize thin layers of tissues covered with a previous split-thickness skin grafts. If undermined, they necrose.
4. Split-thickness skin grafts will not take on bare cortical bone. A meshed graft will usually take on cancellous bone surface if some healthy granulation tissue has formed. Such a graft will not tolerate any abrasive friction.
5. Skin and soft tissues are under some elastic tension. They contract when mobilized. Consequently, flaps should be planned to allow a 10%–20% reduction in dimension.
6. Bone grafts require a normally vascularized, unirradiated recipient bed with good full-thickness soft tissue coverage. A free bone graft placed between one side (normal side) and flap will usually succeed. A free bone graft between two *recent* flaps usually fails.
7. A free cortical bone graft will usually span a 1- to 2-cm defect. Defects over 4 cm require a mesh of bone chips or a myo-osseous vascularized bone graft.
8. Exposed bone will die, become infected, sequester, and slough.
9. If there has been active osteomyelitis of adjacent bone within a year, a subsequent free bone graft will usually become infected and fail.

effort. There must be abundant external and internal tissue. In order of complexity, a small defect (less than 4–5 mm diameter) can usually be closed with "turnover local flap." Larger defects, 5 mm to 3 cm in diameter, can be closed with split-thickness lined rotational flaps, lined shoulder flaps, or forehead flaps. Large defects need large thoracoacromial flaps or myocutaneous flaps. (see Chap. 6). Lip defects are discussed in chapter 12; appropriate techniques are selected.

Inadequate Size or Mobility of the Tongue

After a more extensive glossectomy, primary transfer of full-thickness flaps to an intraoral location has been employed frequently to create mobile soft tissue.[5] These flaps are easiest to install at the time of resection. If the residual tongue is pulled over to close an oral defect, it is overextended and tethered down anteriorly, laterally, or both. Elevation and front-back mobility are lost. Some authors use split skin at the time of resection.[6] We have been discouraged by the high failure rate. Occasionally tongue is used to close the oral cavity after small resections. For these patients we have preferred to do a simple tongue release after 6 weeks. A tongue release improves both speech and deglutition following small resections. If more than 25% of the tongue mass has been removed, we have found no significant improvement in speech when pre- and post-release tapes of standard test phrases are blindly evaluated by uninvolved speech therapists using quantitative criteria. In selected instances it constitutes a sulcus-deepening procedure for placement of dentures. Methods are described by Corso[4] and others.[7] A tongue release cannot be done when the external skin and subcutaneous tissues are not at least 8–10 mm thick; where there has been full-dose therapeutic irradiation; or where a mandibular prosthesis, a bone graft, or a bare mandible will be exposed if an incision is made to free the tongue.

A full-thickness transfer flap is sometimes required for oral lining to mobilize the tongue and/or to allow mandible reconstruction. The principle is to recreate the original surgical defect and then inset an appropriate local or distant flap. The effort of doing a late secondary procedure emphasizes the advantages of preplanned reconstruction at the time of primary surgery.

Inadequate Oropharyngeal Opening

When the asecnding mandibular ramus, oropharynx, and palate have been widely resected, the lateral tissues can be made to fall into the defect to close the tissues without too much tension. If such a closure with lateral tissues is selected, a significant cosmetic concavity will be produced. A more zealous attempt to close a wider gap without bringing in additional tissue can leave a miniiorophmyngeal communication. This severely impairs both speech and swallowing. A primary pedicle flap of adequate dimension is a more desirable alternative. Late correction should follow the principles of recreating the initial defect and then transposing a distant myocutaneous flap of sufficient surface and bulk.

Anterior Mandibular Support for the Tongue

More than half of floor of the mouth cancers are at or near the midline. When the anterior arch of the mandible is removed, lack of support precludes any residual tongue function. The tongue heals in a lowered, everted, contracted position. The sequence of problems is shown in chapter 13. If mandible preservation or marginal bone resection is not possible, we insist on some other means of reconstruction or support in postresectional closure. Simple wires are better than nothing, but they are unstable and erode through soft tissues rapidly. We have used a simple wire-silastic prosthesis with good temporary success and 75% long-term retention.[8] Myo-osseous mandibular bone advancement (see Chap. 6)[9] and prosthetic devices of all sorts have served. It is important that the tongue be supported in the healing process, as emphasized in chapter 13. Even if support fails after 2–3 weeks, rehabilitation and reconstruction are easier and safer because the residual tongue need not be uncoiled from the lower fixed position. Some healing in a supported position allows swallowing in the absence of a mandible, but continuous drooling occurs. Mandibular support can be reestablished by one of the methods discussed in the chapter on reconstructive techniques. It is usually better to set the mandibular reconstruction back slightly, accept a mild overbite, and have better tongue motility with good soft tissue coverage. Small mandibular defects (2 cm) can be spanned by free autologous iliac bone grafts. Tantalium or a plastic mesh tray and cancellous bone chips are reliable for defects to 4 cm in size. For larger spans, vascularized myo-osseous reconstruction[9] is probably required. The larger grafts are harder to install with good coverage. They are difficult to immobilize, and failure is common. If "pepper granules" of hemosiderin are found in recipient bone ends (indicative of smoldering osteomyelitis), if there are purulent collections, or if oral communications are recognized, it is best to not complete the proposed reconstruction. Infection is too often a consequence.

Loss of Functional Division Between Oral and Nasal Cavities

Repair of most postoperative hard palate defects requires the assistance of a good maxillofacial prosthedontist. The prosthedontist should have had the opportunity to examine the patient *preoperatively* and to make reference castings to help in designing and fabricating an appropriate obturator with or without dentures. Preoperative consultation will aid decisions about tooth retention and tissue closure requirements (see Chap. 11, Part III). If sound teeth can be retained as anchor points, there is a wider range of options for stable prostheses. There is a spectrum of techniques for increasing oral competence with increasingly extensive tissue defects.[10–14] Techniques can extend from a simple nub on a partial plate to a full maxillary denture that acts as a base support for nasal and soft tissue prostheses. All maxillary prostheses are custom molded from dental materials. The clinician should be aware that the defect will change shape over a period of time. Consequently, prostheses need revision every 2–3 months in the first year. It is better to reserve a very expensive final prosthesis until the defect is no longer changing size.

Functional soft palate defects allow regurgitation into the posterior nares during swallowing. The typical "cleft palate" speech is also a problem. Many soft palate defects can be minimized by a semiobturator plate.[10] Surgical soft tissue adjustments or pharyngeal flap procedures can help overcome vellopalatine incompetence. The requirements for dental rehabilitation and dental prostheses are outlined in Part III of chapter 11.

Achieving Accurate Occlusion of the Teeth After Unilateral Unreconstructed Mandibulectomy

When one lateral or ascending ramus has been resected, the contralateral side is pulled medially by the unopposed force of the pterygoid muscles. The temporalis force tends to rotate the mandible inward. On occlusion, the lower jaw is medial and slightly rotated. For an edentulous person this is not distressing. For a patient with teeth, the prosthedontist can fabricate appliances with a lateral flange that realigns the mandible and remaining teeth on occlusion.[10]

What are Some of the Options for Cosmetic Revisions With Z-Plasty?

Many procedures require incisions that cannot be ideally placed. The vertical limb of most neck dissections is a typical example. Contracture and "webbing" are common. A thoracoacromial flap brought up to the neck will undergo contracture along the vertical limb. An inset flap will have a different skin color and texture. Well-placed multiple Z-plasties will release the contracture and serve to blend mismatched skin areas. The Z-plasty is designed at 60° angles to minimize tip ischemia. Large inset pedicles can be made less obvious by feathering the edge judiciously with Z-plasties, which then lie in the line of natural skin creases. A word of caution—do not mobilize more than one third of the edge of an inset flap at any one time. The major blood supply to the flap comes from lateral cutaneous connections.

Defatting Bulky Pedicle Flaps

Large flaps with too much soft tissue bulk can be defatted after spontaneous healing. Since there is significant fatty tissue resorption after flap transfer, it is best to wait 3–6 months before surgical adjustment.

Other secondary procedures are described in chapter 6.

HOW USEFUL ARE EXTERNAL PROSTHETIC REPLACEMENTS?

Many patients with extended maxillectomy, orbital exenteration, or loss of an ear or nose along with supporting bony structures are best rehabilitated with a specifically designed prosthesis. A good maxillofacial prosthetist must be an amalgam of dentist, anatomist, artist, sculptor, and cosmetologist. He must also be an impeccable craftsman. Each defect must be custom fitted and a prosthesis made to match remaining features. The surgeon should be involved and cooperate in revision of the defect if necessary to improve fit, mechanical security, or blend. Since fitting and matching require several iterations to get it right, direct consultation is desirable even if the patient must travel to a distant city for the consultation. Preoperative consultation, photographs, molds, pictures, and measurement data make the postoperative fitting much better and easier. In the surgical planning it should be remembered that a prosthesis is constructed to fill a *defect.* A prosthesis cannot fit on top of a bulky flap that is already bulging beyond normal contours.

Many times the best prosthesis is a high-quality wig or a longer hair style that can be adjusted to cover numerous scalp, forehead, or ear defects. A pair of attached or separate stylish eyeglasses with a light-colored tint can obscure lines around the nose, ears, and eyes and help secure a prosthesis.

Women patients usually use cosmetics with skill. Men usually resist cosmetic use. If men can be helped, they become skilled in makeup use. It covers many minimal defects.

WHAT ARE THE OPTIONS FOR ACHIEVING BETTER SPEECH?

When one discusses speech impairment one thinks of sign language and written messages. In the modern world the telephone is a major link for emergency and distance communication.

There are several levels of speech impairment. One should consider the problems of the patient in specific detail in order to target precisely the rehabilitation efforts.

First: There may be an intact functional larynx with oropharyngeal dysfunction. Such patients have a strong sound production mechanism but have problems in gating the sounds, adding resonance, and adding the oropharyngeal complex sounds.

Second: There may be some impairment of laryngeal function. A unilaterally paralyzed cord prevents all but breathy, weak sound production.

Third: The larynx may be absent with few oropharyngeal defects.

Fourth: There may be extensive laryngopharyngeal resection. In these patients it may be difficult to restore esophageal deglutition. Esophageal speech is an impossibility.

Other factors such as pulmonary disorders, myoneural impairment, problems with deglutition, velopharyngeal dysfunction, and auditory disorders may affect the success of rehabilitation. Senility, emotional disorders, hiatus hernia, colostomy, and the presence of metastatic disease may block rehabilitation.

Speech evaluation is best done by comparison with preoperative studies. High-quality recordings should be made of the patient undertaking the following speech activities:

1. Reading a standard passage of connected discourse.
2. Producing items on a standardized articulation test.
3. Providing a sample of conversational speech.
4. Producing items on a speech intelligibility test.

This allows an analysis of the manner of speech formation (stops, fricatives, glides, nasals, vowels, etc); the place of articulation [labial *(p* and *b)*, alveolar tip, *(t* and *d);* the ability to form diphthongs *(ai, au, ju)*, etc]; and finally, the voicing and projection. In addition to the recordings, the patients or family should complete a communication profile that evaluates speech in five situations: (1) at home, (2) with friends, (3) at work, (4) on the telephone, and (5) in complex situations, such as in stores, in taxis, or asking directions of strangers. The Northwestern Communication Profile for Head and Neck Cancer Patients has been used by many workers to appraise the effectiveness of speech rehabilitation techniques. Examples of recorded text and the profile are detailed for the interested reader by Weinberg et al.[15]

One major problem for clinicians is evaluating the effectiveness of different speech methods and monitoring progress in speech rehabilitation. Good quantitative data are needed. Within any one institution, the speech therapists are fairly good at identifying improvement or lack thereof. Comparing data between institutions or speech methods is more a matter of faith than science. The more precise and demanding the criteria, the less satisfactory the result.

What Rehabilitation Is Available for Patients With a Unilaterally Paralyzed Vocal Cord?

For many patients, liquid Teflon injection brings the paralyzed cord closer to midline, allowing phonation. A compromise must be reached between optimum apposition and glottic airway constriction. High-quality telephone voice amplifiers are available for people who must communicate by telephone.

What Methods of Speech Production Are Open To a Laryngectomee?

Weinberg collected 53 reprinted articles that can serve as a basis for more extensive reading.[16] This can be coupled with the recent review of prosthetic speech rehabilitation.[15] The traditional first line of rehabilitation is esophageal speech. This is speech produced by taking air into the esophagus and producing sound vibrations as the air is released in the glossopharyngeal area. Pitch can be varied slightly. It is a "rough" lower pitched voice. It is rarely satisfactory to women. Sounds are shaped in a normal way by oropharyngeal structures. Good function of the esophageal sphincters and pharyngeal musculature is required. Considerable air enters the gastrointestinal tract in most esophageal speakers. Because the technique loads the stomach and intestine with swallowed air, this method works poorly with patients with hiatus hernia, gastrectomy, colostomy, or ileostomy. The current mainstay is to use one of the tracheoesophageal shunts, as discussed in chapter 16.

Another approach is for patients to use an externally applied electronic vibratory device to generate pharyngeal buzzing sounds. Voice pitch is monotonous and has a mechanistic sound. Both esophageal speech and the use of the artificial larynx require much practice by highly motivated patients. A skilled coach is required to improve sound production, timing, and clarity. The difference between a high degree of success and a poor result is 20% technical and 80% patient motivation and intellect.

Various other methods have been used on a trial basis to achieve voice rehabilitation. They were discussed in chapter 16 by Dr. Maisel and in the proceedings of a recent Roswell Park symposium,[15] which reviewed the alternatives and the more experimental procedures for patients who would not be esophageal speech candidates. Some techniques involve controlled tracheoesophageal fistulas with and without prosthetic valves. This vents endobronchial air through the upper esophagus and pharynx without the necessity of swallowing air. Other methods incorporate an external fistula with a sound-producing appliance connected to the tracheostomy. The work of Shedd, who used an external reed fistula, is directed toward helping the patient who has had a more extensive pharyngolaryngectomy. Esophageal speech is an impossibility for most such patients with extended resections.

Other operative techniques are outlined in chapter 16. They include the crichohyoidopexy (Piquet), partial reconstruction at the time of resection (Labayle), tracheal elevation (Serafini), and primary microplastic vocal shunts (Mozolewski). All require incorporation of planned operative techniques at the time of resective surgery. The number of evaluable patients is small. Some surgeons are attempting to construct a neoglottis at the time of resection. The methods show promise, but a significant number of patients require reoperation because of phonatory or deglutitional problems. Reports of all these techniques are by the proponents and are generally favorable. Again, good comparative data are scarce.

Finally, we are seeing the beginnings of surgically implanted, externally powered, parapharyngeal sound generators. These devices are at a relatively primitive stage of development. They still appear bulky. Control and pitch mechanisms have much room for technological refinement.

One might reasonably expect that the near future will see refinements in preservative and neoglottic reconstructive techniques. Implantable medical electronics may simplify options in the more distant future. For the present, esophageal speech, and esophageal speech using the Panje or the Blom-Singer shunt, are the most commonly employed methods of achieving speech capability (see Chap. 16).

All patients should be encouraged to join a laryngectomee support group. Such groups are found in every major area and can be contacted through the American Cancer Society.

OCCUPATIONAL REHABILITATION

Many patients have retired before their treatment so that rehabilitative efforts are directed at the tasks of nonemployment, independent living. The previously employed, younger, nonderelict head and neck cancer patient needs help. If cure can be effected, the usual patient still has communication problems and some changes in appearance. Chapter 1 gave the usual definitions of disability. Occupational rehabilitation can be carried out in several ways: by skills with rehabilitation and retraining; by redirecting the patient's career to circumstances where he can function effectively; by altering the previous employer's attitudes so that the patient may perform his old job, or a related job, with some restructuring or assistance. The occupational counselor is many times most effective in acting as an ombudsman between employee and employer. Occupational rehabilitation takes an objective inventory of the patient's skills and can many times serve to redirect the patient to excellent alternative employment. A person skilled in occupational rehabilitation can help motivate the patient, direct his efforts, and serve as a valuable resource. The entire care team should assist in patient motivation and encouragement.

REFERENCES

1. Edgerton M.T.: Opportunities for reconstruction at the time of cancer surgery on the head and neck, in *Symposium on Cancer of the Head and Neck.* New York, American Cancer Society, 1957, pp. 244–247.
2. Miller A.J.: Deglutition. *Physiol. Rev.* 62:129–184, 1982.
3. Conley J.J.: The crippled oral cavity. *Plast. Reconstr. Surg.* 30:469–478, 1962.
4. Corso P.F.: Rehabilitation of patients with oral cancer. *Surg. Cin. North Am.* 47:1147–1161, 1967.
5. Shons A.S., McQuarrie D.G.: Cervical-pectoral flaps in the treatment of advanced oral cancer. *J. Surg. Oncol.* 7:213–218, 1975.
6. Fister W.H., Sharp G.S.: Intraoral use of the free split thickness skin graft in commando type procedures. *Am. J. Surg.* 106:709–711, 1963.
7. Slanety G.A. Jr., Rankow R.M.: Intraoral use of split thickness skin grafts in head and neck surgery. *Am. J. Surg.* 104:721–726, 1962.
8. McQuarrie D.G.: Immediate functional restoration of the mandible after surgical treatment of advanced oral cancer. *Arch. Surg.* 102:447–449, 1971.
9. Browne G.: Chapter 6, this volume.
10. Hickey A.J., Diane J.B.: Prosthetic treatment and rehabilitation: Use in patients with cancer of the head and neck. *Curr. Probl. Cancer* 2(10):1–37, 1978.
11. Desjardins R.P., Laney W.R.: Prosthetic rehabilitation after cancer resection in the head and neck. *Surg. Clin. North Am.* 57:809–822, 1977.
12. Healy J.E. (ed.): *Ecology of the Cancer Patient.* Washington, D.C., Smithsonian Institution, Interdisciplinary Communication Associates, 1970.
13. Robinson J.E., Niiranen V.J. (eds.): *Maxillofacial Prosthetics: Proceedings of an Interdisciplinary Conference* Washington, D.C., U.S. Public Health Service publication No. 1950, 1966.
14. Aramany M.A., Matalon V.: Prosthetic management of postsurgical soft palate defects. *J. Prosthet. Dent.* 24:304–311, 1970.
15. Weinberg B., Logemann J.A., Blom A.: Evaluation of surgical and prosthetic speech methods: An assessment protocol, in Shedd D.P., Weinberg B. (eds.): *Surgical and Prosthetic Approaches to Speech Rehabilitation.* Boston, G.K. Hall & Co., 1980.
16. Weinberg B.: *Readings in Speech Following Total Laryngectomy.* Baltimore, University Park Press, 1980.

31 / Immunotherapy of Head and Neck Cancer: Past Failures and Future Prospects

NORMAN T. BERLINGER, M.D., PH.D.

THE RATIONALE for the immunotherapy of human cancer is based on several assumptions. First, human tumors possess antigens unique to the tumor cell. These antigens ought to be displayed on the cell surface so that they may be readily recognized by immunocompetent cells. Second, these antigens ought to be relatively strong immunogens capable of eliciting a vigorous immune response. Third, the elicited immune response must be an effective one that results in lysis of the tumor cell. Some immune responses to neoplasia can theoretically protect the tumor cell, such as the blocking antibody response that results in the production of antibodies that combine with and mask tumor cell surface antigens but do not cause cell injury. It should be noted that these assumptions have been mainly derived from animal models of induced neoplasia rather than from instances of spontaneous neoplasia in humans. As such, these assumptions may not be strictly true.

The era of modern immunotherapy began early in the 1970s with the reports that nonspecific bacillus Calmette Guèrin (BCG) therapy appeared to prolong the survival of patients with acute myelogenous leukemia. (BCG is a strain of *Mycobacterium bovis* with attenuated virulence for man.) Subsequently, numerous studies of patients with various solid tumors were undertaken to ascertain whether increased survival could be observed with systemic BCG therapy. Nearly all studies were disappointing, with the exception perhaps of studies in patients with ovarian carcinoma and patients with non-Hodgkin's lymphoma who had received chemoimmunotherapy. The only clear benefit from BCG alone is observed with intralesional injection of melanoma nodules.

Among the disappointing studies are those conducted in patients with squamous cell carcinoma of the head and neck. Donaldson[1] originally reported good results with methotrexate, BCG, and isoniazid in the treatment of advanced head and neck cancer. He observed greater than 50% regression of the tumor mass in 81% of 16 patients. The responses in the uncontrolled study were interpreted to be much better than the historical results observed by other investigators using methotrexate alone. Subsequently, several randomized trials showed no evidence that combining BCG with methotrexate would significantly increase the response rate, duration of the response, or survival relative to treatment with methotrexate alone in patients with advanced squamous cell carcinoma of the head and neck.[2, 3] Another randomized trial examined the effect of adding BCG to a five-drug chemotherapy regimen consisting of bleomycin, Adriamycin, CCNU, vincristine, and nitrogen mustard in the treatment of patients with recurrent head and neck cancer.[4] Although the overall response rate for the two treatment groups was the same, the group that also received BCG therapy survived nearly twice as long (30.5 weeks) as the group that received chemotherapy alone. Nevertheless, this study is criticized on the basis that there were a number of drug-related deaths in the group receiving chemotherapy only, and therefore the survival data may not be representative.

In general, most trials that employ adjunctive BCG to treat head and neck cancer report only failure to obtain any significant benefit. The reasons for this are unclear, but several considerations seem relevant here. It is well recognized that a massive tumor burden may cause nonspecific immunotherapy to fail. Analysis of animal models of squamous cell carcinoma seem to indicate that a small or limited tumor burden is associated with successful BCG therapy.[5] Although patients with head and neck cancer often are assumed to have a limited tumor burden, due to the alleged infrequency of distant metastases,[6] this may not be the case at all, because there is evidence that these patients with advanced cancers frequently demonstrate distant metastases.[7] A second theoretical explanation for the failure of nonspecific immunotherapy is that the host with a head and neck cancer is severely immunologically compromised. BCG can be considered a relatively weak immunostimulant. The characteristic severe deficiencies of cellular immunity seen with head and neck cancer may not be sufficiently reversed or affected by BCG. It is also possible that BCG may induce an immune response that is highly specific rather than nonspecific, since BCG has been found to share some antigenic determinants with certain animal and human tumors. This might explain why immunostimulatory effects are observed with the chemically induced hepatocarcinoma of guinea pigs and human melanoma but not with other histologic types of cancer. Finally, the BCG preparations used in clinical trials are admittedly impure. Various degrees of immunostimulation could be expected with various preparations of BCG. Investigations are currently being performed to identify the immunologically active components of BCG. So far, two have been identified. One has been termed P3 and is an esterified disaccharide. The other is termed CWS (cell wall skeleton) and is an esterified polymeric polysaccharide. Both of these BCG fractions exert immunostimulatory effects. The purification of these fractions might allow the preparation of a more pure BCG vaccine with better adjuvant effects. At this time, however, there is no indication that these fractions will be useful for the treatment of head and neck cancer.

Corynebacterium parvum originally seemed to be another promising form of nonspecific immunotherapy. *C. parvum* was reported to cause regression of pulmonary metastases from osteogenic sarcoma and hypernephroma and to prolong the survival of patients with carcinoma of the breast and small cell carcinoma of the lung. Also, *C. parvum* seemed to act synergistically with concurrent radiation therapy or chemotherapy. Furthermore, *C. parvum* vaccine contains no living organisms, in contrast to BCG, and thus there is no risk of infection.

As with BCG, the clinical trials with head and neck cancer were disappointing. A trial of adjuvant *C. parvum* given subcutaneously or intramuscularly to patients with squamous cell carcinoma of the tongue or floor of the mouth showed no significant increase in survival.[8] Another trial reported by Cheng et al.[9] showed that a schedule of both subcutaneous and intravenous *C. parvum* given with radiation therapy did not significantly improve survival for patients with advanced head an neck cancer. In fact, there was some indication among the group with the earlier stage cancers that the administration of *C. parvum* was associated with decreased survival. This may have been a real effect attributable to *C. parvum*, since this vaccine is also known to cause suppression of some immune functions. Another trial reported by Vogl et al.[10] showed no increase in survival, response rate, or response duration for patients with advanced unresectable head and neck cancer when *C. parvum* was given with weekly methotrexate. All available data indicate that nonspecific immunotherapy with *C. parvum* does not benefit patients with head and neck cancer.

Most of the earlier trials of the immunotherapy of various human cancers involved BCG, the methanol extractable residue of BCG, or *C. parvum*. The experimental design and results of these studies contained inherent flaws because of the variable composition of the agent. As mentioned earlier, quantifying the amount of the immunoactive component was nearly impossible. This was a serious problem since accurate observation of dose-response relationships was virtually impossible. Furthermore, animal studies of these bacterial vaccines showed that certain doses were immunostimulatory whereas other doses could actually suppress certain in vitro indicators of immunity. In addition, significant problems arose with toxicity. Decreased patient tolerance of the bacterial vaccine excluded some patients from the studies.

As a consequence, interest grew in immunoactive compounds that had easily quantifiable doses and better defined immunoactive properties. One such compound was levamisole. Levamisole was introduced in 1966 as an antihelminthic drug. Early observations in mice suggested that it augmented the protective effect of a *Brucella* vaccine and thus exerted some type of immunopotentiating action.

Since that time, nearly 50 controlled reports have described the role of levamisole as an adjunct in cancer therapy. Some limited benefit has been observed in patients with advanced cancers of the breast and lung. The results of trials with head and neck cancer are inconsistent and even contradictory. Mussche and Kluyskens[11] evaluated a small number of patients with potentially curable cancer of the larynx or hypopharynx. After surgery or radiation therapy, 12 patients were randomly assigned to receive levamisole and 12 to receive a placebo. After nearly 2 years from the date of definitive treatment, 50% of the control group had a recurrence of the cancer, whereas only 20% of the group receiving levamisole had a recurrence. The report seems to be flawed, however, by the small number of patients studied. In a series of 65 evaluable patients, Wanebo et al.[12] showed no significant difference in the time of recurrence with levamisole and only a favorable but statistically insignificant trend for the rate of recurrence. In a series of 154 evaluable patients, Olivari et al.[13] found no significant difference in the overall recurrence and death rates with levamisole. There was a significantly higher rate of recurrence with levamisole for stage I and II patients. These investigators felt that these results preclude the use of levamisole in early stage disease. The best summary of these three studies is that levamisole does not seem to be of much benefit to patients with head and neck cancer.

Naturally, such studies as these generated much pessimism about the ultimate effectiveness of immunotherapy in human cancer. Intensive study of murine tumor models raised serious questions about the rationale for the use of immunotherapy for human cancer. Experimental tumors induced by chemicals or oncogenic viruses are, in general, highly antigenic and elicit a specific T lymphocyte rejection mechanism. On the contrary, spontaneous murine tumors are only weakly antigenic and do not elicit a specific T lymphocyte rejection mechanism. It is argued, and probably correctly so, that human malignant neoplasia is immunologically more like the spontaneous cancers in mice. A minority of human tumors are known to be induced by chemicals or viruses, and very few human cancers have well-defined and easily detectable tumor-associated antigens.

Three important developments in immunobiology have rekindled interest in and provided new rationales for the immunotherapy of human cancer. First, studies of the complex immune regulatory mechanisms that result in suppression of an immune response reveal that patients with cancer may not always be strictly immune deficient or inert, but rather they may have suppressed immunity. This provides a new strategy for the manipulation of the immune system. Second, there was definition of nonspecific immune effector cells that seem to be intimately related to the genesis or progression of malignancy. These included the natural killer (NK) cell and the activated macrophage. These cells may provide powerful defenses against malignancy, whether or not the tumor demonstrates strong tumor-associated antigens. Third, the development of processes for producing monoclonal antibodies resulted in the production of monospecific rather than oligospecific antibodies. These antibodies can probe the surface of the neoplastic cell for subtle antigens that were previously undetectable and can exploit these subtle differences for tumor specific forms of immunotherapy based on highly specific antibody reactivity. In short, there has been a dramatic reversal from the pessimism about tumor immunology and immunotherapy. Traditional concepts emphasized the reactions of highly specific cellular effectors. New concepts emphasize nonspecific cellular effectors and highly specific antibodies.

Excessive and inappropriate suppression of immune responses has been detected in mice bearing spontaneous mammary adenocarcinomas and in mice bearing tumors induced by methylcholanthrene or by the Maloney sarcoma virus. This suppression seemed to be mediated by the monocyte (macrophage). Berlinger et al.[14] were the first to describe the same process for humans with a variety of solid tumors. In fact, about 60% of patients with squamous cell carcinoma of the oral cavity, larynx, or pharynx demonstrate excessive circulating suppressor monocytes that significantly impair lymphoproliferation.[15] Balch et al.[16] and Berlinger[17] have both shown that these suppressor monocytes produce increased amounts of prostaglandin E_2 (PGE_2), and this PGE_2 appears to be the suppressor signal that decreases lymphoproliferation. Interference with PGE_2 production could logically be expected to prevent suppression of lymphoproliferation. This has indeed been shown to be true in vitro by Maca and Panje.[18] Furthermore, PGE_2 is known to suppress several other important immune processes relevant to neoplasia. PGE_2 can suppress NK cell activity, the tumoricidal functions of activated macrophages, and the secretion of lymphokines.

Several small uncontrolled trials[19, 20] of oral indomethacin, which interferes with PGE_2 synthesis, have shown regression or stabilization of disease in some patients with head and neck cancer. Nevertheless, Blitzer and Huang,[21] using a rat model of squamous cell cancer, have shown that oral indomethacin can be associated with an increased incidence of metastases. Although all these observations must be considered preliminary, it seems clear that dissection of the role of prostaglandins in the modulation of immune responses may well yield some effective pharmacologic ways of interfering with tumor growth.

Immunocompetent cells produce soluble molecules that are crucial for cell-cell communication and for regulation of the immune response. When produced by lymphocytes, these substances are called lymphokines, and when produced by monocytes, they are called monokines. Earlier, only limited quantities of these substances were available for study and then only in impure forms. Recombinant DNA technology, however, has made available relatively larger quantities of purer materials.

Notable among the lymphokines is interleukin 2 (IL-2). This lymphokine is produced by inducer T cells and exerts a dramatic enhancing effect on cellular immunity.[22] Specifically, IL-2 increases cytolytic T cell function in nude mice and also increases NK cell and macrophage immunity in normal and immunodeficient mice. Already, studies using monoclonal antibody markers[23] have shown patients with head and neck cancer to be deficient in a subset of T cells that produce IL-2. An unpublished study has documented improved in vitro immune responsiveness for head and neck cancer patients with IL-2. Clinical trials with recombinant DNA-derived human IL-2 are now under way for a variety of human diseases involving deficient cellular immunity. These developments should be watched with great interest.

Monoclonal antiodies directed against human tumors are produced by heteroimmunizing mice with human tumor cells and then fusing B lymphocytes from the immunized mice with mouse myeloma cells. The result is a hybrid myeloma cell that secretes an antibody determined by the B cell with only one antigenic specificity derived from the tumor cell. These so-called hybridomas are heterogenous since different B cells possess different antigenic specificities, but the individual hybridomas can be separated by cloning. These hybridomas are nearly immortal since they can be serially passaged in tissue culture, a factor that theoretically makes the supply of antibody limitless.

Extremely pure and highly specific monoclonal antibodies have already been prepared for human cancer of the ovary, colon, pancreas, lung, and prostate, and for malignant melanoma and acute lymphocytic leukemia. Zenner has prepared monoclonal antibodies against human laryngeal cancer.[24] Obviously, monoclonal antibodies may well find utility as a marker for diagnosis and for monitoring recurrence by detecting circulating tumor antigens in a manner more specific than for carcinoembryonic antigen. Similarly great are the potential implications for the immunotherapy of cancer by serologic means. Early studies give a clear indication that complement-mediated cytotoxicity of human melanoma cells is enhanced in vitro by using two monoclonal antibodies against different epitopes of melanoma antigen p97.[25] Furthermore, the specificity of monoclonal antibodies may be exploited for nonimmunologic killing of tumor cells by coupling chemotherapeutic agents or toxins to the antibody. When the drug or toxin is endocytosed, a lethal reaction can occur. The potent toxin, ricin, has been coupled to monoclonal antibodies to form so-called monoclonal immunotoxins which in vitro can kill human colon carcinoma cells or cultured laryngeal carcinoma cells.[26]

The prospects for the immunotherapy of cancer appear bright again, owing to a new understanding of tumor cell-immune cell interactions and an explosive development of new technologies. Immunopharmacology has become a discipline unto itself and will provide many new immunoactive drugs, of which indomethacin is a mere prototype. Recombinant DNA technologies will yield large quantities of cytokines with powerful immune modulatory effects. Monoclonal antibodies will dissect the surface antigenic display of tumor cells with precision, with the real possibility of yielding powerful forms of serotherapy or immunotoxin therapy. The least that can be expected of all this is an incisive test of Burnet's immune surveillance theory of neoplasia.

REFERENCES

1. Donaldson R.C.: Methotrexate plus Bacillus Calmette-Guérin (BCG) and isoniazid in the treatment of cancer of the head and neck. *Am. J. Surg.* 124:527–534, 1972.
2. Papac R., Minor D.R., Rudnick S., et al.: Controlled trial of methotrexate and Bacillus Calmette-Guérin therapy for advanced head and neck cancer. *Cancer Res.* 38: 3150–3153, 1978.
3. Buechler M., Mukherji B., Chasin W., et al.: High dose methotrexate with and without BCG therapy in advanced head and neck malignancy. *Cancer* 43:1095–1100, 1979.
4. Richman S.P., Livingston R.B., Gutterman J.V., et al.: Chemotherapy versus chemoimmunotherapy of head and neck cancer: Report of a randomized study. *Cancer Treat. Rep.* 60:535–539, 1976.
5. Kleinschuster S.J., Rapp H.J., Leuker D.C., et al.: Regression of a bovine ocular carcinoma by treatment with a mycobacterial vaccine. *JNCI* 58:1807–1814, 1977.
6. Roberts J.C., Thompson R.W., Bagshaw M.: Patterns of distant spread of head and neck cancer. *Cancer* 33: 127–133, 1974.
7. O'Brien P.H., Carlson R., Steubner E.A., et al.: Distant metastases in epidermoid cell carcinoma of the head and neck. *Cancer* 27:304–307, 1971.
8. Szpirglas H., Chastand C.I., Bertrand J.C.: Adjuvant treatment of tongue and floor of mouth cancers. *Recent Results Cancer Res.* 68:309–317, 1979.
9. Cheng V.S.T., Suit H.D., Wang C.C., et al.: Clinical trial of *Corynebacterium parvum* (intra-lymph node and intravenous) and radiation therapy in the treatment of head and neck carcinoma. *Cancer* 49:239–244, 1982.
10. Vogl S.E., Schoenfeld D.A., Kaplan B.H., et al.: Methotrexate alone or with regional subcutaneous *Corynebacterium parvum* in the treatment of recurrent or metastatic squamous cancer of the head and neck. *Cancer* 50:2295–2300, 1982.
11. Mussche R.A., Kluyskens P.: Prognosis of primarily treated localized laryngeal carcinoma ameliorated through levamisole treatment. *Oncology* 37:329–335, 1980.
12. Wanebo H.J., Hilal E.Y., Strong E.W., et al.: Adjuvant trial of levamisole in patients with squamous cancer of the head and neck: A preliminary report. *Recent Results Cancer Res.* 68:324–333, 1979.
13. Olivari A.J., Glait H.M., Guardo A., et al.: Levamisole in squamous cell carcinoma of the head and neck. *Cancer Treat. Rep.* 63:983–990, 1979.
14. Berlinger N.T., Lopez C., Good R.A.: Facilitation or attenuation of mixed leukocyte culture responsiveness by adherent cells. *Nature* 260:145–146, 1976.
15. Berlinger N.T., Hilal E.Y., Oettgen H.F., et al.: Deficient cell-mediated immunity in head and neck cancer patients secondary to autologous suppressive immune cells. *Laryngoscope* 88:470–475, 1978.
16. Balch C.M., Dougherty P.A., Tilden A.: Excessive prostaglandin E_2 production by suppressor monocytes in head and neck cancer. *Ann. Surg.* 196:645–650, 1982.
17. Berlinger N.T.: Deficient immunity in head and neck cancer patients due to excessive monocyte production of prostaglandins. *Laryngoscope* (in press).
18. Maca R.D., Panje W.R.: Indomethacin sensitive suppressor cell activity in head and neck cancer patients pre- and post-irradiation therapy. *Cancer* 50:483–487, 1982.
19. Panje W.R.: Regression of head and neck carcinoma with a prostaglandin-synthesis inhibitor. *Arch. Otolaryngol.* 107:658–663, 1981.
20. Hirsch B., Johnson J.T., Rabin B.S., et al.: Immunostimulation of patients with head and neck cancer. *Arch. Otolaryngol.* 109:298–301, 1983.
21. Blitzer A., Huang C.C.: The effect of indomethacin on the growth of epidermoid carcinoma of the palate in rats. *Arch. Otolaryngol.* 109:719–723, 1983.

22. Gillis S.: Interleukin-2: Biology and biochemistry. *J. Clin. Immunol.* 3:1–13, 1983.
23. Dawson D.E., Everts E.C., Burger D.R., et al.: Assessment of immunocompetent cells in patients with head and neck squamous cell carcinoma. *Ann. Otol. Rhinol. Laryngol.* (in press).
24. Zenner H.P.: Monoclonal antibodies against surface antigens of laryngeal carcinoma cells. *Arch. Otorhinolaryngol.* 233:161–172, 1981.
25. Hellstrom I., Brown J.P., Hellstrom K.E.: Monoclonal antibodies to two different determinants of melanoma antigen p97 act synergistically in complement-dependent cytotoxicity. *J. Immunol.* 127:157–161, 1981.
26. Zenner H.P.: Selective killing of laryngeal carcinoma cells by a monoclonal immunotoxin. *Ann. Otol. Rhinol. Laryngol.* (in press).

Index

B

D

F

J

K

L

O

U

V

W

X

Y

Z